CURRENT THERAPY IN PLASTIC AND RECONSTRUCTIVE SURGERY

Head and Neck

Surgical Titles in the Current Therapy Series

Callaham:
Current Therapy in Emergency Medicine
Cameron:
Current Surgical Therapy
Charles, Glover:
Current Therapy in Obstetrics
Ernst, Stanley:
Current Therapy in Vascular Surgery
Fazio:
Current Therapy in Colon and Rectal Surgery
Foley, Payne:
Current Therapy of Pain
Garcia, Mastroianni, Amelar, Dubin:
Current Therapy of Infertility
Garcia, Mikuta, Rosenblum:
Current Therapy in Surgical Gynecology
Gates:
Current Therapy in Otolaryngology—Head and Neck Surgery
Grillo, Austen, Wilkins, Mathisen, Vlahakes:
Current Therapy in Cardiothoracic Surgery
Jay:
Current Therapy in Podiatric Surgery
Long:
Current Therapy in Neurological Surgery
Marsh:
Current Therapy in Plastic and Reconstructive Surgery
Parrillo:
Current Therapy in Critical Care Medicine
Resnick, Kursh:
Current Therapy in Genitourinary Surgery
Rogers:
Current Practice in Anesthesiology
Spaeth, Katz:
Current Therapy in Ophthalmic Surgery
Trunkey, Lewis:
Current Therapy of Trauma
Torg, Welsh, Shephard:
Current Therapy in Sports Medicine

CURRENT THERAPY IN PLASTIC AND RECONSTRUCTIVE SURGERY

Head and Neck

JEFFREY L. MARSH, M.D.

Professor of Surgery
Plastic and Reconstructive
Washington University School of Medicine
Medical Director
Cleft Palate and Craniofacial Deformities Institute
Children's Hospital
St. Louis, Missouri

1989

B.C. Decker Inc • Toronto • Philadelphia

Publisher

B.C. Decker Inc
3228 South Service Road
Burlington, Ontario L7N 3H8

B.C. Decker Inc
320 Walnut Street
Suite 400
Philadelphia, Pennsylvania 19106

Sales and Distribution

United States and Puerto Rico
The C.V. Mosby Company
11830 Westline Industrial Drive
Saint Louis, Missouri 63146

Canada
McAinsh & Co. Ltd.
2760 Old Leslie Street
Willowdale, Ontario M2K 2X5

Australia
McGraw-Hill Book Company Australia Pty. Ltd.
4 Barcoo Street
Roseville East 2069
New South Wales, Australia

Brazil
Editora McGraw-Hill do Brasil, Ltda.
rua Tabapua, 1.105, Itaim-Bibi
Sao Paulo, S.P. Brasil

Colombia
Interamericana/McGraw-Hill de Colombia, S.A.
Apartado Aereo 81078
Bogota, D.E. Colombia

Europe
McGraw-Hill Book Company GmbH
Lademannbogen 136
D-2000 Hamburg 63
West Germany

France
MEDSI/McGraw-Hill
6, avenue Daniel Lesueur
75007 Paris, France

Hong Kong and China
McGraw-Hill Book Company
Suite 618, Ocean Centre
5 Canton Road
Tsimshatsui, Kowloon
Hong Kong

India
Tata McGraw-Hill Publishing Company, Ltd.
12/4 Asaf Ali Road, 3rd Floor
New Delhi 110002, India

Indonesia
P.O. Box 122/JAT
Jakarta, 1300 Indonesia

Italy
McGraw-Hill Libri Italia, s.r.l.
Piazza Emilia, 5
I-20129 Milano MI
Italy

Japan
Igaku-Shoin Ltd.
Tokyo International P.O. Box 5063
1-28-36 Hongo, Bunkyo-ku,
Tokyo 113, Japan

Korea
C.P.O. Box 10583
Seoul, Korea

Malaysia
No. 8 Jalan SS 7/6B
Kelana Jaya
47301 Petaling Jaya
Selangor, Malaysia

Mexico
Interamericana/McGraw-Hill de Mexico, S.A. de C.V.
Cedro 512, Colonia Atlampa
(Apartado Postal 26370)
06450 Mexico, D.F., Mexico

New Zealand
McGraw-Hill Book Co. New Zealand Ltd.
5 Joval Place, Wiri
Manukau City, New Zealand

Panama
Editorial McGraw-Hill Latinoamericana, S.A.
Apartado Postal 2036
Zona Libre de Colon
Colon, Republica de Panama

Portugal
Editora McGraw-Hill de Portugal, Ltda.
Rua Rosa Damasceno 11A–B
1900 Lisboa, Portugal

South Africa
Libriger Book Distributors
Warehouse Number 8
"Die Ou Looiery"
Tannery Road
Hamilton, Bloemfontein 9300

Southeast Asia
McGraw-Hill Book Co.
348 Jalan Boon Lay
Jurong, Singapore 2261

Spain
McGraw-Hill/Interamericana de Espana, S.A.
Manuel Ferrero, 13
28020 Madrid, Spain

Taiwan
P.O. Box 87–601
Taipei, Taiwan

Thailand
632/5 Phaholyothin Road
Sapan Kwai
Bangkok 10400
Thailand

United Kingdom, Middle East and Africa
McGraw-Hill Book Company (U.K.) Ltd.
Shoppenhangers Road
Maidenhead, Berkshire
SL6 2QL England

Venezuela
McGraw-Hill/Interamericana, C.A.
2da. calle Bello Monte
(entre avenida Casanova y Sabana Grande)
Apartado Aereo 50785
Caracas 1050, Venezuela

NOTICE

The authors and publisher have made every effort to ensure that the patient care recommended herein, including choice of drugs and drug dosages, is in accord with the accepted standards and practice at the time of publication. However, since research and regulation constantly change clinical standards, the reader is urged to check the product information sheet included in the package of each drug, which includes recommended doses, warnings, and contraindications. This is particularly important with new or infrequently used drugs.

Current Therapy in Plastic and Reconstructive Surgery ISBN 1–55664–083–8

Library of Congress catalog card number: 88–72309

10 9 8 7 6 5 4 3 2 1

CONTRIBUTORS
Volume 1

BRUCE M. ACHAUER, M.D.

Associate Professor, University of California College of Medicine, Irvine, California
Outpatient Therapy of Burns

RICHARD E. ALBIN, M.D., Ph.D., F.A.C.S., F.A.A.P.

Director, The Craniofacial Center, Denver, Colorado
Maxillary and Mandibular Surgery for Cleft Lip and Palate

BERNARD S. ALPERT, M.D., F.A.C.S.

Assistant Clinical Professor of Surgery, Division of Plastic and Reconstructive Surgery, University of California, San Francisco, School of Medicine; Chief, Department of Plastic Surgery, Davies Medical Center, San Francisco, California
Free Flap Contouring of Facial Asymmetries

HANS ANDERL, M.D.

Professor, Clinic for Plastic and Reconstructive Surgery, University of Innsbruck, Austria
Craniosynostosis Syndromes: Surgery in Infancy

RAVELO V. ARGAMASO, M.D., F.A.C.S.

Professor of Plastic Surgery, Albert Einstein College of Medicine of Yeshiva University; Attending, Montefiore Medical Center, Attending, Bronx Municipal Hospital and Head, Plastic Surgery, North Central Bronx Hospital, Bronx, New York
Postpalatoplasty Velopharyngeal Incompetency

STEPHAN ARIYAN, M.D., F.A.C.S.

Professor of Surgery, Yale University School of Medicine; Attending Plastic Surgeon, Yale-New Haven Hospital, New Haven, Connecticut
Functional Neck Dissection

WILBUR L. BAIRD, M.D.

Assistant Professor, Emory University School of Medicine; Emory University Affiliated Hospital, Atlanta, Georgia
Free Flaps in Craniofacial Surgery

JOSEPH C. BANIS Jr., M.D.

Associate Professor of Surgery, University of Louisville School of Medicine; Staff, Humana Hospital-University, Norton Hospital, Kosair Children's Hospital, Jewish Hospital, Baptist Hospital, Veterans Administration Medical Center, Louisville, Kentucky
Scapular Osteocutaneous Free-Flap Mandibular Reconstruction

BRUCE S. BAUER, M.D., F.A.C.S.

Assistant Professor of Surgery, Northwestern University Medical School; Chief, Division of Plastic Surgery, Children's Memorial Hospital, Chicago, Illinois
Alveolar Bone Grafting: Early

RUSSELL W. BESSETTE, D.D.S., M.D.

Director and Associate Professor, Division of Plastic and Reconstructive Surgery, State University of New Yørk at Buffalo School of Medicine, Buffalo, New York
Temporomandibular Joint Dysfunction

ALBERT F. BORGES, M.D., F.A.C.S.

Plastic Surgeon, Department of Plastic and Reconstructive Surgery, Fairfax Hospital, Falls Church, Virginia; Formerly Chief of Plastic and Reconstructive Surgery, Havana University Hospitals, Havana, Cuba
Scar Revision

HARRY J. BUNCKE, M.D., F.A.C.S.

Clinical Professor of Surgery, Division of Plastic and Reconstructive Surgery, University of California, San Francisco, School of Medicine; Chief, Department of Microsurgery, Davies Medical Center, San Francisco, California
Free Flap Contouring of Facial Asymmetries

GARY C. BURGET, M.D.

Clinical Assistant Professor, Section of Plastic and Reconstructive Surgery, The University of Chicago, Chicago, Illinois
Surgical Restoration of the Nose

JOHN H. COCHRAN Jr., M.D.

Instructor of Plastic Surgery, University of Colorado Health Sciences Center School of Medicine; Chief of Plastic and Reconstructive Surgery, Saint Joseph Hospital, Denver, Colorado
Synthetic Biomaterials for Soft Tissue

I. KELMAN COHEN, M.D.

Professor of Surgery and Chairman, Plastic and Reconstructive Surgery, Medical College of Virginia, Virginia Commonwealth University, Richmond, Virginia
Keloid

CLAUDE C. COLEMAN Jr., M.D., F.A.C.S.

Clinical Professor of Surgery, Medical College of Virginia; Chief of Plastic and Reconstructive Surgery, Henrico Doctor's Hospital, Richmond, Virginia
Squamous Carcinoma of the External Auditory Canal

GUSTAVO A. COLON, M.D., F.A.C.S.

Associate Professor, Plastic and Reconstructive Surgery, Tulane University School of Medicine; Director, Surgi-Unit Plastic Surgery Ambulatory Surgical Facility, New Orleans, Louisiana
Office Surgery

GEORGE C. CORMACK, M.A., F.R.C.S.(Edin)

Formerly Lecturer in Anatomy, University of Cambridge, Cambridge, England
Fasciocutaneous Flaps

EUGENE H. COURTISS, M.D.

Assistant Clinical Professor of Surgery, Harvard Medical School, Boston; Consultant in Plastic Surgery, Massachusetts General Hospital, Boston, Massachusetts, and Chief, Division of Plastic Surgery, Newton-Wellesley Hospital, Newton Lower Falls, Massachusetts
Facelift: Indications for Suction Lipectomy

ROLLIN K. DANIEL, M.D., F.A.C.S.

Division of Plastic Surgery, Hoag Memorial Hospital Presbyterian, Newport Beach, California
Electrical Injury
Rhinoplasty: The Bony Vault

ROBERT J. DEMUTH, M.D.

Associate Professor of Surgery and Acting Director, Division of Plastic Surgery, Oregon Health Sciences University, Portland, Oregon
Role of the Plastic Surgeon in Mohs' Micrographic Surgery

JOHN DEVINE Jr., M.D., F.A.C.S.

Associate Professor of Plastic Surgery, University of Miami School of Medicine; Chief, Plastic Surgery, Veterans Administration Hospital, Miami, Florida
Male Pattern Baldness

RICHARD ELLENBOGEN, M.D.

Director, Ellenbogen Plastic Surgical Institute, Los Angeles, California
Natural Facelift

RAY A. ELLIOTT Jr., M.D., F.A.C.S.

Clinical Professor of Surgery, Division of Plastic Surgery, Albany Medical College of Union University, Albany; Attending Plastic Surgeon, Albany Medical Center Hospital, St. Peter's Hospital, Memorial Hospital and Child's Hospital, Albany; Consultant, Veterans Administration Medical Center, Albany, New York, Sunnyview Hospital and Rehabilitation Center, Schenectady, New York, and Southwestern Vermont Medical Center, Bennington, Vermont
Protruding Ears

ELOF ERIKSSON, M.D.

Professor of Surgery, Harvard Medical School; Chief of Plastic Surgery, Brigham and Women's Hospital, and Children's Hospital, Boston, Massachusetts
Acute Care of Thermal Burns

ROBERT M. FAGGELLA Jr., M.D., M.S.S., F.A.C.S.

Clinical Associate Professor, University of California School of Medicine, Davis, California; Attending Physician, Sutter Community Hospitals, Mercy Hospital of Sacramento, University of California Davis Medical Center, Sacramento, California
Surgical Correction of Drool

JACK FISHER, M.D.

Assistant Clinical Professor, Department of Plastic Surgery, Vanderbilt University School of Medicine; Associate Professor, Department of Surgery, Meharry Medical College School of Medicine, and Associate, HCA Center for Research and Education, Nashville, Tennessee
Hypopharynx and Cervical Esophagus Reconstruction

JACK C. FISHER, M.D., F.A.C.S.

Professor of Surgery, University of California, San Diego School of Medicine, Head, Division of Plastic Surgery, UCSD Medical Center, and Chief, Section of Plastic and Reconstructive Surgery, Veterans Administration Medical Center, La Jolla, California
Radiation Injury

ROBERT S. FLOWERS, M.D., F.A.C.S.

M.D., Medical College of Alabama, Birmingham, Alabama; Chief and Director, Plastic Surgery Center of the Pacific Inc., Honolulu, Assistant Clinical Professor of Plastic Surgery, University of Hawaii School of Medicine, Honolulu, Hawaii
Cosmetic Surgery of the Oriental Face

SIMON FREDRICKS, M.D., F.A.C.S.

Senior Surgeon, Houston Plastic Surgery Associates; Chief of Plastic Surgery, St. Luke's Episcopal Hospital; Clinical Professor of Plastic Surgery, Baylor College of Medicine and University of Texas Medical Branch, Houston, Texas
Facelift: Male Patients

G. GREGORY GALLICO III, M.D., F.A.C.S.

Assistant Clinical Professor, Harvard Medical School; Assistant Surgeon, Massachusetts General Hospital, and Consultant, Shriners Burns Institute, Boston, Massachusetts
Grafting with Skin Substitutes

PETER E. GOODKIN, M.D.

Clinical Professor of Dermatology and Director of Mohs Micrographic Surgery, Oregon Health Sciences University, Portland, Oregon
Role of the Plastic Surgeon in Mohs' Micrographic Surgery

MARK GORNEY, M.D., F.A.C.S.

Associate Clinical Professor, Stanford University School of Medicine, Stanford, and University of California School of Medicine, San Francisco, California
Rehabilitation of the Cleft Lip Nose
The Septum in Rhinoplasty: Form and Function

MARK S. GRANICK, M.D., F.A.C.S.

Director, The Graduate Head and Neck Center; Staff Surgeon, Graduate Hospital and Germantown Hospital, Philadelphia, Pennsylvania
Parotid Tumors: Diagnostic Procedures and Radiotherapy

RICHARD O. GREGORY, B.S., M.D., F.A.C.S.

Clinical Faculty, Department of Health Sciences, University of Central Florida, Orlando; Staff, Orlando Regional Medical Center, and Florida Hospital, Orlando, Florida
The Laser in Plastic Surgery

JOSEPH S. GRUSS, M.B., F.R.C.S.(C)

Associate Professor of Plastic Surgery, Department of Surgery, University of Toronto Faculty of Medicine; Head, Division of Plastic Surgery, Sunnybrook Medical Centre, Toronto, Ontario, Canada
Internal Fixation in Facial Fractures: Principles
Internal Fixation in Facial Fractures: Specific Anatomic Aspects

JACK P. GUNTER, M.D.

Clinical Associate Professor in Plastic Surgery, and Clinical Associate Professor of Otolaryngology, The University of Texas Health Science Center; Attending Surgeon in Plastic Surgery, Presbyterian Hospital, Dallas, Texas
Deviated Nose

DWIGHT C. HANNA, M.D.

Clinical Professor of Surgery (Plastic), University of Pittsburgh School of Medicine; Staff (Emeritus), and Former Director, Western Pennsylvania Hospital, Pittsburgh, Pennsylvania
Parotid Tumors: Diagnostic Procedures and Radiotherapy

ROBERT A. HARDESTY, M.D.

Assistant Professor, Division of Plastic Surgery, Loma Linda University School of Medicine; Chief, Plastic Surgery, Jerry L. Pettis Memorial Veterans Administration Hospital, Loma Linda, California
Major Craniofacial Defects: Role of Free Tissue Transfer

FREDERICK R. HECKLER, M.D., F.A.C.S.

Clinical Associate Professor of Surgery (Plastic), University of Pittsburgh School of Medicine; Head, Division of Plastic Surgery, Allegheny General Hospital, Pittsburgh, Pennsylvania
Local Flaps on the Face

PETER HEECKT, CAND. MED.

Department of Plastic, Reconstructive and Hand Surgery, Burn Center, Munich-Bogenhausen Hospital, Munich, West Germany
Craniosynostosis Syndromes: Surgery in Infancy

PETER T. HETZLER, M.D.

Instructor, Pennsylvania State University College of Medicine; Chief Resident, The Milton S. Hershey Medical Center, Hershey, Pennsylvania
Soft Tissue Expansion

FRANK HÖPNER, M.D.

Professor, Department of Paediatric Surgery, Munich-Schwabing Hospital; Staff, Academic Teaching Hospital, Technical University, Munich, West Germany
Craniosynostosis Syndromes: Surgery in Infancy

PAUL S. HOWARD, M.D.

Assistant Professor of Plastic Surgery, University of Alabama School of Medicine, Birmingham, Alabama
Male Pattern Baldness

NICHOLAS T. ILIFF, M.D.

Associate Professor of Ophthalmology and Plastic Surgery, The John Hopkins School of Medicine, Baltimore, Maryland
Surgical Anatomy of the Orbit
Post-traumatic Enophthalmos

IAN T. JACKSON, M.D., F.R.C.S., F.A.C.S.

Professor, Mayo Medical School; Head, Section of Plastic and Reconstructive Surgery, Mayo Clinic, Rochester, Minnesota
Cranial Base Tumors

JONATHAN S. JACOBS, D.M.D., M.D.

Assistant Professor, Department of Plastic Surgery, Eastern Virginia Medical School; Chief, Department of Plastic Surgery, Sentara Medical Center Hospital, President of the Virginia Society of Plastic and Reconstructive Surgery, Norfolk, Virginia
Temporomandibular Joint Dysfunction

GLENN W. JELKS, M.D.

Assistant Professor of Surgery (Plastic), New York University Medical Center; Attending Staff, Bellevue Hospital, Manhattan Eye, Ear and Throat Hospital, Veterans Administration Hospital, and New York Eye and Ear Infirmary, New York, New York
Ocular Adnexal Reconstruction: The Tarsoconjunctival Flap

JAMES E. JONES, D.M.D., M.S., M.S.D.

Associate Professor of Pediatric Dentistry, Indiana University School of Dentistry, Indianapolis, Indiana; Robert Wood Johnson Dental Services Research Scholar 1987–89, Harvard School of Dental Medicine, Boston, Massachusetts
Alveolar Bone Grafting: Later

M. J. JURKIEWICZ, M.D., F.A.C.S.

Professor, Department of Surgery, Emory University School of Medicine; Chief, Section of Plastic Surgery, Emory Clinic, and Chief of Surgery, Veterans Administration Medical Center, Atlanta, Georgia
Scalp Defects

BERNARD L. KAYE, M.D., F.A.C.S.

Clinical Professor of Surgery (Plastic), University of Florida College of Medicine at Jacksonville; Formerly Chief of Plastic Surgery and Member, Active Staff, Baptist Medical Center, Jacksonville, Florida
Facelift: Avoidance and Treatment of Problems

MARK E. KRUGMAN, M.D.

Associate Adjunct Prrofessor of Plastic Surgery and Otolaryngology, University of California College of Medicine, Irvine; Attending Head and Neck Surgeon, Harbor-UCLA Medical Center, Los Angeles, California
Nonmicrosurgical Reconstruction of Postablative Head and Neck Defects

LAWRENCE C. KURTZMAN, M.D.

Clinical Instructor, Department of Plastic and Reconstructive Surgery, Eastern Virginia Medical School, Norfolk, Virginia
Mandibular Fractures

BYROM G. H. LAMBERTY, M.A., M.B., B.Chir., F.R.C.S.

Consultant Plastic Surgeon and Associate Lecturer, University of Cambridge, Cambridge, England
Fasciocutaneous Flaps

DAVID L. LARSON, M.D.

Professor and Chairman, Department of Plastic and Reconstructive Surgery, Medical College of Wisconsin, Milwaukee, Wisconsin
Surgical Treatment of Cancer in the Neck

GREGORY S. LA TRENTA, M.D.

Assistant Professor of Surgery (Plastic), Cornell Medical Center; Attending Surgeon, The New York Hospital, and Manhattan Eye, Ear, and Throat Hospital, New York, New York
Maxillary Osteotomies

DAVID C. LEBER, M.D., F.A.C.S.

Clinical Associate Professor of Surgery, The Milton S. Hershey Medical Center, Pennsylvania State University College of Medicine, Hershey, Pennsylvania; Staff Physician, Department of Surgery, Section of Plastic Surgery, Harrisburg Hospital, Harrisburg, Pennsylvania
Microtia: Autogenous Framework
Constricted Ears

JAMES A. LEHMAN Jr., M.D.

Professor of Plastic Surgery, Northeastern Ohio Universities College of Medicine, Rootstown, Ohio; Attending Plastic Surgeon, Children's Hospital Medical Center of Akron, and Akron General Medical Center, Akron, Ohio
Mandibular Osteotomies

MICHAEL B. LEWIS, M.D.

Associate Professor of Surgery, Tufts University School of Medicine; Surgeon, Chief of Plastic Surgery, New England Medical Center, Boston, Massachusetts
Timing and Technique of Cleft Palate Repair

VICTOR L. LEWIS Jr., M.D.

Associate Professor of Clinical Surgery, Northwestern University Medical School, Chicago, Illinois
Neurofibromatosis

EDWARD A. LUCE, M.D.

Professor of Surgery, University of Kentucky College of Medicine; Chief, Plastic Surgery, University Hospital and Veterans Administration Hospital, Lexington, Kentucky
Laryngeal Carcinoma

STEVEN D. MACHT, M.D.

Associate Clinical Professor of Plastic Surgery, George Washington University School of Medicine and Health Sciences, Washington, D.C.
Malignant Melanoma

WILLIAM P. MAGEE Jr., D.D.S., M.D.

Associate Professor, Eastern Virginia Medical School; Staff, Norfolk General Hospital and Children's Hospital of the King's Daughters, Norfolk, Virginia
Mandibular Fractures

HAROLD R. MANCUSI-UNGARO Jr., M.D., F.A.C.S.

Associate Professor of Surgery, University of New Mexico School of Medicine, Albuquerque, New Mexico; Chief, Division of Plastic Surgery, and Director, Regional Burn Center, University of New Mexico—Bernalillo County Medical Center, Albuquerque, New York
Skin Grafts

ERNEST K. MANDERS, M.D.

Associate Professor, Division of Plastic and Reconstructive Surgery, The Milton S. Hershey Medical Center, Pennsylvania State University, College of Medicine; Chief, Division of Plastic and Reconstructive Surgery, The Milton S. Hershey Medical Center, Hershey, Pennsylvania
Soft Tissue Expansion
Male Pattern Baldness

PAUL N. MANSON, M.D.

Professor of Plastic Surgery, The Johns Hopkins School of Medicine; Director of Plastic Surgery, The Maryland Institute of Emergency Medical Services System, Baltimore, Maryland
Surgical Anatomy of the Orbit
Post-traumatic Enophthalmos

JEFFREY L. MARSH, M.D.

Professor of Surgery, Plastic and Reconstructive, Washington University School of Medicine; Medical Director, Cleft Palate and Craniofacial Deformities Institute, Children's Hospital, St. Louis, Missouri
Hemangioma

W. EARLE MATORY Jr., M.D.

Assistant Professor, Department of Anatomy, Graduate School of Biomedical Sciences, University of Massachusetts Medical School; Assistant Professor, Division of Plastic and Reconstructive Surgery, University of Massachusetts Medical Center, Worcester, Massachusetts
Special Problems in the Black Face

LEO McCAFFERTY, M.D.

Assistant Professor of Plastic Surgery, University of Miami School of Medicine, Miami, Florida
Male Pattern Baldness

JOSEPH G. McCARTHY, M.D.

Lawrence D. Bell Professor of Plastic Surgery, New York University School of Medicine; Director, Institute of Reconstructive Plastic Surgery, New York University Medical Center, New York, New York
Craniosynostosis Syndromes: Surgery in Infancy and Childhood

FREDERICK J. McCOY, M.D.

Clinical Professor of Surgery (Plastic), University of Missouri School of Medicine; Chief, Division of Plastic Surgery, Truman Medical Center, Chief, Section of Plastic Surgery, Children's Mercy Hospital, and Attending Plastic Surgeon, Menorah Medical Center, and Research Medical Center, Kansas City, Missouri
Facial Fractures in Children

IAN A. McGREGOR, D.Sc., Ch.M., F.R.C.S., F.R.A.C.S., F.A.C.S.

Director, Plastic and Oral Surgery Unit, Canniesburn Hospital, Bearsden, Glasgow, Scotland
Surgical Approach to the Mouth

STEPHEN H. MILLER, M.D.

Plastic Surgeon, Hospital of the Scripps Clinic, La Jolla, California
Role of the Plastic Surgeon In Mohs' Micrographic Surgery

MAMDOUH A. MOTTALEB, M.B., B.Ch., M.Sc.

Fellow in Plastic Surgery, Pennsylvania State University College of Medicine; Staff, The Milton S. Hershey Medical Center, Hershey, Pennsylvania
Soft Tissue Expansion

WOLFGANG MÜHLBAUER, M.D.

Professor, Academic Teaching Hospital, Technical University, Munich; Department of Plastic, Reconstructive and Hand Surgery, Burn Center, Munich-Bogenhausen Hospital, Munich, West Germany
Craniosynostosis Syndromes: Surgery in Infancy

JOHN B. MULLIKEN, M.D.

Associate Professor of Surgery, Harvard Medical School; Director, Craniofacial Center, Division of Plastic Surgery, Children's Hospital, and Brigham and Women's Hospital, Boston, Massachusetts
Bilateral Complete Cleft Lip

IAN R. MUNRO, M.D., M.A., M.B., B.Chir., F.R.C.S.(C)

Director, Humana Craniofacial Institute; Humana Hospital-Medical City Dallas, Dallas, Texas
Hemifacial Microsomia

THOMAS A. MUSTOE, M.D.

Assistant Professor of Surgery, Division of Plastic Surgery, Washington University School of Medicine; Attending Plastic Surgeon, Barnes Hospital, Jewish Hospital of St. Louis, Children's Hospital, St. Louis, Missouri
Evaluation of the Patient with Head and Neck Cancer

FOAD NAHAI, M.D., F.A.C.S.

Associate Professor of Surgery, Emory University School of Medicine; Associate Professor of Surgery, Department of Plastic and Reconstructive Surgery, Emory Clinic, and Crawford W. Long Memorial Hospital of Emory University, Atlanta, Georgia
Free Flaps in Craniofacial Surgery

CHARLES L. NELSON, D.D.S.

Associate Professor of Oral and Maxillofacial Surgery, Indiana University School of Dentistry; Attending Staff, Indiana University School of Dentistry and Indiana University Hospitals, Indianapolis, Indiana
Alveolar Bone Grafting: Later

SEIICHI OHMORI, M.D.

Former Professor of Plastic Surgery, University of Tokyo; Director (Emeritus), Tokyo Metropolitan Police Hospital, and Director, Ohmori Institute for Aesthetic Plastic Surgery, Senior Consultant of Ohmori Institute for Aesthetic Plastic Surgery Clinic, Tokyo, Japan
Microtia: Silastic Framework

JOHN M. OSBORN, M.D., F.A.C.S.

Clinical Associate Professor, University of California School of Medicine, Davis, California; Attending Physician, Sutter Community Hospitals, Mercy Hospital of Sacramento, Sacramento Medical Center, University of California Davis Medical Center, Sacramento, California
Surgical Correction of Drool

DOUGLAS K. OUSTERHOUT, D.D.S., M.D.

Clinical Professor of Surgery (Plastic), University of California School of Medicine; Attending, St. Francis Memorial Hospital and Ralph K. Davies Medical Center and Consultant, Letterman Army Hospital, San Francisco, California
Craniosynostosis Syndromes: Surgery in Adolescence
Feminization of the Skull

ROBERT W. PARSONS, M.D.

Professor in Surgery and Pediatrics, The University of Chicago Pritzker School of Medicine, Chicago, Illinois
Pierre Robin Sequence

RONALD W. PIGOTT, B.A., M.B., F.R.C.S., F.R.C.S.I.

Honorary Lecturer in Plastic Surgery, University of Bristol; Consultant Plastic Surgeon, South Western Regional Health Authority, Bristol, United Kingdom
Cleft Lip Nasal Deformity: Early Correction

PETER RANDALL, M.D.

Professor of Plastic Surgery, University of Pennsylvania School of Medicine; Senior Surgeon, Children's Hospital of Philadelphia, Philadelphia, Pennsylvania
Unilateral Cleft Lip

ANDREW M. REED, Ph.D.

Director, Polymer Technology; Staff, Matrix Medica Inc., Wheat Ridge, Colorado
Synthetic Biomaterials for Soft Tissue

RILEY S.REES, M.D.

Associate Professor, University of Michigan Medical School; Chief of Surgery, Veterans Administration Hospital, Ann Arbor, Michigan
Spider Bites

BRUNO RISTOW, M.D., F.A.C.S.

Chief, Division of Plastic and Reconstructive Surgery, Pacific Presbyterian Medical Center, San Francisco, California
Forehead Lift: Composite Musculoaponeurotic Grafts

NECITA ROA, M.D.

Associate Professor of Anesthesiology, Washington University School of Medicine, and Associate Professor of Anesthesiology in Oral and Maxillofacial Surgery, Washington University School of Dental Medicine, St. Louis, Missouri
Anesthesia for Cosmetic Surgery

MARTIN C. ROBSON, M.D.

Truman G. Blocker Jr. Professor of Surgery and Microbiology; Chief and Director of Plastic Surgery, University of Texas Medical Branch and Director of Surgical Services, Shriners Burns Institute, Galveston, Texas
Infected Soft Tissue Wounds

RODNEY J. ROHRICH, M.D.

Assistant Professor of Plastic Surgery, University of Texas Health Science Center; Chief of Plastic Surgery, Parkland Memorial Hospital, Dallas, Texas
Deviated Nose

LEONARD R. RUBIN, M.D., F.A.C.S.

Professor of Clinical Surgery (Plastic), State University of New York at Stony Brook Health Sciences Center School of Medicine; Director, Residency Training Program and Director, Nassau County Medical Center, Stony Brook, New York
Reanimation of the Paralyzed Face by Contiguous Muscle Transfers

A. MICHAEL SADOVE, M.D., F.A.C.S.

Associate Professor of Surgery, Plastic Surgery Section, Indiana University School of Medicine; Chief, Plastic Surgery Section, James Whitcomb Riley Hospital for Children and Attending Staff, Indiana University Hospitals, Indianapolis, Indiana
Alveolar Bone Grafting: Later

KENNETH E. SALYER, M.D., F.A.C.S., F.A.A.P.

Chairman and Director, International Craniofacial Institute, Humana Advanced Surgical Institutes, Dallas, Texas
Synthetic Biomaterials for Bone

BERND SCHAARSCHMIDT, M.D.

Department of Anaesthesiology, Munich-Schwabing Hospital, West Germany
Craniosynostosis Syndromes: Surgery in Infancy

ANDREAS SCHMIDT, M.D.

Department of Plastic, Reconstructive and Hand Surgery, Burn Center, Munich-Bogenhausen Hospital, Munich, West Germany
Craniosynostosis Syndromes: Surgery in Infancy

RICHARD CARLTON SCHULTZ, M.D., F.A.C.S.

Clinical Professor of Surgery (Plastic), University of Illinois College of Medicine, Chicago, Illinois
Skull Defects

ARTHUR G. SHIP, M.D., D.M.D.

Associate Clinical Professor, Plastic Surgery, Albert Einstein College of Medicine of Yeshiva University; Attending Plastic Surgeon, Montefiore Medical Center, and Doctors Hospital, New York, New York
Blepharoplasty

DAVID S. SOUTAR, Ch.M., F.R.C.S.(Edin), F.R.C.S.(Glasg)

Consultant Plastic Surgeon, West of Scotland Regional Plastic and Maxillofacial Surgery Unit, Canniesburn Hospital, Bearsden; Consultant Plastic Surgeon, Western Infirmary, Glasgow, Scotland
Radial Forearm Flap in Head and Neck Reconstruction

MELVIN SPIRA, M.D.

Professor and Head, Division of Plastic Surgery, Baylor College of Medicine; Chief, Plastic Surgery Service, The Methodist Hospital and Veterans Administration Hospital, Houston, Texas
Cartilage Grafting

SAMUEL STAL, M.D.

Assistant Professor, Division of Plastic Surgery, Baylor College of Medicine; Chief of Plastic Surgery Services, Texas Children's Hospital, Co-Director, Cleft Palate and Craniofacial Center, Texas Children's Hospital, and Chief of Plastic Surgery Services, Texas Institute for Research and Rehabilitation, Houston, Texas
Cartilage Grafting

WILLIAM M. SWARTZ, M.D.

Associate Professor and Chief of Plastic Surgery, Tulane University School of Medicine; Plastic Surgeon, Charity Hospital at New Orleans, Children's Hospital, Touro Infirmary, and Southern Baptist Hospital, New Orleans, Louisiana
Scapular Osteocutaneous Free-Flap Mandibular Reconstruction

PAUL TESSIER, M.D.

Private Practice, Paris, France
Mandibulofacial Dysostosis

GORDON R. TOBIN, M.D.

Professor of Surgery, University of Louisville School of Medicine, Louisville, Kentucky
Lip Reconstruction

JEAN-FRANCOIS TULASNE, M.D.

Private Practice, Paris, France
Mandibulofacial Dysostosis

KARIN VARGERVIK, D.D.S.

Professor, Department of Growth and Development and Director, Center for Craniofacial Anomalies, University of California School of Medicine, San Francisco, California
Craniosynostosis Syndromes: Surgery in Adolescence

ESTHER VERTESY, M.D.

Department of Paediatric Surgery, Munich-Schwabing Hospital, West Germany
Craniosynostosis Syndromes: Surgery in Infancy

LARS M. VISTNES, M.D., F.R.C.S.(C)

Professor of Surgery, Stanford University School of Medicine, Chairman, Division of Plastic and Reconstructive Surgery, Rehabilitative Medicine, Stanford University Medical Center, Stanford, California
Anophthalmic Orbit

R. CHRIS A. WEATHERLEY-WHITE, M.D.

Associate Clinical Professor of Surgery (Plastic), University of Colorado School of Medicine, Denver, Colorado
Timing of Cleft Lip Repair

JAMES H. WELLS, M.D., F.A.C.S.

Formerly Assistant Professor of Plastic Surgery, The Johns Hopkins University School of Medicine; Vice-Chief of Surgery, Memorial Medical Center, Long Beach, California
Interviewing the Patient

MENACHEM R. WEXLER, M.D.

Professor, Plastic and Maxillofacial Surgery, Hebrew University Hadassah Medical School; Head, Department of Plastic and Maxillofacial Surgery, Hadassah University Hospital, Jerusalem, Israel
Down Syndrome Face Reconstruction

LINTON A. WHITAKER, M.D.

Professor of Plastic Surgery, University of Pennsylvania School of Medicine; Chief of Plastic Surgery, Hospital of the University of Pennsylvania and Director, Craniofacial Program, Children's Hospital of Philadelphia, Philadelphia, Pennsylvania
Craniosynostosis

H. BRUCE WILLIAMS, M.D.

Professor of Surgery and Director, Plastic and Reconstructive Surgery, McGill University Faculty of Medicine; Director, Plastic Surgery, Montreal General and Montreal Children's Hospitals, Montreal, Quebec, Canada
Lymphangioma

S. ANTHONY WOLFE, M.D., F.A.C.S.

Clinical Professor of Plastic and Reconstructive Surgery, University of Miami School of Medicine, Miami, Florida
Orbital Dystopias

VERNON L. YOUNG, M.D.

Associate Professor, Washington University School of Medicine, St. Louis, Missouri
Major Craniofacial Defects: Role of Free Tissue Transfer

HARVEY A. ZAREM, M.D.

Professor (Emeritus), UCLA School of Medicine, Los Angeles, California
Injectable Collagen

RONALD G. ZELT, M.D., C.M.

Resident, Division of Plastic and Reconstructive Surgery, McGill University Faculty of Medicine; Staff, Royal Victoria Hospital, Montreal, Quebec, Canada
Electrical Injury

JÖRG ZENKER, M.D.

Department of Neurosurgery, Munich-Bogenhausen Hospital, Munich, West Germany
Craniosynostosis Syndromes: Surgery in Infancy

BARRY ZIDE, M.D., D.M.D.

Assistant Professor of Surgery (Plastic), New York University Medical Center, Bellevue Hospital Center, and Manhattan Eye, Ear and Throat Hospital; Attending Surgeon, New York Eye and Ear Infirmary, New York, New York
Maxillary Osteotomies

RONALD M. ZUKER, M.D., F.R.C.S.(C), F.A.C.S.

Associate Professor of Surgery, Department of Surgery, University of Toronto Faculty of Medicine; Head, Division of Plastic Surgery, The Hospital for Sick Children and Staff Plastic Surgeon, Toronto General Hospital, Toronto, Ontario, Canada
Microvascular Management of Facial Palsy

CONTRIBUTORS
Volume 2

JAMES L. BAKER Jr., M.D., F.A.C.S.

Adjunct Professor of Surgery, College of Health, University of Central Florida, Orlando, Florida; Active Staff, Orlando Regional Medical Center, and Courtesy Staff, Winter Park Memorial Hospital, and Florida Hospital of Orlando, Florida

Augmentation Mammoplasty: A Personal Approach

ROBERT W. BERNARD, M.D.

Chief (Emeritus), Plastic Surgery, White Plains Hospital, White Plains, Chief, Plastic Surgery, Northern Westchester Hospital, Mount Kisco, and Chief, Plastic Surgery, United Hospital, Port Chester, New York

Reduction Mammoplasty

PATRICIA E. BURROWS, M.D., F.R.C.P.(C)

Assistant Professor, Radiology, University of Toronto Faculty of Medicine; Staff Physician, Department of Radiology, The Hospital for Sick Children, Toronto, Ontario, Canada

Vascular Problems in the Hand

H. HOLLIS CAFFEE, M.D., F.A.C.S.

Associate Professor, University of Florida College of Medicine, Gainesville; Chief, Plastic Surgery Service, Gainesville Veterans Administration Hospital, Gainesville, Florida

Augmentation Mammoplasty: Biology of Capsule Contracture

RICHARD W. CLEMENT, M.D.

Assistant Professor of Surgery, Plastic and Reconstructive, Washington University School of Medicine, St. Louis, Missouri

Gynecomastia

BENJAMIN E. COHEN, M.D., F.A.C.S.

Assistant Clinical Professor, Division of Plastic Surgery, Baylor College of Medicine; Academic Chief and Director, Plastic Surgery Residency Program, St. Joseph Hospital, Houston, Texas

Surgical Options and Aesthetic Considerations

I. KELMAN COHEN, M.D.

Professor of Surgery and Chairman, Plastic and Reconstructive Surgery, Medical College of Virginia, Virginia Commonwealth University, Richmond, Virginia

Immediate Breast Reconstruction

LAWRENCE B. COLEN, M.D.

Assistant Professor of Surgery (Plastic), Dartmouth Medical School; Staff Surgeon, Dartmouth-Hitchcock Medical Center, Hanover, New Hampshire

Diabetic Foot

R. EVAN CRANDALL, M.D.

Private Practice, St Louis, Missouri

Implants in the Hand and Wrist

A. LEE DELLON, M.D.

Associate Professor, Plastic Surgery and Neurological Surgery, The Johns Hopkins University School of Medicine; Attending Hand Surgeon, Curtis Hand Center, Union Memorial Hospital, Baltimore, Maryland

Interruption of Nerve Function

BARRY FERNANDO, M.D.

Resident, Department of Plastic Surgery, Washington University Medical Center, and Barnes Hospital, St. Louis, Missouri; Private Practice, Paradise Valley, Arizona

Chest Reconstruction
Implants in the Hand and Wrist
Painful Hand Syndrome

JACK C. FISHER, M.D., F.A.C.S.

Professor of Surgery, University of California, San Diego School of Medicine, Head, Division of Plastic Surgery, UCSD Medical Center, and Chief, Section of Plastic and Reconstructive Surgery, Veterans Administration Medical Center, La Jolla, California

Who Can Benefit from Prophylactic Mastectomy?

ALAN E. FREELAND, M.D.

Professor of Orthopaedic Surgery, University of Mississippi Medical Center, Jackson, Mississippi

Internal Fixation of Metacarpal and Phalangeal Fractures

LOUIS A. GILULA, M.D.

Professor of Radiology, Washington University School of Medicine; Co-Director, Musculoskeletal Section, Edward Mallinckrodt Institute of Radiology, St. Louis, Missouri
Radiologic Examination

BURT M. GREENBERG, M.D.

Attending Plastic Surgeon, Northshore Hospital and Long Island Jewish Hospital, New York, New York
Chronic Traumatic Lower Extremity Wounds: Free Muscle Transfer and Skin Graft

DAVID C. HARDY, M.D.

Assistant Professor of Radiology, Edward Mallinckrodt Institute of Radiology, Washington University School of Medicine, St. Louis, Missouri
Radiologic Examination

CARL R. HARTRAMPF Jr., M.D.

Clinical Professor, Emory University School of Medicine; Private Practice, Atlanta Plastic Surgery, P.A. Atlanta, Georgia
TRAM Flap

VINCENT R. HENTZ, M.D.

Associate Professor of Surgery, Stanford University School of Medicine; Chief, Division of Hand and Upper Limb Surgery, Stanford University Hospital, Stanford, California
Phalloplasty

T. RODERICK HESTER Jr., M.D.

Associate Professor of Surgery, Plastic and Reconstructive, Emory University School of Medicine, Emory University Affiliate Hospitals, Atlanta, Georgia
Augmentation Mammoplasty: Polyurethane-Covered Mammary Implant

CHARLES E. HORTON, M.D., F.A.C.S.

Professor, Medical College of Hampton Roads, Norfolk, Virginia
Hypospadias

DENNIS J. HURWITZ, M.D.

Clinical Associate Professor of Surgery (Plastic), University of Pittsburgh School of Medicine; Attending Staff Surgeon, Montefiore Hospital, Children's Hospital of Pittsburgh, Eye and Ear Hospital of Pittsburgh, and Presbyterian-University Hospital, Pittsburgh, Pennsylvania
Perineal Defects

MICHAEL E. JABALEY, M.D.

Clinical Professor of Surgery (Plastic), University of Mississippi School of Medicine, Jackson, Mississippi
Internal Fixation of Metacarpal and Phalangeal Fractures

JOHN R. JARRETT, M.D., F.A.C.S.

Clinical Instructor in Plastic Surgery, University of Oregon Health Science Center, Portland; Department of Surgery, Sacred Heart Medical Center, Eugene, Oregon
Prophylactic Mastectomy

MORTON L. KASDAN, M.D., F.A.C.S.

Assistant Clinical Professor, University of Louisville School of Medicine, Louisville, Kentucky
Occupational Hand Dysfunction

JOHN G. KENNEY, M.D., F.A.C.S.

Associate Professor of Plastic and Maxillofacial Surgery, University of Virginia Medical Center, Charlottesville, Virginia
Gender Dysphoria

NEIL E. KLEIN, B.A., M.D.

Assistant Professor of Surgery, University of Southern California School of Medicine, Los Angeles, California; Chief, Division of Plastic Surgery, Rancho Los Amigos Medical Center, Downey, California
Pressure Sores

KENNETH E. KORBER, M.H.S.

Research Assistant Experimental Instructor, Microsurgery Laboratory, Division of Plastic Surgery, Washington University School of Medicine, St. Louis, Missouri
Use of Leeches in Plastic Surgery

BRUCE A. KRAEMER, M.D.

Assistant Professor of Plastic and Reconstructive Surgery, Washington University School of Medicine, St. Louis; Staff Plastic Surgeon, Barnes Hospital and St. Louis Children's Hospital, Chief of Plastic Surgery, St. Louis Regional Medical Center, St. Louis, Missouri
Use of Leeches in Plastic Surgery

DONALD R. LAUB, M.D., F.A.C.S.

Associate Clinical Professor of Plastic Surgery, Stanford University School of Medicine, Stanford, California
Phalloplasty

DONALD R. LAUB Jr., M.S.

Medical Student, Medical College of Wisconsin, Milwaukee, Wisconsin
Phalloplasty

JOHN R. LEWIS Jr., M.D.

Clinical Professor of Surgery (Plastic), University of Kentucky College of Medicine, Lexington, Kentucky, Associate Clinical Professor of Surgery (Plastic), Emory University School of Medicine, Atlanta; Director, Institute of Aesthetic Plastic Surgery, Member of Hospital Staff, Metropolitan Hospital, West Paces Ferry Hospital, Crawford W. Long Memorial Hospital of Emory University, Piedmont Hospital, and Grady Memorial Hospital of Emory University, Atlanta, Georgia
Abdominoplasty

JOHN WILLIAM LITTLE III, M.D.

Professor and Director, Division of Plastic Surgery, Georgetown University Medical Center, Washington, D.C.; Consultant, National Cancer Institute, National Institutes of Health, Bethesda, Maryland
Nipple-Areola Reconstruction

SUSAN E. MACKINNON, M.D., F.R.C.S.(C), F.A.C.S.

Associate Professor, Department of Surgery, University of Toronto; Staff Plastic Surgeon, Chief, Hand Service, Sunnybrook Medical Centre, Toronto, Ontario, Canada
Nerve Compression Syndromes

RALPH T. MANKTELOW, M.D., F.R.C.S.(C)

Professor, Department of Surgery, and Chairman, Division of Plastic Surgery, University of Toronto Faculty of Medicine; Head, Division of Plastic Surgery, Toronto General Hospital, Toronto, Ontario, Canada
Microsurgical Muscle Transfer for Upper Extremity Motors

HALLENE MARAGH, M.D.

Assistant Professor of Plastic Surgery, Eastern Virginia Medical School; Full Attending Physician, J.K.T., M.D., Ltd., Norfolk, Virginia
Brachial Plexus Injuries

MARTHA S. MATTHEWS, M.D.

Assistant Instructor, Medical College of Hamptom Roads, Norfolk, Virginia
Hypospadias

G. PATRICK MAXWELL, M.D.

Assistant Clinical Professor, Department of Plastic Surgery, Vanderbilt University School of Medicine; Associate Professor, Department of Surgery, Meharry Medical College School of Medicine and Director of Research, HCA Center for Research and Education, Nashville, Tennessee
Latissimus Dorsi

JAMES W. MAY Jr., M.D.

Associate Clinical Professor, Harvard Medical School; Chief of Plastic and Reconstructive Surgery and Hand Surgery Service, Department of General Surgery, Massachusetts General Hospital, Boston, Massachusetts
Chronic Traumatic Lower Extremity Wounds: Free Muscle Transfer and Skin Graft

ROBERT M. McFARLANE, M.D., M.Sc., F.R.C.S.(C), F.A.C.S.

Professor and Chief, Division of Plastic Surgery, University of Western Ontario Faculty of Medicine; Head, Division of Plastic Surgery, Victoria Hospital Corporation, London, Ontario, Canada
Dupuytren's Disease

TIMOTHY A. MILLER, M.D., F.A.C.S.

Professor of Surgery, UCLA School of Medicine; Chief of Plastic Surgery, Wadsworth VA Hospital, Los Angeles, California
Lymphedema

WILLIAM D. MORAIN, M.D.

Professor of Surgery (Plastic), Dartmouth Medical School; Staff Surgeon, Dartmouth-Hitchcock Medical Center, Hanover, New Hampshire
Diabetic Foot

FOAD NAHAI, M.D., F.A.C.S.

Associate Professor of Surgery, Emory University School of Medicine; Associate Professor of Surgery, Department of Plastic and Reconstructive Surgery, Emory Clinic, and Crawford W. Long Memorial Hospital of Emory University, Atlanta, Georgia
Infected Vascular Prostheses

HENRY W. NEALE, M.D., F.A.C.S.

Professor of Surgery, University of Cincinnati College of Medicine; Director, Division of Plastic, Reconstructive and Hand Surgery, University of Cincinnati Medical Center and Director, Burn Reconstructive and Plastic Surgery, Shriners Burn Institute, Cincinnati, Ohio
Reconstruction of Burns of the Trunk and Breast

MICHAEL G. ORGEL, M.D., F.A.C.S.

Associate Professor of Surgery (Plastic), University of Massachusetts Medical School; Attending Plastic Surgeon, Berkshire Medical Center, Pittsfield, Massachusetts
Rectal Sphincter Reconstruction

CALVIN R. PETERS, M.D.

Associate Clinical Professor of Surgery (Plastic), University of Florida College of Medicine, Gainesville, and University of South Florida College of Medicine, Tampa, Florida
Exstrophy

PAUL G. PIN, M.D.

Instructor of Surgery (Plastic and Reconstructive), Washington University School of Medicine, St. Louis, Missouri
Role of Physical Therapy
Extensor and Flexor Tendon Injuries

WILLIAM E. POWERS Jr., M.D.

Attending Plastic Surgeon, Kaiser Foundation Hospital, Sacramento, California
Replantation Surgery

RICHARD P. RAND, M.D.

Resident, Department of Plastic and Reconstructive Surgery, Emory University School of Medicine, Atlanta, Georgia
Infected Vascular Prostheses

ROGER E. SALISBURY, M.D., F.A.C.S.

Professor of Surgery and Chief, Plastic and Reconstructive Surgery, New York Medical College; Chief, Plastic and Reconstructive Surgery and Director, The Burn Center, Westchester County Medical Center, Valhalla, New York
The Burned Upper Extremity

ROBERT R. SCHENCK, M.D.

Director, Section of Hand Surgery and Associate Professor, Departments of Plastic and Orthopedic Surgery, Rush-Presbyterian-St. Luke's Medical Center, Chicago, Illinois; Senior Attending Staff, Rush-Presbyterian-St. Luke's Medical Center, Chicago, Illinois
Fingertip Injuries

PAUL L. SCHNUR, M.D., F.A.C.S.

Clinical Lecturer in Surgery, University of Arizona College of Medicine; Instructor, Tucson Hospital, Medical Education Program, Tucson, Arizona
Augmentation Mammoplasty: Ancillary Measures

WILLIAM W. SHAW, M.D., F.A.C.S.

Associate Professor of Surgery (Plastic), New York University School of Medicine; Chief of Plastic Surgery, Bellevue Hospital, New York, New York
Microvascular Free Flaps
Replantation Surgery

DAVID J. SMITH Jr., M.D.

Associate Professor of Surgery, Section Head, Plastic Surgery, University of Michigan Medical School, Ann Arbor, Michigan
Ganglions and Other Benign Tumors of the Hand

SCOTT L. SPEAR, M.D., F.A.C.S.

Associate Professor and Deputy Director, Department of Plastic Surgery, Georgetown University School of Medicine, Washington, D.C.
Intradermal Tattooing

THOMAS R. STEVENSON, M.D., F.A.C.S.

Assistant Professor of Surgery, Section of Plastic Surgery, University of Michigan Medical School, Ann Arbor, Michigan
Restoration of Stable Soft Tissue Coverage in Wounds of the Foot

BAHMAN TEIMOURIAN, M.D.

Associate Clinical Professor, Georgetown University School of Medicine, and Faculty Member, George Washington University, Washington, D.C.; Chairman, Department of Surgery, Suburban Hospital, Bethesda, Maryland, and Chairman, Department of Plastic Surgery, Southern Maryland Hospital, Clinton, Maryland
Suction Lipectomy: Body Contouring—Suction Versus Scalpel

JULIA K. TERZIS, M.D., Ph.D., F.R.C.S.(C)

Associate Professor of Plastic Surgery, Eastern Virginia Medical School; Director, Microsurgical Research Center, Eastern Virginia Medical School, and Staff, J.K.T., M.D., Ltd., Norfolk, Virginia
Brachial Plexus Injuries

GORDON R. TOBIN, M.D.

Professor of Surgery, University of Louisville School of Medicine, Louisville, Kentucky
Vaginal Reconstruction

JOSEPH UPTON, M.D.

Assistant Professor of Surgery, Department of Surgery, Harvard Medical School, Boston, Massachusetts
Pollicization for the Aplastic Thumb

PAUL M. WEEKS, M.D.

Professor of Surgery (Plastic and Reconstructive), Chief, Division of Plastic and Reconstructive Surgery, Washington University School of Medicine, St. Louis, Missouri
Role of Physical Therapy
Extensor and Flexor Tendon Injuries

MICHAEL J. YAREMCHUK, M.D.

Assistant Professor of Plastic Surgery, Harvard Medical School, Boston; Plastic Surgeon, Massachusetts General Hospital, Boston, Massachusetts, Former Assistant Director of Plastic and Maxillofacial Surgery, Maryland Institute for Emergency Medical Services Systems (MIEMSS), Baltimore, Maryland
Acute Flap Coverage of Open Fractures of the Lower Extremity

VERNON L. YOUNG, M.D.

Associate Professor, Washington University School of Medicine, St. Louis, Missouri
Chest Reconstruction
Implants in the Hand and Wrist
Painful Hand Syndrome

ELVIN G. ZOOK, M.D.

Professor of Surgery and Chairman of Plastic and Reconstructive Surgery, Southern Illinois University School of Medicine, Springfield, Illinois
Nailbed Injuries

RONALD M. ZUKER, M.D., F.R.C.S.(C), F.A.C.S.

Associate Professor of Surgery, Department of Surgery, University of Toronto Faculty of Medicine; Head, Division of Plastic Surgery, The Hospital for Sick Children and Staff Plastic Surgeon, Toronto General Hospital, Toronto, Ontario, Canada
Vascular Problems in the Hand

PREFACE

One may ask, as I did upon being invited to edit these volumes: is there a need for yet another book on plastic and reconstructive surgery?

Plastic surgeons are distinguished by their originality in conception and finesse in execution. They are a restless breed, preferring untrod paths to worn byways. Being unrestricted by anatomic region or system, their explorations often have yielded insights and techniques readily adopted by sister surgical specialties. This fluidity, which is plastic surgery's strength, makes creation of a contemporaneous text difficult, given the usual lag time between manuscript preparation and publication. In addition, the familiar encyclopedic text, which is cumbersome to produce, may bury creativity beneath historical review and therapeutic ecumenism.

The opportunity, therefore, to invite a large number of active contributors in the field of plastic and reconstructive surgery to write personalized submissions for prompt publication was intriguing. These contributors were chosen for their expertise, as demonstrated by recent presentations, study courses, or articles. They were instructed to submit succinct statements of personal preferences for solutions to problems confronted by practicing plastic surgeons. At publication, the first chapter received will be twenty months old and the last five months old. Publication of subsequent volumes every three years should maintain the currency of the contents and express the diversity of management opinions.

The successful production of this book was made possible by the promptness of the authors, the cooperation of my editor, Mary Mansor, the efficiency of my publisher, Brian C. Decker, the attention of my secretary, Karen Lask-McDonagh, and the tolerance of my wife, Rebecca, and my daughter, Kohli. I thank them all for participating in this project.

Following the invitation to edit, I did conclude that the uniqueness of this book, with respect to the currency and individualization of contents, did make the effort worthwhile. I hope that you, the reader, concur.

Jeffrey L. Marsh, M.D.
St. Louis, Missouri

CONTENTS

VOLUME 1

General Principles

Head and Neck

Trauma

Facial Palsy

Cleft Lip and Palate

Craniofacial Deformities

VOLUME II

Breast

Postmastectomy Reconstruction

The Trunk

Genitourinary Structures

GENERAL PRINCIPLES

INFECTED SOFT TISSUE WOUNDS

MARTIN C. ROBSON, M.D.

Infection in clinical surgical practice has been defined as the product of the entrance, growth, metabolic activities, and resultant pathophysiologic effects of microorganisms in the tissues of the patient. Man's biologic state is not germ-free even in the absence of clinical infection. Some contamination always exists in soft tissue. There is a delicate balance between the factors of host resistance and the actions of a great many species of bacteria, all with the potential to cause infection. If equilibrium remains stable, host resistance factors will eventually overcome any contamination of the wound. However, if equilibrium is upset, either by an impairment in the host defense mechanisms or by an increase in the bacterial inoculum, clinical infection may result.

A major advance in management of the contaminated or infected soft tissue wound has been our understanding that the mere presence of organisms in the wound is less important than the level of bacterial growth. Clinical and experimental data have shown that a level of bacterial growth greater than 100,000 (10^5) organisms per gram of tissue for most bacterial species is necessary to cause wound infection and the potential for invasive sepsis.

DEFINITIVE DIAGNOSIS OF INFECTION

Definitive diagnosis of infection is made by the presence of purulent material draining from the wound or spreading inflammation beyond normal inflammation of healing. It can also be made from the number of bacteria per gram of wound tissue. Quantitative cultures of tissue biopsies that reveal greater than 10^5 bacteria per gram of tissue, or the presence of beta-hemolytic streptococci, suggest clinical infection.

Quantitative bacteriologic cultures can help to differentiate between the contaminated and the grossly infected wound. They also give an endpoint on which to determine management of a soft tissue wound. The presence of 10^5 or fewer bacteria per gram of tissue in the absence of beta-hemolytic streptococci has been shown to allow direct wound closure, successful application of skin grafts, and closure of the wound by pedicle flaps. A quantitative tissue culture is obtained by cleansing the wound surface, removing a tissue specimen, aseptically weighing, flaming, and homogenizing it after tenfold dilution with thioglycolate. Serial tube dilutions and pour plates or backplating can then yield an accurate colony count per gram of tissue.

Such detailed analyses are of little value in determining immediate wound management since they require 24 to 36 hours for completion. However, the important information derived from this technique can be obtained in 15 minutes with the rapid slide method. A specimen is removed from the wound, weighed, diluted, and homogenized as before, but a 0.02 ml aliquot of the suspension is then placed on a glass slide and Gram stained. The slide can then be examined under a microscope. If even a single organism is seen on the slide, the bacterial count in the original biopsy will be greater than 10^5 organisms per gram of tissue. If no organisms are seen on the slide, the bacterial count will be 10^5 or fewer per gram of tissue. Definition of the bacterial balance then allows management of the soft tissue wound. This technique has been successful in our practice for over 15 years.

Qualitative bacteriology is also important. When a tissue biopsy is removed, a portion of tissue should be qualitatively analyzed under both aerobic and anaerobic conditions. This allows for identification of species and antibacterial sensitivities. The antibacterial sensitivities should be performed for both systemic and topical antimicrobials. One important reason for qualitative analysis is to identify those wounds that are contaminated or infected by the beta-hemolytic streptococci. As mentioned previously, these organisms can result in infection and prevent satisfactory wound management if they are present in soft tissue at any level. The specific vagaries of these organisms have been described elsewhere.

PRESUMPTIVE DIAGNOSIS OF CONTAMINATION AND/OR INFECTION

Although quantitative and qualitative analyses of tissue biopsies are the best way to give definitive diagnosis, presumptive diagnoses can also be made. The first useful information for presumptive diagnosis is the exact history of the wounding event. For instance, it is well-known that all traumatic wounds are contaminated, at least to the extent that bacteria can always be identified by cultures performed on tissue biopsies of specimens. In a series of 80 wounds that were presented to an urban emergency department, 20 percent yielded at least 10^5 organisms per gram of tissue.

The circumstances of the wounding and the character of the wounding agent may provide important clues for presumptive diagnosis. There is an obvious difference between the potential bacterial inoculation of a laceration caused by a knife and a crush laceration received from dirty industrial machinery, often covered by grease. Knowledge of the level of bacterial inoculation that can be caused by specific injuries is useful. It is well-known that dry glass supports bacterial growth very poorly. Therefore, a laceration from a car windshield is unlikely to leave heavy contamination in the wound. Conversely, if the same windshield has been in rainy conditions for several days, it is likely to have a much higher surface bacterial level at the time of injury. It was previously reported that 62 percent of all wounds that were presented to an emergency department contained less than 100 organisms per gram of tissue at the time of repair. Eighteen percent of the wounds contained between 100 and 100,000 (10^5) bacteria and 20 percent contained greater than 10^5 bacteria per gram of tissue at the time of repair. From this, one would expect that approximately 80 percent of wounds presenting to an emergency department could be handled as if not heavily contaminated, and closed primarily.

The plastic surgeon often faces specific wounds about which a great deal is known. Among these are bite wounds received by animals and humans. Recently, 546 animal bites were reviewed. Since 475 of these were caused by dogs, it appeared worthwhile to understand the bacterial level in the dogs' mouths at the time of biting. To study this, dogs were evaluated both on meal-eating and meat-eating diets. It was found that dogs eating exclusively a meal diet had bacterial levels of 10^4 to 10^5 per milliliter of saliva, whereas dogs eating a meat diet had bacterial levels of 10^7 to 10^8 bacteria per milliliter of saliva. It is obvious from these data that learning something about the dog is useful for prediction of proper management of a bite wound.

Although there has been some question as to the level of contamination caused by dog bites—hence the recent study—there is no question about the bacterial level in human mouths. It has long been appreciated that the bacterial level in human saliva is 10^7 to 10^8 bacteria per milliliter. Therefore, human bite wounds are not in bacterial balance from the time of injury. In addition, the heavy level of beta-hemolytic streptococci make these wounds inappropriate for management as clean wounds.

Just as there is knowledge about specific traumatic wounds, there are also quantitative data regarding elective wounds. It is well-known that 10^4 bacteria fall into a one-meter-square operating field per hour. Prolonged operations, which are becoming more frequent in plastic surgery, are thus attended by heavy bacterial contamination within the operating theater. The many published studies of increased infection rates from operations exceeding 6 hours attest to the quantitative relationship between bacteria and the host.

Time is another important factor in predicting a wound's bacterial imbalance. In the emergency department study previously cited, the mean time since injury of patients with less than 10^2 bacteria per gram of tissue in their wounds was 2.2 hours. The mean time since injury increased to 3 hours in patients who had 10^2 to 10^5 bacteria per gram of wound tissue. In patients who presented to the emergency department with greater than 10^5 organisms per gram of tissue even before being treated, the mean time since wounding was 5.17 hours. More important, only those in the last group, with more than 10^5 bacteria per gram of tissue, developed clinical infection that prevented primary healing. Surgeons have always considered that wounds had a "period of grace" or "golden period" during which time they could be closed with lesser fear of infection. From these data it appears this period of grace is the time required before a given inoculum into the wound reaches the apparently critical level of greater than 10^5 bacteria per gram of tissue.

Many systemic and local factors control the amount of time that an inoculum requires to multiply to critical levels. Among these is the location of the wound on the body. The location is important because of the blood supply. A facial wound with its attendant excellent blood supply would be expected to handle a given inoculum for a longer period of time than the area at the juncture of the middle and lower thirds of the leg, overlying the tibia, where the relatively sparse blood supply might allow more rapid bacterial proliferation. The period of grace would thus be different for these two areas and explains why different surgical specialists have their own definitions of the safe period between wounding and wound closure. These problems can easily be identified and defined by quantitative bacteriology.

The final step in presumptive diagnosis is determination of the amount of necrotic tissue or debris in the wound. Any necrotic tissue allows for increased bacterial proliferation. Similarly, blood clots and foreign bodies greatly decrease the body's ability to handle a given bacterial load. These deterrents to effective host defense can help predict an imbalance in the wound equilibrium. If these local wound factors are not controlled, circumstances are then produced in which a normally subinfectious inoculum of bacteria can multiply to levels sufficient to produce infection.

TREATMENT OF THE ACUTELY CONTAMINATED WOUND

It was previously stated that all traumatic wounds are contaminated to a degree. If the specific cause of the wound suggests a high level of contamination, or if a prolonged period of time has elapsed since wounding, one would expect the bacterial level to be greater than 10^5 bacteria per gram of tissue. In such wounds a tissue biopsy with rapid slide determination is useful. However, if the wound is seen early and the history suggests minimal contamination, a rapid slide test is neither needed nor justified from a cost-effective point of view. Management of the acutely contaminated wound is undertaken with the goal of reestablishing the bacterial balance, if indeed it is weighted in favor of the bacteria, and managing the wound as if it were a clean one. The mainstay of management is sharp debridement. This could be stated as the *sine qua non* of contaminated wound management. All debris and nonvitalized tissue should be excised. The edges of the wound should be freshened and, when possible, made perpendicular to facilitate closure.

Irrigation may be an important adjunct to sharp débridement. Low pressure wound irrigation removes little but surface contamination even with voluminous amounts of solutions. Therefore, irrigation should be high pressure and intermittent. In an experimental animal system, the pulsating jet lavage was shown to remove significantly more bacteria and result in fewer wound infections than the more conventional low pressure irrigation. If the wound is small with minimal contamination, a modification of the pulsating jet lavage can be constructed using a syringe with 19-gauge needle. Again, this is most efficiently delivered in an intermittent pressure technique so as to let the normal elasticity of soft tissue assist in removal of bacteria and foreign bodies.

Systemic antibiotics are of little use in treatment of the acutely contaminated wound. Systemic antibiotics have practical and potential value only if a therapeutic blood or, more important, tissue level can be achieved within the first 4 hours after wounding. This is almost impossible in the acutely contaminated traumatic wound. In elective wounds in which acute contamination is predicted, prophylactic antibiotics are of documented value. Again, tissue levels are most important and, therefore, the amount and timing of antibacterial prophylaxis is important. When antibiotics are begun *after* the time required for bacterial lodgement, infection rates may be higher than when no antibiotics are used. Surgical debridement and freshening of the wound may render this restriction less rigid and make antibiotics more effective. However, recent data about the role of inflammatory mediators suggest that once vasoconstricting mediators are present, wound penetration of antibiotics may be less efficient. Therefore, debridement and adjunctive irrigation must remain the mainstays of treatment of the acutely contaminated wound.

Once bacterial balance has been reestablished, wound closure can proceed as for a clean wound. As stated previously, a tissue biopsy is unnecessary unless the history of the event or the time since wounding are such as to make one suspect heavy contamination. However, if the wound presents late, or the history suggests heavy contamination, a rapid slide of a tissue biopsy is justified following debridement and adjunctive irrigation. If this test suggests that there are 10^5 or fewer bacteria per gram of tissue, wound closure can proceed. However, if the test suggests greater than 10^5 bacteria per gram of tissue, the wound can be temporarily left open for delayed closure. The principles learned in military surgery are equally operative in potentially contaminated civilian wounds, i.e., when in doubt, it is probably always safer to leave a wound open. It has been repeatedly shown that delayed closures can be performed as easily as those for acute clean wounds if the level of bacteria has been sufficiently reduced to reestablish the bacterial balance.

TREATMENT OF THE CHRONICALLY CONTAMINATED WOUND

Pressure sores, vascular ulcers, and thermal burns are examples of chronically contaminated wounds. All chronic open wounds contain tissue bacterial flora. The common characteristic of such wounds is granulation tissue, which does not occur in the absence of bacteria. Germ-free animals do not form luxurious granulation tissue, nor is it found beneath the surface of a successfully closed wound. Granulation tissue has been likened to a pyogenic granuloma, and successful closure of these wounds is predicated on the surgeon's ability to control the bacterial flora and reestablish the bacterial balance.

It has been shown in blinded studies that it is clinically impossible to predict bacterial balance in a chronic granulating wound. In some wounds, the sign of creeping epithelium from the wound edges has been a useful sign in predicting when a wound can be successfully closed. However, statistically, the best method has been the use of quantitative bacteriology on a tissue biopsy. When wounds have greater than 10^5 bacteria per gram of tissue, or the presence of beta-hemolytic streptococci, they cannot be successfully closed. Therefore, the goal of management in these chronically contaminated wounds with granulation tissue is to decrease the bacterial count in the granulation tissue to 10^5 or fewer bacteria per gram of tissue. In a series of 50 skin grafts applied to chronically contaminated wounds, regardless of the technique used to prepare the granulations for grafting, a bacterial count of 10^5 or fewer bacteria per gram of tissue on the day of grafting resulted in 94 percent successful skin graft take, as opposed to 19 percent when the bacterial counts were over 10^5 bacteria per gram of tissue on the day of grafting.

Management of these wounds consists of various techniques to decrease the bacterial count. Meticulous surgical debridement again is the mainstay of treatment. Any necrotic tissue within the wound must be removed. Systemic antibiotics have been shown to be of no use in lowering the bacterial count in chronically contaminated wounds. Conversely, cream-based topical antibacterials, such as silver sulfadiazine or mafenide acetate, do penetrate to the depths of such wounds and have a direct effect on bacterial growth. The agar well technique for determining sensitivities of the bacteria to topical antibacterial creams has been very useful in my opinion.

An additional technique to lower the bacterial count is the use of temporary biologic dressings for cleansing and temporary closure of the wound. Since true bacterial control is only achieved by wound closure, this technique is both reasonable and of documented value. Allograft skin and amniotic membranes have been shown to be more effective than xenograft skin to decrease the bacterial counts in chronically contaminated wounds. However, the true control of infection in a granulating wound is closure of the wound by autologous tissue. Once the wound is in bacterial balance, with 10^5 or fewer bacteria per gram of tissue, closure by direct approximation, skin graft, or flap can be predictably successful. Successful closure by one of these methods eradicates the remaining bacteria in the wound.

TREATMENT OF THE INFECTED WOUND

The grossly infected wound can be one in which purulent material is obtained from the wound, or one in which there is surrounding cellulitis and inflammation beyond that appropriate for normal wound healing. The treatment of these two clinical presentations is different. For the wound with spreading cellulitis and no loculation of material or drainage, systemic antibiotics can be useful. If the wound is not opened, extreme vigilance is required so as not to miss an unapparent loculation. If the wound quickly responds to the systemic antibiotics, closure may be maintained.

If there is drainage of purulent material, or the suspicion of loculated purulent material, the wound should be opened. It is important not to get too concerned about the purulent material within the wound. It should be irrigated from the wound, and a tissue biopsy obtained from the wall of the abscess. In reported studies, the wound biopsy revealed the causative organism in 87 percent of cases. However, cultures of the purulent exudate often revealed multiple organisms and not those responsible for tissue invasion. It is my personal opinion that a Gram stain of any purulent material may be of use to identify clostridia when they are present. Culture of the purulent material is not as useful as culture of tissue from the wound wall. The fact that tissue biopsies usually yield a single bacterial species is very helpful if systemic antibiotics are chosen in the treatment of the abscess.

Once the wound is open, and a biopsy has identified the causative organism, the goal is to reestablish the bacterial balance in the wound. The techniques for this are the same as those for a chronically contaminated wound. Topical antimicrobials and temporary biologic dressings are useful.

Once the wound has been shown to be in bacterial balance, and the bacterial level has been lowered to 10^5 bacteria per gram of tissue or less, delayed closure can be performed. In a series of delayed closures based on bacterial counts, incisional abscesses were reclosed with a 96 percent success rate. In localized incisional abscesses that have been drained and are being treated as chronically contaminated wounds, systemic antibiotics are not used. They are reserved only for those wounds in which infection appears to be spreading through the subcutaneous tissue even after drainage of the wound and debridement of the infected soft tissue.

SUGGESTED READING

Heggers JP, Velanovich V, Robson MC, et al. Control of burn wound sepsis: a comparison of *in vitro* topical antimicrobial assays. J Trauma 1987; 27:176–179.

Krizek TJ, Robson MC, Kho E. Bacterial growth and skin graft survival. Surg Forum 1967; 18:518–519.

Robson MC. Infection in the surgical patient: an imbalance in the normal equilibrium. Clin Plast Surg 1979; 6:493–503.

Robson MC, Duke WF, Krizek TJ. Rapid bacterial screening in the treatment of civilian wounds. J Surg Res 1973; 14:426–430.

Robson MC, Heggers JP. Delayed wound closures based on bacterial counts. J Surg Oncol 1970; 2:379–383.

Robson MC, Heggers JP. Surgical infection I. Single bacterial species or polymicrobic in orgin? Surgery 1969; 65:608–610.

Robson MC, Heggers JP. Surgical infection II. The B-hemolytic streptococcus. J Surg Res 1969; 9:289–292.

SPIDER BITES

RILEY S. REES, M.D.

BROWN RECLUSE BITES

Loxoscelism is the syndrome of the clinical effects related to cutaneous bites of Loxosceles spiders (Fig. 1). Spiders of this genus, which includes the "brown recluse," are a more significant health hazard than the feared black widow (Fig. 2) because they cohabit with man and are abundant in the southern and midwestern United States. Although they are noted for the localized cutaneous necrosis induced by their venom, systemic loxoscelism with disseminated intravascular coagulopathy, renal failure, and hemolysis occurs and can be fatal.

Historical Perspective

Although loxoscelism was thought to be a recent problem, the first case was documented in 1929, when a Kansas physician identified envenomation by a *Loxosceles refuscens* spider. Later, a subgroup, *Loxosceles reclusa* (brown recluse), was separated from *L. refuscens* spiders. In all probability, the original case report was of a bite from a brown recluse spider. Other bites of Loxosceles species were reported as early as 1872, but they were thought to be due to the tarantula found in west Texas. Other Loxosceles spiders, *L. laeta* and *L. deserta*, have been reported to induce skin necrosis in patients. The active venom components are probably similar in all spiders and many times the distinction between the 13 North American species is subtle.

Loxosceles Species

Loxosceles is a medium-sized spider with an overall leg length of 18 to 30 mm. The color of the cephalotho-

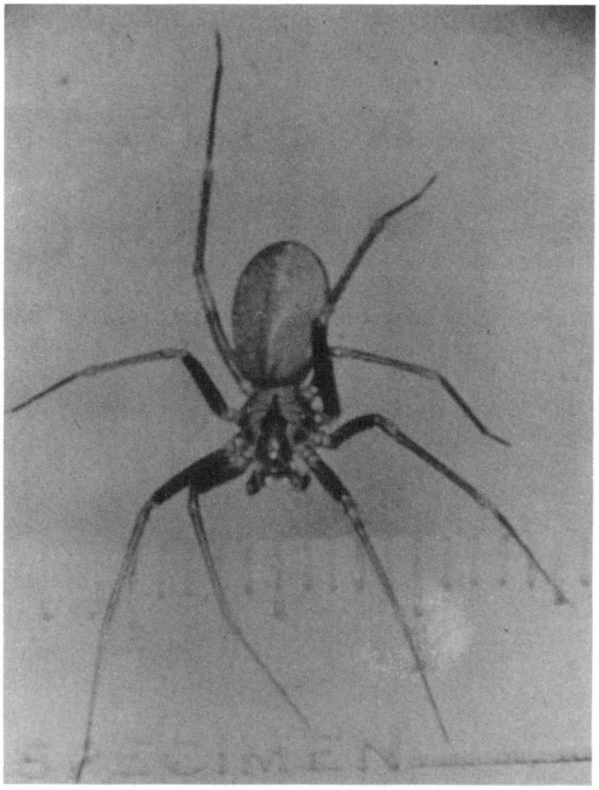

Figure 1 Brown recluse spider. They have a violin on the dorsal cephalothorax and vary from brown to fawn in color. They are found usually alone and typically not in a web.

rax and abdomen varies from fawn to dark brown and appears to be related to the diet of the spider. The unique characteristic of Loxosceles spiders is a violin shaped figure on its back which can be identified either on a dead specimen with a magnifying glass or on the live spider within a glass jar where it can't get out. It is critical for the clinician to identify the spider because therapy depends on the accuracy of the diagnosis. Loxosceles spiders are found in undisturbed environments where it is hot and dry. They are frequently found in abandoned homes, barns, or wood piles where they hunt at night. In residences, they are found in attics, closets, or garages because they can hide without detection. Although the spider is shy, it will attack if it feels threatened. A common instance of this forced aggression occurs when the victim-to-be puts on infrequently-used clothes and traps the spider in sleeves or pant legs. Sometimes the only manifestation of a brown recluse infestation is the identification of molts or exoskeletons on boxes, furniture, or wood piles. Their webs are small, flocculant, and are associated only with the female's egg sac. Although the spider usually hibernates in the winter, it may continue to be active in heated homes. Consequently, people are bitten when doing spring cleaning or when taking out Christmas decorations. These spiders live long lives and can be kept in captivity for as long as 5 years.

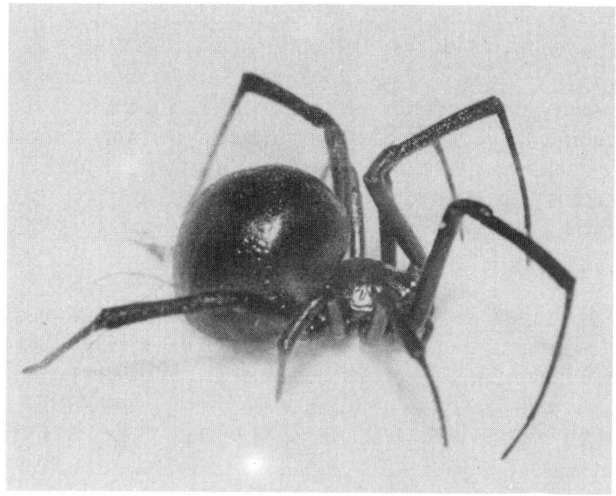

Figure 2 Typical black widow spider. Note the large abdomen and posture of the legs. These spiders have a shiny, sepia black appearance and a red "hour glass" on the ventral abdomen.

Loxoscelism

Clinical Manifestations

The broad spectrum of clinical manifestations of loxoscelism makes diagnosis and treatment difficult. Many bites resemble trivial pustules, whereas others produce large areas of skin necrosis. Some patients develop significant systemic reactions that can be life-threatening. These reactions can be divided into two broad categories: cutaneous loxoscelism and systemic loxoscelism.

Cutaneous loxoscelism is induced by a spider bite. Injury to the skin results from cell membrane damage which is initiated by a venom protein, sphingomyelinase D. Initially, the bite may be felt as a sting; however, the clinical evolution of the cutaneous lesions takes 12 to 24 hours. This timing is important, because it suggests when the bite occurred and separates it from infections or allergies. Classical bites produce itching, redness, and pain accompanied by either a pustular abscess or a purple discolored area in the bite site. Curiously, bites of the lower extremities tend to be purple and discolored and those of the upper extremity are more pustular in the clinical expression. In more severe cases, gravitationally dependent spread of venom and blister formation are noted. These lesions evolve into eschars, many with abscesses beneath them, and are quite painful. Typically, the eschars are very slow to heal.

The systemic form, termed "systemic loxoscelism," accompanies the bite in 20 percent of cases. Elevated temperature, confluent scarlatiniform rash, leukocytosis, arthralgias, chills, malaise, nausea, vomiting, and weakness represent the constellation of systemic reactions. Rarely, hemolytic anemia and hemoglobinuria occur. These reactions are particularly dangerous in children. The development of systemic symptoms occurs within 24 hours and is most severe with large cutaneous lesions. Hemolytic anemia typically is Coombs positive; however, the Coombs-negative type can occur. This complication is usually seen in combination with disseminated intravascular coagulation and renal failure. When the clinical lesion is not impressive, diagnostic confusion with liver failure, leptospirosis, and sepsis can occur.

Loxosceles Venom

Studies into the mechanism of the various actions of venom components have been limited by the small amounts available, the different procedures used to purify it, and the great variability of preparations used to study its biochemical and biological effects. The venom is now known to be a hemolysin and cytotoxin with 8 to 9 major protein bands and 3 to 4 minor bands by gel-electrophoresis. The venom has a number of identified enzyme activities. Hyaluronidase accounts for the "gravitational spread" produced by the bite. Sphingomyelinase D activity, a phospholipase, is the probable cause of dermonecrosis. The dermonecrotic sphingomyelinase D fraction has a molecular weight (MW) of 32,000 and requires Ca^{++} for activity.

Numerous studies of the pathogenesis of both local and systemic effects of the *Loxosceles* venom have been undertaken. Despite this, the underlying mechanisms of venom action are poorly understood. Evidence points to the venom producing a unique form of tissue injury. The constellation of the clinical syndrome occurs in response to the predictable activity of venom found in the spider's venom sacs.

Treatment

The treatment of brown recluse bites with corticosteroids injected locally or systemically, as done previously, is of questionable benefit. Antihistamines have been reported effective against itching, although they have little effect on the evolution of the clinical lesion. Many clinicians have suggested surgical excision of the bite site, but we have not found it effective.

In our experience, the best initial treatment is continuous local application of ice compresses, and systemic dapsone and antibiotics. Our current regimen includes ice, elevation, and immobilization of the bite site for 2 to 3 days until the pain subsides. We administer antibiotics (erythromycin 250 mg four times daily) and dapsone, a leukocyte inhibitor. Dapsone is given in 100 mg doses twice daily, and hematocrits are followed closely. Glucose-6-phosphate deficiency has been reported with dapsone therapy, but we have not seen it in our patients. Dapsone therapy is continued until the wound heals or the erythema resolves.

Experimental antivenom raised in rabbits has been used. The product is an IgG-specific polyvalent antibody, which can be injected into the wound site. It is directed against the sphingomyelinase activity of the venom and must be used within 48 hours of the bite. Combination therapy with dapsone, ice, antibiotics, and antivenom may be the most effective therapy.

When skin necrosis occurs, wounds require local wound care and debridement. After the eschar is removed, Travase ointment is applied for 7 to 10 days until the wound is clean. A skin graft is used, and no attempt is made to close the wound primarily.

BLACK WIDOW BITES

The black widow spider, genus *Latrodectus*, is both the most common and the most feared spider in North America. The genus "*Latrodectus*" comes from the Greek meaning "secret biter." It belongs to the family Therididа or "comb-footed" spiders. Although these spiders are found throughout the world only *L. mactans, L. variolus*, and *L. hesperus* are found on the North American continent. The female spider or the "black widow" has a shiny, sepia color with a red dot on the abdomen. Typically, the red dot resembles an hour-glass in mature females. The male is unobtrusive, brown in color, and is nonvenomous. Since these spiders only live over one winter, size depends on age and habitat. However, most black widows do not exceed 2.5 cm. These spiders are ground dwellers and are usually not found higher than six feet above the ground. They are often noted in bricks or dens, around foundations and hollow stumps or, classically, in the outhouse.

The bite of the black widow is initially painless, and there is no cutaneous lesion. In order for a clinical diagnosis to be made, the patient must recognize that he or she was bitten by a black widow spider. The venom is alpha-lactrotoxin (MW = 130,000) and affects neurotransmission of cholinergic, noradrenergic, and aminergic nerve terminals.

Clinical Presentation

Widow bites are more common in the southwestern United States where the dry, arid climate allows better growth and development. Within an hour of envenomation the victim complains of cramps and muscle spasms which usually begin at the bite site and abdominal rigidity. Reported associated symptoms include clammy skin, feeble pulse, stupor, and slurred speech. Victims often have headache, dysphagia, hypersalivation, bronchorrhea, nausea, vomiting, facial edema, fever, and diaphoresis. A severe, uncontrolled hypertensive crisis is the most feared complication of black widow bites.

Treatment

Treatment of this unusual problem is predicated on correct diagnosis, so it is important to recognize whether the patient was in the right environmental situation to be bitten. Patients who have moderately severe symptoms should be treated with tetanus toxoid, ice compresses, and local wound care. The muscle spasm should be treated with slow intravenous infusion of 5 to 10 ml of a 10 percent calcium gluconate solution. For children, the dose is 1 ml per kilogram. This may be repeated every 2 hours as necessary. Methocarbamol, 1 g given over a 5 to 10 minute period, has also been thought effective. Usually this therapy must be supplemented with diazepam or narcotics for pain. Calcium therapy is usually helpful in treating the hypertensive crisis, although use of sodium nitroprusside, nifedipine labetal, hydralazine, or diazoxide may be necessary.

Antivenom Therapy

Black widow equine antivenom is available from Wyeth Corporation, but is associated with an unusually high risk of serum sickness. Patients with uncontrolled hypertension and seizures, small children, the elderly, and pregnant women represent the only possible indication for its use. Since the reported mortality from black widow bites does not exceed 5 percent, even in the severest forms, antivenom should be used with discretion. Use of antivenom requires preobligatory skin testing with local intradermal injection of one-tenth of 1 ml of the product. Antivenom (2.5 ml) diluted in 50 ml of normal saline is given via intravenous infusion. Rarely is more than one ampule required.

The effects of the black widow bite are self limited. The patient requires observation until asymptomatic; obviously, in high risk patients such as children, the elderly, and pregnant women, hospitalization is indicated.

OTHER SPIDERS

Ten other spiders have been associated with clinically significant human bites. A short description of each is presented in the following paragraphs. The treatment is symptomatic: immobilization and/or elevation, systemic analgesics, antihistamines, tetanus prophylaxis, and antibiotics.

Orb Weavers

Argiope aurantia, known as the golden orb weaver or the black or yellow garden spider, is common in the west coast and the eastern United States. *Argiope aurantia* is only one of six species found in the United States. It is a large, brightly-colored spider that strays from its large symmetrical orb web. The cephalothorax of the female may be greater than 2.5 cm with a leg spread up to 7.5 cm. The body of the female is black with bright yellow or orange spots. Local pain, followed by 0.5 cm of induration and surrounded by 3 cm of erythema has been described after human envenomation. Oral diphenhydramine, antihistamines, triamcinolone, and local steroids produce pain cessation within 30 minutes. No further follow-up has been described. Bites by a related species, *A. argentata*, cause local pain, erythema, and vesicle formation, which resolves within 24 hours (except for the bite marks). Although, from clinical reports, the venom appears to be cytotoxic, research indicates that it has neurotoxic effects in vitro.

Sack Spiders

T. tranquillus, also known as the broad-faced sack spider, is a fairly common medium-sized spider, which has been observed by several authors to enter houses in late summer and fall. At other times it is found in grass and leaf litter, scavenging for dead spiders and insects. Generally, the bites occur inside or near houses when the spider is threatened or disturbed. The bite causes mild local reactions without necrosis. All bites result in localized pain and usually some edema. One bite was treated with parenteral penicillin for secondary infection of the face. Most bites involve the female of the species. No systemic effects have been reported.

Green Lynx Spider

Peucetia viridans, the green lynx spider, is a diurnal hunting spider whose bite results in a burning sensation, pruritus, erythema, and induration. One case report describes a pustule-like lesion with localized swelling. This patient was treated with Benadryl, ACTH, and tetanus immunization 30 to 40 minutes after the bite, but developed a 3-mm ulcerated wound, which may have been the result of excoriation. No necrosis was reported in the three other documented cases. *P. viridans* is translucent green, with red eyes and joints. The female has an average length of 16 mm. The green lynx is common across the southern United States.

Jumping Spiders

Bites by the black jumping spiders of the genus *Phidippus* may be sharp, painful, and cause ulceration. One patient was bitten twice on the dorsum of the hand by *P. formosus*. The acute pain lasted 5 minutes, but was replaced by a dull, throbbing pain. A small 2-mm ulcer surrounded by erythema and induration developed within several hours. By the second day, the swelling encompassed the whole hand but gradually resolved over 9 days. Pruritus, which was the chief complaint, responded to methdilazine. Phidippus spiders may be greater than 10 mm in length.

Jumping spiders have the keenest eyesight of all spiders, which allows them to see for a distance of several centimeters. They live in silk bags spun in crevices. Fifty or sixty species live in North America. *H. ecclesiasticus* is commonly known as the parson spider. Its bite produces pruritus, arthralgia, malaise, and nausea after 1 hour. Locally, the bite results in induration and erythema and is treated with an anti-inflammatory agent, steroid cream, and bed rest. Resolution of the signs and symptoms has been seen after 9 days. No necrosis has resulted. The jumping spider belongs to the family of running spiders, with strong legs and elongated bodies. It is widely distributed throughout the United States and lives under rocks, rubbish, and in houses.

Tegenaria agrestis

Recently, *Tegenaria agrestis,* a spider found in Idaho, Oregon, and Washington, has been implicated in necrotic arachnidism. Experimental envenomation of rabbits by live male spiders resulted in cutaneous necrosis. Autopsy revealed petechial hemorrhages on the surfaces of the lungs, liver, and kidneys. Based on laboratory studies, the bite of the male has significantly greater local and systemic effects than the female. *T. agrestis* has been implicated in 22 cases of human envenomation. Victims developed a small area of induration surrounded by 50 to 120 mm of erythema, followed by vesiculation 15 to 35 hours later. Within 24 hours, these vesicles ruptured with many forming eschars. Systemic symptoms included headache, lethargy, and hallucinations. Four patients saw the spider bite them; two of the patients caught and killed the spider. Unfortunately, these patients did not save the spider for identification. One patient identified a live *T. agrestis* specimen as the biter. *T. agrestis* was found in abundance when the premises were inspected.

T. agrestis is commonly found in association with man-made structures such as housing foundations, wood piles, and railroad ties. It is a moderately large (10 to 15 mm), nondescript brown spider.

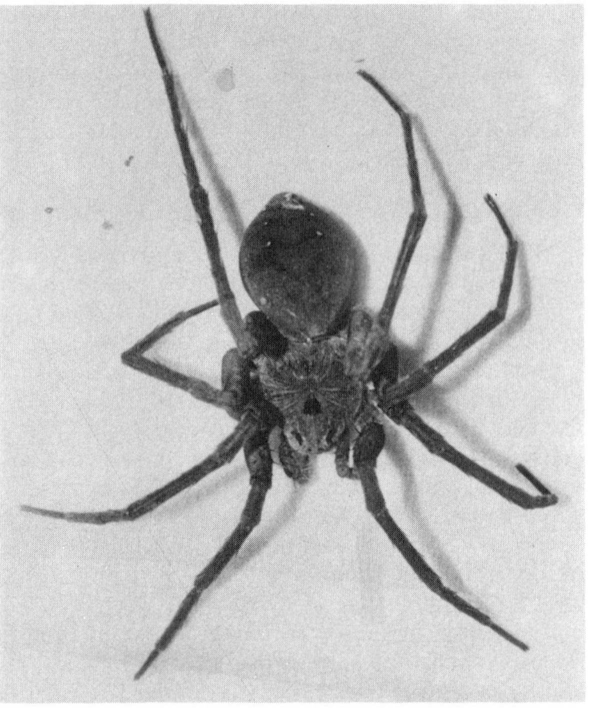

Figure 3 An example of an American wolf spider. Note the large size and robust appearance.

Wolf Spider

American wolf spiders are common diurnal hunting spiders, which are robust in appearance with stout legs, large bodies, and large chelicera (mandibles). Because of their size, they are able to inflict bites that sometimes bleed and are always painful. These spiders are aggressive hunters and frequently attack any movement near their den.

Typically, these spiders are large (up to 3.5 cm), brown in appearance, with fine fur-like hair over the body and legs (Fig. 3). They are often found in gardens, garages, or open porches where they are close to the insect food source.

The bite is painful, red, and associated with malaise, headache, nausea, and dizziness. Treatment is symptomatic with ice compresses, antihistamines, and systemic antibiotics for local infections.

SUGGESTED READING

Gertsch WJ. American spiders. 2nd ed. New York: Von Nostrand Reinhold, 1979:184–192 and 223–241.

King LE, Rees RS. Spider bites and scorpion stings. In: Robert Pakel, ed. Conn's current therapy. Philadelphia: WB Saunders, 1987.

Rees RS, King LE. Arthropod bites and stings. In: Fitzpatrick TB, Eisen AZ, et al, eds. Dermatology in general medicine. 3rd ed. New York: McGraw-Hill, 1986.

Williams HE, Breene RG, Rees RS. The black widow spider: PB1193, University of Tennessee Institute of Agriculture, 1986.

Williams HE, Breene RG, Rees RS. The brown recluse spider. PB1191, University of Tennessee Institute of Agriculture, 1986.

SKIN GRAFTS

HAROLD R. MANCUSI-UNGARO Jr., M.D., F.A.C.S.

Skin grafting offers the surgeon a means of achieving primary closure of a wound when the nature or size of the defect will not permit a simple approximation of its edges. Skin grafting must be approached as one method in the spectrum of achieving primary wound closure. The skin graft suffers from many of the same limitations as direct suture closure, i.e., hematoma, dead space, foreign bodies, and infection all contradict the use of a skin graft to close the wound. Indications for a skin graft fall within a continuum of techniques for wound closure that begins with suture approximation and culminates with free microvascular transfer of composite tissues. Similarly, the methodology of skin grafting progresses through a sequence from split thickness to full thickness. Given the appropriate indications, proper planning, skilled execution, and suitable postoperative care, a skin graft may succeed when a more elaborate method would fail.

THERAPEUTIC ALTERNATIVES

Indications

The blood supply for a skin graft must develop from the wound bed on which it is placed. Hence, the primary requisite and indication for a skin graft is an open wound with a viable bed. The wound may be either the result of a fresh surgical excision or the granulating bed of an old wound. In terms of the wound's depth, dermis, fat, fascia, muscle, peritenon, cancellous bone, as well as the raw surfaces of internal viscera, can all support a skin graft. With grafting, as with other methods of primary closure, the wound should not be infected. As demonstrated by Liedburg et al and Krizek et al, the appearance of the bed matters not as much as the quantity of bacteria contained in the tissues. A bacterial count of less than 10^5 bacteria per gram of tissue must be established prior to effecting closure of a contaminated wound in order to assure success. Unless the skin graft is to be placed on a fresh, clean, or clean-contaminated surgical wound, a wound biopsy with quantitative bacteriologic studies is indicated. When time permits, a formal colony count showing no streptococci and less than 10^5 other bacteria per gram of tissue insures success 98 percent of the time. In more acute situations, the rapid slide technique popularized by Robson and Heggers can achieve a 95 percent success rate. An alternative to biopsy, particularly in evolving wounds, is to demonstrate effective adherence of a biologic dressing. Although homograft remains the standard by which other biologic dressings are judged, the adherence without suppuration of xenograft, amnion, or a biosynthetic (e.g., Biobrane) can be used to demonstrate an uninfected bed. In such cases, the permanent autograft simply replaces the biologic substitute.

The general indications for a skin graft arise out of the nature of the wound itself. A graft reestablishes a stable epithelial cover on a wound that is too big to close primarily. The closure is restricted in that it provides limited dermis in the case of split-thickness grafts and dermis without subcutaneous tissue with full-thickness grafts. In some cases, a graft may temporize when a more complex closure with a flap carries too great an operative risk. Whereas a failed graft can be retried from an alternative or reharvested donor site, a flap donor site cannot tolerate compromise. For example, an acute crush injury to a hand or finger may eventually require mobilizing composite tissue for final reconstruction. Skin grafting the same area confirms the absence of infection and allows associated soft tissue injuries to demarcate, heal, and mature.

Most of the time, skin grafting is synonymous with split-thickness skin grafting. The split-thickness graft provides an epithelial closure, and its donor site heals as a partial thickness wound. Thus, large areas of skin epithelium can be obtained and transplanted. Once the donor site has healed, it can usually supply additional grafts. Certain qualities of skin, particularly its suppleness, are provided by the dermis. Hair and hair follicles, too, are properties of the dermis. When these qualities or characteristics are important in closing a wound, full-thickness skin must be employed, although occasionally a thick split-thickness graft may suffice. Such thicker grafts also decrease proliferation of scar tissue and contraction of the recipient wound bed. Full-thickness grafts, therefore, are often employed on the face, especially on the nose and lower eyelid, where texture, pliability, and appearance all contribute to function. Although thicker grafts offer certain advantages, disadvantages include a lesser chance of success since more tissue must assume a vascular supply. Furthermore, the donor sites for the thicker grafts must be overgrafted or themselves closed since their epidermal elements have been lost with the transplant.

Contraindications

Absolute contraindications arise from the absence of proper indications. A nonviable or infected bed results in failure. Residual or ongoing necrosis, desiccated tissues, or persistent bleeding requires further attention before grafting. Fibroblasts and endothelial cells neither jump nor swim. For vascularization to occur, the living tissue of the recipient bed must remain in immediate proximity to the graft. Similarly, the bed must consist of appropriate tissue. Whereas peritenon provides a vascular bed, a tendon does not, nor does cortical bone. As with any wound closure, the bed may be contaminated but not infected. Local defense mechanisms will overcome a bacterial load of 10^4 organisms per gram of tissue. In this regard, the skin can serve to "clean up" a contaminated wound. Conversely, a bacterial count greater than 10^5 organisms constitutes a contraindication.

Relative Contraindications

A skin graft should not be used if an alternative method of wound closure will serve the patient's needs better. For example, why graft a wound when manipulation of the adjacent tissues by undermining, mobilizing, and advancing will bring about a primary closure? A parallel situation arises in the case of a superficial second degree burn. If the would will heal in 14 to 21 days, a graft usually proves inappropriate and untimely. Even certain full-thickness defects should be allowed to heal by secondary intention, though they may take longer to heal. Contraction and epithelialization from the edges may restore contour or other qualities superior to that provided by a graft. Small finger tip avulsions and scalp avulsions afford just two examples. In the scalp, contraction will reapproximate hairbearing tissues, while in the finger tip contraction will draw together specialized sensate tissues. In larger defects, proper contour and other skin qualities, such as hair, texture, or durability, as well as timeliness, dictate the application of more complex techniques such as flap closure and transplantation of composite tissues.

Occasionally, the lack of an appropriate donor site or a resulting donor site deformity may prohibit the use of a skin graft. In the case of split-thickness grafts, donor site deformity usually consists of altered pigmentation (commonly decreased or bleached effect) and, sometimes, hypertrophic scarring. Either event seldom condemns sites outside of the head and neck. To blend in with facial tones, split-thickness grafts for the face must be harvested from skin above the clavicle. Hence, the possible sequela of altered pigmentation must be considered when the donor site cannot be hidden by clothing or might be bared by prevailing fashion.

RESULT OR APPEARANCE

Color

Although relative hues can be anticipated, the final color of a mature graft or mature donor site cannot be predicated with certainty. Analogous areas tend to match. As noted, grafted skin from above the clavicle retains the pinkness or blush of facial tones, whereas skin from other areas acquires a sallow, tan, or even bronzed tint in comparison. This tint becomes especially obvious when the grafts are side by side or on the face itself. Accordingly, skin grafts to the face should come from adjacent areas. Taking donor site morbidity and disfigurement into account, split-thickness grafts to the face best come from the scalp, whereas nonhairbearing full-thickness grafts can be taken from behind the ear or along the clavicle (Fig. 1).

No matter what the location, even juxtaposed donor and recipient sites will not match perfectly. Noticeable deviations in shade develop as the wounds mature. If wounding stimulates pigment production, tanning ensues; however, injury may diminish production, in which case bleaching results. Concurrently, the wound bed undergoes contraction, drawing the cells and their deposits of melanin closer together, perhaps offsetting, perhaps accentuating pigmentation. Racial differences compound the problem, although darker skinned peoples tend to hyperpigment (Fig. 2).

Texture

In terms of texture, split-thickness grafts tend to assume the characteristics of the recipient site, whereas full-thickness grafts retain those of the donor site. Full-thickness grafts include the dermis. With dermal thickness and suppleness come sweat and apocrine glands that lubricate the skin and allow it to retain moisture. Thus, a retroauricular graft should conform to and match a lower eyelid, whereas palmar or plantar skin remains dry and calloused. In contrast, split-thickness grafts conform to their recipient site. Any thickness or stratification comes through scar deposition, but scar can respond to local stresses of motion and tension. Similarly, the quality of lubrication results from the adjacent spread of local oils and secretions. For instance, a split-thickness graft suits an upper eyelid or responds to the intraoral environment, whereas an expanse on the dorsum of the hand tends to chap if not treated with emollients.

Hair Growth

Hair follicles lie deep in the dermis. Therefore, only full-thickness grafts grow hair. Again, the characteristics of the donor site are retained. The transplantation of hair by grafting requires meticulous attention to the pattern and direction of that growth, lest the transplant not conform. Split-thickness grafts, even from the scalp, do not grow hair since they do not transplant the dermis that contains the follicles. However, at times, the stratum of graft holds shafts of hair and retains the impression of previous hair growth.

THE RECIPIENT SITE—TIMING OF THERAPY

The Fresh Wound

Following excision of a lesion, the fresh surgical wound can be grafted as soon a hemostasis is secured. The surgeon must assume that all the usual requisites for primary closure have been met. In addition, the patient must be able to accept immobilization of the grafted body part.

A persistently oozing surface, a coagulopathy, and inadequate immobilization of an anesthetized, uncooperative patient, all mitigate against immediate skin graft-

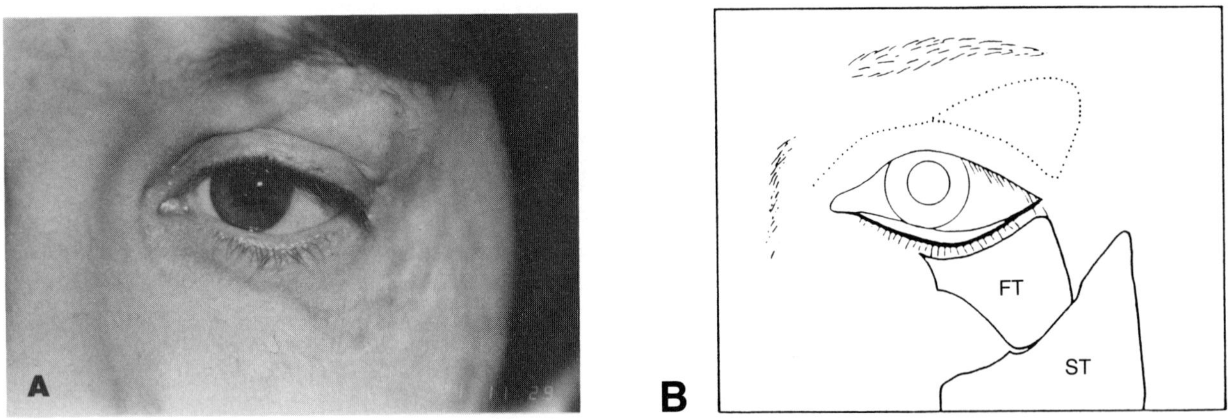

Figure 1 *A* and *B*, Full-thickness (FT) retroauricular skin was grafted to replace the lower eyelid while split-thickness (ST) skin from the scalp was used to resurface the cheek.

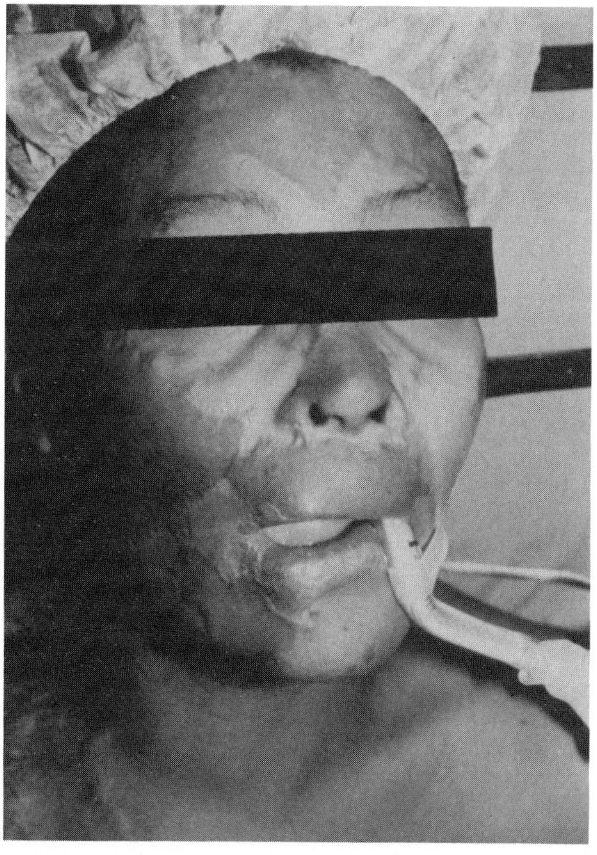

Figure 2 Hyperpigmented split-thickness skin grafts from nonadjacent donor sites became hyperpigmented in this black woman.

ing. In such cases, coverage of the wound can be temporized with a biologic dressing, such as porcine xenograft or human allograft. Indeed, exposure of the raw wound surface to the biological dressing's collagen often induces hemostasis by activation of the extrinsic clotting cascade. In addition, a standard occlusive dressing may serve, providing it maintains the wound's integrity and protects it from contamination and desiccation.

Whatever the dressing, grafting can be performed, usually at the bedside, as soon as the restrictions are satisfied. In most cases, the graft can be harvested at the time of excision and stored in the refrigerator. When refrigerated in sterile saline or balanced salt solution, the graft remains viable for several days. Alternatively, it can be "stored" on the donor site by replacing it after harvesting. Removal within 24 to 48 hours requires analgesia and sedation but not anesthesia or instrumentation.

The Surgically Debrided Wound

In theory, the surgically debrided wound should behave as a freshly excised wound, assuming the debridement was adequate. In practice, the level of residual bacterial contamination or the further demarcation of devitalized tissue requires discrimination. Gunshot wounds exemplify the distinction.

Skin grafting permits delayed primary closure of wounds requiring wide debridement. One standard method for preparation and timing remains that reported by Churchill following experience with over 25,000 casualties in World War II with a 95 percent success rate. After surgical debridement in the operating room, a dry sterile and occlusive dressing is placed on the wound for 5 days. On the fifth day, the dressing is aseptically taken down in the operating room, and the wound is inspected. Providing the wound shows no overt purulence or infection and assuming the need for minimal further debridement, the wound is then grafted. The occlusive technique permits a predictable result within an anticipated schedule, one seldom found with alternative methods of wound management.

Granulating Bed–Contaminated Wound

The granulating wound will accept a skin graft as soon as the bacterial count within the tissue itself is less than 10^5 per gram; qualitative culture of the surface remains irrelevant. The "ready" appearance of the bed is related to the relative proportion of capillary endothelium to fibrous connective tissue, since the latter predominates in older or more mature wounds. Preparation of the bed should be aimed toward stimulating capillary growth while controlling bacteria. Frequent dressing changes appear to do both.

Wet-to-dry dressings draw particulate matter, and probably bacteria, into their interstices by capillary action as they dry; mechanical removal pulls off adherent tissue, thereby debriding and freshening the surface. The addition of antiseptics, such as hypochlorite (Dakin's solution) or iodophor, may serve to control bacterial growth in the dressing and on direct contact with the wound's surface. In comparison, topical antibiotic creams achieve varying degrees of tissue penetration over the duration of their application and control of the growth of bacteria within the depths of the injury. A soluble preparation of mafenide penetrates deeper than a suspension of silver sulfadiazine. Alternatively, the antibiotic can be delivered once incorporated into xenograft tissue. Although the biologic dressing will not adhere to an infected wound, even without antibiotic, it may serve to optimize local host responses that serve to limit bacterial growth. At worst, the biologic dressing serves as a substitute for conventional dressings, debriding with subsequent changes. Adherence of a xenograft (unlike cotton dressings) signals control of bacterial growth and the suitability of the wound for autografting.

PRINCIPLES OF TREATMENT APPROACH

Donor Sites

The surgeon must consider both esthetic and practical aspects in choosing a donor site. From a practical standpoint, the donor site must provide an ample amount of suitable skin. Esthetically, the donor site should not remain as a stigma to the patient nor an embarrassment to the surgeon. For instance, in a major burn injury, donor sites can be precious and few. While almost any site may have to be taken, it is ideal to spare the lower legs in women. For minor defects, although the anterior thigh is readily available, it is often exposed and readily noticeable and, thus, should be avoided. Less obvious and more acceptable sites include the lateral buttock, the posterior buttocks, the pubic escutcheon, and even the scalp (Fig. 3).

Practical considerations for donor sites include the amount of skin necessary, ease of exposure in the operating room, the need to reharvest donor sites, and donor site morbidity. In burn patients or for large defects, the thighs, lateral buttocks, and lower torso become the usual donor sites when available. When possible, the posterior thighs are spared in favor of the lower torso, in order to keep the patient from having to lie on the donor site. In elderly patients, however, the back, buttock, and posterior thigh provide thicker dermis and may prove a safer donor site. These sites even allow reharvesting, although they are more difficult to expose in the operating room and more cumbersome to dress.

Like so many aspects of surgery, hemostasis of the donor site has become a ritual to many surgeons. Spontaneous hemostasis rarely presents a problem for first-time donor sites, unless the graft is unusually thick. Most of the time, wrapping the donor site with a dry surgical towel proves sufficient. If a porous dressing, such as fine mesh gauze, is used, the wound can be dressed immediately, and the towel can be placed directly on top. After several minutes the towel should be saturated with saline and irrigated free from the underlying dressing or exposed donor site to be dressed. A blood loss of less than 150 ml per square foot (1,000 sq cm) can be expected.

Hemostasis is compromised when donor sites are reharvested. The deeper dermis has larger vessels, and it is inflamed from previous surgery. Hemostasis can also be jeopardized by preceding antibiotic therapy with certain cephalosporins or semisynthetic penicillins. In such cases, topical thrombin diluted to 1,000 U per milliliter helps stop bleeding. While it can be applied in compresses, a spray applicator dissipates the relatively expensive hemostatic agent over a larger area. Clots left behind by the thrombin should then be gently teased away with forceps or a damp surgical sponge. Although some surgeons suggest using epinephrine or norepinephrine with or without thrombin, vasoconstrictors have been shown to impair wound healing and seem superfluous.

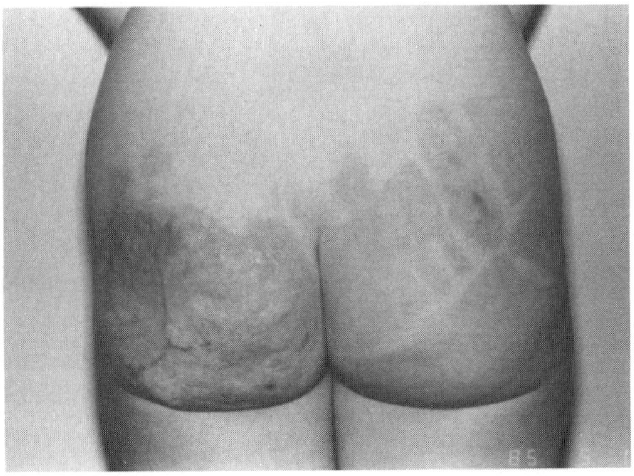

Figure 3 Availability versus concealability: the right buttock provided ample skin to resurface the burn of the left buttock. The donor site remains as hidden as the recipient.

Once hemostasis has been achieved, the donor site requires a simple, reliable, and comfortable dressing. Probably no other aspect of wound care has received more commercial attention and deserved less, since a single layer of fine mesh gauze laid over the donor site and allowed to air dry will suffice. Petrolatum added to the gauze, a semipermeable membrane in place of the gauze, or even an occlusive dressing decreases the rate of drying and diminishes the pain associated with exposure. Agents such as scarlet red or bismuth tribromphenate (Xeroform) have been shown to optimize the rate of epithelialization, while certain topical antibiotics such as mafenide acetate and silver sulfadiazine have been shown to retard healing. Yet, nothing retards healing as much as infection. Sometimes silver sulfadiazine-impregnated gauze is a useful dressing when donor sites are taken adjacent to healing burns. In comparison, although complex and expensive, semipermeable dressings may ease the discomfort of a donor site, they tend to accumulate fluids in the dressing-wound interface, which can serve as a medium for bacterial growth. The subsequent increased risk of infection together with their inflated costs offsets any advantages.

Donor sites dressed with a single layer of medicated fine mesh gauze should be protected from bed linens and left exposed to air until dry. The drying process can be accelerated by exposing the site to the light of a 40-watt bulb placed approximately 3 feet away for about 20 minutes several times a day. A more intense heat source risks burning the donor site. It also may dry the surface of the gauze before it dries the surface of the wound and may allow fluid to accumulate under the dried gauze, thus predisposing to infection.

Therapeutic Options

Split-Thickness Grafts

Split-thickness skin grafts can be thick or thin, meshed or sheet (nonmeshed). The thicker the graft, the more durable and supple it is, and the more dermis it contains. The quantity of dermis appears to limit scarring and secondary contraction of the wound bed. The thinner the graft, the more certain the "take," and the less tissue is required to assume a new blood supply. The thinner the graft, the more dermis left to the donor site, the less likely the donor site is to scar, and the more times the donor site can be reharvested. After all, the quantity of dermis appears to be finite; it does not regenerate; it reepithelializes from the epidermal elements, sweat glands, and hair follicles contained within. The deeper into the dermis a graft is taken, the less of those epithelial elements remain, the slower the wound heals, and the more likely that scarring and contraction will intervene.

The technique of meshing a graft, cutting a pattern into it so it can unfurl like chicken wire, was devised to expand available skin to cover wider areas when donor sites are precious and few, such as in a major burn. Grafts can be meshed and expanded 1.5:1, 2:1, 3:1, 4:1, 6:1, even 9:1. When expanded, the interstices of the mesh fill in over time by the migration of epithelial cells, accompanied by a relative amount of scarring and contraction. As a result, areas so grafted forever carry the waffle pattern of the mesher. Scant or precarious donor sites continue to be the primary indication for meshing a graft. Particularly in the elderly, whose thin dermal architecture make both procuring the graft and healing the donor site difficult, the blemishes left by the mesher can be overlooked. Even then, a 1.5:1 mesh usually suffices, and more than 3:1 is hardly necessary. While a 1.5:1 mesh reepithelializes in about 10 days, a 3:1 mesh requires 14 days, and a 6:1 about 3 weeks. Thus, donor sites can usually be reharvested or alternative sites can be found in less time than it takes a 3:1 mesh to fill in.

Some surgeons claim that meshing enhances the chances for a graft's success. They cite better drainage of serum and blood, as well as increased conformation to irregular surfaces. Suffice it to say that if hemostasis appears marginal, grafting can be temporized with a biologic dressing. Whereas a sheet graft requires more attention to detail, serum collections can be drained through the graft via small incisions or needle aspirations. Such "pie-crusting" of the graft also can help it conform, and a thinner graft conforms better than a thicker graft. A meshed graft requires less care, but it leaves a waffle pattern: "diamonds are forever!" (Fig. 4).

Full-Thickness Grafts

For full-thickness grafts, donor sites must be selected to match the characteristics of the skin desired, and few options remain. Hairbearing skin usually comes from the scalp. Truly nonhairbearing skin comes from behind the ear. Larger expanses of full-thickness skin with sparse hair can be harvested from over the clavicle and the groin crease.

In general, donor sites for full-thickness grafts are designed to enable primary closure by edge-to-edge approximation. However, larger defects can be closed with a split-thickness skin graft. Such an option assumes that the importance of obtaining a full-thickness graft outweighs the deformity left by a split-thickness graft whence it came.

TRICKS AND TRAPS

The Dermatome

Split-thickness grafts can be obtained with a handheld knife (e.g., Ferris-Smith, Cobbett, Goulian), a manu-

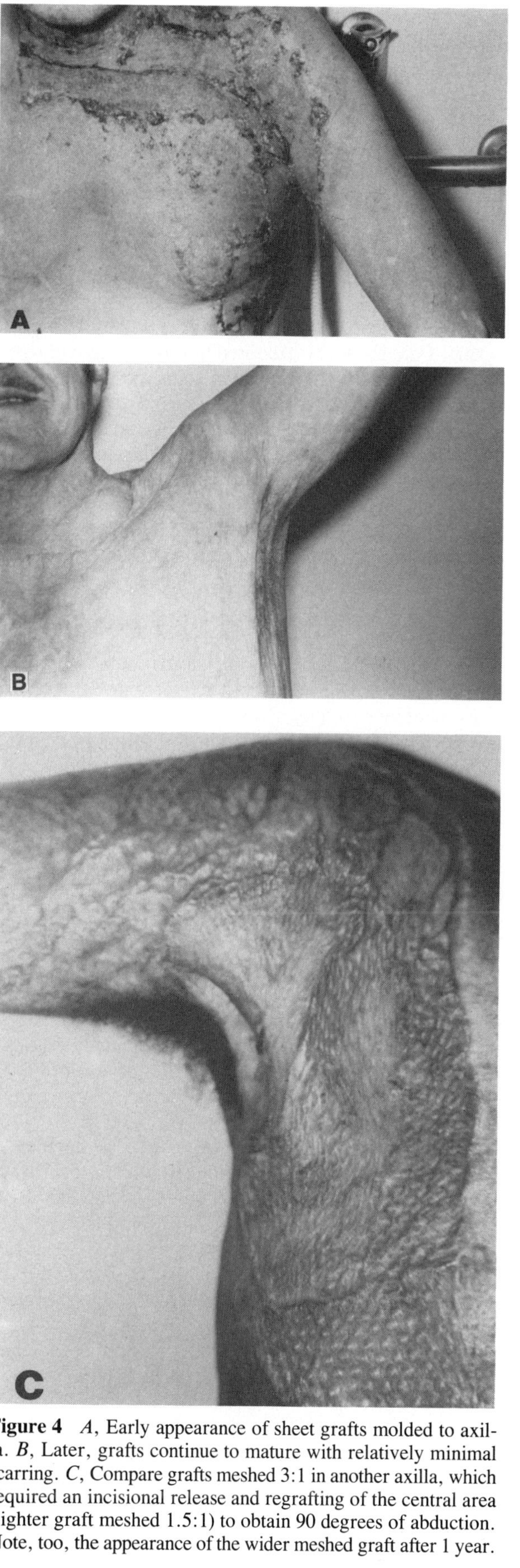

Figure 4 *A*, Early appearance of sheet grafts molded to axilla. *B*, Later, grafts continue to mature with relatively minimal scarring. *C*, Compare grafts meshed 3:1 in another axilla, which required an incisional release and regrafting of the central area (lighter graft meshed 1.5:1) to obtain 90 degrees of abduction. Note, too, the appearance of the wider meshed graft after 1 year.

al dermatome (e.g., Reese, Padgett), or a mechanized dermatome (e.g., Brown, Padgett). Proficiency becomes a matter of practice. For the occasional graft and for the novice, the Padgett electric dermatome provides the most consistent and reproducible results. Graft width is established through a choice of blade guards, and depth is set by a cam adjusted according to a reference scale. One simply has to maintain proximal tension on the skin as the dermatome is passed over the skin.

Donor Site Preparation

Donor sites should be prepared as with any surgical wound. Care should be exercised to rinse the area of soap, which may cause the dermatome to stick. Whereas a manual dermatome requires an adhesive to fix the skin to its drum, all others demand a lubricated surface. Saline often suffices, and a surgical antiseptic such as povidone-iodine may be preferred in contaminated areas. Unless an adjacent wound contradicts its use, a thin layer of mineral oil, followed by a flush with saline, works best with the Padgett electric dermatome.

Securing the Graft

Once the graft has been separated from its donor site, the skin undergoes primary contraction: it shrinks because of its inherent elasticity. Surgical staples provide a rapid and easy way to affix the graft to its recipient site and help overcome the force of such primary contraction. Unfortunately, the staples eventually require removal—a process which can be time consuming for the surgeon and uncomfortable for the patient. Therefore, the number of staples should be minimized. Often, if the grafts are thin and ample, they can be allowed to lie in place with minimal or even no surgical fixation. Indeed, they rapidly become affixed to the underlying surface by the wound's own coagulum.

In certain instances, for example resurfacing facial cosmetic units, epidermal-to-epidermal approximation must be nearly perfect to minimize the potential for a ridge of scar. A fine running suture of chromic gut provides such approximation and eliminates the need for eventual suture removal.

Grafts can be treated open or closed. The open technique requires attention and protection from local trauma, i.e., evacuating fluid collections while not disturbing the remainder of the graft. Hence, a closed technique is easier and, correspondingly, more popular.

With the closed technique, the graft is protected from the overlying dressing by a nonadherent layer—routinely a petrolatum impregnated gauze. If available, a nonwoven, porous plastic film (e.g., N-terface) works best. The nonadherent layer is then overwrapped with a moist gauze dressing, which molds itself to the wound's contour. Because the graft must be immobilized, joint surfaces must be splinted.

Concave surfaces or surfaces that cannot be overwrapped require a tie-over bolster. To create a bolster, sutures are placed at the periphery of the graft. They may be the same sutures used for surgical fixation. When staples are used, the same staples can be placed so as to bisect and affix the tie-over sutures. The bolster is fashioned from wet cotton wadding laid directly on the nonadherent layer. (If petrolatum gauze is used, the cotton should be wet with glycerine or mineral oil.) Fixation sutures are then tied over the bolster from opposite poles of the wound. An assistant can help tying the sutures by securing the first throw of the knot with a smooth Webster needle holder.

POSTOPERATIVE CARE

Postoperative Dressings

If the operative dressing remains intact and immobilized, changing it only serves to disturb the graft, unless the graft's situation can be improved. Graft "take," the development of a blood supply, requires 3 to 5 days. During those few days, the cells within the graft survive by imbibition; they obtain nutrients through the wound's fluids. However, they cannot survive on imbibition much beyond 5 days, and fluid accumulation under a graft prohibits the ingrowth of blood vessels. Therefore, the dressing of a sheet graft should be taken down and the graft inspected on or about day three. At that time, any clots or fluid accumulations must be aspirated; blebs or blisters must be incised and drained by rolling the contained fluids toward the point of drainage with cotton applicators.

In small children and uncooperative patients, the dressing should be left alone for at least 5 days, unless infection or another problem is apparent. Similarly, meshed grafts (by their very nature) drain spontaneously and require no attention until they take—about 5 days.

Lubrication

Sheet split-thickness grafts have a relatively stable epithelium at about a week, full-thickness grafts at about 10 days, and meshed grafts whenever their interstices have closed. At that time a schedule of regular lubrication should be started, two to three times a day. While petrolatum-based lotions maintain a lubricated appearance, they may in fact serve to dissolve the natural skin oils. Therefore, vegetable-based or animal-based emollients are preferred. Indeed, Crisco works well with few allergic reactions and minimal strain on the pocketbook, although it does tend to become rancid in the summer.

Support and Pressure

Grafts require protection from shear forces for at least 2 to 3 weeks. The vasculature of a fresh graft remains fragile for many months. Therefore, areas subject to abrasion should be lubricated then protected with soft dressing. An elastic dressing such as Ace bandages or tubular elastic should be placed over most grafts. Certainly, grafts on legs must be pressure wrapped whenever they are de-

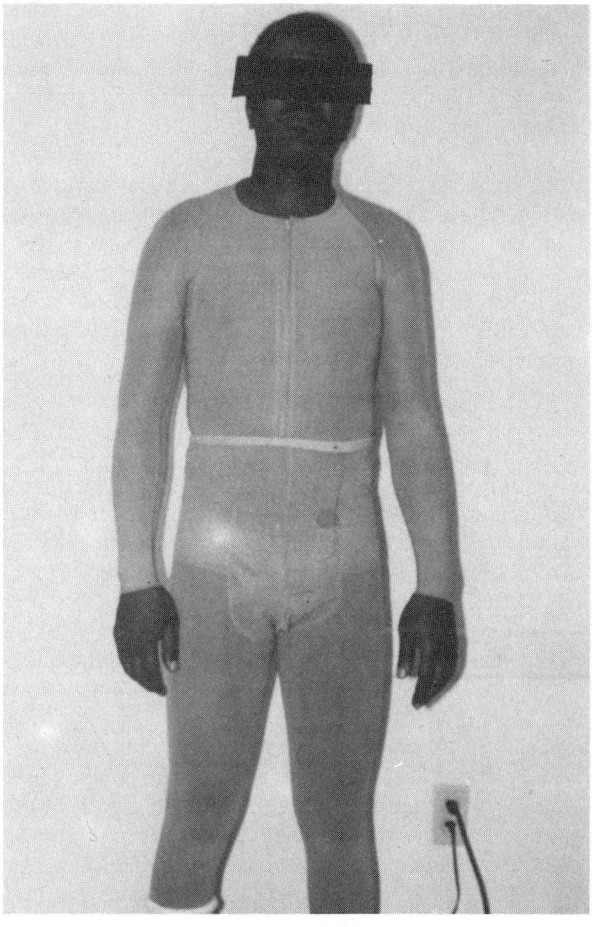

Figure 5 Custom-made elastic pressure garment by Jobst minimizes burn scar hypertrophy.

pendent. Failure to do this causes rupture of fine vessels and bleeding into the graft.

Observation of pressure-wrapped extremities led to the conclusion that scar responds to pressure. Hence, whenever possible, pressure dressings should be employed to minimize the effect of hypertrophic scarring on the graft's ultimate appearance. Once the graft has attained a suitable toughness, elastic bandages can be replaced with custom-made elastic garments such as those manufactured by Jobst (Fig. 5).

Grafts take time to mature. Maturation includes scarring of the bed, remodeling and softening of that scar, resolution of the fine vasculature with loss of hyperemia and a gradual return to relatively normal pigmentation. During the period of maturation, defects may occur in the graft. Pores may be plugged or overgrafted, fine vessels may rupture, and dry skin may chap and crack. Any of these events may lead to fine blister formation and areas of breakdown. These areas can be treated with a topical antiseptic such as Mercurochrome or povidone-iodine which allows the area to desiccate and reepithelialize from the edges. Larger areas of breakdown must be further protected from the trauma of dressing changes. Common surgical sense dictates that some sort of nonadherent or medicated dressing such as Xeroform or Unna's boot paste gauze should be applied and gently changed as necessary.

Eventually, the graft matures, softens, and blends with its surroundings. Small grafts require no further special attention. However, large expanses of graft always require at least intermittent extra lubrication. They never quite replace the original.

SUGGESTED READING

Churchill ED. The surgical management of the wounded in the Mediterranean theater at the time of the fall of Rome. Ann Surg 1944; 120:268–283.

Evans DG, Miles AA, Niven JSF. The enhancement of bacterial infections by adrenalin. Br J Exp Pathol 1948; 29:20–39.

Krizek TJ, Robson MC, Kho E. Bacterial growth in skin graft survival. Surg Forum 1967; 18:518–519.

Liedberg NCF, Reiss E, Artz CP. The effect of bacteria on the take of split thickness skin grafts in rabbits. Ann Surg 1955; 142:92–96.

Miles AA. Non-specific defense reactions in bacterial infections. Ann NY Acad Sci 1956; 66:356–369.

Robson MC, Heggers JP. Bacterial quantification of open wounds. Milit Med 1969; 134:19–24.

OUTPATIENT THERAPY OF BURNS

BRUCE M. ACHAUER, M.D.

All burn patients will at some time require outpatient management. Approximately 95 percent of all burns are classified as minor and can be treated entirely on an outpatient basis. Admission criteria have been suggested by the American Burn Association and the American College of Surgeons (Table 1). In addition, admitting factors (Table 2) need to be considered. Many burn patients who are admitted spend only 1 or 2 days in the hospital where they receive fluid resuscitation; they can be subsequently managed best as outpatients. Also, some patients may initially be treated as outpatients, but complications develop and they then require admission. The goal is to deliver to outpatients care equal to the standard available in the modern burn center, and to coordinate inpatient and outpatient care transition as smoothly as possible for the patient's benefit. A burn center with an active outpatient program is ideally suited to perform this service. The "minor" burn patient may still develop hypertrophic scarring and may have delayed healing and contractures. He is just as likely as a major burn patient to develop post-traumatic stress disorder. Economic implications, particularly time off work, can be tremendous even for the patient with a minor burn. If all the knowledge and resources regarding burn care are applied to the minor burn, tremendous reduction in morbidity can be realized.

TABLE 1 Criteria of Burn Injury

	American Burn Association		*American College of Surgeons*	
Severity	*Adults Degree (%)*	*Children Degree (%)*	*Adults Degree (%)*	*Children Degree (%)*
Minor	2nd <15	2nd <10	2nd <15	2nd <10
	3rd < 2	3rd <10	3rd <15	3rd <10
Moderate	2nd >15–25	2nd >10–20	2nd 15–25	2nd 10–20
	3rd <10	3rd <10	3rd 15–25	3rd 10–20
Major	2nd >25	2nd >20	2nd >25	2nd >20
	3rd >10	3rd >10	3rd >10	3rd >10

Inherent in any decision to treat a burn on an outpatient basis is evaluation by a knowledgeable examiner, who should make certain there are no special problems such as hydrofluoric acid burn, electrical burn, or medical, social, or psychological complications.

Electrical cord burns, particularly in children, can be managed on an outpatient basis, but parents need to be carefully instructed as to the risk of bleeding from the labial artery and how to control this. Chemical burns need copious irrigation. Hydrofluoric acid burns need calcium injections and, possibly, calcium arterial infusions. Tar burns appear dramatic. People often go to great lengths to try to remove the tar immediately. We find this is not essential. Gradual removal is satisfactory. It is important to cool the tar burn immediately to eliminate the burning.

The evaluation should also include routine history, taking details of the injury, the patient's past medical history, allergies, and medication. Tetanus prophylaxis should be given as for any other injury. Antibiotic prophylaxis is not given. Attention must be paid to adequate pain control as these injuries are often extremely painful. Potent oral narcotics, as well as the help of understanding nurses, therapists, and psychologists, are needed.

WHERE TO TREAT

Outpatient burn injuries are handled either in the doctor's office, emergency room, hydrotherapy unit within physical therapy, or, probably least commonly, in the hydrotherapy unit associated with the burn center. In our burn center, a burn and wound service for the outpatient treatment of burns has been established. This is housed in a separate facility and staffed by nurses and physical therapists who are an integral part of the burn team.

This approach has many advantages. The burn wound is seen and each dressing performed by an experienced person. The facility personnel observe wounds each day and note any complications such as infection or delayed healing. Physician time is not used for actual dressing changes, which is cost-effective. Additionally, there is consistent observation by the same personnel. With this arrangement, there is excellent coordination when evaluation by a surgeon is needed. Services of the psychologist and therapist are also invoked when the need becomes apparent. Splinting and scar control (pressure garments) are instituted as soon as needed. Because of their constant experience with burn patients, the staff are very attuned to the normal wound healing process. They are alerted if, for example, there is a delay in returning to work. Questions are asked about symptoms of post-traumatic stress disorder. These include difficulty in sleeping, nightmares, flashbacks, irritability, and loss of libido. Usually these patients have an extreme fear of returning to the scene of the injury. Early detection of post-traumatic stress disorder is crucial to treating this common and highly curable problem.

WOUND CARE

A great deal of research has been done on the initial care of the burn wound. Millions of dollars are spent on various preparations, artificial skins, and agents to improve healing. Despite this, the basic biology of wound healing has not been altered. The major therapeutic efforts are to keep the wound clean and free of infection, remove dead tissue, and not interfere with the normal healing process. There are many ways to accomplish these goals.

Most burn wounds require an *active mode* of treatment. Typical burns are mixed injury, with some areas of deeper or full-thickness injury and surrounding areas of deep partial and light partial-thickness burns. The deeper areas require some debridement and the more superficial areas require protection from drying and desiccation. An active mode of treatment is undertaken for these common types of burns. This consists of daily hydrotherapy and washing with a laparotomy pad (Fig. 1). Loose skin is sharply debrided. Silver sulfadiazine ointment-impregnated gauze strips are applied (Fig. 2). These are covered with tubular net dressings (Fig. 3). Patients are then instructed to reapply the ointment in the evening since it becomes dry after several hours. Patients are seen daily. As the wound heals and the patient is capable of self care, he or she can then be seen every other day, three times a week, or once weekly. The use of silver sulfadiazine is not crucial; however, its use has become the standard of the industry and, since burned *in*patients have it applied

TABLE 2 Admitting Factors

All electrical burns greater than 1,000 volts because there is a high incidence (30%) of delayed arrhythmias.
Patients with complicating medical conditions such as diabetes and chronic obstructive pulmonary disease (COPD).
Very young (younger than 3) and very old (over 60).
Moderate or major burn.
Patients whose environment prevents adequate care at home.
Burns of the hands, eyes, ears, face, and perineum.
Inhalation or electrical injury.
Fracture or other major trauma.
Poor risk (intercurrent disease).

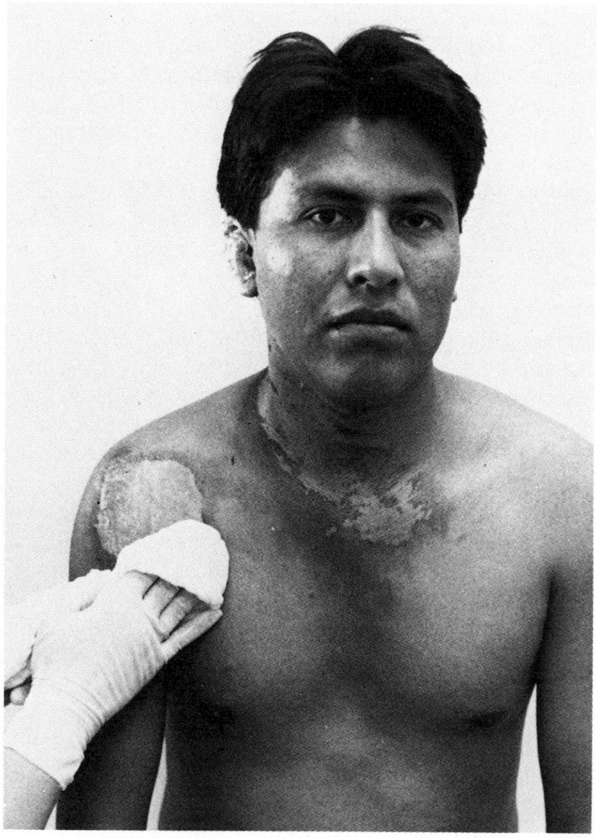

Figure 1 The burn wound is cleaned daily. A laparotomy pad is ideal for this purpose.

routinely, it is simpler to use a standard form of treatment for all burn patients. As healing progresses, the staff should be aware that silver sulfadiazine could interfere with epithelialization. Any bland ointment or antibiotic-type ointment can be used at this stage. It should be emphasized that absorption of topical agents can occur through the burn wound. For example, a small pediatric patient with a moderate burn could absorb toxic levels of Neosporin ointment, leading to otic toxicity.

Many patients are candidates for a *passive mode* of burn wound care. These are patients who have a superficial injury, without necrotic skin that requires debriding. There is essentially no drainage or infection. Such injuries include eschar-free full-thickness burns and relatively clean partial-thickness burns. Many burns move into this category after a few initial dressing changes. It is appropriate to cover these wounds with a membrane-type dressing. Examples of such dressings include Biobrane, Hydron, and a new product currently being evaluated, Dimac.

Biobrane is an ultra-thin silicone membrane with an attached nylon fabric to promote adherence. The entire material is then coated with collagen. It comes in several forms, some with perforations, and is also available as a glove. Biobrane is used in many burn centers as a temporary skin substitute. We have found it useful in a variety of situations.

Hydron is a film of poly-2-hydroxyethyl methacrylate polymerized with polyethyl glycol. It has recently been made available commercially after extensive clinical trials. Excellent patient comfort and epithelialization have been reported.

Dimac is a newly developed drug delivery system composed of polyethylene glycol 400 (PEG), poly-2-hydroxyethyl methacrylate and dimethyl sulfoxide. When the components are mixed, they form an elastic, flexible sheet that adheres to dry surfaces and conforms closely to body contours. When incorporated into the delivery system, silver sulfadiazine is released in a sustained fashion. A preliminary study in patients with partial-thickness burn injury indicated that Dimac with silver sulfadiazine (2 percent), applied for 1 to 4 days, as well as twice daily dressings with Silvadene cream, controlled wound bacterial levels.

Other types of burn wound coverings include

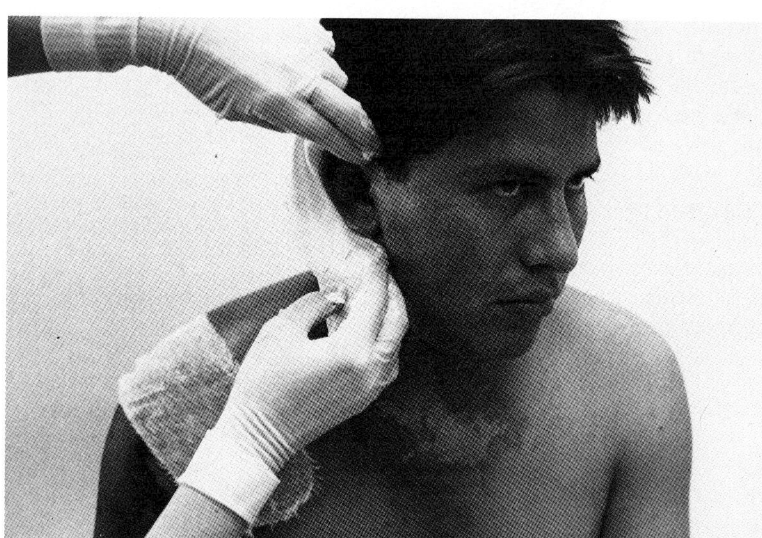

Figure 2 Silver sulfadiazine-impregnated gauze strips are then laid over the burn wound.

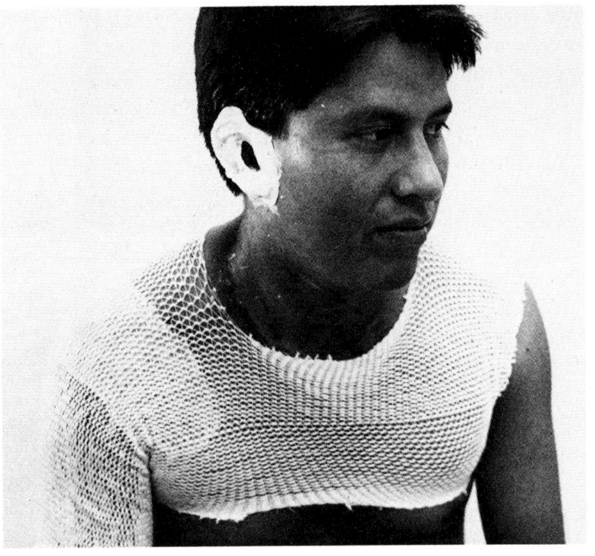

Figure 3 Elastic tubular net dressing is applied in a custom-made fashion to hold the gauze in place. This provides for maximum comfort and activity. Areas on the neck are healed and left undressed. An alternative for the ear is Sulfamylon cream. Some clinicians feel this is superior for preventing auricular chondritis.

xenograft (pigskin) and amnion, which many find useful. An example of porcine xenograft is E-Z Derm. The pigskin is aldehyde cross-linked and can be stored at room temperature for up to 1 year. It is combined with antimicrobial silver. Amnion is available from the obstetrical department and can be processed economically.

Many learned discussions have been held about the proper management of burn blisters. Proponents of leaving blisters intact note the excellent wound healing that occurs beneath the blister fluid. When the fluid is removed, there is desiccation of the underlying dermis and deeper extension of the injury. However, the above discussion shows that from a practical standpoint it is impossible to clean the burn wound actively and debride the dead tissue without disturbing the blisters. In the passive mode, the blisters can be left intact or the fluid aspirated. If one is in a remote setting, or the burn is not being treated by experienced personnel, it is best to leave the blisters intact or aspirate the fluid.

FOLLOW-UP

The major shortcoming of many modes of outpatient burn therapy is lack of follow-up. Small wounds being treated in an emergency room are seen by different examiners until the wound is healed; then the patient is discharged. If one is not sensitive to the complications of burn wounds, a likely assumption may be that once epithelialization has occurred the care is completed. In fact, the major complications of burns occur later, with scar maturation. Wounds that are not healed within three weeks postinjury should be examined by a surgeon and a decision made regarding skin grafting. Once a burn wound has healed, the patient should be examined at one-, two-, and three-month intervals and the presence of any hypertrophic scarring noted. If there is any sign of hypertrophic scarring, the patient should be fitted for a custom-made compression garment for an appropriate period. Silicone inserts beneath the garment to apply pressure to difficult areas also help to minimize scarring. Another form of treatment is application of topical steroids, with the steroid-impregnated tape Cordran often being useful.

Patients need to be instructed in the proper long-term care of burn scar management. The scar will lack normal lubrication and the continuous application of a lanolin-containing ointment is important. The wounds will remain hypersensitive to sun exposure for several months, and patients are instructed to stay out of the sun or wear opaque clothing or make-up and use sun block. They are told they may have sensitivity to extremes of heat or cold and certain chemicals.

Photographic records are kept for the patient's benefit. Correspondence is maintained with the Worker's Compensation carrier about return to work and any limitations of function or chemical heat exposure on the job. Again, questions are asked specifically about symptoms of posttraumatic stress disorder. Minor burns need major league care!

SUGGESTED READING

Davies JWL. Synthetic materials for covering burn wounds: progress towards perfection. I. Short term dressing materials. Burns Incl Therm Inj 1983–1984; 10:94–103.

Davies JWL. Synthetic materials for covering burn wounds: progress towards perfection. II. Longer term substitutes for skin. Burns Incl Therm Inj 1983–1984; 10:104–108.

Martinez SE. Outpatient burns. In: Achauer BM, ed. Management of the burned patient. Norwalk: Appleton-Century-Crofts, 1987:109.

Pruitt BA, Levine NS. Characteristics and uses of biologic dressings and skin substitutes. Arch Surg 1984; 119:312–322.

Tavis MJ, Thornton J, Danet R, Bartlett RH. Current status of skin substitutes. Surg Clin North Am 1978; 58(6):1233–1248.

Warden GD. Outpatient management of thermal injuries. In: Boswick JA, ed. The art and science of burn care. Rockville: Aspen Systems Corp, 1987:45.

Warden GD, Kravits M, Schnebly A. Burn rounds: the outpatient management of moderate and major thermal injuries. J Burn Care Rehab 1981; 2:159–161.

ACUTE CARE OF THERMAL BURNS

ELOF ERIKSSON, M.D.

Over the past four decades, survival from a thermal burn injury has increased greatly. This has mainly been the result of improved understanding and treatment of the complications of thermal burns. In 1970, Janzekovic refocused interest on the burn wound by suggesting early tangential excision. Since that time the early pathophysiology of the burn wound has been studied intensely. However, even if our knowledge has increased, it has not dramatically changed our treatment modalities.

This chapter deals with some of the aspects of the acute care of thermal burns. Many excellent reviews of this topic have been published during the past several years.

PATHOPHYSIOLOGY

The burn injury immediately starts a pronounced local inflammatory reaction, and in major burns the effects of this reaction will spread to the entire body. Some of the mediators are illustrated in Figure 1. A progression of the area of tissue necrosis from the time of the burn up to 48 hours postburn has been documented.

There have been many surgical and medical attempts to halt this progression. Immediate excision of the eschar appears logical, but entails some practical problems such as operating room scheduling and availability of cross-matched blood. Local cooling or administration of various anti-inflammatory agents have been used in order to stop or reverse the progression of the injury. Cooling appears beneficial, but can only be used in small and medium size burns because of the risk of hypothermia. Inhibitors of different inflammatory mediators seem to have some effect in blocking parts of the inflammatory response. There is currently no commonly accepted protocol available for pharmacologic treatment of the early progression of the burn injury.

DIAGNOSIS

The diagnosis of a burn and its prognosis depend mainly upon five factors. These are: (1) age of the patient, (2) the area of the burn, (3) depth of the burn, (4) associated injuries, and (5) the preexisting co-morbidity.

Age

Because of a larger surface-to-volume ratio in the small child, and a sometimes greatly decreased physiologic reserve in the very old, these two age groups show a higher mortality for a burn of a certain surface area. For instance, in a patient older than 70, a burn greater than 40 percent of body surface area (BSA) has a statistical mortality risk of 100 percent.

Area

The total body surface area of the burn expressed in percentage of body surface area is best described in a chart by Lund and Browder (Table 1). Note that if this diagram is not combined with a careful drawing, the surface area of small and medium size burns may be greatly overestimated.

Depth

No reliable, objective way of assessing burn depth is available. The fluorescence of intravenous fluorescein, measurement of evaporation, thermography, ultrasound, and photometric methods have all been found to be of limited value in the diagnosis of burn depth. A careful history, combined with the examination of the burn wound by an experienced surgeon at the time of admission, is still the best method.

In the very superficial burn (first degree), the skin is typically red and tender without blistering.

In the partial thickness burn (second degree), blisters are usually present. They may be intact or broken. The skin surface is usually very tender, but in a deep, partial thickness burn, sensation may be absent. Typically, the skin is red and blanches on compression, and there is rapid capillary refill.

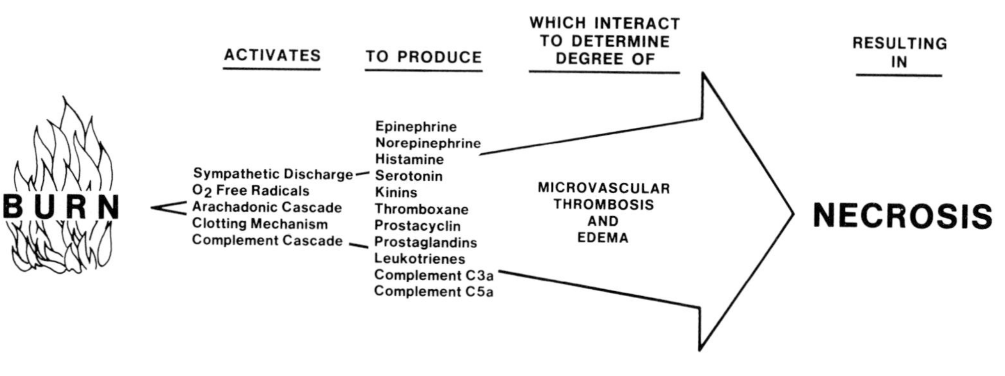

Figure 1 Diagram of the inflammatory process that is activated by the burn. (From Hurt A, Eriksson E. Management of the burn wound. Clin Plast Surg 1986; 13(1):59.)

TABLE 1 Chart for Estimation of Burn Area

Area	*Birth–1 yr*	*1–4 yr*	*5–9 yr*	*10–14 yr*	*15 yr*	*Adult*	*Partial thickness 2°*	*Full thickness 3°*	*Total*
Head	19	17	13	11	9	7			
Neck	2	2	2	2	2	2			
Anterior trunk	13	13	13	13	13	13			
Posterior trunk	13	13	13	13	13	13			
Right buttock	2½	2½	2½	2½	2½	2½			
Left buttock	2½	2½	2½	2½	2½	2½			
Genitalia	1	1	1	1	1	1			
Right upper arm	4	4	4	4	4	4			
Left upper arm	4	4	4	4	4	4			
Right lower arm	3	3	3	3	3	3			
Left lower arm	3	3	3	3	3	3			
Right hand	2½	2½	2½	2½	2½	2½			
Left hand	2½	2½	2½	2½	2½	2½			
Right thigh	5½	6½	8	8½	9	9½			
Left thigh	5½	6½	8	8½	9	9½			
Right leg	5	5	5½	6	6½	7			
Left leg	5	5	5½	6	6½	8			
Right foot	3½	3½	3½	3½	3½	3½			
Left foot	3½	3½	3½	3½	3½	3½			
						Total			

From Lund CC, Browder NC. The estimation of areas of burns. Surg Gyn Obstet 1944; 79:352. By permission of Surgery, Gynecology and Obstetrics.

In the full-thickness burn (third degree), the eschar may be white or charred black. It does not blanch on compression, nor is there any capillary refill. There is usually minimal or no sensation of the skin.

Associated Injuries

In thermal burns that result from fire in a closed space, smoke inhalation injuries frequently add to the morbidity and mortality. Explosions and falls are sometimes part of the accident and, in these cases, closed head injuries, intra-abdominal injuries, major soft tissue trauma, and fractures must be ruled out. The presence of, for instance, intra-abdominal hemorrhage and subsequent hemorrhagic shock can be concealed by the symptoms of the burn injury and its treatment with opiates for analgesia.

Co-morbidity

During the early period of resuscitation and, later, during surgical procedures and possible septic episodes, there is significantly increased stress upon major organ systems. If, for instance, there is a decreased cardiac, pulmonary, renal, or hepatic reserve, the patient has a lesser chance to survive the burn.

TRIAGE

The diagram in Figure 2 was published by Dr. Wachtel and summarizes our guidelines for the triage of the burned patient. In 1987, the majority of hospitalized burns required treatment in specialized burn care facilities. Ambulatory management often requires the patient to be seen frequently, at least during the first week postburn.

FLUID MANAGEMENT

The burn injury initiates a massive inflammatory reaction, locally in the area adjacent to the coagulated tissue and also in unburned areas of the body. The composition of the edema fluid after the burn is similar to a 60 percent concentration of cell-free plasma. It has been shown that, frequently, as much as 50 percent of the fluid loss takes place in areas remote from the burn. Many formulas have been used in the resuscitation of burns (Table 2). I prefer to use the following modification of the Parkland formula:

I. First 24 hours:
   1. Start Ringer's lactate at maximum rate.
   2. Adjust to urine output of 30 to 60 cc per hour in adults and 1 cc per kilogram per hour in infants.

II. Second 24 hours:
   1. Colloid at 0.3 to 0.5 ml per kilogram per burn percentage.
   2. D_5W to maintain same urine output as above.

It is desirable to keep total plasma protein concentration at approximately 6 g per deciliter. When the total protein content of plasma drops down from 6 to 5 g per deciliter, formation of edema increases drastically. Because of this and other studies, there appears to be a move towards giving colloid during the first 24 hours to patients who require a large amount of resuscitation. This results in a smaller total amount of resuscitation fluid and a lesser increase in lung water.

NUTRITION

When there is no need for immediate surgery (such as escharotomies), and the patient is neither nauseated nor

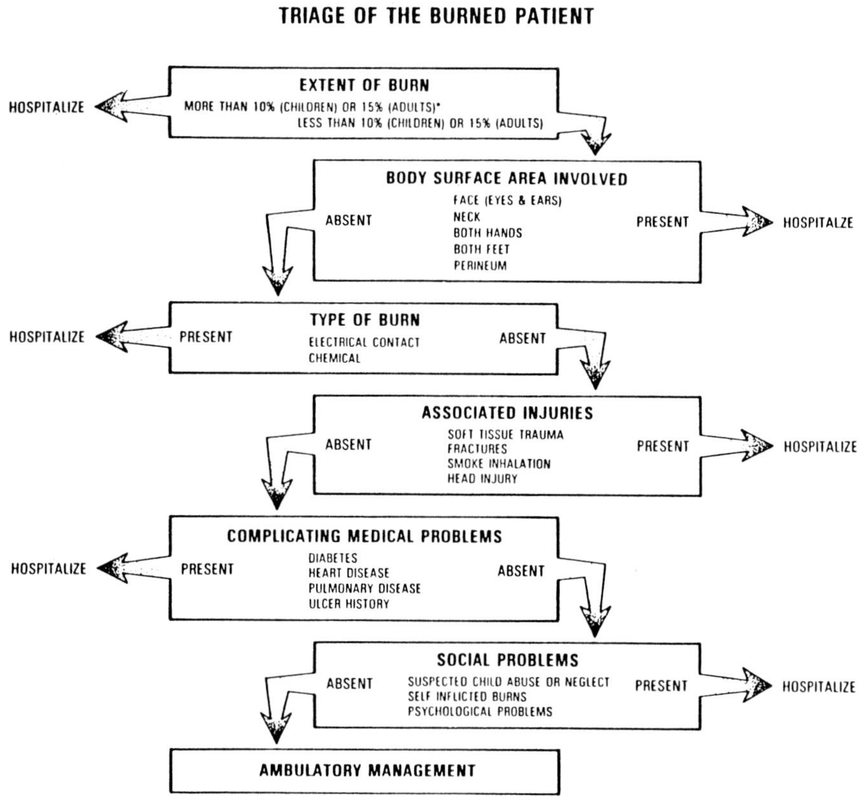

* % TOTAL BODY SURFACE AREA INVOLVED WITH 2° AND 3° BURNS

Figure 2 Decision tree for triage of burn patients. (From Wachtel TL. Epidemiology, classification, initial care, and administrative considerations for critically burned patients. Crit Care Clin 1985; 1(1):11).

going to need immediate transportation to another facility, I prefer to start oral feedings on the day of admission. The patient is encouraged to take a high protein, high calorie diet. When the patient cannot eat, a No. 12 French silicone feeding tube is inserted transnasally and continuous tube feedings are started. Usually, an infusion rate of 150 or even 175 cc per hour can be tolerated within 2 to 3 days. A lactose-free formula with the standard protein content can be used initially. After 1 week, the patient can usually tolerate the high protein formulas, when necessary.

When the patient cannot tolerate enteral feedings in sufficient amounts, I prefer to supplement nutrition with peripheral hyperalimentation. If these two in combination do not supply the patient with an adequate caloric intake, central hyperalimentation is started. In both peripheral and central hyperalimentation, it is attempted to give approximately 50 percent of the calories as carbohydrates, 25 percent as amino acids, and 25 percent as lipids. When central hyperalimentation is used, the site of the intravenous access is changed every 4 days. The standard formulas for caloric needs appear to overestimate the caloric intake. However, when frequent operative procedures limit oral intake, it is usually not possible to give the patient a too-large average daily number of calories. The advent of computerized equipment to measure and calculate caloric expenditure has simplified the accurate assessment of nutritional requirements.

BURN WOUND MANAGEMENT

Any significant burn becomes covered with an eschar, which may be either excised or allowed to separate spontaneously. Immediately after the burn, the eschar contains heat-denatured proteins and various other substances that have been released from the injured cells. After 1 to 2 weeks, the eschar, as well as the burned wound, is contaminated or even colonized with microorganisms. From a surgical standpoint, burn wound management calls for debridement of the eschar and skin graft closure before the wound becomes infected. Until the eschar can be excised, the contamination by microorganisms is minimized either by topical antibacterials (the commonly used method in the United States), or by exposure to warm, dry air, which is common practice in many other parts of the world. I prefer early excision, i.e., a start on debridement of the eschar within 72 hours after admission and an attempt to have the entire eschar removed within 1 week. When donor sites are available, the wounds are skin-grafted at the same time. Usually, the extremities are debrided first, with tourniquets used for control of bleeding. After this, the anterior chest and abdomen and, later, the back are debrided. I prefer to debride the face last except in two situations. One is when the burn is clearly of full thickness, in which case it is preferred to excise and graft the head and neck areas first. The other excep-

TABLE 2 Burn Resuscitation Formulas

	First 24 hours	*Second 24 hours*
Evans formula: "Rule of 50"	Colloid—1 cc/% burn/kg wt	½ of 1st 24 hr crystalloid
	Saline—1 cc/% burn/kg wt	½ of 1st 24 hr colloid
	D_5W for insensible losses (2,000 cc)	D_5W for insensible losses
Brooke Formula	2 cc/% burn/kg weight (adult)—lactated Ringer's	Colloid 0.3—0.5 cc/% burn/kg weight
	3 cc% burn/kg weight (children)—lactated Ringer's	
	½ in the first 8 hr	
	½ each of next 8 hr	
Parkland Formula	4 cc/% burn/kg weight	Colloid 0.3—0.5 cc/% burn/kg weight
	½ first 8 hr	
	¼ each next 8 hr	
Hypertonic Formula	300 mEq Na, 200 mEq DL lactate, 100 mEq Cl infused at a rate sufficient to maintain a urine output of 30 ml/hr	⅓–½ of first day requirements
HALFD Formula	1. 240 mOsm sodium, 120 mOsm of each chloride and lactate	
	2. 1.5 g albumin/liter infused at a rate sufficient to maintain mean arterial pressure of 60 torr	
	End point of resuscitation—urine output 40 ml/hr	
	Pulse pressure $\geq$40 torr	
	Declining serum lactate	
	Abrupt rise in serum sodium	
	Abrupt drop in serum potassium	
	Post-end point resuscitation	
	¼ normal saline with 12.5 g albumin/liter	
Brigham Burn Budget	10% body weight with colloid	
	½ first 12 hr	
	¼ second 12 hr	
	¼ second 24 hr	
	Renal 1,200 cc/day (½ normal saline)	
	Pulmonary loss 1,500–5,000 cc/day (D_5W)	
	Skin loss 1,000–4,000 cc/day (Ringer's lactate)	

From Thornton JW. Resuscitation. In: Achauer BM, ed. Management of the burned patient. Norwalk: Appleton Lange, 1987:69.

tion is when the eyelids are involved and the corneas are becoming exposed. In this case, the eyelids are debrided and grafted early. In most deep, partial-thickness burns, the face will reepithelialize spontaneously with, typically, an epithelium of better color and texture than that of grafted skin.

While waiting for the burn wound to be excised and grafted, it is covered with a topical antibacterial. I prefer Silvadene in all areas except for ears, where Sulfamylon is used because of better penetration. The cream is removed and reapplied every 12 hours. Other burn centers use silver nitrate or Betadine. The advantages and disadvantages of the above agents are listed in Table 3. There appears to be no benefit from using topical antibacterials in burns smaller than 5 percent BSA. Tetanus prophylaxis is given upon admission. No systemic antibiotics are given.

ESCHAROTOMIES

In circumferential extremity burns and, occasionally, in neck and trunk burns, escharotomies are required immediately upon admission. Due to constriction by the eschar, tissue pressure increases and reduces circulation to the tissue. Initially, there is cyanosis and an abnormally short capillary refill time due to venous obstruction. Later, the patient complains of paresthesia, or even complete loss of sensation. If the compartment pressures increase, there is an eventual obstruction of the arterial pulse. When a compartment syndrome has been diagnosed, either clinically, or by the use of an inserted wick pressure catheter, there is a need for immediate midaxial escharotomies. When the vascular compromise by the eschar has been of long duration, release of circulation by escharotomies produces a reactive hyperemia of the whole extremity with subsequent formation of muscle edema. This situation is similar to the revascularization of a limb after vascular occlusion, where there is frequently the need for fasciotomies in order to release the muscle compartments. If this condition is not recognized, the entire muscle compartment, or even the entire extremity, may be lost. When the compartment pressure is higher than 30 cm of water— and definitely when higher than 35 cm of water— immediate escharotomies are indicated.

DEBRIDEMENT

Enzymatic debridement of the eschar may be carried out during certain circumstances. The inactivated enzyme of *Bacillus subtilis* (Travase), or a mixture of streptokinase and streptodornase applied in aqueous solution in a saturated piece of gauze can be used. Pain, and in some cases early sepsis, may complicate this type of treatment. In major burns, the area of application of the enzymatic agents is usually limited to 15 percent of the total body

TABLE 3 Commonly Used Topical Antibacterials

	Mafenide Acetate Cream (Sulfamylon Burn Cream)	*Silver Nitrate Soaks*	*Silver Sulfadiazine Cream (Silvadene)*
Form of treatment	Exposure	Occlusive dressings	Exposure or single layer dressing
Concentration of active agent (%)	11.1	0.5	1.0
Advantages	Penetrates eschar; wound readily visible; compatible with treatment of associated injuries; no gram-negative resistance identified; motion of involved joints is maintained.	No hypersensitivity; painless except at time of dressing change; no gram-negative resistance; reduces heat loss from wound; most compatible with hypertonic resuscitation regimen.	Painless on application; wound readily visible when cream is applied without dressings; compatible with treatment of associated injuries; motion of involved joints is maintained.
Limitations	Painful for 20–30 minutes after application to second degree burns; accentuates post-burn hyperventilation; hypersensitivity noted in 7% of patients; delays spontaneous eschar separation.	No penetration of eschar; marked transeschar loss of Na^+, K^+, Ca^{++},Cl^-; methemoglobinemia (rare); dressings limit motion of involved joints; discolors unburned skin of patient, skin of attending personnel and any environmental objects in contact.	Poor penetration of eschar; bone marrow suppression with neutropenia; hypersensitivity (infrequent); resistance of many *Enterobacter cloacae* and of some *Pseudomonas* sp.; delayed eschar separation.

From Pruitt BA. The burn patient. II. Later care and complications of thermal injury. Curr Prob Surg 1979; 16(5):8.

surface area. When the eschar has been removed, the wound is temporarily treated with a topical antibacterial agent until it is covered with an autograft or biologic dressing. Enzymatic debridement has the advantage of eliminating the need for surgical removal of the eschar, and it preserves the surviving dermis to a maximal degree by not digesting viable tissue.

Early removal of the eschar by tangential excision with a guarded knife has been suggested. Thin layers of epidermis and dermis are excised until arterial bleeding is encountered in all areas. Full-thickness excision of dermis and epidermis down to subcutaneous fat can also be carried out. A third method for removal of the eschar is excision down to fascia. I usually favor tangential excision on the extremities, while excision down to fascia is most useful on the trunk. Skin graft take appears to be better if the recipient bed consisted either of some dermis or some fascia. Grafting onto subcutaneous fat is undertaken only if there is a need for padding over a joint or bony prominence, or if the contour in an area of esthetic concern will be greatly altered by the removal of subcutaneous fat. It is preferable to do the skin grafting in conjunction with the excision in order to avoid a second procedure for application of the skin grafts. Usually, adequate hemostasis can be achieved at the time of debridement. In geriatric patients or those with very large burns, survival priorities usually dictate an excision down to fascia. Harvested skin grafts are usually meshed and expanded three or four times before application. The function of mesh-grafted areas appears to be as good as that of sheet-grafted areas. However, in areas of significant esthetic concern, such as face and hands, sheet grafts are preferred because of their better appearance.

BURN WOUND COVERAGE

When the eschar has been excised and sufficient amounts of autograft are not available, the wound is temporarily covered with a skin substitute. Several factors, such as experience, organization, availability, and price usually dictate the choice of skin substitutes. My preference now is Biobrane.

If the wound has been autografted, the graft is either covered with an ointment gauze or, if the autograft has been expanded four times or more, it is covered with Biobrane. Several layers of gauze are then applied and, finally, a splint is used to immobilize the graft area. Usually, the knee is splinted in extension and the foot in dorsiflexion. In the hand, the MP joints are flexed 70 to 90 degrees and the IP joints are splinted straight. The thumb is maximally abducted and opposed. The wrist is kept in 30 degrees of dorsiflexion, the elbow is kept straight, and the shoulder joint is usually maintained in 120 degrees of abduction. The splinting is done not only for immobilization, but also for protection of important functions. Deviations from the above rule are common; for instance, in the grafted burn wound of the palm of the hand, where the hand is splinted in full extension in order to avoid flexion contractures.

POSTOPERATIVE CARE

Autografts are usually inspected on the third day postoperatively. If there is reason to suspect heavy drainage or hematoma, they may be inspected earlier. If Biobrane is used to cover the grafts, it is usually only necessary to remove the dressing down to the Biobrane, through which the graft can be inspected. Small incisions in the Biobrane usually makes it possible to evacuate hematomas and seromas. After this, a new gauze dressing and new splint are applied and the wound is inspected daily. Usually, the Biobrane starts peeling off after 8 to 10 days; it is trimmed back and subsequently removed. If unepithelialized portions remain when the Biobrane is removed, the wound is covered with an ointment-impregnated gauze and a dry dressing, which is changed daily. Once the wound has epithelialized, it can usually be left open and treated against dehydration with a lubricating skin cream.

SUGGESTED READING

Achauer BM, ed. Management of the burned patient. Norwalk: Appleton Lange, 1987.
Artz CP, Moncrief JA, Pruitt BA Jr, eds. Burns. A team approach. Philadelphia: WB Saunders, 1979.
Boykin JV, Eriksson E, Pittman RN. In vivo microcirculation of scald burn and the progression of postburn dermal ischemia. Plast Reconstr Surg 1980; 66:191-198.
Hurt A, Eriksson E. Management of the burn wound. Clin Plast Surg 1986; 13:57-67.
Wachtel TL. Epidemiology, classification, initial care, and administrative considerations for critically burned patients. Crit Care Clin 1985; 1:3-26.
Wise DL, ed. Burn wound coverings. Vols I and II. Boca Raton: CRC Press, 1984.

GRAFTING WITH SKIN SUBSTITUTES

G. GREGORY GALLICO III, M.D., F.A.C.S.

TABLE 1 General Requirements for the Design of a Skin Graft Substitute

Available "off the shelf"
Flexible and adherent
Seal for water and protein
Barrier against bacterial invasion
Durable wound surface

Split-thickness skin grafting is one of the oldest and most useful techniques in plastic surgery. For small, open wounds split-thickness autografts may be harvested from another area of the body and employed to close a wound and to protect the patient from invasion of bacteria and loss of water vapor. However, when the area of skin loss exceeds 50 percent of the body surface area, there is, obviously, insufficient intact donor skin to cover the wound in one operative procedure. The donor skin may be cut before it is applied to form a mesh that can be spread to cover a larger wound with full epithelialization of the interstices by 7 to 10 days. However, in practice this technique of meshing the skin to expand its area of coverage does not facilitate wound coverage so significantly that repeated harvesting of the same donor sites as they regenerate is not required. This repeated harvesting leaves portions of the wound open for a long time thereby inviting sepsis. Traumatic skin degloving injuries, congenital absence of skin (aplasia cutis congenita), giant congenital nevi, and especially large thermal burns, may all require such a large amount of skin graft that available skin graft donor sites will not suffice. In such cases, a temporary or permanent skin substitute is needed. This chapter describes some of the methods currently available to close wounds either temporarily or permanently with natural or synthetic skin substitutes.

DESIGN OF SKIN SUBSTITUTES

What characteristics of skin would be desirable to reproduce in a skin substitute? What features of the normal anatomy and physiology of skin are necessary to provide a skin substitute that produces early coverage of the wound, inhibition of water and protein loss, prevention from bacterial invasion, and long-term, durable protection from trauma? (Table 1).

Human skin is composed of two layers, epidermis and dermis, which are anatomically and functionally dependent on each other. The epidermis is comprised of multiple layers of keratinocytes, which are attached to the underlying papillary dermis by a basement membrane. The deepest layer of the epidermis, immediately juxtaposed to the basement membrane, consists of the basal cells. These basal cells differentiate through the malpighian layer to produce the stratum corneum, the outermost keratinized layers of cells and the protective layer of skin. The epidermis is firmly attached to the dermis by the basement membrane, but is not vascularized. The basal cells and differentiating keratinocytes obtain their nutrients by diffusion from the dermal vasculature through the basement membrane.

The epidermis functions as a barrier, and its barrier capability resides in the stratum corneum, the outer layer of anucleate, cornified cells. This keratinized layer prevents the entry of bacteria and toxic materials and the loss of water and electrolytes. An ideal skin substitute must provide an immediate barrier to water vapor loss and bacterial invasion—the most important attributes to duplicate in a skin substitute. The normal epidermis also contains appendages and organelles, such as hair follicles and sweat glands. These skin appendages provide lubrication, in the case of the sebaceous glands, and heat regulation, in the case of the sweat glands. Patients who have large areas of their bodies covered with split-thickness skin grafts, which have few if any organelles, do not have exceptional difficulty with heat regulation or skin lubrication. In addition to the predominant cell population of keratinocytes, the epidermis contains "passenger cells" such as melanocytes, Langerhans' cells, and Merkel's cells. Neither the appendages nor the "passenger cells" are necessary to the barrier function of the skin and would be superfluous in a skin substitute.

The dermis lies below the epidermis and is composed of collagen fibrils and glycosaminoglycans joined together in an architecture, which is not amorphous and which is thought to contribute to the viscoelastic properties of skin. However, its exact architecture and, therefore, the need in a skin substitute for such an architecture, is not clear. The dermis supports the nonvascularized epidermis through the basement membrane and provides nourishment through diffusion.

Except for its role as supporter of the epidermis, the function of the dermis is more difficult to define than that of the epidermis. The best evidence of its role in a free graft is provided by clinical experience. Surgeons have long known that the more dermis transferred with a skin graft, the more primary skin graft contraction, and the less secondary wound contraction and scar in the final wound bed. In addition, they know that the more dermis that remains after split-thickness skin graft harvesting or burn injury, the more rapid the epithelialization, and the less dense the ultimate scar obtained. A thin skin graft provides an early wound barrier, but may be expected to provide a skin surface in the long-term that is susceptible to minor trauma and that results in significant cicatricial wound contraction. Thus, an ideal skin substitute would contain not only an epidermis to provide a barrier, but also a dermis to provide support and to minimize wound contraction.

SKIN SUBSTITUTES

Skin substitutes may be categorized as either biologic or synthetic, temporary or permanent. Biologic skin substitutes are direct natural products or are cultivated from natural products. Synthetic skin substitutes are completely produced in the laboratory from man-made materials. Obviously, some imprecision of categorization is possible since skin substitutes may contain both natural and synthetic components and since some synthetic components, though man-made, may be identical to biologic materials.

Skin substitutes may be further categorized as either temporary or permanent depending on whether they are designed to remain on the wound for only a short period of time or to remain as a permanent replacement for skin (Table 2). Temporary skin substitutes may require physical removal or may be biodegraded in situ. Some skin substitutes have portions which are temporary and portions which are permanent.

WOUND PREPARATION

Regardless of the material to be used for wound closure, the essential step that determines surgical success is proper wound preparation. The burn wound is the model for this discussion, but the tenets described can be generalized to traumatic or surgical wounds. All necrotic eschar must be debrided before grafting. This debridement is most efficiently carried out by direct excision. When the wound is relatively small, the excision can be carried out in a tangential fashion. Using either a free-hand graft-cutting knife (e.g., the Watson knife) or a motorized dermatome, the surgeon removes the eschar in strips going deeper with each stroke. The eschar is removed until there is a clean, bleeding surface; any tissue that does not bleed must be excised. For a deep second-degree burn, the final bleeding surface will be the deep dermis, which provides an excellent bed for skin grafts. However, third-degree burn wounds require the removal of the entire thickness of the skin, leaving a bed of subcutaneous fat. Skin grafts and skin substitutes "take"* less well on fresh fat than on dermis or muscle fascia. This fresh fat may be best dressed for 5 days until the surface has formed granulation tissue, which provides a more sure bed for the graft. When third-degree burns cover a large body surface area, a full-thickness excision of skin and subcutaneous fat may provide the best graft bed in the shortest time with the least blood loss. The detriment to fascial excisions is the late cosmetic effect of the grafted wound. Because of the poor appearance of these fascial excisions, most surgeons strive to perform tangential excisions where blood loss is not a major risk.

The freshly excised wound can be covered with a skin graft or a skin substitute. If a temporary skin substitute is used at this time, it will have to be removed at a later date and the wound prepared again for the final permanent skin layer. If the temporary graft has adhered well to the wound, it may be simply stripped away to produce a clean, bleeding surface. However, if areas of poor adherence have allowed a layer of hypertrophic, contaminated granulation tissue to develop, then this layer must be removed. The contaminated granulation tissue may be removed tangentially, similar to the original excision. These tissues may also be completely removed back to the deeper fibrotic layers by scraping them away with a broad-edged tool, such as a periosteal elevator. After hemostasis, fresh beds should be an excellent surface for skin graft or skin substitute. Skin substitutes "take" less well in general than standard split-thickness skin grafts, and the bed for application should be the best the surgeon can provide.

TABLE 2 Categorization of a Skin Substitute*

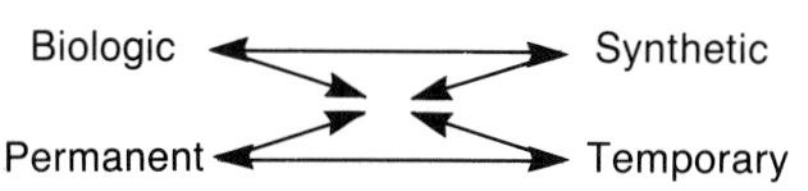

* Skin substitutes can be either of biologic or synthetic origin and can remain on the wound temporarily or permanently.

HUMAN ALLOGRAFT

In World War II, Brown and McDowell advocated the use of human cadaver skin allografts as an emergency, temporary dressing for burn wounds. They also noted that such grafts would only "survive from 3 to 10 weeks," but realized that if "these grafts could be gotten to survive, one the greatest problems in plastic surgery would be solved." Unfortunately, Gibson and Medawar documented shortly thereafter that skin allografts would be immunologically rejected. Despite rejection, however, skin allografts have been widely employed as a temporary wound coverage

* The "take" of a standard skin graft is defined as the vascularization of that graft. In the case of skin substitutes, which may not be vascularized, "take" is best defined as tight adherence to the wound at 1 week.

material. Allograft skin "takes" on an open wound surface as does an autograft. The allograft becomes vascularized and initially fulfills the barrier role of a skin substitute in that it prevents bacterial invasion and slows the loss of water, electrolytes, and protein from the wound. The adherence of the allograft sterilizes the underlying wound. Development of a skin bank where frozen cadaver skin is available at all times has allowed an aggressive approach to the therapy of massive burn wounds involving early excision of the entire burn wound and temporary coverage with cadaver allograft until autograft donor sites are available. However, the use of human allografts has been hampered recently by the possibility of the transmission of AIDS.

ALLOGRAFTS AND IMMUNOSUPPRESSION

Burke performed the first clinical evaluation of the use of immunosuppression to prolong the allograft survival in three children with burn wounds covering 91 percent, 81 percent, and 91 percent of body surface area. Immunosuppression was effected with oral azathioprine and was continued until allograft skin covered less than 20 percent of the burn wound. The medication was continued for 30, 31, and 49 days; the allografts evidenced no signs of rejection while immunosuppression was continued. The patients survived and were discharged from the hospital 28, 24, and 28 weeks after burning. Achauer has also administered Cyclosporine A (CsA) to one burn patient who received allografts from disparate donors onto excised burn wounds. These allografts appeared by meshed pattern and pigment differences to remain permanently on the wounds even after CsA was stopped. The lesser toxicity of CsA made this work very promising, but the advent of the AIDS epidemic may have dampened enthusiasm.

SUBSTITUTES FOR DERMIS

Gibson and Medawar noted that immune rejection of a skin allograft seemed to be primarily directed at cells within the epidermis and dermis with little rejection of the collagen within the dermis. Following this lead, Grillo and McKhann transplanted dermis (whose cells had been killed by freezing and thawing or by exposure to cyanide) to open wounds on the flanks of congenic strains of mice. However, just as Gibson and Medawar had seen in their patient, the dermal implants were slowly resorbed over 4 to 6 weeks by a "massive invasion by fibroblasts and capillaries," not distinctly immunologic in nature. Grillo and McKhann had hoped that the collagen matrix would provide a framework to direct invading fibroblasts and to orient the collagen produced. Unfortunately, the allograft collagen was replaced by scar. Heck and Cuono have separately attempted to use human allograft dermis as a free graft covered with epithelial sheets. In the short-term, they have demonstrated that this dermis remained, but long-term persistence has not been documented.

SYNTHETIC SKIN

The most successful synthetic membrane to act as a temporary barrier and to provide a permanent collagen scaffold was developed by Yannas and Burke. Their matrix was produced by covalently linking bovine collagen and glycosaminoglycans (GAGS), chondroitin 6-sulfate, and expanding the material into a sponge-like lattice with a fibril size of approximately 7 μ and a pore size of approximately 150 μ. Burke and Yannas believe that this bilayer membrane when placed on the wound undergoes direct invasion of the collagen-GAGS sponge by fibroblasts.

In practice, the artificial dermis of Burke and Yannas can be applied to a clean wound bed with a reasonable expectation of adherence. Because it is a foreign body, the surgeon may anticipate it to be susceptible to infection, and poor "take" will result more frequently than with split-thickness autograft. Synthetic skin is provided in a sealed envelope packaged in preservative, which must be washed away with Ringer's lactate before the sheet is sutured firmly to the wound. The Silastic surface provides an immediate water vapor barrier. Without contamination, the collagen sponge adheres to the wound, and granulation tissue invades the pores, thereby incorporating the collagen into the wound. After 3 to 6 weeks the Silastic layer can be easily separated away and the vascularized collagen sponge overgrafted with meshed split-thickness skin graft. The collagen sponge will be degraded and replaced. Although Burke and Yannas hypothesize that the lattice structure of the sponge will guide its own replacement with a neodermis of host collagen, the long-term architecture has not been easily differentiated from scar. The use of the artificial dermis is illustrated in Figure 1.

TISSUE CULTURED EPITHELIAL AUTOGRAFTS (CEA)

Human epithelial cells, keratinocytes, can be serially grown in tissue culture by providing fibroblast support to produce coherent sheets of cells, which can be used as a skin graft substitute. When applied to full-thickness wounds on nude mice, a naturally immunosuppressed experimental model, such grafts differentiate into an epithelium of human origin. Such sheets of autologous epithelial cells can be placed on open wounds on patients and produce a permanent skin.

The epithelial cells are grown in tissue culture from a small biopsy specimen of split- or full-thickness skin, 2 to 3 cm^2, harvested from an unburned area, such as axilla or groin. The epithelium is separated with scissors from the underlying collagen and disaggregated in trypsin to form a single-cell suspension. Aliquots of the suspension are inoculated into rectangular flasks containing a monolayer of lethally irradiated 3T3 cells. The cultures are fed with a medium supplemented with fetal calf serum, hydrocortisone, insulin, transferrin, triiodothyronine, choleragen, adenine, and epidermal growth factor and are

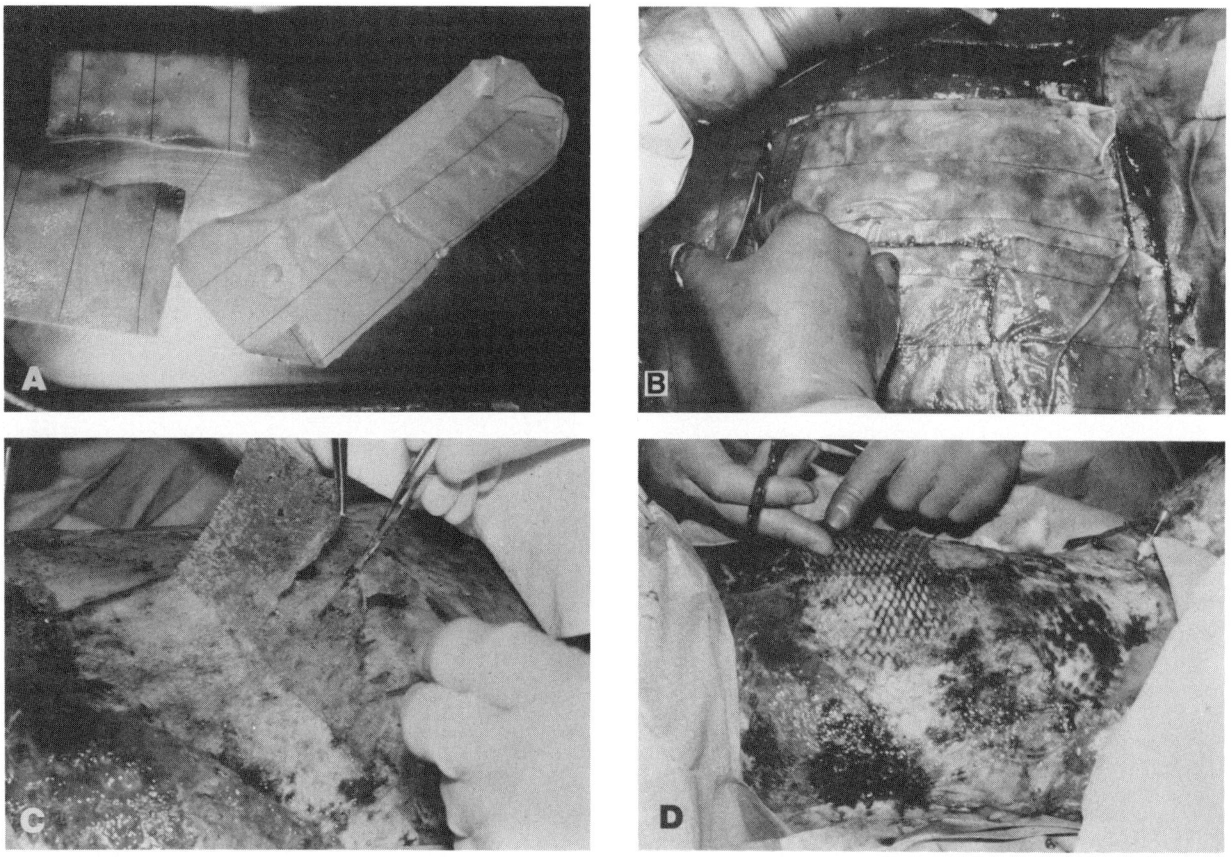

Figure 1 *A*, The artificial skin of Burke comes as a sheet packaged in preservative. *B*, The sheet of collagen sponge-GAGS is sutured to the prepared wound bed. *C*, After 3 to 6 weeks the outer Silastic layer can be stripped away. *D*, The vascularized collagen sponge can be overgrafted with thin split-thickness skin grafts.

incubated for 10 days at 37° C. Secondary cultures are prepared from primary cultures by trypsinization and transferred to culture flasks for another 10 days. When the secondary cultures become confluent at approximately 3 weeks from the initial biopsy date, the epithelium is detached as a coherent sheet with the enzyme, Dispase II, attached to a rectangle of petrolatum gauze with surgical clips, covered with serum-free medium, and transported to the operating room in a cooled, sealed chamber containing 10 percent CO_2.

CEA are fastened to the wound bed with skin staples or sutures. A sheet of wide-mesh nylon gauze (bridal veil) is stretched and stapled over the grafts. A bulky, dry gauze dressing is wrapped or sutured over the nylon mesh. On the extremities, a circumferential wrap of coarse mesh gauze (Kling) holds the CEA firmly. Because of blood loss, heat loss, and anesthetic requirements, it is practical to graft a maximum of approximately 20 percent body surface area (BSA) at one operation. The patients receive systemic antibiotics for 5 days after surgery. If the dressing remains dry, it is not removed until the seventh day; if a purulent exudate develops, dry dressing changes are begun sooner. At 1 week, all the dressings and the gauze carriers are removed. Saline, nonadherent dressings are then changed regularly. If surface infection is suspected at any time, topical antibacterials, 0.05 percent silver nitrate or dilute acetic acid, are applied to the dressings. Such topical antibiotics may be toxic to the epithelial cells sooner than 1 week in vivo. The techniques of grafting with CEA are illustrated in Figure 2.

One week after grafting, when the dressings are removed, the epithelium can be seen as a diaphanous, white layer on the wound surface. At this time the histology shows a differentiated epithelium with a stratum corneum (Fig. 3). On early excised wounds, the "take" of the epithelial grafts may be expected to be in the range of 70 to 90 percent. Only in surgically sterile wounds does "take" exceed 90 percent. When the patients are septic or hemodynamically unstable, or when the wounds are heavily contaminated with bacteria, the "take" of the epithelial grafts is poor. Areas which have not been successfully covered by the first grafting can be regrafted at 2 weeks—the grafts are either visible at that time or they are not there. In sick patients with major burns, it is not uncommon for two or three grafting procedures to be required to cover a large area. In healthy, freshly-excised wounds, one operation usually effects coverage.

After the initial dressings have been removed, the epithelial grafts will be adherent as separate islands on the wound. These islands epithelialize toward each other to cover the interstices and produce a confluent epithelial surface. The rate of this epithelialization is dependent on

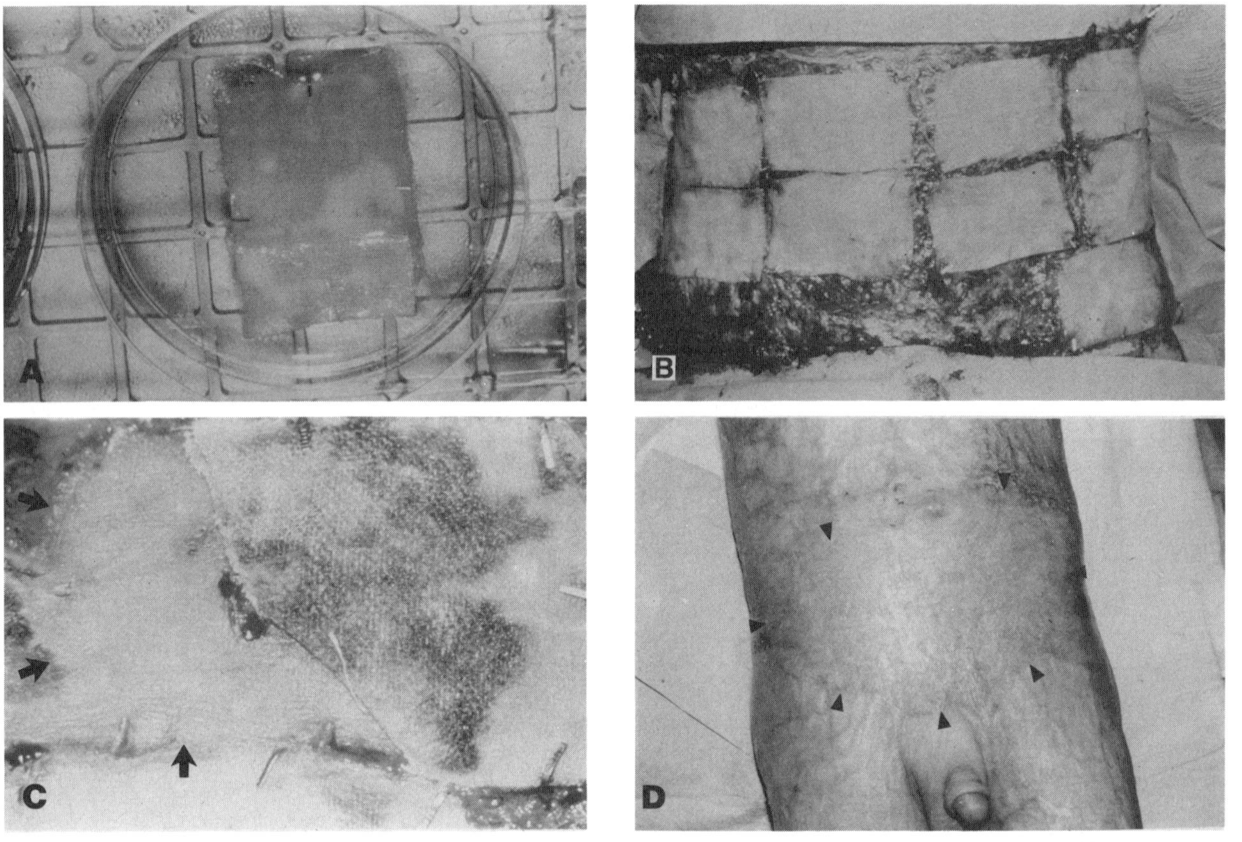

Figure 2 *A*, Human epithelial cells are grown into sheets in tissue culture. *B*, The sheets of epithelial cells are sutured to the prepared wound bed. *C*, After 1 week the gauze carrier can be removed leaving the epithelium adherent to the wound (arrows delineate cultured cell margin). *D*, The epithelium will remain on the wound as a permanent skin replacement (arrows indicate cultured cell area).

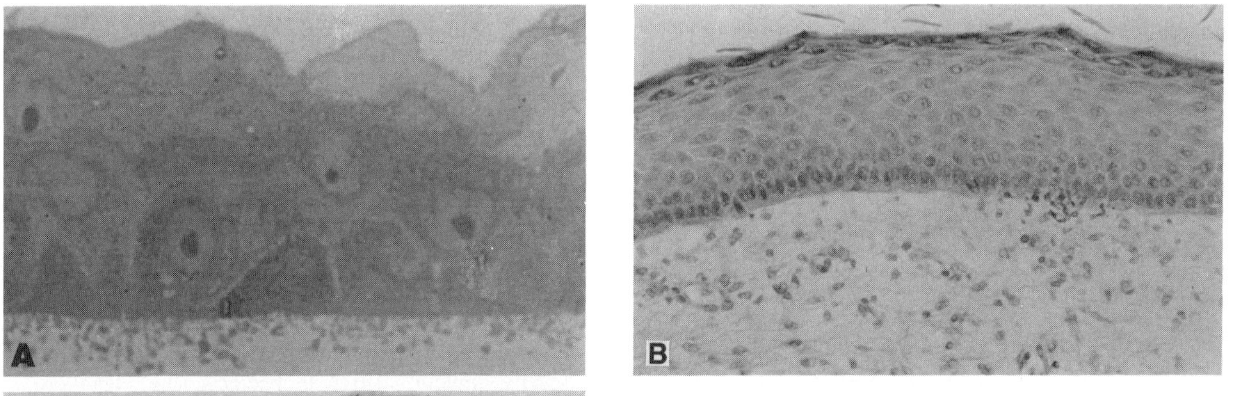

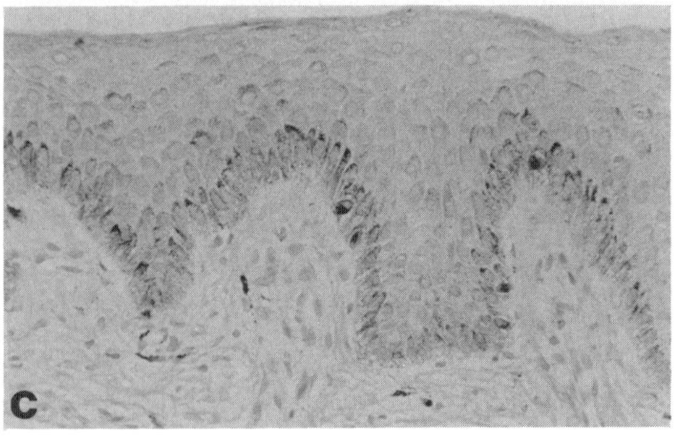

Figure 3 *A*, The cultured epithelium consists of several layers of basal cells. *B*, After 1 week on the wound, the basal cells have differentiated into a multilayered epithelium. *C*, In time the epithelium develops a basement membrane, anchoring fibrils, and rete ridges and pegs.

patient and wound conditions. This rate of epithelialization appears to be slower than one would expect with split-thickness skin graft. During the first several months after grafting, the cultured epithelial surface may form spontaneous bullae which break to produce small wounds, but thereafter, the epithelium will become stable.

CULTURED EPITHELIAL ALLOGRAFTS

Neonatal foreskin is commonly available, and can be grown and transferred as a tissue-cultured epithelial allograft. Such allografts could be maintained in tissue culture to provide a steady supply ready at any time to be placed on a patient immediately after burning. Preliminary analysis of these allografts indicates that they are rejected between histoincompatible pairs. Although tissue-typing has not been found to be influential in the past in prolonging standard skin graft "take," pure epithelial cell grafts, devoid of Langerhans' cells may react differently. Moreover, cultured epithelial cells could undergo antigenic modulation in culture making it conceivable that an antigenically "null" skin could be available "off the shelf" as a universal skin substitute. Obviously, the major advantage of cultured epithelial allografts at this time is that they can be provided with absolute assurance that they are free of the AIDS virus. Such cultured epithelial allografts may be useful in providing temporary coverage where standard allograft can no longer be used. That they adhere to the wound may make them preferable to synthetic materials.

CONCLUSION

Skin has been transplanted for centuries, and split- or full-thickness skin autograft has proved itself the "gold standard" of skin substitutes. Skin allografts, however, can substitute for missing skin quite well in the short-term, and new immunosuppressive techniques may make them a long-term substitute. Unfortunately, passenger viruses, such as the AIDS virus, may limit their use. To provide both temporary wound coverage and perhaps a permanent neodermis, which will inhibit wound contraction and produce a supple skin, biosynthetic membranes, such as the artificial dermis of Yannas and Burke, have been successfully used on large burn wounds. However, the persistence of the neodermis beyond the acute wound phase has not yet been documented, and such a dermis substitute does not solve the problem of a dearth of epidermis. Cultured sheets of autogenous epithelial cells have proved themselves capable of acting as a permanent, durable skin substitute. Further work will address the provision of a dermis and the role of cultured allografts.

The author wishes to acknowledge the collaboration in much of the work described in this chapter of Nicholas E. O'Connor, M.D., Carolyn C. Compton, M.D., Howard Green, M.D., Olaniyi Kehinde, B.S., John P. Remensnyder, M.D., and Susan Briggs, M.D.

SUGGESTED READING

Banks-Schlegel S, Green H. Formation of epidermis by serially cultivated human epidermal cells transplanted as an epithelium to athymic mice. Transplantation 1980; 29:308–313.

Cuono CB, Langdon R, Birchall N, Barttelbort S, McGuire J. Composite autologous-allogeneic skin replacement: development and clinical application. Plast Reconstr Surg 1987; 80:626–635.

Gallico GG III, O'Connor NE, Compton CC, Kehinde O, Green H. Permanent coverage of large burn wounds with autologous cultured human epithelium. N Engl J Med 1984; 34:448–451.

Green H, Kehinde O, Thomas J. Growth of cultured human epidermal cells into multiple epithelia suitable for grafting. Proc Natl Acad Sci USA 1979; 76:5665–5668.

Heck EL, Bergstresser PR, Baxter CR. Composite skin graft: frozen dermal allografts support the engraftment and expansion of autologous epidermis. J Trauma 1985; 25:106–112.

O'Connor NE, Mulliken JB, Banks-Schlegel S, Kehinde O, Green H. Grafting of burns with cultured epithelium prepared from autologous epidermal cells. Lancet 1981; 1:75–78.

Yannas IV, Burke JF. Design of an artificial skin. I. Basic design principles. J Biomed Mater Res 1980; 14:65–81.

Yannas IV, Burke JF, Gordon PL, Huang C, Rubenstein RH. Design of an artificial skin. II Control of chemical composition. J Biomed Mater Res 1980; 14:107–132.

ELECTRICAL INJURY

RONALD G. ZELT, M.D., C.M.
ROLLIN K. DANIEL, M.D., F.A.C.S.

Few injuries are more traumatic and incapacitating than severe electrical burns. Whereas low-voltage injuries are primarily a local wound problem, contact with high voltage is characterized by explosive entry and exit lesions and massive thermal damage to tissue. Despite the continual introduction of new techniques in burn care, the fundamental concepts of managing electrical burns have not changed significantly in the past 50 years. Periodic evaluation, sequential debridement, and delayed reconstruction remain the standard clinical approach. Although the concept of immediate resection and skin grafting was recommended as early as 1929, difficulties in differentiating damaged tissue from normal tissue, and significant risks of "progressive necrosis" and infection have prevented widespread implementation of early reconstruction.

Reliable statistics on the incidence of electrical injury are difficult to obtain and are plagued with problems of interpretation. It is important to remember the considerable range of severity of injury in electrical trauma. Accident statistics that fail to differentiate between low- and high-voltage contact tend to perpetuate controversy surrounding the etiology, evolution, and management of electrical lesions.

LOW-VOLTAGE INJURY

Management of low-voltage injuries varies significantly, but generally requires local wound care and functional rehabilitation only. Initial treatment should include the identification of all affected areas, adequate pain control and tetanus prophylaxis. Systemic antibiotics are not indicated in the early postinjury period unless the burns are complicated by gross contamination. Patients undergo sterile dressing changes two or three times daily with topical application of antibiotic creams or ointments.

Patients with minor injuries are treated conservatively, and any residual scarring is dealt with on an elective basis at a later date. More severely injured patients are taken to the operating room on the second day following injury for definitive debridement and wound coverage. Under general anesthesia, the wound is examined carefully so that all affected structures can be identified. The cutaneous insult is excised full thickness. All muscles and neurovascular structures in the surrounding area are identified and carefully assessed for injury. Functional and aesthetic considerations dictate the type of wound closure, with skin grafting or local skin flaps used as necessary.

The prognosis of low-voltage injuries varies and is generally site dependent. Low-voltage injuries to the mouths of young children may result in severe scar contractures and tragic oral deformities. Less severe injuries are more often a cosmetic problem, and return of function is generally good. It must be emphasized that although the cutaneous lesion often appears insignificant, associated deep tissue injury is common and must be suspected in all cases of low-voltage injury.

HIGH-VOLTAGE INJURY

In contrast to low-voltage accidents, high-voltage injuries (over 1,000 volts) are frequently devastating occurrences that result in marked local and systemic alterations. The vast majority of injuries occur in male utility workers. Approximately 50 to 75 percent of these cases involve the upper extremity, usually caused by grasping a charged object. The remaining sites of injury are dictated by the point of current grounding and commonly involve the contralateral upper extremity, the lower extremity, the thoracoabdomen, or the scalp. The inherent difficulties in treating these injuries result from a basic uncertainty of the pathophysiology of the wound and the specter of progressive necrosis.

Cutaneous Injury

The demarcation between viable and nonviable skin is usually distinct following high-voltage injury. Skip lesions, known for their appearance proximal to viable regions, are most frequently seen overlying flexion and extension creases. Previously thought to be caused by external arcing of electrical energy, skip lesions are now believe to result from the thermal by-product of current flowing across joints which is made up of electrically resistent tissues, i.e., tendon and bone. The cutaneous margins following electrical injury remain distinct and do not undergo progressive necrosis.

Muscular Injury

Deep Injury. Universal to all clinical reports is an obvious lack of correlation between the damage to skeletal muscle and the overlying cutaneous injury. Frequently, small skin lesions are observed in association with more extensive muscle involvement. Lesions involving the hand or distal forearm may extend proximally into the arm for distances up to 30 cm beneath viable skin.

Also of clinical importance is extensive injury to the deep aspect of muscles or muscle groups. The deeper aspects of individual muscles are often damaged more proximally than their superficial surfaces. This undoubtedly represents what is referred to as the deep, "hidden" component of muscle injury. Deep muscle groups in the forearm and in the arm also reveal more proximal damage. Interestingly, the level of injury on the superficial aspect of a deep muscle usually corresponds to the level of injury on the deep aspect of the overlying more superficial muscle. The result is a "cone" of tissue injury with its apex extending proximally for considerable distances beneath viable skin and muscle.

Choke Points. When an upper extremity sustains electrical injury, some specific areas show more extensive injury than the surrounding tissue. These areas are the wrist, cubital fossa, and possibly the axilla (Fig. 1). Common to these is a decreased cross sectional area which is composed predominantly of highly resistant bone and tendon. Clinically, these areas show a propensity for increased tissue injury. These critical areas demonstrate three significant findings: (1) muscular injury extends both distally and proximally from them; (2) they often do not correspond to the level of vascular injury; and (3) the most proximal "choke" point appears to correspond to the level of peripheral nerve injury. In the lower extremity, the ankle, and knee also appear to demonstrate these characteristics.

Progressive Muscular Injury. The uncertainty of progressive necrosis has plagued the treatment of electrically-injured patients and has provided the foundation for two contradictory management protocols. Some investigators feel that an ongoing tissue necrosis of muscular or vascular origin leads to prolonged sloughing of tissues following the initial insult. Strategies for treatment concentrated on multiple debridements and deferral of definitive treatment as long as possible to enable the progressive necrosis of tissues to stabilize. Others believe that the injuries sustained by the passage of electrical energy occurred as the result of the initial contact. Proponents of this theory advocate early excision and wound coverage. The authors strongly believe that the inability to appreciate and detect the deep muscular injury associated

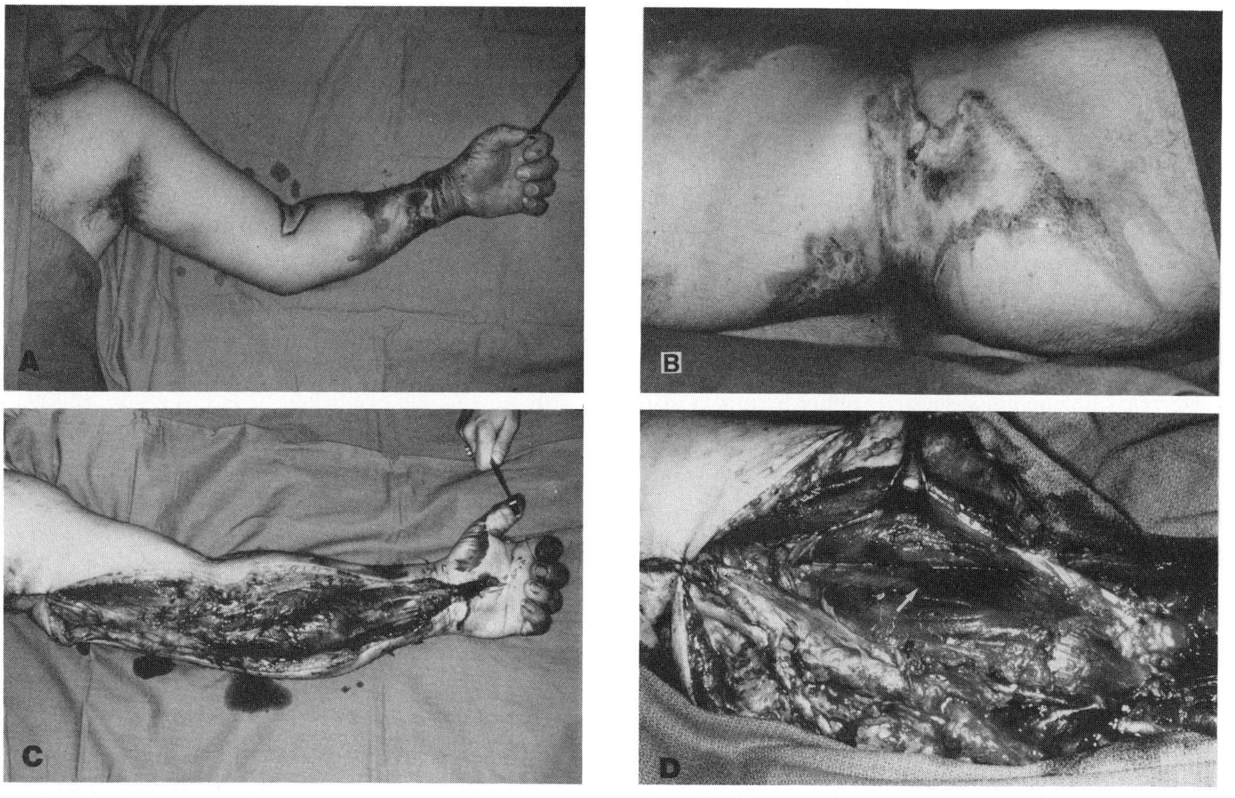

Figure 1 *A*, High-voltage electrical injury with mummification to the midforearm level. Note near-circumferential injury at cubital fossa "choke" point. *B*, Exit lesion on the lateral thoracoabdomen extending into right buttock. *C*, Fasciotomies of all muscle compartments is completed to the level of the axilla. *D*, A high-risk area is assessed in the early postinjury period. The biceps is retracted superiorly off the underlying brachialis muscle. The brachialis and undersurface of the biceps were found to be necrotic to the midforearm level (arrow).

with high-voltage electrical injuries results in delayed tissue sloughing and the appearance of "progressive necrosis."

Vascular Injury

The pattern of injury to the vascular system is a critical determinant of ultimate tissue survival and limb reconstruction. Major vascular trunks thrombose abruptly with little preobstructive aneurysmal formation and marked pruning of small vessels in areas sustaining significant muscular injury. There often is significant segmental narrowing in the large vessels, especially at the "choke point" level, which may predispose to later occlusion. There does not appear to be a progressive vascular injury.

Peripheral Nerve Injury

Although some nerve recovery is noted following extensive electrical injury, permanent nerve damage is common. There usually is a sharp demarcation of conduction loss along affected peripheral nerves acutely. This loss neither recovers nor shows signs of progression in the early postinjury period. More common than previously believed, the levels of vascular and peripheral nerve injury are frequently unrelated, i.e., the level of vascular patency is often consistently more distal than the level of nerve conduction. Conduction loss is usually found just proximal to the most proximally damaged choke point and roughly corresponds to the line of demarcation between viable and nonviable muscle in the surrounding area.

Treatment

The flow of electrical energy within the body appears to be anatomically determined and not simply a random event. This enables certain patterns of injury to be predicted depending upon the involved region of the body. Once critical areas are carefully investigated, the extent of injury can readily be appreciated and treated. The authors believe the management of a high-voltage electrically-injured patient should be completed in four stages: (1) initial resuscitation; (2) primary evaluation and decompression; (3) diagnostic evaluation; and (4) definitive debridement and wound coverage. Our management of the more common upper extremity injury thus proceeds as follows.

Initial Resuscitation

Achievement of cardiopulmonary stability dominates the primary management of high-voltage electrical injuries. As occurs with thermal burns, the injured extremity is initially of secondary importance. Following the establishment and maintenance of an adequate airway, cardiovascular evaluation should include continuous electrocardiographic (ECG) and blood pressure monitoring, as well as cardiac enzyme analysis. As demonstrated by clinical experience, fluid regimens established for thermally injured patients correlate poorly with the extent of injury and fluid requirements of the electrically injured patient. Urine outputs of 60 to 100 ml per hour must be maintained for the initial 24 hours following electrical injury to protect the kidneys from hemochromogens and acute tubular necrosis. Fluid and electrolyte requirements should be tailored to serial blood chemistries and diuretics, such as mannitol, should be used whenever inadequate renal function is suspected. Initial treatment also includes tetanus immunization and management of coexisting injuries.

Initial Evaluation

The patient is taken to the operating room following resuscitation and stabilization. In order to decompress affected muscle and neurovascular structures, fasciotomies of appropriate muscle compartments must be completed regardless of whether circumferential skin injury or distal pulses are present. Since muscle damage and edema may occur for great distances proximally beneath viable skin, the proximal extent of the fasciotomy incision is of critical importance. Certainly injuries to the hand must be decompressed into the forearm. When the wrist is involved, a complete forearm fasciotomy is essential. In an injury that involves the distal third of the forearm, the possibility of involvement of the distal biceps, triceps, and brachialis muscles must be anticipated. This involvement necessitates decompression of the upper arm compartments.

Evaluation of the affected extremity is begun distally in a systematic fashion with muscles and muscle layers assessed in the hand, forearm, and arm. Attention is directed towards known choke points, (wrist, cubital fossa, and axilla). Peripheral nerves should be decompressed when nerve entrapment from edema is suspected, especially at the carpal tunnel. Once this preliminary evaluation is completed, the wounds are dressed sterilely, and the patient monitored in an acute care facility.

Diagnostic Evaluation

During the 3 or 4 days following decompression, objective testing and general treatment options are considered. The cutaneous injury is examined daily under sterile conditions. Margins of viability should be determined early without difficulty; sharp demarcation between viable and nonviable skin can be identified subjectively and is usually distinct. At the present time, no reliable objective means exists of assessing the viability of the electrically injured skeletal muscle in a nonoperative setting. Pilot studies using magnetic resonance imaging and electrical impedance analysis have revealed encouraging results and, even when obtained in the early postinjury period, appear able to predict ultimate muscle viability. Plain roentgenographic films and computed tomography (CT) scanning have yet to prove helpful.

Standard or digital subtraction angiography is performed to assess vascular injury. Areas of concern include the patency of large and nutrient vessels and the identification of areas of segmental narrowing. Affected vascular segments are isolated areas of vasculitis, which may be predisposed to vascular thrombosis or bacterial invasion.

An accurate assessment of both motor and sensory function is recorded based on several clinical examinations during the postfasciotomy period. Although such preliminary evaluations may correlate poorly with ultimate neural recovery, they nonetheless are critical to the preoperative planning of wound debridement and coverage.

Following the evaluation of skin, muscle, and neurovascular structures, the major reconstructive options are considered.

Definitive Debridement And Wound Coverage

Depending upon the severity of initial injury, the definitive debridement need not be delayed longer than the third to fifth day. Excision of devitalized tissue should begin distally and continue proximally following a proper evaluation of skin and individual muscles, nerves, and vessels.

The cutaneous margins of viability, having been assessed preoperatively, should be confirmed. Nonviable skin is debrided full thickness to the underlying fascia.

The skeletal musculature of the upper extremity should be evaluated through the fasciotomy incisions in a systematic order: intrinsic hand musculature, superficial and deep forearm flexors, superficial and deep forearm extensors, and arm musculature. During the evaluation of both muscles and muscle groups, the following five critical questions must be answered: (1) Is there deep injury in the muscle or muscle group being examined?; (2) Does the proximal portion of the muscle or muscle group show evidence of injury?; (3) Has the entire radial aspect of the forearm been evaluated?; (4) Have all muscles in the periosseous areas been evaluated?; and (5) Have all choke points been evaluated carefully for muscular injury both distal and proximal to the joint being examined?

At this time, grossly necrotic muscle appears pale in color, does not bleed when stabbed with a scalpel, and does not contract on electrical stimulation. Although viable muscle may not contract when stimulated, viable muscle usually is normal in color and bleeds bright red blood when stabbed. Objective testing for an instantaneous assessment of muscle viability is lacking at present. However, the key to debridement of these injuries is the proper identification of areas at highest risk for electrical injury. Using subjective techniques of assessment, the majority of necrotic muscle can be identified. We feel that the patterns of injury are anatomically determined and, therefore, critical areas of skin, muscle, nerve, and vessel injury can be predicted in most cases. The key to successful treatment of electrical injuries is following a systematic method of evaluating the muscular and neurovascular injury. Following this protocol ensures evaluation of high-risk areas in an orderly fashion and greatly reduces the risk of discovering necrotic tissue postoperatively.

Angiographic evidence of vascular injury outlines areas of severe muscular injury as evidenced by the occlusion of nutrient vessels. Distally thrombosed vessels should be debrided and more proximal segmentally affected areas assessed.

Subjective assessment of peripheral nerves often reveals minimal abnormalities in the early postinjury period. Nerve conduction studies are indicated to appreciate the level of conduction loss in the major nerve trunks. Immediate recovery of neural function frequently does not occur although long-term recovery cannot be excluded. Debridement of peripheral nerves thus is determined by the extent of distal injury to surrounding tissues and their reconstructive potential.

Wound coverage should be completed at the time of definitive debridement to minimize bacterial colonization and cover vital structures. Skin grafting is sufficient for coverage of nonvital structures. Exposure of neurovascular tissue and tendon most often requires skin or muscle flap coverage. However, the design of local flaps is most often hindered by injury to the surrounding tissues. Free tissue transfers, in the form of muscle or myocutaneous flaps, are ideally suited for reliable coverage of large defects. Particular attention must be directed towards the site of microvascular anastomosis in relation to angiographic evidence of segmental narrowing. Where possible, the anastomosis should be placed above the most proximal area of narrowing. Amputation is frequently required in major injuries and should be performed early to minimize infection and prolonged morbidity.

The ultimate prognosis of high-voltage injuries varies considerably; mortality rates range from 2 to over 15 percent. Strict attention must be given to coexisting injuries and complications involving the respiratory, gastrointestinal, cardiovascular, urinary, and central nervous systems. Bacterial colonization and sepsis are a major cause of patient morbidity and necessitate diligent wound care, serial quantitative bacterial analysis, and intelligent use of topical and systemic antibiotics. The patient's functional recovery is greatly enhanced by early, aggressive physical and occupational therapy. Rehabilitation is frequently prolonged in severely affected patients and psychological assistance is often required.

SUGGESTED READING

Baxter CR. Present concepts in the management of major electrical injury. Surg Clin North Am 1970; 50:1401–1418.

Butler ED, Grant TD. Electrical injuries, with special reference to the upper extremities. Am J Surg 1977; 134:95–101.

DiVincenti FC, Moncrief JA, Pruitt BA. Electrical injuries; a review of 65 cases. J Trauma 1969; 9:497–507.

Hunt JL, Sato RM, Baxter CR. Acute electric burns—current diagnostic and therapeutic approaches to management. Arch Surg 1980; 115:434–438.

Laberge LC, Ballard PA, Daniel RK. Experimental electrical burns: low voltage. Ann Plast Surg 1984; 13:185–190.

Luce EA, Gottlieb SE. "True" high-tension electrical injuries. Ann Plast Surg 1984; 12:321–326.

Mann RJ, Wallquist JM. Early decompression fasciotomy in the treatment of high-voltage electrical burns of the extremities. S Med J 1975; 68:1103–1108.

Marshall KA, Fisher JC. Salvage and reconstruction of electrical hand injuries. Am J Surg 1977; 134:385–387.

RADIATION INJURY

JACK C. FISHER, M.D., F.A.C.S.

This discussion is written for plastic surgeons faced with a patient who suffers the chronic tissue destructive consequences of radiation injury. This is a problem that remains as common today as at any time in the past, despite advances in the technology for administering high energy radiation therapy. The clinical problem, the biologic effects of ionizing irradiation, specific tissue sequelae, and some guiding principles for the practicing reconstructive surgeon will be concisely defined.

THE PROBLEM

Therapeutic administration of ionizing irradiation remains an integral part of cancer treatment and will likely continue until a more specific solution is found. Despite invention of the Tumor Board responsible for combining the best features of radiation, surgery, and chemotherapy, extraordinary disagreement remains commonplace between surgeons and radiation oncologists.

"Radiation is most effective when tissue oxygen has not been interrupted by the surgeon's knife," asserts the radiologist. "Wound healing is compromised and the options for reconstruction are limited at best following radiation," declares the surgeon.

How best to choose between or else integrate excision and high energy cell destruction? Which specialty treats first? Given complications, which therapist is responsible? No one can decide. Meanwhile, patients can genuinely suffer from these unresolved issues.

Worst of all, polarization of the two camps precludes anticipation of certain inevitable consequences of irradiation. Most often, cancer patients cured of their malignancy reach the reconstructive surgeon only after months and sometimes years of postradiation misery. Clearly we must do better for patients whose cancer is best controlled by radiation or by a combination of surgery and radiation therapy.

WHAT IS IONIZING IRRADIATION?

Think of two radiation sources: the electromagnetic spectrum and atomic particles.

In the first case, photons propagated by wave motion are characterized according to frequency and wavelength. At the low energy end, microwaves and radiowaves have long wavelengths and low frequency. At the high end, x-rays and gamma rays exhibit short wavelengths and high frequency. In between are infrared, ultraviolet, and visible light. All of these travel at a single velocity, 186,282 miles per second, but penetrating power varies widely.

Particulate radiation refers to discrete atomic particles generated either by decay of naturally-occurring radioactive substances or by acceleration of electrons or protons in a cyclotron. This kind of irradiation is characterized according to the type of particle involved. Unlike electromagnetic radiation, particulate radiation does not travel at uniform velocity.

Ionizing radiation is termed "high energy" because its units are far greater than the binding energies of valence electrons. For example, molecular binding energies are 5 to 10 electron volts whereas x-rays and gamma rays generate 1 million electron volts (meV) of energy!

BIOLOGIC EFFECTS OF IRRADIATION

Ionizing irradiation can inflict cell death or partial injury by direct or indirect means. Whenever a cell's nucleus serves as the target for a high energy gamma ray, a lasting interruption of cellular function results. Indirect effects include secondary ionization of cell water with concurrent liberation of free radicals.

Molecules, intact or fragmented, become highly reactive once ionized. Their unstable secondary products, known as free radicals, are strong oxidizing and reducing agents, which can crosslink and thereby cripple macromolecules such as DNA and RNA. Free radicals can also bind with cell membranes, thereby blocking certain surface attachment functions.

As early as 1906, observers noted a greater x-ray effect on cells with increased reproductive activity. Later, it became apparent that cancer cells sustained greater injury than normal cells.

Plastic surgeons have traditionally attributed most of their postirradiation wound complications to vascular injury. Indeed, microvascular injury is apparent after radiation exposure despite the fact that endothelium is not especially radiosensitive. Vacuolization, focal necrosis, subintimal hyaline sclerosis, and endothelial proliferation are all seen eventually. Clinically, granulation fails to form, contraction stops, and grafts do not take. Yet intravenous fluorescein shows abundant capillary uptake, and bleeding is vigorous at the time of debridement. Therefore vascular injury cannot be the sole explanation.

Atrophy is an appropriate term for describing what clinicians see when they examine a radiation wound. A general absence of fibroblast proliferation and collagen deposition can be seen by inference from histologic studies and from direct quantitative analysis of irradiated fibroblasts grown in culture.

Ordinarily, collagen turns over continuously in any wound healing site. Apparently this is not the case within an irradiation field; parenchymal cells (particularly fibroblasts) are gradually depleted, which might explain why these wounds develop many years after exposure.

Ionizing energy is also a potent mutagen, an effect sustained not only by somatic cells, but by germinal cells as well. Carcinogenesis has also been a recognized effect of high energy electron exposure, not only from x-rays and gamma rays, but also from the somewhat slower ultraviolet spectrum. Furthermore radiation effects are known to be cumulative, a fact not well understood by early radiation workers who eventually developed skin cancer and other malignancies.

SPECIFIC TISSUE EFFECTS

Historically, the skin surface has displayed most prominently the destructive potential of ionizing radiation. Acute changes like erythema, epilation, and hyperpigmentation are less apparent now that more powerful sources can penetrate the skin with less damage. However, the late chronic changes seen in x-ray-damaged skin may be undiminished: telangiectasia, hyperkeratosis, and eventually cancer.

The oral cavity is particularly vulnerable to radiation damage. The salivary glands decrease their function very soon after exposure. This is a partial loss during the early months following treatment, but it can be progressive over time. Very few studies have evaluated salivary function beyond six months.

Dry mouth is not a casual aftermath of cancer treatment. Taste and continued dental hygiene are very closely related to salivary function. Ironically, patients with oral cavity carcinoma select x-ray as the treatment least threatening to their well-being, but they will often express a different viewpoint months and years after therapy.

Nearly all patients in our civilized, sucrose-dependent society are likely to experience some dental instability at the time of planned irradiation. Extraction of carious teeth prior to x-ray is no longer recommended; careful restorative dental care is the essential alternative.

Chronic damage of the anterior chest wall and of the breast should have become less frequent over past decades. Instead, the frequency of complications following irradiation may be rising. Why? A period of fascination with adjuvant radiation for breast carcinoma led to countless disabling ulcerations of the chest wall. Ionizing energy was applied soon after mastectomy, and the result was often attributed to both modalities. Delayed healing after surgery alone is rarely a problem, and therefore the influence of high energy tissue effects is unquestioned.

More recently, popularity of primary radiation as the sole means for treating breast carcinomas has resulted in an initial series of papers claiming minimal risk of complication, likely to be followed by an increasing frequency of patients with disabling postirradiation changes of the breast.

The principal indication for pelvic irradiation is cancer of the uterine cervix. Survival following treatment of early stage disease (I and IIA) is no better following surgery than after x-ray; therefore, most patients choose radiation over radical hysterectomy. No one has ever measured total morbidity following pelvic irradiation. Gynecologists, urologists, orthopaedists, and general surgeons all recognize a steady increase of problems related to ionizing damage to the bowel, bladder, hip joint, and vagina. A survey of sexual function and marital stability after pelvic irradiation shows a high percentage of problems.

Reports of gastrointestinal, urologic, musculoskeletal, neurologic, and even cardiovascular damage following ionizing energy exposure are a regular part of the published medical literature. Reconstructive surgeons will likely experience ample opportunity to apply their skills to reconstruction of these extraordinarily difficult problems.

PRINCIPLES OF RECONSTRUCTION FOR THE RADIATION WOUND

Based on our understanding of what is happening or failing to happen at a cellular level in postirradiation defects, it is possible to define principles for reconstructive management of these wounds:

1. Because we are not yet in a position to accurately predict injury, nor is it commonplace to anticipate tissue breakdown, most patients with a radiation wound come to us for treatment very late. Their predominant symptoms are pain, and their overwhelming need is relief of pain. Although the surgical steps required to achieve the patient's goal seem forbidding, most patients will comply.
2. Patients with chronic radiation wounds harbor a lingering fear of recurrent cancer. Most patients are wrong, but some will be correct. Don't overlook this eventuality. Biopsy radiation wounds, even for no other reason than to convince your patients that no cancer is present. This will always serve to buoy spirits before the surgery begins. Even in the presence of recurrent cancer, reconstruction can often be justified because of the painfulness of these lesions.
3. Before embarking on the surgical adventure, always anticipate for your patient the nature of the challenge ahead. Explain why healing potential is reduced and why complications and delays are the rule, not the exception. A wise reconstructive surgeon prepares the patient to expect progress slowly. Radiation wounds are brought under control in months and years, not in days and weeks.
4. Avoid definitive debridement well in advance of surgical closure. Remember that the excised but still exposed radiation defect is not likely to granulate nor will it show signs of contraction or epithelialization. This explains why the wounds are there in the first place. Admittedly, the untidy and neglected wound requires local attention in advance of surgical repair. However, the major excision should be completed at the same time that a flap is ready for coverage of the resulting defect.
5. The zone of radiation damage is always more widespread than you think, certainly more than overt clinical signs would indicate, and wider still than the additional margin our very best surgical judgment would include. For this reason especially, use of the local random pattern flap is treacherous and leads often to failure.
6. Skin grafts aren't very reliable either. Remember: no granulations, no capillary proliferation, and few if any fibroblasts behaving as we would want them to. What chance then do skin grafts have?
7. If random pattern flaps and skin grafts are worthless, what can be used? The arterial flap is at least a possibility, although not a fully reliable one. Remember that larger arteries can show radiation damage as well. The tip of an arterial flap is often dependent on a healthy subdermal plexus for success. Therefore, select and apply these flaps with great care.
8. Any flap brought into a radiation defect must include its own vascular pedicle, and that pedicle should be permanent, not temporary. J. Barrett Brown introduced the permanent pedicle principle not long after World War II and it remains valid today.
9. The myocutaneous or fasciocutaneous flap offers more security, but complications are still possible. For example, a viable flap may have difficulty adhering to the radiation defect, especially if it has not been excised immediately prior to flap transfer.
10. The microvascular free flap is another option, but it requires an adequate recipient vessel. A preoperative arteriogram can be useful prior to formulating a final plan.
11. The omentum is also an excellent source of abundant highly vascular tissue. It may be transferred with vascular pedicle intact or as a microvascular flap. Skin grafts take readily to a viable surface of omentum.
12. For a very few patients, conservative management may be the prudent choice. Whenever pain is not predominant and the patient or spouse is attentive to wound care needs, the balance may be in the direction of omitting surgical care.
13. Once again, remember to provide emotional support to your patient throughout the course of treatment. Reaching the acceptable outcome requires patience, your own and that of your patient!

AVOIDING THE PROBLEM

Surgeons can reduce the frequency of complications following therapeutic irradiation by discouraging use of ionizing energy for benign skin disease or for treatment of keloid scars. Also, our participation on tumor boards affords us opportunity to consider the long-standing effects of radiation. We can demand of editors that reports of cancer treatment outcome include late follow-up with definition of morbidity, not just mortality.

The reconstructive surgeon can devote time to persuading other specialists on the cancer treatment team that radiation injuries can be anticipated and should be treated earlier than has been our habit in the past. Far better to resurface a wound showing progressive atrophy than to wait until wound breakdown leads to the full spectrum of disability. The reconstructive surgeon must begin treatment of the radiation defect with full knowledge of the challenge that awaits. Success is more likely for those who prepare very well for these most difficult wound healing problems.

SUGGESTED READING

Dunlap CE. Effects of radiation. In: Anderson WAD, ed. Pathology. 5th ed. St. Louis: CV Mosby, 1966:166.

Goldman M. Ionizing radiation and its risks. West J Med 1982; 137(6):540–547.

Kitagawa T, Glicksman AS, Tyree EB, Radiation effects on skin and subcutaneous tissue. Radiat Res 1961; 15:761–766.

Larson DL, Lindberg RD, Lane E, Goepfert H. Major complications of radiotherapy in cancer of the oral cavity and oral pharynx. A 10-year retrospective study. Am J Surg 1983; 146(4):531–536.

Palmer JA, Vernon PC, Cummings BJ. Gracillis myocutaneous flap for reconstructing perineal defects resulting from radiation and radial surgery. Can J Surg 1983; 26(6):510–512.

Peled IJ, et al. Tensor fascialata muscular cutaneous flap for abdominal wall reconstruction. Ann Plast Surg 1983; 11(2):141–143.

SCAR REVISION

ALBERT F. BORGES, M.D., F.A.C.S.

Contrary to frequent statements in medical literature, the quality of the scar that results from uneventful healing of a wound is determined not so much by minute details of surgical technique as by the location of the wound, the course or direction it follows in relation to the relaxed skin tension lines (RSTL) (Fig. 1), and its length. It is important to keep these factors in mind when deciding whether or not to revise an unsatisfactory scar and what would be the best scar revision technique.

If the direction and length of a scar are so important, we conclude that even a relatively satisfactory antitension line (ATL) long scar should improve if submitted to an indicated scar revision procedure.

Skin tension pulling on the scar is the fundamental cause of an unsatisfactory scar. The greater the skin tension at right angles to the scar the worse the scar will be. Skin tension is greater on: (1) most scars not on the face; (2) scars that do not follow the RSTL; (3) scars that have resulted from the loss of integuments by avulsion, slough, excision, or burns, and (4) scars in younger persons.

Two to three months after injury is the best time for scar revision. By then the depth of the wound has healed sufficiently, and the soft tissue is not swollen and has reacquired adequate circulation. Although the scar will mature and improve spontaneously in 1 to 3 years, there is no reason to submit the patient to the mental anguish of disfigurement during that time when it is clear that if the patient desires the best possible result, a scar with unsatisfactory direction will eventually require revision. Moreover, the improvement from revising a young scar is much greater and obvious to the patient than that obtained from revising an old, matured scar.

FUSIFORM SCAR REVISION

Fusiform scar revision (FSR) is the simple excision of a scar and subsequent closure of the wound thus created.

Indications

FSR is mainly indicated in unsatisfactory scars that closely follow the RSTL. It can also improve scars that do not follow the RSTL, but greater improvement may be obtained here using the zigzag revision procedures (Z- and W-plasties).

Contraindications

The most important contraindication for FSR is an attempt to revise a wide and/or hypertrophic scar that had

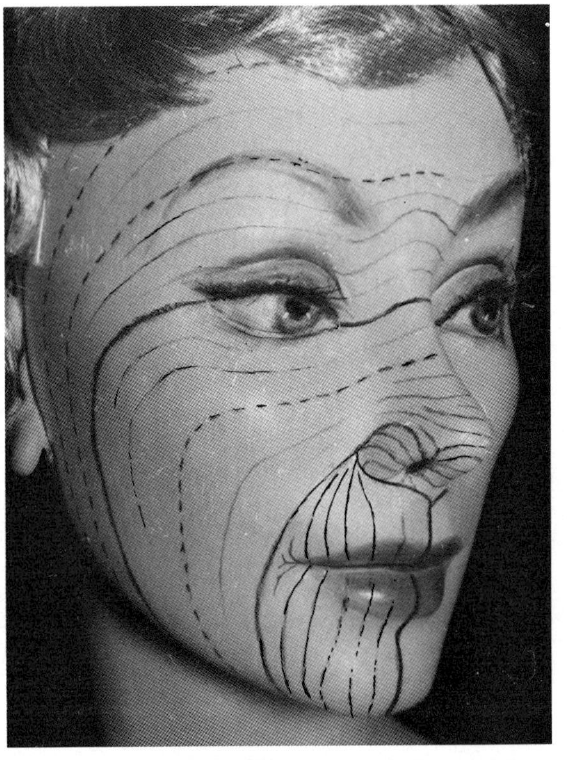

Figure 1 The relaxed skin tension lines (RSTL) on the face. Note that they run transversely on the glabella and nose, obliquely downward lateral to the eyelids, across the inferior border of the mandible, and longitudinally on the anterior aspect of the chin.

resulted from the uneventful healing of a wound by primary intention. The bad scar cannot be blamed on poor surgical technique. It is almost impossible to obtain a very wide, flat, or hypertrophic scar by poorly suturing a wound, even if done on purpose. The wide scar, as previously stated, is due to skin tension at right angles to the scar. Since excision of the scar and careful suturing of the resulting skin defect will not decrease the surrounding skin tension, the result may be as bad, or perhaps worse, than prior to revision. Extensive undermining, closure in layers, subcuticular or intradermic nonabsorbable suturing, immobilization, and protracted use of Steri-Strip, will not prevent the scar from widening.

Technique

When a scar is to be removed within a fusiform-shaped segment of tissue, the long axis of the excision should follow or run closely to the RSTL in regions where the RSTL are straight (e.g., forehead), but in curved RSTL regions (e.g., cheeks) it should be on a *straight* tangential line to the RSTL that runs through the center of the scar.

Z-PLASTIC SCAR REVISION

The Z-plastic scar revision (ZSR) is the use of the well-known Z-plasty procedure for the improvement of linear ATL scars. When this technique is applied to an ATL scar, there may be the following beneficial effects:

1. *Improvement of the scar's direction in relation to the RSTL.* The direction of scars slanted over 60 degrees from the RSTL is improved following transposition of the Z-plasty's triangular flaps.
2. *Division of the scar into smaller components.* Three or more continuous Z-plasties used on a scar divide it into smaller postoperative segments, thereby reducing the bowstring tension effect of long scars.
3. *Leveling effect.* The ZSR achieves an excellent leveling effect, superior to that of the W-plasty. It raises depressed scars on convex areas and lowers raised linear scars on concave areas. This leveling effect is achieved by adding skin in the direction of the original scar, taken from skin lying in the opposite direction.
4. *Halving in depth and surface.* The postoperative zigzag scar will not coincide in depth with the deep subcutaneous scar (halving in depth). Moreover, due to the zigzag superficial halving effect the postoperative scar has more cohesion than the original straight scar because of more tissue contact due to the new scar's greater length, still spread over the same area.
5. *Camouflaging effect.* Postoperatively there would be intermingling of scar tissue with unscarred normal skin, thus making the scar more difficult to see.
6. *Accordion-like elasticity.* ZSR changes an inelastic, contracted, long ATL straight scar into a zigzag pattern with an accordion-like elasticity.

Indications

The ZSR is indicated for: (1) ATL scars on eyelids, lips, nasolabial folds (Fig. 2), and in nonfacial regions regardless of the angle of inclination to the RSTL; (2) most other ATL scars on the rest of the face (forehead, nose, temples, cheeks, and chin) at an angle less than 35 degrees to the RSTL; (3) very depressed scars, including severe trapdoor deformity (Fig. 3), or elevated ATL scars anywhere and of any length; (4) ATL small (about 1 to 1½ cm) facial scars; and (5) areas with multiple scarring.

Contraindications

The ZSR should not be performed on scars that follow the RSTL closely, or on many wide and/or hypertrophic scars in regions of high skin tension that are not depressed or that do not bowstring across joints. In such cases the ZSR produces little or no esthetic improvement.

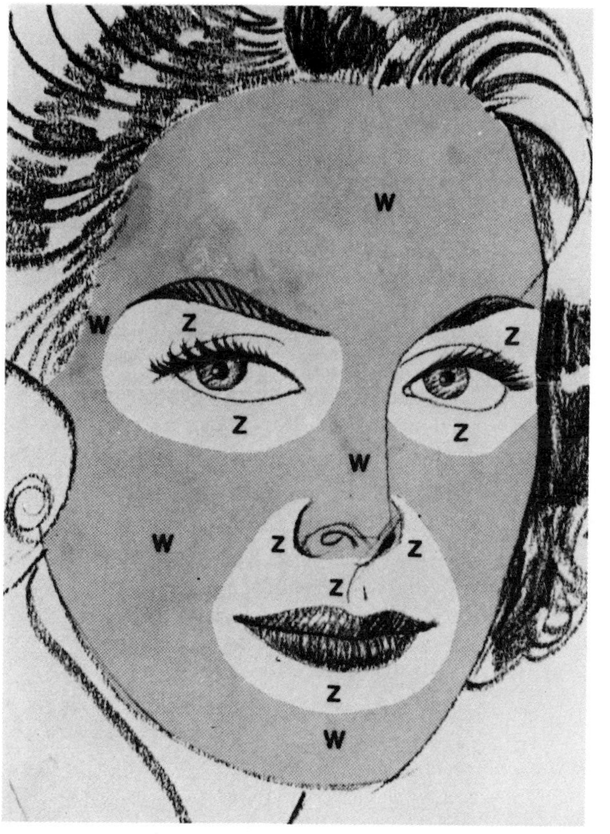

Figure 2 Antitension line scars inclined over 35 degrees from the RSTL on the forehead, nose, temples, and cheeks are best revised by the W-plasty. On the eyelids, lips, and nasolabial folds the Z-plasty scar revision is preferred, as it is also for those unsatisfactory scars of less than 35 degree inclination from the RSTL on the rest of the face.

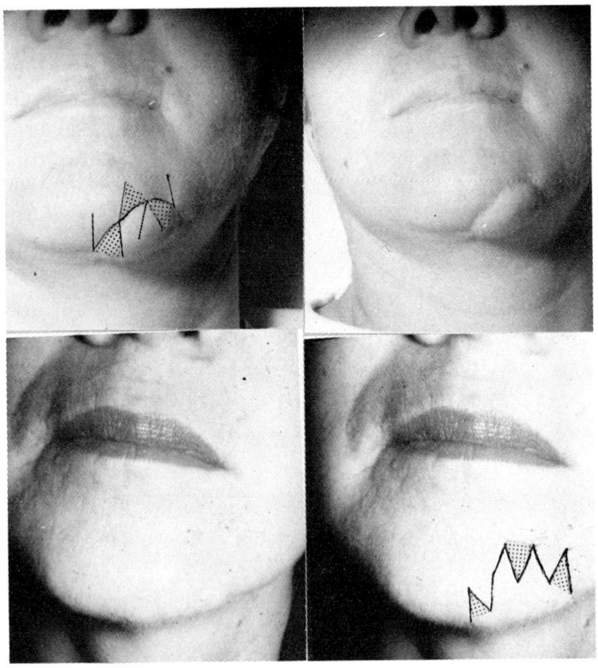

Figure 3 Very depressed trapdoor-type scar on the chin. Treatment of choice is the multiple Z-plasty. The medial and lateral Z-plasties have limbs following the RSTL. The middle Z-plasty, with diagonal lying over the scar at right angles to the RSTL, has limbs at 60 degrees.

Technique

The ZSR consists of making one or more Z-shaped or reversed Z-shaped incisions with the middle segment over the scar, raising the juxtaposed triangular flaps of skin, and transferring them to the angle at the base of the opposite raised triangular flap (Fig. 4).

All three segments of the Z-plasty, diagonal and limbs, should be equal in length. On the face each segment should measure from 1 to 1½ cm; in nonfacial areas they should measure 3 cm or more. The limbs of the Z should exactly follow the RSTL when the scar's inclination is 60 degrees or less. The closer a scar is to the RSTL, the more acute are the angles of the Z-plasties, and vice versa. After transposition of the flaps the limbs again exactly follow the RSTL, which is the best direction for any scar in order to obtain a pleasing esthetic result. Scars over 60 degrees would have limbs at 60 degrees from the diagonal.

When performing the ZSR, the scar in most cases should *not* be excised unless it is very depressed, in which case only a thin sliver is removed. If the scar requires excision, which occurs very rarely, this can easily be done after the flaps have healed and the revised scar has had time to mature. This applies particularly to wide and/or hypertrophic scars that connote excessive skin tension. Therefore, no part of the scar should be excised; it should be included in the flaps of the Z-plasty to prevent further increase in skin tension. Frequently, hypertrophy spontaneously flattens out after the ZSR of a hypertrophic scar. Moreover, if the scar were excised, the width of the triangular flaps that were preoperatively drawn would become very thin and difficult to suture, and the results would not be as satisfactory.

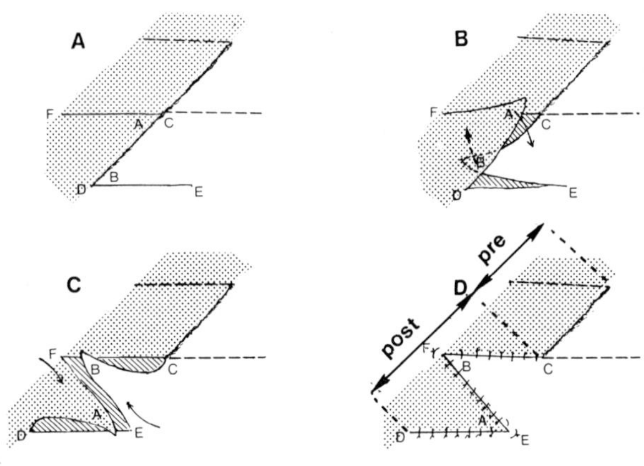

Figure 4 Z-plasty revision on oblique scar. Only the lower Z-plasty has had its flaps transposed so that the addition of tissue in the direction of the scar can be seen (post) and compared to the Z-plasty (pre) that has not yet had its flaps transposed.

W-PLASTY

The W-plasty is the revision of linear scars in which an ATL scar is first excised within pinking shears types of skin incisions on each side; the resulting skin defect is closed by straight advancement of its borders.

This procedure was first described 30 years ago. It was developed to take advantage of the benefits of the ZSR—improved scar direction and division into smaller segments—yet forestall two of its drawbacks—postoperative sequential bulgings and depressions, and displacement of neighboring anatomical landmarks. The W-plasty breaks up the scar into smaller components, thus relieving bowstring effect and redirecting malaligned scars, and has some halving effect in surface and depth as well as a substantial camouflaging effect.

Indications

The W-plasty is indicated in long ATL scars running at an angle greater than 35 degrees from the RSTL and situated on the forehead (Fig. 5), nose, temples, cheeks, and chin. A W-plasty with larger segments can also be used successfully in the abdominal wall to correct unsatisfactory wide longitudinal surgical elective wound scars. It would have been better if the surgeon had originally used a zigzag elective surgical incision instead of the straight ATL elective surgical incision!

Contraindications

The W-plasty is contraindicated, or inadvisable because of the small improvement obtained in some cases compared to results using the ZSR, in: (1) unsatisfactory, nonfacial scars except on the abdominal wall; (2) scars that closely follow the RSTL (35 degrees or less); (3) wide and/or hypertrophic scars; (4) scars on the eyelids, lips,

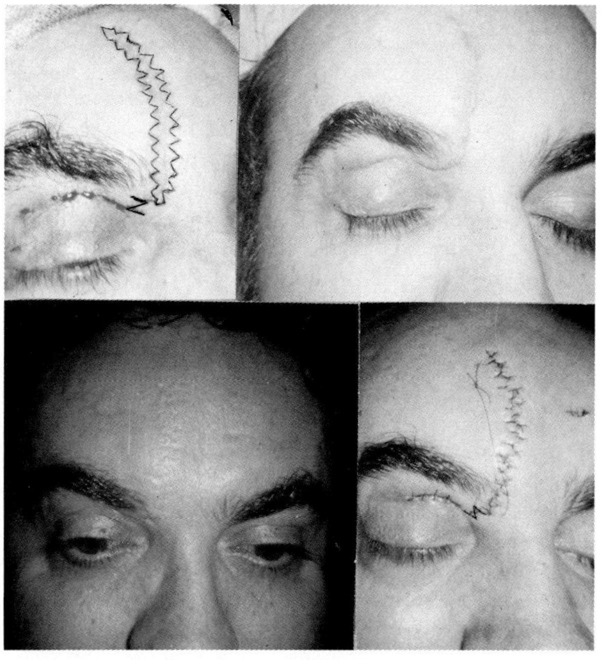

Figure 5 U-shaped facial scar involving the forehead and right upper eyelid. Treatment consisted of a long W-plasty to the segment on the forehead, small Z-plasty to that segment on the eyelid that ran about 35 degrees from the RSTL, and fusiform scar revision to the rest of the scar on the eyelid that followed closely the RSTL.

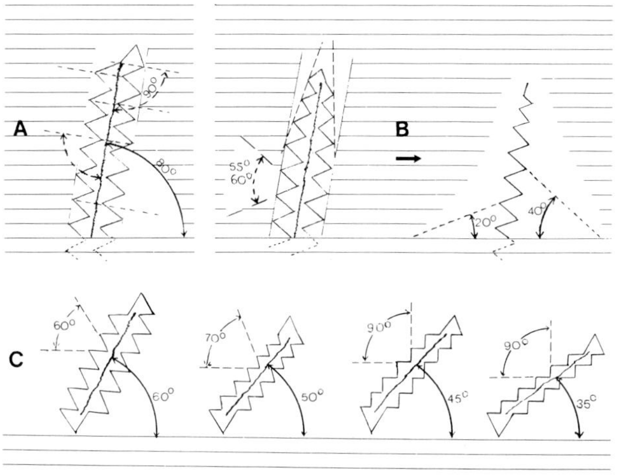

Figure 6 *A*, W-plasty revision on vertical or almost vertical scar. Note that the base of the commissure triangle is at right angles to the scar and that the tip or corresponding angles should also be in a line at right angles to the scar. Angles should be approximately 55 to 60 degrees. The segments are between 5 to 7 mm. *B*, The last triangles of the W-plasty may be made with shorter segments to prevent the formation of dogears. *C*, Stair W-plasty on scars inclined 60 degrees or less. As the scar's inclination decreases, the angles should be increased up to 90 degrees so that half of the segments (the larger ones) exactly follow the RSTL.

and nasolabial folds; (5) very depressed or elevated ATL scars; and (6) scars smaller than 1 to 1½ cm.

Technique

Zigzag incisions are made on each side of the ATL scar. The segments measure approximately 6 mm in length. They should be shorter towards the end to prevent formation of dogears. The end or commissure triangles should have their bases at right angles to the scar, one of the sides straddling the end of the scar and the other away from the scar (Fig. 6). Angles should be approximately 55 to 60 degrees on scars with inclination between 90 and 60 degrees to the RSTL. Scars with inclination from 60 to 35 degrees should have triangles with one of the segments exactly following the RSTL (stair W-plasty). This requires angles greater than 60 degrees. Scars with inclination of 45 to 35 degrees should have angles of 90 degrees.

SUGGESTED READING

Borges AF. Elective incisions and scar revision. Boston: Little, Brown, 1973.

Borges AF. Facial scar revision. In: Brent B, ed. The artistry of reconstructive surgery. St. Louis: CV Mosby, 1987:425.

Borges AF. Scar analysis and objectives of revision procedures. Clin Plast Surg 1977; 4:223–237.

Borges AF. Unfavorable results in scar revision. In: Goldwyn R, ed. The unfavorable result in plastic surgery. Boston: Little, Brown, 1984:197.

Borges AF. Zigzag incisions for improved exposure and scarring. Clin Orthop 1979; 145:202–207.

KELOID

I. KELMAN COHEN, M.D.

Keloids are raised collagenous scars that occur in skin after injury or that may occur spontaneously. In contrast to hypertrophic scars, keloids extend beyond the confines of the original injury and invade adjacent tissue (Fig. 1). Keloids rarely regress and recur frequently. Although much more common in dark-skinned races, keloids do occur in Caucasians. A family history of the disease is often noted, but no distinct genetic pattern has been found.

Therapy should be based on patient needs. Pain, burning, and itching may be relieved by antihistamines, such as Benadryl (50 mg orally) at bedtime. The effectiveness of H_2 blockers is unclear. Intralesional triamcinolone (40 mg per cc—no more than 2 cc) every 6 weeks may also relieve these symptoms, but dermal atrophy and local skin hypopigmentation may occur. Rarely should any surgical modality be used for these symptoms alone because of the high incidence of recurrence.

If the lesion causes either an aesthetic or functional disability, several therapeutic modalities have been suggested. If the lesion is relatively small, intralesional corticosteroids alone may produce enough lesion regression to give patient satisfaction (Fig. 2). Surgical excision alone often leads to recurrence of the lesion. However, in spite of the risk of recurrence, excisions may be required to eliminate the excessive collagen bulk and to allow for other adjunctive therapy. Some authors have advocated perioperative low dose radiotherapy, but I oppose such treatment because malignancy could develop at the treatment site in later years and because many keloids recur even after radiotherapy. Although intralesional triamcinolone administered before, during or after surgery may prevent recurrence, the evidence supporting efficacy is weak. Recent claims that laser excision of keloids prevents recurrence is undocumented. Likewise, the benefits of cryotherapy have never been well documented.

Several authors have suggested that post-excision pressure prevents recurrence. Although benefits of this treatment are undocumented, there can be no harm in trying this modality as long as excessive pressure, which could result in skin necrosis, is avoided.

Surgery may be indicated for either aesthetic or functional reasons. When the lesions are disfiguring, the aesthetic aspects take on severe socioeconomic connotations, and, although the risks of recurrence may be great, surgery with adjunctive treatment such as steroids and/or pressure may offer some hope to the patient for a lesser deformity. Simple surgical debulking of the lesion may allow for more effective use of corticosteroids to control lesion growth.

There is no particular magical technical formula for keloid excision. The type of suture, intraoperative steroids, or electrocautery mean nothing in terms of recurrence. I frequently close the wounds with a running subcuticular suture to avoid the possibility of suture marks that could evolve into more keloids. Some authors have suggested that a rim of keloid tissue be left for support and prevention of further growth. There are no data to support this concept. Usually, I excise the entire lesion. There is always the question of donor site keloid if a split-thickness skin graft is required. At times, this risk must be taken. However, expansion of tissue adjacent to the keloid frequently obviates the need for split-thickness skin grafts and negates the chance of a keloid forming at the donor site.

Postoperative use of corticosteroids is important in either preventing or at least controlling regrowth. This is especially helpful in earlobe keloids when they are treat-

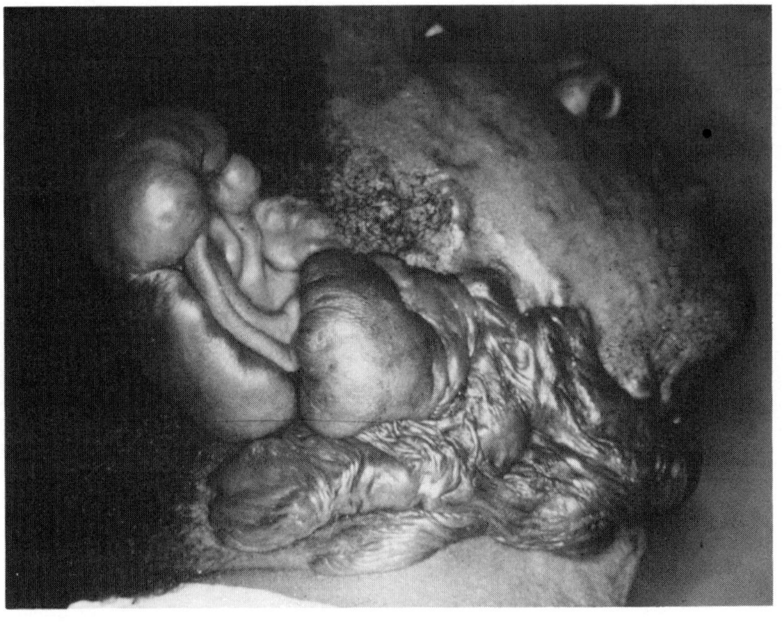

Figure 1 A facial keloid extends beyond the confines of the original injury and invades the adjacent normal tissue.

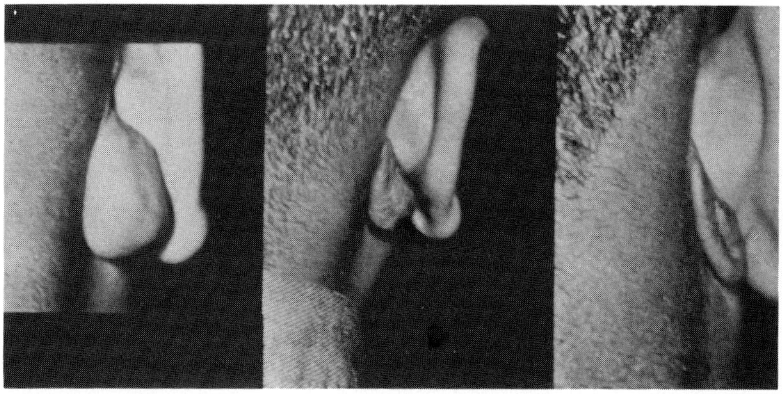

Figure 2 Keloid behind the ear of an 11-year-old patient. It regressed following four monthly intralesional injections of triamcinolone acetonide. (Courtesy of Dr. Lynn Ketchum, et al. The treatment of hypertrophic scar, keloid and scar contracture by triamcinolone acetonide. Plast Reconstr Surg 1966; 38:209.)

ed postoperatively with intralesional triamcinolone at the first sign of any skin thickness in the excision site; recurrence may be avoided. Patients should be followed at least every 8 weeks until the lesion is controlled and should then return for reinjection at the first sign of thickening.

Perhaps most important from the onset is to inform patients that keloid formation is not a disease where either cause or cure is defined, that control, not cure, is the best that can be hoped for, and that control may only be obtained with a very cooperative patient.

SUGGESTED READING

Cohen IK, McCoy BJ. The biology and control of surface over-healing. World J Surg 1980; 4:289–295.

Griffith BH. The treatment of keloids with triamcinolone acetonide. Plast Reconstr Surg 1966; 38(3):202–208.

Ketchum LD, Smith J, Robinson DW, Masters FW. The treatment of hypertrophic scar, keloid and scar contracture by triamcinolone acetonide. Plast Reconstr Surg 1966; 38(3):209–217.

Murray JC. Pollack SV, Pinnell SR. Keloids: a review. Clin J Am Acad Dermatol 1981; 4(4):461–470.

Peacock EE, Madden JW, Trier WC. Biologic basis for the treatment of keloids and hypertrophic scars. S Med J 1970; 63:755–760.

THE LASER IN PLASTIC SURGERY

RICHARD O. GREGORY, B.S., M.D., F.A.C.S.

The laser, which was developed for medicine in the late 1950s, has become an increasingly important tool for physicians. Recently, plastic surgeons have adapted use of the laser for many disorders in plastic surgery that previously had no treatment or were only poorly treated by conventional techniques. Nevertheless, the laser should be considered only another tool in the armamentarium of the plastic and reconstructive surgeon.

The laser is basically a transformer of electrical energy into light energy. As it does this, it can span the electromagnetic spectrum from the ultraviolet to the infrared. The light produced by the laser has special qualities in that it is monochromatic, coherent, and collimated. These unique qualities of laser light allow it to interact with the tissue in a predictable manner. The laser can react with the tissue in two ways: photobiochemically and thermally.

The photobiochemical effects of the laser include specific effects on ultracellular structures such as mitochondrial cell membranes. At present, an experimental application in plastic surgery is photodynamic therapy (PDT); a specific treatment being investigated for cancer. Almost every other application of the laser involves production of heat in the tissue.

Light as it strikes any substance, including tissue, can produce three patterns of interaction: (1) it can be transmitted, i.e., it passes through the tissue without effect, (2) it can be scattered or reflected, meaning that the tissue bends the light rays, and (3) it can be absorbed. Absorption of light energy by tissue produces a thermal effect on the tissue. Absorption is specific for the type of tissue pigment or chromophore, such as hemoglobin, water, and other tissue components. Although the specific chromophore's absorption of laser light at different wavelengths is well-known, the fact that tissue is not homogenous makes the laser light-tissue interaction less predictable than desired. As heat builds up in the tissue due to absorption of the laser light, specific effects on the tissue are seen. Protein coagulates at about 60° C. This means that irreversible damage is produced at this level and, probably, even at lower temperatures. Water boils at 100° C, thus forming gas bubbles within tissue heated to this temperature. At 120° C, charring and eventual carbonization and vaporization occur, and solid tissue is converted to a gas plume of smoke and tissue fragments.

The three main types of lasers presently available for medical use are the carbon dioxide (CO_2) laser, the argon laser, and the neodymium/YAG (Nd/YAG) or YAG laser. Each of these lasers has specific effects because of its wavelength.

The CO_2 laser emits light at 10,600 nanometers (nm) in the far infrared range. It is primarily a vaporizing or cutting laser, but can coagulate small vessels (less than

0.5 mm in diameter) and tissue. It is generally a high-power laser and, at present, is delivered by an articulated arm attached to the laser itself, which makes it somewhat cumbersome.

The argon laser emits light in the blue-green portion of the spectrum at 488 nm and 514 nm. These wavelengths are absorbed heavily by hemoglobin, as well as other pigments. Thus, this lower power laser is used primarily for coagulation and treatment of superficial vascular lesions.

The YAG laser, which will soon receive approval for clinical use in cutaneous surgery, emits laser light at 1,060 nm in the near infrared. Its energy is delivered by a fiberoptic bundle and has qualities of both the carbon dioxide and argon laser. It both penetrates comparatively deeply and is absorbed heavily by hemoglobin and water. Although, in the past, the YAG laser found little application in plastic surgery, the recent development of sapphire crystal tips for the laser handpieces and fibers has resulted in its increasing use in plastic surgery for a variety of tasks.

The goal of the laser therapist—to maximize the heat effect on the target tissue while minimizing the damage to the surrounding structures—is a concept similar to the therapeutic index of drug administration. This goal is achieved in most instances by using the highest practical power density (concentration) and the shortest exposure time that achieves the desired results. This inverse relationship between power density and exposure time allows the therapeutic effects to be seen, while at the same time it restricts the heat absorbed by the tissue surrounding the target tissue, thereby limiting the adverse effects.

Categories of laser treatments are discussed below, with the generalized treatment parameters that are commonly used by a number of therapists. Each therapist must determine the optimal parameters compatible with the experience of the operator, the lasers available, and the individual patient. A treatment that might give an excellent result on one occasion, or even in one anatomic area of an individual patient, may lead to untoward results on another occasion, or in another area on the same patient.

SOLID TUMORS

Solid tumors may be subclassified with respect to neoplasia as benign or malignant, and with respect to size as small or large. Every lesion in which there is any suspicion of malignancy should be biopsied prior to treatment with the laser. Since histologic monitoring of margins to ensure complete resection of the tumor is difficult after laser treatment, use of the laser on malignant cutaneous lesions is, in most cases, not indicated.

Benign cutaneous tumors appropriate for treatment with the laser include among others, warts, keratoses, polyps, condylomata, molluscum, and neurofibromata. In general, these lesions are best vaporized with the CO_2 laser, or, when large enough, they can be excised with the laser. Warts can be vaporized to the basement membrane with good results, low recurrence (less than 15 percent), and little pain. Mosaic warts, condylomata, and similar conditions likely to involve intervening tissue that appears to be clinically uninvolved, may require wide treatment of normal-looking tissue plus several retreatments. The deep extensions of neurofibromata require that these lesions be "cored out" to prevent recurrence.

Oral mucosal lesions, such as leukoplakia, gingival hyperplasia, and papillomata, are readily vaporized with the laser and heal in most instances without much scar. Biopsy of these lesions before treatment is advisable to rule out malignant degeneration that may alter the treatment plan.

Most vaporization or cutting of tissue is accomplished with the CO_2 laser in the focused mode, with either pulsed or continuous laser beam. Spot size may vary from 0.2 to 2 mm and power from 1 to 15 watts.

SCARS

Hypertrophic scars and keloids have been treated with both CO_2 and argon lasers, either by perforation of the scar with many small holes or by excision of the keloid. Much speculation as to the mechanism of action has been offered, but no firm scientific evidence is available. Recurrence rate, especially in refractory lesions, is lower than with other treatments, but intralesional steroids and pressure devices should be employed post treatment as with any modality. Excision of the lesions is accomplished with the CO_2 laser at high-power density (small spot size and high power), while perforation technique requires very high-power density with short pulse duration to limit the heat build-up in surrounding tissues. The perforations are spaced far enough apart to leave tissue between the impact sites undisturbed.

SUPERFICIAL VASCULAR LESIONS

Superficial vascular lesions include port wine stain, telangiectasias, and spider angiomata (Fig. 1). Treatment of these lesions is frequently accomplished with the argon laser in a pulsed or continuous mode. The lowest power and largest spot size that can cause minimal blanching of the vessels is probably the most effective and least damaging to the normal tissue. Cooling of these areas before and during treatment may limit thermal damage to normal skin architecture. In general, the older the patient, the darker the lesion because of increased hemoglobin content and, consequently, the better the results of laser treatment. The complications of scarring from laser therapy are far less frequent in older patients and, thus, some therapists do not treat pediatric patients for these lesions. Many individual factors must be considered, however, and in some instances, it is entirely appropriate to treat younger patients. Test areas, i.e., small, relatively obscure portions of the vascular lesions are treated to allow both the therapist and patient to determine the benefits versus risk. However, there is considerable variability in response to laser therapy even within a single lesion. Rarely is the ideal goal achieved of complete blanching of the lesion without adverse effects on the surrounding tissue.

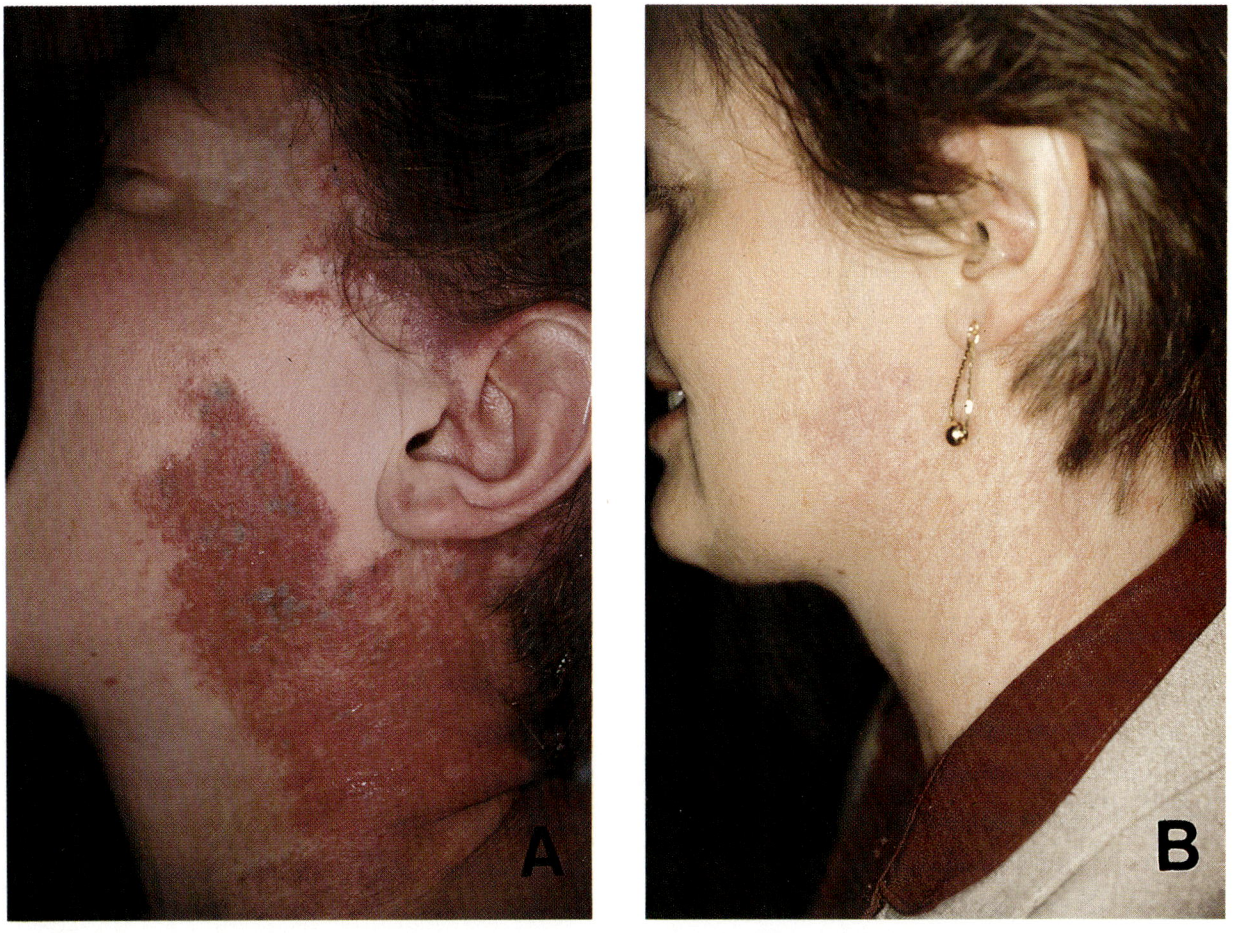

Figure 1 *A*, A 35-year-old patient with port wine stain present at birth is shown during treatment with argon laser. Notice the blanching at laser impact site. *B*, The patient after three treatments, 2 years later, demonstrates an ''average'' result. Note the depigmentated areas, which will improve, and the deeper residual vessels.

The argon laser with 0.2 to 2 mm spot size, 1 to 3 watts power, and 0.2 second to continuous pulse duration is commonly used for superficial vascular lesions.

Superficial telangiectasias of the legs have not been consistently and effectively treated with the laser up to now. Frequently, pigment remains within the vessels of these lesions.

VASCULAR LESIONS

Capillary cavernous hemangiomas and arteriovenous malformations that are deep and have widely dilated vessels are best treated by excision. The CO_2 laser may be a useful adjunct in reducing the blood loss associated with this surgery (Figs. 2 and 3).

Strawberry capillary hemangiomas that occur in the neonatal period and progress to large, deep hemangiomas will spontaneously involute in 80 percent of cases, according to the literature. Nevertheless, many of the remainder can have disastrous consequences, with impairment of the airway, eyesight, or facial features. Psychological trauma associated with the 80 percent that do shrink spontaneously but leave sequelae, has led investigators to treat these lesions with the argon laser when they first appear, usually within the first few days of life. This can be done with little or no anesthesia. Long-term follow-up of these treated lesions is not available, but present results indicate that the growth of many of them can be prevented if treated very early by shrinking the capillary component with the argon laser, using the laser parameters given previously.

INFLAMMATORY LESIONS

Inflammatory conditions treatable by laser include granuloma faciale, pyogenic granuloma, adenoma sebaceum associated with tuberous sclerosis, and rhinophyma. Such lesions may be treated either with the argon laser for those more dermal in nature or the CO_2 laser for those that are extradermal. Remarkable results may be obtained by sculpturing the rhinophyma with the CO_2 laser.

INFECTED LESIONS

Since the laser sterilizes tissue as it vaporizes it, contaminated ulcers, e.g., pressure ulcers and neurotrophic ulcers, can be débrided with the CO_2 laser. While this approach has no known salutary effects on ulcer healing,

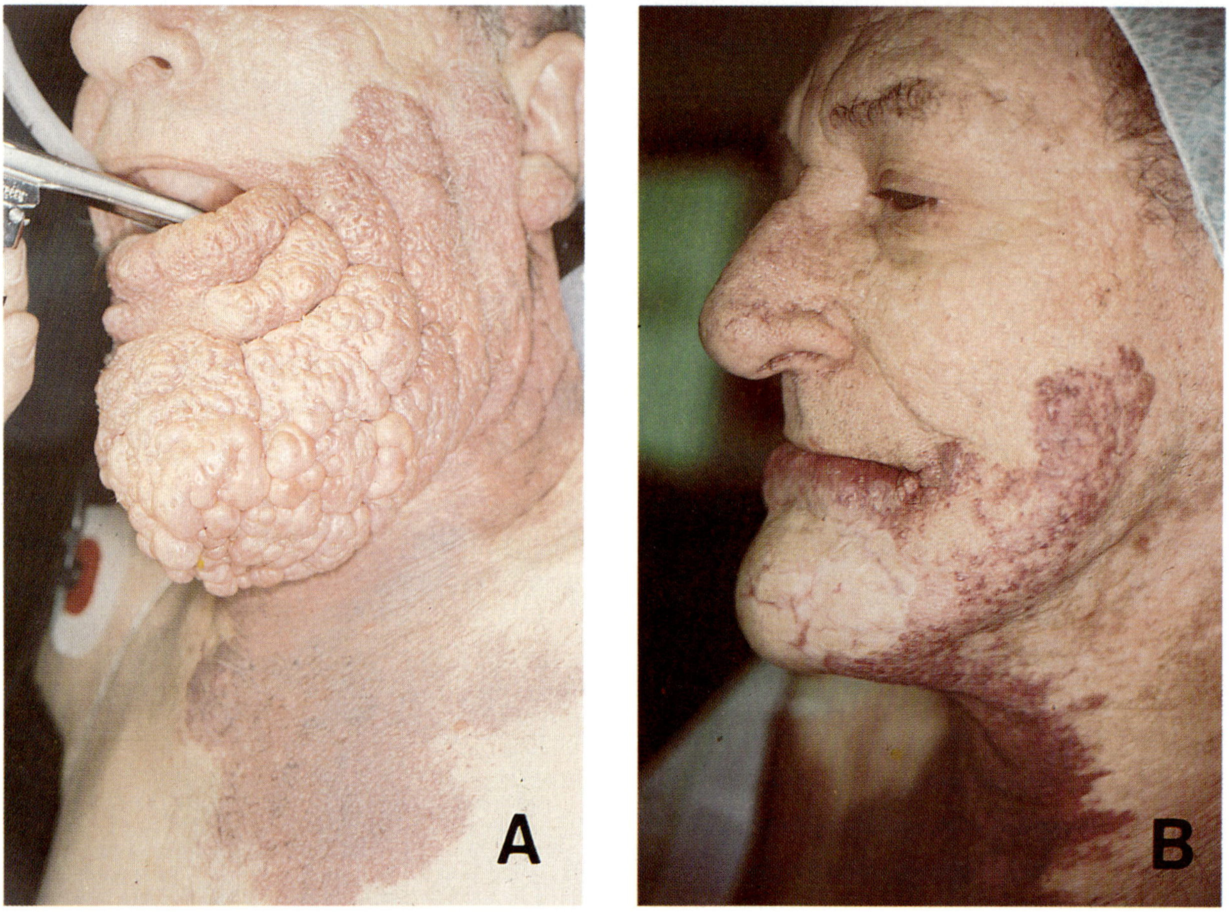

Figure 2 *A,* A 70-year-old patient suffered proliferation of port wine stain that was present at birth. The enlargement started in middle age and consisted of an infected vascular mass. *B,* He is shown 18 months later after two excisions and skin graft. He desired no treatment for the flat port wine stain.

laser biostimulation healing of chronic wounds currently is being investigated. Hidradenitis suppurativa of the inguinal, perineal, and axillary areas, as well as other infected tissues, can be advantageously excised, debrided, or excavated with the CO_2 laser. For such applications, the CO_2 laser should be used the same as in the vaporizing mode (10 to 20 watts power, 1 to 2 mm spot, continuous pulse).

TATTOOS

Both decorative and traumatic tattoos can be removed with the laser. Traumatic tattoos are vaporized with either the CO_2 or argon laser, under magnification, according to pigment and depth. Decorative tattoos can be removed equally well with either the CO_2 or argon laser. As in the other laser treatments, scarring always results, sometimes becoming hypertrophic or frank keloid. More than one treatment is usually necessary to achieve the optimal result with tattoos. Adjunctive therapy, which includes tissue cooling with treatment, and postoperative topical steroids and pressure, is indicated.

NEW DEVELOPMENTS IN LASER THERAPY

New laser instruments, wave lengths, and treatment techniques are constantly being developed. For this reason, the serious laser therapist should attend courses and meetings and keep up with pertinent current literature.

New laser instrumentation for plastic surgery, now in various stages of development and marketing, includes: YAG laser with sapphire tips; "yellow light" tunable dye laser that emits at 577 nm; and a laser emitting at 532 nm. This list is not exhaustive, but the above items should be available in the near future.

The YAG laser, wavelength 1,060 nm, penetrates more deeply than CO_2 or argon and coagulates better than either. Its primary drawback has been tissue damage surrounding the area of impact, but this has been largely overcome by sapphire crystals attached to the fiber, thus converting it to a contact-type surgery that focuses the light. The power required, therefore, is reduced, as is the tissue damage. This instrument can dissect flaps and cut tissue comparably to the cutting cautery, but with less tissue damage.

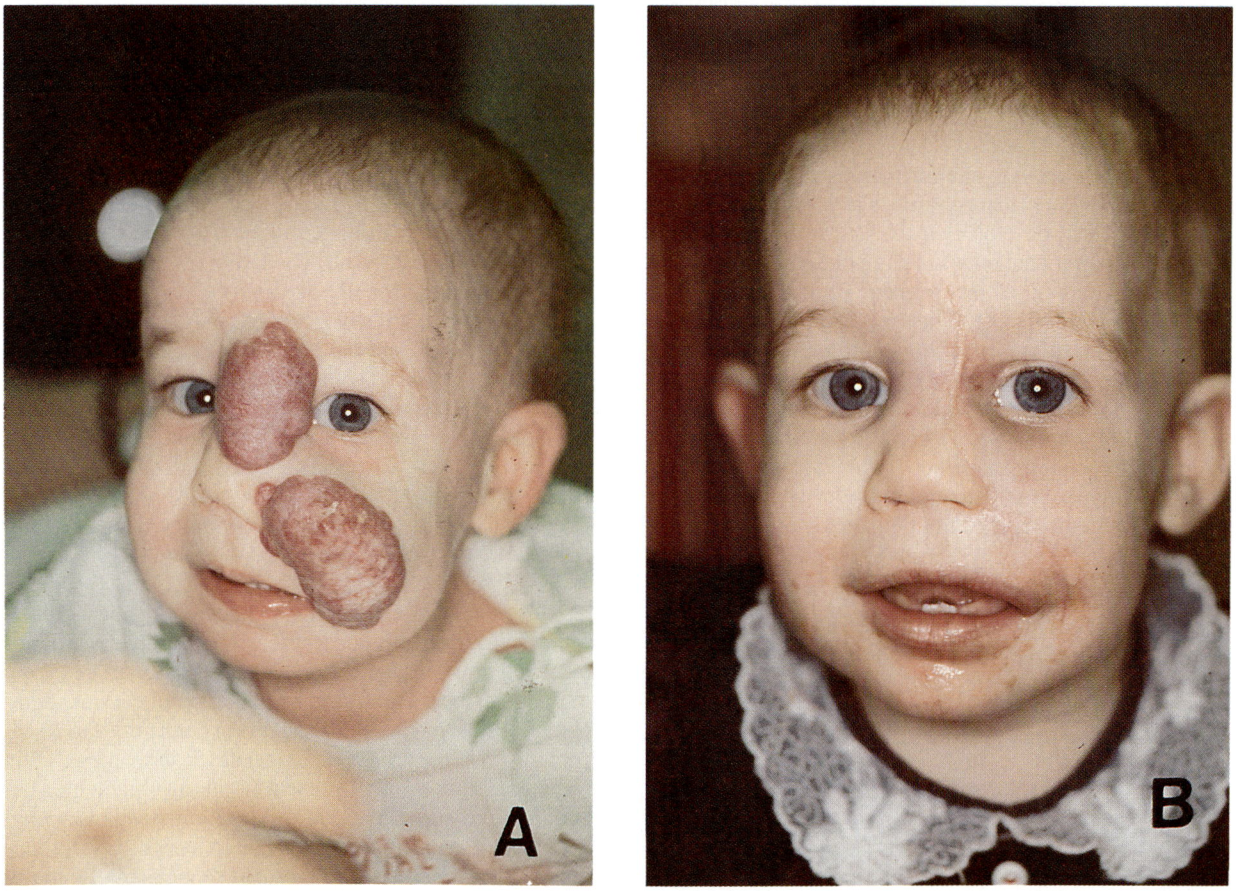

Figure 3 *A*, A 1-year-old patient had extensive hemangioma of the face. *B*, The child is shown 1 year after excision with the CO_2 laser. The scar was still immature after 18 months.

Hemoglobin absorbs light better at a wavelength higher than that emitted by the argon laser (488 to 514 nm). Thus, the tunable dye laser, set at 577 nm, preferentially targets hemoglobin while affecting melanin and xanthophyll to lesser degrees. This laser, which is useful for treating port wine stains and other superficial telangiectasias, should cause less scarring and pigmentary changes than the argon laser.

The laser that emits at the wavelength of 532 nm is a hybrid YAG laser that offers some advantages over the CO_2 and argon lasers.

Photodynamic therapy is an experimental therapy for cancer that uses the laser as a dye activator. The dye, given intravenously or topically, is selectively retained in malignant tissue and couples the laser light energy to highly energized and toxic molecules within the tumor, thereby causing the tumor cells to die. PDT technology is still in an early phase of development, which may preclude its general clinical availability for some time. Nevertheless, this promises to be an extremely useful tool in the treatment of many types of tumors.

Laser tissue welding, or fusion, is being investigated as an alternative to suture fixation of vessels, nerve, and skin. The clinical usefulness of this technique in plastic surgery has yet to be substantiated.

There is growing enthusiasm to use the laser in cosmetic surgery applications, particularly by physicians not fully trained in plastic surgery. The benefits of laser blepharoplasty, for example, accrue primarily to the operators, who frequently can be identified in the media promoting their wares, with little, if any, advantage to the patient. As has been stated, "If you don't need the laser, don't use it."

The parameters recommended herein are meant as guidelines only. The surgeon must acquire the training, knowledge, and experience necessary to evaluate and treat the individual patient.

SUGGESTED READING

Apfelberg DD, et al. Evaluation and installation of surgical laser systems. New York: Springer-Verlag, 1986.

Arndt KA, Noe JM, Rosen S. Cutaneous laser therapy principles and methods. New York: John Wiley & Sons, 1983.

Gregory RO, Goldman L. Applications of photodynamic therapy in plastic surgery. Lasers Surg Med 1986; 6:62–66.

Henderson DL, Cromwell TA, Mes LG. Argon and carbon dioxide laser treatment of hypertrophic and keloid scars. Lasers Surg Med 1984; 3:271–277.

Hobby LW. Argon laser treatment of superficial vascular lesions in children. Lasers Surg Med 1986; 6:16–19.

Hyata Y, Dougherty T. Lasers and hematoporphyrin derivatives in cancer. Tokyo: Igaku-Shoin, 1983.

HEMANGIOMA

JEFFREY L. MARSH, M.D.

Hemangiomas are malformations of the red blood cell-containing vascular system. They may be fully expressed at birth, develop over the first few months of life or become significant only in the second or third decades. They range in area of involvement from trivial spots to entire limbs and viscera. They may be of cosmetic concern only or may present a threat to life through obstruction of the naso-oropharynx or exsanguination. The challenge for the care provider is to predict accurately the natural history for a patient's specific lesion and to recommend appropriate management. This chapter presents a personal approach to hemangiomas derived from an experience with management of 86 patients over the past 10 years.

EXPRESSION OF THE HEMANGIOMA

A variety of classification schemas have been published for hemangiomas. Although those systems based upon histologic examination purport to have better prognostication than those based upon clinical examination, in my experience, biopsy has not been a useful tool. I find the combination of the physical appearance of the lesion and the chronology of its development to be a satisfactory means of prognostication.

An algorithm for management of hemangiomas can be established upon a few key questions: Which tissues are involved? When was the lesion first noted? How has the lesion changed since birth? Does the lesion affect any physical function? Does the lesion cause psychological distress?

Hemangiomas reside within the dermis, the dermis and the subcutaneous tissue, the subcutaneous tissue alone, the subcutaneous and subjacent (fascia, muscle, bone) tissues, or the viscera.

Intradermal Hemangioma

Known as port wine stains, intradermal hemangiomas are present at birth. The surface area of these lesions increases as the individual grows, however the same proportion of surface involvement remains constant from birth to death. In contrast to *neonatal staining* and *salmon patches*, which are two other types of intradermal hemangioma, port wine stains do not lose pigmentation over time. Rather, they tend to become more intense in hue and violescent in color in adulthood. Verrucous excrescences often arise on the surface of port wine stains in adults. While intradermal hemangiomas never impair physical function, they can cause psychological distress. Patients with port wine stains of the head must be screened for Sturge-Weber syndrome; intradermal hemangioma, vascular malformations of the meninges, and seizure disorder.

Capillary Hemangioma

Known as "strawberry birthmarks," capillary hemangiomas usually are not recognized at birth. In retrospect, some parents recall a small area of reddish or bluish discoloration at the site of the subsequent lesion. The capillary hemangioma commonly becomes clinically evident at about 6 weeks of age. The skin becomes bright red, tense, and shiny with the surface raised above that of the uninvolved adjacent tissue. The lesion continues to engorge and expand centrifugally for up to 1 year; however, the extent of most capillary hemangiomas has stabilized by 6 months of age. Between 1 and 4 years of age, most capillary hemangiomas involute. The color of the lesion becomes less intense, progressing from bright red to dull red-purple to grey to cutaneous white, the turgidity decreases and the elevation subsides gradually during this period. While bleeding, ulceration, and suprainfection can occur during the involution of capillary hemangiomas, these problems are more frequent with capillary-cavernous lesions.

The extent of the capillary hemangioma at its maximum stage, and the occurrence of complications determine its sequelae. When the lesion does not exceed 2 cm in diameter, and there have been no complications, complete involution without residual skin deformity can be expected. When the lesion exceeds 2 cm, loose, thin redundant skin is often present at the involuted site. Ulceration and suprainfection produce cutaneous scarring, which can range from insignificant to unsightly. Capillary hemangiomas rarely have physical sequelae. A lesion of the eyelids can interfere with vision, thereby causing amblyopia. Capillary hemangiomas rarely causes psychological problems for the affected child since the lesion usually has involuted before the child could become aware of it. Parents and grandparents, however, have a difficult time with these lesions because they seem to arise from nothing, grow rapidly, and appear ominous in color and configuration.

Capillary-Cavernous Hemangioma

Capillary-cavernous hemangiomas involve the subcutaneous as well as the cutaneous tissues. Their early natural history parallels that of capillary hemangioma: no significant lesion at birth, rapid expansion and engorgement beginning at 6 weeks of age, and continued enlargement for 6 to 12 months. Although these lesions also usually involute, they take longer to do so and often have more complicated courses than do pure capillary hemangiomas. This difference presumably reflects the increased vascular tumor mass of the capillary-cavernous lesion. Bleeding, ulceration, suprainfection, scarring, and residual redundant dystrophic skin often accompany capillary-cavernous hemangiomas.

Patients with these lesions are at risk for platelet entrapment and consumption coagulopathy (Kasabach-Merritt syndrome). I have taken care of two such infants, one of whom had a clear history of antecedent local trauma to the hemangioma while the other did not. Because capillary-cavernous hemangiomas have a subcutaneous volume, they can cause physical impairment due to mass effect. Examples that I have seen include impairment of vision, obstruction of the external auditory canal, obstruction of the nasal airway, obstruction of the oral cavity, and splaying of the metacarpal and phalangal bones. In addition to these direct effects, capillary-cavernous hemangiomas can cause distortion and overgrowth of adjacent tissues, including bone. As with capillary hemangiomas, the psychological sequelae during infancy and early childhood involve the parents and grandparents. The permanent deformities of scar, redundant skin, overgrowth asymmetry, and impaired function can induce psychological problems within the affected individual in subsequent years.

Cavernous Hemangioma

Cavernous hemangiomas have the same natural history as capillary-cavernous hemangiomas except for the cutaneous manifestations. That is, surface bleeding, ulceration, suprainfection, and cutaneous scarring do not occur in cavernous lesions. However, they are subject to consumption coagulopathy (Kasabach-Merritt syndrome). In my experience, cavernous hemangiomas are diagnosed later than those with capillary components, and the proper diagnosis may be delayed for some time due to the vagueness of the soft tissue deformity. The inability to directly observe a component of the lesion makes early separation from the more ominous lesions of visceral hemangiomatosis and arteriovenous malformation difficult.

Cavernous hemangiomas cause physical problems by nature of their location. Because of the absence of cutaneous manifestation, they seem to be less disconcerting to parents. Psychological sequelae in the affected individual depend upon persistent physical manifestations of the lesion.

Visceral Hemangiomatosis

Visceral hemangiomatosis is a systemic disorder in which multiple tissues, including visceral organs, are invaded by hemangiomatous vessels. Patients with visceral hemangiomatosis may have cutaneous involvement, usually of the capillary-cavernous type. Patients may present with limb deformity or cavitary (intra-abdominal or thoracic) masses. These lesions usually do not involute, but may become exceedingly problematic due to mass effect, overgrowth, hemorrhage, and consumption coagulopathy. The physical and psychological sequelae of visceral hemangiomatosis can be formidable.

Arteriovenous Malformation

Arteriovenous malformations usually are not evident at birth. Classically, an area of intradermal staining begins to engorge in association with dilation of regional vessels in the teen years. Sometimes a history of antecedent local trauma is noted; however, the significance of trauma in the natural history of congenital arteriovenous malformations, as opposed to traumatic arteriovenous fistulae, is uncertain. Once the arteriovenous malformation opens, the area of involved tissue expands. Local heat increase, a palpable thrill, and an auscultatable bruit may be detected. These malformations cause progressive deformity that can be both physically and psychologically incapacitating.

MANAGEMENT

Intradermal Hemangioma

Intradermal hemangiomas of the face are treated preferentially with the medical laser. There still is debate regarding the proper timing for laser therapy due to reports of unfavorable scarring in children younger than the midteens. In our institution, if a suitable area for a test patch is present laser treatment is offered in the preschool years. The advantage of this approach is minimization or elimination of the psychosocial sequelae of the lesion. The disadvantages are the need for general anesthesia and the possibility of hypertrophic scarring. Camouflage makeup is a reasonable solution for the patient who has not had or does not want laser therapy. Resection of small port wine stains that are amenable to resurfacing with adjacent tissue expanded flaps is indicated in some cases. I do not perform resection and skin graft resurfacing as the esthetic results are no better than the original lesion in the patients I have seen.

Capillary Hemangioma

Capillary hemangiomas usually are observed in anticipation of their involution by about age 4 years. Nonintervention requires counseling of the parents with interval support as needed. I show parents sequential photographs of infants with hemangiomas similar in size and location to their child's so that my advice can be credible. It is most disheartening to see a child mutilated by an ill-advised attempt to remove a hemangioma that would have involuted spontaneously without sequelae.

The only adjunctive maneuver without known morbidity that may facilitate the maturation of capillary and capillary-cavernous hemangiomas is compression therapy. The efficacy of compression for hemangiomas has been questioned and is unclear. I still recommend compression when the hemangioma is not extensive enough to warrant steroid administration, when it involves tissue I do not wish to resect, e.g., the breast or hand, and is in a location amenable to compression. Most of these lesions are capillary-cavernous rather than pure capillary hemangiomas.

A second adjunctive maneuver is laser therapy. Some authors assert that, at 6 weeks to 6 months of age, laser treatment of engorging capillary hemangiomas stops the engorgement. Since the natural history of a single hemangioma is impossible to know for certain and since the proponents of early laser therapy advise treatment of intradermal discolorations before they engorge (when possible), it is difficult to know whether the absence of progression was due to the laser or to the predestined course of the hemangioma. Further experience with this approach is necessary before it can be endorsed.

Some capillary hemangiomas are candidates for intervention. Parents may decide that they want the lesion removed even though there is a high probability of involutions. If surgical removal can be done without producing an unesthetic scar or regional distortion, then an operation is a reasonable choice. Some hemangiomas are in difficult hygiene areas—the neck, axillae, and perineum. When such lesions ulcerate, surface care is compromised by the local fat rolls of the infant and by perineal soiling. Having struggled with such problems, I now advise parents of infants with nonulcerated hemangiomas in such locations to have them resected electively (Fig. 1). This recommendation assumes that there is adequate local tissue for wound closure and that the scar will lie within favorable skin creases. When the extent of the lesion precludes simple excision and closure—as often is the case perianally—I use topical antibacterial agents, frequent bathing, and air exposure for management. Should the infant develop signs of systemic sepsis, hospitalization and parenteral antibiotics would be indicated. However, I have never seen this happen.

The only absolute indication for intervention with a capillary hemangioma occurs when the lesion interferes with a vital function. For capillary hemangiomas, this really means vision. A lesion of the upper eyelid can produce amblyopia (Fig. 2). I have all patients with such lesions evaluated and followed by a pediatric ophthalmologist with whom I work routinely. If patching cannot improve vision, then intervention is indicated. Ophthalmologic authors seem to favor intralesional steroid for periorbital hemangiomas. I have no personal experience with intralesional steroid periorbitally but have been disappointed in its use elsewhere. I favor resection and skin graft resurfacing when feasible. When there is a cavernous component as well, the involvement may include the levator. In such cases, two-stage management may be necessary: resection of the hemangioma followed by management of the eyelid ptosis.

Capillary-Cavernous Hemangioma

Capillary-cavernous hemangiomas often require intervention. I cannot estimate what percentage of capillary-cavernous hemangiomas come to therapy since my patients are preselected by the referring physicians. It is rare for me to see an early engorgement; most patients arrive after their lesions have been observed for several months. Progressive enlargement, especially of a lesion in a critical area, prompts consultation. When the history is clear (a negligible lesion at birth followed by rapid and continuing engorgement beginning at 6 weeks of age), and there is impairment of a vital part or involvement of a significant portion of the face, I recommend systemic steroid therapy (Fig. 3). I have identified the following series of empirical criteria that must be fulfilled for steroid therapy to be effective: (1) the infant must be under 6 months of age at the initiation of the steroid; (2) the steroid must be continued in pharmacologic doses until the infant is at least 6 months of age; (3) alternate day therapy is used; (4) the initial dose must be large (40 mg prednisone every other day for infants under 3 months, 60 mg for those older); (5) the initial dose is administered for 1 month, the dose is decreased by 10 mg per month until a daily dose of 10 mg is reached, and the final month's dose is 5 mg; (6) the parents must be capable of understanding the implications of pharmacologic steroid administration. I recommend that the prednisone be crushed and administered in a small amount of apple sauce or jelly to a hungry baby on an empty stomach. The mother should wait 15 to 30 minutes before nursing the child to minimize the possibility of regurgitation of the medication.

Both my clinical nurse and I explain the significance of steroid therapy, including the risks attendant to its abrupt cessation, to the parents and give them the American Medical Association's (AMA) drug information sheet for steroids. The fact that the infant has been started on pharmacologic steroid therapy and the dosage schedule also are communicated in writing to the child's pediatrician. Since the child cannot receive live vaccines while on

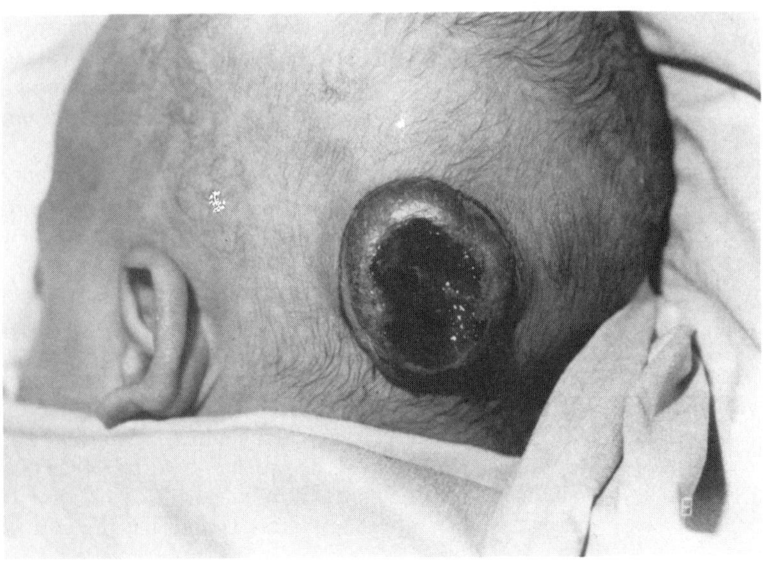

Figure 1 Ulcerated capillary hemangioma: 5-month-old boy with recent onset of ulceration, bleeding, and superficial infection of a capillary hemangioma of the scalp. The infant had four additional hemangiomas that were quiescent. The scalp hemangioma was excised and the defect closed directly.

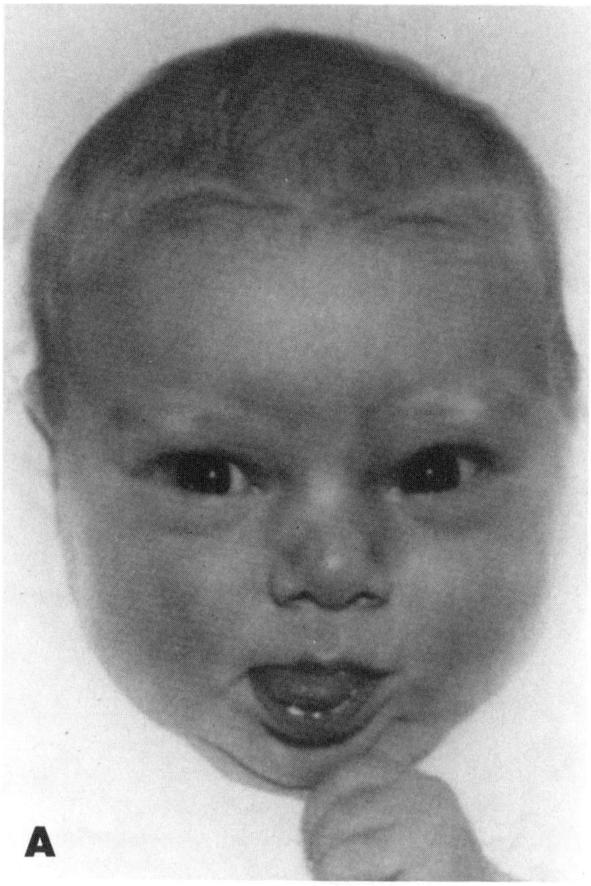

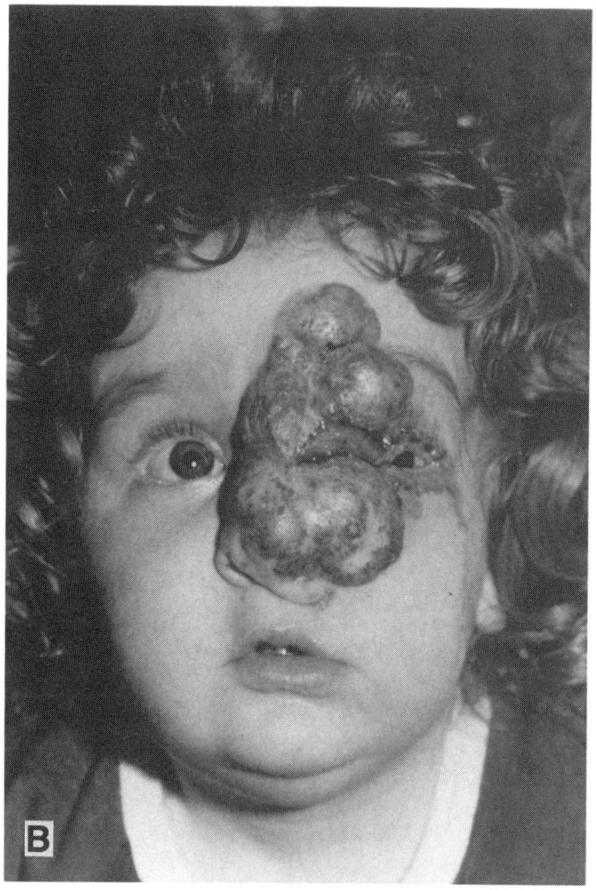

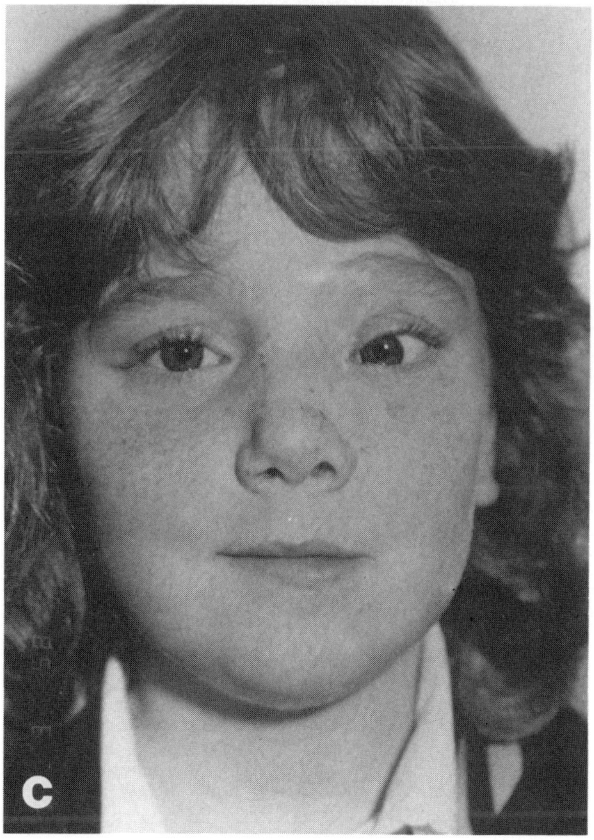

Figure 2 Capillary hemangioma. *A*, Birth picture. There is minimal cutaneous staining of the medial left orbital region. *B*, At 19 months of age with obstruction of vision of the left eye secondary to ulceration and suprainfection of the hemangioma. She had received prednisone, initial dose 40 mg every other day from 2 to 7 months of age. Steroid was resumed at 8 months of age due to ulceration and continued until 16 months of age. Due to persistent ulceration and visual embarrassment, the decision was made to resect the lesion. *C*, At 7 years of age. The hemangioma site was initially grafted with split-thickness skin from the buttock. The left upper eyelid was debulked twice over the next 20 months to open the left palpebral fissure. The left periorbital area and nose were resurfaced with retroauricular skin, in conjunction with resection of residual hemangioma of the nasal tip and Z-plasty of the left medial canthus, at 4½ years of age. There is residual deformity of the left medial canthus and medial upper lid. In spite of this management, she has a dense amblyopia with myopia and astigmatism of the left eye. While there is no ocular deviation in primary gaze, her left inferior oblique muscle is overactive and the left superior oblique underactive.

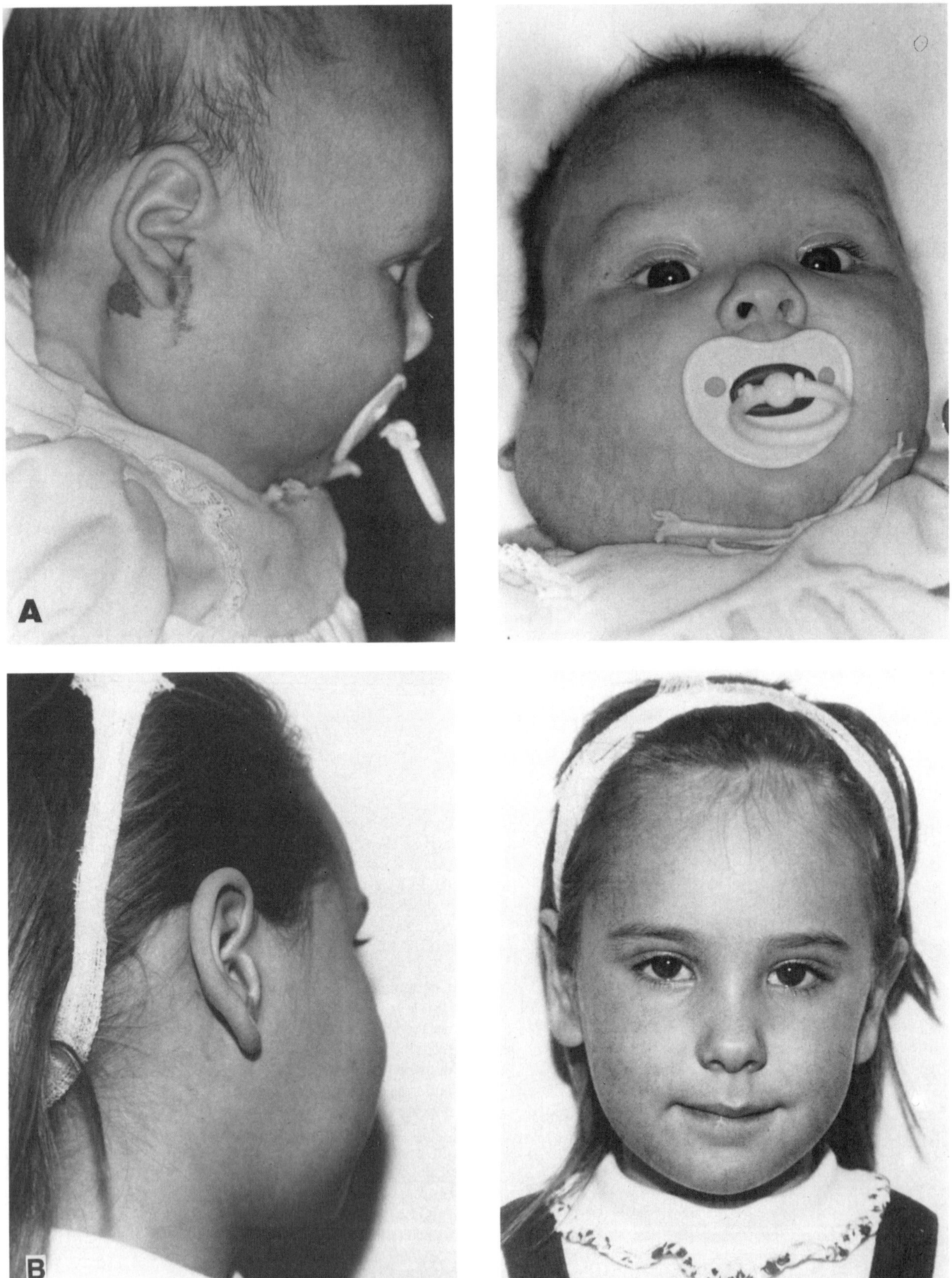

Figure 3 Capillary-cavernous hemangioma. *A*, A 2-month-old girl with a capillary-cavernous hemangioma of the right parotid region with stenosis of the external auditory canal. She initially was treated with prednisone, 30 mg every other day. She received alternate day steroid from ages 2 to 8 months. *B*, Appearance at 5 years of age.

steroid, the normal immunization sequence is altered and must be updated when the steroid is discontinued. It is important that efforts be made to prevent the infant on steroid from being exposed to chicken pox. Should exposure occur, a crash taper of steroid is begun and hyperimmune globulin is administered to the infant. I have had two such cases over the past 10 years: one developed a mild eruption without central nervous system involvement; the other had no clinical symptoms whatsoever. Since neither patient had rebound enlargement of the hemangioma, the steroids were not resumed. Rebound enlargement can occur when the steroid is tapered too abruptly. In my experience, once rebound occurs it cannot be halted even though high-dose steroid is resumed. The administration schedule advocated above was derived empirically from personal experience with rebound cases.

Since I adopted this regime in 1979, none of my patients has had rebound. None of the infants has become cushingoid on this regime; growth and mental development have proceeded normally in the steroid treated patients. Some mothers do relate consistent mood changes in the infant depending upon whether the day is an administration day or not. No child has had to be hospitalized for administration of the steroid due to a concurrent viral syndrome with emesis or diarrhea; however we inform parents of this possiblility. No child has had addisonian crisis. After the dosage has been 5 mg for 1 month, the prednisone is discontinued. I advise the parents that steroid supplementation for severe viral syndromes, operations, or major injury is indicated for 6 months after cessation of the treatment. I do not obtain endocrinologic testing to assess the function of the adrenal axis.

Steroid administration is important to the management of platelet trapping and consumption coagulopathy (Kasabach-Merritt syndrome). Of the two cases I have taken care of, one developed in a 2-month-old infant with no history of trauma (Fig. 4). Low dose steroids (12 mg daily) had been administered without effect; the consumption ceased after the dosage was increased to 40 mg every other day. The second infant had responded dramatically to high dose steroid, but had been tapered rapidly, as is recommended in the literature. The infant sustained trivial local trauma to the hemangioma which was in the cheek, bled into the lesion, and then developed consumption coagulopathy. The hematologic status stabilized on 40 mg of prednisone every other day. The hemangioma, however, remained engorged in spite of resumption of high dose steroid. His face remains asymmetric today, 8 years later, even though he underwent one attempt at debulking at 6 years of age, which included left facial skin resection and suspension, left zygoma debulking, and resection of Bichat's fat pad.

Capillary-cavernous hemangiomas can be resected, when indicated, using bipolar cauterization (Fig. 5). I inject the dermis beneath the proposed incision with 1:200,000 epinephrine solution. After vasoconstriction has occurred, I incise the skin with a scalpel and then use the bipolar cautery to shell out the hemangioma. Many of these lesions are quite discrete. When the hemangioma penetrates tissues that the surgeon does not want to discard (e.g., the levator palpebrae superioris muscle), the bipolar cautery is used to divide the hemangioma through its bulk. I even have placed skin grafts onto such a bed, the periorbital musculature, with satisfactory take (see Fig. 2). In such a case, I prefer to use skin from a distant site (e.g., the groin), thereby preserving the precious retroauricular and superior eyelid skin for definitive reconstruction, which occur at around age 5 years.

Management of the infected, bleeding hemangioma can be problematic. Whereas parents of infants with uncomplicated hemangiomas are informed of the possibility of these events, it seems that they arise in children I have never seen before. Reassurance regarding the magnitude of blood loss (I've never seen it be significant in a capillary-cavernous hemangioma) and instructions in topical wound care are the order of the day. If the ulcer reepithelializes within a few weeks, and there are no untoward sequelae of the breakdown, I recommend continued observation. If, however, the ulcer does not heal in the face of adequate management, or if the inflammatory process has caused a local problem, such as eyelid ptosis with impairment of vision, then I recommend excision with either primary closure or skin grafting as indicated.

A more difficult problem with less probability of successful resolution is the residual deformity of untreated or inadequately treated facial capillary-cavernous hemangiomas (Fig. 6). Children so affected may have scarred skin with uneven surface and varied texture, redundant soft tissues, proptosis and dystopia, and skeletal asymmetry. A variety of reconstructive techniques are necessary to achieve the best result possible. Small areas of scarred skin can be resected with direct closure; larger areas benefit from tissue expansion of adjacent uninvolved skin. Although I only use skin grafting when sufficient local tissue is not available, grafts are first choice solutions for the eyelids. Ptosis of the facial skin and subcutaneous tissue can be managed either with direct excision or with modified rhytidectomy. Displacement of the ocular globe requires craniofacial surgical techniques, which include orbital decompression and transposition. Involvement of the intraorbital tissues with hemangioma often results in a permanent increase in the volume of the orbital contents even after involution of the hemangioma is completed. The collagenous residue of the hemangioma frequently transgresses the muscle cone, encasing the muscles and nerves, making resection hazardous if not ill advised. Expansion of the orbit is the safer procedure in these cases. Correction of skeletal asymmetries due to osseous overgrowth beneath the now involuted hemangioma ranges from surface recontouring in younger children to maxillary and mandibular osteotomies in adolescents and adults. Although improvement can be made in the appearance of affected individuals, the final result is never as good as that obtained by effective use of steroids within the first 6 months of life.

Cavernous Hemangioma

Cavernous hemangiomas usually are treated expectantly. The majority involute by midchildhood. In my

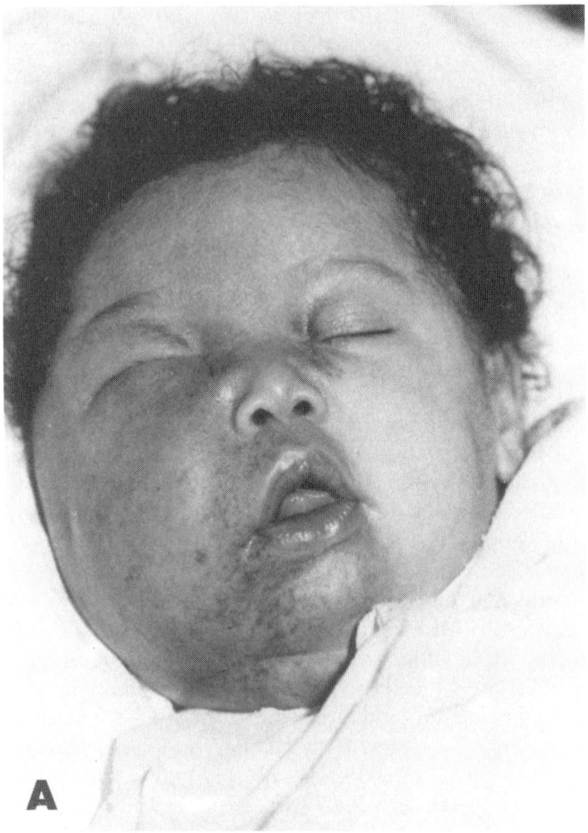

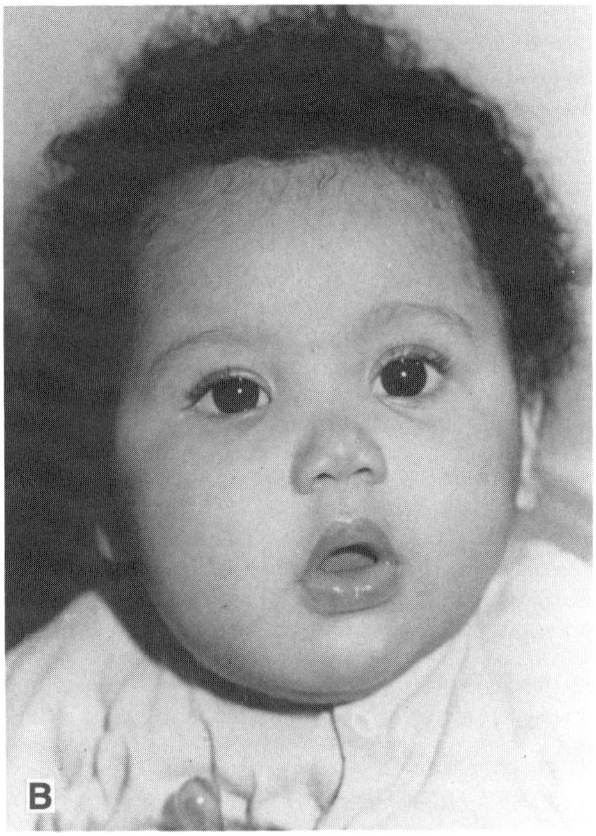

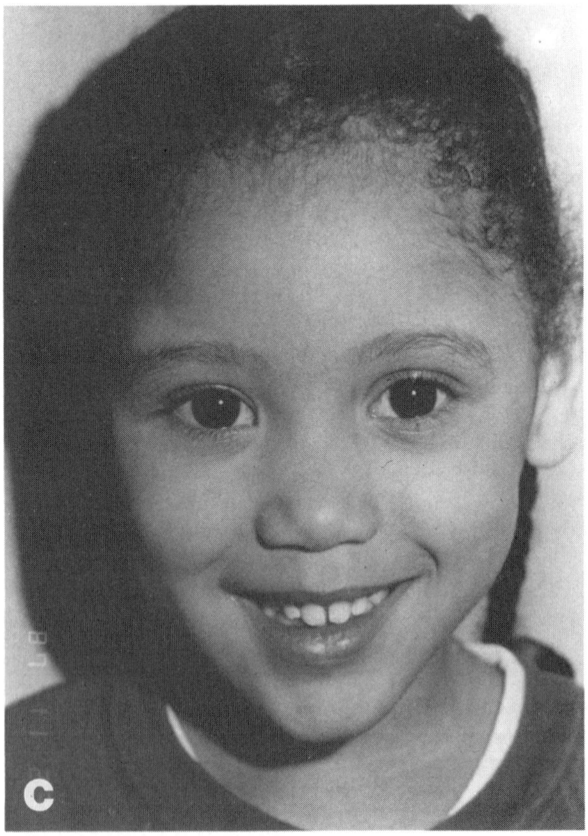

Figure 4 Kasabach-Merritt syndrome. *A,* A 2-month-old female admitted to hospital with acute ecchymotic engorgement of her right face. Her mother had noted progressive enlargement of the right face over the previous month. The infant had been treated with antibiotics for "facial cellulitis," although there had been no fever. On admission, her platelets and fibrinogen were decreased, prothrombin time and fibrinogen split products were increased. An initial daily dose of 12 mg of prednisone had no effect upon the coagulopathy. The patient was transferred to the plastic surgery service and the steroid dose increased to 40 mg every other day. The platelet count rose to 34,000 from a low of 14,000. She never had signs of hemorrhage beyond the face. *B,* Appearance at 6 months of age. The prednisone was discontinued at 10 months of age. *C,* Appearance at 3 years of age. There is minimal facial symmetry with intact facial nerve function.

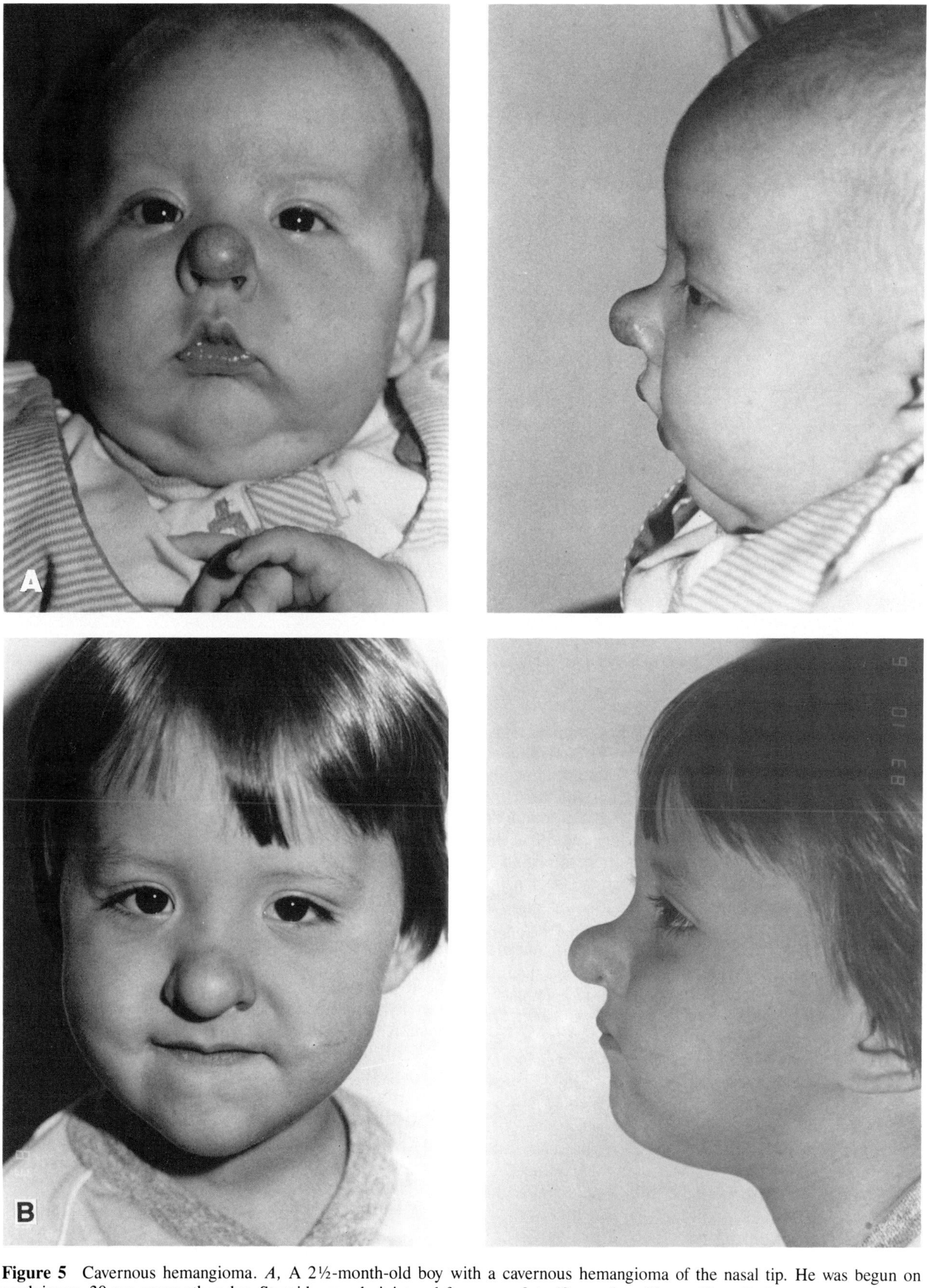

Figure 5 Cavernous hemangioma. *A,* A 2½-month-old boy with a cavernous hemangioma of the nasal tip. He was begun on prednisone, 30 mg every other day. Steroid was administered from ages 2 to 10 months without effect. *B,* Appearance at 4 years of age without involution of the hemangioma.

Figure continues on following page

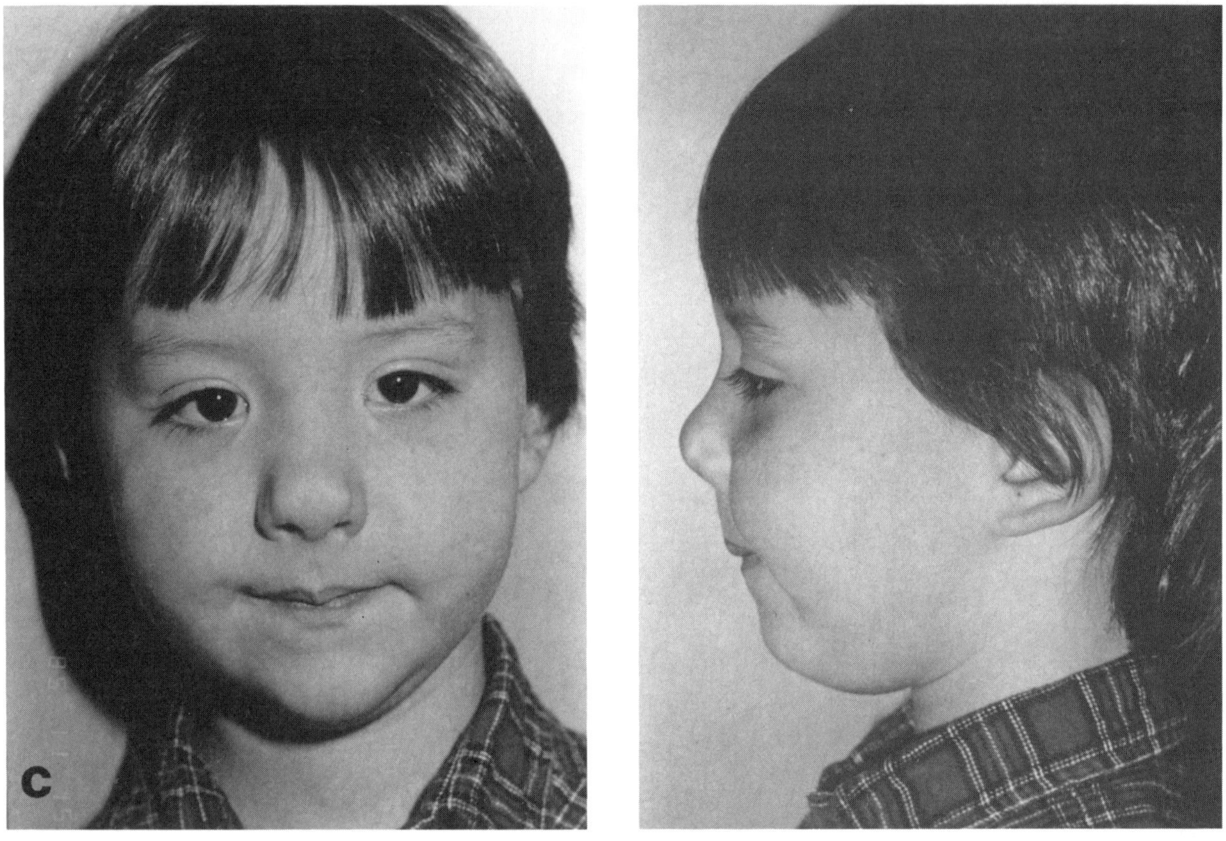

Figure 5 (continued) *C*, Two years after nasal debulking via an "open" rhinoplasty approach using the bipolar cautery resection technique.

experience, those that do not prove to be lymphangiomas rather than hemangiomas. Preliminary work with computed tomography (CT) and magnetic resonance imaging (MRI) scanning suggests that it may be possible to distinguish between these two types of vascular malformations. MRI scanning has been helpful in delineating the extent of the lesion and specifically defining its relationship to the facial muscles of expression. Although the facial nerve cannot be imaged on either MRI or CT scans since its fascicles enter the muscles of expression on their deep surface, vascular malformations superficial to those muscles can be excised directly without nerve injury. Surgical intervention should be reserved until the child is at least 5 years of age since many of the lesions will involute. The risk of facial nerve injury is high when surgery is performed before the hemangioma has matured because of poor visibility within an excessively bloody field. This is especially true when a preauricular parotidectomy-type approach is used. I have performed sural nerve interpositional grafting, including intratemporal exposure of the main trunk, for a facial nerve that was divided during such an operation elsewhere when the child was 2 months old.

Visceral Hemangioma

Visceral hemangiomatosis usually is managed by pediatric rather than plastic surgeons. The resurfacing expertise of the plastic surgeon may be requested by the pediatric surgeon when portions of body cavitary walls are involved in continuity with underlying viscera.

Arteriovenous Malformation

Arteriovenous malformations are curious in that they often are not manifest until the teen years. It has been speculated that this may be related to the change in endocrine balance much as the disappearance of maternal estradiol seems to unleash the expansion of capillary and capillary-cavernous hemangiomas in infants. The combination of engorged veins, increased local heat, thrill and bruit, and overgrowth is an ominous one. Once an arteriovenous malformation has been diagnosed the best management is total extirpation. Unfortunately, the anatomic locus of the malformation may make extirpation incompatible with life or at least so it often seems to the care providers. The decision to amputate a child's limb or to sacrifice an orbit and its contents is difficult not only for parents to make but for surgeons to advise for a nonmalignant disorder. Although benign histologically, arteriovenous malformations behave as if they were locally invasive neoplasms. As time passes, these same children have increasing problems with tissue breakdown, major hemorrhage requiring multiple transfusions, and nonutility of the involved part. Furthermore, surgical extirpation becomes increasingly complicated as the individual be-

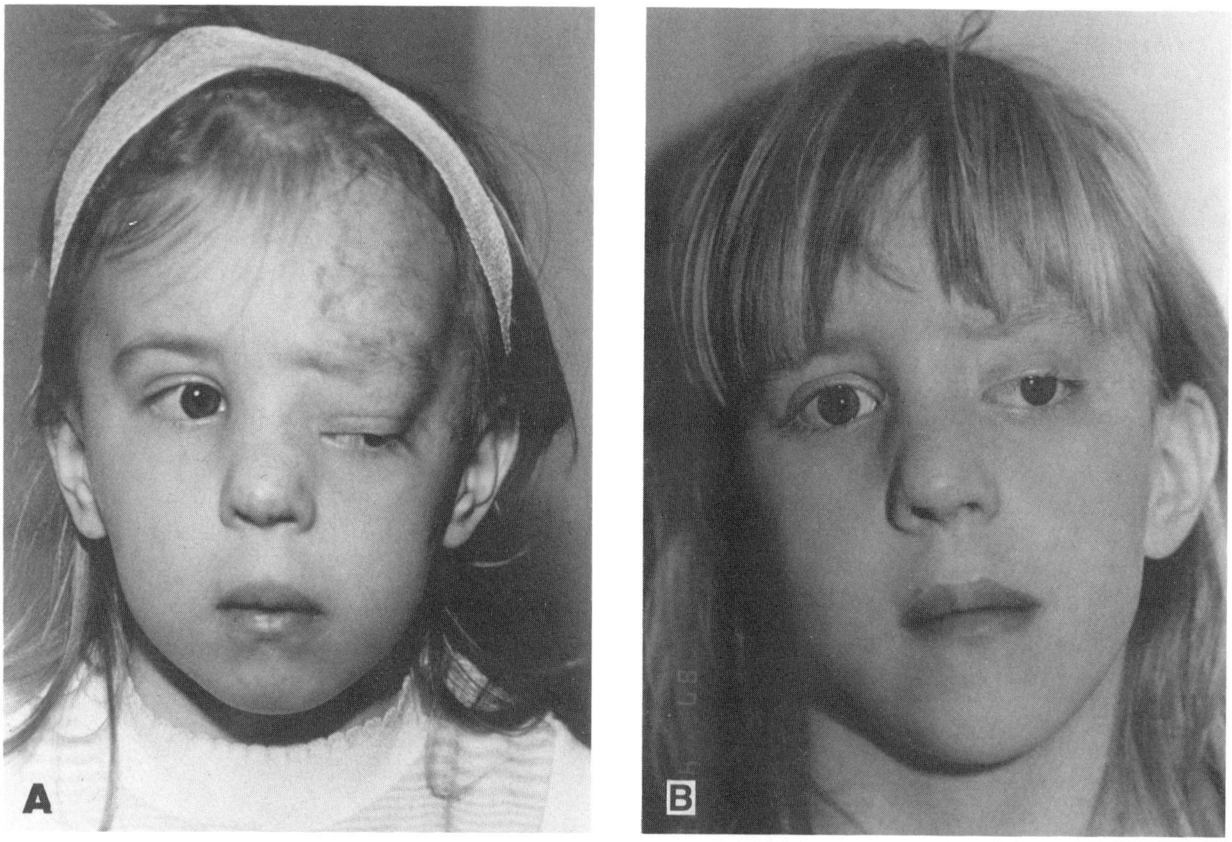

Figure 6 Late sequelae of capillary-cavernous hemangioma. *A,* A 3-year-old girl with scar and residual pigment of the left forehead and orbital region, eyelid ptosis, proptosis and caudal dystopia, and amblyopia secondary to an inadequately treated capillary-cavernous hemangioma. Elsewhere, she received two 1-month courses of steroid at 3 and 10 months of age with regression followed by recurrent engorgement after cessation of steroid. *B,* Appearance at 7½ years of age, status post lateral decompression of the left orbit, elevation of the left globe with autogenous rib graft, medial canthoplasty, debulking of the left upper eyelid and resection of redundant tissue of the left forehead. Although the vertical dystopia has been corrected, there is persistent proptosis and residual eyelid ptosis.

comes larger. In spite of the preceding argument, I have yet to definitively treat an arteriovenous malformation in a young child: the resections I have performed and participated in have been in adults with complicated case histories (Fig. 7). It is not known whether it is better to remove a major body part from an infant before the individual incorporates that part into awareness or to wait until the ravages of the pathology are so apparent to the patient that sacrifice of the involved part is a welcome relief.

Techniques less than total extirpation have proven unrewarding except when used as adjunctive measures to definitive resection. Interruption of arterial feeders, either by direct ligation or angiographic embolization, temporarily decreases flow to the malformation. Soon, however, recanalization and recruitment of new arterial supply occur with enlargement of the involved tissue volume. An additional problem with attempts at definitive embolization therapy has been major tissue loss. Embolization with agents that are currently investigational may prove more successful in the future. At this time, I use arteriography and embolization as preparatory maneuvers for surgical extirpation. The literature is unclear as to the appropriate time interval between embolization and operation. I prefer to do both within the same hospitalization.

CONCLUSIONS

Management of hemangiomas should be based upon the expected natural history of the lesion, the location of the lesion, and the presence of complicating factors. In my experience, physical examination has been satisfactory to classify hemangiomas for prognostication. Those which are expected to involute, capillary and capillary-cavernous hemangiomas, should be observed unless they develop complications or are still present at age 5 years. Those capillary and capillary-cavernous hemangiomas that impair vital functions or deform major structures can be treated with systemic steroid providing that the patient is

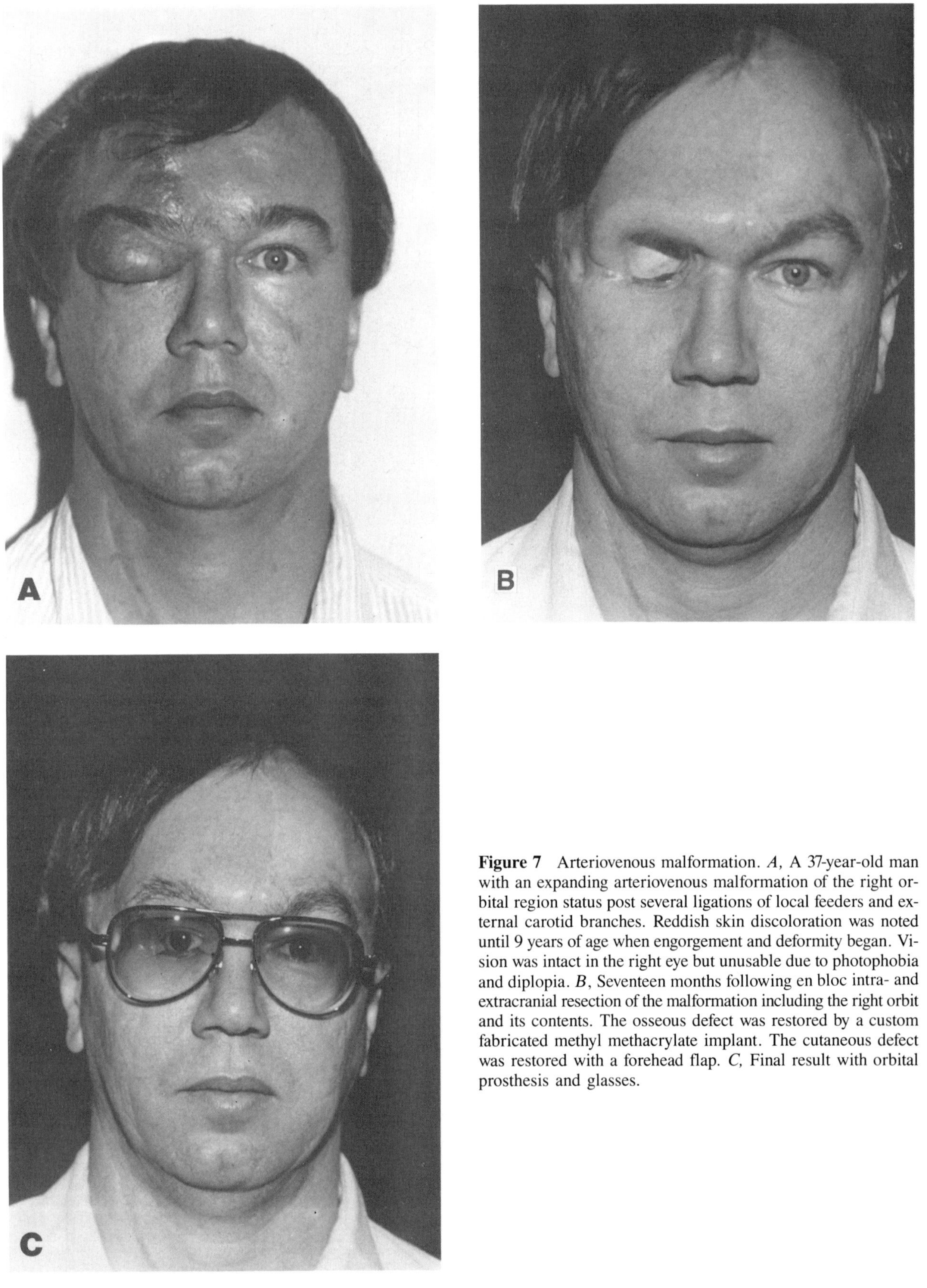

Figure 7 Arteriovenous malformation. *A*, A 37-year-old man with an expanding arteriovenous malformation of the right orbital region status post several ligations of local feeders and external carotid branches. Reddish skin discoloration was noted until 9 years of age when engorgement and deformity began. Vision was intact in the right eye but unusable due to photophobia and diplopia. *B*, Seventeen months following en bloc intra- and extracranial resection of the malformation including the right orbit and its contents. The osseous defect was restored by a custom fabricated methyl methacrylate implant. The cutaneous defect was restored with a forehead flap. *C*, Final result with orbital prosthesis and glasses.

under 6 months of age. Intradermal hemangiomas can be treated with laser therapy, however the possibility of hypertrophic scar in childhood must be appreciated.

SUGGESTED READING

Edgerton MT. The treatment of hemangiomas with special reference to the role of steroid therapy. Ann Surg 1976; 183:517–532.

Kasabach HH, Merritt KK. Capillary hemangioma with extensive purpura. Am J Dis Child 1940; 59:1063–1070.

Mulliken JB, Glowacki J. Hemangiomas and vascular malformations in infants and children: a classification based on endothelial characteristics. Plast Reconstr Surg 1982; 69:412–420.

Sasaki GH. Hemangiomas and vascular malformations: an update on diagnosis and management. In: Habal MB, et al, eds. Advances in plastic and reconstructive surgery. Vol. 3. Chicago: Year Book, 1987:211–232.

Thompson H. Cutaneous hemangiomas and lymphangiomas. Clin Plast Surg 1987; 14:341–356.

LYMPHANGIOMA

H. BRUCE WILLIAMS, M.D.

Lymphangiomas are hamartomas of the lymphatic system. The lymphatic system is a vast network of endothelial-lined vessels that develops embryologically along with the venous system and maintains this relationship throughout life.

EMBRYOLOGY

The two theories of embryologic origin are: (1) centrifugal, and (2) centripetal. The centrifugal theory, as outlined by both Sabin and Lewis, supports the concept that the lymphatic vessels are outgrowths of endothelium that extend from the lymph sacs and veins into the surrounding mesenchyme. The centripetal theory of Huntington and McClure suggests that the primitive lymphatic channels develop in the mesenchymal tissue and make contact later, after coalescing with the venous system.

The lymphatic system in the embryo consists of two paired jugular lymph sacs, the cisterna chyli, the retroperitoneal lymph sac, and the two paired posterior sacs. The jugular lymph sacs appear during the sixth week of embryonic development between the internal jugular and subclavian veins. Extensions of lymphatics from these sacs develop into the head, neck, and upper extremities. The cisterna chyli is dorsal to the aorta and appears at about the eighth week of gestation (23 mm stage). The retroperitoneal lymph sac is located at the root of the mesentery; its embryologic appearance is at about the same time as the cisterna chyli. Paired posterior lymph sacs form at the bifurcation of the femoral and sciatic veins; they link together by the ninth week (30 mm stage) of embryonic development. The thoracic duct forms from the inferior right and superior left lymphatic draining systems with the interconnecting portion crossing at the level of the fourth to sixth vertebrae. The thoracic duct drains into the junctional area of the internal jugular and subclavian veins. After the ninth week of embryonic development, the jugular lymph sacs and the cisterna chyli cease to enlarge and eventually become mere dilatations of the thoracic duct.

Embryonic errors in development of the lymphatic system lead to a variety of congenital malformations. Peripherally, lymphatics are present at the subepithelial and subdermal levels, with numerous communications for drainage to the subcutaneous level. From there, lymph flows proximally through connecting channels and the main trunks. Lymph nodes, interspersed along the length of lymphatic vessels and at junctional areas, act as sieves for and add lymphocytes to the lymphatic fluid. It is probable that the clinical conditions of lymphangioma, lymphedema, and lymphangiectasia represent gradations in severity in maldevelopment of the lymphatic system. For example, errors in development at the subepithelial level would result in capillary lymphangiomas, and errors at the subdermal or subcutaneous level would cause cavernous lymphangiomas. Similarly, cystic hygromas probably are related to developmental defects in the major lymphatic trunks or sacs. Lymphangiectasia is believed to be a developmental error in the embryo in which the normal regression of connective tissue elements around the lymphatics fails to occur. This leads to an obstruction, or inability to communicate with the larger lymphatics that drain each specific area. Lymphangiectasia, therefore, represents an error in both the development and the connection of embryonic lymphatics. When generalized, many organs, such as the lungs, liver, and intestinal tract, might be involved in addition to the cutaneous changes of lymphangiectasia.

CLASSIFICATION OF LYMPHATIC ABNORMALITIES

Under the classification of Mulliken and Glowacki, lymphatic abnormalities fall within the group of vascular malformations. They may be classified as follows:

1. Lymphangioma: (a) capillary or simplex, (b) circumscriptum, (c) cavernous.
2. Cystic hygroma.
3. Lymphedema.
4. Lymphangiectasia.

APPROACH TO CLINICAL MANAGEMENT

Lymphangioma

Capillary (Lymphangioma Simplex)

This presents as small, clear yellow to pink, thin-walled vesicles, which may be single or multiple. They usually are treated by our colleagues in dermatology with a combination of liquid nitrogen and electrodesiccation. Often, they are a manifestation of a deeper lesion.

Lymphangioma Circumscriptum

This is composed of numerous thin-walled vesicles that usually contain translucent, clear yellow fluid. However, the vesicles may become confluent and the fluid might be pink, red, or black, depending on its blood content. Verrucoid changes may occur in those lesions that undergo chronic irritation. Localized lymphedema also might result, with swelling localized to the area and surrounding tissue.

The main areas of involvement of lymphangioma circumscriptum are the proximal limbs, the axillae, the chest wall, and the groin (Fig. 1). Secondary infection and lymphangitis often occur, particularly in areas of irritation and maceration. If the tongue is involved with a similar lesion, there could be embarrassment of the airway, particularly in the young child.

Treatment. Since lymphangioma circumscriptum usually involves the subcutaneous fat down to the fascial and muscle layers, full-thickness excision is required before eradication is achieved. When only superficial removal is done, recurrence and apparent spread of the malformation often results. This was pointed out by Whimster (1974) and confirmed in a number of other publications. Complete surgical excision often results in large skin and soft tissue defects that require skin grafting procedures.

In most cases, conservative methods should be attempted, with surface cleansing and disinfection with bacteriostatic soaps, detergents, or appropriate topical antibiotics. Systemic antibiotic therapy is indicated when lymphangitis supervenes.

Cavernous Lymphangioma

Cavernous lymphangiomas may occur in any area of the body. They vary in size from less than a centimeter to lesions many centimeters in diameter. They present as soft, easily compressible, subcutaneous masses that fluctuate in size without clear lines of demarcation. Lymphangiomas can involve the skin and mucous membranes, with extension into muscle, the mediastinum, the retroperitoneal area and, rarely, bone. When the bone is involved, secondary deformities result in some patients. Microscopically, cavernous lymphangiomas are composed of multiple, endothelial-lined cystic elements, filled with clear fluid (Fig. 2).

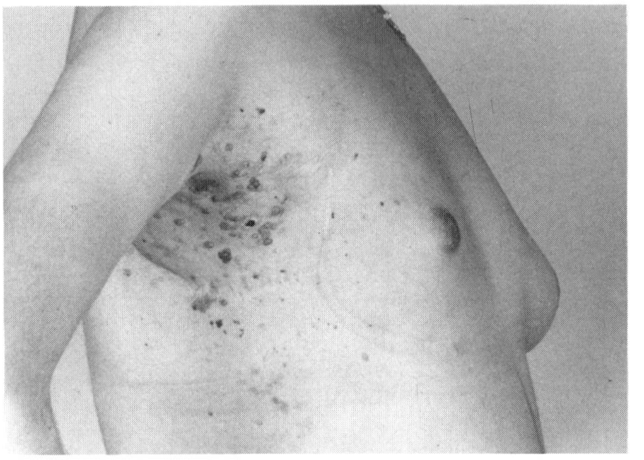

Figure 1 Extensive lymphangioma circumscriptum in axilla and surrounding skin of chest wall and breast. Note variation in vesicles (some are clear, while others are dark and occasionally verrucoid). Complete surgical excision would leave a massive soft tissue defect.

Treatment. Wherever possible, surgical excision is the treatment of choice. Localized cavernous lymphangiomas can be excised satisfactorily, with preservation of vital structures.

Lymphangioma of the Tongue

Extensive, mixed, capillary-cavernous lymphangiomas or lymphangioma circumscriptum of the entire thickness of the tongue can be a difficult management problem. Minor trauma, or even a surgical biopsy, might lead to massive swelling of the tongue with an inability to contain the structure within the oral cavity. Superimposed lymphangitis may result from infection and potential airway problems must be anticipated. Conservatism is the treatment of choice in the early years of life, with watchful waiting and appropriate antibiotic therapy when indicated. Even massive enlargement of the tongue can be treated conservatively and gradual resolution of the swelling results in most cases. Surgery should be delayed until

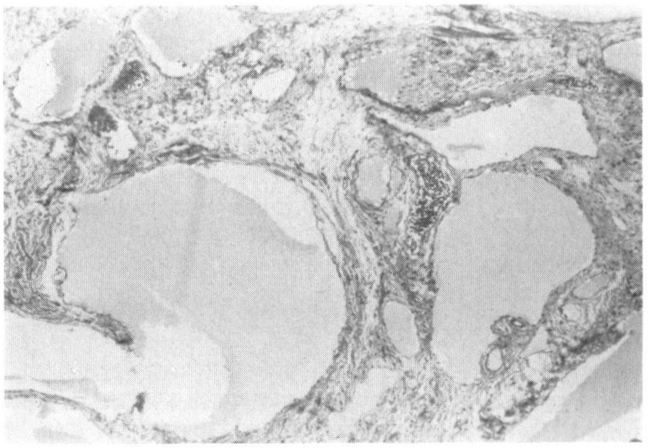

Figure 2 Histologic section of a cavernous lymphangioma. Note small and large cystic spaces lined with endothelium and filled with clear fluid.

the child is older (4 to 5 years) to lessen the chances of airway problems postoperatively.

Cystic Hygroma

Cystic hygromas result from an error in development between the collecting lymphatics and the venous system. They are most commonly seen in the cervical region, the axilla, or groin (Fig. 3). In contrast to much that has been written in the literature, in my experience, many large cystic hygromas regress or involute spontaneously. Therefore, it is my recommendation that surgery be delayed for several years unless vital structures are impinged upon. Even though the size of the lesion can be alarming, both to the parents and to the treating medical personnel, spontaneous resolution often occurs, possibly from collapse of the lymphatic abnormality. When first seen, I recommend careful evaluation of the lesion both clinically and radiologically, and usually include computerized tomography (CT) scans. When in doubt as to the extent of cervical lesions, I recommend laryngoscopy be performed to rule out involvement of the upper respiratory tract. When there is no airway involvement, conservatism is the treatment of choice. I often perform a small surgical biopsy of the cervical lesion, usually taken just below the earlobe, to confirm the diagnosis. The histology of the biopsy shows a thick-walled cystic lesion with many muscle fibers in the cyst wall (Fig. 4). Although I have seen a significant number, I have not performed major extirpative surgery on any cystic hygroma in a child during the past 10 years.

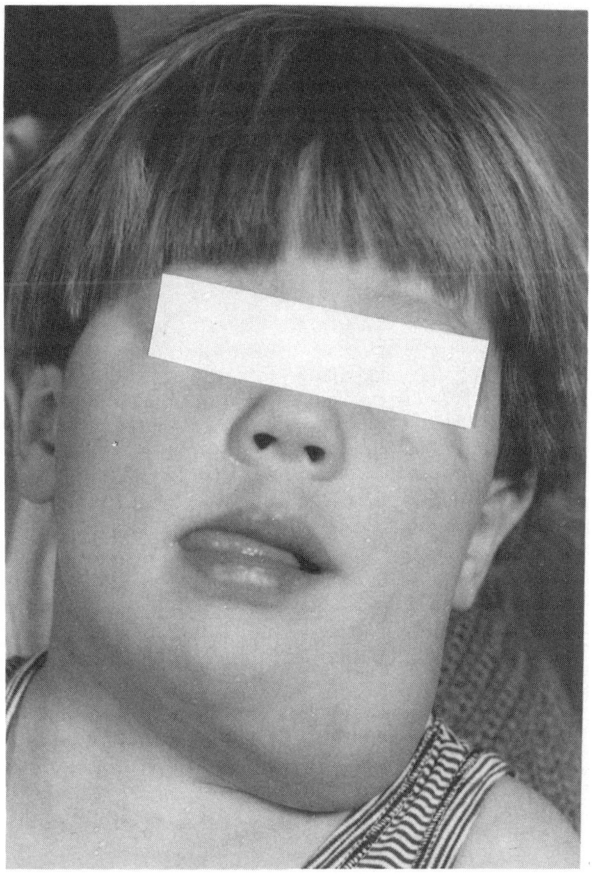

Figure 3 Photograph of a 2½-year-old boy with cystic hygroma on the left side of the neck with extension into floor of the mouth. Involution is expected in many of these lymphatic malformations.

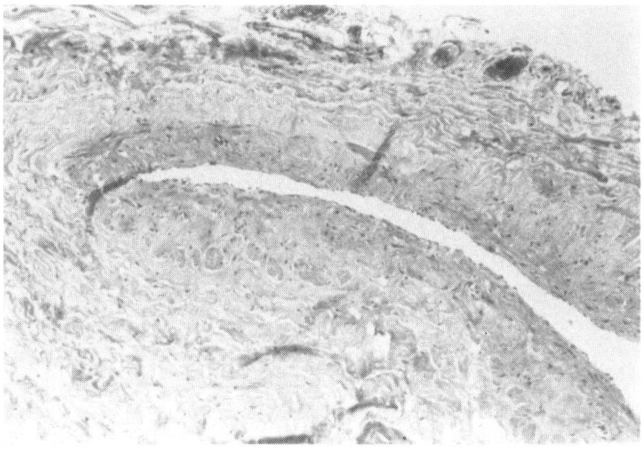

Figure 4 Biopsy from wall of cystic hygroma. Note the thick-walled structure that contains muscle fibers.

Lymphedema

Localized lymphedema might be seen in relation to confluent lymphangiomas or with lymphangioma circumscriptum. Generalized hypoplasia of the lymphatic system in an extremity results in lymphedema with varying degrees of severity. It might be seen as the familial variety at birth (Milroy's disease), be evident at puberty (lymphedema praecox), or appear later in life (lymphedema tarda). All forms of lymphedema represent a gradation in the severity of hypoplasia of the lymphatic drainage system. Elevation, elastic garments, local skin care, and sometimes, compression pumps are of value in many patients.

Marked lymphatic hypoplasia with massive edema of both lower extremities and the genitalia is occasionally seen. The only method of treatment in these advanced cases is surgical excision, with replacement of the skin either from the lymphedematous extremity, whenever possible, or with large skin grafts taken from elsewhere in the body. The penis and scrotum can be reconstructed in two stages after excision of the massive lymphedematous tissue cover (Fig. 5). Usually, massive hydroceles are present around each testicle in severe forms of this disease. It is of interest to note that the posterior scrotum is usually free of lymphedema due to its different lymphatic drainage. It often can be used in reconstruction for partial coverage of the testes and gives a better permanent cosmetic result.

Lymphangiectasia

The most advanced form of lymphatic hypoplasia is seen in lymphangiectasia with a generalized underdevelop-

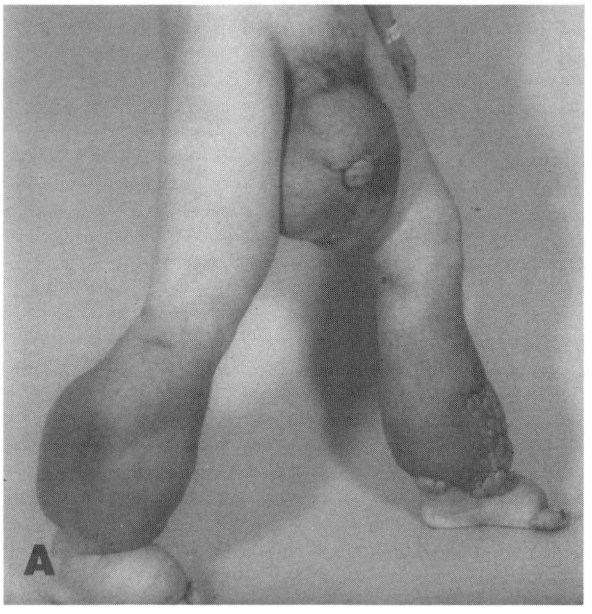

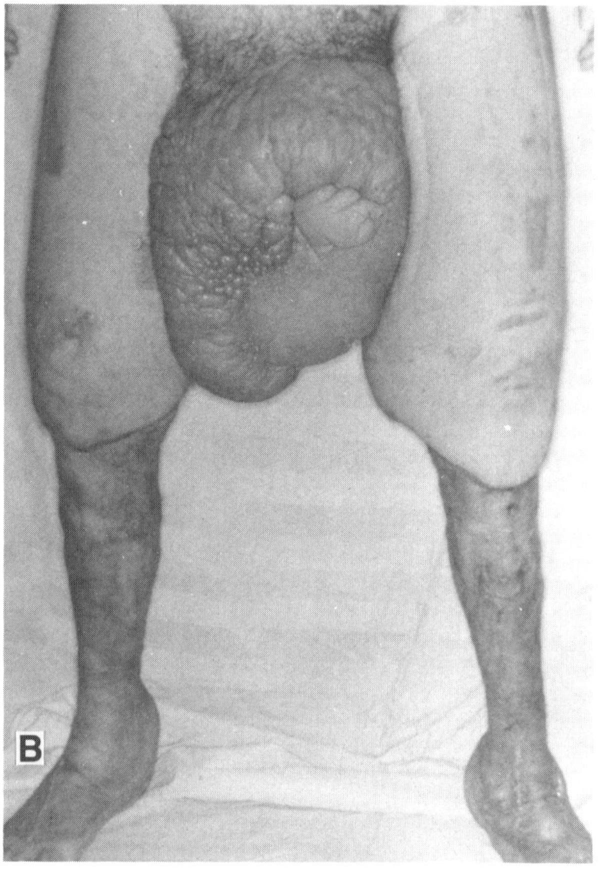

Figure 5 *A,* A 22-year-old man has advanced lymphedema that involves both lower extremities and genitalia. Surgical excision and replacement with skin grafts is the treatment of choice in such cases. *B,* Patient's postoperative appearance 6 months following surgery on both legs (below knees). Reconstruction of genitalia and debulking of lower thighs will be completed with additional surgery.

ment of the system. Prognosis is poor in the advanced stage and patients present with short stature, massive ascites, malabsorption from the gastrointestinal tract, chronic pulmonary insufficiency, and lymphedema of all four extremities and genitalia. Surgical excision of massive areas of lymphedematous involvement, such as that seen in the genitalia, gives some symptomatic relief.

SUGGESTED READING

Bauer BS, Kernahan DA, Hugo NE. Lymphangioma circumscriptum —a clinicopathological review. Ann Plast Surg 1981; 7:318–321.

Huntington GS, McClure CFW. The anatomy and development of the jugular lymph sac in the domestic cat. Am J Anat 1910; 10: 177–179.

Lewis FJ. The development of the lymphatic system in rabbits. Am J Anat 1905; 5:95–97.

Mulliken JB, Glowacki J. Hemangiomas and vascular malformations in infants and children: a classification based on endothelial characteristics. Plast Reconstr Surg 1982;1 69:412–417.

Sabin FR. On the origin of the lymphatic system from the veins and the development of the lymph hearts and thoracic duct in the pig. Am J Anat 1902; 1:367–370.

Whimster IW. The pathology of lymphangioma circumscriptum. Br J Dermatol 1976; 94:437–442.

Williams HB. Vascular neoplasms. Clin Plast Surg 1980; 7:397–411.

Williams HB. Embryology and classification of lymphatic abnormalities. In: Williams HB, ed. Symposium on vascular malformations and melanotic lesions. St. Louis: CV Mosby, 1983:175.

Williams HB. Facial bone changes with vascular tumors in children. Plast Reconstr Surg 1979; 63:309–316.

MALIGNANT MELANOMA

STEVEN D. MACHT, M.D.

Melanoma is increasing in frequency second only to lung cancer in women. While the true cause remains unknown, the most likely source is sun exposure and heredity. The incidence of melanoma in Australia and America seems to parallel proximity to the equator. The most commonly affected sites are the exposed areas. However, as with most epidemiologic data, significant exceptions exist. Why unexposed areas are susceptible is not known, nor are the reasons why intermittent sun exposure is a greater risk than constant exposure. Trauma, chemical induction, and hormonal stimulation are occasionally cited as causes—most often in anecdotal cases—however, nearly every prospective review fails to find a statistical correlation.

DIAGNOSIS AND PROGNOSIS

Excisional biopsy is best when the lesion is less than 2 cm in diameter. If the lesion is larger, incisional biopsy should include the thickest-appearing part of the tumor, the most typical, and the transition of normal skin to tumor. The pathology report should indicate the diagnosis, the tumor thickness, level of invasion, and any other information that might affect prognosis, i.e., mitosis, lymphocytic infiltration, or ulceration, etc. One should be careful of the patient who arrives with a single slide and a diagnosis. It is good practice to request the block of tissue to allow a second pathologist independently to confirm the diagnosis and, equally important, determine thickness of the lesion. One must question reports that are inconsistent; such as, 3.0 mm-thick lesions that are Clark Level II, or 0.45 mm lesions that are Level IV. Frozen section diagnosis, used in some countries, should be discouraged. The histopathologic diagnosis can be very difficult at times and thickness measurements may be unreliable.

There are significant shortcomings in all histopathologic techniques that predict prognosis. The most useful method is that described by Dr. Breslow whereby the tumor thickness is measured from the top of the granular cell layer to the deepest portion of the tumor, or from the ulcer base if present. Errors may occur if the thickest portion of the tumor is not sampled, or the tissue is severely beveled. Other problems may arise if an inexperienced pathologist overmeasures a lesion adjacent to a hair follicle, or includes normal nevus cells below the melanoma when it arises within a nevus. Dr. Clark's technique lacks reproducibility in situations where the papillary-reticular dermal junction is difficult to find. This typically occurs in sun-damaged skin, but may be found normally in other parts of the body. Further disagreement occurs on the exact number of cells needed to constitute an increase in level when the bulk of tumor is more superficial. Please note that neither Breslow's nor Clark's method is valid in the presence of recurrent or metastatic disease. There are several controversial areas where the thickness measurement *may* not correlate with prognosis. Regressed, ulcerated, desmoplastic, and amelanotic melanomas may do worse than equally thick lesions. Tumors in the BANS (back, arm, neck, and scalp) area may also carry a more unfavorable prognosis. Lentigo malignant melanoma may do better. My personal experience is consistent with the BANS and lentigo tumors despite literature to the contrary.

METASTATIC WORK-UP

At this point, it is prudent to classify lesions into one of three groups: low risk—less than 0.76 mm thick; high risk—more than 3.0 mm thick; and intermediate risk—between 0.76 and 3.0 mm thick. Once the diagnosis and assessment of risk are made, the patient should have examination of the entire skin surface, with palpation of axillae, inguinal region, and neck for adenopathy. Synchronous tumors can occur. More likely, there will be atypically pigmented lesions elsewhere on the body. Any patient with melanoma is at increased risk for developing still another melanoma.

Minimal systemic work-up should include a chest x-ray study and liver function tests for lower risk lesions (less than 0.76 mm thick). Many studies document the extremely low yield of a metastatic work-up in the asymptomatic patient; however, pressure from patient and referring physician often prevails. My preference is to obtain a computed tomography (CT) scan of brain, chest, abdomen, and pelvis, in addition to radionuclide bone scan in those patients for whom a major resective procedure is planned. Special attention is given to the first echelon of likely metastasis. For example, in head and neck lesions, the chest CT scan will include the supraclavicular region, and in lower extremity lesions, the pelvic CT scan will include the femoral triangle. These areas would not normally have been included. Communication with the radiologist is imperative. Monoclonal antibody and gallium total body scans have been recommended as a screening tool, as has technetium for localization of lymphatic drainage. The value of these has yet to be proven.

Controversy remains regarding width of excision, inclusion of fascia, method of reconstruction, prophylactic lymph node dissection, and limb isolation-perfusion with chemotherapy. Systemic adjuvant immuno- or chemotherapy is beyond the scope of this summary and should be considered experimental.

Wide excision of skin has been suggested since the early 1900s, based on the finding of tumor cells 5 cm from satellite lesions, *not* primary tumors. Several authors indicate that width of excision has had no bearing on outcome; others cite the virulent behavior of melanoma as justification. The rationale for wide excision is to prevent local recurrence. This has been shown to increase in thicker lesions when margins are less than 2 cm. The finding of atypical melanocytes in normal skin surrounding melanomas has also prompted wide excision. Truncal lesions are usually excised with the greatest margins, but still have the worst prognosis. There is only one prospective, randomized study with concurrent controls that exists for margins of excision. This study has indicated that for tumor thicknesses less than 2.0 mm, margins of 1 cm are as safe as 3 cm. Many surgeons believe that wider excisions are helpful in that subgroup of patients destined to have local recurrence. We do not yet know how we can prospectively identify this group. My recommendation is for about 1 cm margin for lesions less than 0.76 mm, but less is certainly justified around vital areas, such as the face. Most often this involves an excision under local anesthesia. Flaps and grafts are almost never done. As the thickness of the lesion increases, so does the margin of normal skin. The greatest margin is in areas where esthetics are of less concern. Most of the higher risk group will undergo 3 cm-margin resections. Based on mapping of local recurrences, the ellipse of normal skin is greatest toward the draining lymph node area. On the trunk, single, double, or even triple rhomboid flaps are used. Extremities may require skin grafting, but local flaps are preferred when feasible. Several older studies indicate the fascia to be beneficial either as a tumor barrier, or, conversely, as an aid in the eradication of microscopic disease. No reasonable study exists to settle this matter and my recommendation is to take it—or leave it—as a matter of convenience.

GRAFT VERSUS FLAP

Standard teaching has suggested that all melanomas should be treated with split-thickness skin grafts so as to herald recurrent disease when it is still presumably curable. Again, no study indicates a detriment to survival by immediate reconstruction. As in much of plastic surgery, the patient is given the option of the best reconstructive effort that utilizes the best tissue available. It should be borne in mind that local recurrence does happen, but is not inevitably fatal; in fact, some studies suggest 50 to 65 percent survival rates even with lymph node metastasis. Local recurrence may require reexcision of the operative site. If grafting is planned, one should consider showing the patient a picture of how it will look. No matter how well the procedure is described preoperatively, the patient always seems surprised. As a rule, I inform the patient of the controversy surrounding margins of excision. I present the extremes—wide versus narrow excisions—make a recommendation of how I would like to do it; then allow the patient to provide input as to the treatment. With experience, one will encounter melanomas that behave aggressively despite the widest of excisions. When this occurs after use of conservative margins, the question of adequate excision always lurks. This problem seems more manageable when the patient has had input into the decision.

LYMPHADENECTOMY

No one argues the benefit of lymphadenectomy (LND) when palpable disease exists. Whether or not prophylactic node dissection improves survival is less clear. Unlike other areas of melanoma treatment, the prospective, randomized study does exist and fails to show benefit when compared to a control group who underwent lymphadenectomy only when metastatic disease became evident. Unfortunately, these studies were flawed. When these studies are reviewed together with several retrospective studies that indicate significant improvement in survival and disease-free interval, the surgical community is still unsure. My recommendation is for prophylactic node dissection in lesions thicker than 1.5 mm with predictable nodal drainage. I may perform LND for lesions that are as thin as 1.0 mm but are still Clark level IV, for those that directly overlie the nodal basin, and for patients whom it may be difficult to follow up. Retrospective studies indicate benefit only for a subgroup of lesions from 1.5 mm to between 3.0 and 4.0 mm thickness. The thicker lesions are found to have a poor prognosis that is not improved by lymphadenectomy. I have a problem abandoning this higher risk group of patients. Since no study indicates that node dissection patients do worse, I prefer to offer my patients LND despite the poor outlook. LND at the very least will "stage" the patient for consideration of adjuvant treatment. Based on published studies, it appears that a subgroup of patients will do well with almost any conservative treatment; another subgroup will do poorly in the face of the most radical surgery; and still another subgroup may benefit from our treatment choice. Unfortunately, we do not yet know how to identify this last group. Extremity lesions in the highest risk group are considered for hyperthermic limb isolation-perfusion.

Questions about timing of operation arise frequently. There is little to be gained by waiting once the diagnosis and operative decision is made. On the other hand, several studies have indicated that several weeks' delay from biopsy to treatment had no adverse effect on outcome.

LIMB PERFUSION

Prophylactic limb perfusion seems to be regaining popularity. The world's largest experience shows a definite benefit if perfusion is performed in a prophylactic setting for lesions thicker than 1.5 mm. Unfortunately, this group compares its results to historical controls. Nearly every medical center that treats melanoma now gets at least 10 to 15 percent improved survival rates from the same (if not more) conservative surgical treatment used 20 years ago. The reasons for this are unclear, but the biologic behavior of melanoma seems to be improving. Possibly tumors are seen earlier in their course due to increased patient awareness. Most centers that utilize limb perfusion will do so for recurrent or extremely high-risk lesions. Our practice is to perfuse lesions greater than 3.0 mm thickness, local recurrence, satellitosis, in-transit metastasis, or palpable metastatic disease. Agents most commonly used are L-PAM and DTIC. As of this writing, L-PAM is not available for intra-arterial use due to FDA restraints, despite its availability for over 20 years. Complications are quite rare, but are most often due to atherosclerotic disease at the arteriotomy site or systemic leakage of the chemotherapeutic agent. Local control of disease is clearly improved with perfusion—whether overall survival is increased has yet to be proven.

FOLLOW-UP

Patient follow-up is extremely important. Eighty percent of patients who fail their initial treatment present within 2 years of diagnosis. The remainder recur at a rate of 1 percent each year over the next 20 years. The lower-risk lesion patients are followed every 3 months for the first 2 years, then yearly. Usually a direct skin and lymph node examination is sufficient with a chest x-ray film and SMA-12 yearly. The higher-risk lesions are followed more closely. Patients are encouraged to do monthly self-examination and are given published material from the American Cancer Society regarding this. Other suspicious lesions are excised. In situations where numerous nevi are present, or difficult to evaluate, we obtain full-body photographs (known as our dysplastic mole series) from the medical photography section of our medical school.

RECURRENT DISEASE

Management of recurrent or metastatic disease is always difficult, both technically and emotionally. Melanoma is probably the most unpredictable cancer known to man. On the negative side, local recurrence will appear either in the scar or adjacent to it and may herald eventual systemic involvement. Not uncommonly, a subcutaneous nodule appears greater than 5 cm from the initial incision. More often, disease will present as lymphadenopathy, or in lung, liver, brain, or bone. The prognosis decreases the farther one gets from the primary site and if solid organs are involved. Pigmented recurrences in the scar do better than subcutaneous masses greater than 5 cm from the primary site. Major resections should be considered as should limb isolation-perfusion for extremity recurrences. On the positive side, several series of long-term palliation have been reported with tumor resections in brain, lung, and liver. Melanoma seems to have the closest link to immune modulation of all cancers. New protocols surface every week and should be considered after standard treatment has been exhausted. An oncologist should be consulted.

Melanoma management will always remain controversial. An understanding of the controversies allows the clinician and patient to embark on a reasonable treatment course. Fortunately, successes will occur ten times more frequently than failures.

SUGGESTED READING

Breslow A. Thickness, cross-sectional areas and depth of invasion in the prognosis of cutaneous melanoma. Ann Surg 1975; 172:902–908.

Cascinelli N, Vanderesch EF, Breslow A, et al. Stage I melanoma of the skin: the problem of resection margins. Eur J Cancer 1980; 16:1078–1085.

Clark WH. Clinical diagnosis of cutaneous melanoma JAMA 1976; 236:484–485.

Krementz ET. Regional perfusion. Cancer 1986; 57:416–428.

Milton GW. Prophylactic lymph node dissection in clinical stage I cutaneous malignant melanoma: results of surgical treatment in 1319 patients. Br J Plast Surg 1982; 69:108–120.

Olsen G. Removal of fascia—cause of more frequent metastasis of malignant melanoma of the skin to regional lymph nodes? Cancer 1964; 17:1159–1168.

Sim FH. A prospective randomized study of the efficacy of routine elective lymphadenectomy in the management of malignant melanoma. Cancer 1978; 41:948–956.

Veronesi U. Inefficacy of immediate node dissection in Stage I melanoma of the limbs. N Engl J Med 1977; 297:627–637.

CARTILAGE GRAFTING

SAMUEL STAL, M.D.
MELVIN SPIRA, M.D.

Appropriate selection of graft or implant material for facial soft tissue augmentation presents a challenge due to the many materials available. The ideal implant would be biocompatible, readily available, and would produce little or no donor site morbidity. Although no single material can be considered ideal in all cases, autogenous cartilage graft material offers an effective and reliable way to fill soft tissue defects, as well as camouflage underlying irregularities in the head and neck region. It can act as a rigid structure to maintain soft tissue, as well as recontouring overlying skin to modify form. Cartilage grafts are nourished by diffusion of tissue fluids into its matrix. The minimal metabolic requirement of chondroblasts greatly enhances initial graft take and ultimate survival. Cartilage easily can be carved and shaped and does not require functional use to retain bulk as does bone. Cartilage is also relatively tolerant of stress. Unlike bone grafts, cartilage grafts can survive well in subcutaneous pockets with only a thin cutaneous cover.

The removal of cartilage creates a new donor wound. Warping, displacement, and infection are all potential problems, however, careful attention to detail can minimize these factors and allow a reasonable solution to difficult reconstruction needs. Personal techniques for autogenous graft harvesting, specific usage, as well as fixation of such grafts are discussed in this chapter.

COMMON DONOR SITES

Donor site sources vary depending on the degree of deformity and individual patient history (previous surgery, age, trauma). Each site has its own advantages and disadvantages, including particular morbidity. The costal chondral rib, concha of the ear, and nasal septum are the most commonly used cartilage donor sites.

Rib

Rib cartilage is favored when large quantities of graft material are required. Clinical examples include augmentation of maxillary hypoplasia, total ear reconstruction, and subtotal or major nasal reconstruction. The seventh, eighth, and ninth ribs are easily accessed through a modified inframammary incision. The rib cartilage is of the rigid hyalin type and is especially useful for maintaining support to the tip of the nose and for large onlays to the maxilla. To comply better with the stresses inherent in cartilage and to minimize problems of warping when cartilage is modified, careful selection of the appropriate recipient shape is necessary. The seventh rib cartilage is relatively straight and is more appropriate for nasal dorsum augmentation, whereas the eighth is slightly curved and is ideal for malar and maxillary onlay. The extensive availability of graft material makes this site ideal in patients whose cartilage is exhausted from other sources. The rib also is an acceptable donor site in a growing child where harvesting nasal septal cartilage would be unacceptable.

Rib is the cartilage of choice when I want more rigid support, such as in maintaining tip support with a columellar strut. In patients with severe bilateral cleft lip deformities, there often is secondary tethering of the nasal tip and absence of the nasal spine and caudal septum. Rib cartilage can be fashioned to extend the septum after soft tissue columella lengthening (Fig. 1). The addition of cartilage helps support the tip and places the entire nose in a more favorable environment for normal growth and development. In patients with good occlusion, but who have maxillary hypoplasia, a solid piece of rib cartilage is ideal and superior to smaller plumping grafts for maxillary augmentation. Experience with bone grafts on the anterior maxilla documented marked resorption, whereas cartilage grafts seem to have maintained reasonable size and form.

Many people avoid this technique because "it seems like a lot of work" with increased operative time, large and unsightly scars, and the potential morbidity of pneumothorax. These objections may be true when almost total removal of the rib chondral cartilage is necessary, such as in an ear reconstruction; however, by modifying the harvesting technique, more than adequate amounts of cartilage can still be taken in a safe effective manner with minimal problems. Our group has almost exclusively used this donor site over the past 4 years in approximately 150 cases where there was a need for more cartilage than could be obtained safely from the nose or ear. The patients ranged in age from 2 to 60 years, with the majority having a cleft lip, craniofacial or traumatic facial deformity.

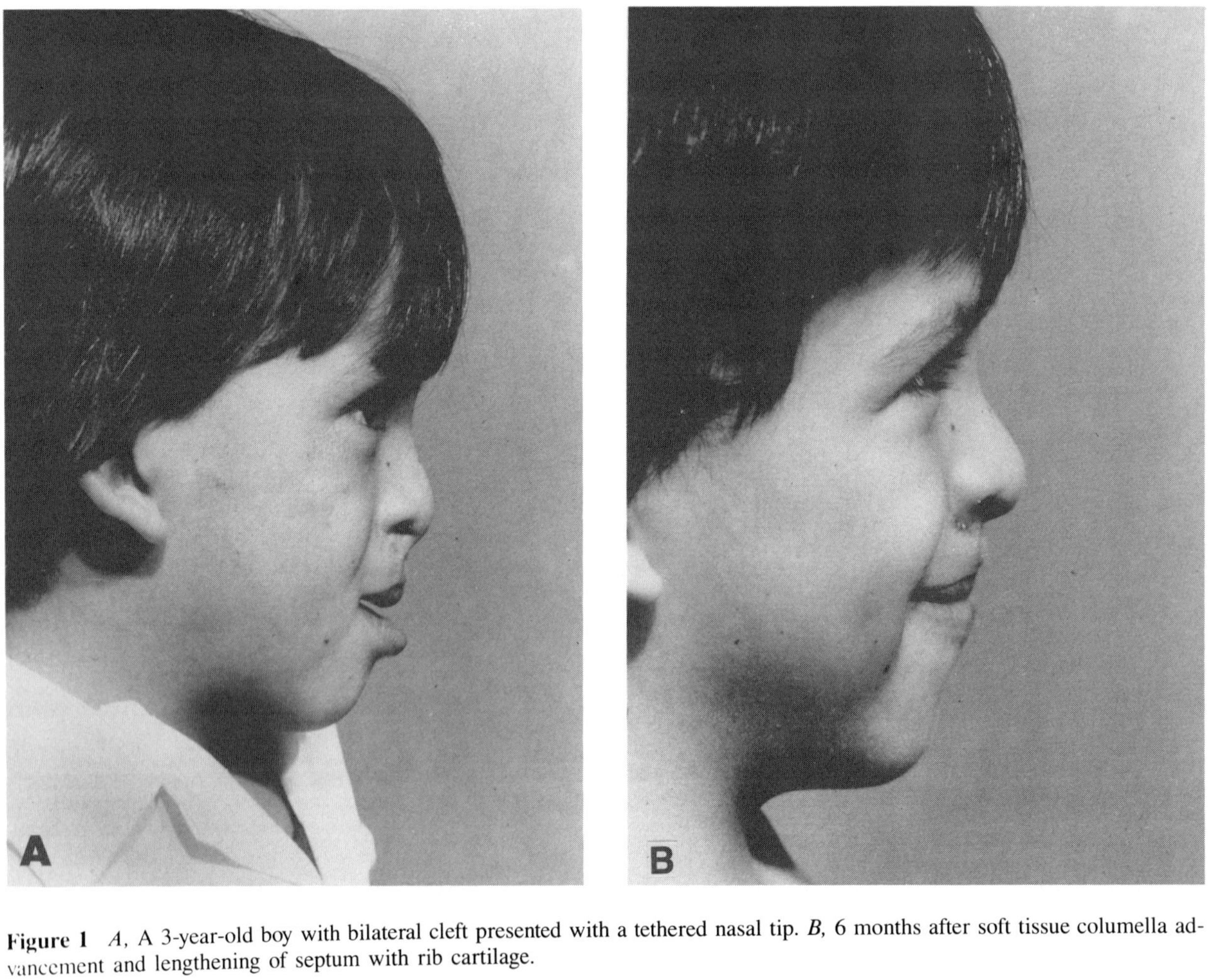

Figure 1 *A*, A 3-year-old boy with bilateral cleft presented with a tethered nasal tip. *B*, 6 months after soft tissue columella advancement and lengthening of septum with rib cartilage.

Surgical Technique

The costal cartilage is approached through a small (3 to 4 cm) oblique incision directly over the seventh and eighth cartilaginous ribs, approximately 6 cm from the midline. This minimally disturbs the underlying rectus muscle. The harvest can be done simultaneously in conjunction with a second surgeon elevating soft tissue planes in the face in preparation for the graft. Harvest access is made easier by using a self-retaining retractor, and one assistant moves a retractor to facilitate exposure. Since the parietal pleura and deep perichondrium are so intimate, it has proven easier to remove subtotal portions of the cartilage along with its anterior perichondrium. A No. 66 beaver blade facilitates a right-angle cut and helps delineate only the outer or ventral-most three-fourths of the cartilage. After the necessary amount of cartilage is removed, the wound is closed anatomically in three layers without a drain, and a light pressure dressing is applied.

Since the cartilage has already been sheared of its deep perichondrium during harvest, the only superficial anterior layer remains to be removed using an No. 11 blade. The middle portion of the cartilage, which is relatively straight, remains for use. The cartilage shavings, which have been removed, are both excellent filler for soft tissue defects and onlay grafts to the alar cartilage, as they assume a configuration and thickness very similar in appearance and consistency to nasal alar cartilage. When crushed in the Cottle bone crusher, these shavings also serve as an excellent overlay for camouflage. In static areas, such as in the premaxilla, large pieces can be used relatively unmodified with simple feathering of the edges for better configuration (Fig. 2). The bone crusher and the Rubin morselizer are useful as adjuncts to help modify the shape of the cartilage.

The biggest problem I have seen with rib cartilage occurs when it has been used as a large segment to augment the nasal dorsum. Even after complete cross sectional carving on a relatively straight middle portion, I found early warping of large grafts to be the rule and not the exception (Fig. 3). In cases of severe saddling or nasal dorsum hypoplasia where considerable augmentation is necessary, I routinely use cranial or rib grafts. These grafts are applied with intimate contact to the proximal nasal bones and are fixated with interosseous wires. I tend to use more rib bone grafts of late because of the abundant rib cartilage accessible through the same harvest incision. Cartilage grafts help enhance bony nasal reconstruction by augmenting and increasing tip projection, thus allowing the creation of a contoured double break and supratip concavity. The subtotal approach of harvesting rib cartilage takes approximately 20 to 25 minutes to obtain the graft and close the wound. Unused cartilage may be banked in the original wound. Postoperative discomfort in our series was minimum with no evidence of hematoma. This result is significant since 46 of our patients were 5 years of age or younger. All scars seen were acceptable. No pneumothoraces were diagnosed when the subtotal ap-

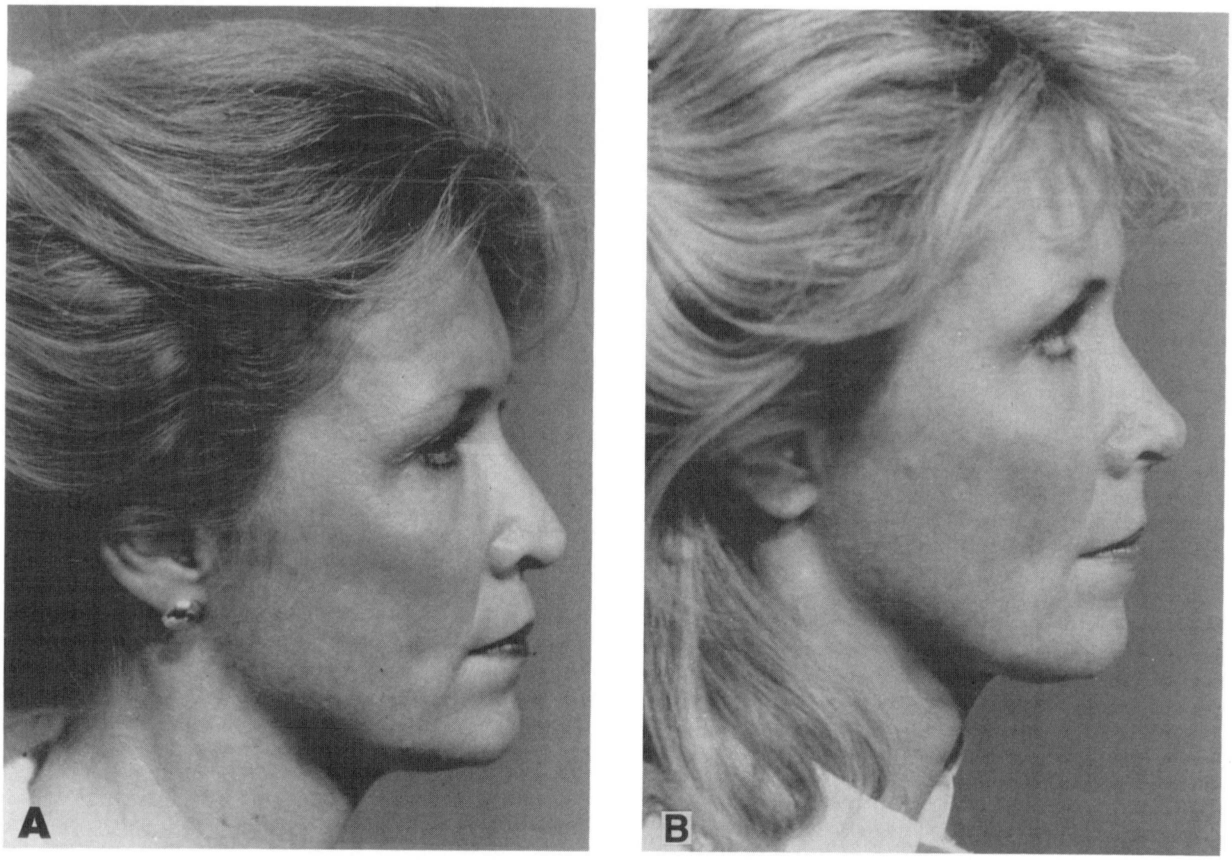

Figure 2 *A*, A 42-year-old woman unhappy with her nose-lip relationship. *B*, 6 months after only cartilage graft to anterior maxilla.

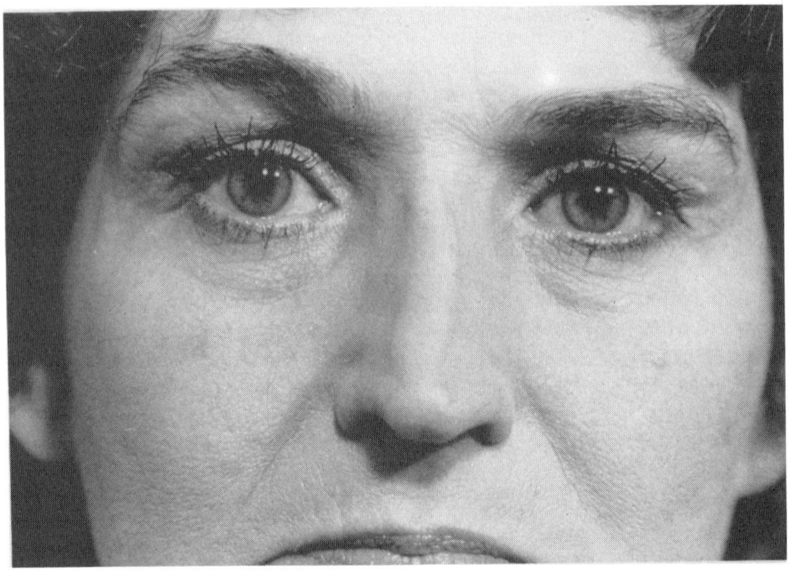

Figure 3 A large rib cartilage graft was placed on the nasal dorsum 3 months postoperatively. Subsequent warping occurred.

proach was used. Full-thickness removal of cartilage has a marked increase in postoperative discomfort as well as complications.

Septal Cartilage

After reduction rhinoplasty, there is often residual cartilage from the resection of the caudal and dorsal septum, as well as from the resection of the cephalic margins of alar cartilages. Due to the lack of rigidity and unpredictable amounts of cartilage from these sites, the surgeon cannot count on these sites as a primary harvest source. Nasal septal cartilage, on the other hand, is an excellent anatomic area for the harvesting of cartilage. Generous amounts may be harvested from the quadrangular cartilage, posterior to an imaginary line connecting the osteocartilaginous junction with the nasal spine, without jeopardizing septal support. Care must be taken to preserve at least 1 to 1.5 cm struts of the dorsal and caudal margins of the septal cartilage to maintain a supporting structure. In a primary rhinoplasty, sufficient amounts of septal cartilage may be removed conservatively to create both a reasonable onlay dorsal graft (4 × 1 cm) and tip grafts (0.1 × 1 cm). In a patient with a previous septoplasty, a review of the operative report might give some clue as to the extent of the septal resection that was performed. The patient must understand preoperatively the possible need for utilizing another source of cartilage if septal cartilage is unavailable.

The septal cartilage is of the rigid hyaline type and is ideally suited for use in the nose. A large (4 × 1 cm) fusiform shaped graft can be modified to distend the skin and create the illusion of a straight smooth dorsum. This is especially helpful after a reduction rhinoplasty to help restore dorsal continuity by covering the open roof and overlie any irregularities. In some cases, the septal cartilage can be used flat after the edges have been modified or feathered. As time passes, the overlying skin thins, exposing edges that were left too sharp (Fig. 4). Accurate placement and fixation are essential to minimize graft movement. By grooving either the posterior or ventral side of the cartilage, a bend can be created forming an A-frame or a U-frame shape (as described by Gunter), compatible with the patient's own aesthetic lines and dorsal width (Fig. 5). It is sometimes helpful to introduce these grafts

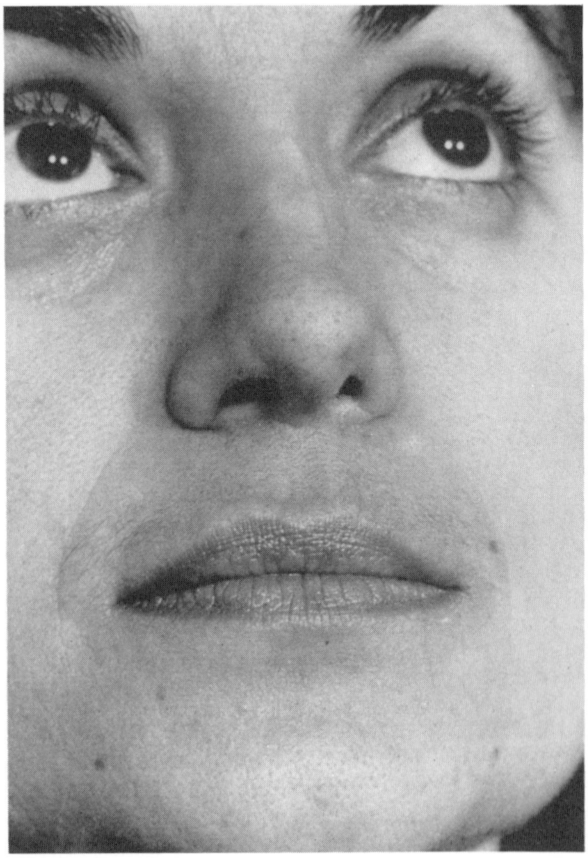

Figure 4 Status 4 years after septal cartilage graft to dorsum with inferior malposition and over-defined edges.

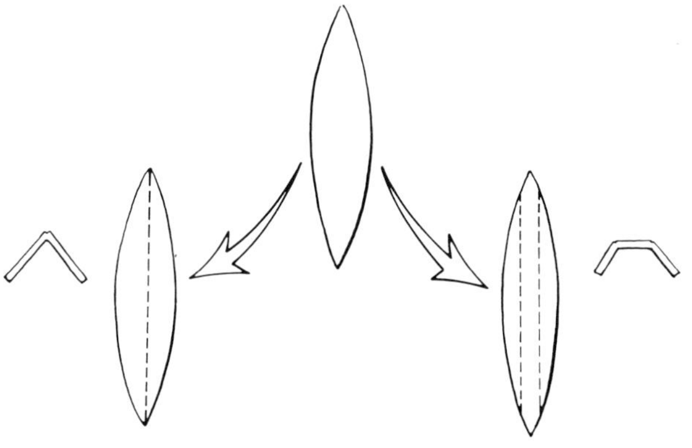

Figure 5 Technique of recontouring septal cartilage for dorsal onlay (redrawn from Gunter, personal communication).

with a suture that is brought out through the skin with a large Keith needle. The suture may be left in place for another week tied over a Telfa bolster helping to maintain the graft in position.

Cartilage also can be used to create tension on the overlying skin in patients with rounded, droopy, poorly defined nasal tips. Increased nasal tip projection can be achieved by placing the graft over the lower lateral cartilages at the most anterior leading edge. This cartilage must be shaped and placed carefully in a preplanned position. The rectangular (Peck graft) is used to increase projection with a multi-layered graft. The larger shield (Sheen graft) is placed in a slightly different plane, not only enhancing projection, but also creating aesthetic high points for definition.

Septal cartilage, accessed through a transfixation incision, is also a good sturdy source of material to act as a batton or strut in the columella. This graft may be inserted retrograde and placed between the feet of the medial cura. The strut can also be simply inserted through a small sublabial stab incision after a midline pocket has been created. This is a very helpful tool when used not to create projection but to maintain it. Such a graft is used ideally for patients in whom a lack of tip support is commonly seen, such as the cleft nose, the non-Caucasian nose, and the older patient with tip laxity.

The ideal material to markedly enhance the acute nasolabial angle is rib cartilage. However, when a small amount of augmentation is necessary, layered pieces of septal cartilage allow a modest plumping in this area. A septal cartilage strut may also be anchored to the septum to augment the retruded or "hanging columella."

Surgical Technique

After preparation of the mucosa with cotton saturated with topical anesthetic (4 cc of 4 percent cocaine), Xylocaine 0.5 percent is injected using a 25-gauge 2½ inch needle with the bevel end down. This is injected ideally in the subperichondrial plane forcing the fluid to hydraulically separate the perichondrium from the cartilage. The injection may extend the entire area of dissection without risk of ischemic necrosis. The subperichondrial plane is identified using a sharp Cottle elevator, which is excellent for beginning the dissection. A Freer or blunt edged elevator is used for the remainder of the dissection of the mucoperichondrial flap. It is helpful to begin dissection from anterior to posterior above, then to sweep down posteriorly, dissecting forward under direct vision. The mucoperichondrium is bluntly teased away while the decussated fibers found in the anterior and inferior border of the septum and vomer are cut. After dissection of one side of mucoperichondrium, the contralateral side of the graft to be removed is elevated only. This dissection can be helped by placing the tip of the fifth digit of the nonoperating hand in the contralateral vestibule to exert stabilizing pressure. The cartilage is cut and the blunt end of the elevator used to complete the transsection of the cartilage without perforating the mucosa on the other side. The septal cartilage can be removed separately or in conjunction with the perpendicular plate of the ethmoid using serrated cartilage scissors. Before removal of the cartilaginous segment, the lining must be carefully delineated with a Freer elevator to avoid perforation. Interrupted mattress sutures of 4–0 plain catgut help adhese the mucoperichondrial flaps and close the incisions. This is necessary to avoid hematoma by closing the dead space. The use of septal splints made up of Teflon or Silicone (Xomed) is also an excellent way to apply additional gentle pressure to coapt the mucoperichondrium as well as maintain support.

External Ear

The cartilage of the ear is elastic and somewhat different from the hyaline cartilage of the nose and rib. However, with appropriate carving or sculpting, stacking, or simply rolling the cartilage on itself, a sturdy graft may be created that gives effective form and support. As long as the antihelical fold is not transgressed, minimal changes occur in the ultimate appearance of the ear after the entire cymba and cavum concha have been removed. This can yield segments of cartilage up to 4 cm long. Because of the curvature peculiar to the ear, appropriate selection of donor grafts must be customized since the more the graft resembles part to be reconstructed, the better. With slight modification, curved concha will resemble the lower lateral cartilage, but it is too thin as a columella strut without appropriate layering. Single pieces of cartilage are difficult to use for anything except camouflage or overlay. When these grafts are to create tension, multiple layers must be used. It is difficult to create a large dorsal graft with ear cartilage that will maintain its shape over a long term. Hence, the ear is considered a secondary donor site for this purpose. For cartilage it is probably most useful for filling in small contour irregularities and for filler or camouflage overlay in conjunction with septal cartilage grafts.

When harvesting grafts from the ear, it is important to minimize oral and nasal contamination by using separate instruments and by changing gloves when going to the ear. I have seen this with two patients who lost the graft secondary to infection.

Surgical Technique

Ear cartilage grafts can be harvested easily through either anterior or posterior incisions. When the maximum amount of cartilage is needed, an anterior incision, placed at the base of the antihelix, is preferred. The anterior skin and underlying soft tissue are infiltrated with 0.5 percent Xylocaine with epinephrine. The incision is carried down to the appropriate plane. Separating the anterior perichondrium from the cartilage helps to preserve at least one layer of the perichondrium to better maintain support of the donor site. The Cottle elevator is used to elevate the perichondrium from the cartilage. The cartilage is then incised full-thickness through and through including the posterior perichondrium over the proposed area of resection. A Brown-Adson forceps is used to grasp the cartilage, thus avoiding traumatic laceration. After hemostasis, the skin is reapproximated with a 6–0 plain suture. A dressing is required to coapt the flap and prevent accumulation of fluid. Though mini flap drains and mastoid dressings work well, a simple bolster type dressing using petrolatum gauze and 2–0 silk sutures, maintained for 3 to 5 days, is more tolerable for the patient. In most patients, the scar is obscured in the shadow at the base of the antihelix.

Ear cartilage can also be accessed through a posterior incision. This approach is more ideal for small pieces to be used for onlay grafting. The natural curve of the concha allows for excellent configuration for multiple small onlay grafts for the nasal tip or dorsum.

The ear remains the primary source for composite grafts of skin and cartilage. These grafts are invaluable for correcting defects of the eyelid, nasal lining, and alar rim. Grafts as large as 2 × 1.5 cm can be removed safely from the root of the helix, concha, or tubercle and still achieve primary closure (Fig. 6).

When more cartilage than is necessary is removed, it is ideal to bank it under the hairbearing postauricular area. A small area of scalp is shaved and a 1-cm incision is made and a pocket is developed superficially. The wound is closed with a 4–0 plain catgut. Stored grafts can be helpful in secondary and tertiary reconstructions. Similarly, rib cartilage donor sites offer an ideal area to replace excess in the original bank without making an additional incision.

Fixation

Immobilization of the cartilage graft is important to its success. Autogenous tissue becomes incorporated into the body— unlike synthetic materials, which are surrounded by a capsule. When the initial fixation is secure, migration is unlikely. Ideally, it is best to create as precise a subcutaneous pocket as possible. However, if the pocket is too small, the implant may be distorted. An overly large pocket allows shifting and malposition. Accurately marking the extent of the pocket on the external skin prior to anesthetic infiltration is helpful. This is especially critical in the nasal tip where accurate placement of the pock-

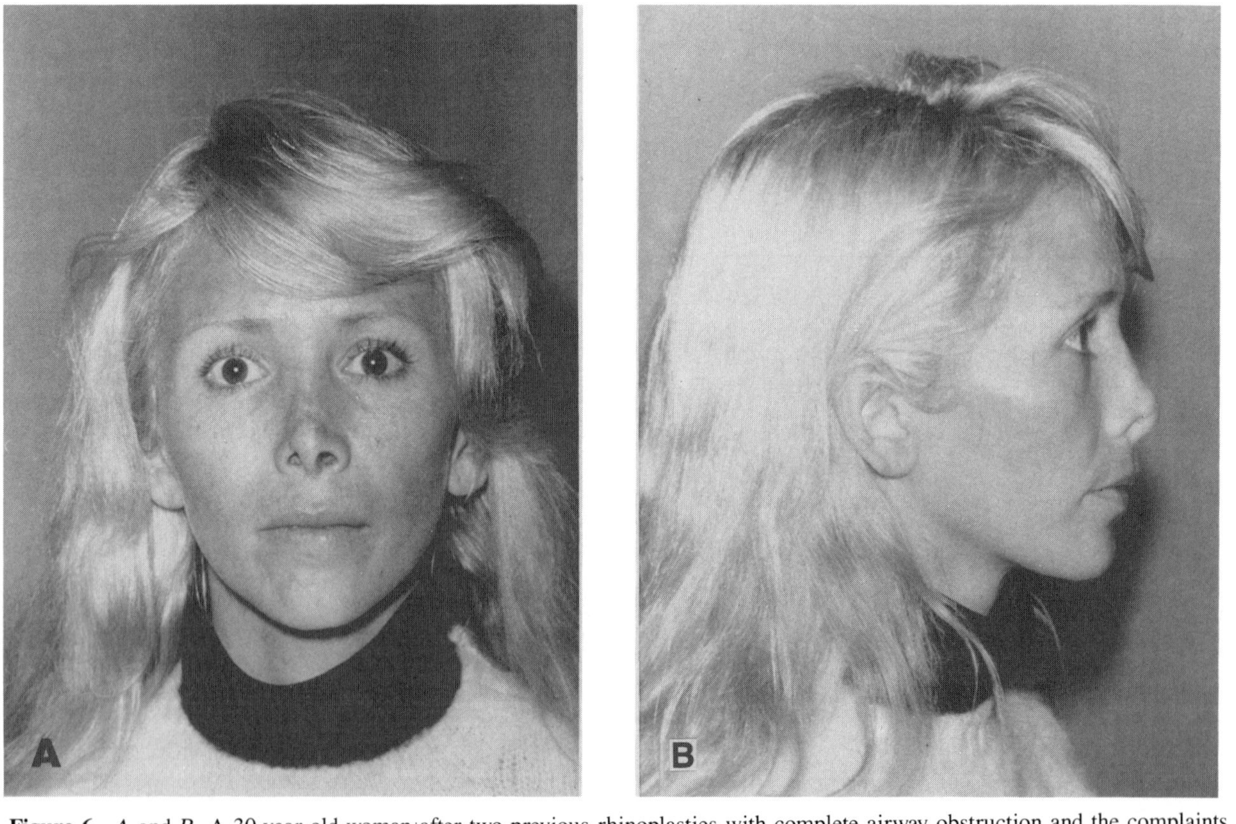

Figure 6 *A* and *B*, A 30-year-old woman after two previous rhinoplasties with complete airway obstruction and the complaints of her nose being too small and asymmetric.

Figure continues on opposite page

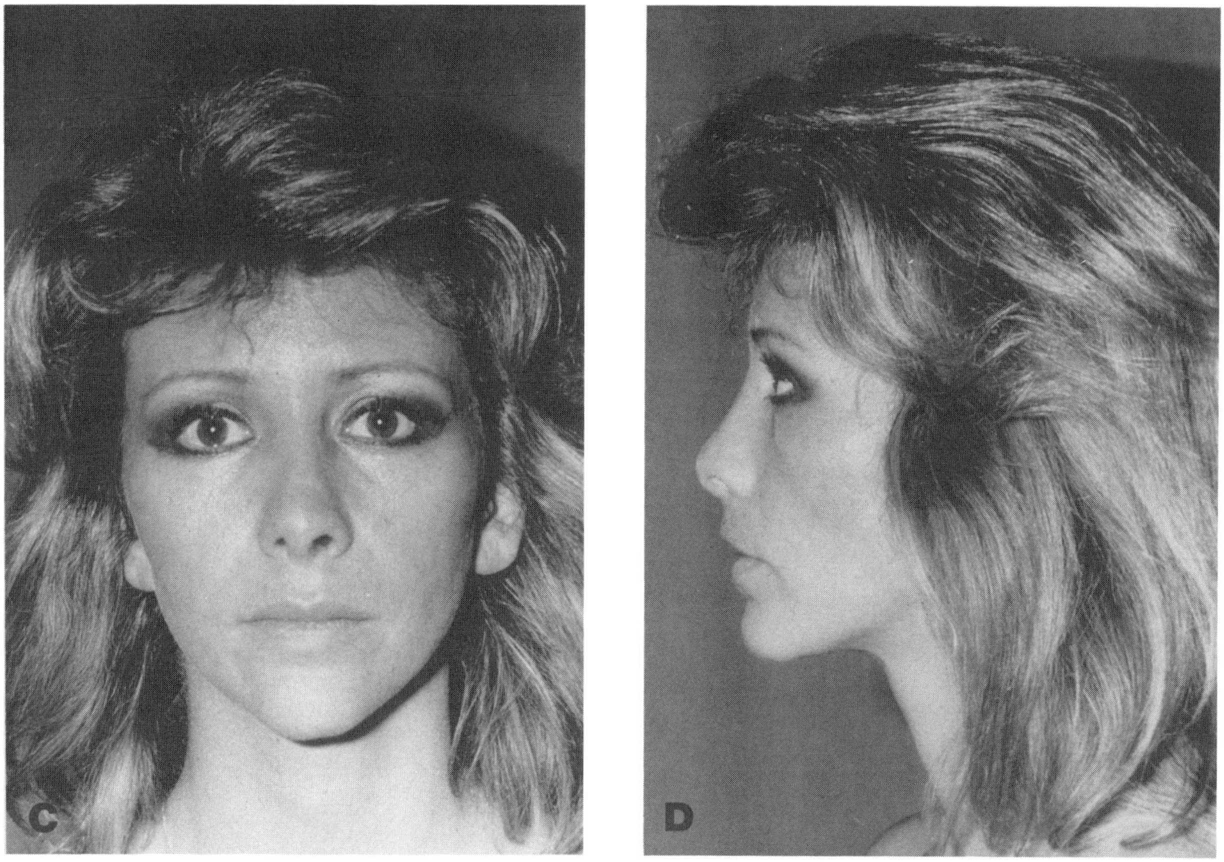

Figure 6 (continued) *C,* and *D,* 6 months after multiple cartilage grafts from nasal septum and ear and composite graft of ear skin and cartilage to increase vestibular lining, augment and overlay dorsum, as well as increase tip projection and camouflage irregularities.

et is necessary for accurate projection. When the pocket is too large, an absorbable suture brought out through the skin may be used to retain cartilage grafts in place. It may be necessary to suture pieces of cartilage together when trying to layer grafts. This should be done with an atraumatic needle and absorbable suture (4–0 plain catgut). Another method of achieving fixation that looks promising is the use of tissue glues. Cyanoacrylates, in particular histoacryl R, have been used in experimental animals and have shown no demonstrable cartilage damage or local tissue toxicity. I have used these adhesives in onlay tip grafting, as well as onlay maxillary grafting, with good initial success. This approach requires obtaining autologous blood 5 days before surgery to allow accumulation of sufficient fibrin for creation of the tissue glue. Pooled autograft thrombin, which is commonly used in Europe, has not been cleared by the FDA in this country.

Warping

In my experience, warping occurs as an early phenomenon. In the majority of patients, it occurs within 10 days of implantation and, in most of the remainder, within 3 months. It is noted that breaking the cartilage by crushing is a significant factor in those autografts in that over time, they undergo significant resorption and modification with fibrous ingrowth. Every effort should be made to select the most appropriate configuration necessary for reconstruction rather than remodeling.

Cartilage Alternatives

In a recent national survey on cartilage implantation, the majority of surgeons responding use autogenous cartilage. Those who still use preserved homograft cartilage, use alcohol and Merthiolate as the most common preservatives. A similar infection rate was noted between autologous and preserved cartilage grafts (15 percent and 19 percent respectively). However, the mean absorption rate for autologous grafts was 23.7 percent, which was significantly lower than that for preserved grafts. Other surgeons throughout the country sterilize human autologous cartilage by exposing it to 3 million rad of gamma radiation from a cobalt source. A recent 3-year study of 145 implants with radiated homologous costal cartilage for facial contour reconstruction showed an infection rate of 4.1 percent. An interesting finding was that the implants inserted transorally did not have a statistically different infection rate from ones inserted percutaneously. The partial resorption rate was only 1.4 percent. Frequency of graft loss was only 2.8 percent. Radiated homologous cartilage seems to offer an alternative when autologous cartilage is not available.

Autogenous cartilage remains a versatile material for facial augmentation. Careful preoperative planning and basic sound surgical techniques yield good results when appropriately used. Additional time spent in harvesting the appropriate graft minimizes morbidity both in the donor and the recipient site.

SUGGESTED READING

Donald PJ, Col A. Cartilage implantation in head and neck surgery: report of a national survey. Otolaryngol Head Neck Surg 1982; 90:85–89.

Peck GC. The onlay graft for nasal tip projection. Plast Reconstr Surg 1983; 71:27–37.

Ronis ML, Harwick JD, Fung R, Dellavecchia M. Review of cyanoacrylate tissue glues with emphasis on their otorhinolaryngological applications. Laryngoscope 1984; 94:210–213.

Schuller DE, Bardach J, Krause CJ. Irradiated homologous costal cartilage for facial contour restoration. Arch Otolaryngol 1977; 103:12–15.

Sheen JH. Achieving more nasal tip projection by the use of a small autogenous vomer or septal cartilage graft. A preliminary report. Plast Reconstr Surg 1975; 56:35–40.

Sheen JH, Sheen A. Aesthetic Rhinoplasty. Vol. 1. 2nd ed. St. Louis: CV Mosby; 1987.

SYNTHETIC BIOMATERIALS FOR SOFT TISSUE

JOHN H. COCHRAN Jr., M.D.
ANDREW M. REED, Ph.D.

Synthetic biomaterials are essential components of the therapeutic armamentarium of the present day reconstructive surgeon.

Although autogenous tissue is preferable in nearly all situations where it is available and the morbidity of the donor is not too great, synthetic materials are efficacious in many situations. Major uses are as implantable materials, dressing materials, and suture materials. Knowledge of specific features of each material can help a surgeon select the best material for each situation. For the purposes of this article, the term synthetic biomaterial will be defined as a synthetic polymeric material (plastic) that has been designed specifically for use in medical applications. In many cases, manufacturers of medical devices have been extremely careful in choosing the correct biomaterial for the specific application for which the device is destined.

Materials that are to be used as implants, or contact broken skin, ideally should be biocompatible, nontoxic, and nonmutagenic. Similarly, they must be free of toxic leachable additives such as plasticizers, colorants, and stabilizers. They should elicit minimal immune response and not increase the rate of infection.

Devices that are designed to degrade over a predetermined period of time should have well-defined degradation products. The biologic fate and effect of these degradation products should also be known.

In reconstructive surgery today there are three main areas in which one encounters synthetic biomaterials:

1. Suture materials, e.g., degradable and permanent.
2. Wound dressings, e.g., semiocclusive dressings.
3. Implantable devices, e.g., breast, chin, nose, malar region, etc.

Each synthetic material has specific physical characteristics such as strength, elasticity, flow, moldability, carvability, flexibility, hydropermeability, hydroplasticity, porosity, and gas permeability. These properties will be mentioned where the particular characteristic affects the surgeon's choice of materials. Surgeons must be able to evaluate the data and claims of the companies that have a commercial interest in the product, so that they can select a material that is both efficacious and has minimal drawbacks for the particular situation being considered.

SUTURE MATERIALS

As the practice of surgery entered the twentieth century, the primary sutures used were silk, cotton, and catgut. In the last 3 decades, the work of the polymer chemist has given the surgeon a much wider variety of sutures from which to choose (Table 1).

Selection of the type of suture to use in a particular clinical setting should be based on a knowledge of the structure, functional characteristics, and limitations of each material.

Selection of the size of suture material and needle should be on the basis of the smallest size that provides the necessary strength to secure the desired repair.

The naturally-occurring suture materials (silk, cotton, catgut) have seen their applications limited by the development of synthetic materials with superior features. These earlier materials, along with steel filament, represent what we can describe as traditional materials.

Silk is the easiest material to handle, and has good tensile strength. Silk causes a marked reaction when implanted, and the antigenic response limits its use. Silk is useful as a temporary suture during any procedure and its ease of use makes it ideal for tie-over bolster dressings. It is also used by some surgeons in the oral cavity, as it is easy to tie and stays longer than degradables.

Catgut (chromic and plain) was the basic absorbable suture for some time, but has now been replaced in most situations by synthetic sutures. These synthetic materials have greater strength and slower degradation. Catgut is

TABLE 1 Types of Synthetic Sutures

Polymer Type	*Trade Name*
Polyester	Mersilene Tevdek Ethibond
Nylon	Supramid
Polypropylene	Prolene
Polyglycolic acid	Dexon
Polyglycolic acid/polylactic acid copolymer	Vicryl
Polydioxanone	PDS

still used in certain oral and ophthalmic surgery where rapid healing is expected and rapid degradation is desired.

Stainless steel is a very strong and nonreactive suture that can be very effective in certain buried repairs, such as tendons, where suture strength is critical. It is, however, a difficult material with which to work and many surgeons prefer other synthetic materials.

Nylon and polypropylene are the primary sutures used for skin closure. Nylon is nonreactive and strong, but it is slightly springy, stretches moderately, and requires four knots to tie securely. It makes a fine material to close skin in a running, interrupted, or subcuticular manner. Braided nylon is easier to use and stronger than monofilament. It is used primarily to close dura. Nylon tends to lose tensile strength on long-term implantation.

Polypropylene is similar to nylon, but is a little springier and has the lowest coefficient of friction for tissues. Polypropylene may thus be the best suture to use for a subcuticular pullout repair.

Polyester fiber sutures include products like Mersilene, Ethibond and Tevdek. These are strong, nonabsorbable sutures that undergo some encapsulation. They can be used for closures that require strong, permanent repairs such as ligaments and cartilage.

Supramid is a polyfilament suture with an external sheath of caprolactam that has some practical advantages based on its structure. The polyfilament construction makes it a very strong suture, and the external sheath allows it to go through tissue like a monofilament. It is a good choice for buried repairs such as tendons.

Absorbable sutures of the polyglycolic/lactic acid family of polymers (Dexon, Vicryl, etc.) degrade over a longer and more predictable time period than catgut. The mechanism of degradation of these polymeric devices is predominantly by chemical hydrolysis. The resulting degradation products are naturally-occurring metabolites and are easily expelled from the body by normal processes.

Polyglycolic/lactic acid sutures maintain their strength for a minimum of 30 days, but are physically present for up to 90 days or more. If they are placed too near the skin, or become exposed, they may "split" through the wound.

Polydioxanone (PDS) is a more recent member of the synthetic degradable suture product line. The material is supplied as a monofilament (as opposed to the braided polyglycolic/lactic acid type sutures). The monofilament is rather stiff and may actually penetrate through the healing surface with time. Its acceptance along with other newer sutures will be evaluated with time.

SYNTHETIC WOUND DRESSINGS

The development of improved synthetic dressing materials has only occurred in the past few years. Although some advances have been made in understanding the role of dressings in wound healing, the state of the art is still quite basic. The future should hold some substantial advances in both understanding and evaluation of improved wound dressings.

Historically, scientists looked carefully at the organ to be duplicated before evolving pulmonary replacement (respirators), renal replacement (dialysis), or cardiac replacement (ventricular assist devices). This seemingly basic philosophy has only been applied to skin replacement (synthetic dressings) in recent years.

For many years, wounds were left open, covered with dry or nonadherent gauze, or painted with drying agents. The evolution of an understanding of the microenvironmental influences that normal skin and idealized synthetic dressings should share has led to an increasing acceptance of moist wound-healing therapy (Table 2).

Many authors feel that ideal dressings should have certain basic characteristics that are much like those of human skin. A first generation of synthetic dressings evolved in recognition of the fact that open wounds, gauze, nonadherent gauze, and ointments did not fulfill these criteria. These are the dressings currently available to the clinician. As the true heterogeneity of the wounds becomes more fully appreciated, subsequent generations of dressings will provide therapeutic features tailored to different situations.

Homograft skin is certainly the best coverage for full-thickness defects and "takes" by mechanisms that are well understood. Temporary biologic dressings can be either homograft (allograft) such as placental or cadaver skin, or heterograft (xenograft) such as porcine skin.

Synthetic dressings can provide a covering to allow full-thickness wounds to heal to the point of being able to accept a graft, or allow partial-thickness wounds to heal completely.

Polyurethane film dressings with adhesive were the first widely-used synthetic dressings (Op-site, Tegaderm). These dressings provide a sterile barrier, plus a wound-healing environment that allows wounds to heal at an acceptable rate with little pain. These dressings absorb little wound exudate, and have a rather low moisture vapor transport so they tend to pool fluid beneath them. This pool may require drainage or it could become a source of infection.

A newer development in film dressings consists of a silicone rubber film with a nylon mesh and a layer of reconstituted collagen (Biobrane). This dressing has a low absorptive capacity, but a high moisture vapor transport so that pooling under the dressing does not present a significant problem, and the healing is efficient with little pain. The exact role of each of these structural components is not clear.

TABLE 2 Environmental Wound Dressings

Dressing Type	*Trade Name*	*Manufacturer*
Hydrocolloid dressings	DuoDERM	Convatec, Inc.
	Restore	Hollister, Inc.
	Comfeel Ulcus	Coloplast, Inc.
	Ulcer Dressing	Johnson & Johnson
Hydrogel dressings	Vigilon	C.R. Bard, Inc.
	Spenco Second Skin	Spenco, Inc.
Film dressings	Op-Site	Smith & Nephew, Ltd.
	Tegaderm	3M Company
	Biocclusive	Johnson & Johnson
	Biobrane	Woodruff Labs, Inc.
Foam dressings	Epi-Lock	Derma-Lock Medical Co., Inc.
	Lyofoam	Ultra Labs, Ltd.

Hydrogel and hydrocolloid materials have become popular synthetic dressings. Hydrocolloid dressings (e.g., DuoDERM, Restore) consist of a polymeric foam substrate with one side covered with a gelatin, pectin, carboxymethylcellulose, polyisobutylene, and mineral oil mixture. These dressings manage exudate by absorption into the dressing, and they have a very low moisture vapor transport rate. In some formulations, the gelatin dissolves after a few days' contact with the wound. These types of dressing are used widely and have proven to be effective, especially when used on chronic wounds of the buttock and lower extremity.

Hydrogel dressings, constructed from polyethylene oxide with a film backing sheet, are available (e.g., Vigilon, Spenco Second Skin). They manage exudate by absorption and have little moisture vapor transmission. Although the gel does not dissolve into the wound, they do not have the adhesive advantages of the hydrocolloids.

Polyurethane foams have been developed as semiocclusive dressings (e.g., Epi-Lock, Lyofoam). These dressings have the ability both to absorb exudate and to transport water by vapor transmission. These dressings work well on clean or sterile wounds such as donor sites and dermabrasions. They may also be used on chronic wounds.

In general, there are no dressings that can be left on infected or contaminated wounds without frequent changing. These wounds may do better with wet gauze dressings that are changed frequently.

Colonized wounds that are not invasively infected and are of a chronic or acute etiology can be managed by cleaning and application of any of the semiocclusive dressings. These dressings are changed every 2 to 5 days or more, depending on the level of the contamination and clinical response.

Clean or sterile wounds can be managed by most of these dressings. The polyurethane films and foams both provide an optimal environment for healing when simply left on the wound and monitored until healed. Ease of use and presence of adhesive are factors of varying importance to individual surgeons.

The future of synthetic dressings holds great hope for the reconstructive surgeon. The use of a membrane as a vehicle to deliver cultured skin cells is an exciting application. Additional research is ongoing to incorporate hormonal growth factors on membrane surfaces. Finally, dressings that incorporate antimicrobial compounds or antibiotics for use on more contaminated wounds will become available. The evolution of these changes should bring the researchers' findings to the clinician for practical patient application.

IMPLANTABLE DEVICES

Implantable devices are those manufactured from biomaterials and designed for long-term stable implantation. These materials are designed as permanent replacements, or enhancements, for reconstruction of breast, chin, nose, malar region, or other soft tissue, as well as for bone or cartilaginous replacement. Autologous materials are generally preferable to alloplasts, but often are not available in sufficient quantity, or the donor site morbidity is of sufficient concern to cause the surgeon to look for alternatives such as synthetic biomaterials.

The fundamental properties of implants, including such issues as biocompatibility and toxicity, have previously been mentioned. In permanent implants, however, one also needs to take into consideration such factors as long-term stability, mechanical reliability, and carcinogenicity.

Specific clinical applications require versatility in the type of polymer used. For instance, there may be a need for different sizes, which are readily available through standard manufacturing processes, or there may be a requirement for different shapes. These needs are met by custom-made implants or by implants that can be carved or modified at the time of surgery.

Because of the long-term nature of these implants, two areas of concern become more important when synthetic dressings or sutures are used. The first is the body's reaction to the polymer, which includes such responses as inflammation, fibroplasia, and long-term scar formation or contracture. Many of these responses are not significantly altered by the material because they are a natural physiologic body response to foreign materials. However, there have been many reports in the literature that suggest the chemical composition of a biomaterial, e.g., electrical charge, degree of hydrophilicity and surface morphology (porosity), can greatly modify the body's response to these materials when implanted. The second concern is the effect the body may have on the implanted material. Ideally, there should be minimal change in the biomaterial, but in certain cases controlled degradation may be desirable. In cases where degradation is neither specifically controlled nor fully understood, then the body's response to a material requires careful observation.

Certain general surgical principles continue to apply after many years of experience in the placement of implantable plastic materials into patients. In spite of advances in biocompatibility and tissue tolerance, these principles must be carefully kept in mind and observed. The primary concern in placing alloplastic materials into patients is to ensure that there is adequate soft tissue coverage by viable, well-vascularized tissue. Violation of this principal has caused many implants to extrude and fail in the past, but awareness of it has increased the surgeon's utilization of such procedures as muscular or fascial covering over implants to ensure that they stay in place, covered by healthy, stable tissue. A second principle is the need to be aware of the specific chemical characteristics of implant materials and the resultant features of clinical application that make each more efficacious in a specific situation. Finally, careful observation for sterility of technique is of utmost importance in any alloplastic implantation, as these materials can significantly modify the body's ability to respond to certain levels of bacterial inocula.

Specific classes of biomaterials are identified herein and their individual clinical applications discussed and compared. The most widely used class of polymers is the polydimethylsiloxane family, known as the silicones. Variations in the configuration of these polymers can create material that are fluids of varying viscosities, adhesives, gels, or rubbers. The lower molecular weight polymers are silicone fluids. The viscosity is increased with increasing molecular weight. An increase in the level of crosslinking creates a modification and makes the material more rigid, thereby resulting in a gel or, ultimately, a rubber-type consistency. In the silicone gels that are often seen as central portions of implantable mammary prostheses, there is both gel-like crosslinked silicone and silicone fluid. The fluid is the material that is considered responsible for transmembrane "silicone bleed."

Silicone, in its rubber form as a Silastic sheet, is a standard of comparison for bioreactivity as the material that evokes minimal reaction of the body to its presence. This reactivity varies with the purity of the material and also changes with the state of the material, e.g., gel or liquid. These polymers have persisted as the safe and standardly-used material for mammary augmentation and other soft tissue prostheses where biocompatibility and durability are important. Newer materials are being developed and are being used clinically that have been designed to be even more tissue-compatible. This has been achieved by modifications of surface or by limitation of silicone liquid bleeding.

Although polyester materials are more reactive than silicone, because of their tensile strength and compatibility with tissue ingrowth, they can be used as a mesh (Mersilene) for soft tissue or fascia reconstructions. Polyester is also used in suture material for long-term stabilization of wounds such as otoplasties and tendons. Polyethylene is used primarily as a high-density mesh (Marlex). This is a strong material that, after implantation, also allows fibrous tissue ingrowth for anchoring stability. This material is used for fascia, ligament, and tendon reconstruction due to its strength and biocompatibility.

The fluorocarbon polymers such as polytetrafluoroethylene (Teflon) are available under several trade names (e.g., Gore-Tex, Proplast). Proplast, which has been available for several years, has been modified for different applications. This material can be used as a sheet for implantation in areas such as the orbital floor that require a flat material. It can also be used as a block, which is readily carved for intraoperative modification, and has been used for reconstruction of bony defects or esthetic enhancement of areas such as the malar complex. Because of the dark color (black) of Proplast I, it was modified in recent years, by the addition of aluminum oxide to the compound to create a lighter color (white), so that it could be placed more superficially. This material has enjoyed success over many years' experience. Its surface porosity seems to be a significant factor in its ability to be fixed securely in the tissues (due to tissue ingrowth), and to be well tolerated. A final recent modification of this material was its combination with hydroxylapatite, which theoretically provides bone mineral and osteoconductive characteristics that may allow its utilization and acceptance adjacent to bone. Experience with this material is minimal at this time, and it will need to be evaluated more fully. Gore-Tex surgical membrane (microporous polytetrafluoroethylene) has only recently become available to the reconstructive surgeon. This material is soft and pliable and is being used in facial reconstruction. It is similar to Gore-Tex patches that have been used in cardiovascular surgery as pericardial closure devices and vascular grafts.

Polyurethanes are another group of polymers with certain common characteristics, but which also have significant variation in their structure and characteristics based on individual chemical and structural conformations. These materials can be used as sheets or films, as thicker foams, or as elastomeric materials with varying elastic qualities.

In recent years, the polyurethane family has come under close scrutiny for implant use. Such episodes as the failure of polyurethane pacemaker leads and reports of delaminating coatings around breast implants have cast a cloud over these materials.

Although it is beyond the scope of this chapter to discuss the vast area of polyurethane chemistry, it is possible to say that not all materials termed polyurethanes are identical either in physical properties or in the body's response to such materials when implanted.

Polyurethanes, and more specifically polyetherurethanes, are highly biocompatible, both for soft tissue and as blood-contact materials. They have excellent physical properties such as elasticity, flexibility, and tear resistance. As with all polymeric materials, under certain conditions polyurethanes may undergo various chemical reactions. An important reaction in practical terms is that of hydrolysis, i.e., the action of an aqueous environment on the polymer. This is particularly highlighted by the well-known fact that polyesterurethanes are highly susceptible to hydrolysis, with subsequent loss of physical properties. Polyetherurethanes, however, are much more stable than their polyesterurethane counterparts. The correct choice of polyurethane for a particular application is crucial if the desired properties of the implants are to be attained and ultimately maintained on long-term implantation.

SUGGESTED READING

James JH, Watson ACH. The use of Op-Site a vapor permeable dressing on skin graft donor sites. Br J Plast Surg 1975; 28:107–110.

Lawrence JD. The physical properties of a new hydrocolloid dressing. In: Ryan TJ, ed. An environment for healing: the role of occlusion. Royal Society of Medicine, International Congress and Symposium Series, 1985; 69.

Lelah MD, Cooper SL. Polyurethanes in medicine. Boca Raton: CRC Press, 1986.

Reed AM, Gilding DK. Biodegradable polymers for use in surgery–poly(glycolic)/poly (lactic acid) homo and copolymers: 2. In Vitro Degradation. Polymer 1981; 22:494–498.

Turner TD. Semiocclusive and occlusive dressings. In: Ryan TJ, ed. An environment for healing: the role of occlusion. Royal Society of Medicine, International Congress and Symposium Series, 1985:5.

Williams DF, ed. Biocompatibility of clinical implant materials. Vols. 1 and 2. Boca Raton: CRC Press, 1981.

Winter GD. Epidermal wound healing under a new polyurethane foam dressing (Lyofoam). Plast Reconstr Surg 1975; 56(5):531–537.

Woodroof EA. Biobrane, a biosynthetic skin prosthesis. In: Wise DL, ed. Burn wound coverings. Vol. 2. Boca Raton: CRC Press, 1984:1. 1984:1.

SYNTHETIC BIOMATERIALS FOR BONE

KENNETH E. SALYER, M.D., F.A.C.S., F.A.A.P.

Esthetic surgeons, who are primarily concerned with contour change of the bony structure of the face, readily select synthetic materials because of their ease of use and relatively low complication rate. As a surgeon who primarily deals in surgery of the cranial and facial bones, I prefer the use of autogenous bone when there is esthetic or reconstructive need for contouring the face. This is consistent with most reconstructive craniofacial surgeons who prefer direct bone remodeling with the addition of autogenous split cranial, rib, and/or iliac bone as the main source for replacement or augmentation. In this chapter I will describe my preference for the use of various materials available today for replacement of the craniofacial skeleton (Fig. 1).

ALTERNATIVE MATERIALS

A rapidly expanding number of biomaterials offer good alternatives to autogenous bone. The following discussion is based on my experience and preference for these materials. Many factors come into play in the selection of the material for face or cranial-region bone replacement: the age of the patient; the presence or absence of irradiation in the recipient site; other potential healing problems; the degree of contour change desired; the mobility of the region; the anatomy of the region; the biocompatibility of the implant; the nature of the implant and its potential for replacement or biodegradation; implant tissue reactivity; the chemistry, physiology and biostructure of the implant; the history and clinical evaluation of the material; the surgeon's experience with the implant; and the patient's and surgeon's preference. The experience and background of the surgeon appear to be key items, which markedly influence the eventual choice.

On a theoretical biologic basis, hydroxyapatite (produced by the replamineform process introduced by Interpore International) offers an improved material for ingrowth of living host bone into uniform pores in the implant (Fig. 2). One of the disadvantages of hydroxyapatite is that the material is rather difficult to contour and handle (Fig. 3). Both an advantage and disadvantage, is the lack of resorption of this material which necessitates an accurate prediction of the adjacent tissues and their subsequent remodeling.

Proplast II, a white material composed of Teflon and alumina is also a frequently used contour material since many surgeons have responded favorably to it. A combination of hydroxyapatite and Proplast has been offered by Vitek as Proplast HA (hydroxyapatite). This material deserves consideration. Injectable Teflon, methyl methacrylate, Silastic, polyethylene, and polypropylene are other possible materials offering modern day bioscience advantages.

Theoretically, temporomandibular joint (TMJ) replacement is desirable; however, long-term results for this procedure have not been satisfactory. Alloplastic TMJ replacement is in an evolutionary process. The current state-of-the-art is the Type VK2 TMJ prosthesis marketed by Vitek. Further evaluation and assessment of such prostheses may be needed, since all TMJ prostheses in current use have undergone a series of changes within a relatively short period following their introduction.

Treated and untreated autogenous tissue, such as freeze dried or lyophilized, still remain the best choice for bone replacement. Alternatives to autogenous tissue that should be considered are lyophilized cartilage, radiated homograft cartilage, xenograph cartilage, cadaver

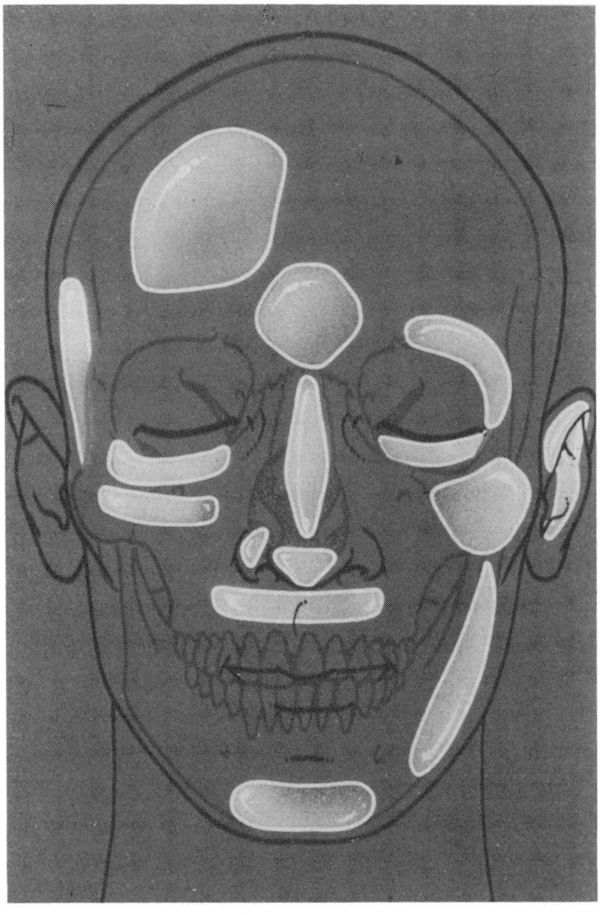

Figure 1 Multiple implant sites for commonly used alloplastic or autogenous implants.

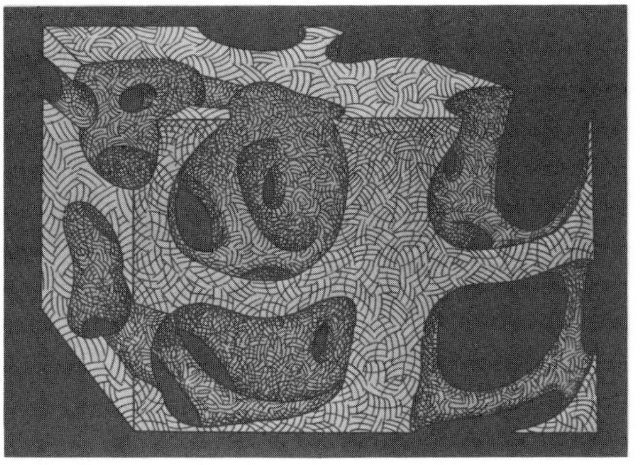

Figure 2 Illustration of the porous structure of Interpore 200. This material, produced by a replamineform process from the coral genus *Parietes*, is made up of 60 to 80 percent of space. This space allows for uniform ingrowth of bone into the porous hydroxyapatite structure.

bone, and demineralized bone paste. Each of these offers advantages and disadvantages as a bone replacement material.

Preferred Approach

Surgical exposure of the craniofacial skeleton is best obtained through a coronal incision for the upper face and zygomatic arch region, an intraoral approach through the upper labial sulcus for zygoma and maxilla, and an intraoral approach through the lower labial sulcus for mandible. The intraoral approach, which is preferred since it eliminates scars on the face, should be performed in combination with the use of antibiotics, as well as antibiotic impregnated implants, to minimize infection.

Location of Implant

I believe that all bone replacement implants should be placed next to bone. Once the periosteum is elevated, and the implant is ideally placed below it, the implant is stabilized by the periosteum and the overlying muscle, fascia, and skin. Special consideration is necessary for the chin region, where implants of Silastic and other materials have been associated with erosion of the bone, presumably as a result of implantation below the periosteum. For this reason, implants placed above the periosteum were thought superior. However, new implants made of hydroxyapatite and Proplast HA may be implanted below the periosteum for chin augmentation, since bone grows into these implants.

ALLOPLASTIC MATERIALS

Porous Hydroxyapatite (Calcium Triphosphate)

I first became aware of porous hydroxyapatite (manufactured by Interpore 200, Interpore International Irvine, CA) during a biomaterials meeting at Clemson University in 1972. The material was developed by White of Pittsburgh State using the replamineform process. We

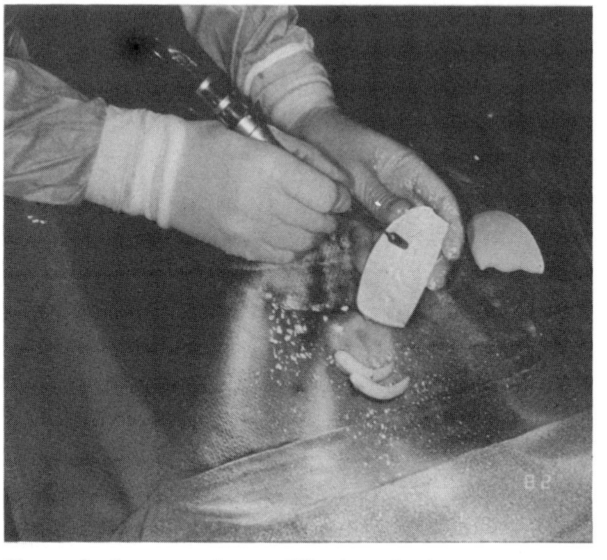

Figure 3 Intraoperative modification of a large segment of porous hydroxyapatite using a diamond bur for shaping and contouring.

became interested in the material because of the potential for a bone-like substitution in craniofacial surgery, and a number of experiments were conducted in our laboratories.

Porous hydroxyapatite is initially harvested in the South Seas as calcium carbonate coral of the genus *Parietes*. This coral has a uniform porosity of 180 to 200 microns. With the replamineform process, coral is transformed into hydroxyapatite, but the physical structure of the original uniform interconnecting pores of coral is maintained. The uniform porosity enables bone regeneration and vascularization to occur throughout the implant. Research using this process has led to its commercial development, and to the availability and involvement in this material by Interpore 200 (Interpore International). I conducted the first clinical study of this material as an onlay graft in maxillofacial surgery. During experimentation in 1982 to 1983, 45 implants were used and compared to 23 bone grafts; complications were minimal. One patient had extrusion using granules in combination with a sliding genioplasty. No other cases reported loss of the implant in this series of patients (Fig. 4).

Porous hydroxyapatite is somewhat difficult to handle because it is easily fractured. However, it can be contoured with a diamond bur or carefully carved with a scalpel (see Fig. 3). To eliminate small particles and fragments, the wound should be thoroughly washed prior to implantation. Carving or contouring should be done on the back table away from the surgical wound because of potential contamination by the particles. With this material, careful contouring should be performed before implantation to eliminate sharp edges or ridges that will not remodel because of minimal resorption. Preformed implants can be designed by a computer using CT scan data (Fig. 5). In animal studies up to 48 months post insertion, Holmes demonstrated that there is only 1 percent resorption per year. In comparison, rib onlay bone grafts undergo up to 30 to 40 percent resorption during the same time period. Hydroxyapatite is available commercially in multiple block shapes and sizes; and implants of specific design can be fabricated.

In our series of patients, this material has done well and has been followed up to 5 years post implantation without significant complications. It should be noted that these implants were used in a carefully selected group of patients without soft tissue problems, such as previous radiation or vascular disease. Good surgical judgment is needed when using this material. We do not believe that it is as good as bone but in certain cases it offers a good alternative for the reconstructive surgeon.

Porous hydroxyapatite has been used in a series of patients as an inlay material with miniplate fixation or other types of fixation with fairly good results even when exposed to open sinuses.

Interpore 200 has also been used in dentistry to prevent interdental bone resorption, being a good substitute material for bone because of minimal resorption. It also has been used clinically in more than 1,000 patients for alveolar ridge augmentation. Longitudinal follow-up has shown a high extrusion rate. For this reason, Interpore International does not recommend the continued use of this

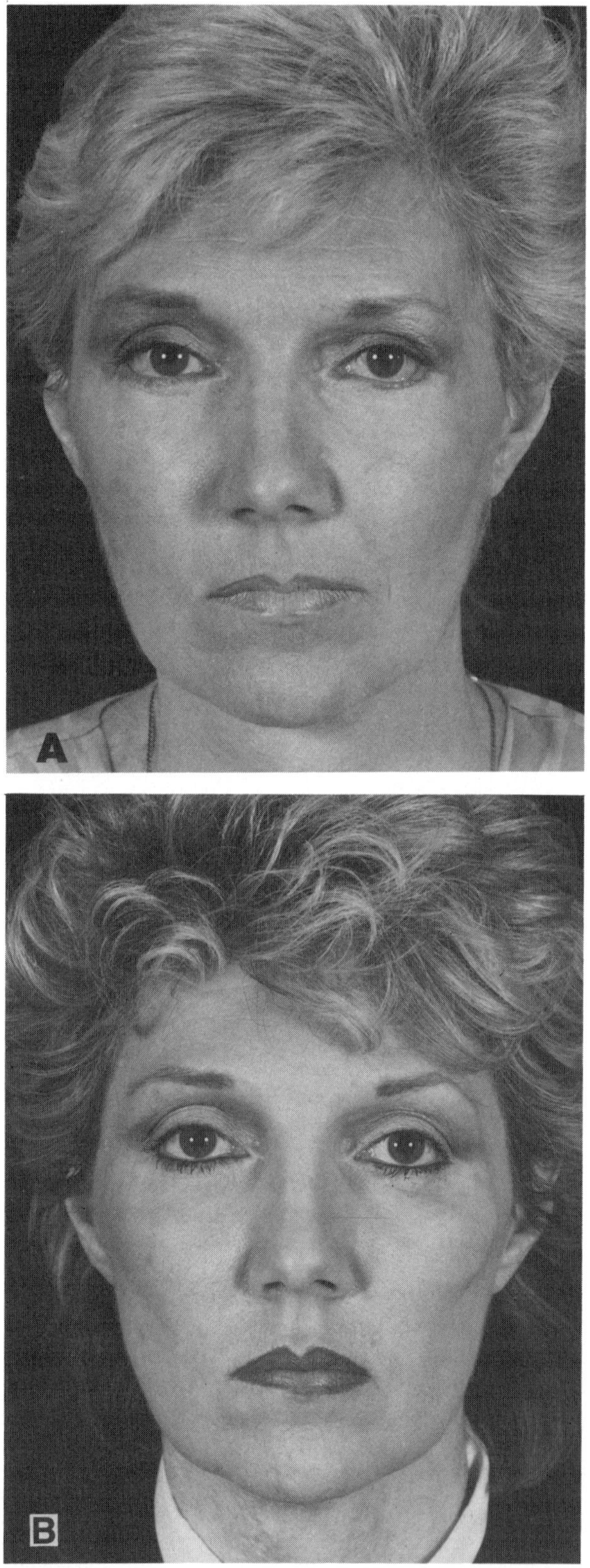

Figure 4 *A*, Preoperative frontal view of a patient with traumatic injury resulting in malar displacement treated by methyl methacrylate left malar augmentation. *B*, Postoperative view following porous-hydroxyapatite inlay malar implant designed by the computer from a CT scan using the CAD-CAM system for production of this implant.

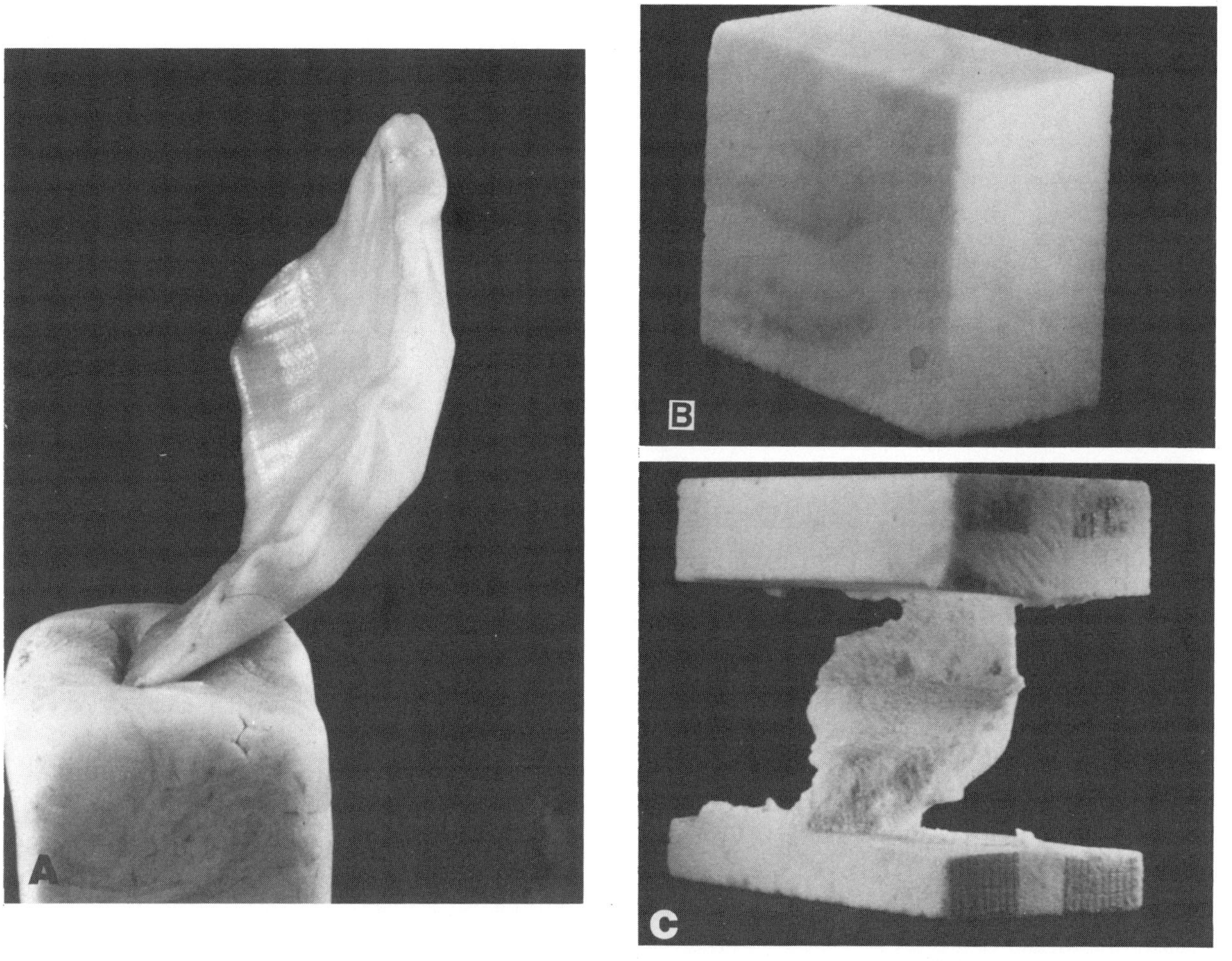

Figure 5 *A*, The plastic template constructed by a computer using 3D reconstruction from a CT scan to fashion the new implant. *B*, A block of coral that is to be carved by the computer for the patient in Figure 4. *C*, The malar implant has been machined using a CAD-CAM system driven by a computer to make a new cheek implant using the normal side flipping the mirrored image over to determine the exact contour and shape for the deformed left cheek enabling removal of the old inadequate implant and insertion at the same time of the new computer generated implant.

material for alveolar ridge augmentation. Clinical judgment regarding soft tissue coverage is important. Although this material has not done well as an alveolar implant in dental surgery its failure may be due to poor soft tissue coverage, rather than to the material per se. Initial clinical studies performed by selected expert surgeons yielded good results up to 2 years postoperatively. Hydroxyapatite deserves further evaluation and should be considered one of the best biomaterials available today in plastic surgery for facial bone replacement.

Proplast I and II

Proplast was initially marketed by Vitek as Proplast I; this alloplast was black in color and was composed of porous carbon with an added Teflon molecule. This material has been improved by combining Teflon and alumina to produce a white alloplast, Proplast II. This substance has had favorable reports by Whitaker and Freeman as a craniofacial onlay material. The complication rate has been minimal when used as a maxillary onlay. There has been an increased rate of complications when the material is used in the mandible, and for this reason, Whitaker discontinued its use in mandibular reconstruction. His overall complication rate is only 2 percent.

Proplast is available in a number of shapes and forms for implantation. Proplast is porous in volume by 70 to 90 percent, with a pore size ranging from 50 to 400 microns. It is soft, with a low modulous of elasticity and easy wetability. It is resilient, autoclavable, and easily carved. Extensive experience has shown the material to be chemically inert, biocompatible, and nonallergenic. Proplast II is rapidly stabilized to adjacent structures by ingrowth of vascularized fibrous tissue.

The Proplast package insert suggests that the material be impregnated with antibiotic solution before implantation. In practice, this recommendation has minimized secondary infection. Proplast is commercially available as chin, periorbital rim, nasal dorsum, zygomatic malar, zygomatic orbital rim, and mandibular angle implants; custom implants can also be manufactured. The advantage of this material is its easy insertion when wet because of its pliability. Thousands of Proplast implants have been utilized with a low complication rate, particularly for malar and maxillary augmentation.

Proplast Hydroxyapatite

A new material, which may offer specific advantages, combines porous hydroxyapatite and Proplast II and is marketed as Proplast (hydroxyapatite) HA. This material improves certain characteristics of hydroxyapatite but gives up the replamineform structure of Interpore 200. It looks, feels, and adapts much like Proplast II. Both substances contain an ultraporous polymer base with 70 to 90 percent porous volume and both are lightweight with a low modulus and softness similar to tissue. Also, like Proplast II, it is wetable and thus may be impregnated with antibiotics. It also allows for pliability and sculpturing with a sharp scalpel.

The theoretical advantage of adding the hydroxyapatite is that it is an osteoconductive material, as compared to Proplast, which allows only for fibrous tissue ingrowth. This material is available in block and sheeting, in preformed implant shapes for chin, malar, and custom implants, as well as a temporomandibular joint. Proplast HA can be bonded to metal mesh or other material that expands its potential utility. Time and further experience are necessary to confirm or reject these theoretical ideas regarding this new material. As an onlay material, it deserves evaluation.

Teflon Injection

Although not currently available because of FDA disapproval, injectable Teflon has been used for augmentation in and around the palate and posterior pharyngeal region primarily to adjust small defects in velopharyngeal closure. This material demonstrates a fair amount of mobility and migration, which is probably the reason why it has not been approved.

Solid Hydroxyapatite Calcitite

Solid hydroxyapatite calcitite (Calcitek, Inc., San Diego, CA) utilizes a solid form of modular solid segments of hydroxyapatite. In my opinion, it has less appeal than porous hydroxyapatite. It acts primarily as a spacer without bone ingrowth.

Methyl Methacrylate

Methyl methacrylate (Cranioplast, Codman and Shuntleff Inc., Randolph, MA) has been utilized by most neurosurgeons for cranioplasties. This material has been proven an acceptable space filler with no associated resorption and a low complication rate in secondary cranioplasties. In craniofacial surgery, it has been my experience and that of others that this material is not readily resistant to infection or trauma and may erode through soft tissue and become exposed with secondary infection. Methyl methacrylate is easily used because it can be shaped at the table. It is, however, thermic in that it generates a considerable amount of heat at the time of hardening and adjacent tissues need thermal protection. In my opinion, this material should not be used during major craniofacial surgery or in patients such as children or adolescents, whose facial bones are growing. In the mainstream of craniofacial surgery, this material has received little attention or use with a few exceptions. We have seen patients who required removal of their implant, which technically can be very difficult. Also, infection in primary or secondary major craniofacial cases or even long term after correction, is a potential hazard with this material. Therefore, use of this material in craniofacial surgery is not recommended.

Lyophilized Cartilage

Lyophilized cartilage is currently not available in the United States. It has been popularized by Obwegeser over the past 20 years, and it has been documented by Sailer who wrote his thesis and published a monograph on this material. It may be used as an inlay or an onlay grafting material in craniomaxillofacial surgery. It is a good material for contouring and may be cut with the dermatome or knife blade and used for soft tissue augmentation—particularly as a layering material in facial asymmetries. It does not have a memory and is not distorted by cutting or carving as is autogenous cartilage. Lyophilized cartilage does demonstrate some resorption but not to a major degree. It is rubbery in consistency and it may be easily carved. This is a proven material in contour reconstruction of the face, which offers promise and which will be available soon in the United States. My experience with this material, although limited, has been very favorable, and I predict a bright future for it as a contour material. It would not be satisfactory as an ear framework because of subsequent volume change. It does have promise as a bone replacement material and has demonstrated calcification in experiments by Sailer.

Radiated Homograft Cartilage

With a few exceptions, experience in Europe with radiated homograft cartilage has been extensive compared to the United States. Bardach has used this contour material in the faces of children and adults, with overall good results. Bardach initiated the use of this cartilage while in Europe and continued to use it at the University of Iowa when he moved to the USA. The material has also been utilized at the University of Michigan with favorable results. I have used radiated homograft cartilage on a number of occasions as a bone filler, when bone was resorbed or became infected, when there was a potential high-risk of repeated infections in an implantation site where organisms linger in the tissues for years. In a number of cases, this material acted as a good salvage material for permanent contour and filling of craniofacial defects. In contouring, the material demonstrates minimal problems of rejection and is recommended as a satisfactory space filler for bone.

Xenograph Cartilage (Chem RX)

The evaluation of xenograph cartilage was originally reported by Ersek. Although supported to date primarily by one investigator, the use of chemically treated bovine cartilage may offer an alternative material as a potential augmentation source. I have no experience with this material. Ersek has done research and clinical investigation and believes very strongly that it is a worthwhile material. It is currently undergoing investigations for potential approval by the FDA. Further evaluation is indicated before it could be recommended for use but it has good potential.

Cadaver Bone

I have had no experience utilizing cadaver bone. This nonliving bone is treated by various methods and acts as a lattice formation or space filler for new bone formation. I recently operated on a patient who had banked bone implanted in his mandible following a traumatic deformity. At the time of surgery, the bone demonstrated very little bleeding from the surface, however, a sagittal split of the mandible was performed and secured with lag screws. It gave a marked esthetic improvement, and the patient to date has done well.

Demineralized Bone Paste

Demineralized bone paste has been developed over a number of years by Mulliken and by the research group in Boston lead by Glowacki. This material is composed of living osteoblasts derived from treated homograft materials, which provide osteogenic cells capable of regenerating bone. This material has not been widely used or evaluated outside of Boston, and no structurally strong form of the material has been developed to date.

Demineralized bone paste can be used alone or in combination with materials such as porous hydroxyapatite, which provides a porous structure for bone regeneration. This combination could offer theoretical advantages as a graft that provides a structural supporting matrix combined with cells that have osteogenic capabilities. When implanted in the shark, a nonbone-forming animal, Glowacki has shown demineralized bone paste to be osteogenic.

Silastic

Prefabricated Silastic or Silastic 382, which is cured at the time of the surgical procedure, has been used in the craniofacial region. More recent long-term follow-up of patients receiving Silastic implants has documented a great propensity for this material to migrate. Silastic is nonreactive to adjacent tissues and is nonadherent. It is prone to loss secondary to trauma and has the potential for development of pocket infection and implant extrusion. At this time, I do not recommend this material for use as a craniofacial bone replacement.

Polyethylene or Polypropylene

In the mid 1970s, we had the opportunity to evaluate both of these porous materials in experimental animals. As materials for facial contour, they are relatively pliable and soft, and are readily contoured, cut, and adapted. A large series of patients reported by Rubin had a very low extrusion rate. Although better materials appear to be on the market, these porous materials are superior to some of the nonporous materials available today. I have no clinical experience with polyethylene or polypropylene.

Polyetherurethane and Polyethylene Terephthalate Cloth

Over the last 10 years Habal has gained experience with polyetherurethane and polyethylene terephthalate cloth mesh with autogenous bone grafts. His results have been very favorable. In noninfection-prone areas, he recommends this approach when large segments of bone replacement are needed. Other investigators have very little experience with this material. It deserves consideration and further evaluation by others.

SUGGESTED READING

Ersek RA, Denton DR. Silver impregnated porcine xenografts for treatment of meshed autographs. Ann Plast Surg 1984; 13:482–487.

Glowacki J, et al. Applications of the biological principle of induced osteogenesis for craniofacial defects. Lancet 1981; 1:959.

Habal MB, Leake DL. The biologic basis for the cascade of the bone morphogenetic pathway; experimental and clinical correlation, in craniomaxillofacial reconstruction. In: Maneksha RJ, ed. Transaction of the ninth international congress of plastic and reconstructive surgery. New Delhi: Tata McGraw-Hill, 1987:180–181.

Holmes RE, Salyer KE, Hanusiak WM. Bone regeneration in onlay replamineform hydroxyapatite implants. Transactions of the Society for Biomaterials 1978; 2:180–181.

Rubin LR. Polyethylene as a bone and cartilage substitute: a 32 year retrospective. In: Rubin LR, ed. Biomaterials in reconstructive surgery. St. Louis: CV Mosby, 1982:275.

Sailer HF. Transplantation of lyophilized cartilage im maxillofacial surgery. New York: Karger, 1983.

Salyer KE, Holmes R, Johns D. Replamineform porous hydroxyapatite as bone substitute in craniofacial osseous reconstruction. J Dent Res 1977; 56:B173.

Whitaker LA. Aesthetic augmentation of the malar-midface structures. Plast Reconstr Surg 1987; 80(3):337–346.

White EW, White RA, Weber JN: Replamineform: a new process for preparing porous ceramic, metal and polymer prosthetic materials. Science 1972; 176:922–924.

FASCIOCUTANEOUS FLAPS

GEORGE C. CORMACK, M.A., F.R.C.S.(Edin)
BYROM G. H. LAMBERTY, M.A., M.B., B.Chir., F.R.C.S.

Since Pontén's first description of a fasciocutaneous flap in 1981, the anatomy of the fasciocutaneous system has been documented by ourselves and by others. As a result, we now recognize three basic patterns of skin blood supply: (1) direct subcutaneous vessels, as in an axial skin flap; (2) the musculocutaneous system; and (3) the fasciocutaneous system. Flaps based on the fasciocutaneous system of perforators may combine the essential elements of skin, deep fascia with arterial plexus, fascial intermuscular septum with perforators, and compartmental artery from which the perforators arise, in various forms. Some of these combinations are illustrated in Figure 1.

Early fasciocutaneous flaps were either like Pontén's flaps (basically as in Fig. 1A) or like the Chinese radial forearm flap (as in Fig. 1C), but detailed modifications of these fundamental types have evolved. This process of improvement continues with a resultant increased choice of fasciocutaneous flaps, and this has given rise to the concept of *flap refinement*. Where these avenues of development will lead in the future is a matter of great interest, but already it is apparent that one road is taking us away from the fascia plus skin combination towards increased use of purely fascial flaps. In this chapter, we shall deal mainly with the established fasciocutaneous flaps and will present our views on where they may be clinically appropriate.

THERAPEUTIC ALTERNATIVES

It is no longer acceptable to select any one of a number of available flaps at random (perhaps a more appropriate definition of the term "random flap") merely to obtain skin cover over a defect without due regard to the merits or disadvantages of that particular flap. In choosing a flap, several factors need to be considered.

Requirements of the Flap in Terms of Reconstruction

The basic requirement of the majority of flaps is to provide stable epithelial cover, although we also need to

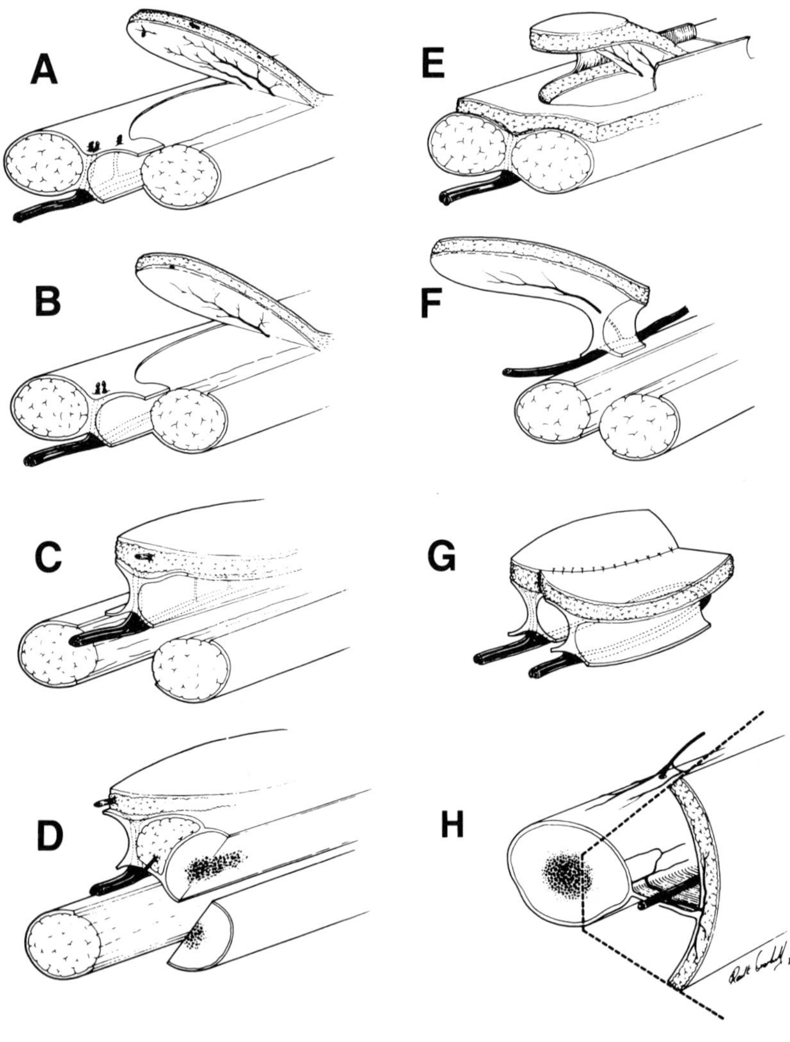

Figure 1 A schematic diagram illustrating the various forms that the fasciocutaneous flap may take. *A*, Flap dependent for arterial input on multiple vessels in the deep fascial plexus; *B*, flap dependent on a single large perforator at the level of the deep fascia; *C*, multiple perforators reaching skin along an intermuscular fascial septum and removed in continuity with the compartmental artery from which they arise; *D*, as *C*, but with a segment of bone receiving its blood supply from the same compartmental artery via branches to muscles that attach to bone; *E*, a refinement of *A* in which the skin is confined to an island on a subcutaneous and deep fascia pedicle; *F*, a modification of *B* where the single perforator is removed in continuity with a segment of the artery from which it arises (to provide a larger diameter vessel for free flap anastomosis); *G*, a modification of *C* where a long, narrow skin island is divided transversely to create a wider, shorter flap without interfering with the vascular pedicle; *H*, another method of raising an osteofasciocutaneous flap when a compartmental artery lying on a fascial septum supplies both periosteum and overlying skin.

consider the possibility of compound reconstructions additionally involving either muscle, tendon, or bone.

If, for example, all that is needed is thin supple skin to cover an exposed tendon, then a locally transposed fasciocutaneous flap may be ideal. Conversely, if a massive defect with gross tissue destruction requires cover, then a locally transposed fasciocutaneous flap is adequate in terms of skin, but a musculocutaneous or free flap is more appropriate. However, the placing of a bulky musculocutaneous free tissue transfer on a dorsal hand defect with exposed tendons is a poor choice of flap as opposed to, for example, a reverse fasciocutaneous radial forearm flap, a reverse posterior interosseous artery flap, or possibly purely fascial versions of either of these covered by split skin grafts.

Flap Reliability

We need to know how reliable a flap is in terms of its length to breadth survival. Put another way, how large is the defect to be covered and will the flap which we have selected be adequate to cover that defect? Take, for example, a defect over the elbow. A small defect might adequately be covered by the small anconeus musculocutaneous flap and a large defect by a radial forearm fasciocutaneous flap, whereas an intermediate defect is more appropriately closed by a reverse radial or ulnar recurrent island fasciocutaneous flap. This is an example of what would be termed flap refinement. The radial forearm flap is adequate cover for all these defects, but in the first instance, it is an unnecessarily large procedure for a small defect; it is ideal for the larger defect and is adequate, but less than ideal for the intermediate defect. How much more elegant to use the reverse island radial (or ulnar) recurrent fasciocutaneous flap with direct skin closure of the donor defect as opposed to the relatively more conspicuous grafted secondary defect of the radial forearm flap and the inevitable loss of the radial artery.

Vascular Anatomy

A detailed knowledge of vascular anatomy is essential to the successful raising of many flaps. We need to know not only the anatomy of the vascular pedicles and their possible variations, but also the anatomy of the perforating vessels supplying the skin. For example, in raising the reverse anterior tibial artery fasciocutaneous island flap on the lower leg, careful planning is required. Basing the skin paddle over the smaller or less constant perforators emerging between tibialis anterior and the extensors is likely to lead to a higher incidence of flap necrosis than if the flap is raised on the larger perforators of the anterior peroneal septum. In this context, it is often possible to identify the positions of the larger perforators when the flap is raised, but it should be noted that raising this type of flap involves the same techniques as raising a flap for a free microvascular tissue transfer, since the only difference between this reverse islanded pedicled flap and a free tissue transfer is that the pedicle is not ultimately divided. A surgeon should bear these considerations in mind before embarking upon such procedures.

The Donor Defect

The acceptability of a donor defect may in itself dictate our choice of flap where several flaps might be appropriate in terms of the reconstruction. Consideration of the donor defect is not entirely in cosmetic terms. For example, fractures of the radius have been reported after raising the radial forearm flap with a bone segment. Similarly, the resultant loss of muscle function from raising a muscle or musculocutaneous flap may be unacceptable. We may also need to bear in mind the possibility of delayed healing of a grafted secondary donor defect as, for example, sometimes occurs with the dorsalis pedis flap. Consideration should be given to the possibility of obtaining direct closure of a secondary defect as opposed to having to use a split-skin graft. If direct closure means that the flap has to be long and narrow while the defect to be reconstructed is broad and short, the maneuver in Figure 1G may be appropriate.

Secondary Considerations

The choice of a particular flap may be dictated by considerations of a more general nature. Facilities for microsurgery may not be available, thereby limiting the possible choice of flap and overriding some of the criteria already discussed. When establishing the aims of treatment, we should also give consideration to the patient's lifestyle and his or her attitudes to the treatment. Complicated repairs giving ideal results are to be applauded and recommended where resources and circumstances permit, but less perfect results may be acceptable where the socioeconomic background of the patient or lack of facilities dictate against more complex repairs.

Choice of flap for skin cover or compound reconstruction must, therefore, be the result of balanced consideration, and it follows that didactic recommendation of this or that flap for a particular defect is inappropriate. This chapter concerns only the relatively "new" fasciocutaneous flap, which in its original form was christened the "superflap." Superflap it may be, but all flap reconstructions have their place and we should not lose sight of the fact that these new flaps merely increase our armamentarium and do not displace what has gone before.

We feel it appropriate at this point to comment on the terminology which is being used in some of the current literature. This concerns the use of the term "septocutaneous flap." It refers to a flap in which the source artery, arising from a main artery, reaches the fascia and/or skin via a fascial septum. The term "fasciocutaneous flap" pertains to a flap in which the fascia is raised with the skin paddle. Fasciocutaneous flaps derive their blood supply from fascial septal vessels and to that extent the two terms "septocutaneous" and "fasciocutaneous" are synonymous. Strictly speaking, however, they are different anatomic descriptive terms. More appropriately, therefore, "septocutaneous" is equivalent to "fasciocutaneous perforator."

The remainder of this chapter will outline briefly the fasciocutaneous flaps currently in use and the authors' views as to their respective suitability.

THE TRUNK

Despite the fact that on the trunk there is no true deep fascia of the type forming the intermuscular septa on the limbs, there is one place on the trunk where fasciocutaneous perforators definitely do exist and that is where branches of the circumflex scapular artery emerge from between the muscles attaching to the lateral border of the scapula. These muscles belong, in evolutionary terms, to the upper limb rather than to the body wall musculature, and the perforators fan out over the rather thicker fascia covering infraspinatus. The horizontal and parascapular branches of the circumflex scapular artery may each support elliptical free flaps or the two branches together, dissected back to the circumflex scapular artery, may provide a large area of skin. The parascapular flap may be combined with the latissimus dorsi musculocutaneous flap to provide a large free tissue transplant on one vascular pedicle. The parascapular branch appears to be the more reliable of the two, and its flap has a particular use as a local pedicled transposition flap (Fig. 1B) for release of axillary scar contractures. The donor site may be closed directly with flaps up to 12 cm in width. None of these flaps has the capability of sensory innervation.

THE UPPER LIMB

In the upper limb, the local pedicled flap of choice is, without doubt, a fasciocutaneous flap by virtue of the fact that the arterial supply to the skin of the forelimb is by fasciocutaneous perforators. Muscle flaps in the upper limb are limited to the coracobrachialis, the anconeus, and the flexor carpi ulnaris since these are the only muscles with a dominant proximal vascular pedicle.

The Arm

The upper arm provides us with two useful flap donor sites—the medial and lateral arm flaps. These flaps are based on the fasciocutaneous perforators in the medial and lateral intermuscular septa arising respectively from the superior ulnar collateral artery and the middle collateral artery.

As a free flap donor site, the upper limb provides thin, supple, and (on the medial side) relatively hairless skin. The donor defects can usually be closed directly. Both vessels are consistently large enough (1.5 to 3 mm diameter) for microvascular anastomosis. The lateral flap may be raised with the lateral cutaneous nerve of the arm and therefore has sensory potential.

These flaps are illustrated in Figures 2 and 3. The medial arm flap is of the type shown in Figure 1F, whereas the lateral flap follows the principles of Figure 1C with the potential of incorporating a segment of the lateral supracondylar ridge of the humerus as in Figure 1H.

The Elbow

Defects around the elbow had been difficult to cover with local flaps until the advent of fasciocutaneous flaps. The antecubital fasciocutaneous flap and the more recently described radial and ulnar recurrent fasciocutaneous flaps are all suitable for repair of defects around the elbow. The only locally available muscle flaps are the flexor carpi ulnaris, brachioradialis, and anconeus flaps, all of which have serious limitations.

The antecubital flap is based on a perforator of the radial artery arising on average 4 cm distal to the midpoint of a line joining the humeral epicondyles. This vessel has been named the inferior cubital artery. A flap of up to 17 by 4 cm in the style of Figure 1B can be raised and will reach all points around the elbow. As a free flap, it may be raised with a segment of the radial artery in the manner of Figure 1F (vide infra).

Alternative flaps are the distally based radial and ulnar recurrent flaps; all points around the elbow may be covered between these two flaps. In particular, they are a first choice flap for defects of the antecubital fossa where the inferior cubital artery is damaged or when release of scar contracture requires the insetting of a flap in front of the elbow. These two distally-based island flaps have the added advantage that, with a defect up to 5 cm wide, direct closure of the secondary defect can generally be achieved.

The Forearm

Flap skin cover for the forearm itself is rarely required, but if it is, then a distant flap in the form of either a pedicled groin/abdominal flap or a free flap is required.

As a free flap donor site, the Chinese radial forearm flap has now been proven as one of the most useful and versatile flaps discovered. The skin paddle is nourished by fasciocutaneous perforators from the radial artery that may be removed between elbow and wrist in continuity with the flap. The flap may be used where any thin skin is required and, in particular, it has been used extensively for intraoral reconstruction with or without a segment of radius for mandibular segmental reconstruction. As a free flap, one of the disadvantages of the radial forearm flap is that the larger the skin paddle becomes, the shorter the free vascular pedicle remaining; this may present problems at the recipient site. Increased venous pedicle length can be obtained by dissecting out the basilic or cephalic veins in the upper arm, and increased arterial pedicle length can be achieved by dividing the septum (containing perforators) connecting the distal radial artery and overlying flap, thereby leaving the skin supplied only by the inferior cubital vessel. In this form, the arterial anastomosis is made to the distal end of the radial artery, which then creates a long reverse-flow pedicle. An example of this is illustrated in Figure 4.

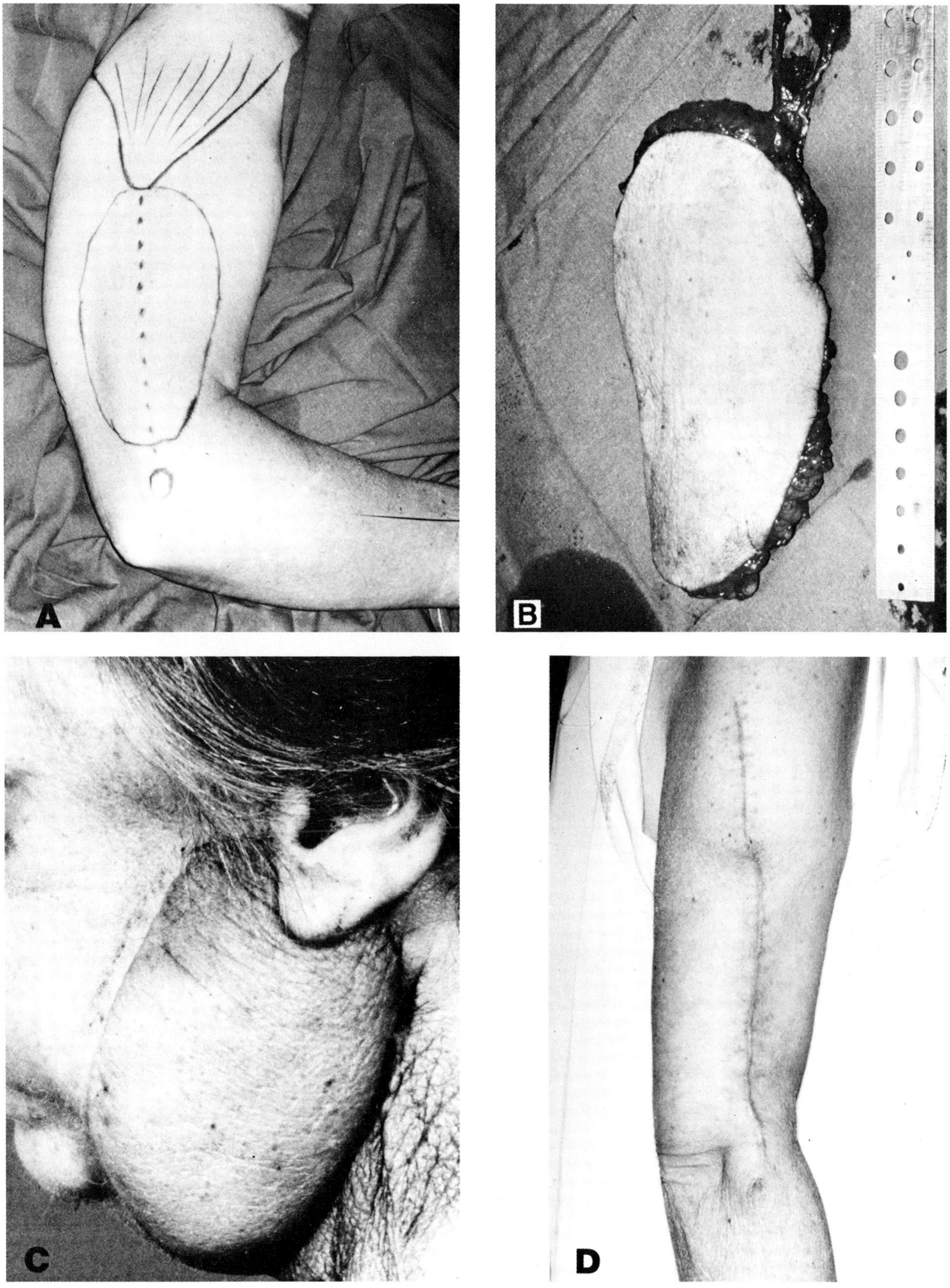

Figure 2 Lateral arm free flap based on middle collateral artery used for facial reconstruction (as in Fig. 1*C*). *A*, The skin paddle marked out on the lateral arm with its upper limit at the insertion of the deltoid. *B*, the flap raised with the middle collateral artery and venae comitans. *C*, The flap in place one month postoperatively. *D*, Direct closure of the donor defect.

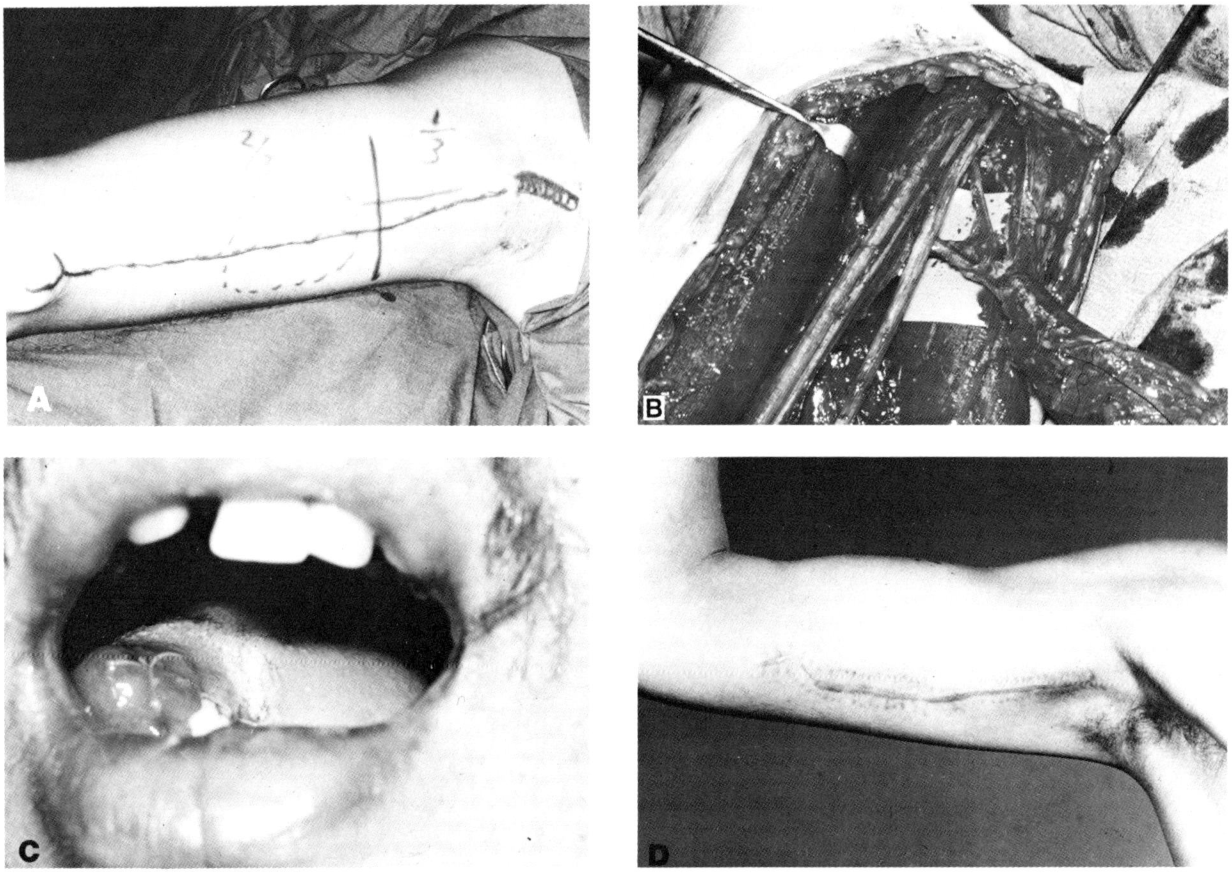

Figure 3 Medial arm free flap based on a large fascial branch of the superior ulnar collateral artery (as in Fig. 1*B*), used for intraoral reconstruction. *A*, The skin paddle marked out in the arm and centered over the medial intermuscular septum. *B*, The flap pedicle illustrating the superior ulnar collateral artery. The median nerve and brachial artery lie anteriorly. *C*, The flap in the oral floor 3 months postoperatively. *D*, Direct closure of the donor defect.

One of the great merits of the radial forearm flap is the ease with which it may be raised, even when including bone. In order to reduce the likelihood of subsequent fracture, it is recommended that oblique saw cuts should be made in the radius so that less than half the cross-sectional area of the radius is removed. The length of radius that can be taken is limited proximally by the insertion of the pronator teres and distally by the brachioradialis. The medial and lateral cutaneous nerves of the forearm give this flap sensory potential.

Although usually used as a free flap, the radial forearm flap may be reverse pedicled for osteoplastic reconstruction of the thumb.

One of the major drawbacks of the radial forearm flap is the donor site defect that is not only cosmetically poor, but may give rise to complications such as exposed tendons. Where a small skin paddle is used, it is preferable to locate this paddle as high as possible on the forearm, not only because of the cosmetic appearance, but because the donor defect then lies over muscle bellies rather than over tendons.

Perhaps one of the main disadvantages of the radial forearm flap is its very simplicity. How many times has this flap been used when perhaps some other flap might have been equally good in terms of functional result and better in terms of donor defect cosmesis? For example, the medial arm flap illustrated in Figure 2, although less easy to raise and perhaps for that reason less reliable, is perfectly adequate for intraoral reconstruction and leaves a much more acceptable donor defect. The radius is popular for mandibular reconstruction, but if we are looking for flap refinement, then the carved and sculpted bone of the pelvis as advocated by Taylor must surely be an improvement, although it appears to require sophisticated molds and preformers and a degree of expertise that not all of us might be able to achieve.

The ulnar forearm flap has found less popularity than its radial counterpart possibly because it is no more versatile than the latter and is a little more difficult to raise. It provides equally thin supple skin with an innervative potential and the added advantage that the skin on the ulnar border of the forearm is less hairy than it is on the radial border.

The posterior interosseous artery flap, either proximally or distally pedicled, is a more difficult flap to raise and its place has not yet been fully established. It may

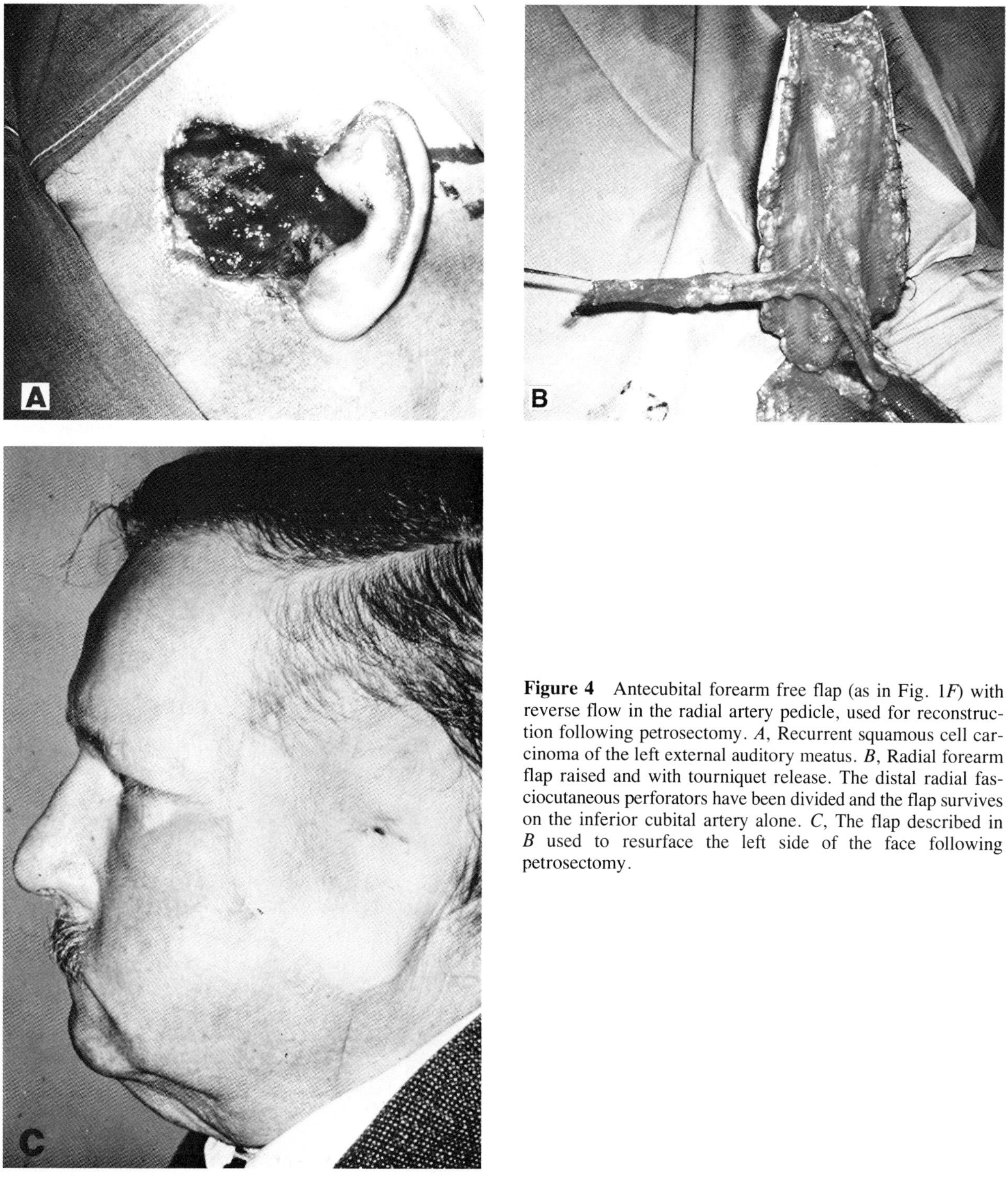

Figure 4 Antecubital forearm free flap (as in Fig. 1*F*) with reverse flow in the radial artery pedicle, used for reconstruction following petrosectomy. *A*, Recurrent squamous cell carcinoma of the left external auditory meatus. *B*, Radial forearm flap raised and with tourniquet release. The distal radial fasciocutaneous perforators have been divided and the flap survives on the inferior cubital artery alone. *C*, The flap described in *B* used to resurface the left side of the face following petrosectomy.

find a limited role in distally pedicled form for reconstruction of small defects on the dorsum of the distal forearm and hand.

THE LOWER LIMB

The Lower Leg

The fasciocutaneous flap is the flap of choice for nonextensive tissue loss with exposed tendon or bone. By nonextensive, we refer, not to the area of skin loss, but rather to the depth and severity of the injury. Where massive soft tissue destruction has occurred, either a local muscle flap or a free muscle transfer is indicated. The superiority of the muscle or musculocutaneous unit over any other flap for cover of contaminated or infected defects has been elegantly demonstrated in the laboratory of Chang and Mathes. Massive destruction of tissue by trauma invariably compromises the fasciocutaneous flaps as a result of local vascular damage either to the perforating vessels or the main limb arteries, and because of edema of the deep fascia and subcutaneous tissues.

Proximally or distally based pedicled fasciocutaneous flaps on the medial or lateral aspects of the leg are made possible by the multiple fasciocutaneous perforating vessels arising from the posterior tibial, anterior tibial, and peroneal vessels. In general terms, vessels on the medial side of the leg are larger and more reliable than on the lateral side, and the medial flap is preferred where a choice exists.

The posterior aspect of the upper calf may also be utilized as a fasciocutaneous flap donor site. The flap is based on superficial sural arteries that arise from the sural arteries before they enter gastrocnemius. The flap may be extended as far distally as the commencement of the Achilles tendon.

Fasciocutaneous flaps on the leg have been criticized on the grounds that the resultant donor defect, which usually has to be grafted, is unacceptable. Critics would suggest that the muscle flap is preferable in this respect, but in our experience, the donor defect in the lower leg is of secondary importance when compared to the ease and simplicity with which these flaps may be transposed without resultant functional loss.

The ankle region is still a problem area in terms of local flap cover. The deep fascia of the leg blends with the retinacula around the ankle joint, and proximally pedicled fasciocutaneous flaps at the level of the malleoli become unreliable. However, the reverse fasciocutaneous island flaps in the lower leg have gone some way towards solving this problem. In particular, the reverse anterior tibial island flap (Fig. 1C) has proved useful and is illustrated in Figure 5. In this flap, venous drainage is by reverse flow in the venae comitantes. This concept of reverse flow in vessels is one which we feel will become more important in the future.

Distally-based pedicled flaps based on perforators from the peroneal artery and of the posterior tibial artery have been described. These may follow the principles of Figures 1A, B, and E. Island cutaneous flaps (Fig. 1C) based on the peroneal artery, with and without fibula, are also possibilities.

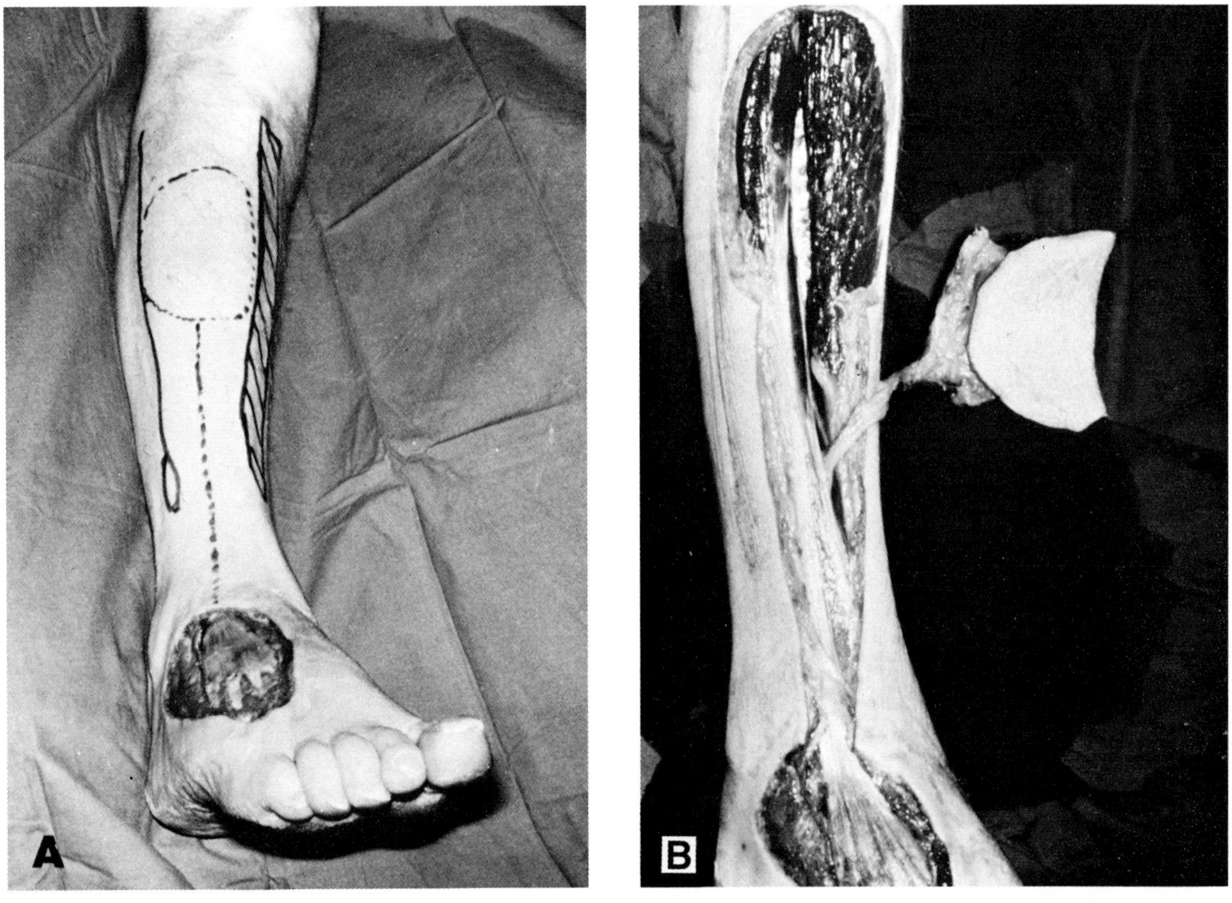

Figure 5 Distally pedicled anterior tibial artery fasciocutaneous island flap used to achieve skin cover of exposed tendons on the dorsum of the foot (as Fig. 1*C*). *A*, Dorsal foot defect with reverse island anterior tibial flap drawn out. The shaded area represents the tibia and the lateral line, the fibula. *B*, The flap raised on its reversed pedicled anterior tibial artery together with the perforators reaching the skin paddle along the anterior peroneal septum.

Figure continues on opposite page

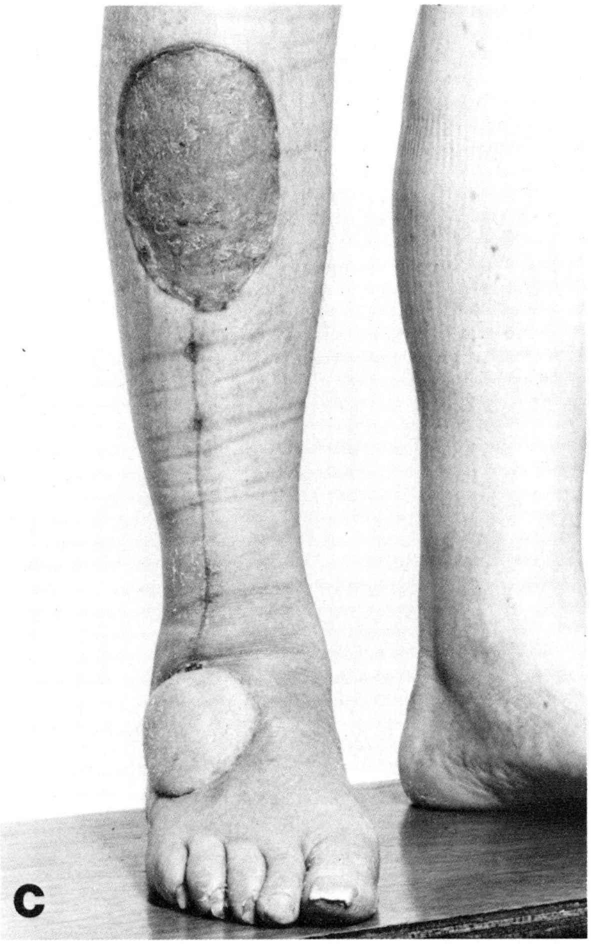

Figure 5 (continued) The flap in position 1 month postoperatively.

The Foot

A fasciocutaneous flap can be raised on the medial plantar artery based on its perforating branches, which emerge along the septum between abductor hallucis and flexor digitorum brevis (Fig. 1C). This flap was originally described as a musculocutaneous flap incorporating the abductor hallucis muscle, but this is not necessary to the vascular support of the skin island; excluding this muscle from the flap confers the advantages of reduced donor site morbidity and elimination of a wad of soft tissue from beneath the flap which, if transposed to a weight-bearing area, would tend to confer a feeling of flap mobility and instability.

Whether the lateral calcaneal flap based on calcaneal branches of the peroneal artery should be classed as fasciocutaneous is uncertain, but we have certainly found it to be a useful local flap, particularly in islanded form, for reconstructing small defects around the heel.

The Thigh

The thigh is unquestionably an area dominated by muscle flaps, and therefore, we do not consider fasciocutaneous flaps of the thigh to be a first choice for local reconstructions. Thigh skin is largely supplied by musculocutaneous perforators, and a thigh defect requiring flap cover is likely to require bulk that cannot be provided by a fasciocutaneous flap.

Two fasciocutaneous free flaps are available from the thigh—the medial and lateral thigh flaps. These conform to the general pattern of Figure 1B.

The lateral thigh free flap is based on the third profunda perforator branch, which passes along the lateral intermuscular septum and fans out anteriorly over the iliotibial tract. Pedicled or islanded flaps may also be based on the first profunda perforator and used for cover in trochanteric or ischial pressure sores. However, since most of these defects are deep, we would prefer a musculocutaneous flap.

Branches of the femoral artery provide the basis for two further free flaps—the medial thigh free flap in its proximal third and the saphenous free flap in its distal third.

The medial thigh flap is based on a perforator passing around the medial border of sartorius in the apex of the femoral triangle. A similar flap, based on perforators from the lateral circumflex femoral artery, has also been described, but we have found this to be an inconstant vessel.

The saphenous free flap is based on the branches of the descending genicular artery, which give it a moderately long pedicle. The flap itself is thin and has the potential for innervation and for direct closure of the donor defect if small. The main disadvantage of this flap is that it requires a careful dissection and a detailed knowledge of the vascular anatomy and its variations. It is little used.

SUGGESTED READING

Acland RD, Schusterman M, Godina M, Eder E, Taylor GI, Carlisle I. The saphenous neurovascular free flap. Plast Reconstr Surg 1981; 67:763–774.

Amarante J, Costa H, Reis J, Soares R. A new distally based fasciocutaneous flap of the leg. Br J Plast Surg 1986; 39:338–340.

Baek S-M. Two new cutaneous free flaps: the medial and lateral thigh flaps. Plast Reconstr Surg 1983; 71:354–363.

Biemer E, Stock W. Total thumb reconstruction: a one-stage reconstruction using an osteo-cutaneous forearm flap. Br J Plast Surg 1983; 36:52–55.

Chang N, Mathes SJ. Comparison of the effects of bacterial inoculation in musculocutaneous and random pattern flaps. Plast Reconstr Surg 1982; 70:1–9.

Cormack GC, Lamberty BGH. The arterial anatomy of skin flaps. Edinburgh: Churchill Livingstone, 1986.

Donski PK, Fogdestam I. Distally based fasciocutaneous flap from the sural region. A preliminary report. Scand J Plast Reconstr Surg 1983; 17:191–196.

Lovie MJ, Duncan GM, Glasson DW. The ulnar artery forearm free flap. Br J Plast Surg 1984; 37:486–492.

Maruyama Y, Onishi K, Iwahira Y. The ulnar recurrent fasciocutaneous island flap: reverse medial arm flap. Plast Reconstr Surg 1987, 79:381–387.

Maruyama Y, Takeuchi S. The radial recurrent fasciocutaneous flap: reverse upper arm flap. Br J Plast Surg 1986; 39:458–461.

Parry SW, Wood JW, Mathes SJ. Vascular anatomy of the upper extremity muscles. Plast Reconstr Surg (In press).

Ponte̗n B. The fasciocutaneous flap: its use in soft tissue defects of the lower leg. Br J Plast Surg 1981; 34:215—220.

Song YG, Chen GZ, Song YL. The free thigh flap: a new free flap con-

cept based on the septocutaneous artery. Br J Plast Surg 1984; 37:149–159.
Taylor GI. Circumflex iliac osteocutaneous flaps. Transactions of the IXth International Congress of Plastic and Reconstructive Surgery 1987.
Wee JTK. Reconstruction of the lower leg and foot with the reverse-pedicled anterior tibial flap: preliminary report of a new fasciocutaneous flap. Br J Plast Surg 1986; 39:327–337.

SOFT TISSUE EXPANSION

ERNEST K. MANDERS, M.D.
MAMDOUH A. MOTTALEB, M.B., B.Ch., M.Sc.
PETER T. HETZLER, M.D.

Soft tissue expansion allows reconstruction of soft tissue defects with tissues like those lost. This is accomplished with minimal donor site deformity. The technique depends upon the progressive distention of a subcutaneous envelope of silicone elastomer. The balloon-like envelope is filled by the injection of sterile isotonic saline into a self-sealing injection port. As the envelope is progressively inflated, the overlying tissues are increased in area. The expanded flaps may then be advanced for a wide range of reconstructive procedures.

Numerous precedents occur in nature for soft tissue expansion. Pregnancy affords an example of gradual distention of soft tissues by an enlarged underlying mass. Afterward there is redundant tissue in the abdominal wall, but the redundancy typically contracts and is largely eliminated. However, were the redundant tissue advanced and supported by underlying tissues, it would maintain its increased area. Controlled soft tissue expansion is precisely analogous to this.

Redundant tissue following massive weight loss is another obvious example of what can be achieved with progressive soft tissue distention. Controlled expansion was foretold by the progressive distention of lips and earlobes, which has been known since ancient times.

Though these examples make the possibility of controlled soft tissue expansion seem obvious, it was not until Dr. Charles G. Neumann first attempted expansion of periauricular skin to reconstruct the upper portion of an auricle that controlled soft tissue expansion was introduced to plastic surgery. Though Neumann presented this in 1956 and published it in 1957, the full implications were not appreciated and the idea was lost.

Dr. Chadomir Radovan devised a totally implantable device, which he used to remove a tattoo in 1976. This ushered in the modern era of soft tissue expansion. A number of manufacturers expressed interest in the new technique and through their efforts a variety of well designed and carefully manufactured soft tissue expanders have become available. Devices today consist of silicone elastomer envelopes with both remote injection ports attached by a tube and injection ports incorporated in the envelope itself. They come in a variety of shapes and sizes (Fig. 1).

The surgeon who employs soft tissue expansion ascends a learning curve. Success in soft tissue expansion depends upon an appreciation of principles and careful planning. The latter is of paramount importance. This chapter describes the principles for planning and safe conduct of soft tissue expansion.

Soft Tissue Expansion Is Not For Immediate Reconstruction

Useful though it is, it is important to realize that soft tissue expansion is a late reconstructive technique. With the exception of expander placement at the time of mastectomy, soft tissue expansion is not a technique that can be used immediately for reconstruction of acute injuries. It should follow skin grafting of a soft tissue avulsion in an extremity, for instance, with late reconstruction being the goal. After extirpation of a malignancy, a period of ob-

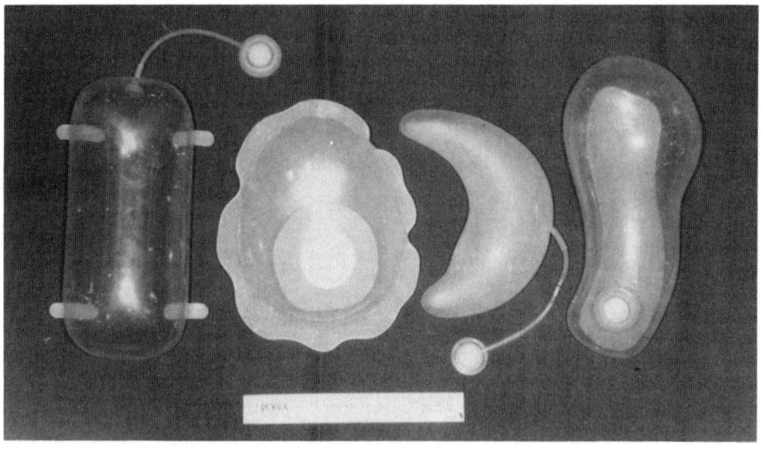

Figure 1 Different expanders now available: from left to right, a backless expander with a remote injection port, an expander with a still backer and an integrated injection port, a croissant expander with a custom base, and a differential expander whose envelope expands more at one end. Surgeons may specify type of injection port, presence or absence of a backer, shape of the base plate, and properties of the envelope.

servation is often required. Here too one would not carry out a soft tissue expansion immediately.

It is particularly important to note that a soft tissue expander should not be inserted next to a malignancy in order to advance an expanded flap at the time of tumor excision. The reasons for this are twofold. First, it is conceivable that one might distribute tumor cells throughout the expander cavity and thereby disseminate the malignancy. Second, intraoperative frozen section determination of the tumor margin might require a larger than anticipated excision, which may leave the expanded flap too small to do the job.

Hemangiomas that have an unstable surface, and particularly those that may have been infected, may best be treated by primary excision and subsequent skin grafting, with repair of the defect by soft tissue expansion to follow when primary healing has been completed. This approach has been fostered by troublesome seromas and hematomas around expanders placed next to hemangiomas. Furthermore, infection may also complicate such placement.

Choose A Suitable Patient

To carry out a soft tissue expansion successfully, stable skin of adequate dimension must be available. Scarred skin, skin graft, and soft tissues that have been irradiated are by and large not suitable for soft tissue expansion. It is particularly important to emphasize that irradiated soft tissue, which appears of good quality, may not survive after its elevation as a flap following soft tissue expansion. Furthermore irradiated tissue tends to be less distensible. The course of expansion is usually prolonged and may require such high pressures that the process of inflation becomes painful. Discomfort is always undesirable.

In addition, a patient must be psychologically stable. A patient who may become reclusive because of extreme self-consciousness is not an appropriate candidate for soft tissue expansion. Likewise, a psychotic patient who does not understand what is going on may not cope with the process of expansion, and his course may thus be complicated.

Soft tissue expansion should be chosen for the patient for whom it offers special advantages. It is ideal for replacing a shortage of skin. Such a shortage may exist because of a previous burn or because a large benign nevus is to be resected. An increase in available skin area may be essential for creating an envelope for breast reconstruction (Fig. 2). For some patients, skin of special qualities such as scalp or beard-bearing skin may be required. In other patients, it might not be possible to form the needed flap because of inadequate donor site dimensions, inadequate vascularity, or because without expanded tissues to close the donor site, the deformity would be unacceptable. Patients who need expanded frontalis muscle for forehead reconstruction are particularly good candidates for soft tissue expansion. Furthermore soft tissue expansion may be used all over the body to minimize donor site defects. For instance, even a cross-leg flap may be raised after expansion. This will allow a longer flap with better vascularity. In addition, the donor site can be closed primarily without a depressed skin graft marking the donor site of the flap.

Soft tissue expansion also offers an additional advantage in that contour deformities can be partially or wholly corrected. By advancing an expanded flap, one can improve the surface appearance, as in replacing an area of skin graft, and also largely eliminate the depressed contour. An expanded flap may also be de-epithelialized at its tip and folded on itself for additional bulk.

Counsel The Patient

All patients must be advised that there will be a change in appearance. In the case of breast reconstruction using soft tissue expansion, this is a salutary change. However, late in the course of expansion, if a large skin envelope is being generated, there can be abnormal infraclavicular fullness, which can make patients self-conscious. Soft tissue expansion over the scalp can often be masked with a hat or scarf as can forehead expansions. Some soft tissue expansions are difficult to hide, however, and the method of coping should be openly discussed with the patient.

In talking to our patients, we encourage them to "go public." They are urged to discuss the process of expansion frankly with anyone curious enough to ask about it. By and large, patients have found their friends and associates and even strangers to be most sympathetic and supportive.

Patients need to be counseled regarding the time required for the completion of expansion and the fact that a number of visits will usually be necessary. Indeed, soft tissue expansion is labor intensive. A patient who cannot afford the time required is not suitable for the technique. It must be emphasized again and again that soft tissue expansion will proceed until an adequate arc of tissue is available for reconstruction. Patients are told that no one fits a formula exactly. Patients must be willing to accommodate schedules to afford the amount of time required for complete expansion before reconstruction.

Many of our patients have enjoyed the convenience of home expansion. Our hospital is located in a rural setting, and it is difficult for many patients to travel the distances between home and clinic. We have found it easy to instruct families and patients in the technique of soft tissue expansion so that it may be reliably and safely conducted at home. Patients and families who indicate an interest in this alternative are given an instructional course over 2 to 3 weeks. The instruction takes them from filling syringes to actually making the injections and monitoring the pressures as they fill the expander. Patients are called periodically and are expected to visit every 3 to 4 weeks during expansion to gauge progress. Some patients are even given paper measuring tapes so that they may monitor their own progress and report it. It has been our experience that granting the patient and his family this independence and confidence makes them ready allies in the treatment program.

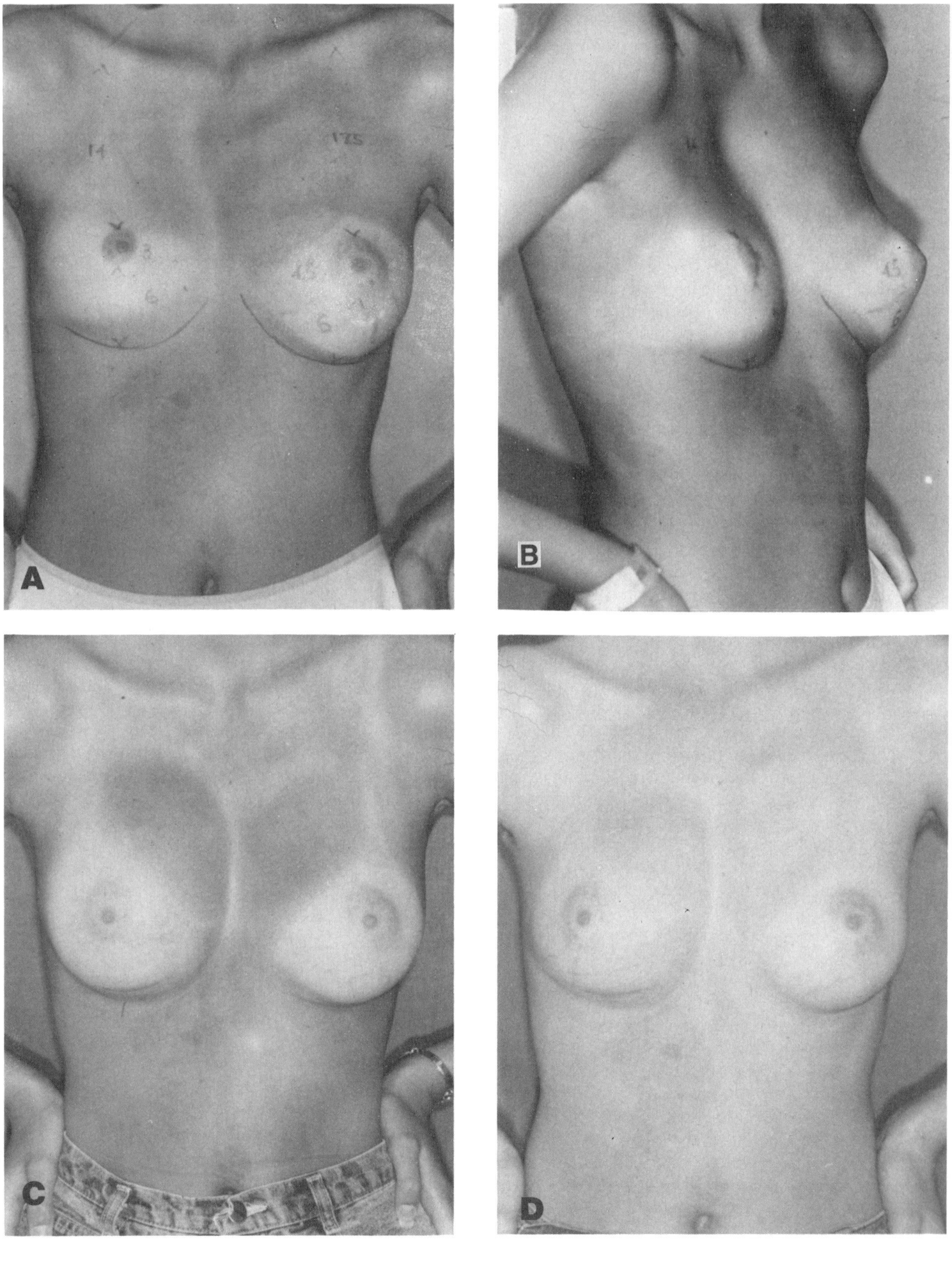

Figure 2 *A* and *B*, A patient with thoracic asymmetry and a hypoplastic right breast. *C*, The right breast expanded with the appearance of stria and increased diameter of the nipple-areolar complex. *D*, The patient with a permanent breast prosthesis in place and carved Silastic filling the area of sternal cavity.

Figure continues on opposite page

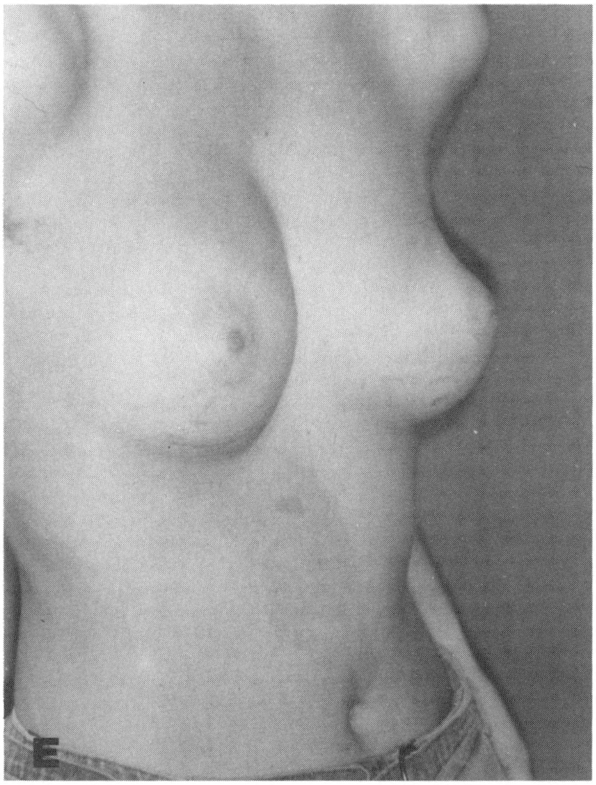

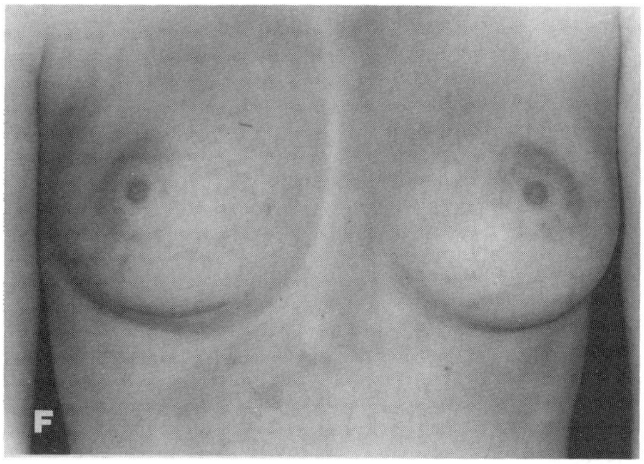

Figure 2 (continued) *E*, Profile view. *F*, Breast symmetry.

Proper Flap Design Is The Key To Success

When creating any flap, three general concerns come to mind first. First, the vascularity of the intended flap must be preserved. It is important to remember the site of the cutaneous arteries supplying the tissue to be expanded. The angiosome concept advanced by Taylor and his co-workers is of value in planning placement of soft tissue expanders. Surgeons should remember that vessels serving angiosomes frequently exit intramuscular septa. Observing this anatomic fact aids the surgeon in fashioning pockets for expanders with circulation to overlying soft tissue intact.

A second concern is where the final scars will lie. For example, if expanding to eliminate burn scar from the anterior abdominal wall, it is better to expand anteriorly and to move the expanded skin laterally to leave the scar closure on the flank. Here it will be less obvious.

In several instances, one should design soft tissue expansion with attention toward what may happen in the future. For example, in expanding about the face or under the scalp of a male, one must keep in mind that with the development of secondary sex characteristics the beard grows and the anterior hairline recedes. One should plan soft tissue expansion for scalp reconstruction for the eventuality that male pattern hairloss may develop. In some situations, it is possible to prevent marked asymmetries caused by loss of hair on one side without comparable loss on the other side of the head. Likewise one must be careful not to expand and advance bearded skin to an unnatural location on the face of a male child.

A variety of flaps may be fashioned with the aid of soft tissue expansion. These include hemispheric flaps, croissant flaps, differential expanded flaps, axial flaps, and distant random flaps. In addition, the technique can be of use for temporary intraoperative expansion to gain added flap length for closure of difficult wounds, such as for a myelomeningocele.

Hemispheric Flaps

Hemispheric flaps are flaps typically generated by today's soft tissue expanders. Even if there is a rectangle with a length similar to the width, the result will be a flap approximating a hemisphere. Hemispheric flaps work well when advanced across the vertex or around the occiput. Here the flap fits the curved surface of the calvarium like a glove. It is more difficult to advance a hemispheric flap across the top of the head or on a flat surface, such as the back, or around a cylindrical surface, such as the arm. Hemispheric flaps have significant limitations. Some surgeons have attempted to overcome these limitations by incising the flaps and unfurling them. This can lead to longer scars and decreased flap vascularity. Planning can be more sophisticated in order to avoid having a hemispheric flap with limited potential for advancement over the trunk or an extremity.

Croissant Flaps

Croissant flaps are generated by a crescent-shaped expander, which half surrounds the defect intended for resurfacing (Fig. 3). The croissant is wider in the middle, hence the arc of expansion is greater there. This is appropriate because the round or elliptical defect requires a greater advancement across the middle than at either end. A mini-

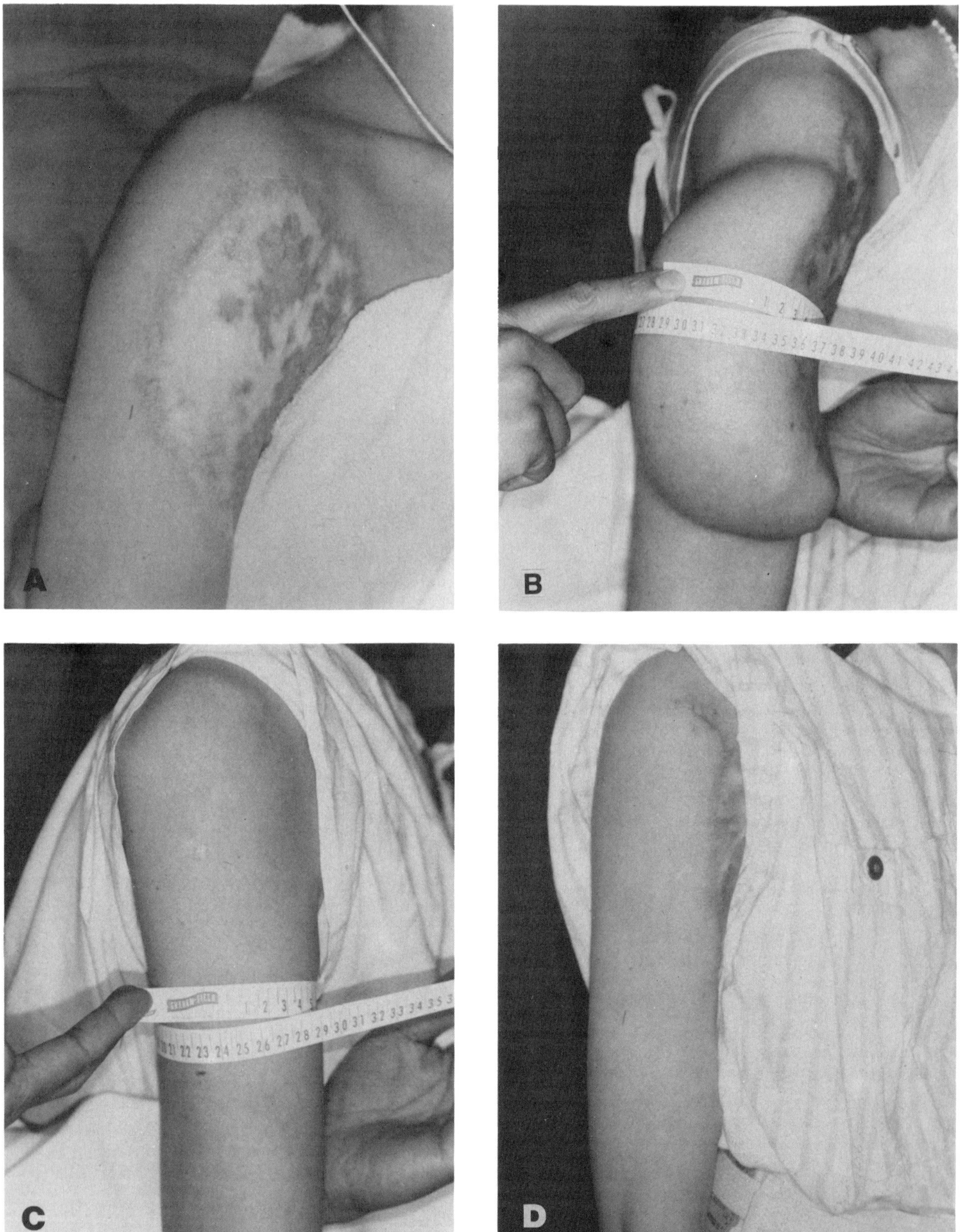

Figure 3 *A*, Burn scar of the upper arm. *B* and *C*, Croissant expander in place adjacent to the burn scar. The tape compares the circumference over the expander with that of the other arm. The difference predicts the advancement possible. *D*, The upper arm after advancement.

mum of scar is generated with this flap for the edge adjacent the expander advances like a handle of a bucket over the mouth of the bucket to approach the far edge of the defect. The chief advantage of the croissant flap is that it half surrounds the defect. Thus one can move the edge of the defect more easily than in the case of a hemispheric flap. The hemispheric flap is restrained by the periphery of the expanded tissue and the unexpanded soft tissue between the periphery of the expansion and the edge of the defect.

Differentially Expanded Flaps

Differentially expanded flaps are formed by asymmetric expansions. In selected situations, surgeons may wish to make one end of a flap larger than another end. One way to achieve this is to carry out a differential expansion. This has proven useful in eliminating male pattern baldness. For this, a soft tissue expander is placed under both the right and left sides of the hairbearing scalp. With expansion, the temporal area is expanded more than the occipital area. The temporal area may then advance further medially and anteriorly to establish a new hairline. In the case of breast reconstruction, differential expanders are being developed to produce more projection caudally with less infraclavicular fullness. It is hoped that this will also generate a larger skin envelope than conventional hemispheric expanders so that ptosis can be achieved in a greater number of patients.

Axial Flaps

Axial flaps of great value may be developed with soft tissue expansion. An example is the expanded median forehead flap used for total nasal reconstruction. This flap is based upon the supratrochlear artery of one side or the other. This flap may be thinned of its capsule and frontalis muscle so that it can be folded with great ease. Prior expansion can afford an axial pattern flap of great dimension, and increased vascularity. Furthermore, the donor defect may be closed primarily.

Distant Random Flaps

Distant random flaps may be prepared using soft tissue expansion with elimination of donor defect and increased length because of enhanced vascularity. It is possible now to create cross-leg flaps from donor sites that parallel the popliteal crease. These sites are much less visible than traditional axial donor sites, which were skin grafted in the past.

Temporary Expansion

Temporary expansion may be of great value in avoiding excessive tension in the closure of selected wounds. We have used this successfully in elongating the skin flaps for midline closure over myelomeningocele repairs. Temporary expansion can be utilized in the operating room with cyclical loading of the skin so that there is a nonelastic deformation, that is, stretching that affords extra length and allows closure without relaxing incisions or other maneuvers to create a longer-length flap.

Expander Ports

Many expander designs are available today. It is possible to obtain expanders with injection ports that are integrated into the envelope or remote from the envelope. Some surgeons prefer remote valves because they feel that perforation of the envelope is less likely if the port is distant on the end of a tube. For other surgeons, carrying out an expansion with a valve integrated into the envelope is more convenient. It is easier to insert an expander and remove it if the filling port is integrated into the envelope.

A remote injection port requires careful positioning away from the envelope if it is to be used. Its removal is always more difficult because it is invested by fibrous tissue. A remote port should not be placed over a bony prominence such as the mastoid where necrosis may ensue with exposure of the port. Furthermore, a remote port should not be placed caudal to the envelope, as in the case of an expander over the trunk, for as the expander grows it may overhang the injection port which makes filling very difficult. Remote subcutaneous ports may be located higher in the subcutaneous fat, off the fascia in fleshy areas such as the thigh. In addition, a suture placed around the tubing may prevent the injection port from pulling back into the larger expander cavity. Redundant tubing may simply be placed under the expander in a gentle curve. Kinking causing difficulty in filling the expander has not been encountered.

Some surgeons prefer soft tissue expanders with stiff backs. This helps in placing some expanders through small incisions, and it helps insure that dissection of the pocket has been adequate. The broader the pocket, the greater the arc of soft tissue expansion, and the more tissue is available. In some cases, backers can impinge on the skin and even lead to exposures. Some surgeons enjoy employing expanders without backers for these can be folded to accommodate irregular shaped pockets.

Manufacturers have accommodated surgeons by making custom implants as required. Custom implants can be fabricated with a template to indicate to the manufacturer the size of the base of the expander. We find it useful to sketch the defect on a piece of exposed x-ray film and to draw on this film the proposed shape of the base of the expander under the adjacent soft tissue which is to be expanded. The pattern can then be cut out and sent to a manufacturer; the type of filling port and the dimensions of the envelope are specified.

Place The Soft Tissue Expander In a Natural Tissue Plane

Incisions for placement of soft tissue expanders should be chosen carefully. Incisions should not be sited in unstable tissue. In areas of abundant vascularity, such as the scalp, incisions can typically be made at the edge of defects. Where the soft tissue is less likely to heal well, it may be prudent to make a remote incision and to dissect a pocket from a distance. There are those who advocate orienting the incision so that it lies radially with respect to the radius of the expander as opposed to lying perpendicular to its diameter (that is, parallel to the edge of the expander). These advocates assert that the tension distributed along the wound is not a force to distract wound edges, whereas an incision parallel to the edge of the expander is more likely to be separated.

In fact, if the soft tissues are closed so that the edge of the expander cannot impinge upon the skin closure, most parallel incisions heal very nicely without exposure during the course of expansion. The surgeon must judge each case on its own merits when deciding which approach will be safest for a given patient.

The soft tissue expander pocket is typically created in a relatively avascular plane. When expanding the scalp, the soft tissue expander should be placed in a pocket that lies under the galea. Dissecting this place causes little blood loss if the pericranium is not torn.

When expanding over the forehead, the surgeon must decide whether frontalis is needed in the expanded flap. The surgeon has the option of expanding above the frontalis or in what is an extension of the subgaleal plane above the pericranium. In breast reconstruction, the surgeon typically expands between the submuscular plane above the rib cage. Over extremities, the pocket is created above the muscular fascia. For expansion prior to placement of calf implants, the soft tissue expander should be placed below the deep investing fascia of the leg and above the muscle. It is possible to expand over the abdominal wall. Here, too, the soft tissue expander should be placed above muscular fascia.

Expansion Should Be Slow and Deliberate

Expansion typically begins 1 to 2 weeks after insertion of the soft tissue expander. The wound should appear to be healing per primum. The sutures need not be out at the time of initiation of expansion.

Especially at the early expansions when the needle is withdrawn, there may be a leakage of seroma. This generally subsides in several minutes. Seromas are more likely to appear when soft tissue expanders are placed in the lower extremity and when they are placed near hemangiomas. When the soft tissue expander is inflated, pressure in the cavity rises and the seroma drains from the needle hole after filling. To avoid the troublesome dribble, one may back the needle out of the injection port after expansion and, with the needle atop the port, aspirate much of the seroma.

If careful attention is given to placement of the injection ports, they will be easy to locate. Injection ports should be located in the superficial subcutaneous tissue and away from pressure points over the body. Integrated ports are typically easy to feel when used in a submuscular plane for breast reconstruction. This is because the flaps are typically thin. If integrated ports are used in the lower extremities, seromas may make them difficult to palpate initially. In this case roentgenography or ultrasonography can help the surgeon localize the injection port. If some fluid has already been injected into the expander, it is often possible to locate the injection port by transillumination with a fiberoptic light source.

It is very important to be aware of pressure changes during soft tissue expansion. Injection of saline should be terminated when the patient begins to complain of a sense of tightness. We know from pressure measurements obtained during inflations that a sense of tightness is appreciated when the intraluminal pressure in the expander ranges from 40 to 50 mm Hg. At 80 mm Hg, the patient becomes uncomfortable, and the transcutaneous oxygen tension falls to 54 mm Hg. Increasing the pressure to over 100 mm Hg causes distinct pain.

It should be noted that the pressure-volume curve becomes very steep as the elastic limit of the overlying soft tissues is reached. Therefore very little increase in volume is gained for tremendous increases in pressure. One should realize this important fact: high filling pressures will not lead to a proportionate increase in total volume injected. In fact it can lead to significant patient discomfort and cause tissue necrosis and exposure of the expander.

In some patients, we have deliberately increased the pressure to over 100 mm Hg for intervals of 10 minutes to cause a nonelastic deformation of the largely collagen capsule surrounding the expander. Then the intraluminal pressure was lowered to physiologic range of 30 to 40 mm Hg. This allowed us to increase the amount of fluid injected for the final resting pressure.

The patient must be appraised of the necessity of continuing the expansion until an adequate arc length of tissue is achieved. It is not surface area that is important, it is the length of the arc of the tissue to be advanced. One can measure the circumference of an extremity and compare it with the pre-expansion circumference or the circumference of the normal extremity at the comparable level.

One can follow expansion by measuring the increase in distance between landmarks. One can also look down on top of the expander with a ruler in hand to measure the width of its base from side to side. Then one measures the arc over the expander and, by subtracting the width of the base, determines the net increase in arc length. The arc length must equal the width of the base of the expanded flap plus the width of the defect. The patient can follow this with the surgeon and, in particular those patients who are conducting home expansion, can keep track and report by phone their progress as they measure it.

Home expansion has proved highly effective. Only those patients who wish to pursue this approach are allowed to do it. It is cost effective both for the physician and the patient. There is minimal traveling back and forth and no more materials are required than would be used typically.

Both patients and doctors need a perspective in judging the suitability of this approach. It should be pointed out that it has been proven to be safe and effective. The whole process may be made simpler for some families by leaving the ports external when expanders with remote ports are used. This may be particularly effective for small children who are afraid of needles. It might be pointed out that some would judge home expansion less dangerous and less complicated than the administration of insulin in diabetes mellitus.

Advancement Should Be Simple

Advancement of an expanded flap may often be achieved under local anesthesia. Scalp expansion is particularly well suited to this approach (Fig. 4). It should be noted that in areas of burn scar, local anesthesia does not diffuse particularly well, and multiple injections may be required. These can be painful and for some patients regional or general anesthesia is preferable. Patient selection is of course important.

Postoperative pain is minimal after a typical flap advancement. The soft tissue expander cavity itself and the expanded flap are not painful; the only pain and discomfort comes from the site that has been prepared to receive the flap. Typically, with good coverage, the recipient site is not painful.

Advancement should be simple. Whenever possible, a simple advancement flap should be used. The surgeon should restrict himself to a minimum of back cuts and sculpting incisions. With proper flap design minimal incisions should be necessary and the scars following advancement should be short.

Before the entire defect or lesion is resected, a trial advancement should be carried out. The farthest advance of the flap should be marked, and then a decision can be made regarding excision. If the flap advancement is shorter than expected, the surgeon can deflate the expander in place and leave it under the advanced flap. Alternatively, he or she may elect to replace the expander with one of a different design or different size. One can expand and advance the same flap several times. This is well tolerated in patients who understand the program and are well motivated toward achieving the significant improvements afforded by soft tissue expansion.

After advancement, showers are prescribed for the first morning after surgery. These are enjoyed by patients and are an important part of wound care. Patients can shower even with drains in place. Most patients do have drains inserted at the time of flap advancement to prevent the accumulation of seroma or hematoma which might prevent firm coaptation of the flap and its bed.

Aftercare Is Required

Some of the aftercare depends on preoperative counseling. Patients should know about the natural history of healing and scar formation. They should know that a wound ridge will be palpable and that scars may widen. Typically we counsel patients that a scar created by the suturing of an expanded flap to adjacent tissue will widen to the same degree as any incision there would.

Ripples or soft tissue redundancies are common and patients are counseled that these will often settle. Dog ears may persist, but, particularly over the scalp, they are usually inapparent and can shrink remarkably in a short

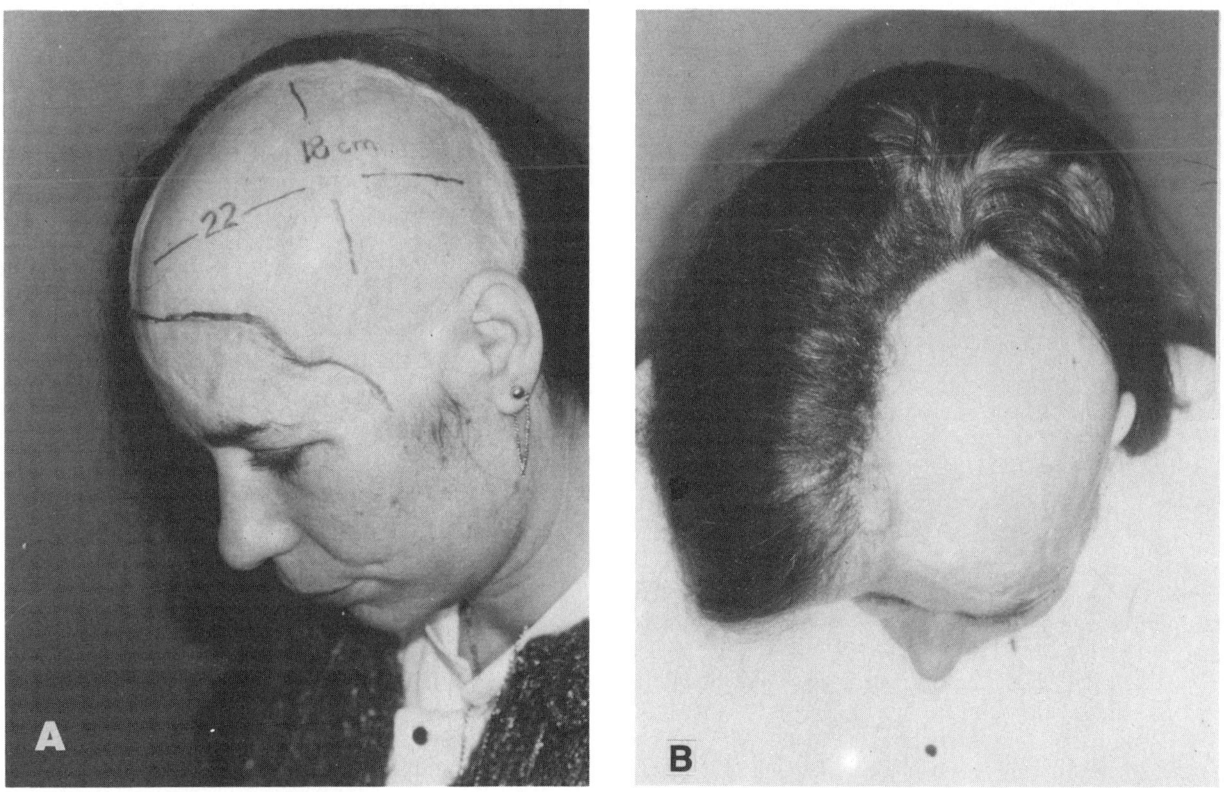

Figure 4 *A,* A large scalp defect after an avulsion injury. *B,* Expansion to a dimension that will allow a wrap-around reconstruction.

Figure continues on following page

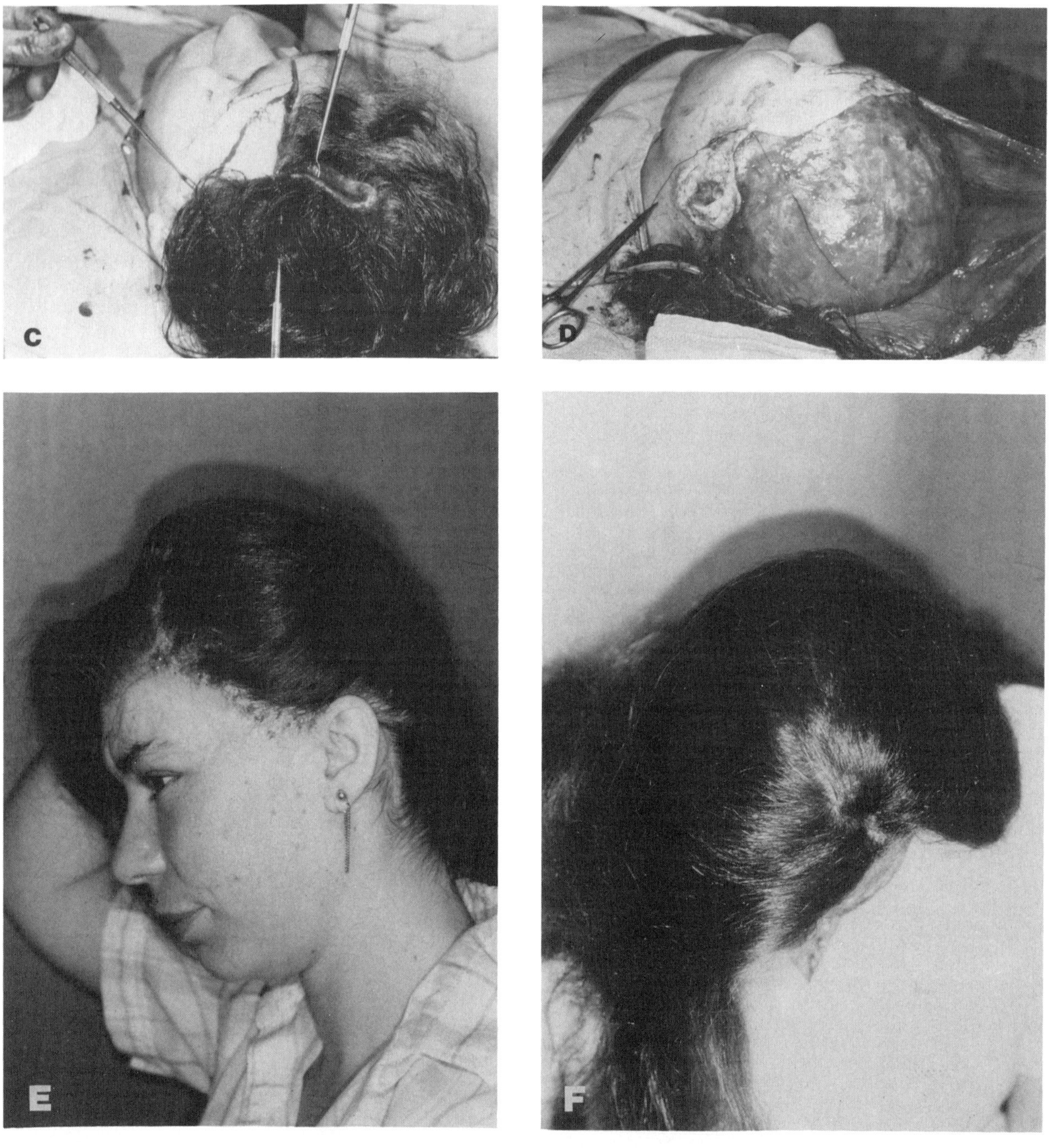

Figure 4 (continued) *C,* Trial advancement under local anesthetic before the skin graft is excised. *D,* The defect prior to coverage. *E* and *F,* The final result showing an acceptable hairline and good hair density.

time. By and large we avoid resection of dogears until some time has passed to allow resolution. Particularly in the scalp, resection of dogears removes good hairbearing tissue and makes longer hairless scars.

All patients should be counseled that scars will widen and revision could be necessary in selected cases.

Some patients have depressions in the skin which resulted from atrophy of subcutaneous fat caused by pressure of injection ports or envelope folds. Typically these depressions will fill out with time and generally do not require an operative treatment early.

COMPLICATIONS

Complications may be divided into minor complications and major complications. Pain, seroma formation, dogears after advancement, and widening of scars are typically minor complications. Pain can largely be avoided by not overdistending the expander at the time of inflation. Seroma formation is usually self-limited. Dogears usually are significantly reduced with time. Scars do widen and, at times, they may require revision. A closure with significant tension increases the chance of significant widening.

Major complications include exposure of the expander, implant failure, and induced ischemia. Placement of the soft tissue expander at or below the knee when an open wound is present will, in all likelihood, be complicated by infection. Infection is infrequent around the head and neck where expanders may be routinely placed without shaving the scalp.

Exposure commonly results from overzealous expansion, an inadequate pocket (so that the baseplate of an expander protrudes through the line of incision), or from peri-expander infection. Incipient exposures due to folds of the soft tissue expander projecting into the overlying subcutaneous fat and skin may be arrested by reducing the volume in the expander to let the area heal. Subsequent careful expansion may be successful. During the time of partial deflation, it may be possible to manipulate the expander and change the site of a projecting fold to another spot.

Implant failure is rare. The surgeon can prove the integrity of the expander by partially filling it with air and immersing it in water or saline prior to implantation. At the present time, the vulnerable point seems to be the site of attachment of the tubing of a remote filling port to the envelope. Soft tissue expanders should not be dangled by their filling port tubing nor should the junction of tubing and envelope be subjected to deliberate tension.

Induced ischemia is possible if the filling pressures are increased to a high level. One should be particularly watchful in patients who have muscle flaps that are undergoing expansion or who have ongoing soft tissue expansion under tissues whose circulation is otherwise abnormal.

BIOLOGICAL IMPLICATIONS OF SOFT TISSUE EXPANSION

One might logically ask where the extra tissue comes from. Is it simply stretched tissue, or is there an actual induction of growth? To be sure there can be thinning of soft tissues and some of the effect is indeed from nonelastic deformation of skin and subcutaneous tissue and from recruitment of adjacent tissue. It does appear, however, that expanded soft tissues do actually increase in mass. Typically expanded scalp, for instance, is not appreciably thinner when one includes the capsule in measuring its thickness.

Austad and Pasyk have demonstrated increased epidermal mitotic activity in skin of animals undergoing soft tissue expansion. Others have suggested there is an actual increase in collagen content in the integument of animals undergoing expansion. From working with patients, one gains the definite clinical impression that there is an actual growth of expanded soft tissues and early laboratory work supports this impression.

The implications for the biology of surgery are of major import. Soft tissue expansion appears to represent an actual induction of tissue growth for the purposes of reconstructive surgery. Manders et al have elongated nerve, ureter, and small bowel using soft tissue expansion. An attempt has been made to expand the bladder as well.

It appears that a nerve can be elongated even if largely by recruitment of an adjacent nerve. The process of expansion does not alter the electrophysiologic or morphometric characteristics of peripheral nerve if the intraluminal pressure does not exceed 40 mm Hg. The technique has been used successfully in nerve reconstruction in human beings.

Smooth muscle has been elongated in the case of the ureter and the small bowel. In the small bowel there has been tremendous hypertrophy, perhaps due to subacute obstruction. Work is progressing towards determining whether short gut syndrome might one day be treated by elongation of the bowel as opposed to reliance on elemental diets or parenteral nutrition.

From preliminary work, it seems that soft tissue expansion is possible for a variety of tissues. This is important, for tissue expansion represents an actual controlled growth of tissues, which can then be used for reconstructive surgery. This offers the plastic and reconstructive surgeon untold possibilities for treatment of heretofore insoluble problems.

SUMMARY

Soft tissue expansion is an elegant technique. A large measure of its elegance is its simplicity. There are many benefits for both patient and doctor alike. Typically the color, texture, and hairbearing characteristics of the expanded flap best match the needs of the adjacent reconstruction. Additionally, the advanced flap is usually sensate and does not become a biscuit-like flap as the cutaneous islands of myocutaneous flaps typically do. The donor site is minimal or undetectable following soft tissue expansion, an additional aesthetic benefit.

Functional benefits are real and deserve mention. The soft-tissues have an increased vascularity, which makes the success of the reconstruction more assured. As indicated above, advanced flaps are typically sensate. Muscle is not sacrificed as a carrier or filler and furthermore in the case of the frontalis muscle, reanimation of the forehead may be gained.

From the doctor's point of view, soft tissue expansion is cost effective. Furthermore it presents a means of reconstruction that has a relatively low morbidity. Should the expansion be compromised or complicated by infection, or threatened by actual exposure, it is a simple matter to remove the expander, let the wound heal, and then return another day for insertion of a second expander. It is important to emphasize that tissue loss seldom occurs during soft tissue expansion or during the process of flap advancement after expansion. As indicated above, many soft tissue expansion procedures can be done with the patient enjoying an outpatient status.

Readers should be aware that soft tissue expanders can be safely reused, although it is not the current practice in the United States of America. The Federal FDA has identified these devices as one time use items. In the developing world, there is a great need for soft tissue expanders, and there they can be recycled with great effectiveness. Soft tissue expanders should be washed after removal and autoclaved with a 21-gauge needle venting the injection port. The expanders should be propped up on a lint-free towel so that no saline covers the point at which the filling port tubing enters the envelope.

When the expander is being prepared for insertion, it should likewise be washed and autoclaved for 15 minutes at 15 lbs per square inch pressure (239°F).

Soft tissue expansion has been boon to many patients. It offers a safe, low-risk means of reconstructing complex defects. The skill of the surgeon is tested in the planning phase of soft tissue expansion more so than in his managing the conduct of expansion or in his advancing the flap. Planning is of paramount importance. A three dimensional appreciation of the defect and the strategies for its repair are essential for success. Typically, the results are extremely gratifying to both patient and surgeon alike.

SUGGESTED READING

Argenta LC, Marks MW, Pasyk KA. Advances in tissue expansion. Clin Plast Surg 1987; 12:159–172.

Austad ED, Thomas SB, Pasyk K. Tissue expansion: dividend or loan? Plast Reconstr Surg 1986; 78:63–67.

Manders EK, Au VK, Wong RKM. Scalp expansion for male pattern baldness. Clin Plast Surg 1987; 14:469–475.

Manders EK, Graham WP, Schenden MJ, Davis TS. Skin expansion to eliminate large scalp defects. Ann Plast Surg 1984; 12:305–312.

Manders EK, Saggers GC, Diaz-Alonzo P, et al. Elongation of peripheral nerve and viscera containing smooth muscle. Clin Plast Surg 1987; 14:551–562.

Manders EK, Schenden MJ, Furrey JA, et al. Soft-tissue expansion: concepts and complications. Plast Reconstr Surg 1984; 74:493–507.

Neumann CG. The expansion of an area of skin by progressive distention of a subcutaneous balloon. Plast Reconstr Surg 1957; 19:124–130.

Radovan C. Tissue expansion in soft-tissue reconstruction. Plast Reconstr Surg 1984; 74:482–492.

Sasaki GH. Intraoperative sustained limited expansion (ISLE) as an immediate reconstructive technique. Clin Plast Surg 1987; 14:563–573.

Taylor GI, Palmer JH. The vascular territories (angiosomes) of the body: experimental study and clinical applications. Brit J Plast Surg 1987; 40:113–141.

HEAD AND NECK | TRAUMA

SCALP DEFECTS

M. J. JURKIEWICZ, M.D., F.A.C.S.

The focus of this chapter is the reconstruction of partial loss of the scalp following trauma or excision of congenital nevocytic nevi and tumors. It is not intended as a guide for the correction of male pattern baldness.

To be successful, the surgeon must keep in mind the anatomy of the scalp; not only its laminated, unyielding character but also its blood supply (Fig. 1). The supraorbital, supratrochlear, temporal, auricular, and occipital vessels that vascularize the scalp all run in the subcutaneous fatty layer, immediately superficial to the galea aponeurotica. They freely anastomose with one another, thus permitting long axial flaps to be raised for advancement or transposition. The scalp is the adult is thick, its layers well defined, and its blood supply robust. In the infant and growing young child, however, the scalp is relatively thin, its layers much less well defined, and its axial blood supply much less robust and, therefore, less dependable.

THERAPEUTIC ALTERNATIVES

In a broad sense, the surgical alternatives in scalp reconstruction include skin grafting and local and distant flaps. Local flaps are preferred as the definitive mode of reconstruction because they not only restore the normal durable scalp cover but also the normal configuration of hairbearing and non-hairbearing scalp. Skin grafts should be thought of as temporary cover in most instances. Distant flaps are required following massive resections for tumor that include resection of the underlying calvaria. In these cases, the revascularized, free, musculocutaneous flap is the first choice, with or without immediate bone grafting. Such cases clearly have to be considered on an individual basis with age, co-morbid factors, and therapeutic objectives taken into account.

In the acute situation that involves avulsion, the scalp should be replaced, whenever possible, by replantation with microvascular anastomoses, using vein grafts when necessary. In our unit, the entire scalp from eyebrows to the nuchal line, with one ear included, has survived on one superficial temporal vessel bridged by vein grafts. A replanted scalp can survive and grow normal hair when revascularized up to 14 hours following avulsion. Attempts at free grafting of avulsed scalp, which has been meticulously thinned, have met with universal failure.

When the patient has partial scalp avulsion and the part is lost, the surgeon should débride, close the defect by skin grafting, and await definitive closure with the use of expanders or mobilized transposition flaps. An alternative tactic within the same basic strategy, is to construct bilateral bipedicle flaps on either side of the defect and use these flaps to close the primary defect. The defects left in the wake of the flap transpositions are skin grafted and then the grafts are excised secondarily.

When the therapeutic objective is closure by local flaps to restore normal scalp appearance and function, the options are: (1) expanders and advancement flaps, (2) expanders and advancement and transposition flaps (Orticochea), or (3) advancement and transposition flaps alone—the Orticochea method.

Age, size and nature of the defect, and co-morbid factors have to be taken into account. For example, the possibility of permanent alteration of the configuration of the skull or of erosion of the calvaria by an expander is an important consideration.

SKIN EXPANDERS

Skin expanders have greatly simplified scalp reconstruction. In most circumstances, simple expansion of the scalp, over approximately 6 weeks, with subsequent removal of the expanders, scoring of the capsule, and closure by simple advancement of the resultant expanded flaps is the primary choice of most surgeons. It must be kept in mind that there will be some thinning of the hair attendant upon the increase in surface area due to the expansion. This thinning can be exacerbated into permanent loss of hair by ischemia. When the expander is being inflated saline is injected to the point of pain, then fluid withdrawn to point of clinically-detectable capillary refill. After 15 to 30 minutes there is again expansion to point of pain followed once more by withdrawal to restore capillary refill.

In the final scalp closure, the tension on the flap must not compromise the axial blood supply. Such tension, when unrelieved, can result in alopecia.

In the younger child one must be aware of the possibility of deformation and erosion of the calvaria. Expansion must be done slowly over time and checked with x-ray films or computed tomography (CT) scan when necessary.

THE ORTICOCHEA METHOD

The use of skin expanders has made the method of scalp reconstruction described by Orticochea irrelevant in some instances, or relevant but forgotten in others. The best advice is to put the method up front in the planning process. In so doing, it may prevent the absurdity of inability to close the defect after expansion, when only advancement flaps were planned. In short, one must plan ahead and discard the complicated when simple advancement flaps will suffice.

The key to understanding Orticochea's method is knowledge of its historical evolution. In 1953, Kazanjian described closure of a scalp defect with a bipedicle, relatively narrow, axial flap that was widened by linear scoring of the galea parallel to the long axis of the flap. The defect in the wake of the sliding flap was dealt with secondarily as suggested by Dufourmental.

Orticochea made a significant contribution to scalp reconstruction by cutting the bipedicle flap on a bias somewhere in its midportion, by lengthening the flaps through scoring of the galea, and, more importantly, by *extensive* mobilization of the scalp (eyebrow to nuchal line or below, over to the ears). The flaps were then used to cover not only the original defect but also the defects left in the wake of the transposition. When these flaps were insufficient, a large advancement flap(s) was added.

Orticochea also advocated cutting the "bucket handle" axial flap 6 to 8 cm in width, which works out well empirically. One must remember Kazanjian's rule: restore the anterior hairline as the first priority in flap design. Also, the axial nature of the flaps to be constructed must be kept in mind. The anatomy of the vessels of the scalp must be known and the flaps designed accordingly.

To understand the method, the original articles should be studied. Study of Figures 1 to 4 accompanying this chapter will also help.

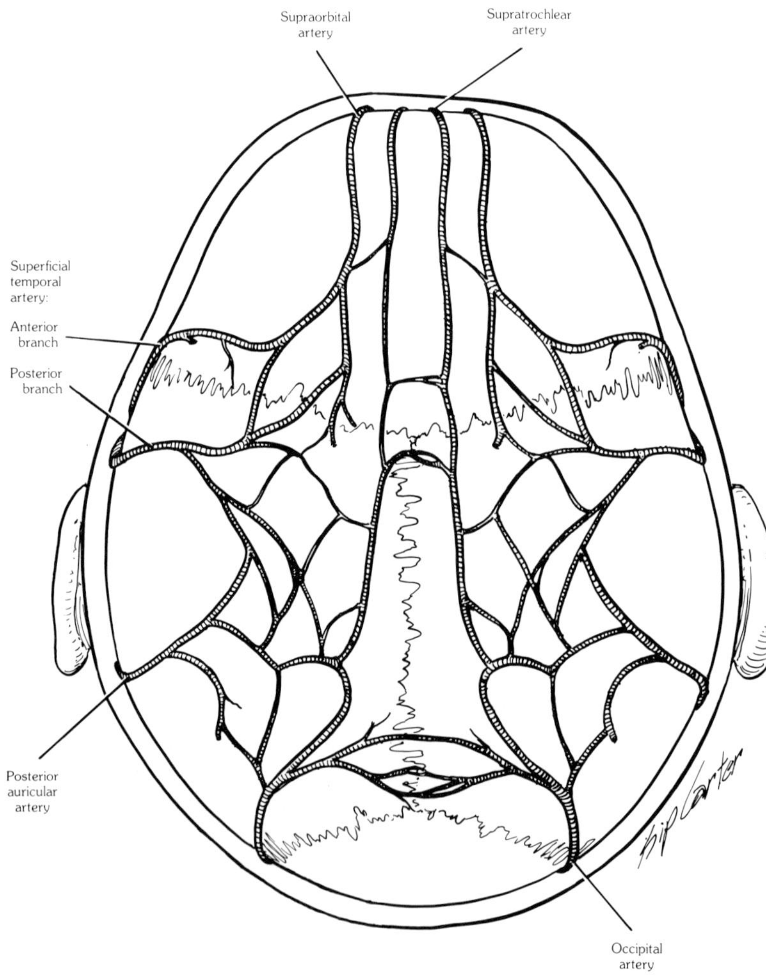

Figure 1 Scalp's vascular anatomy is illustrated. Note the extensive anastomoses across the midline.

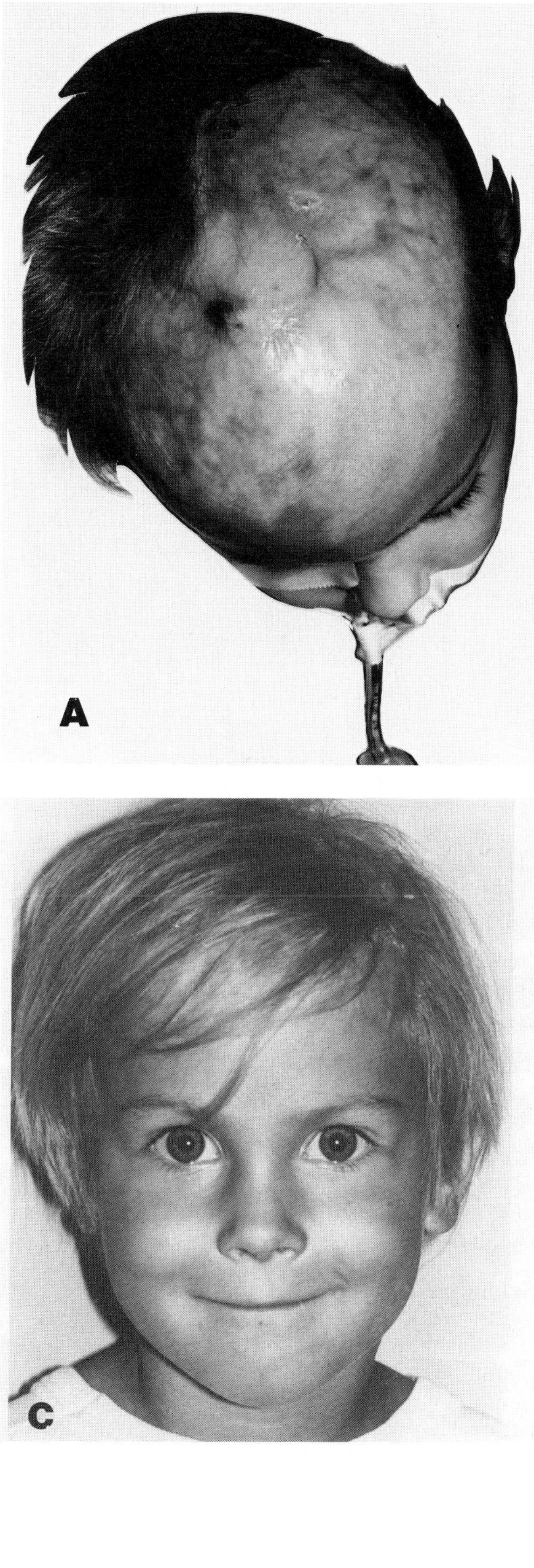

Figure 2 The first stage of scalp repair on a 2-year-old with thermally injured scalp is shown. *A*, Preoperative appearance. *B*, The planned "bucket-handle" bipedicled flap is outlined along the alopecic margin and is based on the left occipital and right temporal arteries. Two weeks prior to transposition, the flap is "delayed" by incising the outlined flap and its oblique transection, but the two flaps are not elevated. *C*, Postoperative appearance.

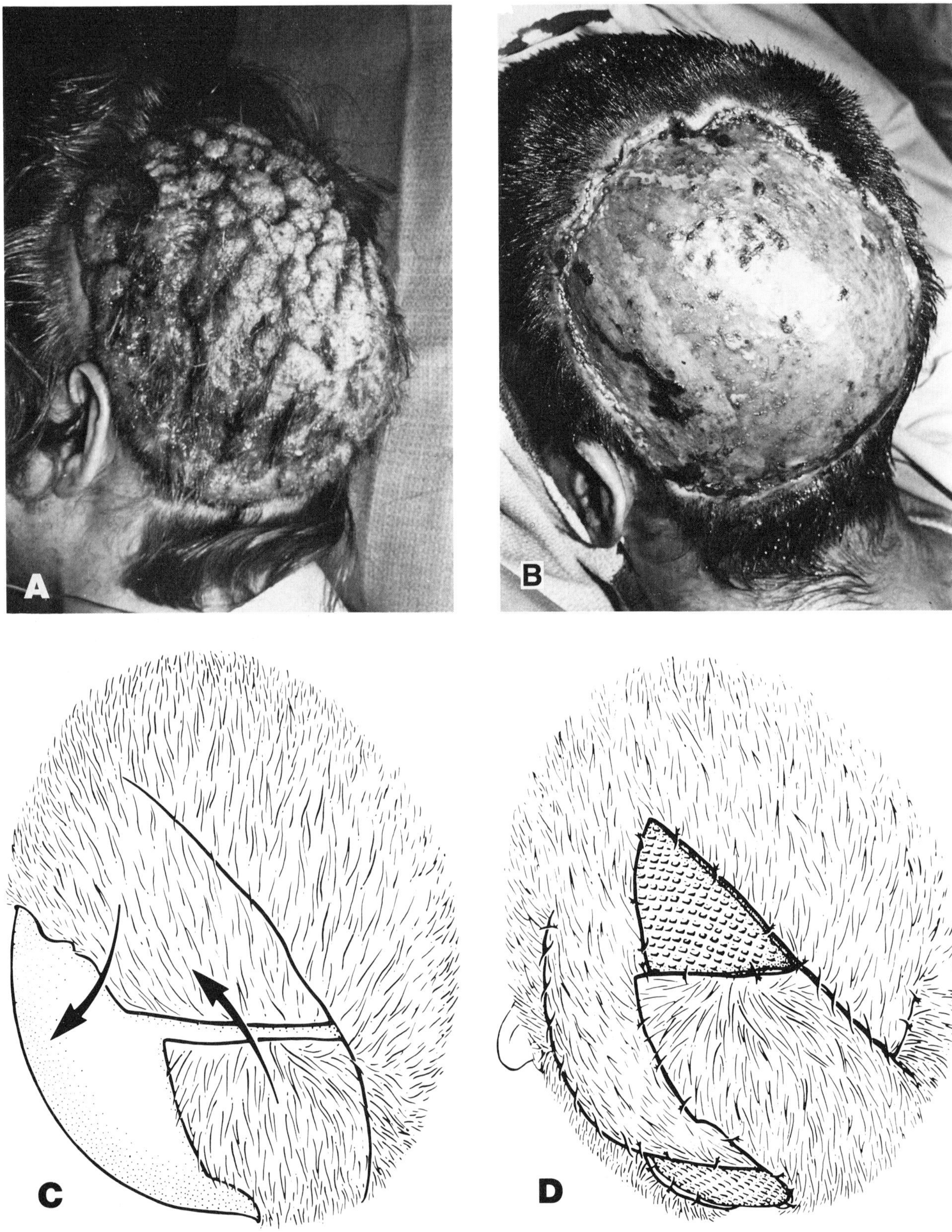

Figure 3 A 12-year-old boy with a fungating scalp tumor. *A,* The infected lesion is shown. *B,* It has been excised and the pericranium temporarily surfaced with a meshed split-skin graft in preparation for the scalp reconstruction. The occipitoparietal defect has a diameter of 27 cm. *C,* Shows how "bucket-handle" bipedicle flap was designed along alopecic margin and based on right occipital and left temporal arteries. It is bisected and mobilized along with the rest of the scalp. *D,* The "bucket-handle" flap is transected and the scalp mobilized along its entire anatomic extent. The galea is scored. These measures are necessary to close a scalp defect of this magnitude.

Figure continues on opposite page

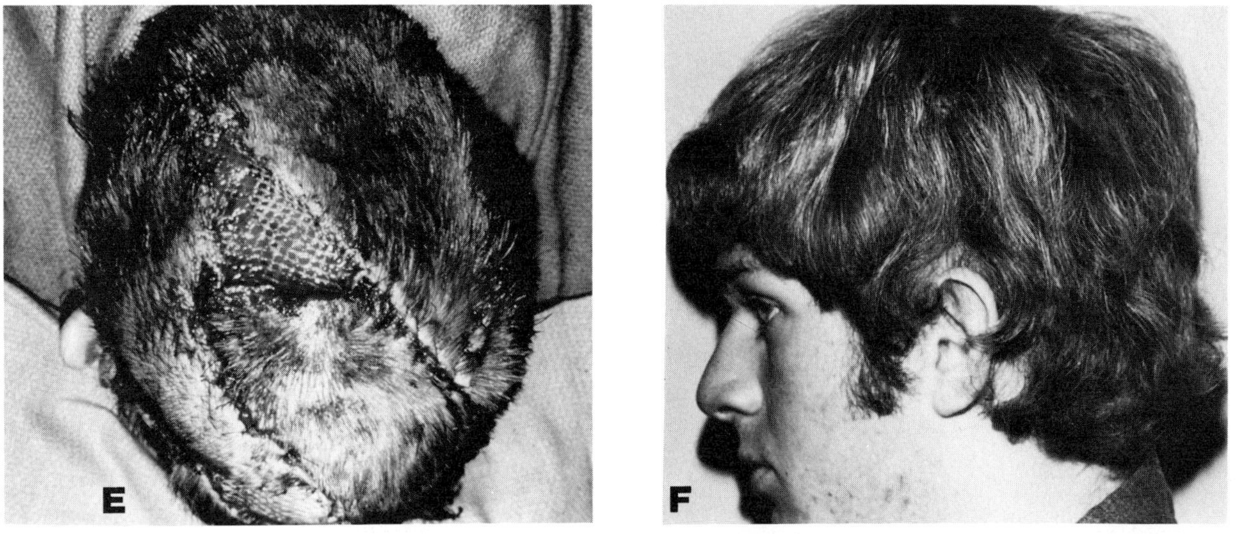

Figure 3 (continued) *E,* For closure, one flap now extended by galeal scoring, is used to obliterate the original occipitoparietal defect; the second flap is used to fill the defect left in the wake of the transposition. The secondary defects are closed with the meshed skin grafts. *F,* The final result after secondary excision of the residual interim skin grafts.

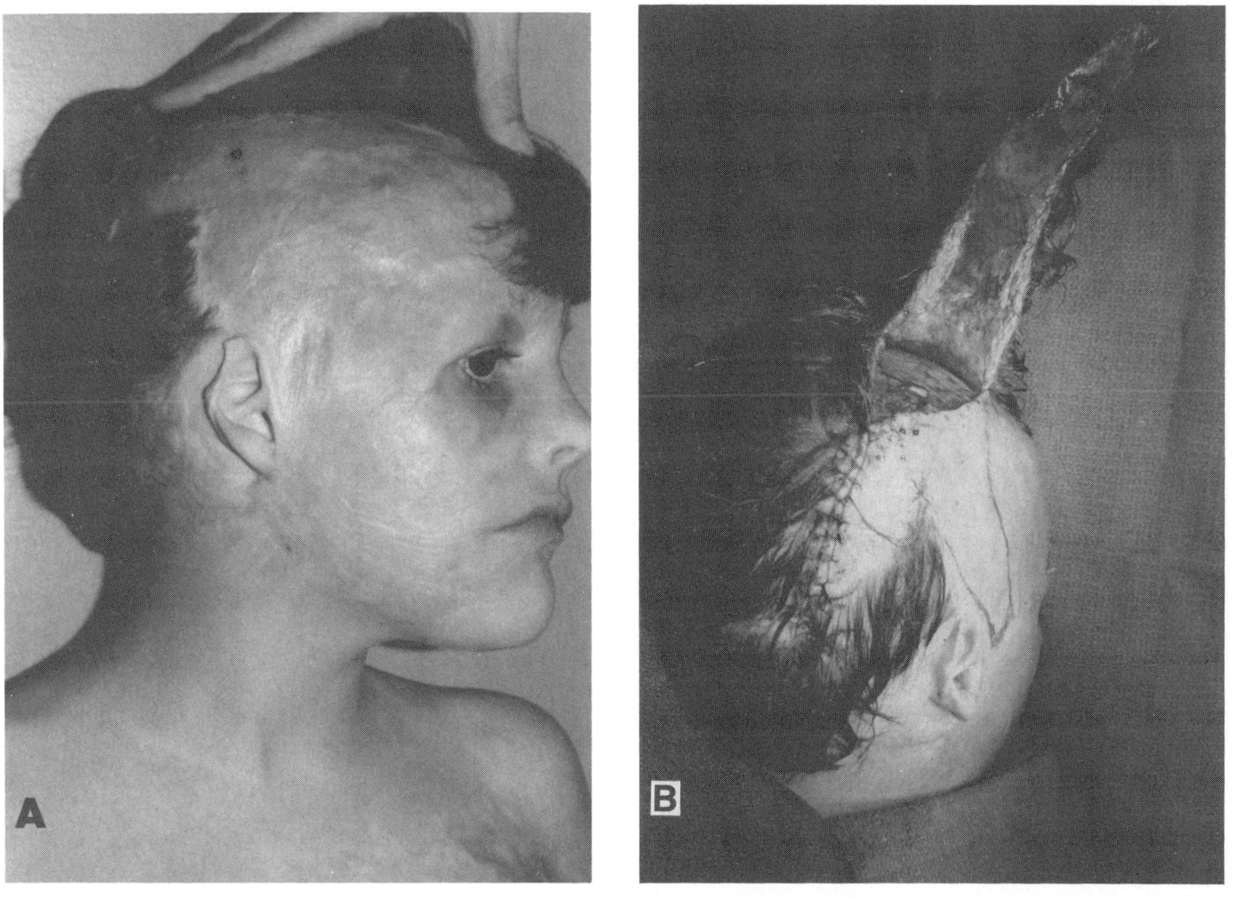

Figure 4 *A,* Preoperative photograph shows the area of burn alopecia, treated by skin grafting, in a 7-year-old boy who had suffered overall full-thickness burns to 30 percent of his total body area 2 years before. *B,* Illustrates design of the flap, previously delayed. The area of the graft to be excised is marked in methylene blue. The remaining small portion of burn alopecia, lateral to the closed suture line, was excised at a later operation.

Figure continues on following page

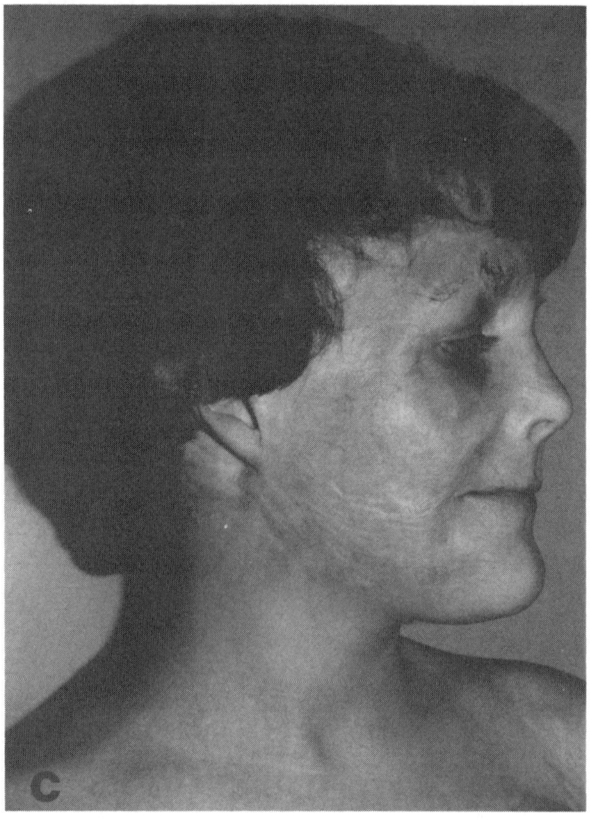

Figure 4 (continued) *C*, The result 3 years later at age 10.

BENEFIT-RISK ANALYSIS OF PREFERRED APPROACH

No study has been made to analyze cost and outcome of one method of scalp reconstruction as opposed to another. The Orticochea method was originally designed as a one-stage approach. As such, it has a distinct advantage over the expansion method, which, of necessity, is a planned two-stage procedure. Although we have successfully closed defects up to 25 cm in diameter by the Orticochea method, we have always had to resort to a secondary procedure in such large defects. The secondary procedure has involved either scar revision or, more frequently, the removal of a small skin graft placed in the secondary defect to avoid excessive tension on the flaps. Therefore, for reconstruction of large scalp defects, both methods, Orticochea's and tissue expansion, involve a two-stage procedure. In my mind, the two methods are complementary not exclusionary.

SUGGESTED READING

Dufourmental L. Plastic operations on the skull. Paris Med 1918; 8:503.

Jurkiewicz MJ, Hill HL. Open wounds of the scalp: an account of methods of repair. Trauma 1981; 21:769–778.

Kazanjian VH. Repair of partial losses of the scalp. Plast Reconstr Surg 1953; 12:325–334.

Manders EK, Schenden MJ, Furrey JA, et al. Soft tissue expansions: concepts and complications. Plast Reconstr Surg 1984; 74:493–507.

Orticochea M. New three flap scalp reconstruction: reconstruction technique. Br J Plast Surg 1971; 24:184–188.

SKULL DEFECTS

RICHARD CARLTON SCHULTZ, M.D., F.A.C.S.

Skull defects, seen predominantly in the frontal area, most commonly result from trauma, infection, electrical or thermal burns, and tumor resection. Their successful reconstruction is, to a large extent, dependent upon the quality of the overlying scalp. Though reconstruction can obviously never be attempted without scalp cover, errors are sometimes made in attempting reconstruction beneath thin unstable scars or skin grafts. Scars of moderate dimensions can be excised, and the surgical defect closed with adjacent scalp flaps. Where donor site defects are of such dimensions that they cannot be closed by extensive undermining, split skin grafts can be used over healthy pericranium distant to the bony reconstruction. To reconstruct massive scalp defects microvascular free flaps are used. These can be designed as musculocutaneous free flaps or muscular free flaps, such as the latissimus dorsi, covered with a split-thickness skin graft. Bony reconstruction can then begin, either at the time of scalp reconstruction or after scalp reconstruction has healed and scars have matured.

Reconstruction of the bony defect can be accomplished either with autogenous material or alloplastic material. Autogenous reconstruction is by far superior and, once healed, eliminates the long-term problems such as late implant movement, exposure, or infection sometimes seen with alloplastic reconstruction.

PREPARATION OF BONY DEFECT

Before either of these materials is used, the recipient site for reconstruction must be surgically prepared. This consists of debridement of any nonviable material, granulation tissue, and scar. Where frontal sinuses are involved, either their function or obliteration must be established before they are covered with reconstructive material. To cover a nonfunctioning, infected, frontal sinus invites subsequent mucocele, pyocele, external purulent drainage or, in the worst case, brain abscess. In any of these events, alloplastic reconstruction invariably fails and reconstruction with autogenous material often requires secondary debridement, sinus exenteration, and regrafting.

AUTOGENOUS RECONSTRUCTION

Depending upon the size and location of the skull defect, autogenous graft donor sites are: ribs, cranium, and ilium. Ribs can be used as full thickness, or they can be split. Their viability is almost assured beneath a healthy scalp flap, and subsequent coalescence of the rib graft can usually be demonstrated by x-ray studies.

Cranial grafts can be taken either from adjacent or opposite portions of the skull, usually from the parietal bone. Cranial grafts also can be taken as full-thickness grafts or split grafts at the level of the diploë. To take a split graft from the calvarium, the periphery of the graft is first outlined with a high speed electrical or air-driven burr, and the shoulders of the periphery of this outline are then burred down to permit appropriate angulation of an osteotome. The bone shavings that result from such burring are saved for subsequent use in the final contouring of the recipient or donor site. When a full-thickness bone graft is taken from the cranium, it is usually also split through the diploë at the back table. The inner surface is replaced into the donor site and the outer surface is used for the recipient site; both segments are then rigidly fixed in place by interosseous wires.

Iliac bone can be a valuable source of donor material. Normally, it is split and either the outer or the inner cortex is used, depending upon the contour desired. The ilium is also an excellent source of large quantities of cancellous material, taken with a bone curette. Such amorphous cancellous material and cortical shavings are useful in obtaining refined bony contour, particularly in the frontal area.

ALLOPLASTIC RECONSTRUCTION

Alloplastic material for skull reconstruction has certain undeniable advantages. It eliminates donor site morbidity; the quantity is unlimited; and the filling of irregular contour defects is technically easier. The alloplastic materials that I have found most useful for skull reconstruction are silicone rubber (Fig. 1), methyl methacrylate (Fig. 2), hydroxyapatite, and bioresorbable ceramic.

SILICONE RUBBER

Silicone rubber can be used either by carving an implant from a medium-hard block of Silastic* or the implant can be custom-made from a moulage of the defect. Custom-made silicone rubber implants can be made from either heat vulcanizing silicone rubber (clean room stock, Dow Corning Corporation*) or room temperature vulcanizing medical grade silicone rubber, Silastic 382.*

Heat vulcanizing rubbers utilize a high viscosity polymer and the resultant raw material is nonflowing; thus it is somewhat difficult for the surgeon to use. Room temperature vulcanizing rubber, on the other hand, uses a less viscous polymer so that the raw rubber is liquid. Room temperature vulcanizing rubber is weaker than the heat vulcanizing types, but it is easier to use and can be molded in situ where heat cannot be tolerated. Both types, once vulcanized, retain a memory of their original form and can be subsequently heat-autoclaved without losing shape.

When prefabricated implants are used, one must be prepared to revise the shape of the implant after it has been autoclaved and the bony defect exposed, despite great attention to detail in their construction. Only at this time can the contact surfaces be ascertained precisely. Revision usually consists of whittling the implant edges to achieve the best possible fit. In such cases, the flexibility of silicone rubber becomes a great asset.

METHYL METHACRYLATE

Cold-curing methyl methacrylate, or bone cement, is formed by mixing a liquid monomer with a powered polymer. The two most commonly used commercial products are Simplex† and Cranioplast.‡ Previously polymerized polymer granules are held together by newly polymerized monomer. Considerable heat is generated as the two elements cure, and the resulting plastic paste is sterile. When fully cured, it becomes a hard, rigid, translucent plastic of low specific gravity (1.8) that can be polished smooth and is impervious to fluids, gases, and bacteria. It can be heated and heat sterilized without change. Solid heat-cured acrylic is nearly identical to cold-curing bone cement both in physical properties and host response characteristics, but it requires multi-staged prefabrication. It can be reduced in size by burring at the time of surgery and can be augmented, as with bone cement, by first painting the surface with monomer. Both of these forms of acrylic are strong, have a similar density to bone, possess a low thermal conductivity, and their electrical conductivity is similar to that of skull. They are well tolerated by soft tissue, bone, and dura, and are radiolucent except when additives are used to make them radiopaque, as in the case of Simplex.

When bone cement is used, unbound monomer is lost by evaporation; therefore, mixing techniques that encourage evaporation are desirable. The mixing time should take about 2½ to 3 minutes. Monomer loss has been shown to be related more to frequency than to duration of stirring. Therefore, the material should be beaten as rapidly as possible during the mixing period before being molded in situ. The mixing and fitting time together can last up to 7 minutes; hardening takes another 7 minutes. The material should be worked until it is tacky before it is implanted. When molded in situ, it should be worked from the center out, so avoiding folding and lapping. This cement becomes progressively stronger up to 1 week. Severe hypotension, severe pyrexia, and cardiac arrest have been reported with the use of methyl methacrylate in orthopaedic surgery, but this has not been observed with

* Silastic: Dow Corning Wright, Arlington, TN 38002

† Simplex: Howmedical International Ltd., Rutherford, NJ 08080

‡ Cranioplast: L.D. Caulk Co., Milford, DE 19663

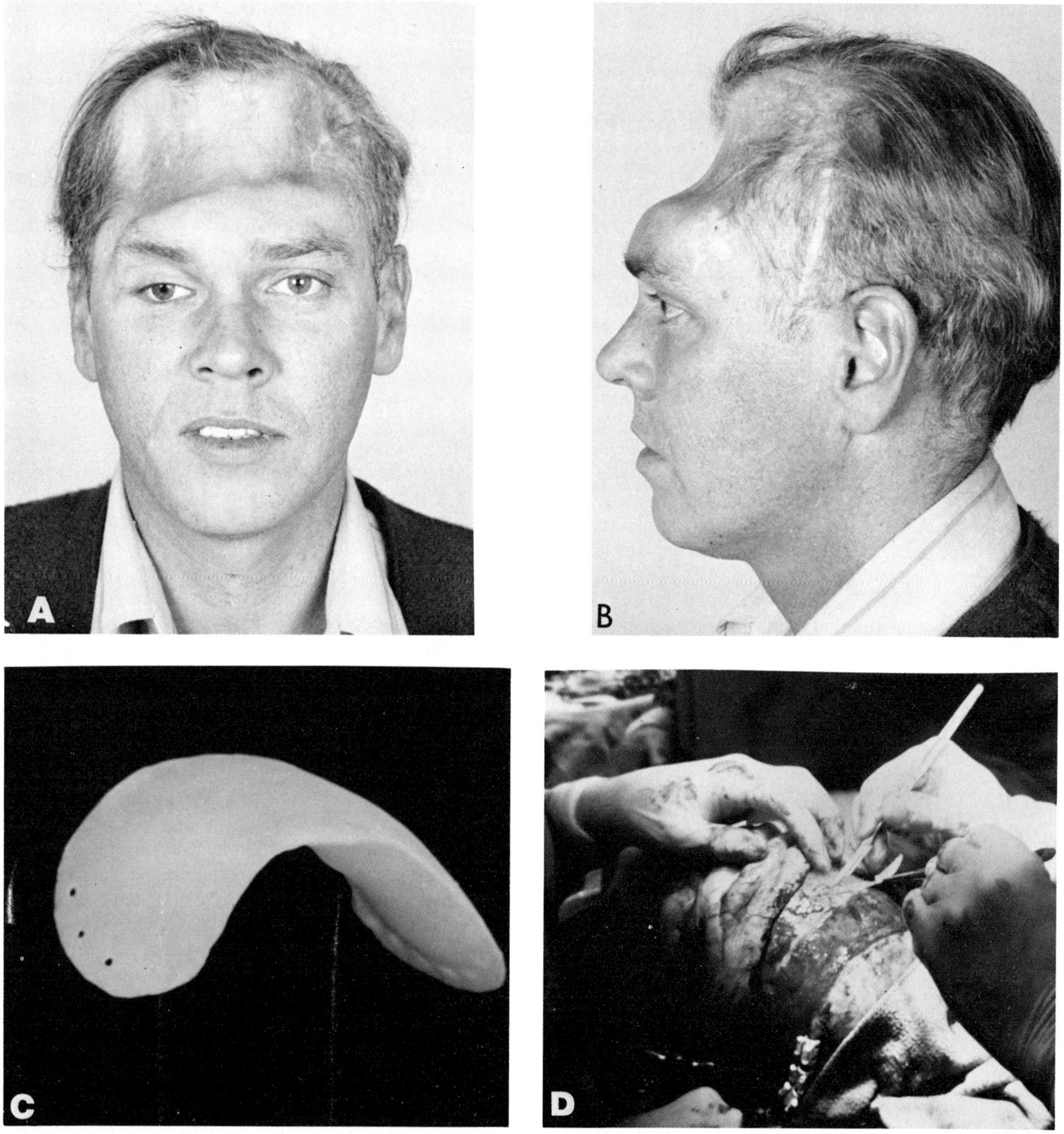

Figure 1 Reconstruction of massive frontal bone defect after several previous failed attempts at reconstruction with metallic implants. *A* and *B* show extent of deformity, *C*, prefabricated silicone rubber implant, *D*, precise fitting of implant by trimming the peripheral edges at the time of reconstruction through bi-temporal forehead flap.

Figure continues on opposite page

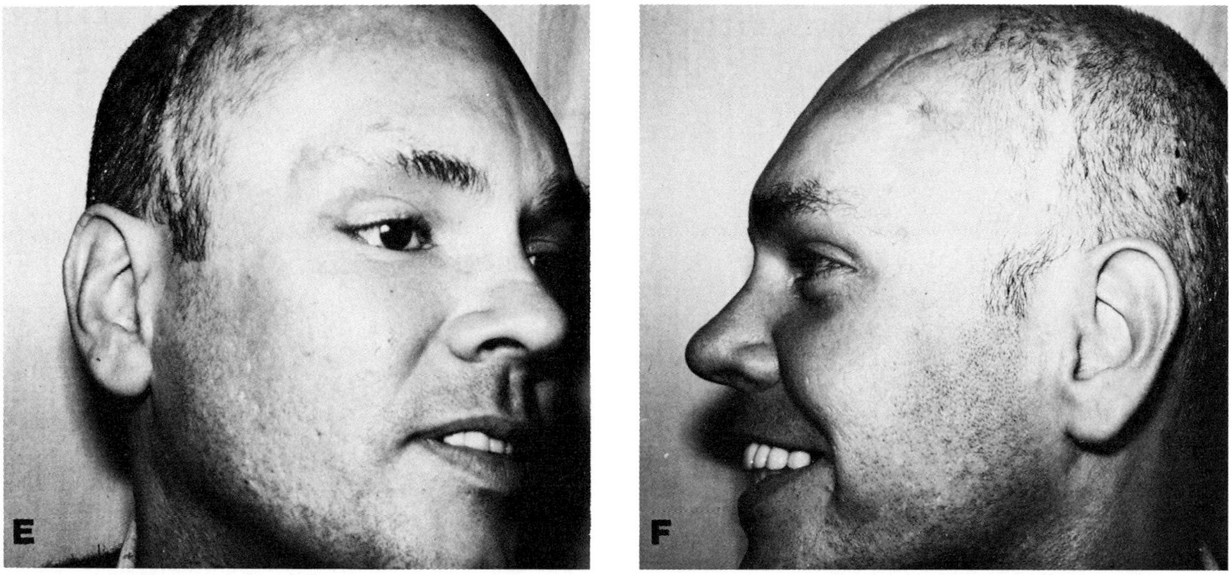

Figure 1 (continued) *E*, and *F*, appearance of patient 1 year after alloplastic reconstruction. (From Schultz RC. Facial injuries. 2nd ed. Chicago: Year Book, 432–433.)

its use in small amounts in facial bone and skull reconstruction.

Specimen failure can occur at the laminations created by the blood-cement interfaces. Such lamination can be minimized by manual pressure on the methyl methacrylate mass as it hardens. The specimen can be even further strengthened by embedding wire mesh into the semisolid cement. This prevents fragmentation should the specimen fracture. Loosening of the specimen can cause a technical failure that can be due to thermal injury from high polymerization temperature on the living bone in contact with the curing cement. The burned bone later resorbs and leaves the specimen slightly too small. This can be minimized by allowing the methyl methacrylate to undergo most of its cure outside the body before it is finally molded in situ. Irrigation with cool saline solution further reduces this excess heat at the interface. To facilitate contouring of the peripheral edges of the methyl methacrylate, a bony shelf is carved out of the adjacent bone with a bone-cutting burr before introduction of the tacky methyl methacrylate. This permits a smoother junction between the methyl methacrylate and the surrounding skull. All preparations at the recipient site, including hemostasis, should be completed before the liquid monomer is mixed with the powdered polymer.

When bone cement is used for reconstruction of defects of the glabella that involve the posterior wall of the frontal sinuses, or for full-thickness defects of the frontal bone, the integrity of the dura is essential before bone cement is introduced. Contact of curing bone cement with cerebral cortex may result in the development of foci of irritation and subsequent seizures.

Hydroxylapatite in polycrystalline form[§] is a high-density nonporous material with a chemical structure that resembles mineral bone. It can be characterized as osteoconductive and osteophylic, but not osteogenic. Over a period of several weeks, hydroxylapatite particles bond to bone, and there is a growth of dense fibrous connective tissue throughout the particles. The material is often mixed with cancellous bone ground to a small particle size, similar to hydroxylapatite particles, to form a uniform mixture. Iliac bone is ordinarily used and the saline-wetted mixture is injected through a small bore syringe. Although hydroxylapatite alone can be injected for contour augmentation, the addition of ground bone seems to enhance adherence and give stability of form to the implant. To reduce particle migration, custom-made implants of this material have been fabricated by the addition of a fibrin adhesive, partially obtained from human plasma. Preformed hard implants can then be used for onlay grafts.

Bioresorbable ceramic[#] (tricalcium phosphate) is available as a white, brittle, hard, but porous, material, although it can also be obtained in granular or powdered form. This material acts as a lattice for osteogenic substitution as it is biologically reabsorbed. The induced osseous proliferation conforms to the size and shape of the ceramic implant. The ceramic material should be sterilized by dry heat or ethylene oxide, and not autoclaved. It tolerates very little bacterial contamination because of its porosity, and should infection appear, the material must be removed. It is available commercially only in relatively small pieces (20 mm square), but can be ordered by weight in any size.

SURGICAL APPROACHES

Access to the skull defect can either be direct or indirect (see Figs. 1 and 2), depending upon the location

[§] Calcitite: Calcitite Inc., San Diego, CA

[#] Synthes: Miter, Inc., Worthington, OH 43085

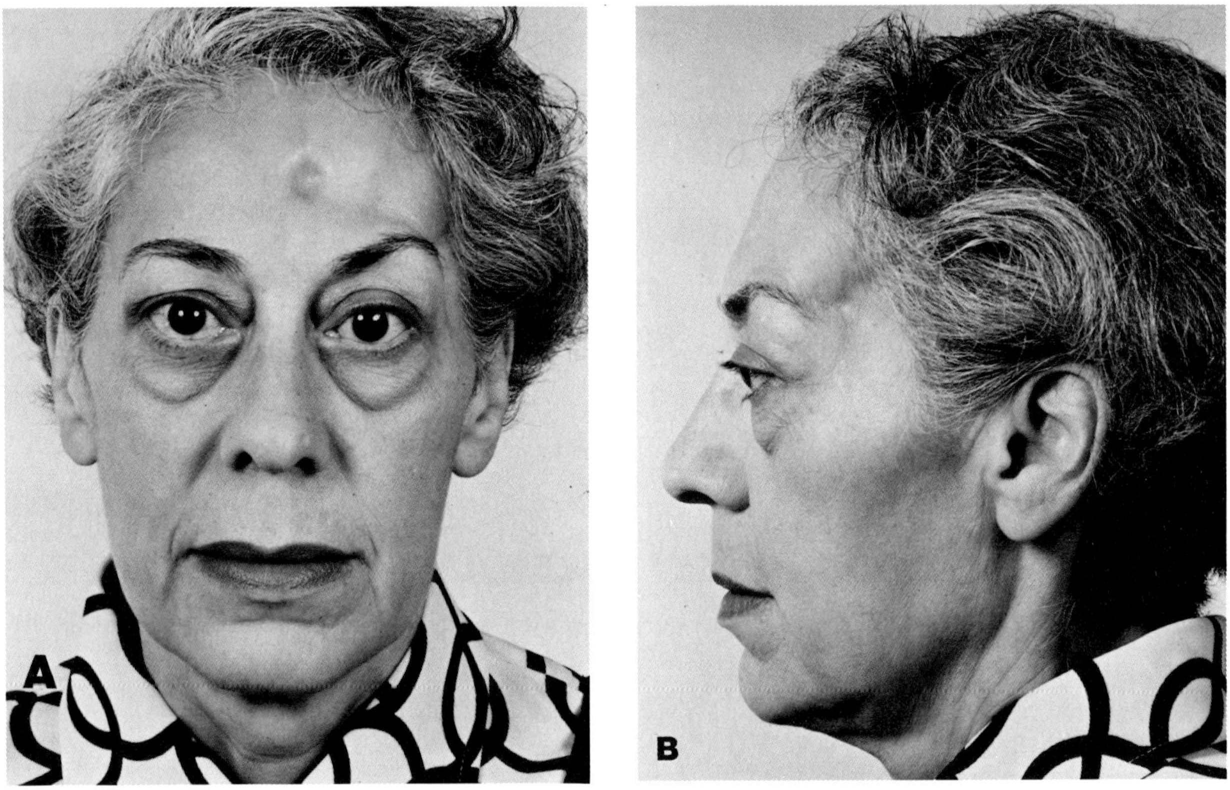

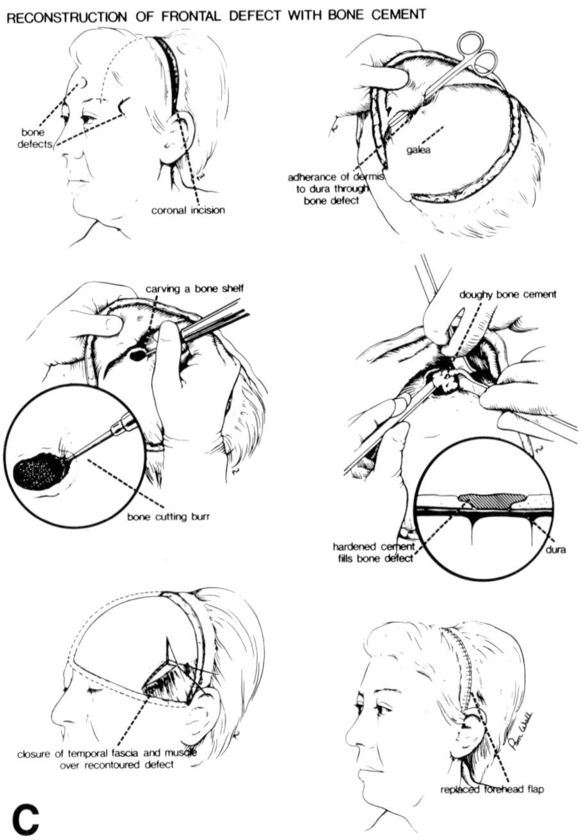

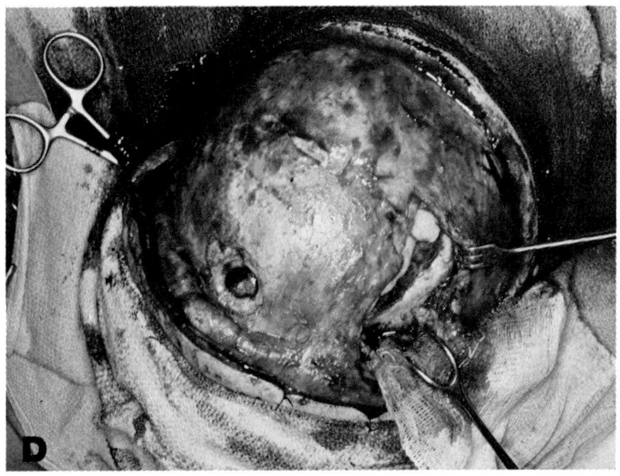

Figure 2 Reconstruction of frontal and temporal skull defects with cold-curing methyl methacrylate. *A* and *B*, appearance of patient following neurosurgical treatment of subdural hematoma, *C*, scheme of procedure performed, *D*, exposure of bony defects through bitemporal coronal approach—note division of temporalis muscle and the development of a bone shelf about the periphery of each bony defect.

Figure continues on opposite page

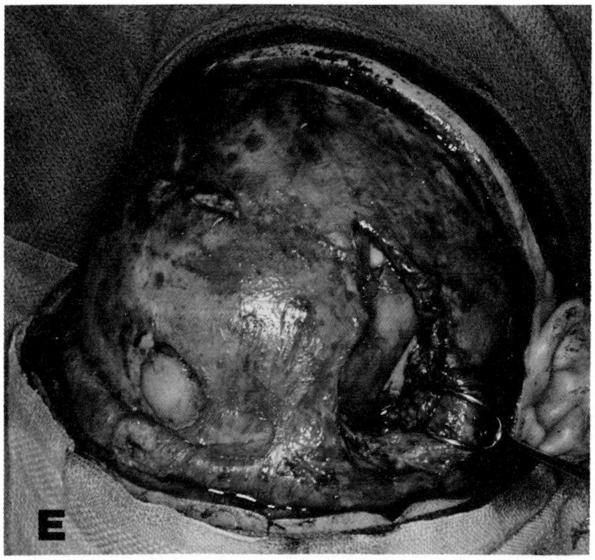

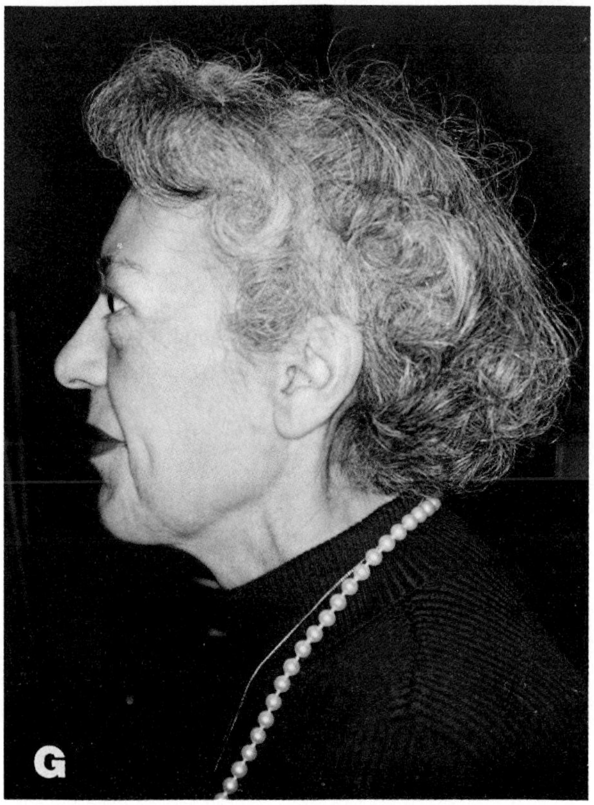

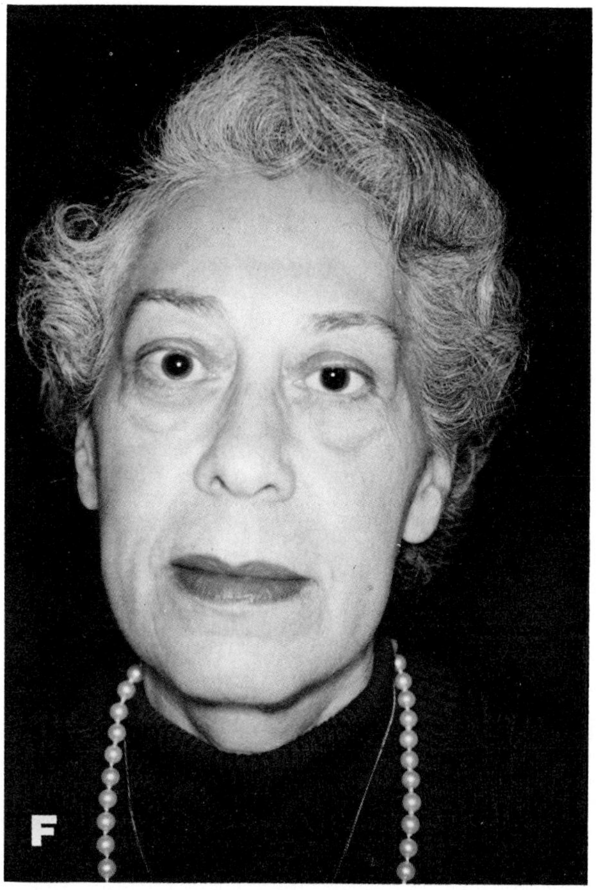

Figure 2 (continued) *E*, bony defects filled with cold-curing methyl methacrylate, *F* and *G*, appearance of patient 2 years following reconstruction. (*A, B, E, F,* and *G* from and *C* modified from Schultz RC. Facial injuries. 2nd ed. Chicago: Year Book, 439–442.)

of the defect and the quality of the overlying skin or scalp. The direct approach to the surgical defect has the advantages of minimal dissection and decreased operative time. When used on the forehead, however, incisions should be planned either to utilize previous scars, to follow normal skin creases, or to blend into facial contour as much as possible. The indirect surgical access is typified by the bitemporal coronal forehead flap. This is the standard workhorse for frontal reconstruction and provides superb exposure so that resultant symmetry of contour can be facilitated. For some defects of the frontotemporal area that do not cross the midline, a hemitemporal forehead flap is ideal. As with the bitemporal coronal flap, the dissection is begun at the subgaleal level and carried over the deep temporal fascia. As the dissection approaches the supraorbital rim, the supraorbital vessels and nerves are carefully dissected free. Sometimes these structures are protected by release of the supraorbital foramen with an osteotome when full exposure of the supraorbital rim is required.

Reconstruction of the skull and frontal contour can be gratifying to both the patient and the surgeon, as demonstrated by the illustrations. The morbidity associated with such reconstruction is surprisingly minimal, and the hospital stay is often as short as 2 or 3 days.

SUGGESTED READING

Braley S. Symposium on synthetics in maxillofacial surgery (the silicones in maxillofacial surgery). Laryngoscope 1986; 78:549–557.

Cabanela ME, Coventry MB, MacCarty CS, et al. The fate of patients with methyl methacrylate cranioplasty. J Bone Joint Surg Am 1972; 54:278–281.

Jarcho M. Calcium phosphate ceramics as hard tissue prosthetics. Clin Orthop 1981; 157:259–278.

Jarcho M, et al. Hydroxylapatite synthesis and characterization in dense polycrystalline form. J Mater Sci 1976; 11:2027–2035.

Peebles DJ, Ellis RH, Stride SDK, Simpson BRJ. Cardiovascular effects of methyl methacrylate cement. Br Med J 1972; 1:349–351.

Schultz RC. Facial injuries. 2nd ed. Chicago: Year Book, 1977:392.

Schultz RC. Restoration of frontal contour with methyl methacrylate. Ann Plast Surg 1979; 3(4):295–303.

Schultz RC. Reconstruction of facial deformities using silicones and acrylics. In: Rubin L, ed. Biomaterials in reconstructive surgery. St. Louis: CV Mosby, 1982:437.

Schultz RC. Clinical experience with biomaterials for reconstruction and augmentation. In: Boretos JW, Eden M, eds. Contemporary biomaterials. Park Ridge, NJ: Noyes Publications, 1984:332

Sessions RB, Wolfe SK, Moiel RH, et al. Wire mesh foundation for methyl methacrylate cranioplasty. Laryngoscope 1974; 84:1020–1030.

INTERNAL FIXATION IN FACIAL FRACTURES: PRINCIPLES

JOSEPH S. GRUSS, M.B., F.R.C.S.(C)

With the advent of regional trauma centers and rapid air transport systems, more patients with extremely complex craniomaxillofacial trauma are now being seen. The problem of high-velocity facial injuries with multiple facial fractures, particularly in the polytraumatized patient, concerns the severity of the bony injury. The majority of these fractures, particularly in the midface, are unstable and often have multiple comminuted segments. Segments of bone are often markedly displaced, or actually dislocated and, in addition, segments and areas of bone may be so severely damaged as to preclude any form of fixation. They may even be missing, having been lost through large skin or mucosal lacerations. Attempts at closed reduction or internal wire suspension of these comminuted areas result in eventual bony collapse and soft tissue shrinkage. The traditional treatment of a bony gap is some form of external fixation to try and maintain the bone segments in position and allow soft tissue healing in anticipation of secondary bone grafting. External fixation techniques maintain the position of mandibular segments, but cannot maintain the position of comminuted midfacial bony segments. The inability to stabilize these midfacial segments results in rapid soft tissue shrinkage and makes secondary bony correction very difficult, or impossible.

The solution to the problems of midfacial bony collapse and soft tissue shrinkage and scarring lies in the early exposure of all fracture segments and their repair by internal fixation techniques. This results in the reestablishment of a normal craniofacial skeletal anatomy and maintains soft tissue expansion during healing of the face. Comminuted or missing bone is replaced by immediate bone grafting. The utilization of these techniques allows the one-stage repair of even the most severe injury, with an insignificant increase in the rate of infection, and prevents the development of secondary deformity that may be very difficult, or impossible, to correct adequately.

PRINCIPLES OF REPAIR

Whenever possible, the facial injuries are repaired immediately, or within the first few days, depending upon the magnitude of coexisting multisystem trauma. Careful coordination and planning of the involved surgical disciplines facilitate early repair. Definitive repair can be delayed for up to 2 weeks, but this increases the difficulty of adequate reduction and fixation. A striking decrease in facial edema and discomfort follows early, rigid, internal fixation and repair. Once the diagnosis of a complex injury has been made, a coordinated approach, based on principles derived from reconstructive craniofacial surgery, is utilized.

Direct Exposure of Fractures

All fractures are exposed directly, so that the degree of comminution and displacement and the pattern of the fractures can be accurately assessed by inspection. Only then can a logical plan for repair be formulated.

Failure to expose all fractures and bone segments adequately results in bone segments being stabilized in an unreduced, or displaced, position because the surgeon can only assess each fracture site individually. This is particularly true in the orbital region, where it is supposed that reduction of fracture segments through small incisions can be easily accomplished without the realization of other fractures and displacements elsewhere in this region. This results in the development of severe secondary deformities, particularly in the orbital and nasoethmoid region.

Reduction and Internal Fixation

All fractures are reduced and internally fixed with meticulous interosseous fixation that links fragments and bone segments to adjacent fragments and to areas of intact craniofacial skeleton until mechanical stability is obtained. The fixation may be interosseous wiring or metal plates and screws.

Primary Bone Grafting

All severely damaged or absent bone is replaced, whenever possible, with immediate bone grafting. Deficits in bony contour can be augmented similarly at the time of initial repair.

These techniques allow repair of even the most severe injuries in one stage and minimize the occurrence of secondary deformities. External fixation techniques are rarely needed, and internal craniofacial suspension wires are never used.

INCISIONS AND APPROACHES

Preexisting lacerations are utilized in combination with planned incisions, as required. All incisions are linked to each other subperiosteally to provide direct visualization of the entire involved facial skeleton. No attempt is made to preserve periosteal attachment to small segments of bone, as this compromises the adequacy of exposure.

The coronal incision is used for access to the upper craniofacial skeleton and zygomatic arch. Direct access to the entire craniofacial skeleton can be obtained by combining the coronal incision with eyelid incisions and an upper buccal sulcus degloving incision.

METHODS OF INTERNAL FIXATION

Interosseous Wiring

Interosseous wiring is adequate fixation for relatively stable and undisplaced fractures, which usually are localized to one area of the craniofacial skeleton. In severely unstable, displaced, and comminuted fractures of multiple areas of the facial skeleton, interosseous wires have been found to be less useful. An interosseous wire provides only two-dimensional stability and cannot prevent rotation around the wire. Even with the use of multiple wires, movement of bony segments persists. In many of our earlier cases fixed with extensive interosseous wiring and bone grafting, the early correction obtained on the operating table was not maintained consistently when soft tissue and bony healing progressed. At the present time, interosseous wire fixation is primarily utilized for comminuted segments of the cranium and in repair of the infraorbital rim in certain selected cases where adjacent segments have been rigidly fixed with miniplates.

Lag Screws

The lag fixation principle is achieved by drilling a hole in the outer, or more proximal, bone to a diameter that approximates the outer diameter of the screw threads. The inner, or more distal, hole is drilled with a diameter that approximates the inner, or core, diameter of the screw. This principle can be used with either self-tapping or tapped screws. The screw glides through the outer hole without any form of fixation. As it enters the distal bone segment, the screw threads engage this bone, either by cutting threads in a self-tapping system, or by engaging along precut threads in a tapped system of fixation. When the head of the screw, engages in the proximal segment, with the screw threads engaged in the distal segment, and the screw is tightened, the outer and inner bone segments are lagged together, thereby producing direct interfragmentary compression of the bone. Since rotation of bone is still possible around a single lag screw, usually more than one lag screw is needed for adequate bony fixation. This is the most sophisticated and rigid of all forms of bony fixation. Lag screw fixation is ideally applied to oblique fractures in various areas of the midface and mandible. It can be used in combination with miniplates in the midface, and compression and reconstruction plates in the mandible. In addition, lag screws are the ideal form of fixation for bone grafts.

Miniplates and Screws

Specially designed miniplates and screws have revolutionized the care of upper and midfacial injuries. These can secure accurate reduction with three-dimensional stability for repaired bone and bone segments, without the risk of secondary relapse. Self-tapping screws should always be used in the thin midfacial bone. The use of long miniplates with multiple screws is the ideal method of fixation for long, comminuted segments. The miniplate is fixed at each end to relatively stable bone segments; then each comminuted segment is anchored to the plate by multiple miniscrews. Miniplates have proved to be the ideal method of fixation at the frontozygomatic suture line, the zygomatic arch, the nasoethmoid orbital region, and the anterior maxillary buttresses. In addition, they are the ideal method of fixation of various bone grafts; in particular, bone grafts to the lateral orbit and cantilever grafts to the nose.

Compression Plates

Dynamic compression plates that produce compression at the fracture site are ideal for fixation of mandibular fractures. These compression plates are manufactured to be much stronger than miniplates in order to counteract the deforming forces that act on the mandible. Their purpose is to allow primary bone healing of the fracture site. As in all plate and screw fixation, at least two screws are needed on either side of the fracture site to prevent rotation around a single screw.

Reconstruction Plates

The reconstruction plate is a specially designed plate that is bendable in three-dimensions to mimic the shape of the mandible. Reconstruction plates are ideally suited to stabilized long segments of comminuted, or segmental, fractures of the mandible, or to bridge bony gaps in the mandible such as following gunshot wounds. Their use is frequently combined in the same patient with the use of miniplates, lag screws, and compression plates.

PRINCIPLES OF FIXATION

The zygomatic arch is the key to the repair of complex orbitozygomatic and midfacial injuries. The position of the zygomatic arch between its temporal attachment posteriorly and zygomatic body and lateral orbit anteriorly predetermines the position of the lateral and midfacial bones. A careful review of our early patients, treated with extensive midfacial fixation and immediate bone grafting without zygomatic arch fixation, has shown late flatness of the zygomatic bodies and midface and an obvious shortening of the zygomatic arch in a significant number of them, both clinically and on x-ray film. In all complex orbitozygomatic and midfacial fractures that show a shortening or loss of projection of the zygomatic arch on axial computed tomography (CT) scanning, it is essential first to stabilize the zygomatic arch. Careful stabilization of the zygomatic arch itself, with the use of miniplates and lag screws in combination with miniplate fixation at the frontozygomatic suture line, produces exact restoration of correct zygomatic body and lateral orbital wall projection in relation to the cranial base. This produces an intact outer facial frame. The inner facial frame, which is composed of the orbital rims, naso-orbital ethmoid, and maxillary buttresses, then can be repositioned exactly within the outer facial frame to produce an exact three-dimensional anatomic reconstruction with normal midfacial projection.

All fractures are exposed and reduced, with each fragment linked to its adjacent fragment until all links in the chain are restored. With an intact mandibular arch, correct maxillary and mandibular occlusion is reestablished first. Reduction and repair is commenced with the zygomatic arch and lateral orbit. This results in reconstruction of an outer facial frame with restoration of vertical and transverse facial height. Anterior, posterior, or horizontal facial height and projection are reestablished by reduction and fixation of the inferior and medial orbits, nasoethmoid, nose, and central maxillary fractures within this previously established facial frame.

When fractures of the mandibular symphysis, or body, are present, continuity of the mandibular arch is reestablished by rigid internal fixation with the use of lag screws, compression, or reconstruction plates. It is essential in the repair of all facial fractures that involve the upper or lower dental arch, to reestablish the correct occlusion prior to the application of plate or screw fixation. Failure to do this maintains stabilized segments with an incorrect occlusion that is impossible to correct secondarily by orthodontic means.

PRIMARY BONE GRAFTING

All severely damaged or missing bone is replaced, and contour deficits are augmented, whenever feasible, by immediate bone grafting. Only in the presence of a heavily contaminated or infected wound, or in the absence of adequate soft tissue cover, may the bone grafting be delayed. In certain cases, such as gunshot wounds with extensive bone and soft tissue loss, simultaneous primary replacement of the missing soft tissue and bone can be performed with safety. In our experience, bone grafting performed at the time of the original repair always gives a superior result compared with secondary bone grafting, which is usually compromised by soft tissue shrinkage and scarring.

In the majority of patients with craniofacial trauma, split calvarial bone grafts have become the primary source of graft material. However, these are difficult to use and contour in extensive orbital wall defects, or when there is extensive bone loss, such as in gunshot wounds. In these situations, I combine the use of split calvarial grafts with split rib grafts. Rib grafts are easier to bend and shape to large contour deficits of the orbital cavity and very large defects in the maxilla and zygomatic regions and skull.

Split skull and split rib grafts yield a readily available source of bone grafting material and are associated with minimum morbidity. These grafts have an exceptional ability to survive, even when portions of the graft are exposed to the air percutaneously or through the mucosal lining of the nose or oral cavity. The risk of possible graft exposure in patients with severe soft tissue and bony injuries should not preclude use of these materials. Bone grafts, especially in the midface and nasal area, maintain soft tissue expansion and projection, even if they become partially exposed. In this situation, they act as an internal splinting mechanism and maintain the normal stretch and position of the soft tissue during soft tissue healing and scar maturation. Bone grafts used to reconstruct the anterior wall of the frontal sinus, medial wall and floor of the orbit, and anterior wall of the maxilla survive adequately even though they are placed over an open cavity with vascularized soft tissue coverage on one side only. The failure to use bone grafts results in rapid shrinkage of soft tissue, which makes subsequent reconstructive efforts difficult and often inadequate.

Adequate fixation of bone grafts is essential as inadequate fixation predisposes to infection or resorption. Bone grafts are stabilized, whenever possible, using lag screws or miniplates. The addition of lag screw fixation to bone grafts has added a new dimension to the stability of midfacial reconstruction. Bone grafts, either calvarial or rib, that are stabilized with lag screws undergo minimal resorption. Bone grafts used to reconstruct the orbital cavity require no form of fixation and are merely wedged into place and held in place by the orbital contents.

SUGGESTED READING

Gruss JS, MacKinnon SE, Kassel EE, Cooper PW. The role of primary bone grafting in complex craniomaxillofacial trauma. Plast Reconstr Surg 1985; 75:17–24.

Gruss JS. Naso-ethmoid-orbital fractures: classification and role of primary bone grafting. Plast Reconstr Surg 1985; 75:303–315.

Gruss JS. Fronto-naso-orbital trauma. Clin Plast Surg 1982; 9:557–589.

Merville L. Multiple dislocations of the facial skeleton. J Maxillofac Surg 1974; 2:187–200.

Merville LC, Derome P. Concomitant dislocations of the face and skull. J Maxillofac Surg 1978; 6:2–14.

INTERNAL FIXATION IN FACIAL FRACTURES: SPECIFIC ANATOMIC ASPECTS

JOSEPH S. GRUSS, M.B., F.R.C.S.(C)

ORBITOZYGOMATIC FRACTURES

Injuries to the midface may result in fractures of the orbitozygomatic complex. These fractures may be isolated, or may be combined with other midfacial injuries. Orbitozygomatic fractures are wrongly termed tripod fractures and should always be considered as quadripod fractures, as the fourth site of fracture, the zygomaticomaxillary buttress is one of the keys to the understanding and management of unstable zygomatic fractures. This lateral buttress acts as a direct antagonist to the pull of the masseter muscle and forms the structural support to the zygoma itself. Fractures of this buttress allow the zygomatic body to tilt downward and inward, thus resulting in late depression of the zygomatic prominence. Two-point fixation of the frontozygomatic suture line and inferior orbital rim does not prevent downward rotation of the zygomatic body. Direct exposure by means of an upper buccal sulcus incision of this buttress, and direct anatomic reconstruction with miniplates or bone grafts, does prevent this complication. When the fracture has involved the zygomatic arch and resulted in loss of anteroposterior projection of the zygoma, it is essential to stabilize the zygomatic arch as well. Miniplates are used to stabilize the frontozygomatic suture line, zygomatic arch, and zygomaticomaxillary buttress (Fig. 1). The final point of fixation on the inferior orbital rim can be stabilized with the use of a miniplate (Fig. 2), or interosseous wire. In many cases, an interosseous wire is preferable as a miniplate may be felt through the thin eyelid skin. Inadequate treatment of orbitozygomatic fractures is the commonest cause of secondary deformity following facial fractures. Coexisting orbital wall fractures should always be suspected, particularly in the medial, inferomedial, and lateral walls. These deficits should be carefully outlined and totally reconstructed with immediate bone grafting to prevent the late occurrence of enophthalmus and oculo-orbital displacement.

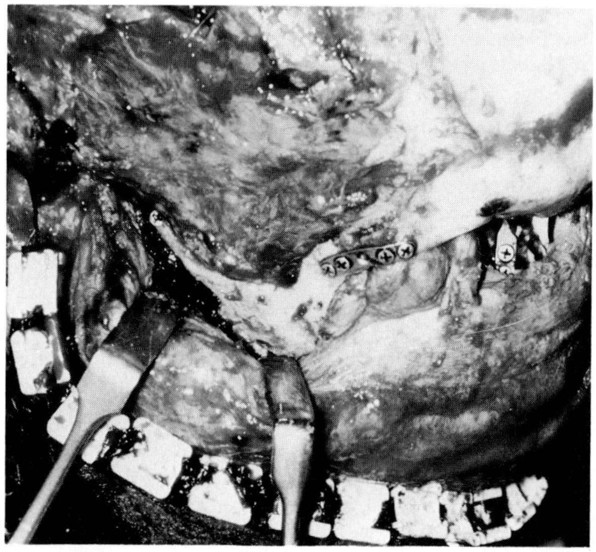

Figure 1 Exposure of upper face through a coronal incision shows exposure of zygomatic arch in fixation at the frontozygomatic suture line, with miniplate and lag screw fixation of zygomatic arch to the temporal bone posteriorly. This approach repositions the fractured zygomatic bone exactly and reconstructs an outer facial frame. On the right, miniplates can be seen as they reconstruct the nasoethmoid region.

NASOETHMOID ORBITAL FRACTURES

A direct blow to the midface may result in fractures of the bony nasoethmoid orbital complex and injury to the adjacent soft tissues. These injuries may be confined to the nasoethmoid orbital complex, but, more frequently, are associated with other facial fractures and often complicated by multisystem trauma. The injuries result in severe cosmetic and functional deformity due to collapse of the nose, ethmoids, and medial orbits and are accentuated by coexisting injury to the medial canthal ligaments and nasolacrimal apparatus. Extension into the anterior cranial fossa, with concomitant dural tear, cerebrospinal fluid rhinorrhea, and cerebral injury, may be life-threatening.

Nasoethmoid orbital fractures are the most challenging of all craniofacial fractures to treat due to the intricate anatomy of this region and the difficulty of fracture fixation. Inadequate initial treatment often results in severe deformity that may be extremely difficult, or impossible, to correct adequately. Optimal management involves ear-

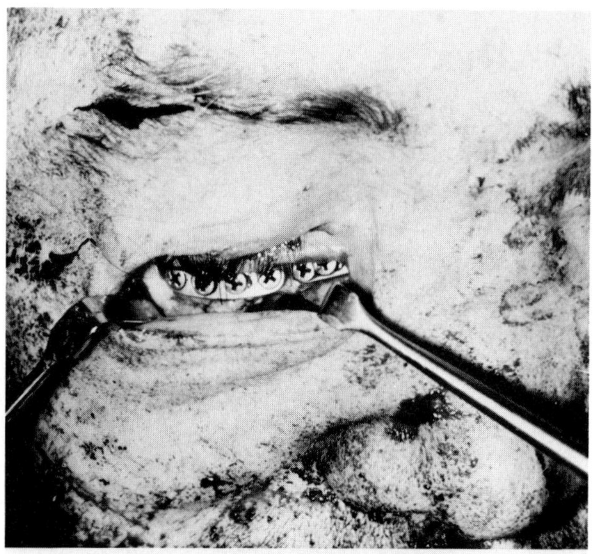

Figure 2 A complex midfacial and multiply-comminuted orbital fracture is exposed through a subciliary muscle-splitting incision. Fractures are stabilized with multiple miniplates and screws.

ly surgical exploration and meticulous bony and soft tissue repair that utilizes the principles learned from reconstructive craniofacial surgery. It is essential to understand that the nasal bones, vomerine bone, perpendicular plate of the ethmoid, and ethmoid labyrinth are thin and predisposed to comminuted fractures. Conversely, the nasal process of the frontal bone and frontal process of the maxilla are strong and comminution is rare. The medial wall of the orbit, however, is extremely thin and invariably comminutes. Telecanthus is nearly always produced by the splaying apart of the nasomaxillary buttress, which is displaced laterally and downward, taking the medial canthal ligament with it. It is extremely rare for the ligament to be actually lacerated or avulsed from the bone. Correct anatomic repair of the nasomaxillary buttress allows restoration of a correct intercanthal distance. Attempts to hold this segment in place with multiple interosseous wires rarely has been successful in my experience. The stabilization of this segment with miniplates, both above (thereby attaching it to the region of the frontal bone and frontal sinus) and below (attaching it to the infraorbital rim), results in a three-dimensionally stable reconstruction with restoration of a correct intercanthal distance (Figs. 3 and 6). The miniplate can be placed adjacent to the canthal ligament itself, which should be isolated in all cases during medial rim and orbital wall dissection. It is essential not to strip the ligament off the bone during this dissection as it will then have to be rewired to the nasal bone. A transnasal canthopexy, in my experience, rarely gives a perfectly natural-appearing medial canthal region. When there is loss of distal nasal support, a cantilever bone graft should be used to restore nasal projection and prevent soft tissue shrinkage. A split calvarial bone graft is preferred, and this is cantilevered by means of a miniplate and fixed to the anterior portion of the frontal bone. The degree of cantilevering can be varied by adjustment of the angle of the bend in the miniplate. Split calvarial grafts, rigidly fixed and cantilevered in this fashion, rarely undergo resorption and produce an excellent long-term nasal reconstruction.

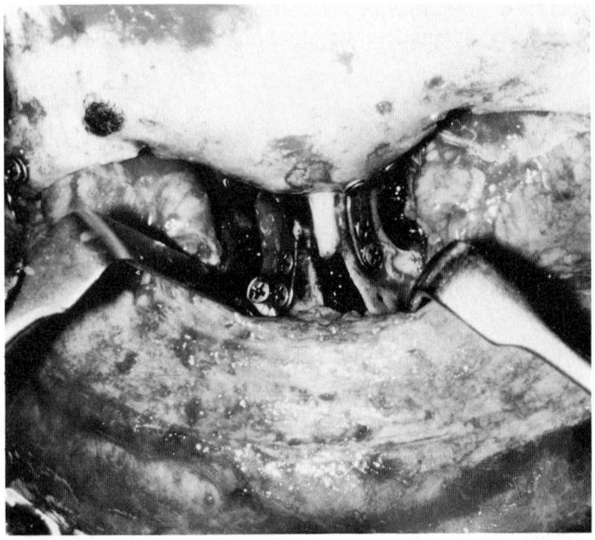

Figure 3 Exposure of naso-orbital ethmoid region through coronal incision, with careful repair of medial orbital walls and rims through miniplates attached to frontal bone. Correct contouring of miniplates in this area repositions the frontonasal buttress exactly and reconstructs an exact intercanthal distance by maintaining the attachment of the canthal ligaments to these segments.

COMBINED INJURIES OF THE CRANIUM AND FACE

Various technical factors are important in the reconstruction of this region.

1. With severe comminution of the cranial vault, it is essential first to stabilize the cranium with rigid interosseous fixation. The facial bones can then be stabilized and fixed to the now intact cranial vault.
2. With massive comminution, or actual loss of cranial bone, a reverse order of fixation is used. The facial fractures are fixed first, and the face is stabilized to the residual cranial vault. The amount of missing bone can now be assessed and replaced with primary bone grafting with either split cranial or split rib grafts being used.
3. Inadequate reconstruction of the supraorbital ridge commonly leads to flatness in this region. The use of a full-thickness rib graft, or the stacking of bone grafts in layers, prevents this.
4. Injury to the orbital roof may result in isolated fractures, comminuted fractures, or areas of bone destruction or loss. Concomitant loss of the posterior wall of the frontal sinus results in direct communication between the anterior cranial fossa and orbit. The orbital roof should always be reconstructed in this situation to separate the two cavities. When the posterior wall of the frontal sinus is intact, it is not necessary to reconstruct small defects of the orbital roof. However, failure to reconstruct larger defects, even with the posterior wall of the frontal sinus intact, may lead to herniation and entrapment of orbital contents and possible enophthalmus and diplopia.
5. When the frontal sinus injury is associated with severe injury at the base of the frontal sinus, with direct communication between the ethmoids and frontal sinus, a pericranial, galeal, or galeofrontalis flap is inserted into the frontal sinus and placed along the floor of the sinus to separate the nasal and cranial cavities.

Fractures of the cranial vault are not under the influence of muscle pull and tension, as opposed to fractures that influence the toothbearing areas of the craniofacial skeleton. Thus, the same degree of rigid internal fixation is not essential in this area. Interosseous wires play a useful part in the management of comminuted area of cranial bone. However, miniplate fixation has proved extremely useful in the management of significantly large and segmental fractures of the cranial vault. Long miniplates can be exactly contoured to the shape of the skull and individual fragments can be lagged to the plate, with specially designed miniscrews that are only 3 mm and 4 mm in length so as to prevent them entering the cranial cavity and damaging the dura. My preference now, in the face of markedly comminuted segments of the anterior cranial vault, is to replace these primarily with split calvarial grafts held in place at selected sites with miniplates. This gives an exact reconstruction of a normal cranial skeletal contour and greatly minimizes the occurrence of secondary deformity (Figs. 4, 5, and 6).

MAXILLARY FRACTURES

The paired nasomaxillary, zygomaticomaxillary, and pterygomaxillary buttresses maintain the position of the maxilla in relation to the cranial base, above and the mandible, below. Exact anatomic reconstruction of the four anterior buttresses, namely the nasomaxillary and zygomaticomaxillary buttresses, allows exact repositioning of the maxilla in its correct anteroposterior position in relation to the cranial base and allows reconstruction of the exact vertical height and horizontal projection of the maxilla (Fig. 7). No reconstruction of the posterior buttress is needed because the four anterior buttresses will maintain correct position of the maxilla. The intact mandible provides an additional buttress in relation to the cranial base, and the reestablishment of normal maxillary and mandibular occlusion provides additional support to the reconstructed maxilla.

The anterior maxillary buttresses are exposed through an upper gingival buccal sulcus degloving incision (Fig. 8). All unstable buttresses are repaired with miniplates, and missing buttresses are replaced with bone grafts fixed in place with lag screws. When the fractures that cross the buttresses are low and situated close to the toothbearing bone, care must be taken not to place screws through the teeth apices. In this situation, it may be necessary to use small bone grafts to reinforce the buttress repair, as the lag screws can be placed exactly between the teeth apices.

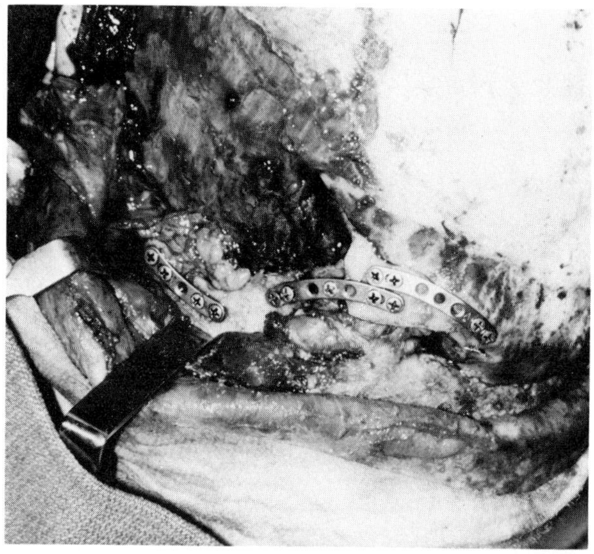

Figure 5 Split calvarial bone grafts are used to reconstruct the anterior wall of the frontal sinus and are held in place with miniplates. Miniplate is also used to repair zygomatic arch fracture.

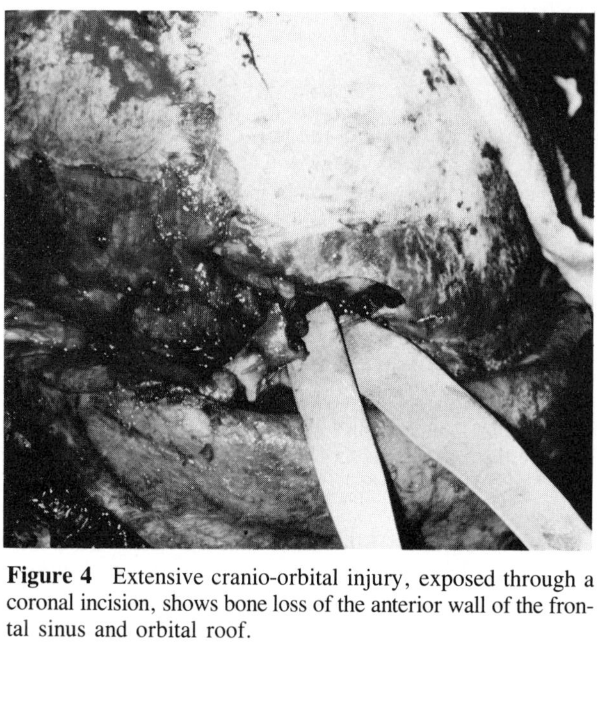

Figure 4 Extensive cranio-orbital injury, exposed through a coronal incision, shows bone loss of the anterior wall of the frontal sinus and orbital roof.

COMPLEX MANDIBULAR FRACTURES

Internal fixation of mandibular fractures by use of compression plating, lag screws, and reconstruction

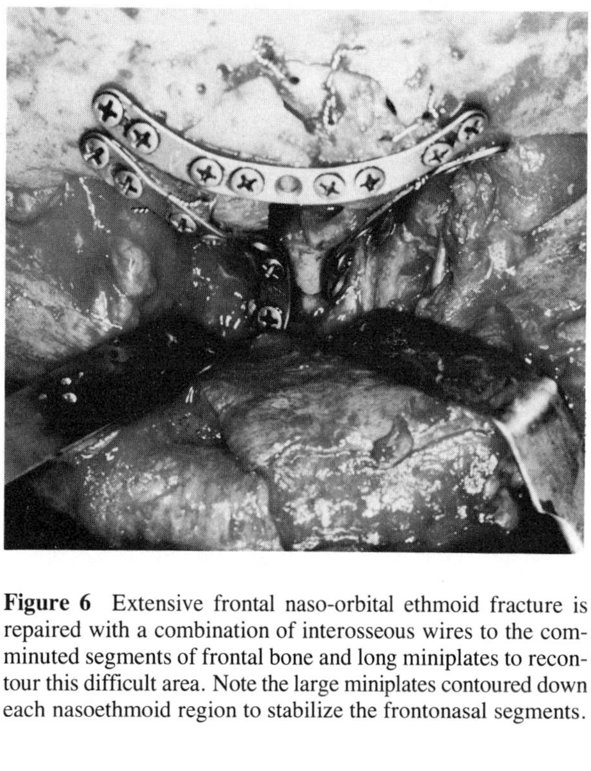

Figure 6 Extensive frontal naso-orbital ethmoid fracture is repaired with a combination of interosseous wires to the comminuted segments of frontal bone and long miniplates to recontour this difficult area. Note the large miniplates contoured down each nasoethmoid region to stabilize the frontonasal segments.

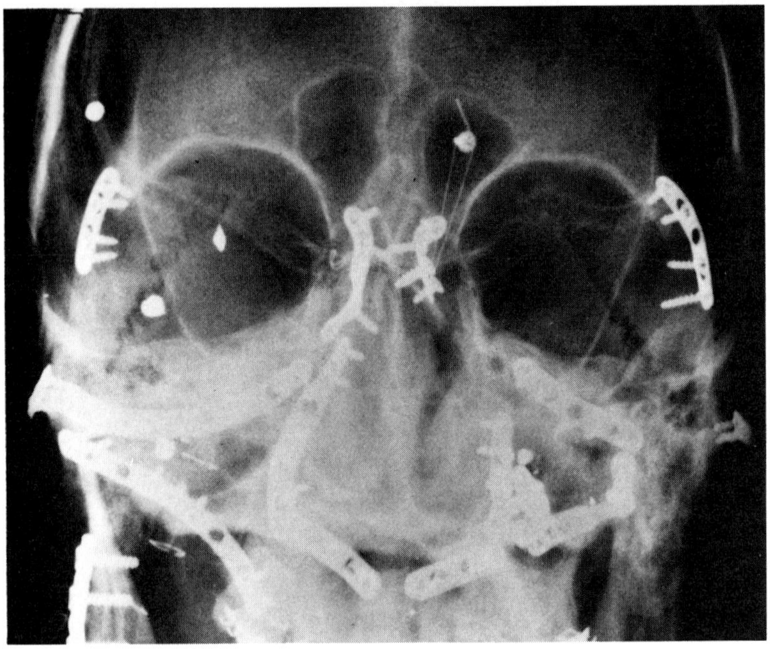

Figure 7 Extensive craniomaxillofacial injury was repaired in a three-dimensional fashion with multiple miniplates and screws. Note the miniplates that stabilize both frontozygomatic areas and zygomatic arches, both orbital rims, and all maxillary buttresses.

plates has revolutionized the care of the complex mandibular injury. These techniques are particularly useful in the care of the polytraumatized patient with associated head injuries and cervical spine fracture. In addition, they facilitate stabilization in the comminuted or segmental fracture, or the mandibular fracture with bone loss.

Airway management is facilitated by using rigid internal fixation techniques with plates and screws. In midfacial or mandibular injuries in the multiple trauma patient, or combined injuries of the midface and mandible, the orotracheal tube can be pushed to the side, thereby allowing temporary intermaxillary fixation to establish the correct occlusion. Following rigid internal fixation of the mandible and midface with plates and screws, in combination with immediate bone grafting where necessary, the intermaxillary fixation can often be released. This allows endotracheal intubation to be maintained postoperatively until a patent airway is assured. Tracheostomy is only needed in the patient with bilateral condylar neck fractures, where the position of the mandible has to be maintained in relation to the maxilla. The ability to repair multiple facial fractures without the need for intermaxillary fixation has revolutionized the care of the multiple trauma patient. This allows early fixation of the facial fractures and facilitates airway management in the early postoperative phase, without the need for tracheostomy in the majority of cases.

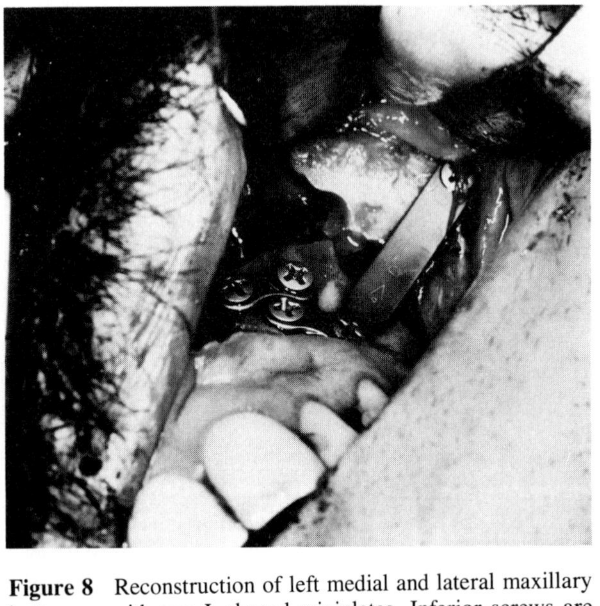

Figure 8 Reconstruction of left medial and lateral maxillary buttresses with two L-shaped miniplates. Inferior screws are placed carefully to avoid apices of teeth roots.

GUNSHOT WOUNDS

Gunshot wounds of the face often present as formidable wounds that offer a great challenge to the reconstructive surgeon. Frequently, there is both bony and soft tissue loss with the bony loss usually the more severe. This may be further complicated by concomitant injuries to the oral cavity, nasal passages, orbits, cranial cavity, and their contents. Lessons and techniques learned in the management of complex facial trauma by using craniofacial surgical techniques, immediate bone grafting, and rigid internal fixation with plates and screws in the midface and mandible can be successfully applied to the management of severe gunshot wounds of the face. Extensive bone loss is replaced with rib and cranial grafts, stabilized with lag screws and miniplates. The use of extensive miniplate and lag screw fixation in the midface, and large reconstruction plates in the mandible, to bridge bone gaps facilitates stabilization and reconstruction in these areas in combination with the bone grafts. Soft tissue repair can be by means of various local or regional flaps, or, in massive soft tissue loss, by means of a free, vascularized, omental flap that can be wrapped around the bone grafts. Total nasal reconstruction, with use of tissue-expanded forehead skin, provides an ideal method of nasal reconstruction once initial midfacial reconstruction projection has been obtained.

SUGGESTED READING

Antonyshyn O, Gruss JS. Complex orbital trauma: the role of rigid fixation and primary bone grafting. Plast Reconstr Surg 1988; 7:61–92.

Gruss JS, Mackinnon SE. Complex maxillary fractures: Role of buttress reconstruction and immediate bone grafts. Plast Reconstr Surg 1986; 78:9–22.

Rosen HM. Miniplate fixation of LeFort I osteotomies. Plast Reconstr Surg 1986; 78:748–754.

Schilli W, Ewers R, Niederdellman H. Bone fixation with screws and plates in the maxillo-facial region. Int J Oral Surg 1981; 10(suppl 1): 329–332.

Spiessl B. Principles of rigid internal fixation in fractures of the lower jaw. In: Spiessl B, ed. New concepts in maxillofacial bone surgery. New York: Springer-Verlag, 1976.

SURGICAL ANATOMY OF THE ORBIT

PAUL N. MANSON, M.D.
NICHOLAS T. ILIFF, M.D.

SURGICAL ANATOMY OF THE ORBIT

Three basic structures determine globe position: (1) the bony orbit; (2) the ligament system; and (3) orbital fat.

Bone

The bony orbit is an anteriorly based, roughly quadrilaterally-shaped pyramidal space that is oriented slightly superiorly and medially. The size of the orbital rim is approximately 30 mm vertically by 40 mm horizontally (Fig. 1). Immediately behind the rim, the orbit widens with the widest orbital diameter being 8 to 10 mm posterior to the rim. Beyond the rim, the middle section of the orbit is roughly circular being 30 mm by 30 mm. Because the pyramidal structure of the orbit is oriented slightly medially and superiorly, the apex of the orbit and the optic foramen are located almost directly posterior to the medial orbital wall. The orbital floor is convex in its middle and posterior thirds and concave in its anterior third. Posterior to the globe, the floor bulges upward. The effect of this slope is that the orbital floor inclines superiorly at an approximately 30-degree angle.

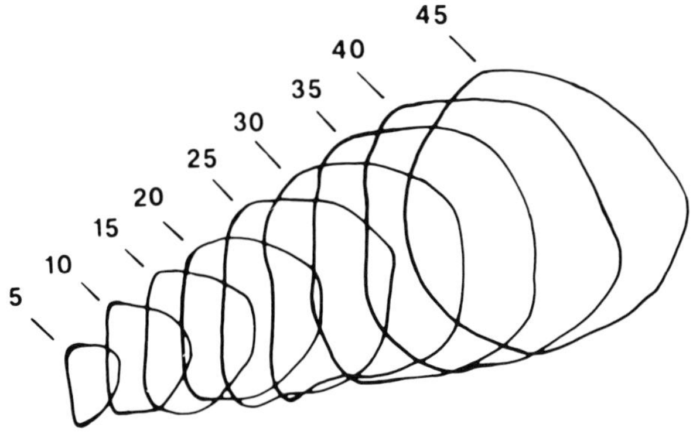

Figure 1 Dimensions of the bony orbit. The relative dimensions of the bony orbit are seen in this artist's diagram where sequential coronal sections of orbital volume are illustrated. © JHU

The medial orbital wall also bulges inward posterior to the globe. Thus, the middle sections of the medial orbital wall and the orbital floor deviate inward behind the globe and meet each other at a 45 degree angle, thus reducing the retrobulbar orbital volume. This middle section of the orbit, especially inferiomedially, is the critical section for orbital volume reduction. The anterior section is critical for globe support. Paradoxically, it is the exact reconstruction of the middle section (inferiomedial orbit) that is the most difficult and the critical determinant of anteroposterior globe position following soft tissue mobilization.

The orbital floor is a thin plate of bone perforated by the infraorbital nerve. The nerve crosses the orbital floor traveling anteriorly and medially, first in a groove, then becoming a canal. The nerve emerges into the groove from the posterior portion of the inferior orbital fissure. Anteriorly, the nerve exists from the anterior surface of the maxilla about 10 mm beneath the inferior orbital rim in line with the medial corneoscleral limbus in primary gaze. The maxillary sinus lies beneath most of the orbital floor; its roof is 0.5 to 1 mm in thickness. The roof of the sinus ends posteriorly about 7 mm anterior to the optic foramen. The weakest spot in the orbital floor is medial to the infraorbital groove or canal. The weakest section of all the internal orbital walls is located medially in the lamina papyracea of the ethmoid bone.

Functional Bone Anatomy

The bony orbit can be divided into thirds, both with regard to sections of the rim and to the anteroposterior divisions of the orbit (Fig. 2). The superior section of the rim is the supraorbital segment; medially is the nasoethmoidal section and, inferiorly and laterally, the zygoma.

With regard to the anteroposterior orbit, the anterior third (0 to 10 mm) consists of strong bone and is the orbi-

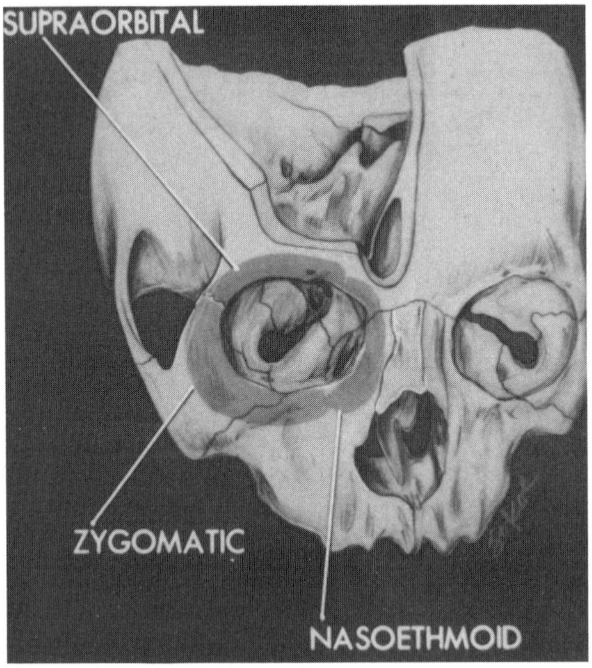

Figure 2 Divisions of the orbital rim. The orbital rim is divided into three sections: superiorly, the supraorbital section; medially, the nasoethmoidal section; inferiorly and laterally, the zygoma. © JHU

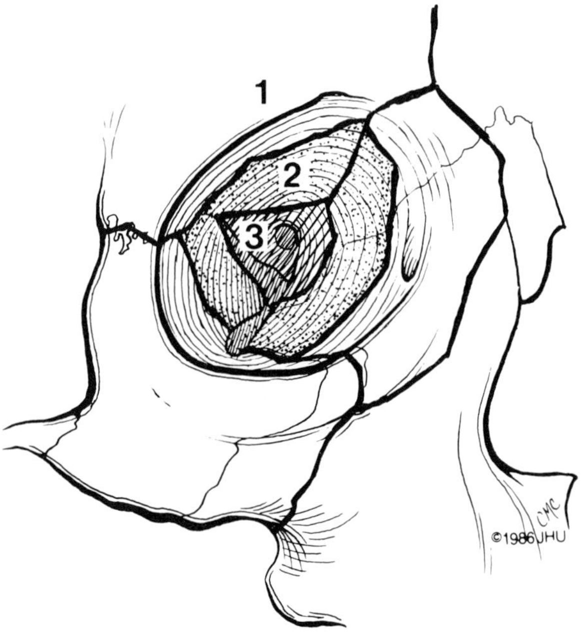

Figure 3 Anteroposterior divisions of the orbit. The orbit, from anterior to posterior, is also divided into three sections: (1) Anteriorly is the rim; (2) the middle section, where orbital fractures commonly comminute the bone, is the important section for enophthalmus correction; (3) posteriorly, fracture displacement is less common as thicker bone surrounds the optic canal and superior orbital fissure. © JHU

tal rim (Fig. 3); the middle third (10 to 38 mm) is a thin section where isolated orbital "blow-out" fractures occur; posteriorly, (38 to 45 mm) the orbital bone is again thicker and protects the superior orbital fissure and the optic foramen. In fractures, the anterior and middle sections displace; the middle segment crumbles, absorbing the shock and sparing the posterior segment from severe displacement.

Ligaments

The thickness and number of ligaments vary from anterior to posterior within the orbit's soft tissue. Anteriorly, the medial and lateral canthal ligaments form a suspensory network connected to the eyelids and tarsal plates (Fig. 4). Lockwood's ligament extends from Whitnall's tubercle to the posterior limb of the medial canthal ligament and forms a sling underneath the globe for vertical support. Both the medial and lateral canthal ligaments have anterior and posterior limbs (Fig. 5). The posterior limbs keep the eyelids tangent to the globe, while the subsequent limb in each case is responsible for the drape and architecture of the canthal ligament. Laterally, extensions of the levator sling also attach to Whitnall's tubercle with Lockwood's ligament and the posterior limb of the lateral canthal ligament (Fig. 6).

Whitnall's ligament, in the superior portion of the orbit, extends from the trochlea to the superolateral orbital rim extending through the orbital and palpebral lobes of the lacrimal gland. Whitnall's ligament and Lockwood's ligament form a superior and inferior "sling" for the globe (see Fig. 6). Posteriorly, fine ligaments attach diffusely from the orbital walls to the internal structures of the orbit including the extraocular muscles (see Fig. 5). In the posterior portion of the orbit, the ligaments become thinner. There is no distinct ligament linking the superior, medial, inferior, and lateral rectus muscles (see Fig. 5). Fine ligaments intersperse fat and soft tissue diffusely, but there is no clear anatomic boundary between the intramuscular fat compartment and the extramuscular fat compartment in the posterior orbit. These ligaments extend throughout the fat putting orbital soft tissue into smaller spaces and restricting displacement. Most of the fat in the posterior orbit is intraconal or intramuscular.

Course of Extraocular Muscles

Extraocular muscles in the anterior half of the orbit are located a short distance from the walls of the orbit and are cushioned by a small amount of extramuscular cone fat. Check ligaments extend discretely in an anterior direction and diffusely in a posterior direction from the muscular sheaths to the orbital walls. Posteriorly, the muscles travel adjacent to the orbital walls. To avoid muscle injury, surgeons must be aware of these relationships in the repair of blow-out fractures in the posterior portion of the orbit. The inferior oblique and inferior rectus muscles are usually visualized in blow-out fractures, inferiorly, and the superior oblique and medial rectus muscles, medially. The lateral rectus muscle is immediately present adjacent to

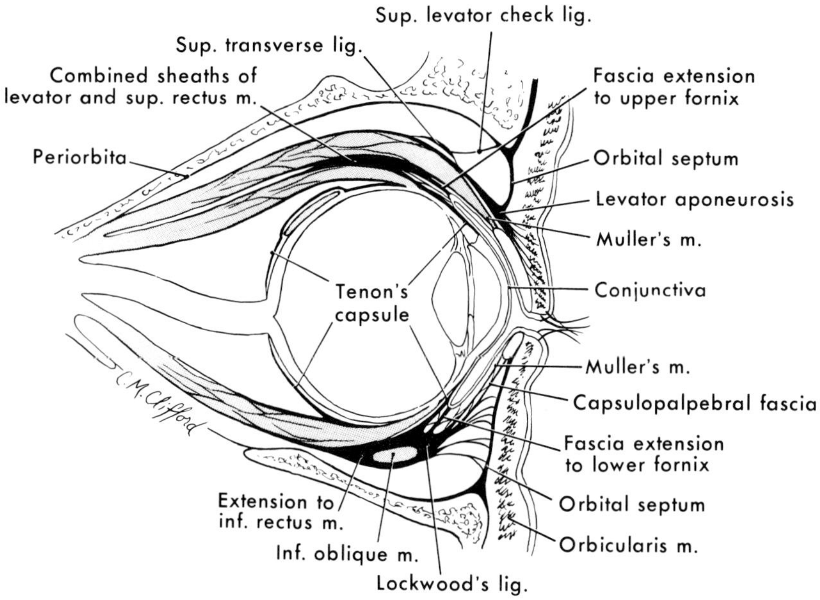

Figure 4 Sagittal section of orbital ligaments in the plane of the optic nerve. The distribution of the ligaments providing globe support is seen in this parasagittal section in the plane of the optic nerve. Condensations of ligaments are seen inferiorly (Lockwood's ligament) and superiorly to provide a "sling" for globe support. (Reprinted from Manson PN, Clifford CM, Su CT, et al. Mechanisms of global support and post-traumatic enophthalmos: I. The anatomy of the ligament sling and its relation to intramuscular cone orbital fat. Plast Reconstr Surg 1986; 77:193–202.)

the greater wing of the sphenoid. Superiorly, the levator palpebral superioris is encountered beneath a small cushion of orbital fat. Inferiorly, in dissections of the orbital floor the nerve to the inferior oblique is also vulnerable (traveling next to the inferior rectus muscle). A small vascular coupling exists between the infraorbital neurovascular bundle and the inferior rectus in the mid portion of the orbital floor. This coupling must often be sectioned in dissections of the floor to provide visualization for repair of blow-out fractures in the posterior portion of the orbit.

Orbital Fat

The volume and quantity of intramuscular orbital fat is an important determinant of globe position. In the posterior orbit, most fat exists within the muscle cone as intramuscular fat. In the anterior orbit, some fat exists outside the muscle cone along the roof and floor.

Superiorly, this sausage-shaped extramuscular orbital fat isolates the superior extraocular muscles from the orbital roof. In orbital fractures, dystopia of the globe allows this fat to prolapse away from the upper lid, thereby creating a "supratarsal hollow." When one pushes up on the globe and the contents of the anterior and middle thirds of the orbit, this fat is displaced forward and the hollow disappears. Upper lid fullness is created by the presence of fat in the superior portion of the orbit against the upper eyelid.

Studies have demonstrated no significant change in globe position with loss of extramuscular cone fat (for example, following blepharoplasty). Loss of intramuscular cone fat produces enophthalmus and is a major mechan-

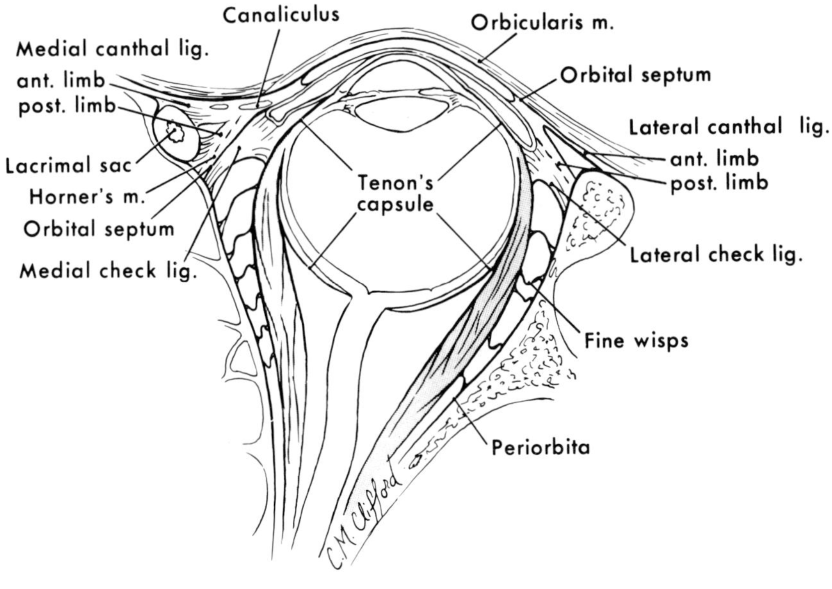

Figure 5 Transverse section indicates the distribution of orbital ligaments as seen in transverse section. Anteriorly, the canthal ligaments have both anterior and posterior limbs. Smaller "check" ligaments extend from the muscles to the orbital walls immediately behind the canthal ligaments. The size of the ligaments decreases dramatically from anterior to posterior. These fine ligaments diffusely connect orbital soft tissue structures. (Reprinted from Manson PN, Clifford CM, Su CT, et al. Mechanisms of global support and post-traumatic enophthalmos: I. The anatomy of the ligament sling and its relation to intramuscular cone orbital fat. Plast Reconstr Surg 1986; 77:193–202.)

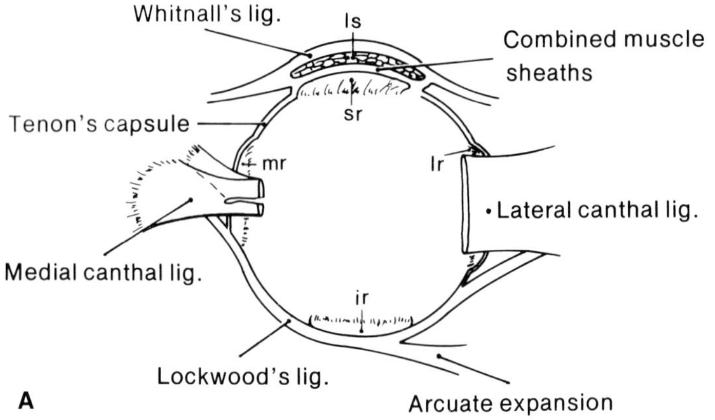

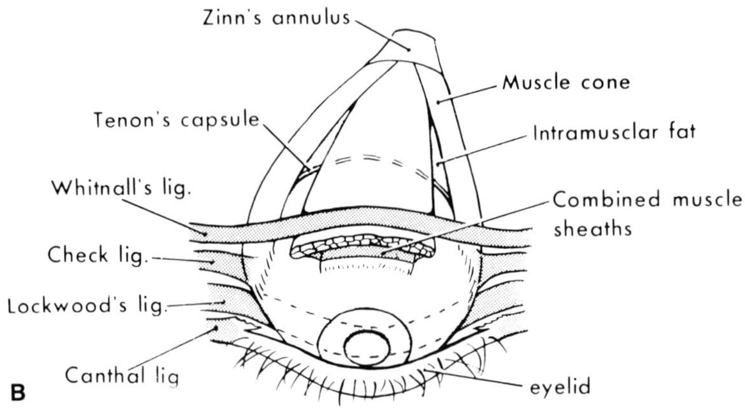

Figure 6 Concepts of the ligament "sling" for the globe. *A*, The anterior sling for the globe is indicated in this section. It consists of the medial and lateral canthal ligaments, Lockwood's ligament and Whitnall's ligament with extensions of the levator sling. *B*, The extraocular muscles and intraconal fat also provide forward support for the globe. They attach to the anterior ligament sling. The removal of intramuscular cone orbital fat produces globe displacement posteriorly (enophthalmus).

(Reprinted from Manson PN, Clifford CM, Su CT, et al. Mechanisms of global support and post-traumatic enophthalmos: I. The anatomy of the ligament sling and its relation to intramuscular cone orbital fat. Plast Reconstr Surg 1986; 77:193–202.)

ism of enophthalmus in conditions such as Romberg's disease or "shrinking sinus" syndrome. When fat from the intramuscular cone compartment is displaced to the extramuscular cone, it does not contribute to globe support, and a change of globe prominence occurs. An important mechanism of enophthalmus in orbital fractures is soft tissue disorganization and fat displacement. Since the ligament sling is not strong in the posterior portion of the orbit, intramuscular cone fat is relatively easily extruded to the extramuscular cone after rupture of fine ligaments. This allows a change in globe position. Several studies have emphasized that fat atrophy is not the usual mechanism of post-traumatic enophthalmus, as the quantities of soft tissue usually remain the same post injury.

Orbital Landmarks for Dissection

A knowledge of the important landmarks of the bony orbit is necessary for safe orbital surgery. Specifically, the location of the superior orbital fissure from both the superior rim and the lateral rim, and the location of the optic foramen from the medial, superior, and inferior rims should be noted and constantly kept in mind. (Fig. 7). When an orbital rim is depressed posteriorly, this fact must be integrated into normal measurements in order to provide safe guidelines for surgical dissection.

Measurement of Eye Position

Comparative globe position is most accurately evaluated by clinical examination; the patient should be assessed from the frontal and "inferior" or "worm's eye" position. Measurements of globe position relative to the inferior and lateral rims are also helpful. Normally, in Caucasians, the cornea should be aligned tangentially to a line drawn between the normally positioned superior and inferior orbital rims in the midpupillary line. If the cornea is 2 mm in front of this line, the condition is termed "exophthalmus," and if it is 2 mm behind this line, the condition is termed "enophthalmus." The position of the cornea relative to the lateral orbital rim is measured and compared with the normal side; in fact, this is the basis for the Hertel exophthalmometer reading. The Hertel exophthalmometer notes the distance between the pupils then measures the prominence of the cornea relative to the lateral orbital rim. The image of the cornea is superimposed on a millimeter scale with a system of mirrors. The Leude exophthalmometer measures the prominence of the cornea from either the lateral orbital rim or the inferior orbital rim with a millimeter rule. These measurements provide a relative index of globe position. In reality, globe position would be most accurately evaluated with a measurement from the apex of the orbit to the anterior margin of

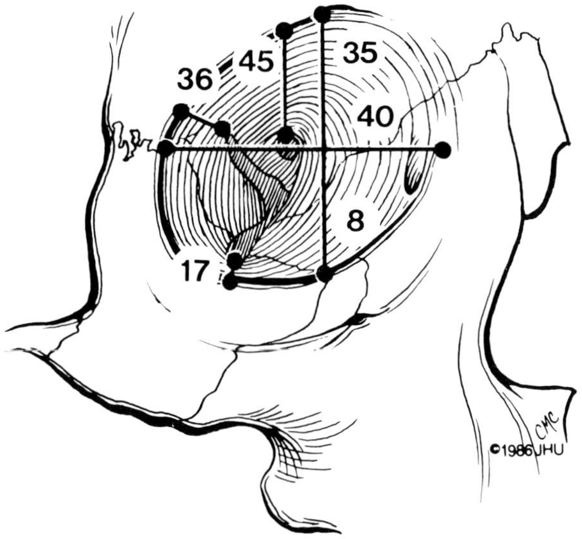

Figure 7 Landmarks for orbital dissection. The landmarks for safe orbital dissection are illustrated. The location of the optic foramen, superior orbital fissure, and inferior orbital fissure must be constantly used as guides for safe orbital dissection in the posterior half of the orbit. © JHU

the globe on a computed tomography (CT) scan. For such a measurement, CT scans must be carefully taken with the patient's head unrotated or angled to avoid error.

Physical Examination

It is important to measure the dimensions of the orbital rim both on clinical examination and plain radiographs. These measurements should be compared with the normal side, when it is present. The position of the medial and lateral canthal ligaments is recorded and any disparity of anterior, lateral, or inferior positioning is noted. Lateral canthal deformity usually consists of inferior, medial, and posterior displacement. The medial canthus is usually displaced anteriorly, inferiorly, and laterally. The palpebral fissure is thus shortened and becomes more rounded with blunting of the angles. The amount of lid ptosis relative to the brow and globe is measured. The length of the palpebral fissure should be measured and compared with the normal side. Approximation of the lid to the globe should also be noted. Poor approximation disrupts the tear film and can contribute to a loss of corneal clarity and thus visual acuity.

Significant enophthalmus is usually accompanied by major fractures of the orbital rim, in addition to the middle orbit. Many patients who pursue correction of enophthalmus have displaced zygomatic, nasoethmoidal, or supraorbital fractures. Thus, enophthalmus correction must be combined with rim osteotomies for an accurate single-staged correction.

Globe Center Versus Pupillary Position

It is important to note not only the position of the globe, but also the absence or presence of globe rotation. Pupillary position may not be an accurate index of globe position in the presence of rotation, and the surgeon should attempt to define a "globe center" position in his mind as he is evaluating eye position. Pupillary position measurements must be corrected for globe rotation. Most often, the globe is displaced posteriorly, medially, and inferiorly. Pupil position (or globe center when rotation is present) relative to the midlines of the face, midline of the nose and lateral orbital rim is determined. Periorbital and maxillary sensation should be evaluated as should tear secretion. Specifically, the lacrimal system's patency into the nose should be confirmed. When the lacrimal system is not patent, but the patient has no symptomatic tearing, reconstruction of the lacrimal system need not be contemplated. Many patients have a deficiency of tear secretion, which renders them asymptomatic despite lacrimal duct obstruction.

Ophthalmic Examination

An ophthalmologic consultation should be obtained by everyone undergoing enophthalmus correction. Inherent in any extensive orbital surgery is risk to the visual system. Documentation of the preoperative status of that system is essential. Using this examination as a baseline, the surgeon may detect adverse changes at an early and reversible stage and act to reduce the possibility of permanent iatrogenic damage. Furthermore, undocumented pre-existing damage that is discovered intraoperatively or postoperatively may be erroneously considered to be a result of surgery and may lead the surgeon to modify his operative or postoperative management in a manner detrimental to the optimal result. A preoperative comprehensive ophthalmologic consultation includes vision testing, evaluation of pupillary response and external examination of the lids and the globe. Precise and extensive extraocular motility evaluation is important and includes deviations in all fields of gaze in addition to limitations of excursions and diplopia fields. Abnormalities of tear function and patency of the lacrimal system are determined. The ophthalmic evaluation concludes with slit lamp microscopy and fundus exam.

When at all possible, vision evaluation should be done using the patient's best refractive correction. Trauma and corrective surgery can both induce or modify refractive error. Pupillary response is extremely important. A patient with 20/20 vision may still have an afferent pupillary defect, which indicates optic nerve injury. Documentation of existing nerve injury prior to surgery is obviously advantageous, and should be an accurate assessment of pupillary response.

Extraocular motility is significantly affected in major orbital fractures. The presence or absence of diplopia is, of course, of primary importance to the patient. However, measurable deficiencies in motility may be present in the absence of significant diplopia. Diplopia may be minimized by eyelid ptosis, decreased vision in one or both eyes, suppression of an image, or ignoring an image. Correction of enophthalmus may move the globe against contracted fibrotic muscles. Globe rotation toward the most severely affected muscle can occur, and the relative strabismus angles and limitations of gaze change. Ten percent of patients who undergo surgical treatment of enophthalmus can no longer fuse, suppress, or ignore the second image and develop diplopia.They may experience clinically significant exacerbation of pre-existing diplopia. These possibilities must be discussed with patients prior to surgery.

Fundus examination notes possible atrophic changes in the optic nerve. Vascular pulsation and evidence of other vascular abnormality are also noted. Optic atrophy may be subtle and may be present with 20/20 vision. Retinal pathology is recorded.

Correction of enophthalmus poses little risk to the lacrimal excretory system. However, frequently medial canthal abnormalities are present and can be managed concurrently. Presence or absence of lacrimal obstruction in the common canalicular area must be noted. There is risk to this area at the time of medial canthal dissection and medial canthal ligament suturing. A patient's lacrimal system requires meticulous protection at surgery. Preoperative determination that the system is irreparably damaged allows the surgeon freedom to be more aggressive in the area of the lacrimal sac and medial canthus.

Psychological Evaluation

Most patients who have post-traumatic enophthalmus have a complicated history of previous surgical treatment. They are frequently unhappy with previous results. Often their accidents are involved in lawsuits. The patients reaction to the injury and to their deformity should be evaluated. The family's reaction to the patient's problems and the family's perception of the problem should also be confirmed. One should not hesitate to obtain a psychiatric consultation for any complex patient situation; however, there is no substitute for adequate time personally spent with the patient and family discussing the condition and the surgery to make sure that expectations are realistic.

Radiographic Evaluation

Plain radiographs are useful to identify the dimensions of the orbital rim. The intact side may be compared with the injured side. Radiographic dimensions of the orbital rim should confirm the clinical measurements.

A thorough CT scan of the frontal bone, orbital roof, medial and lateral orbit and zygoma, nasoethmoidal area, and infraorbital rim should be obtained. The frontal, ethmoidal, and maxillary sinuses must be completely visualized. Sinus opacification should be excluded as a source of potential or existing low-grade infection prior to operative correction. Orbital CT scan should include both axial and coronal sections. Seldom are "reconstructed" cuts as illuminating as true coronal sections. One is frequently unable, in axial sections, to identify the exact position of the floor and to compare subtle changes in diameter of the internal orbit, which are responsible for globe malposition. The exact anatomy of bony displacement must be identified and used as a plan for correction.

Three-Dimensional CT Scanning

Three-dimensional CT scans are helpful in conceptualizing changes in orbital volume and rim position and in providing an overall composite view of orbital deformity. Such composite reconstructions help in conceptualizing the movements necessary in the malar eminence, zygomatic arch, nasoethmoidal area and orbital roof. There is no substitute, however, for thin section axial and coronal cuts in orbital reconstructive surgery.

SUGGESTED READING

Bite U, Jackson IT, Forbes GS, et al. Orbital volume measurements in enophthalmos using three-dimensional CT imaging. Plast Reconstr Surg 1985; 75:502–507.

Koorneef L. Sectional anatomy of the orbit. Amsterdam: Aeolus Press, 1981:1–29.

Koorneef L. Spatial aspects of the orbital musculo fibrous tissue in man. Amsterdam: Swets and Zeitlinger, 1977.

Manson PN, Clifford CM, Su CT, et al. Mechanisms of global support and post-traumatic enophthalmos: I. The anatomy of the ligament sling and its relation to intramuscular cone orbital fat. Plast Reconstr Surg 1986; 77:193–202.

Manson PN, Grivas A, Rosenbaum A, et al. Studies on enophthalmos: II. The measurement of orbital injuries and their treatment by quantitative computed tomography. Plast Reconstr Surg 1985; 77:203–214.

POST-TRAUMATIC ENOPHTHALMOS

PAUL N. MANSON, M.D.
NICHOLAS T. ILIFF, M.D.

Post-traumatic enophthalmos is a condition that was formerly poorly understood. Its mechanisms have recently been greatly clarified by the widespread use of computed tomography (CT) and more extensive open reductions of orbital fractures. Recent anatomic and clinical research have provided insight into the mechanisms of the condition. The mechanisms provide a basis for surgical correction using craniofacial techniques of exposure to achieve soft tissue repositioning and an anatomic reconstruction of the bony orbit.

Enophthalmos is defined as a backward displacement of the globe into the bony orbit. Usually, the globe also is displaced downward and slightly medially. In 1889, Lang suggested that enlargement of the orbital cavity was the usual mechanism of enophthalmos. In 1943, Pfeiffer further analyzed post-traumatic enophthalmos and suggested severai other possible mechanisms. He postulated that fat atrophy, as well as enlargement of the bony orbit, were involved. Additional mechanisms suggested were soft tissue contracture, dislocation of the superior oblique muscle, contraction of the globe, cicatricial contraction of retrobulbar tissues, and rupture of ligaments and fascial bands. Koorneef's identification of the musculofascial fine ligament system within the orbit has allowed further clarification of enopthalmos, fat displacement and ocular motility disorders. Koorneef has suggested that entrapment of fat tethers the fine ligament system that extends throughout orbital soft tissue and might hold the globe in a displaced position and limit the excursion of extraocular muscles.

Of the postulated etiologies, bony orbital enlargement, fat atrophy, disorganization of soft tissue structures (fat displacement), and change in the shape of the soft tissue mass of the orbit have received the most attention in the literature. The advent of computerized studies of bone and soft tissue volumes and three-dimensional computed tomographic imaging techniques have allowed the contributions of each of these mechanisms to be evaluated accurately.

SURGICAL TECHNIQUE

Among some craniofacial surgeons, it is popular to correct enophthalmos by a rather random insertion of bone and cartilage grafts superiorly, medially, laterally, and inferiorly, or by a zygomatic osteotomy. Such treatment does not emphasize the exact anatomy of the bony displacement for each patient. Three studies have compared changes in orbital soft tissue and bone volume after orbital injury resulting in enophthalmos. All three have shown an increase in bony volume (Fig. 1) with relatively constant soft tissue volume for most patients. Thus, fat atrophy is not a principal component of the deformity. Therefore, globe position should be accurately restored by mobilization of the soft tissue and anatomic reconstruction of the bony orbit.

Conceptually, one should concentrate on restoration of (1) proper anatomic dimensions of the orbital rim and (2) proper anatomic dimensions of the internal portion of the orbit. Therefore, for soft tissue mobilization to be effective, the soft tissue contents of the bony orbit must be freed well beyond the area of fracture displacement. This always involves a broad dissection of the entire medial and inferior orbit. Usually, the lateral orbit also must be completely dissected. In some cases, correction also involves the superior portion of the orbit. Such dissection frees the soft tissue that adheres to bone and sinus structures and allows soft tissue to conform to a new shape and position. Enophthalmos corrections thus emphasize change in shape and position of soft tissue as the anatomic basis for correction. To achieve this change, orbital soft tissue must be frequently dissected down to a pedicle that consists of the contents of the posterior third of the orbit (superior orbital fissure and optic foramen).

Surgical Incisions

Two incisions are utilized for reconstruction: the lower eyelid approach and the coronal approach.

The lower eyelid approach may consist of either a subciliary incision, with a skin-muscle flap, or a transconjunctival incision, with division of the lateral canthus (Fig. 2). In the former, an incision is made 2 to 3 mm below the cilia and a skin-muscle flap dissected to the level of the inferior orbital rim. The lateral limb of either incision extends 1 cm directly lateral to the lateral canthus. In a transconjunctival incision, a skin incision 8 to 10 mm in length is made directly to bone, first lateral to the canthus and then dividing the canthus, through the lateral commissure of the eyelids. The lower lid is everted so that the conjunctival surface can be seen, and the lower eyelid retractors are divided 2 to 3 mm below the tarsus.

Dissection continues on the anterior surface of the orbital septum, in the same plane as with the subciliary skin-muscle flap incision, to reach the infraorbital rim. A periosteal incision is made on the anterior aspect of the rim, and subperiosteal dissection is begun laterally on the anterior aspect of the zygoma. The zygomaticofacial nerve may be divided for exposure. The subperiosteal dissection clears the entire anterior face of the malar eminence out on to the zygomatic arch and includes the frontal process of the zygoma (the lateral canthus having been detached).

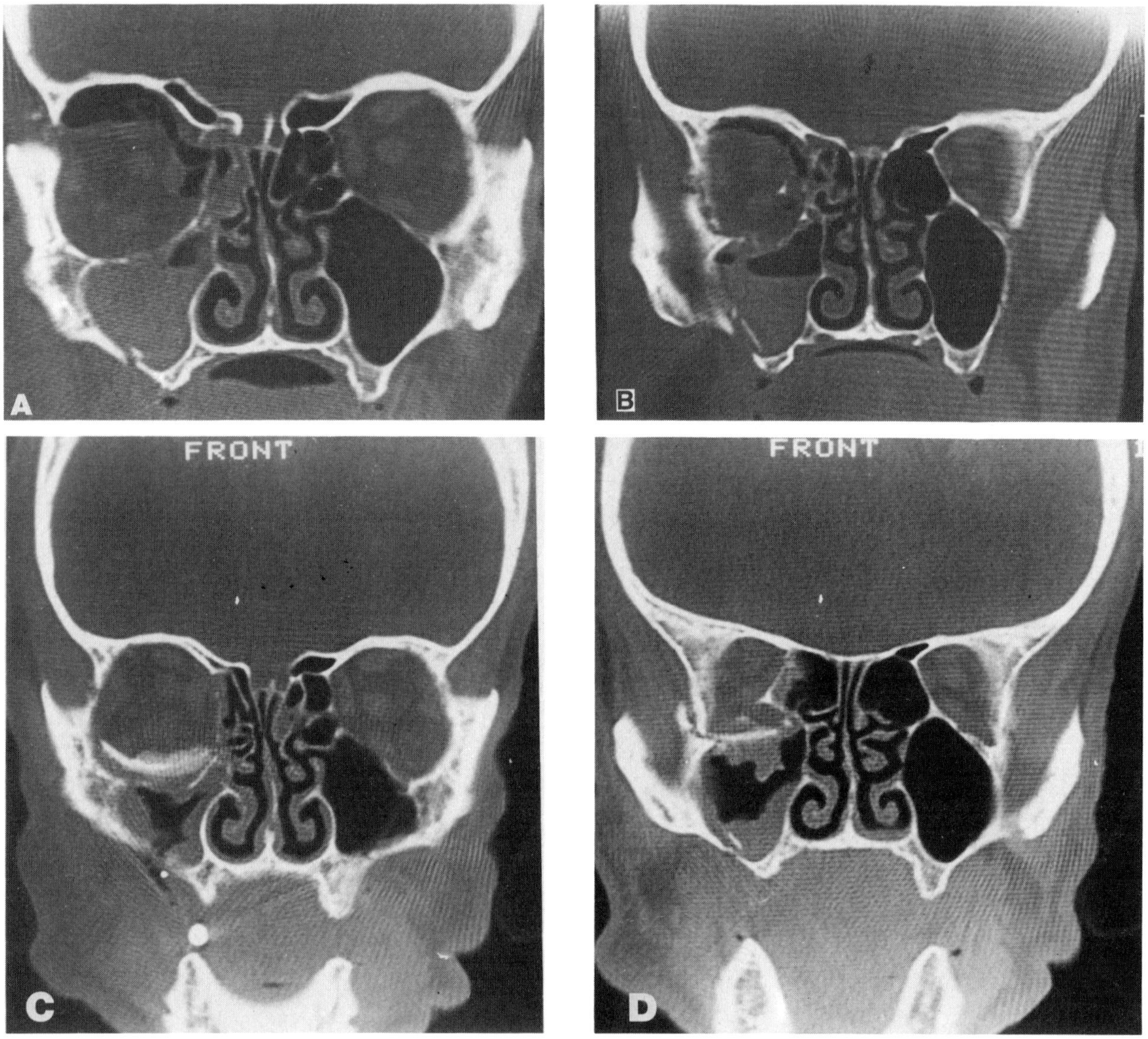

Figure 1 CT scan demonstrating bony orbital enlargement in the middle third of the orbit. Normally, the middle third of the orbit bulges inward behind the globe. *A* and *B*, In enophthalmos, bone and soft tissue have prolapsed into the maxillary sinus and into the nose. *C* and *D*, The soft tissue must be mobilized and bone reconstruction used to hold the soft tissue in proper position. Note bone grafts in posterior, medial, and lateral orbit.

The Infraorbital Nerve

The infraorbital nerve is identified anteriorly by dissection toward the nerve first from the lateral portion of the malar eminence and then medially by dissection of the medial margin of the maxilla and the pyriform aperture. The nerve is easily identified and is protected by a simultaneous medial and lateral approach. It "appears" between the two dissections under the attachment of the levator labii superioris and is protected by careful gentle dissection around the foramen. In order to separate an infraorbital nerve that is adherent to orbital soft tissue in the inferior orbit, it is frequently necessary first to identify the nerve below and anterior to the orbital rim. The nerve is freed with a limited osteotomy of the rim and is then traced to the inferior orbital fissure with neurolysis. In cases where a rim osteotomy is necessary for rim repositioning, the osteotomy may be designed to enter the infraorbital foramen to allow for mobilization of the nerve. The branch of the infraorbital nerve to the anterior maxillary teeth travels in the maxillary sinus wall and should be protected. In the middle section of the orbit following fracture, the infraorbital neurovascular bundle and inferior rectus muscle frequently are adherent when intervening bone has disappeared or been dislocated. Adherent structures are carefully separated by dissection under loupe magnification with microinstruments. Preoperative sensation in the infraorbital nerve should be documented in all divisions, as a partial deficit is usually present. Regarding this sensation, several divisions should be separately noted: the medial nose, upper anterior alveolus, and cheek. The dissected orbital soft tissue is then replaced into the orbit

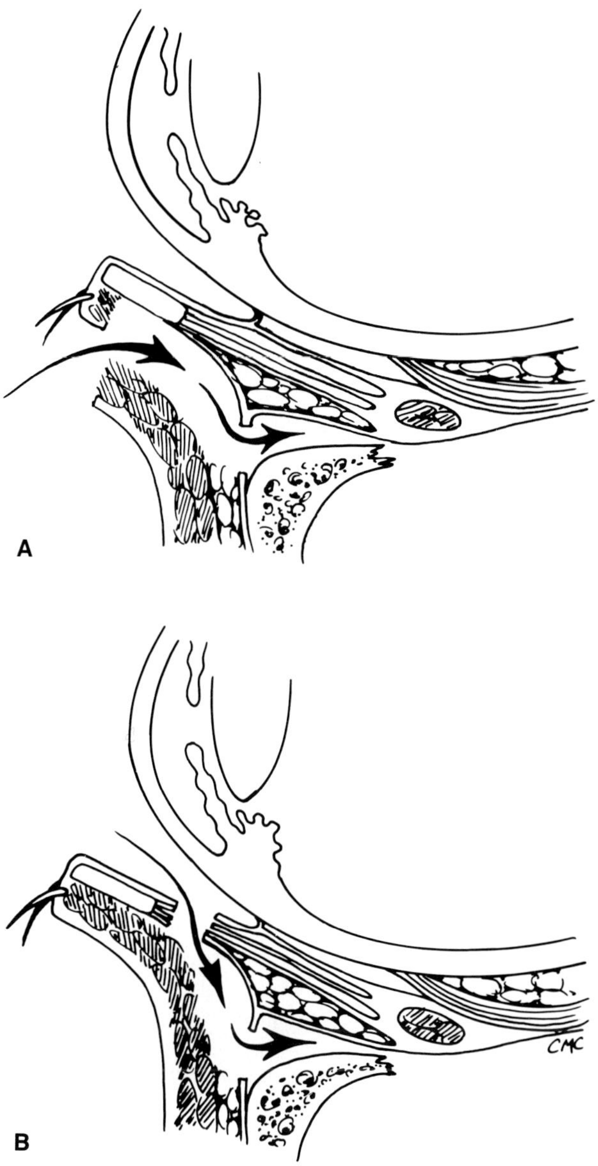

Figure 2 Lower eyelid incisions. *A*, Subciliary incision with skin muscle flap. *B*, Transconjunctival incision accompanying a lateral canthotomy. © JHU

while the nerve is kept caudal to the bone grafts. Bone reconstruction should restore exactly the bony anatomic structure present prior to the fracture.

A lower eyelid incision alone provides adequate exposure for all fractures in the lower third of the medial orbital wall, the orbital floor, and the lateral orbital wall. When nasoethmoidal, superior orbital, or upper medial wall exposures is necessary, a coronal incision is required. A coronal incision is required for fractures of the zygoma with arch deformity and those orbital fractures with extensive lateral wall "blow-out" areas that require arch osteotomy. Although a hemicoronal incision can be utilized, a full coronal incision is esthetically superior, provides better exposure, and is technically easier.

The contents of the superior orbit must be dissected free from the roof to expose the medial and lateral orbital walls. It is necessary to free the periosteal attachments of the entire frontal process of the zygoma and nose to be able to retract the coronal incision far enough inferiorly so that the entire medial orbital wall can be visualized.

Posterior Limits of Orbital Dissection

"Ledges" of Intact Bone

The CT scan should be analyzed to determine the position of intact orbital bone at the posterior margins of the orbital dissection. Usually there are intact "ledges" of bone (see Fig. 1) medially, adjacent to the posterior ethmoid foramen, and inferiorly 35 to 38 mm behind the orbital rim. These "ledges" of bone form the posterior margins of the orbital dissection. They serve as anatomic guides for precise reconstruction of the floor and medial orbital wall. Soft tissue is dissected from adherent bone fragments and sinus mucosa to reach these ledges. They may be approached from within the nose or within the maxillary sinus to avoid injury to eye muscles from dissections within orbital soft tissue ("extra marginal" dissection technique).

Marginal Osteotomy

A marginal or rim osteotomy is frequently required to reposition displaced sections of the anterior orbital rim (Fig. 3). This concept has been popularized by Tessier. It is designed to reposition anatomically any rim section appropriately, and may be done segmentally if desired. The procedure also may be utilized when rim position is normal simply to expose the posterior orbital floor through the maxillary sinus. Visualization of herniated orbital soft tissue in the posterior aspect of the maxillary sinus is facilitated by removing an anterior rim segment. This maneuver allows freeing of incarcerated orbital soft tissue under direct vision and improves visualization of the intact "ledge" of bone in the posterior orbit.

Herniated orbital contents, once freed, are replaced into the normal boundaries of the orbital cavity. In the area of the lateral and inferolateral orbit, buccal fat is frequently in contact with orbital soft tissue. If desired, some of this fat can be included with the orbital tissue in repositioning, thereby effectively increasing volume of soft tissue contents. The temporalis muscle is usually adherent to soft tissue in extensive blow-out fractures involving the lateral orbit. This plane must be dissected and bone grafts must be used to isolate the contents of the orbit from the contents of the temporal fossa and buccal space.

Following dissection, the orbital rim segment is replaced either into its former position or into the position desired to place the rim anatomically. The segment is initially positioned with interfragment wires and then stabilized with plate and screw fixation. If a marginal osteotomy leaves a gap in the maxilla or zygomatic bone, it is filled with an interpositional bone graft (Fig. 4).

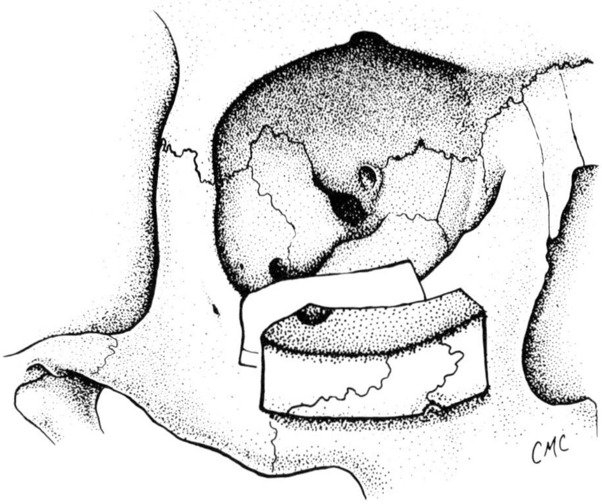

Figure 3 Marginal osteotomy. A section of the orbital rim may be removed either for repositioning or to visualize herniated orbital soft tissue within the maxillary sinus. Such visualization enhances protection of delicate orbital soft tissue contents. © JHU

Total Osteotomy of Sections

In severely displaced fractures, multiple pieces of the rim may need repositioning. In most cases, it is technically simpler (and more stable) to perform marginal osteotomies than to totally osteotomize segments such as an entire zygoma. When an entire zygoma is displaced, a thorough release of the masseter attachments is required before it can be repositioned. (The masseter shortens following inferior displacement of the zygoma, and the zygoma cannot be put into anatomic position without releasing its muscular attachments.)

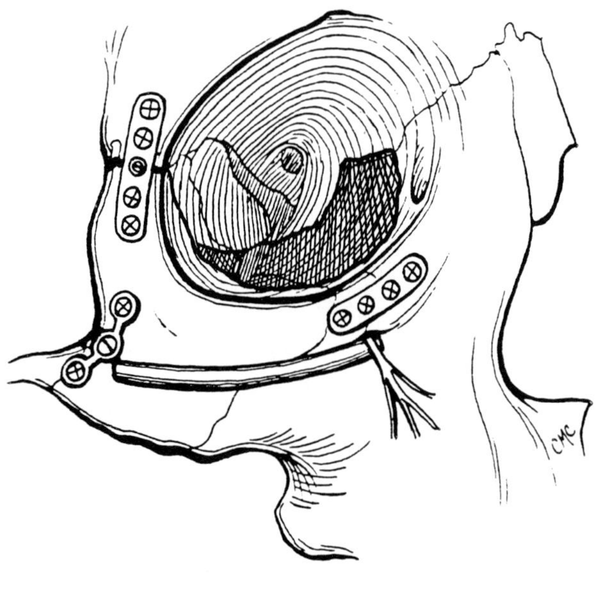

Figure 4 Interpositional bone grafts. Interpositional bone grafts have been utilized to stabilize the position of an osteotomized rim segment. © JHU

Superior Orbital Roof Osteotomy

The usual deformity in fractures involving the superior portion of the rim is an inferior and posterior displacement. This produces downward and forward displacement of the globe. Correction of an inferior orbital fracture in the presence of a displaced superior rim fracture produces exophthalmos and not correct vertical eye position. It is important to correct displacement of the roof in order to satisfactorily position the globe. These fractures must be carefully analyzed both on physical examination, plain films, and CT scans.

MATERIALS FOR ORBITAL RECONSTRUCTION

There are two generic types of materials for orbital reconstruction: artificial materials and bone grafts. Bone grafts may be taken from the calvaria, rib, or iliac crest. Artificial materials include types of silicone, Proplast, polyethylene, and Teflon, and recently titanium for rigid fixation. The only advantages of artificial material are that no donor site is required, and there is no absorption. Artificial materials are more difficult to shape to the exact dimensions required by an orbital reconstruction than are bone grafts. Rigid fixation consists of placing titanium mesh as a framework for bone reconstruction (Fig. 5). While the immediate risk of infection with either bone or alloplastic materials is the same, there is a remote (long-term) risk of infection from alloplastic materials that approximates 2 to 3 percent in most series. Obviously, this risk of remote infection is not present in bone graft reconstructions.

It is currently fashionable to utilize split calvarial bone grafts for orbital reconstruction. Previously, surgeons utilized rib and iliac crest. The theoretical advantage of calvaria is that it resorbs less than other types of bone materials. Its disadvantages are that it is dense, brittle bone and is more difficult to contour into the tight curves required in posterior orbital reconstruction. Bone grafts must be strongly curved to fit the curvature of the posterior orbit. Orbital curvatures of bone are produced by bending the bone with Tessier rib contouring forceps. The basic curve of this forceps is suitable for the anterior portion of the orbit. A curve suitable for the posterior portion of the orbit is fashioned by bending the bone graft around the edges of the jaws of the forceps. Such "tighter" curves are required in the posterior portion of the orbit.

It has been our impression that postoperative displacement of bone grafts is a common problem in extensive orbital reconstructions where large wall defects are spanned with pieces of bone. Insuring against postoperative displacement in extensive posterior defects is difficult without the use of some kind of supporting material. In the last 2 years, titanium mesh has been utilized for orbital fractures that require support of bone grafts in the inferomedial orbit.

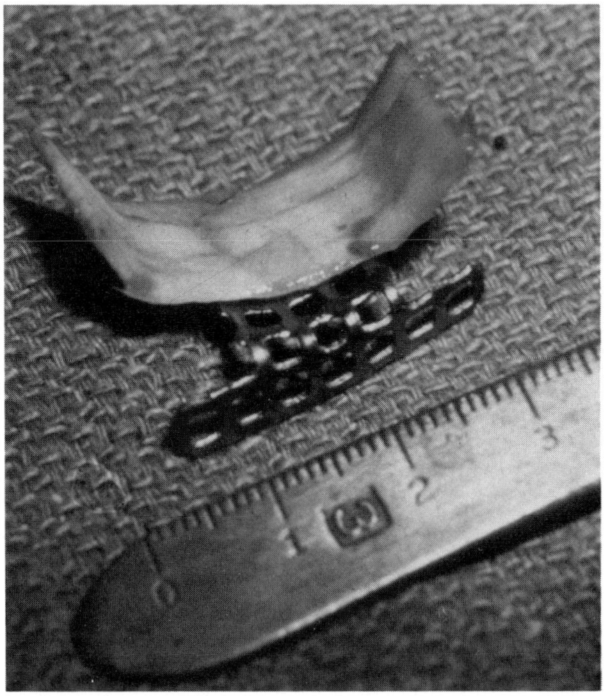

Figure 5 Titanium mesh—bone reconstruction. Rigid fixation utilizing a titanium mesh can be utilized to provide support for bone reconstruction in the manner indicated.

Several preformed metallic internal orbital implants are now under design for use with orbital plate and screw systems. These provide support for bone graft materials and act to prevent postoperative displacement. The most critical area for enophthalmos correction, and thus for support, is the inferomedial part of the orbit. This is the most difficult area to reconstruct with bone grafts, since grafts tend to "settle" inferiorly and medially, enlarging the size of the orbit. The metallic support provides the superior and lateral pressure required to support bone graft reconstruction of the bone "bulge" area behind the globe in the inferomedial orbit (Fig. 6).

EYE POSITION AT SURGERY

In patients having reconstruction, eye position at surgery is frequently used as a guide to correct reconstruction of the bony orbital dimensions. Because of the swelling that occurs during dissection, eye position may need to be distinctly overcorrected anteroposteriorly following proper bony orbital reconstruction. Vertically, however, eye position should be symmetrical. Care must be taken in the analysis of globe position to compensate for any rotation of the globe; the examiner should visualize the true "center" of globe position rather than pupil position. In most orbital reconstructions, the goal is anatomic reconstruction of the bony dimensions of the normal orbit: in the presence of swelling, this may have to be accomplished by overcorrecting eye position anteroposteriorly intraoperatively.

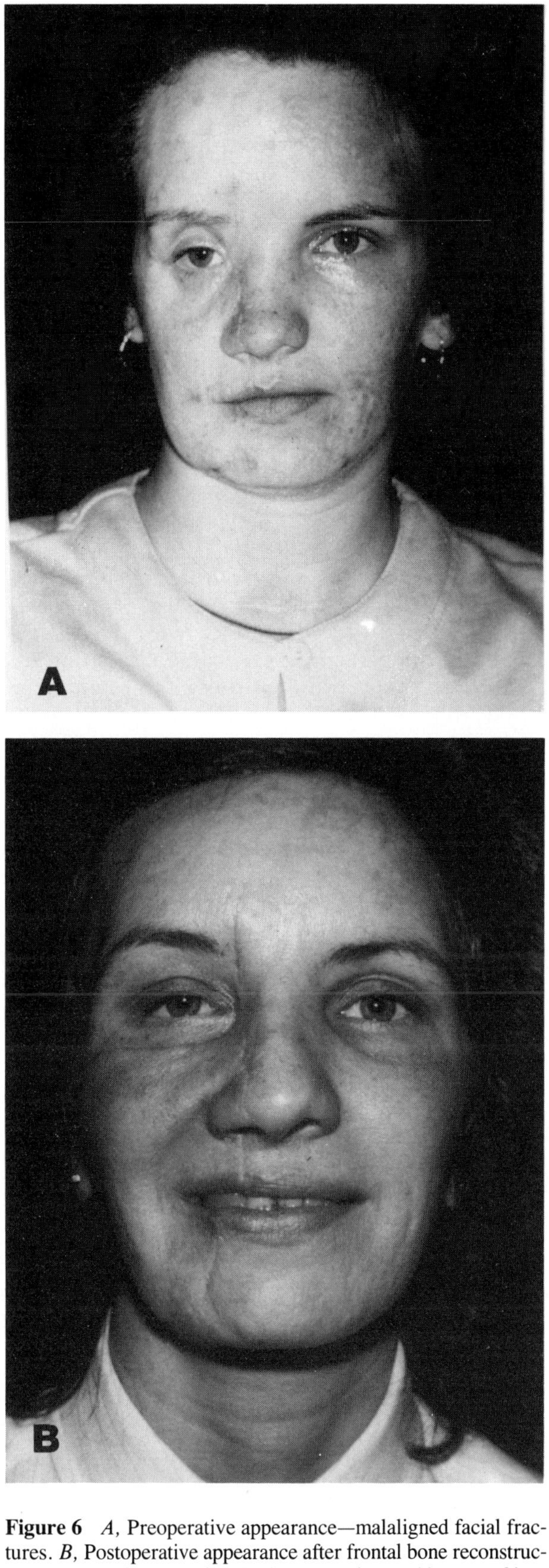

Figure 6 *A,* Preoperative appearance—malaligned facial fractures. *B,* Postoperative appearance after frontal bone reconstruction, zygomatic, nasoethmoidal osteotomies, and bone grafting.

CICATRICIAL CONTRACTURE OF SOFT TISSUES

Release of orbital soft tissue from attachment to displaced bone frequently results in immediate partial correction of eye position. Such correction is unstable; it must be stabilized by filling in any defects between the released soft tissue and bone; otherwise, in the postoperative period, the soft tissue merely readheres to the bone and the globe positional deformity recurs.

In response to an injury, the pyramidal mass of orbital soft tissue tends to reorganize its shape into a spherical, rather than a pyramidal configuration. This follows the principle that, for a given volume of tissue, the smallest surface area is assumed—a sphere. This is the so-called "spherical contracture" of orbital soft tissue. The shape of orbital soft tissue must therefore be changed following bone reconstruction of the orbit.

Following extensive orbital dissection, considerable swelling is often encountered. It is our impression that this swelling is worse if the contents of the inferior orbital fissure are divided (the veins draining orbital soft tissue).

Prolapsed conjunctiva is common postoperatively and must be protected with ointments and eye patches. It is our preference to keep a Frost suture in place for 24 hours or more postoperatively and to release this after some of the swelling has decreased. This suture splints eyelid tissues and assists their redraping and adherence in the proper anatomic position.

REATTACHMENT OF CANTHAL LIGAMENTS

Attachment of medical and lateral canthal ligament should be recreated when it is released in the course of surgical dissection, suturing adjacent to the eyelid commissure with a nonabsorbable suture and anchoring this to an appropriately positioned wire. For the lateral canthus, the reattachment position is the anterior edge of the orbital rim adjacent to the zygomaticofrontal suture; for the medial canthus, the reattachment is posterior and superior to the lacrimal fossa.

REFIXATION OF SOFT TISSUE TO THE CRANIOFACIAL SKELETON

Frequently, a component of the postoperative deformity is the thinning or displacement of overlying soft tissue. Following fracture displacement of the zygoma, the thickest tissue over the malar eminence of the cheek is usually positioned inferiorly. Soft tissue displacement is diagnosed by analyzing the thickness of soft tissue over the malar eminence on axial CT scans. Soft tissue of adequate thickness may be recruited through subperiosteal dissection, then placed into a more favorable position and anchored to the bone reconstruction. This should be accomplished with nonabsorbable sutures.

Soft tissue closure is more accurate when certain fascial layers are surgically closed. Several sutures lateral to the lateral canthus close deep soft tissue in the subciliary or conjunctival orbital incision. No sutures should be placed at the level of the inferior orbital rim since lid shortening will occur. For a coronal incision, the incisions through the temporal fascia and periosteum over the frontal process of the zygoma are closed.

COMPLICATIONS

Undercorrection

In enophthalmos corrections, when a result is obtained that does not equal the desired result, a postoperative CT scan of the orbit should be obtained to identify the cause of the unsatisfactory result. Frequently, an undercorrection in the posterior and inferomedial portion of the orbit will be seen. Displacement of bone grafted materials may have occurred, or perhaps soft tissue position was initially undercorrected. Less commonly, fat atrophy should have required a bony "overcorrection." After 3 to 6 months reoperation may be required.

For some patients, alloplastic materials may be utilized in orbital reconstruction with no worry about bone absorption, which results in an increase in orbital volume. Artificial materials are utilized if there are no communications with sinus mucosa and if the defect is relatively easily filled with a contoured alloplastic implant; otherwise, bone grafts are preferred. It is our preference to utilize calvarial or rib donor sites.

Risks of Orbital Surgery

The risks of orbital surgery include standard surgical complications such as bleeding and infection, both of which are uncommon; they also include damage to vision, double vision, decreased ocular motility, and damage to the lacrimal system. Orbital surgery may damage sensation in facial sensory nerves such as the infraorbital nerve. This may be permanent or temporary, partial or complete.

Decreased Visual Acuity

In most cases, visual acuity is not decreased following enophthalmos correction. In fact, it is frequently improved by better lid globe approximation and better lubrication of the cornea. When visual acuity decreases postoperatively, emergency evaluation and medical treatment are instituted (steroids, diuretics, and head elevation). Decompression of the orbit by removal of bone grafts and drainage of any hematoma should be performed if retinal or vascular compromise is evident. If arterial pulsations are seen in the retina, it may imply impending vascular occlusion. Optic canal decompression should be considered if visual loss is present with normal retinal circulations. One mechanism of postoperative visual loss involves swelling within the optic canal, thereby reducing circulation to the optic nerve. The risk of visual loss and diminished vision ranges between 2 and 3 percent in most series, but should be less in experienced hands.

Diplopia

Diplopia may be produced either by damage to eye muscles, to nerves travelling to the muscles, or by moving the globe forward in the presence of muscle shortening. Release of displaced soft tissue may damage a muscle particularly in the posterior portion of the orbit. It is important to emphasize that extraocular muscles travel close to the edges of the orbital dissection in this area.

When the globe is moved forward in the presence of a contracted (shortened) eye muscle, the globe rotates into the field of this shortened muscle and diplopia may result. Some patients demonstrate a reduction in the speed of ocular movement (ocular motility), as well as the total excursion after extensive orbital dissection. Often this does not produce troublesome diplopia. Forced duction examinations should be performed before orbital dissection, after orbital dissection, and after placement of grafts to confirm free movement of extraocular muscles.

Ectropion

Production of lower lid ectropion is secondary to lid scarring. Ectropion is usually temporary, responding to nonoperative observation. Rarely it may require lid reposi-

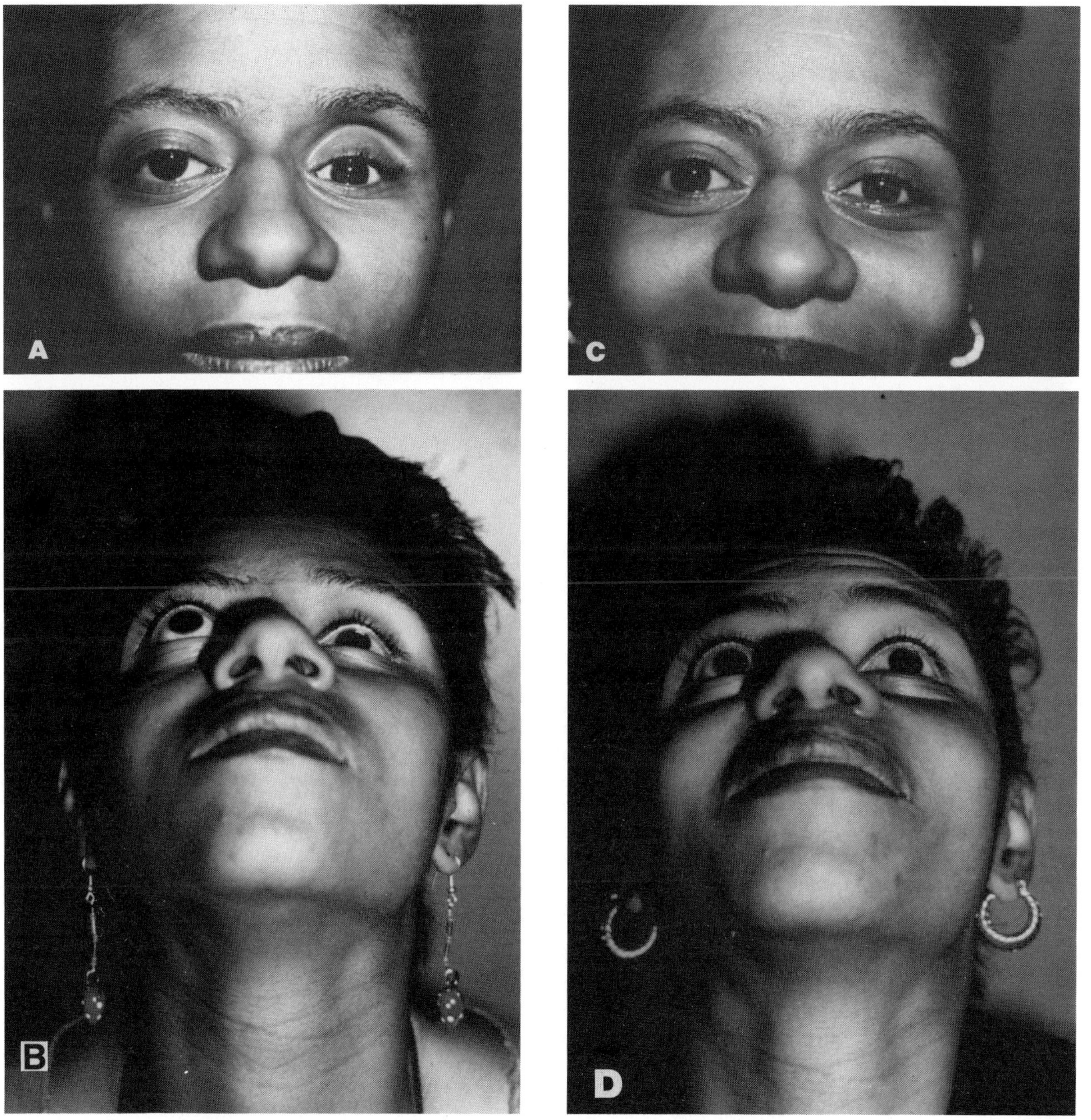

Figure 7 *A*, Frontal view of patient with enophthalmos. *B*, "Worm's eye" view. *C*, Frontal view after correction. *D*, Inferior view after correction.

tioning or skin graft reconstruction. Abnormal posture of the lid should be confirmed preoperatively. Any scarring, shortening, or thickening is noted and pointed out to the patient as increases to the risk of ectropion. The presence of eversion, inversion, or positional abnormalities of the lid should also be noted and dissection keyed to correct rotation and position abnormalities of the lid.

SUMMARY

Correction of enophthalmos is possible and is most accurate if based on an anatomic concept of the bony orbital enlargement. The rim and the internal orbit must be considered separately. The exact areas of enlargement are defined by axial and coronal CT scans and globe displacement measurements. The surgical approach is designed to reduce the bony volume in these areas. Bony volume is most accurately stabilized with bone graft reconstruction following a thorough dissection of the soft tissue, utilizing rigid fixation as support for bone position. Marginal osteotomies of the rim are utilized to increase exposure or to reposition rim segments. An anatomic, rather than a random approach, to enophthalmos correction should be employed. Globe position should be anatomically restored by analysis and treatment according to the principles identified in this discussion (Fig. 7).

SUGGESTED READING

Converse JM. Orbital blow-out fractures—a ten-year survey. Plast Reconstr Surg 1967; 39:20.

Converse JM, Francoise F, Wood-Smith D, Friedland JA. The conjunctival approach in orbital fractures. Plast Reconstr Surg 1973; 52:656.

Kawamoto HK. Late post-traumatic enophthalmos: a correctable deformity? Plast Reconstr Surg 1982; 69:423–430.

Manson PN, Ruas E, Iliff N. Single eyelid incision for exposure of the zygomatic bone and orbital reconstruction. Plast Reconstr Surg 1987; 79:120–125.

Manson PN, Crawley WC, Yaremchuck MJ, et al. Midface fractures: advantages of extended open reduction and immediate bone grafting. Plast Reconstr Surg 1985; 76:1–10.

Manson PN, Ruas EJ, Iliff NT. Deep orbital reconstruction for correction of post-traumatic enophthalmos. Clin Plast Surg 1987; 9:113–121.

Monasterio FO, Rodrequez A, Bernavides A. A single method for the correction of enophthalmos. Clin Plast Surg 1987; 14:169–177.

Tessier P. Inferior orbitotomy—a new approach to the orbital floor. Clin Plast Surg 1982; 9:569–575.

Tessier P. The conjunctival approach in orbital fractures. Plast Reconstr Surg 1973; 52:656.

OCULAR ADNEXAL RECONSTRUCTION: THE TARSOCONJUNCTIVAL FLAP

GLENN W. JELKS, M.D.

Large defects of the central section of the lower eyelid that result from neoplasm excision, trauma, or congenital malformations present challenging reconstruction. The eyelid repairs become more complex if the medial canthal, lacrimal excretory, or lateral retinacular structures are also involved. In 1885, Landolt was the first to employ the tarsoconjunctival flap to reconstruct a defect of the lower eyelid. Hughes, in 1937, popularized the technique and was able to demonstrate adequate functional reconstruction of large lower lid defects. The original technique required a lid-splitting incision at the grey line that caused a high incidence of upper eyelid entropion, trichiasis, and corneal damage. The technique has been modified to maintain at least a 4 to 5 mm lid element in continuity with the lid margin, thereby, virtually eliminating these complications.

Currently, lower eyelid defects are preferentially reconstructed with the tarsoconjunctival flap. Routine use of visual magnification by loupes or the operating microscope, improved suture material, and specifically-designed needles, allow performance of this operation with ease and confidence. The technique requires a thorough knowledge of the anatomy of the eyelids.

The upper and lower eyelids have a layered anatomical orientation with functionally analogous structures. Most superficial is the skin of the eyelids, which is the thinnest of the body. Beneath the eyelid skin is the orbicularis oculi muscle which is divided into palpebral and orbital portions. The palpebral portion is subdivided into the pretarsal and preseptal portions. In the lower lid the tarsus is 4 to 5 mm in height and provides attachments for the orbital septum and lower lid retractor (capsulopalpebral fascia) system. In the upper lid the tarsus has a height of 9 to 10 mm in the central portion. The tarsi provide skeletal support for the eyelids and consist of dense fibroelastic tissue and oil-secreting meibomian glands. Just posterior to the orbital septum is the peripheral orbital fat. In the upper lid this fat is termed the preaponeurotic fat and is a key anatomical landmark. The levator aponeurosis and Müller's muscle are just posterior to the upper lid fat. In the lower lid the lid retractor system, with its occasional smooth muscle fibers, abuts the fat. The palpebral conjunctiva is adherent to these posterior elements.

For convenience, the eyelids can be divided into anterior and posterior segments or lamellae. The anterior lamella consists of the skin and orbicularis muscle and their associated fascial and vascular structures. A marginal artery runs approximately 3.5 mm from the lid margin posterior to the pretarsal orbicularis fibers. This artery, as well as the peripheral arterial arcade of the upper lid (just posterior to the levator aponeurosis at the superior border of the tarsus), is supplied by major branches off the infratrochlear artery medially and the lacrimal artery laterally. The posterior lamella consists of the levator aponeurosis, tarsus, Müller's muscle, and conjunctiva in the upper lid and of the capsulopalpebral fascia, tarsus, and conjunctiva in the lower lid. The levator muscle (the primary elevator of the upper lid) usually becomes aponeurotic at the equator of the globe in the superior orbit. The aponeurosis courses anteriorly to insert into the lower two-thirds of the anterior tarsal plate. The levator muscle provides origin to Müller's muscle, the nonstriated, sympathetically innervated elevator of the upper lid that inserts into the superior edge of the tarsus. The superior transverse ligament of Whitnall is a fascial condensation along the upper aspect of the levator muscular-aponeurotic junction. This ligament attaches medially to the trochlear fascia and laterally to the fascia of the orbital lobe of the lacrimal gland.

When presented with a lower eyelid defect, it is important to contemplate reconstruction of the missing parts by analogous tissues from the opposing upper lid. Therefore, it is imperative that a normal upper lid is present. Attempts at local advancement of lower lid tissue with the assistance of lateral cantholysis and medial displacement should initially be attempted. Other methods of lower eyelid reconstruction, including the Mustardé cheek advancement flap over a septal chondral mucosal graft, may be considered. However, this latter procedure often results in an unstable, thick lower lid with less optimal eyelid function and cosmesis. This procedure may also cause injury to the temporal branch of the facial nerve, eyelid margin instability, and unacceptable facial scarring in the younger patient. The advantage of the Mustardé cheek advancement procedure lies in obtaining a reconstruction in one stage without occlusion of the patient's vision for 3 to 6 weeks.

Use of the upper lid tarsus and conjunctiva, with their own blood supply, allows replacement of missing lower lid tarsus and conjunctiva (posterior lamella) with analogous tissue. The anterior lamella, save for orbicularis muscle, is replaced with a free full-thickness skin graft. The modified lid-sharing procedure produces a dynamic, movable lower eyelid with superior cosmesis and lid function.

The main disadvantage of the tarsoconjunctival procedure is that it requires two stages and occludes the vision of the affected eye for several weeks. The procedure is ideally suited for central lower eyelid defects approximately 5 to 6 mm in vertical dimension.

The tarsoconjunctival flap procedure should, when possible, be performed immediately following resection of neoplasms of the lower lid. Careful attention to fresh tissue histopathologic confirmation of clear margins must be maintained. With the advent of fresh tissue Mohs resection, a close relationship with the ablating surgeon is mandatory. If surgery must be delayed, sterile dressings and ocular protection must be provided until the wound is ready for reconstruction.

The first stage of the tarsoconjunctival reconstruction requires inspection of the lower lid defect and determination of its horizontal and vertical dimensions. Involvement of the lateral canthal or medial canthal structures, including the lacrimal drainage structures, must also be documented. If the defect is irregular, it may be trimmed to make the lid margins perpendicular. The base of the wound should be inspected for the conjunctiva, lid retractors, and residual orbicularis oculi. Figure 1 shows a large, central lower eyelid defect following resection of a basal cell carcinoma in a 40-year-old white female. Notice the rectangular shape of the defect with perpendicular lid defect tarsal edges. In Figure 2 the horizontal dimension of the lower lid defect is transferred to the posterior surface of the upper eyelid, which has been everted with a Desmarres retractor. The portion of the tarsoconjunctival flap used for the repair can be as much as 25 percent narrower than the defect in the horizontal dimension. This is especially true in the older patient with lax lids. However, in the younger patient it is best to place tension on the edges of the lower lid defect in order to adjust the proper lid-globe relationship before measuring the necessary tarsoconjunctival flap width. In Figure 3, the tarsoconjunctival flap has been elevated 4 mm from the lid margin in a horizontal direction to a depth just beneath the tarsus and above the levator aponeurosis insertion. Vertical incisions are then made to allow further dissection of the flap to above the superior border of the tarsus so as to include Müller's muscle in the flap. This muscle is best identified by the high degree of vascularity on its surface. Note the large blood vessels at the superior border of the transposed tarsoconjunctival flap. Inclusion of Müller's muscle with the flap is helpful in assuring a better blood supply to the reconstructed lid. After the tarsoconjunctival flap is dissected and advanced into the defect, the leading margin of the advanced tarsus is attached to the recipient site and conjunctival base with interrupted sutures of 7–0 Vicryl or 6–0 chromic catgut. The knots are tied externally so that they do not irritate the ocular globe. Advance-

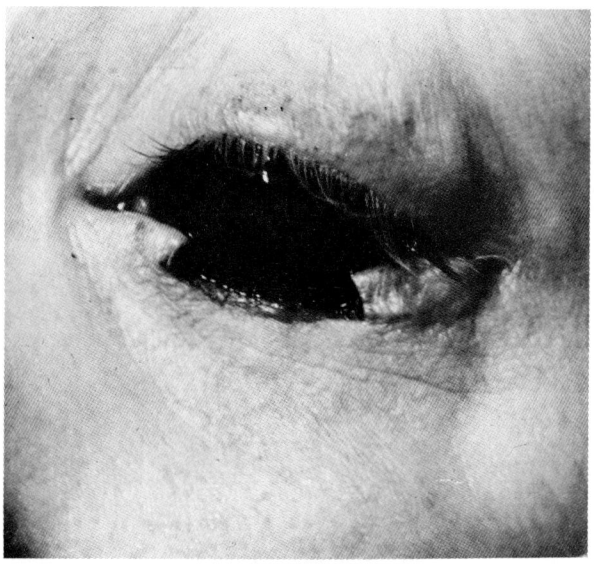

Figure 1 Large, central, left lower eyelid defect following resection of basal cell carcinoma.

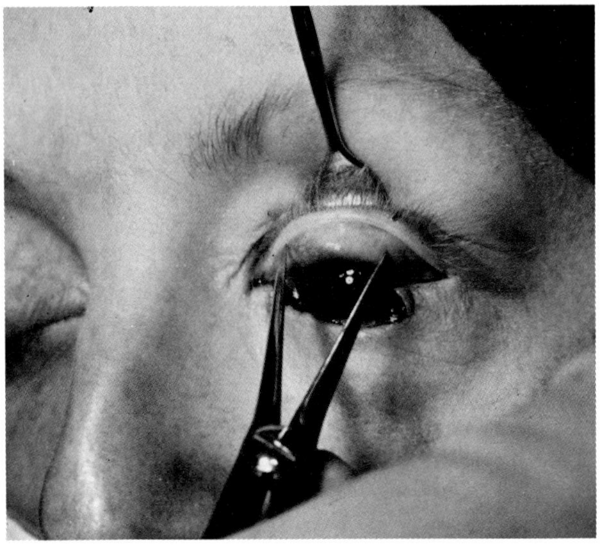

Figure 2 Left upper lid everted, and tarsoconjunctival flap being measured for subsequent transposition.

ment of the lid retractors into the base of the conjunctival closure should also be completed with interrupted sutures. The margins of the tarsal flap are then securely attached to adjacent margins of the lower lid defect by careful apposition of the superior border of the upper lid tarsus to the corresponding lower lid margin level. Thus, the posterior lamella of the lower lid defect is replaced with tarsus and conjunctiva. A rectangular raw area over the tarsus is the only residual defect. This defect is resurfaced by a full-thickness skin graft (Fig. 4) or an advancement flap from the cheek. The choice of a graft or advancement flap is determined by the laxity of the surrounding skin. A full-thickness skin graft is the preferred technique and the donor sites in order of preference are: the opposite upper eyelid, retroauricular sulcus, or supraclavicular area. The graft is neatly fitted into the defect and sutured on all sides with 6–0 silk sutures. The skin graft is covered with a Telfa pad and moist gauze. Eye pads are applied to the reconstructed lid and left undisturbed for 72 hours, at which time the dressing is changed and the wound inspected. Sutures are removed in 1 week and a protective eyepad dressing is worn for 10 days. The tarsoconjunctival flap with skin graft is left in place for 6 to 8 weeks. During this time there is considerable loosening of the vertical contracture of the transposed flap and the upper eyelid becomes more mobile.

The second stage requires separation of the tarsoconjunctival flap and creation of a stable, conjunctival-lined lid margin. Under local anesthesia the flap is divided with a No. 15 Bard-Parker blade over a hemostat or grooved director. Care is taken to protect the cornea during this maneuver. The upper lid is then everted on a Desmarres retractor and the donor bed of the tarsoconjunctival flap is dissected of scar tissue and foreshortened Müller's muscle fibers. This maneuver helps prevent residual upper eyelid retraction, secondary to Müller's muscle advancement. Once the upper lid is released and in stable position, attention is drawn to the new lower lid margin. A 0.5 to 1.0 mm horizontal strip of grafted skin is removed from the superior edge, taking care to preserve the underlying mucosal layer. The mucosal layer is then rolled over the new lid margin and sutured to the newly-created anterior mucocutaneous junction with a running 7–0 Vicryl suture. This maneuver assures conjunctiva covering the new lower lid margin and is essential in preventing marginal entropion and corneal irritation. Any excess conjunctiva tends to keratinize and appear normal in time (Fig. 5). Attempts to reconstruct the eyelashes with eyebrow hair grafting is a technical possibility; however, it is not recommended.

Reconstruction of full-thickness defects of the lower lid can be as simple as local advancement and closure, with or without the use of a lateral canthal release. Occa-

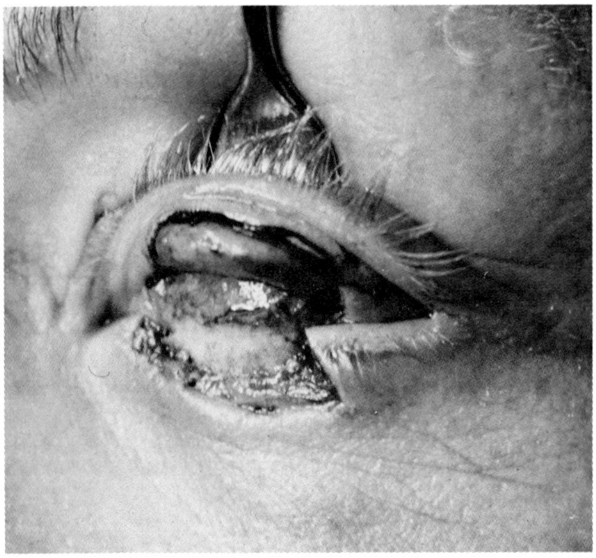

Figure 3 Tarsoconjunctival flap elevated and sutured into the lower eyelid defect.

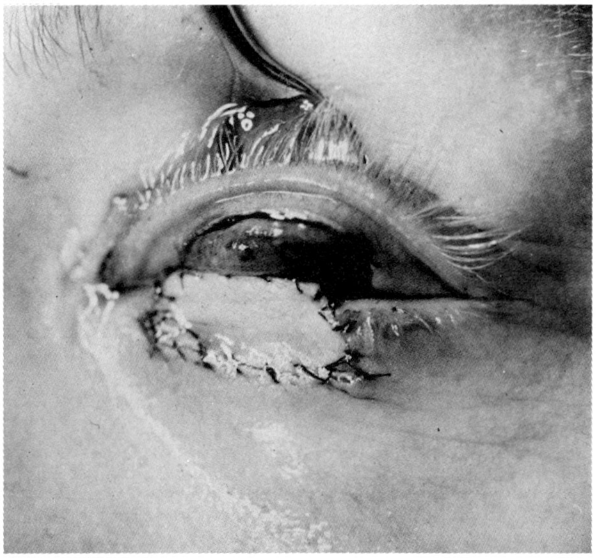

Figure 4 Retroauricular full-thickness skin graft sutured to raw surface of the tarsoconjunctival flap.

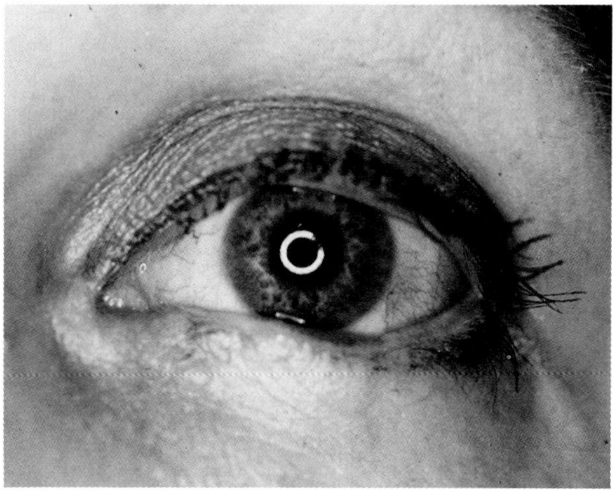

Figure 5 The final result 6 months after division of the tarsoconjunctival flap.

sionally, local rotation flaps from the adjacent upper lid and temporal skin will assist in closing somewhat larger defects. When closure of larger defects, involving two-thirds to three-fourths of the lower lid, is required, the tarsoconjunctival flap can provide a stable, functional, and cosmetically-pleasing reconstructed lid.

SUGGESTED READING

Cies WA, Bartlett RE. Modification of the Mustarde and Hughes methods of reconstruction of the lower lid. Ann Ophthalmol 1967; 7:1497–1501.

Hughes WL. Reconstructive surgery of the eyelids. 2nd ed. St. Louis: CV Mosby, 1954; 120–124.

Landolt M. De quelques opérations pratiquées sur les paupières. Arch Ophthalmol 1885; 5:481–498.

McCord CD, Tanenbaum M, eds. Oculoplastic surgery. New York: Raven Press, 1987:100.

Mustardé JC. Repair and reconstruction in the orbital region. Edinburgh: Churchill Livingstone, 1971:126.

MANDIBULAR FRACTURES

LAWRENCE C. KURTZMAN, M.D.
WILLIAM P. MAGEE Jr., D.D.S., M.D.

The prominence of the mandible explains why it is the second most commonly fractured facial bone, after the nasal bones. The usual causes of mandibular fractures are altercations and motor vehicle accidents; other less common causes include falls, gunshot wounds, and pathologic fractures. The most frequent sites of mandibular fractures are the condyle, angle, and body, with a lower incidence of fractures at the ascending ramus, symphyseal, and parasymphyseal areas. The least frequent areas of fracture are the alveolar segments and the coronoid process.

The primary objective in the treatment of mandibular fractures is to return the dentition to its original occlusal relationship. A definitive knowledge of the basic anatomy and physiology of the dental, bony, and muscular apparatus of the mandible is of absolute necessity.

ANATOMY

The standard classification of maxillomandibular occlusal relationships focuses upon the relationship between the first molars (Angle classification). The maxillary-mandibular midlines, i.e., the spaces between the central incisors, align perfectly in the ideal situation. Although these assessments assume ideal relationships, one should not evaluate occlusion dogmatically. The bottom line is that the teeth should be placed by their preinjury position.

The incisor teeth are used for biting and, therefore, are sharp with a single cusp. They have only one root that is relatively conical in shape. The canine or cuspid teeth are stronger, although they also have a conical root. These are the longest teeth in the dental arch and are more firmly anchored into the alveolar bone. The incisors and cuspids have a prominent cingulum with an undercut beneath this bulging. It is imperative that any circumdental wires on these teeth be placed in this undercut to prevent loosening of the wires. There are two bicuspid teeth in each quadrant. These teeth are firmly anchored in the alveolar bone and are extremely useful in the establishment of adequate dental wiring. There are three molar teeth in each quadrant. The mandibular molars have two roots and the maxillary molars have three roots. These teeth are extremely tenacious unless severe dental disease has disrupted their normal physiology.

Bony Anatomy

The mandible is unique both as the body's only U-shaped bone and in being suspended in space by muscular and ligamentous attachments (Fig. 1). Its sole articulations are the condyles at the temporomandibular joint (TMJ) that articulate with the temporal bones in the glenoid fossae. The mandible is composed of two types of bone: a basal bone that gives it strength and the alveolar bone that anchors the teeth. The alveolar bone is reabsorbed in an edentulous mandible, thereby causing a shortness of the vertical height and loss of the buccal sulcus.

Muscular Anatomy

It is essential to understand the muscular anatomy in order to fully appreciate the pathophysiology and displacement in mandibular fractures. The mandible is unique in the motions that occur at the temporomandibular joint.

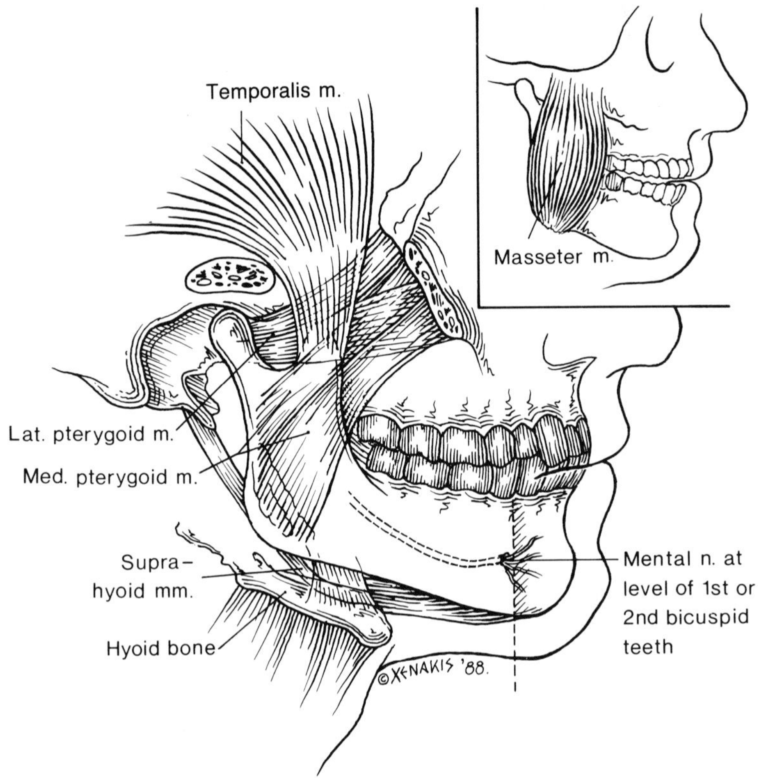

Figure 1 Functional anatomy of the mandible.

In addition to a hinge motion, there is anterior translation that allows wider opening of the mandible. The four major muscles that affect mandibular motion are all innervated by the mandibular branch of the trigeminal nerve. The temporalis muscle, originating from the temporal fossa, inserts on the coronoid process and the anterior surface of the ascending ramus of the mandible. This muscle provides rapid closure of the mandible. The masseter muscle originates from the zygomatic arch and inserts on the buccal aspect of the ramus and proximal body of the mandible. The masseter acts as a powerful mandibular closer. The internal or medial pterygoid muscle forms a sling opposite the masseter. The pterygoid's origin is from the medial aspect of the pterygoid plate, and it inserts at the medial aspect of the mandibular ramus and angle. Its function is similar to that of the masseter in closing the mandible. The lateral or external pterygoid muscle originates from the lateral aspect of the pterygoid plate and inserts onto the joint capsule of the TMJ. The function of the lateral pterygoid is in protrusion, translation, and side-to-side motion of the mandible. The much weaker suprahyoid muscles work with gravity to provide active opening of the mandible. These muscles include the mylohyoid, geniohyoid, and digastric muscles.

An understanding of the forces and direction of pull of these muscles leads to a clear understanding of "favorable" and "unfavorable" fractures (Fig. 2) and, therefore, to an intelligent approach in the treatment of these injuries.

DIAGNOSIS OF MANDIBULAR FRACTURES

Physical Examination

The most common presenting symptoms of mandibular fractures are pain and malocclusion. Other symptoms include ecchymosis, edema, and trismus. Careful, systematic physical examination of the mandible should identify the location of fractures in almost all individuals. After examination, the fracture sites can be confirmed by radiologic examination.

Careful examination begins externally with palpation of the mandible. The fracture sites are typically sensitive and edematous. The condylar region is examined by preauricular and tympanic canal examination. After external evaluation, a detailed and careful intraoral examination is performed. The occlusion is checked initially for comparison to the preinjury occlusion. Careful questioning of the patient and family often provides knowledge of preexisting dental abnormalities. Occasionally dental models have been previously constructed; these can be extremely useful in the current management of the patient. The status of the teeth and alveolus is noted next to identify loose teeth or alveolar fractures and to document the status of dental hygiene, including caries, plaque, and periodontal disease. The intraoral perimandibular mucosa is examined for edema, ecchymosis, or breaks in the

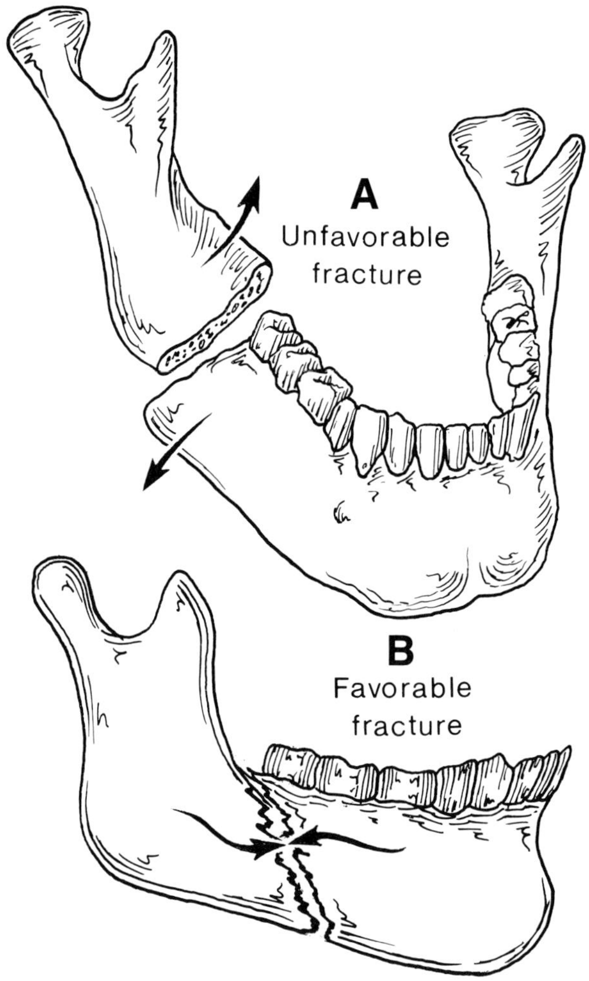

Figure 2 Classic classification of mandibular fractures (useful to understand muscular relationships).

mucosa. Digital palpation may reveal steps in the mandible; careful examination of the basal bone on the lingual and buccal side is performed. Bimanual intraoral-extraoral examination should also be performed to evaluate motion at fracture sites.

Radiologic Examination

Patients with suspected mandibular fractures should undergo a "mandibular series" examination. This includes an anterior-posterior (AP), Townes view, and right and left lateral oblique views of the mandible. Additionally, orthopantographic ("panorex") examination should be obtained when available to provide a basic overall view of the mandible. Most fractures and the status of the teeth can be seen on the panorex. The status of the condyles with respect to the glenoid fossae can also be evaluated on the Townes view.

Since the mandible is so closely adherent to the oral and lingual mucosa, most fractures of the mandible are open, with the exceptions of condylar and subcondylar fractures. With an open fracture into the oral cavity, continued contamination of the fracture site occurs until adequate fracture reduction is achieved. For this reason, it is best to proceed to operative reduction as soon as feasible. Antibiotic coverage during the preoperative and perioperative period is strongly encouraged.

FRACTURE MANAGEMENT

Teeth

Teeth that will produce deleterious effects in the treatment of facial fractures should be extracted. These include the following:

1. a loose tooth in the fracture site;
2. a partially-erupted third molar in the fracture site;
3. end-stage carious teeth with no effective crown;
4. teeth with periapical infection at fracture site, with or without a good crown;
5. any teeth with fractured roots; and
6. nonsalvageable teeth, loosened by periodontal disease.

A partially-erupted third molar at the fracture site should be extracted because its overlapping lip of mucosa harbors a large amount of bacteria in the pocket it creates. This often leads to pericoronitis that, in turn, can lead to postoperative infection if the tooth is not removed. In addition, the removal of this tooth in angle fractures allows placement of a wire through the empty socket for internal fixation when necessary. This can easily be done by an intraoral approach.

Avulsed teeth that are brought with the patient may be replantable. The best results with reimplantation are achieved when the procedure is performed immediately. The avulsed, nonviable tooth will require a root canal. This can be performed acutely, if available, or later in the management. The tooth is replaced into its socket and held in place by one of several techniques including wiring, segmental arch bar, and acrylic bonding to adjacent teeth.

Alveolar fractures can be handled similarly to avulsed teeth. With stable teeth on either side of the alveolar fracture, a segmental arch bar can be used for fixation. Dental bonding to adjacent teeth is also an excellent alternative. Significant alveolar fractures, especially those involving the anterior teeth, are best treated by taking dental impressions and rearranging the segments on the dental models. Acrylic splints fabricated presurgically from the models, then hold the segments in their appropriate positions.

Placement of Arch Bars

In placement of arch bars, there are basic principles that should be understood and firmly followed. The arch bars need to be placed securely around the appropriate teeth. Loosening of the arch bars during intermaxillary fixation leads to improper immobilization with the possibilities of malocclusion and motion at the fracture site. Many types of interdental fixation can be utilized. Erich arch bars are used most commonly. Twenty-five gauge wire is used for circumdental arch bar fixation from the cuspid distally and 28-gauge wire is used on the incisors. Minimally displaced fractures may only require fixation of four teeth per quadrant, extending from the canine to first molar. Placement of arch bars on the central and lateral incisors should be avoided when possible, as extrusion of these teeth can occur easily. Should circumdental wiring be required around the incisors all the incisors should be ligated.

It is best to interrupt the arch bar at the site of each fracture when there are enough teeth on each side of the fracture to allow stable placement of the bar. An arch bar crossing the fracture site, unless perfectly placed, can prevent easy mobilization of the dentition into the premorbid occlusion during fracture reduction. Attainment of premorbid occlusion is the most important aspect in fracture treatment and should not be compromised.

There are many patients with a preinjury dental status that makes them unsuitable for routine intermaxillary fixation: multiple missing teeth, the edentulous mandible, and multiple alveolar injuries. When dentures are available, these can be wired to the mandible and used for fracture reduction and intermaxillary stabilization. For edentulous patients without dentures, the construction of Gunning splints is necessary. In the patient with multiple fractured segments, it often is necessary to obtain dental impressions and to do model surgery for realignment of the segments by cutting the plaster models at each fracture site and articulating the dental arches with wax fixation in the preinjury state. An acrylic occlusal splint then is fashioned for intraoperative use. A lingual splint is often helpful to prevent lingual collapse of the segments.

Types of Mandibular Reduction

Each mandibular fracture must be evaluated individually with respect to fracture site and displacement to determine whether an open or a closed reduction is necessary. The dental arch situation is evaluated to determine how to create a stable anatomic reduction based upon the knowledge of the pull of the muscles of mastication. Closed reduction is indicated when the extent of the fracture is minimal and is not adversely affected by the muscular forces. The converse requires open reduction.

Fixation can be achieved by either external or internal devices. Extraskeletal fixation, such as the Joe Hall Morris device, has some indications:(1) the thin, atrophic mandible when rigid internal plating is unobtainable; (2) in gunshot wounds and in avulsive injuries where there is loss of bony continuity to maintain adequate length; (3) when osteomyelitis occurs requiring removal of rigid internal fixation. The advantages of the extraskeletal fixation include the device being distant from the site of the fracture or contamination, as well as the avoidance of periosteal stripping that might devascularize a fracture fragment. The disadvantages include the use of an external device, scarring of the face, and possible injury to the marginal mandibular branch of the facial nerve and facial artery.

Internal fixation can be achieved with interosseous wiring or with rigid internal fixation plates. Rigid fixation allows for a shorter period or no period of intermaxillary fixation and allows primary bone healing at the fracture site as compared to interosseous wiring. Plates that are made of stainless steel will corrode and, therefore plate removal is recommended after adequate fracture healing. Persons with nickel allergies are unable to tolerate the stainless steel plates. More recently, Vitallium and titanium plates have been introduced. These plates provide advantages over the stainless steel plates, which include better malleability and the ability to leave them in situ unless other indications require removal.

A specific type of internal fixation plate, the dynamic compression plate, is suited especially to the immediate removal of intermaxillary fixation. Patients with seizure disorders or severe respiratory disease are best treated without intermaxillary fixation to insure an adequate airway. Untrustworthy patients, such as psychotics and alcoholics, who are likely to remove their intermaxillary fixation also are ideal candidates for compression fixation.

Lag screw fixation is another type of rigid internal fixation that allows dynamic compression at the fracture site and primary bone healing. Lag screws are especially useful when the mandible is split in a sagittal fashion. A minimum of two lag screws should be used at each fracture site.

FRACTURES OF THE MANDIBULAR CONDYLE

Isolated unilateral or bilateral condylar fractures with no associated maxillary fracture can usually be treated by closed reduction and a 2 to 3 week course of intermaxillary fixation followed by progressive physical therapy to achieve adequate motion (Fig. 3). When a unilateral fractured condyle is associated with a maxillary fracture, the opposite condyle is usually sufficient to stabilize the mandible anteroposteriorly. When bilateral condylar fractures and maxillary fractures occur together, the posterior mandibular height must be kept at proper length to prevent shortening with a resultant anterior open bite. In such cases, the maxilla is stabilized with rigid internal fixation plates; the mandible is maintained in its proper orientation through intermaxillary fixation. The use of plates in these cases often prevents the necessity for open reduction of the condylar fractures.

The isolated unicondylar fracture with minimal displacement and no pain is treated with a dental soft diet as long as the occlusion is unaltered from the premorbid status. This same fracture with mild pain and reproducible occlusion is treated with dental elastics. Intermaxillary fixation becomes necessary when the occlusion is unreproducible.

There are some indications for open reduction of condylar fractures: (1) displacement of the fractured condyle into the middle cranial fossa; (2) the inability to attain adequate occlusion with closed reduction; and (3) lateral or medial extracapsular condylar displacement. Shortcomings of the open approach are the difficulty in exposure,

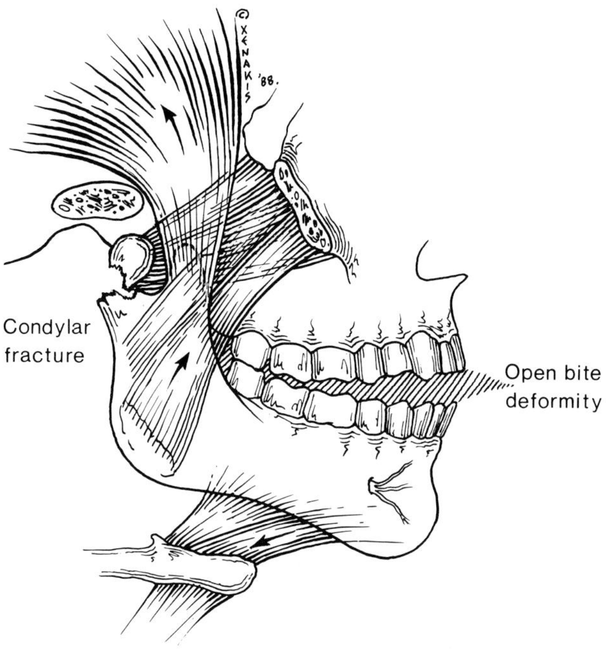

Figure 3 Condylar neck fracture showing displacement and action of muscular forces.

possible seventh nerve injury, and external scarring. Alternatives in fixation include K-wire spearing, interfragmentary wiring, and condylar head replacement. The sequelae of open as well as closed reductions include pain in the TMJ, arthritic changes, and decreased motion in the joint.

FRACTURES OF THE MANDIBULAR RAMUS

Fractures of the mandibular ramus are uncommon. Because of the sling effect of the medial pterygoid and masseter muscles, these fractures are rarely displaced significantly. Most fractures of the ascending ramus can be treated by closed methods with intermaxillary fixation. When reduction is unobtainable, a transmucosal incision can be utilized for open reduction. Fixation may be achieved by interosseous wiring, lag screws, or bone plating. If transoral access for plating is difficult it may sometimes necessitate an external approach. More recently, the use of right-angled instruments and screwdrivers has made the approach to plating these fractures somewhat easier. When plating mandibular fractures, the operator must be acutely aware that the rigid plates are nonforgiving and only perfect bone alignment will produce an excellent occlusal result.

FRACTURES OF THE MANDIBULAR ANGLE

Fractures of the angle of the mandible are one of the most common fractures seen (Figs. 4 and 5). Minimally-displaced fractures can be treated with closed reduction and intermaxillary fixation. More severely displaced fractures, which are not amenable to closed reduction, are approached transorally. After fracture reduction interosseous wires, lag screws, or bone plates can be utilized for fixation. Care must be taken in this area of the mandible not to place these devices through the inferior alveolar artery or nerve.

FRACTURES OF THE MANDIBULAR BODY

Fractures of the mandibular body often are open fractures because of the close association of the mucoperiosteum to the bone. When the dentition is good, these fractures can be treated with closed reduction and intermaxillary fixation. When the muscular forces of mastication work to distract the fracture segments or when there is poor or absent dentition, or both, open reduction often is necessary including the use of stabilizing splints or dentures. Transoral open reduction may be possible in such cases. The interosseous wiring or bone plates are placed on the lower border of the mandible for adequate fixation. Care must be taken to avoid the inferior alveolar nerve and artery as well as dental root tips that can be damaged with the wires or screws. Remember that the tooth root is twice the length of the crown. This may be measured to assure that placement of any hardware is inferior to the root apex.

FRACTURES OF THE MANDIBULAR SYMPHYSIS

Fractures in the symphyseal and parasymphyseal areas have considerable muscular forces pulling on the segments. Once again, the decision regarding closed versus open reduction depends upon the angle of the fracture and the direction of the muscular forces. The greater majority of these fractures are treated by open reduction. Transoral

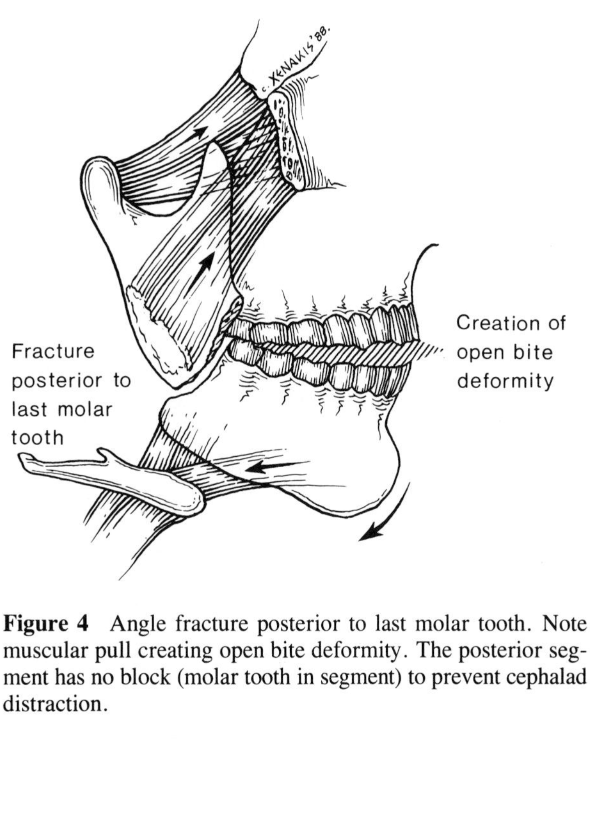

Figure 4 Angle fracture posterior to last molar tooth. Note muscular pull creating open bite deformity. The posterior segment has no block (molar tooth in segment) to prevent cephalad distraction.

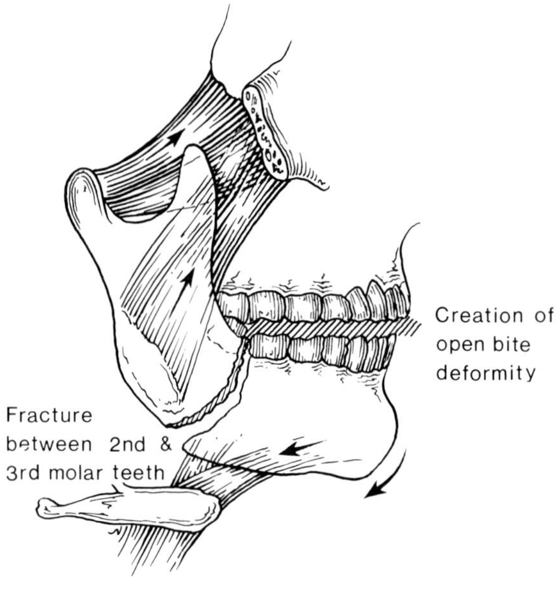

Figure 5 Angle fracture with molar tooth in posterior segment blocking cephalad displacement. Displacing forces on anterior segment create open bite deformity.

open reduction and internal fixation is accomplished easily for these injuries. This can be performed by interosseous wiring or bone plating at the inferior border of the mandible.

FRACTURES OF THE MANDIBULAR CORONOID

Fractures of the coronoid process are extremely rare. Because of the long insertion of the temporalis muscle onto the coronoid and anterior border of the ascending ramus, distraction of a fractured coronoid is uncommon. In the absence of other fractures, no fixation is necessary. Dental elastics may be used if the fracture is painful. The patient typically is kept on a dental soft diet until the pain resolves.

POSTOPERATIVE CARE

With rigid internal fixation (lag screws or compression plates) of a mandibular fracture, postoperative feeding with a dental soft diet begins as soon as the pain from the operation subsides. When the patient is in intermaxillary fixation, a blenderized diet is necessary. Routine oral care with irrigation and dental cleansing is continued regardless of the means of fixation.

The length of time before healing of a mandibular fracture is achieved cannot be determined by radiographic examination. No bony callus is seen even though stable healing has occurred in the early postoperative period. The absence of pain on palpation at the fracture site is the best indication of healing for timing of intermaxillary fixation removal. Condylar fractures usually are healed adequately to allow motion at 2 to 3 weeks post injury. Early motion and physical therapy is of great importance to prevent stiffness at the temporomandibular joint. Angle fractures often require 4 to 6 weeks of intermaxillary fixation until they are adequately healed for motion. Symphyseal and parasymphyseal fractures typically take the longest before intermaxillary fixation can be released, usually 6 to 8 weeks (Fig. 6). After removal of the fixation, mandibular physical therapy must be performed to reverse stiffening of the joints.

In all cases irrespective of fracture site, the intermaxillary fixation is removed once the tenderness on palpation at the fracture site has resolved. The arch bars are left in place for a short period of time to allow the patient to confirm whether the occlusion is reproducible or not. With satisfactory reproducible occlusion, the arch bars are removed. However, when the occlusion is not reproducible, the intermaxillary fixation is replaced for a period of 1 to 2 weeks, when removal is attempted again.

COMPLICATIONS OF MANDIBULAR FRACTURES

In treating mandibular fractures, the key point that cannot be forgotten is that anatomic reduction will follow

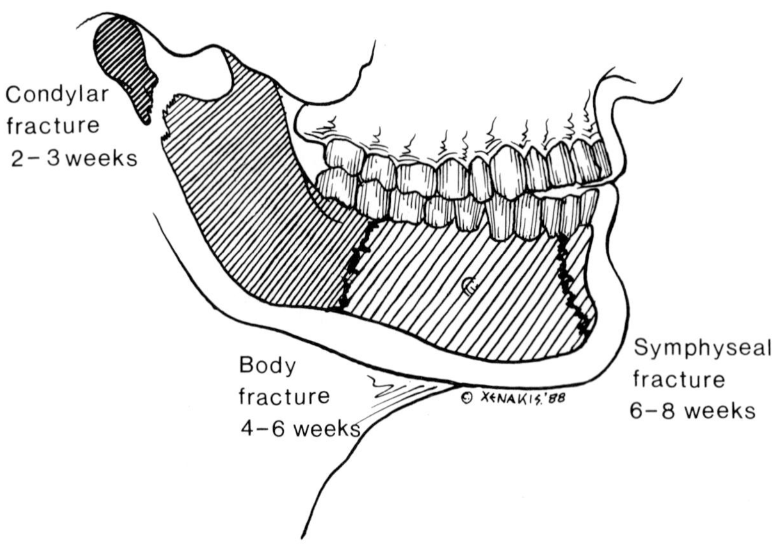

Figure 6 Average length of time for fracture healing with closed reduction or interfragmentary wiring.

the restoration of occlusion. Malocclusion is one of the most common complications of mandibular fractures. The smallest deviation from the preinjury state is noticed by the patient. Minor occlusal disharmony can be treated by orthodontics or dental occlusal equilibration. Major occlusal disharmony may necessitate a secondary mandibular procedure.

Infection of the fracture site can be decreased by early reduction of the fracture and perioperative antibiotics. Infections of the mandible are treated, as elsewhere, with incision and drainage and removal of any nonviable material. Occasionally it is necessary to remove foreign bodies such as wire, screws, and plates. Joe Hall Morris external fixation can prove useful at this time. Compression fixation devices do not necessarily need to be removed in the presence of infection: if they stably fix the fragments without motion, they can be left in place until fracture healing has occurred. Persistent drainage at that time often is cured by removal of the fixation and by curettage of the draining sinus and screw holes.

Nonunion of mandibular fractures can have many causes. Infection is one cause. Another cause is motion at the fracture site secondary to inadequate fixation. With unstable fixation and motion, a fibrous union often occurs. Therefore, any time motion is noted in the postoperative period, tightening of the fixation is indicated immediately. When patient noncompliance occurs after intermaxillary fixation removal, stable rigid internal fixation is necessary. When nonunion is due to bony gaps, bone grafting is necessary.

Temporomandibular joint symptoms are not uncommon following management of mandibular fractures. These can be treated nonoperatively with anti-inflammatory medications and splints as necessary. When progressive degenerative changes of the joint develop, direct surgical intervention in the joint may be necessary.

SUGGESTED READING

Converse JM. Kazanjian and Converse's surgical treatment of facial injuries. 3rd ed. Baltimore: Williams & Wilkins, 1974:142.

Dingman RO, Natvig P. Surgery of facial fractures. Philadelphia: WB Saunders, 1964.

Mathog RH. Maxillofacial trauma. Baltimore: Williams & Wilkins, 1984:124.

Rowe NL, Williams JL. Maxillofacial injuries. London: Churchill Livingstone, 1985:232.

Schultz RC. Facial injuries. 3rd ed. Chicago: Year Book, 1988.

TEMPOROMANDIBULAR JOINT DYSFUNCTION

JONATHAN S. JACOBS, D.M.D., M.D.
RUSSELL W. BESSETTE, D.D.S., M.D.

Recent surveys have estimated that between 4 and 28 percent of the adult population is affected by symptomatology of the temporomandibular joint (TMJ) with a female-to-male ratio of 3 to 1. Young to middle-aged females are most often affected. The common triad of symptoms includes pain in the preauricular area, popping and clicking of the TMJ, and limitation of mandibular movement. The mandible may deviate to the affected side, and the symptoms may be episodic. A strong psychological component has been implicated in many patients. It should be stated at the outset that the majority of patients with these symptoms are best treated by nonsurgical therapy. However, all patients deserve adequate evaluation to eliminate the possibility of organic disease. Conditions of neuralgia, paranasal sinusitis, dental pulpitis, central nervous system neoplasms, and neuritis (such as temporal arteritis) can all masquerade as TMJ syndrome. A complete head and neck physical examination remains the mainstay in evaluation of these patients. However, after a thorough examination, a significant number of patients complain of pain originating at the area of the joint. These patients may require special diagnostic testing reserved for suspected internal derangements of the TMJ.

Most investigators consider malocclusion and long-term microtrauma to be of importance in the etiology of TMJ dysfunction. These may be secondary to either dental occlusal prematurities or overclosure of the mandible. Bruxism with microtrauma to the joint also has been implicated as have direct and indirect joint trauma. These factors are thought to work alone or in conjunction with anxiety to produce masticatory muscle spasm. In order to denote the special role of muscle spasm, the term myofascial pain dysfunction (MPD) syndrome has been proposed. Many investigators believe that the symptoms are secondary to dental malocclusion only and to subsequent muscle spasm. Efforts have been directed toward correcting occlusal function; the vertical dimension of occlusion has been adjusted by either orthodontic or prosthetic means.

When overclosure is felt to be a problem, it seems important to raise the height of dentition, thereby opening the bite and increasing the vertical dimension. As part of the therapy, mandibular opening is limited to hinge movement only, since this eliminates the need for external pterygoid contraction. The construction of splints that disarticulate the occlusion also has been advocated. Splints change the position of the condyle in the glenoid fossa when the jaws are articulated. Therefore, they help interrupt the pain-spasm cycle associated with grinding. Splints may be effective in "capturing" a subluxating disc by repositioning the condyle under the anteriorly positioned disc. Adjunctive treatments for muscle spasm are usually employed. These include heat, ultrasonography, diathermy, exercises that decrease range of motion, and muscle relaxants and anti-inflammatory drugs.

RATIONALE FOR TREATMENT

An individual with a mandibular condylar head that is positioned anteriorly in the glenoid fossa, thereby stretching the posterior attachment, may eventually develop temporomandibular joint dysfunction. On the other hand, if the condylar head is forced posteriorly, as with posterior directed dental contacts, pressure may be exerted upon the disc to dislocate. Many clinicians advocate treatment of asymptomatic clicking or popping (Fig. 1) to avoid eventual symptoms and secondary joint changes. This may be accomplished by splinting, orthodontic therapy, or dental re-alignment by prosthetic manipulation.

TREATMENT

Splints should be designed to recapture the subluxating disc while disarticulating the occlusion. The splint should be constructed so that the condylar head is brought under the posterior meniscal band. Ideally, this eliminates the clicking and presumably allows shortening of the attenuated posterior attachment. Maintenance of splinting in this position for a period of 3 to 6 months frequently eliminates further symptomatology. Some patients become asymptomatic while "functioning" on the posterior band region or even completely off the disc. However, because of stretching and pain about this band, external pterygoid muscle pain may be concomitant. Use of adjunctive muscle relaxant therapy is sometimes helpful. Heat packs, ultrasonography, diathermy, anti-inflammatory drugs, and limited range of motion with either soft diet or periods of liquid diet are advocated.

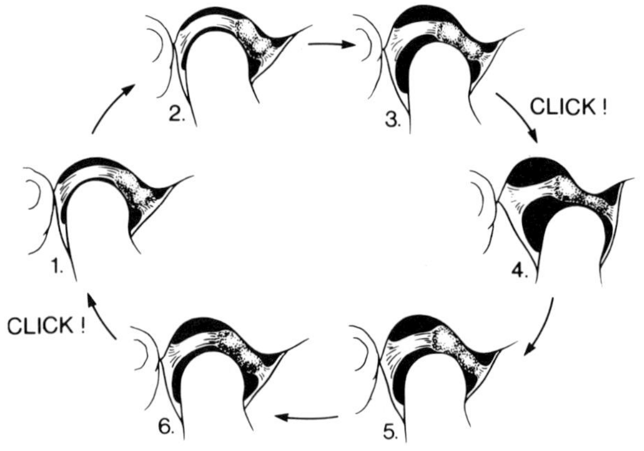

Figure 1 Mechanism of joint clicking. If the thickened posterior band of the articular disc is subluxated, opening produces a click as it is recaptured (between 3 and 4). A reciprocal click may be heard or palpated on closing if the disc again subluxates (between 6 and 1).

Surgical treatment is indicated when both conservative measures have failed to relieve pain and popping and to restore normal range of motion and correctable anatomic changes have been documented. This usually arises with internal derangements that are recalcitrant to conservative therapy (e.g., disc perforation) or in cases of advanced degenerative or rheumatoid arthritis. When degenerative joint disease is seen on plain films or tomograms, more sophisticated imaging (such as arthrography, computed tomography (CT) scanning, or magnetic resonance imaging [MRI]) may not be needed.

Surgical procedures have been designed to attack the problems as they present anatomically. When the articular disc is dislocated anteriorly and prevents opening, arthroplasty is carried out (Fig. 2). A preauricular incision is used to expose the joint capsule. A flap of the lateral capsular elements is raised such that closure is possible after completion of the intra-articular procedure. The articular disc is repositioned by removal of a wedge from the disc and its posterior attachment and then suturing the disc posteriorly. This tents the disc backwards, repositioning it once again over the condylar head. It is important to take the thickened portion of the posterior band with the resected specimen to obviate further difficulties with subluxation. In addition, it is felt that sectioning the posterior attachment helps in relief of pain. Some surgeons combine a high posteriorly angled condylar shave with disc plication. We advocate this only when condylar head pathology warrants it. When disc pathology is severe, total meniscectomy may be appropriate. This procedure had been the standard of care for many years.

If irreversible destruction of the condylar head is found, replacement is carried out. It is important to reconstruct the height of the condylar head either directly or by glenoid fossa augmentation to avoid collapse of ramus height. Multiple methods of joint reconstruction techniques have been advocated. We utilize a Proplast-coated metallic prosthesis, a Silastic sheet interpositional arthroplasty, or an ulnar head prosthesis. The type of prosthesis chosen depends on the clinical situation.

A variety of surgical corrections of internal derangement of the temporomandibular joint have been intermittently popular. The most common procedures have been meniscectomy, condylar shave, and true condylectomy. All authors report satisfactory results. Some have questioned the appropriateness of meniscectomy. They report failure in resolution of pain, deviation to the side of the meniscectomy, and inability to control symptoms when the disease has been longstanding. Long-term changes in the morphology of the condylar head are consistent findings. Indeed, even proponents of meniscectomy admit a small percentage of patients who may go on to ankylosis following this procedure. It seems logical to leave the meniscus as a cushion over the condylar head if it can be repaired in an attempt to return normal joint function. A period of physical therapy is mandatory after any of these procedures to restore joint function.

Proponents of condylectomy have reported similar difficulties with deviation, but more frequently bite col-

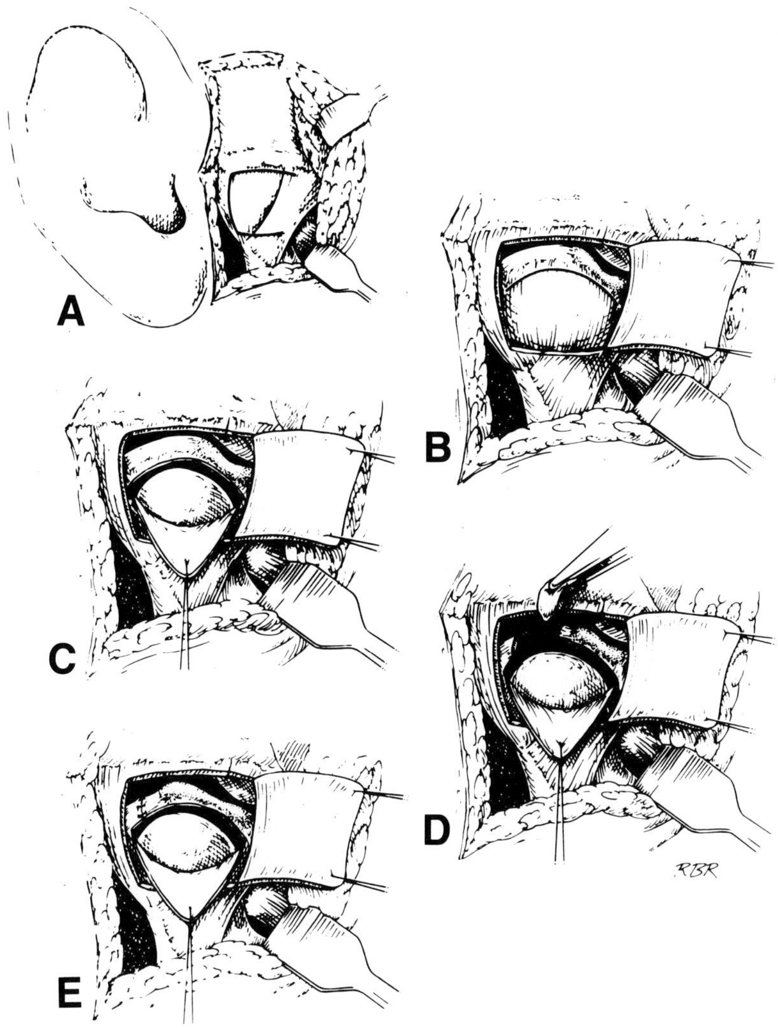

Figure 2 Disc plication procedure. Through a preauricular incision, the joint capsule is exposed under the body of the parotid gland. *A*, An anterior based flap of capsule is raised and access is gained to the upper joint space. *B*, An incision in the disc attachment then allows access to the lower space. *C*, A wedge is removed from the posterior attachment. *D*, This allows plication of the disc in a more posterior position overriding the condylar head. *E*, The joint structures are then repaired in layers using nonresorbable suture.

lapse and worsening symptoms following condylar resection. Condylar shaves frequently have not relieved symptoms. In our experience, the high posterior angled condylectomy in conjunction with disc plication has been the most frequent procedure (Fig. 3). Shortening the posterior attachment and repositioning the disc are the anatomic corrections that we feel restore normal joint function in the great majority of cases, thus eliminating painful symptomatology and joint noise. For this reason, we no longer perform a "high posterior angled condylectomy" on a routine basis. We see no advantage to removing normal condylar head cartilage and bone. When the condylar head is arthritic with bone spurs and osteophytes, then conservative condylar shave is indicated.

Temporalis fascia has been used for repair of the posterior attachment. This has been combined with high condylectomy to restore function and to leave an appropriate amount of joint space. Other repair materials have been advocated, but the use of viable fascia easily available through the same incision seems most appropriate (Fig. 4). Silastic sheet interposition for the meniscus is sometimes well tolerated, but has been found to fracture in some cases.

In patients who require condylar replacement, a number of options are available (Fig. 5). Silastic sheeting is most commonly used, not to restore the shape of the condylar head, but to line the surface of the glenoid fossa. The modified ulnar head prosthesis, readily available in most operating suites, provides an adequate condylar prosthesis. It restores the height of the ramus and can be secured by its "internal" suture to the area of the sigmoid notch so that it remains secure on the stump of the condylar head. The use of this prosthesis has been successful in the great majority of patients who require replacement prosthesis (see Fig. 5B). Certainly, other techniques for condylar head replacement are available and include replacement with autogenous material such as metatarsal head or costochondral grafts. Alloplastic materials, other than silicone, have also been popular. The Proplast-coated metallic prosthesis has been advocated by Kent and provides total replacement when no remnant of condylar head or neck is salvageable. It has been well-tolerated in a majority of patients, but requires an additional operative site (submandibular) for placement. It also entails more involved instrumentation and placement of a larger foreign body.

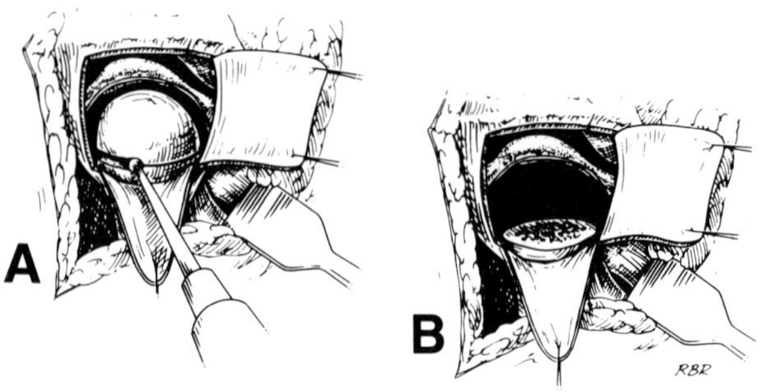

Figure 3 High condylectomy. The condylar head is removed to the area of the neck through a preauricular approach. An attempt is made to leave the attachments of the external pterygoid on the neck intact.

TEMPOROMANDIBULAR JOINT ANKYLOSIS

TMJ ankylosis is a difficult problem for both patient and reconstructive surgeon. The patient experiences difficulty with speech, mastication, oral hygiene, and esthetics and often has chronic pain. The surgeon is faced with a technically difficult problem, which has inherent complications and requires the utmost patient cooperation. Instigation of surgical therapy requires careful, detailed consideration. In 1938, Kazajian classified ankylosis as true or false—false ankylosis being extra-articular, true ankylosis being intra-articular. True ankylosis is more common and is produced by any condition causing fibrous or bony adhesions between condyle and fossa. False ankylosis can be caused by myogenic, neurogenic, and psychological factors, bony impingement, fibrous adhesions, and tumors. Major etiologies of end-stage ankylosis are trauma, intracapsular hematomas, birth deformities, and the arthritides (post-traumatic, postinfectious, and degenerative).

Regardless of etiology, destruction of the meniscus and atrophy of the condyle and fossa cartilage are constant findings. Progressive destruction leads to narrowing of the joint space and formation of thick fibrous scar adhesions that blend with periarticular tissues. Bony changes consist of severe erosions, lipping, osteophytes, and subcortical cysts with irregular condylar contour, flattening, and bony ankylosis.

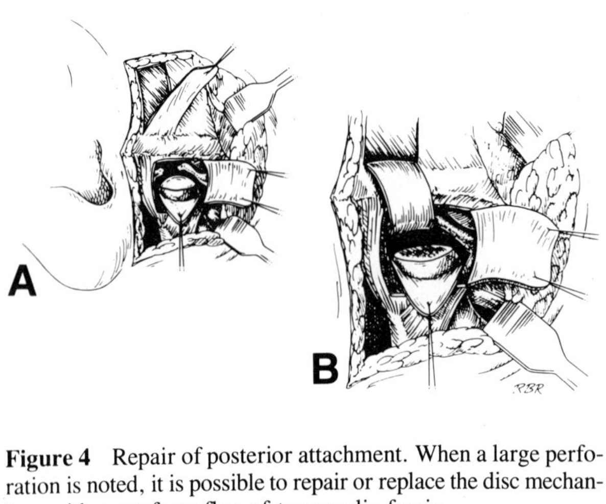

Figure 4 Repair of posterior attachment. When a large perforation is noted, it is possible to repair or replace the disc mechanism with a graft or flap of temporalis fascia.

Patients can masticate despite ankylosis. Rarely does it completely prevent all oral opening. An interincisal opening of 5 mm or less is indicative of complete bony ankylosis.

Facial deformity is often associated with ankylosis. Its severity is related to age at onset and degree of ankylosis. It consists of malocclusion with possible crossbite, incisor malalignment, class II relations with decreased ramus height and anterior open bite. Protrusive function is absent in true ankylosis.

Radiographs are indispensible in the diagnosis of ankylosis. Anteroposterior and lateral tomograms or plain films usually provide adequate information. Panorex, cephalometrogram, and submental vertex views are useful in determining the extent of ankylosis and associated dentofacial deformity. Enlargement of the coronoid process frequently accompanies ankylosis; it must also be diagnosed radiographically.

Dentofacial growth must be analyzed in the growing patient. These patients ideally should have restoration of growth potential to the affected condyle. Currently, costochondral grafting is the most popular and the best available technique short of the use of vascularized bone. However, growth of the graft is unreliable and unpredictable in occurrence and degree.

Condylectomy with gap arthroplasty by artificial or autogenous interpositional material is the basic technique for treating the nongrowing patient. Treatment of acquired dentofacial deformities may be necessary. If ankylosis is not severe, a limited sculpting condylectomy of the condylar head may be adequate to produce joint motion. This minimally disturbs anatomy.

In condylectomy, excision should be as high as possible on the condyle to maintain the joint as close as possible to its normal position. This maintains the class III level of the mandible and minimizes potential for posterior open bite. Interpositional material should be used with any significant excision of the condyle. The most widely accepted material is Silastic rubber in block form. It usually performs well, but has the usual problems associated with a foreign body. Condylectomy at the level of the condylar neck causes loss of ramus height and leaves only simple hinge motion. If this articulation is not balanced with the contralateral side by interposition materials, internal derangements and bony degeneration may occur on the contralateral side. Interpositional arthroplasty maintains posterior facial height and prevents formation of bony and fibrous adhesions, but does not reduce normal anatomy and does not function as a glide and hinge joint.

Joint replacement more closely reproduces normal anatomy and function. Proponents of the condylar replacement made of Proplast-coated Vitallium claim an 87 percent success rate in cases that require functional TMJ rehabilitation. Ninety percent of all successful prostheses used for ankylosis maintain or increase ramus height, incisal opening, and lateral excursions. Therefore, the need

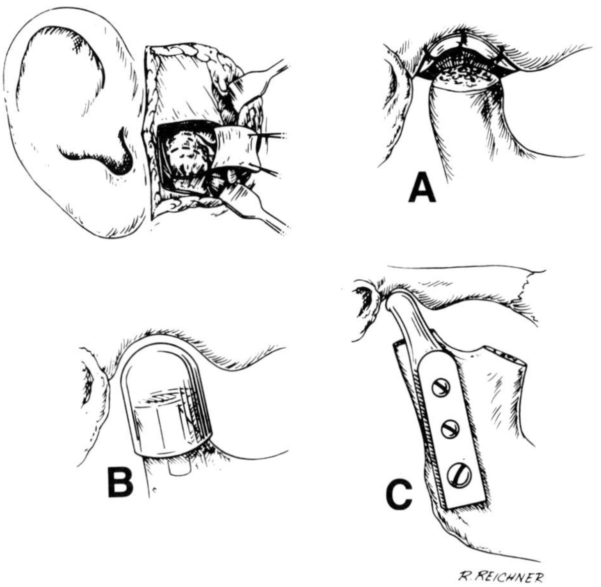

Figure 5 Options for condylar head replacement after resection for ankylosis or severe degenerative disease. *A*, Silastic block arthroplasty is secured to the base of glenoid fossa. *B*, Condylar head is replaced by Silastic ulnar head prosthesis. *C*, Proplast-Vitallium ramus-condyle implant.

for simultaneous correction of the dentofacial deformity and bony ankylosis may be an indication for a metallic condylar prosthesis in the nongrowing patient.

Patients with active primary inflammatory arthritis and severe ankylosis present a special problem. They require condylar reconstruction with simultaneous correction of open bite and retrognathia. A costochondral graft may undergo reabsorption because of ongoing disease. A prosthesis may produce glenoid fossa erosion. Long-term follow-up of joint replacement is not available in these patients.

HYPERMOBILITY AND DISLOCATION OF THE CONDYLE

Acute Dislocation

Acute dislocation of the condylar head occurs with its extension forward past the articular eminence. It may occasionally luxate into the infratemporal fossa. Rapid spontaneous reduction usually occurs; however, the mandible can be repositioned manually with little difficulty. Relocation is accomplished as follows: facing the patient, the operator's thumbs are placed in the buccal sulcus adjacent to the mandibular bicuspids. The fingers of each hand are placed under the inferior border of the mandible body. Downward, anterior, and then posterior pressure is applied to the patient's mandible over several minutes to stretch the spastic elevator muscles and then to relocate the condyle within the fossa. Intravenous sedation prior to manipulation may be necessary.

Recurrent Dislocation

Recurrent dislocation may cause recurrent TMJ pain and degenerative joint changes. Intra-articular injection of sclerosing agents to produce fibrosis of the capsular ligaments (thereby preventing dislocation) has been advocated. This indirect approach is rarely effective. If conservative therapy (i.e., patient training of consistent avoidance of maximum opening) does not control the problem, several surgical procedures are available (Fig. 6). Tightening the capsule by excision of redundant tissue or by plication is the simplest procedure. Mechanical interference in the condylar path may be increased by augmenting the articular eminence with Silastic or autogenous bone. Removal of the articular tubercle prevents locking of the condylar head anterior to the articular eminence. It is effective, technically easy, and the current treatment of choice.

CORONOID ABNORMALITIES CAUSING LIMITED MANDIBULAR MOVEMENT

Abnormalities of the coronoid process may cause limited mandibular motion. Although rare, such abnormalities should be considered when evaluating the TMJ. The etiologies are bilateral or unilateral enlargement of the coronoid process, ossification of the temporalis tendon and muscle after trauma, or ankylosis of the coracoid process to adjacent body structures. All produce similar symptoms and differ only by the history of trauma associated with temporalis ossification. Plain films, tomograms, a CT scan, or MRI are needed to make the diagnosis.

Satisfactory access can be obtained through intraoral incisions. This approach is less likely to injure vital nerves and vessels and maintains better cosmetic results. An incision can be made directly over the external oblique line and carried superiorly along the anterior edge of the ramus up the coronoid process. This incision can be extended downward and forward over the bone to the distal buccal aspect of the second molar and then forward laterally in the gingival sulcus to the first premolar. The periosteum is reflected laterally, exposing the sigmoid notch, the coronoid process, and the tendon of the temporalis muscle. If ossified, a portion of the temporalis tendon or muscle is removed, the ankylosis is removed, or the coronoid process is excised. If the diagnosis was correct, the mandible should open wide with utilization of a mouth prop.

INFLAMMATORY ARTHRITIS

After internal derangement, arthritis is the most common organic TMJ problem. Osteoarthritis occurs most often, followed by rheumatoid arthritis. The TMJ is affected in as many as 50 to 60 percent of patients with rheumatoid arthritis. In one study, 68 percent of these patients have radiographic evidence of TMJ involvement.

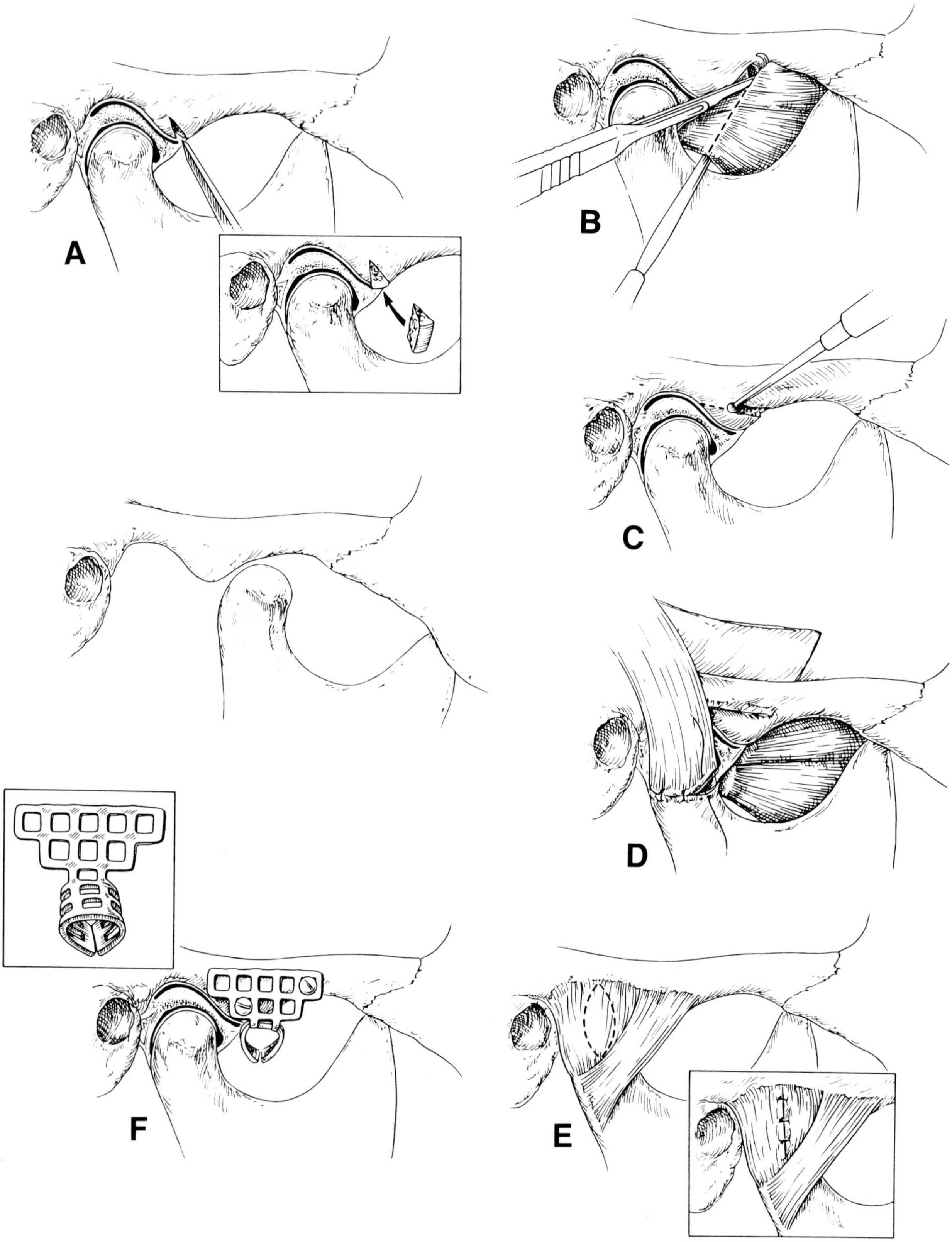

Figure 6 Options for treatment of chronic dislocation. *A*, Wedge bone graft to augment eminence; *B*, external pterygoid myotomy; *C*, eminectomy; *D*, fascial flap to limit translation; *E*, capsulorrhaphy; *F*, Vitallium crib—for eminence augmentation.

However, they rarely have severe handicapping temporomandibular symptoms. The most common symptoms are crepitus, limitation of motion which may become progressive, and pain which is usually mild.

On the contrary, in juvenile rheumatoid arthritis, TMJ and facial growth involvement can be devastating. Progressive resorption of the condyle occurs. The adult condyle may be a mere remnant with shortened ramus height and resulting anterior open bite deformity. In the growing patient, this severely retarded mandibular growth can cause secondary growth deformities of the upper jaw. Treatment consists of surgical corrections of the jaw and of facial deformity to restore occlusion and facial form. When ankylosis is present or when significant temporomandibular joint damage is associated with debilitating pain, the surgical options are gap arthroplasty with interpositional alloplastic or autogenous material, or total joint replacement.

Other diseases may occasionally cause arthritis of the TMJ. These include: familial Mediterranean fever, collagen vascular syndromes (i.e., scleroderma, systemic lupus erythematosus), gout, Sjögren's syndrome, infectious arthritis, and chronic psoriasis. Psoriasis occurs in 1.2 percent of the general population and TMJ psoriatic arthritis in 5.7 percent of patients with chronic psoriasis. Psoriatic arthritis is characterized by the following triad: (1) psoriasis; (2) erosive arthritis; and (3) negative results on a serology test for rheumatoid factor. Involvement of the TMJ in psoriatic arthritis is characterized by episodic, painful, unilateral inflammation, often with a sudden onset. Typically, spontaneous exacerbations and remissions occur. The painful episodes may last for months and are usually associated with the presence of skin lesions. Improvement of the arthritis usually follows improvement of the skin lesions. Radiographs of the TMJ may be normal, but necrosis and osteoporotic changes are often seen. Nonsteroidal anti-inflammatory drugs may be helpful during exacerbation. To our knowledge, only one case of psoriatic arthritis of the TMJ leading to ankylosis has been reported in the English language literature.

INFECTIOUS ARTHRITIS OF THE TMJ

The joint may become infected after an open operation of access procedure (arthrography, aspiration, or injection), by local spread of infection from adjacent regions such as otitis media, mastoiditis, or parotitis, and rarely by hematogenous spread of a distant infection. Septic arthritis is very rare, but carries the potential for serious complications such as osteomyelitis and resulting ankylosis. Strict sterile techniques should be observed in all procedures. When infected, the joint requires incision and drainage with sequestrectomy as indicated and appropriate antibiotics.

AVASCULAR NECROSIS

Avascular necrosis of the mandibular condylar head was thought to be rare. However, new evidence obtained by MRI scanning may prove this to be a much more frequent phenomenon. It may develop several months after an untreated intracapsular fracture or inadvertent devascularization of the head during open reduction of a fracture. Clinical symptoms are pain in the TMJ on the affected side and limited opening of the mouth. Radiographically, the condylar head is characteristically eroded and irregular. Treatment consists of surgical removal of the necrotic condylar head and conservative débridement. Eventual condylar replacement is indicated.

ARTHROSCOPY

Recently it has become apparent that the upper joint space can be visualized by the needle arthroscope. Some workers have advocated arthroscopy and lysis of adhesions as beneficial in the treatment of patients with disc subluxation and dislocation. Scopes have been developed that range in diameter from 1.5 to 2.7 mm and have varied angles of view. They can be inserted by percutaneous puncture, allow for combined influent Ringer's lactate to lavage the joint, and require a separate puncture by a large-bore needle for joint effluent. To date, limited series have been developed, but complications have been infrequent. These, however, include hematoma, transient frontal branch of the seventh nerve damage and entrance into the middle ear. Micro instrumentation, which will allow manipulation of joint structure, is under development.

It is fair to say that only limited application of this procedure either diagnostically or for treatment can be claimed. With improvement in instrumentation and technique, this situation may improve rapidly. There appears to be at least a temporary relief of painful symptomatology associated with joint lavage. However, no claim at long-term relief of a true dislocation can be made. The argon laser has been additionally used to begin instrumentation of the internal joint as well as micro shaves and bone rasps. We look forward to more information about the efficacy of these techniques.

SUGGESTED READING

Bronstein S. Postsurgical TMJ arthrography. J Craniomandib Pract 1984; 2(2):165–171.

Guralnick W, Kaban LB, Merril RG. Temporomandibular joint afflictions. N Engl J Med 1978; 229:123–129.

Kent JN, Misiek DJ, Akin RK, et al. Temporomandibular joint condylar prosthesis: a ten-year report. J Oral Maxillofac Surg 1983; 41:245–254.

Laskin DM. Etiology of the pain-dysfunction syndrome. J Am Den Assoc 1969; 79:147–153.

Lewis RW, Wright JA. Silastic ulnar head prosthesis for use in surgery of the temporomandibular joint. J Oral Surg 1981; 39:572–584.

Manzione JV, Katzberg RW, Seltzer SE, Mellius HZ. Computed tomography of the TM Joint. Radiology 1984; 150:111–115.

Stanson AW, Baker HL. Routine tomography of the temporomandibular joint. Radiol Clin North Am 1976; XIV:105.

FACIAL FRACTURES IN CHILDREN

FREDERICK J. McCOY, M.D.

The devotion of a chapter to facial fractures in children implies that these problems in children are significantly different from those in adults. This is true. The physical characteristics of growing bones such as malleability, the presence of active growth centers, the reduced size or absence of sinus cavities, mixed dentition, and environmental differences in the type of trauma to which they are exposed, constitute special considerations in the diagnosis, management, and potential sequelae that must be addressed.

A primary difference is the cause of facial injuries, summarized in Table 1. Avoidance of injury when presented with a hazardous situation depends upon recognition of the danger and quick, intelligent, agile reaction. This places a child at a disadvantage when exposed to traumatic confrontation. Even so, the incidence of facial fractures in children is relatively small and is usually reported as 6 to 10 percent of all facial fractures treated.

EVALUATION AND RESUSCITATION

When children are injured in vehicular accidents, falls from windows, or through parental abuse, frequently there are associated injuries. In a large series the incidence may be as high as 55 percent and may include central nervous system (CNS) injuries, extremity fractures, closed chest injuries, direct ocular injuries, and severe lacerations with significant blood loss (Table 2). In infants and small children the danger from the *apparent* blood loss may be underestimated. A reduction in blood volume of 20 percent may produce hypovolemic shock. A rapid method of calculation of normal blood volume can be done by multiplying the total body weight in kilograms by 8 percent, which provides the answer in milliliters.

TABLE 1 Etiology

Causative Factors	*Percentage of Patients*
Automobile trauma	
Pedestrian	19.8
Passenger	25.6
Fall while running	11.6
Fights	9.3
Fall from significant height	9.3
Baseball	9.3
Swing	3.5
Bicycle	2.3
Falling object	1.2
Farm accident	3.5
Fall from bed	3.5
Sledding accident	1.2
"Battered Child Syndrome"*	11.6

* The "*Battered Child*" category may overlap other categories depending upon how they were reported by parent.

TABLE 2 Associated Injuries

Injury	*Percentage of Patients*
Central nervous system injuries	
Skull fracture	40.8
Concussion without fracture	31.4
CNS rhinorrhea	14.0
Vertebral injury	2.3
Compound wound other than facial	1.2
Extremity fractures	
Clavicle	2.3
Femur	2.3
Tibia	2.3
Pelvis	1.2
Humerus	1.2
Ocular injury with blinding	3.6
Other injuries	
Major facial wounds	48.9
Minor facial wounds	39.6
Intra-abdominal injury	2.3
Hematuria (transient)	1.2
Closed chest injury	5.8

Establishment of airway, control of hemorrhage, cerebrospinal fluid leak, and fluid replacement are even more critical in children than in adults. An additional problem, peculiar to young age groups in connection with trauma, is a tendency towards vomiting and aspiration. This usually occurs at the scene of the accident and may account for many of the instances of temperature elevation during the first 3 to 5 days. Acute gastric dilation is sometimes seen 72 hours after trauma and requires prompt decompression (Fig. 1).

NASAL FRACTURES

Nasal fractures and septal deformities often begin at birth. The passage through the birth canal frequently dislocates the septal cartilage from the vomerine groove. Unless this is recognized and corrected promptly by the obstetrician or pediatrician, permanent deformity of the septum occurs. Reduction is easily accomplished in the crib by grasping the nasal tip with a gauze sponge and pulling it forward while finger pressure is exerted on the appropriate side.

Because of its prominent position on the face, the nose bears the brunt of many childhood falls and mishaps. Since growing bone is inherently malleable with a tendency toward "green stick" fracture, management is different from adults. Instead of relatively brittle bone that fractures cleanly and then dislocates, young bone tends to bend before breaking and shifting. X-ray films are of little use in the diagnostic evaluation.

Treatment consists of manipulation of each side of the arch with Asch forceps to correct the "bend" while lifting forward. The septum is then relocated in the midline with a forceps blade on either side. It should then be inspected for intraseptal hematoma, which, if present, must be evacuated to avoid the disastrous sequelae of septal abscess.

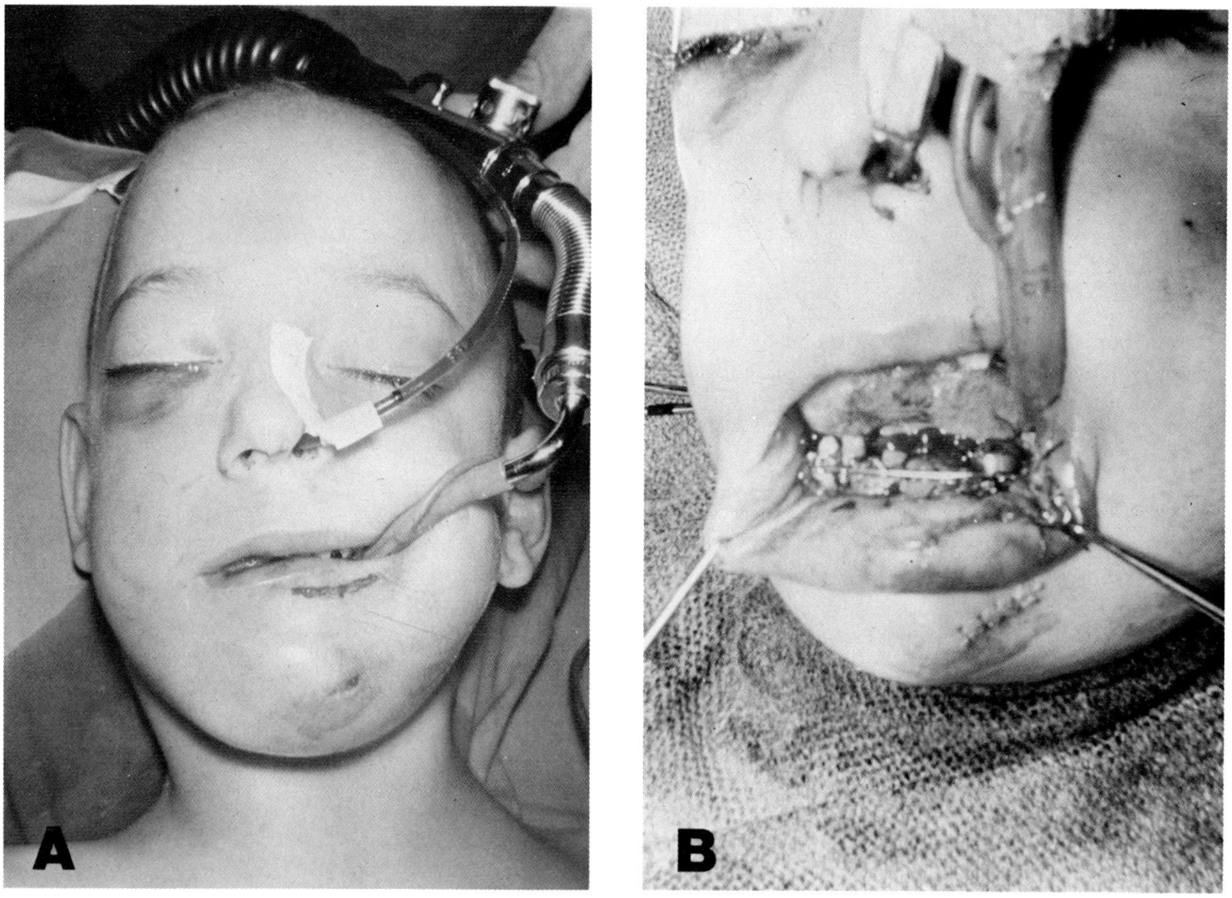

Figure 1 *A*, A 6-year-old boy received compound fractures of the mandible in an auto-pedestrian accident and had a 2-hour loss of consciousness with vomiting and aspiration. *B*, Parasymphyseal comminuted fractures were reduced through a degloving exposure by extending the laceration in the labial sulcus. Two cross wires at the lower border were supplemented by arch bars, circumferential support loops, and wire ligatures at the dental level crossing the alveolar portion of the fracture line, using the first solid teeth on both sides of the fracture—at least one tooth beyond the ones immediately adjacent to the fracture line.

Reduction should be carried out immediately if possible, or as soon as swelling subsides in about 5 days.

Packing should usually be avoided and is potentially hazardous, especially in very young children. Immobilization with a thinly-padded copper splint is preferred.

MIDDLE THIRD FRACTURES

Le Fort I, II, or III fractures are virtually never seen in infants, but are not uncommon after age 14, concurrent with a growing enthusiasm for driving automobiles, motorbikes, and snowmobiles, increased participation in water sports and skiing, and greater likelihood of barroom encounters.

Clinical signs and symptoms of midfacial fractures include: compound wound with visible bone fragments; visible or palpable deformity; abnormal mobility of upper jaw; malocclusion; pain or restriction on opening jaws; ecchymosis and subscleral hemorrhage; diplopia, entrapment, or enophthalmos; epistaxis or CNS rhinorrhea, and infraorbital nerve anesthesia.

High quality x-ray studies are necessary for diagnostic, conceptual, and medico-legal reasons. A complete series would include the following: occipitomental (Water's); posteroanterior (Caldwell); lateral; frontonuchal (Towne); computerized tomograms; submental vertex (for zygomatic arches); posteroanterior and oblique mandibular views, and panoramic mandibular views.

If ophthalmologic examination indicates serious visual disturbance, a modified Stenvers or Rhese view of the optic foramen should be taken.

Treatment

Fractures in children begin to heal quickly, and reduction should be carried out as soon as the patient is stable. Every 24 hours beyond 4 or 5 days significantly increases the difficulty, and after 14 days it may be impossible to achieve complete correction even with heroic effort.

Reduction and fixation of displaced or unstable fragments can only be reliably accomplished by adequate exposure and wiring or plating. A Le Fort I (floating maxilla) fracture requires intermaxillary fixation. The wiring technique exposes the fragments through a buccal incision and wires them directly; or they may be immobilized with Adam's wire suspension at the frontozygomatic junction, infraorbital rim, or zygomatic arch. After intermaxillary elastics have accomplished precise occlusion, they may be replaced by wire ligatures and maintained for 4 weeks.

An alternative method is the use of steel or Vitallium plates across fracture lines in critical support areas. The rigidity provided by this method makes it unnecessary to continue with intermaxillary fixation after occlusal relationships have been achieved. In younger children with mixed dentition, the use of plates and screws in the maxillary buttress areas carries added risk of injury to buds of unerupted teeth.

An obvious, but sometimes overlooked, fundamental principle is the necessity of confirming the *adequacy* of the reduction before fixation is carried out. Failure to do so guarantees a poor result and a difficult or impossible late reconstruction.

ORBITAL FRACTURES

Most fractures involving the zygomaticomaxillary complex involve the walls, roof, or floor of the orbit. The most common signs and symptoms relating directly to the orbit in the order of frequency are as follows: (1) orbital swelling and discoloration; (2) visible or palpable deformity; (3) tenderness over fracture sites; (4) infraorbital nerve anesthesia (cutaneous and/or gingival); (5) diplopia and/or entrapment (present in 15 percent); and (6) crepitus (bony, or air in tissues).

The most consistently reliable indication of orbital floor fracture is infraorbital nerve anesthesia that persists for more than 48 hours.

Treatment

Orbital exploration is carried out through an incision in the lower eyelid 5 mm above the normal level of the infraorbital margin. Some use an alternative conjunctival approach from personal preference. One need not fear the cutaneous scars since they virtually disappear, and there may be less risk, by this method, of postoperative ectropion.

The periorbita is cut at the rim and elevated widely from the floor and, if indicated, from the medial and lateral walls. Retracting the orbital contents gently upwards with a malleable ribbon retractor permits inspection of the entire floor (Fig. 2B). At this point, it is necessary to determine whether there is backward displacement of the rim. If present, it should be reduced and fixed. Wiring is preferred along the inferior and lateral orbital rims because plates are often palpable under the thin, soft tissue covering. The reduction is easily carried out by direct manipulation with a bone hook, or preferably by a cervical sound introduced through a Gillies incision in the temporal area. The maneuver should be done while the orbital floor is kept under direct and continuous observation. This obviates any possibility of sharp bone spicules being forced upward into the vulnerable soft structures of the orbit; and,

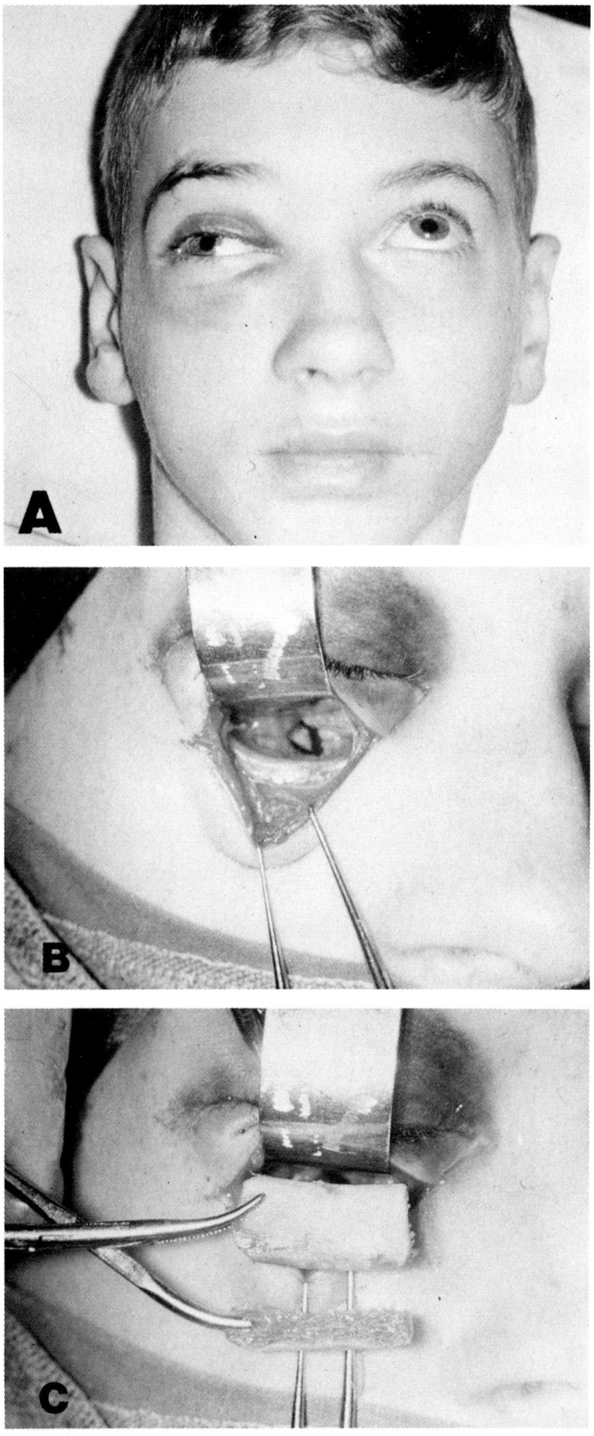

Figure 2 *A*, Boy, 14, injured in schoolyard fight showed uncommon immediate signs of entrapment and diplopia, clouding of antrum, and flattening of the malar eminence. *B*, At exploration and reduction a large defect with extensive comminution developed. The orbital contents were carefully retrieved from the antrum and disengaged from the upturned bone spicules. *C*, The floor was reconstituted with a split rib graft.

equally important, it provides the opportunity to see what effect the forward movement of the displacement rim has had on the floor. In many cases, it may be seen that a fractured, but apparently competent, floor has developed a large defect as the rim moves back to the normal position, leaving behind a collection of telescoped, unstable, comminuted fragments. Some of them may be free and must be retrieved along with orbital fat from the antrum below. It is the reduction of the zygomaticomaxillary fracture itself that has produced the defect. Once rim reduction is completed, the fragments in the floor are tested by pressure for stability.

Reconstitution of the floor may not be required if the defect is less than 6 mm and the adjacent bone is rigid, although it would be prudent in such instances to repair the tear in the periorbita with 4–0 chromic sutures. In most cases the floor must be supported. Split rib grafts are preferred because of their malleability for proper shaping, necessary rigidity, and resistance to infection (Fig. 2C). Alloplastic materials have been abandoned because of higher incidence of complications.

THE NASOETHMOID PYRAMID

A direct impact against the nasal arch may produce telescoping and spreading of the ethmoid area, with widening of the intercanthal distance. Direct open reduction should be carried out through bilateral angled incisions 5 mm anterior to the inner canthus. Dissection is carried straight to bone just anterior to the lacrimal rim, and the periosteum elevated 2.5 to 3 cm posteriorly. The unprotected blades of the Asch forceps are then inserted in the bilaterally dissected tunnels and the spread fragments compressed medially. At the same time forward traction is exerted if needed (Fig. 3). If the fragments appear unstable, a buried transnasal wire offers the most positive fixation (Fig. 4). Externally placed transnasal wires with buttons or plates are only effective for the nasal arch anterior to the lacrimal crest, and may cause skin necrosis. This method has limited usefulness.

MANDIBULAR FRACTURES

Mandibular fractures in children present a problem not seen in adults and older teenagers. In the younger age group the mandible is almost completely filled with teeth in various stages of development. This means that not only is there little bony architecture available for direct wiring or plating, but also the teeth are shaped in such a manner as to make it difficult to apply wire for ligation of the arch bars. When open reduction is performed, the drill holes must be inserted with care below the dental roots or buds in the inferior portion of the mandible. Often the lower arch bar must be secured with circumferential wires in addition to dental ligatures. It is also necessary to supplement the osseous wires with wire compression at the dental level across the fracture line, and teeth are selected just beyond the ones immediately adjacent to the alveolar por-

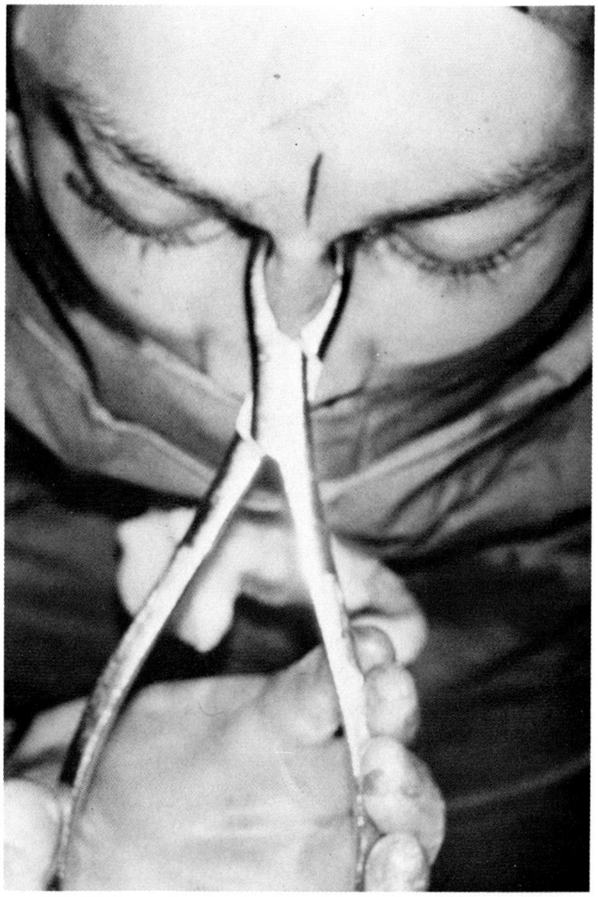

Figure 3 Shows method of reduction of retrodisplacement and widening of the nasoethmoid pyramid with Asch forceps. Wire fixation is usually required as in Figure 4. (From McCoy FJ. Late results in facial fractures. In: Goldwyn RM, ed. Long term results in plastic and reconstructive surgery. Vol. II. Boston: Little, Brown, 1980:491.)

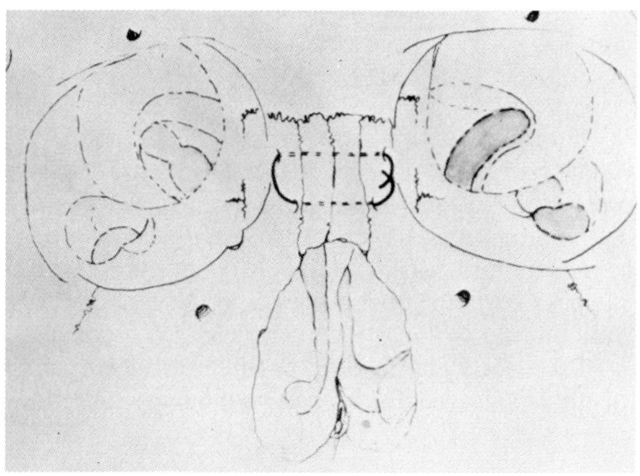

Figure 4 Transnasal wiring is frequently necessary to maintain nasoethmoid reduction. The anterior loop should be placed in, or just anterior to, the lacrimal ridge. The posterior loop is through the lamina papyracea and requires no drill holes. In passing the wire, the medial canthal tendon should be included on both sides.

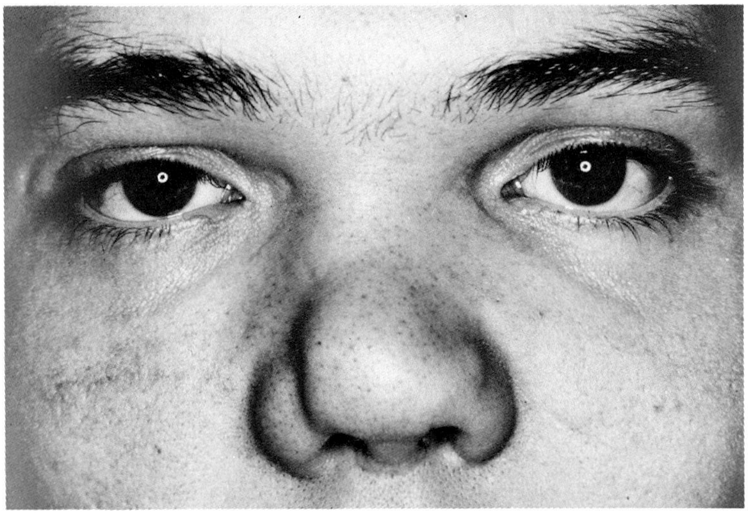

Figure 5 Boy, 15, had a severe injury to the nasal arch and septum at age 4. It was reduced promptly. Despite the absence of any apparent complications, distortion of subsequent growth, involving all nasal components, produced marked deformity. This is probably due to the involvement of the vomerine growth center prior to age 5.

tion of the fracture line in addition to the arch bars. This is especially important in the symphyseal and the parasymphyseal areas and is essential if there are two or more fractures (see Fig. 1). It may also be necessary to support the upper arch bars through drill holes on each side of the pyriform fossa.

Condylar fractures in children may be unilateral or bilateral and are frequently of the green stick variety. In the absence of any occlusal disturbance, limitation to a soft diet is all that is required. If the teeth are out of occlusion, the application of arch bars with elastic intermaxillary fixation is promptly corrective and may be discontinued after 3 to 4 weeks. Follow-up x-ray studies after 10 to 18 months nearly always demonstrate complete condylar remodeling, even with moderately severe initial displacement.

In the absence of supervening infection of bone or soft tissue, ankylosis or growth disturbance is virtually never seen.

DENTAL INJURIES

Injuries to the teeth are common in children with or without fractures to the bony socket. Disruption of the neurovascular supply and to the periodontal ligament can cause discoloration, abscess, or loss of teeth. Even injuries of the primary teeth should receive attention, since their close juxtaposition to the permanent bud endangers the latter's development.

The viability of fractured or subluxated teeth can frequently be salvaged if properly and promptly treated. Delay of more than 30 to 90 minutes could seriously compromise the prognosis, and it is highly advisable to consult with a pediodontist in such cases.

GROWTH DISTURBANCE

The question of growth disturbance has been argued in the literature for many years and a clear concensus is still not apparent. In the study series reported here, 90 patients were followed through age 15 years or older. In only one patient, was a definite growth alteration evident (Fig. 5). In that instance, there was an extensive injury to the vomerine portion of the nasal septum at age 4. It appears that growth centers essential to midface development are most vulnerable prior to age 5. Two other patients who were referred late with severe developmental deformities of the mandible had developed severe ankylosis following extensive soft tissue infection or osteomyelitis.

SUGGESTED READING

Clark KC. Skull, facial bones and maxillae positioning in radiography. 9th ed. London: William Heinemann Medical Books, 1973.

McCoy FJ. Late results in facial fractures. In: Goldwyn RM, ed. Long term results in plastic and reconstructive surgery. Vol. II. Boston: Little, Brown, 1980:491.

McCoy FJ, Chandler RA, Crow ML. Facial fractures in children. Plast Reconstr Surg 1966; 37:209–215.

McCoy FJ, Stark RB. Plastic surgery of the head and neck. Vol 2. Edinburgh: Churchill Livingstone, 1987:1031.

McTigue DJ. Management of orofacial trauma in children. Pediatr Ann 1985; 14:125–129.

FACIAL PALSY

REANIMATION OF THE PARALYZED FACE BY CONTIGUOUS MUSCLE TRANSFERS

LEONARD R. RUBIN, M.D., F.A.C.S.

The previous day he was a captain of industry in excellent health. During the night, he awoke with severe pain in his ear that continued down his left cheek. In the bathroom, his mirror reflected a strange, distorted image. In horror, he saw his face pulled strongly to the left. His left eyelid refused to close over his irritated eyeball, and tears dropped down his cheek. He tried to smile, but his cheek and mouth refused to move up. Saliva drooled from his left lips and little vesicles were present in front of his left ear. His pain was intense. His face was paralyzed! He had suffered a herpes zoster viral attack to his left seventh and eighth facial nerves and exhibited the Ramsay Hunt syndrome.

The pretty 19-year-old girl showed a complete right facial paralysis. She had left for college in September and was now home for Christmas. During the past 3 months she had noticed an ever-increasing lag to her right face when she tried to smile. As she spoke, she drooled saliva and tears rolled down her cheek. Her right mouth would not elevate. The right nasolabial fold was obliterated. Subsequent computed tomography (CT) scans showed an acoustic nerve tumor, which was removed. The seventh facial nerve had been involved. Postoperatively, she was left with a total right-sided paresis.

Both of these persons desperately sought facial restoration to return to their normal status. Unfortunately, complete return to their previously complete facial activity is not possible by any currently available technique. However, near-normal function can be obtained.

WHAT CAN THE DOCTOR OFFER?

He could tell the patient to wait for spontaneous nerve restoration. The frequently seen Bell's palsy is caused by the herpes simplex virus. Near normal restoration of facial nerve function can be expected in most cases. Affected individuals should await return of function for at least 2 years, using high frequency galvanic stimulation twice a day to maintain muscle tone and limit degeneration.

When the Ramsay Hunt syndrome is present, however, total nerve degeneration can be anticipated, and restorative surgery should be considered after the acute symptoms subside.

The acoustic neuroma patient requires study of the operative report. If removal of the tumor was accomplished without cutting the seventh nerve, there is a possibility that new axons might regenerate to the paralyzed muscles. It takes at least 2 years for this to happen. During this time, high frequency galvanic stimulation to the facial muscles must be applied twice a day to limit muscle degeneration.

Patients awaiting return of nerve function must be told about the pathologic processes that occur during the period before restoration. When nerve impulses to the facial muscles are interrupted, the muscles begin to degenerate despite galvanic stimulation. If regenerating axons reach the affected muscles within a reasonable time (4 to 8 months), degeneration is limited and some regeneration can be expected. The problem is found in the scar barrier, interposed at the various levels and particularly at the myoneural junctions in the muscles. The remaining viable muscles may be inadequate to restore normal facial function.

If the facial nerve was injured or cut within the cranium, experience has taught us that spontaneous functional restoration does not occur. By the time regenerated axons reach the facial musculature, these muscles have degenerated beyond the degree necessary to give normal movements. The young lady, therefore, should have surgical intervention.

SURGICAL INTERVENTION

Pros and Cons of Various Techniques

1. Transfer of the twelfth nerve from the ipsilateral side to the seventh nerve stump.
   Advantages: gives some tone to the face when used within several months after paralysis.
   Disadvantages: (1) normal facial movements are impossible, (2) hemitongue paralysis is produced with some speech defects, (3) 25 percent of patients show severe hemitongue atrophy and 25 percent show limited hemitongue atrophy. (I have devised a surgical procedure to restore tongue function. This is based on neuralmuscular renervation using a Z-plasty.)

Conclusion: the twelfth-seventh crossover operation should rarely be used because of limited normal facial movements and hemitongue deformity.

2. Static sling to hike up the paralyzed side.
   Conclusion: It should never be used.
3. Cross-face nerve grafting which must be started soon after paralysis.
   Cross-face nerve grafting has failed to meet expectations. Only 20 percent of regenerated axons penetrate the scar barriers generated by the epineurium. The end result of a paucity of axons, and the degeneration of myoneural junctions and muscles by the time the axons get to their destination, is almost no function. Facial movements are very poor following this technique.
   Conclusion: The results are too poor to be considered.
4. Eleventh nerve crossover.
   The eleventh nerve crossover leaves a winged scapula. The face moves very poorly and only when the shoulder is moved. The tenth and eleventh nerve crossover give some improved tone.
   Conclusion: This procedure has not resulted in satisfactory improvement and should be condemned.
5. Ansa hypoglossal rami to corner of paralyzed mouth.
   Transposition of ansa hypoglossal rami to the corner of the paralyzed mouth gives some tone but does not contribute to facial smile efforts.
   Conclusion: The results do not give a normal facial movement.
6. Cross-face nerve grafting with microvascular muscle transfer to supply a new motor function.
   Cross-face nerve grafting (that accepts the 20 percent axon penetration) is performed. The distal end of the nerve graft is sutured to the motor nerve of the revascularized muscle transfer, such as the gracilis, serratus, pectoralis minor, or extensor hallucis brevis. This procedure brings any one of these muscles to the paralyzed side and sutures it into position to activate the face. Microsurgical methods are used to anastomose blood vessels.
   Conclusion: The pros and cons are discussed in the chapter *Microvascular Management of Facial Palsy.*
7. Transposition of contiguous muscles about the face (the temporalis, masseter, and frontalis).
   The transposition of contiguous muscles has been the most effective treatment for facial paralysis in more than 200 cases I have performed. The only drawback of this approach is the patient's need to concentrate actively on facial movements. Because the temporalis and masseter muscles are innervated by the fifth nerve, a retraining period is needed. However, with correct biofeedback, excellent facial symmetry can be obtained. Normal fifth nerve function to active temporalis and masseter muscles is a prerequisite. The function of a motor nerve is determined by having the patient clench his teeth while the physician palpates the temporalis muscles, above and anterior to the ears. With normal function, the examiner feels the muscles tighten and bulge to a slight degree.
   Advantages: (1) immediate reanimation of the face. There is an early postoperative massive edema that resolves in several months, (2) with constant biofeedback training, normal symmetrical facial movements can be obtained.
   Disadvantages: (1) constant retraining is needed to obtain symmetrical facial movements, (2) the movements are voluntary and the patient must overcome spontaneous overreaction on the normal side, (3) reconstruction, must be carefully tailored to the smile mechanism of the normal side when using the contiguous muscles, (4) eyelid closure is difficult to obtain and requires techniques unrelated to the muscles. These techniques are described later in this paper.

THE NORMAL SMILING MECHANISM

Before any muscle transposition takes place, the normal smile must be studied to obtain symmetrical movements. Muscle contractions about the mouth create the lip movement we call a smile. Figure 1 shows the relative contractile strength of the muscles responsible for variations in smiles. The most common type is the zygomatic major (69 percent). In this pattern, the corner of the mouth is pulled upward and backward toward the zygomatic arch. The canine smile accounts for about 29 percent of smiles. Its pattern results from dominant contractions of the levator labii superior muscles that pull the lip upward to reveal the canine tooth area. The third major smile type is one where all the muscles about the mouth contract and expose both upper and lower dentition (2 percent).

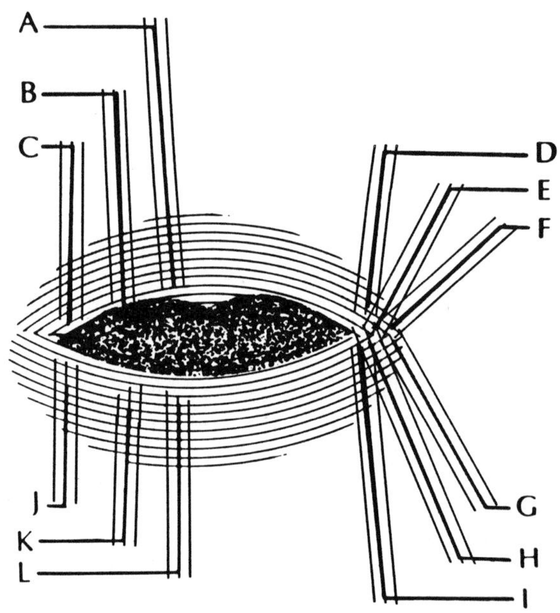

Figure 1 Shows the relationship of muscles about the mouth—the relative strength of different muscles determines the type of smile. A, B, and C are elevators of the upper lip—the levator labii superior is the prime mover. D, E, and F indicate the elevators of the angle of the mouth—the zygomatic major muscle is the strongest. G, H, and I show the depressors of the angle of the mouth and J, K, and L are the depressors of the lower lip.

Variations of the smile are created by the relative strength of the contracting muscles. The muscles are intimately connected with the superficial fascia of the face, commonly known as the superficial musculoaponeurotic system (SMAS). Fibrous filaments pass through the fascia, attached to the muscle on one end and to the overlying dermis on the other. This mechanism creates synchronized muscle movements that produce endless facial expressions.

At present, the temporalis-masseter-frontalis muscle transfer offers the most reliable method for animating a paralyzed face (Figs. 2 to 5). The temporalis muscle, transposed through the cheek, is used to activate the upper lip and the nasolabial fold. Because the muscle is not long enough to reach the desired position, the thick temporalis deep fascia is used as tendons. The anterior one-fourth of the masseter muscle is used to control the corner of the mouth and the lower lip, with fascia used as tendons. Both the temporalis and masseter muscles are innervated by the fifth cranial nerve. About 1 cm width of the frontalis muscle is transposed with temporalis tendons to give some minor activity to the medial end of the paralyzed eyebrow. Reanimation of the eyelids requires separate consideration. I used a strip of temporalis muscle, attached to strips of fascia, threaded through the margins of the upper and lower lids, and finally sutured to the medial canthus. Unfortunately, the procedure does not close the eyelids effectively, and unless the temporalis muscle is voluntarily contracted, the eyelids remain open. This is especially true at night. The solution (described below) is based on passive elevation of the lower eyelid by a fascial strip, and the use of a stainless steel wire spring to give tension and a closing force to the upper eyelid. The upper eyelid is elevated by the levator of the upper lid, which is innervated by the third cranial nerve. When the muscle relaxes (involuntarily), the spring gently closes the lids.

Treatment of the partial facial paralysis is complicated. I have described it in the January, 1986, issue of *Plastic and Reconstructive Surgery.* Through shortening or plicating of weakened muscles after electronic testing, the upper lip can be elevated to the normal level. A 4 cm strip of temporalis muscle can be brought down to aid lip elevation when added muscle power is required. Further lift can be obtained by excision of skin and subcutaneous tissue above and below a new nasolabial fold.

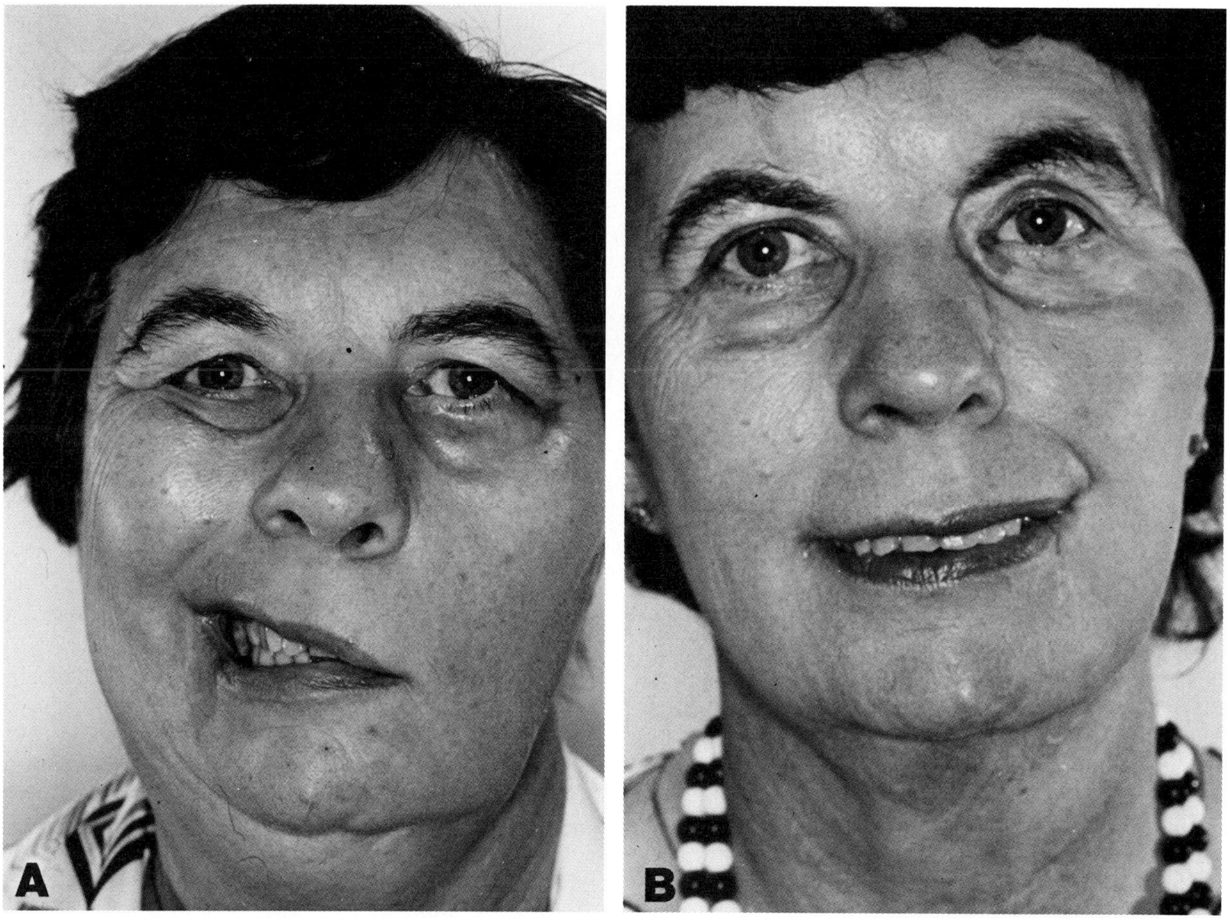

Figure 2 *A,* Preoperative and *B,* Postoperative views of a 46-year-old female patient who was left with a residual facial paralysis after an acoustic nerve tumor was removed. She had a left partial tarsorrhaphy to help close her eyes. Her normal smile was a zygomatic muscle type. The temporalis muscle was used to activate her eyelids and nasolabial fold. The lower lip was controlled by transferring one-third of the masseter muscle to the corner of the mouth and lower lip. Because her normal lower lip depressor was hyperactive, the depressor muscle on the normal side was excised through an incision of the mucosa.

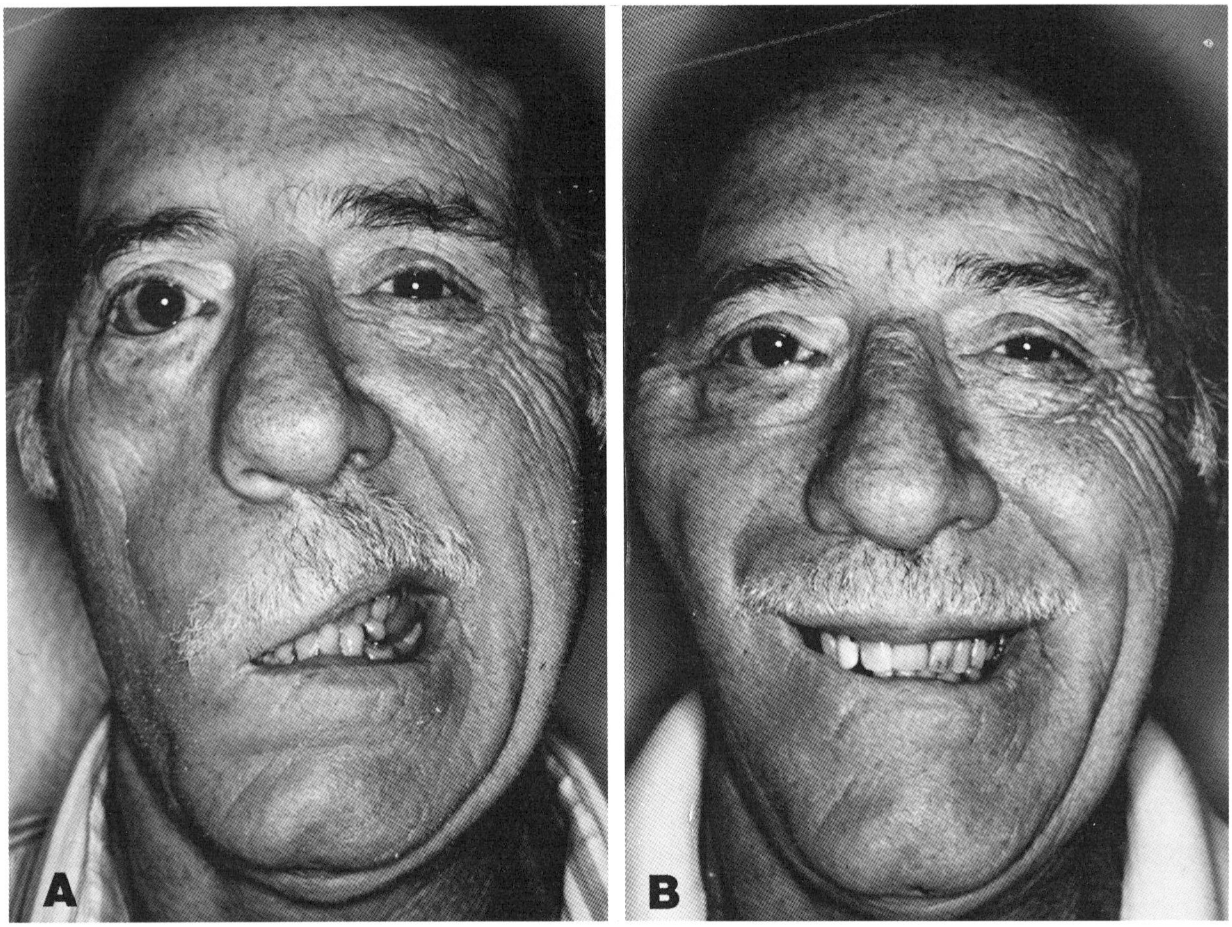

Figure 3 *A*, Preoperative view of a 56-year-old man who had an acoustic nerve tumor removed 25 years previously with residual left facial paralysis. Note how the patient has a marked ectropion from the muscular degeneration. *B*, The postoperative photo shows the therapeutic results of transferring the entire temporalis muscle to activate the upper lip and eyelids. The lower lip was controlled by partial masseter muscle transfer. The patient had a zygomatic major smile, with some canine smile characteristics, on the normal side. The ectropion was corrected by a through-and-through wedge resection performed at the time of the muscle transfer operation.

OPERATIVE TECHNIQUE

Incisions are predetermined as previously described. A subcutaneous tunnel is dissected through the cheek within the deep fascia from the lower border of the incision above the zygomatic arch to the nasolabial incision. The upper lip is dissected along its entire length down to the mucosa and mucocutaneous border. The width of the tunnel through the cheek encompasses the area from along the zygomatic arch to the length of the nasolabial fold. After the anterior half of the masseter muscles are exposed, the tunnel curves medially to expose the corner of the mouth. A separate incision is used to expose the medial border of the frontalis muscle. A tunnel is made through the incision of the paralyzed brow into the upper part of the frontalis muscle. An additional narrow tunnel is dissected along the margin of the lower eyelid laterally to the inner canthus.

The deep temporalis fascia is exposed medially and laterally by blunt dissection: medially, to the vertical extent of the outer canthus and, laterally, to the vertical extent of the midear. A superiorly-based flap of temporalis fascia is dissected off the underlying temporalis muscle almost as high as the superior temporalis line. The superior border is left attached to the temporalis muscle. A horizontal incision is made above the temporal line through pericranium down to bone.

Based inferiorly, a muscle flap of the same width as the fascia is created by vertical incisions and stripped off the bone. The stripping is carried inferiorly to the superior border of the zygomatic arch. The effective length of the muscle, draped over the arch, is elongated by the fascial flap, which acts as tendons. The fascial attachment to the temporalis muscle is reinforced with 4–0 white nylon horizontal mattress sutures.

The temporalis muscle is used exclusively to activate the cheeks, the new nasolabial fold, and the upper lip. White nylon suture (4–0) is used to insert the tendon fascia into the dermis of the dissected lip at the level of the mucocutaneous line and the midlip; the cheek is raised upwards, and the lip sutured under great tension. The upward and backward pull should be strong enough to ex-

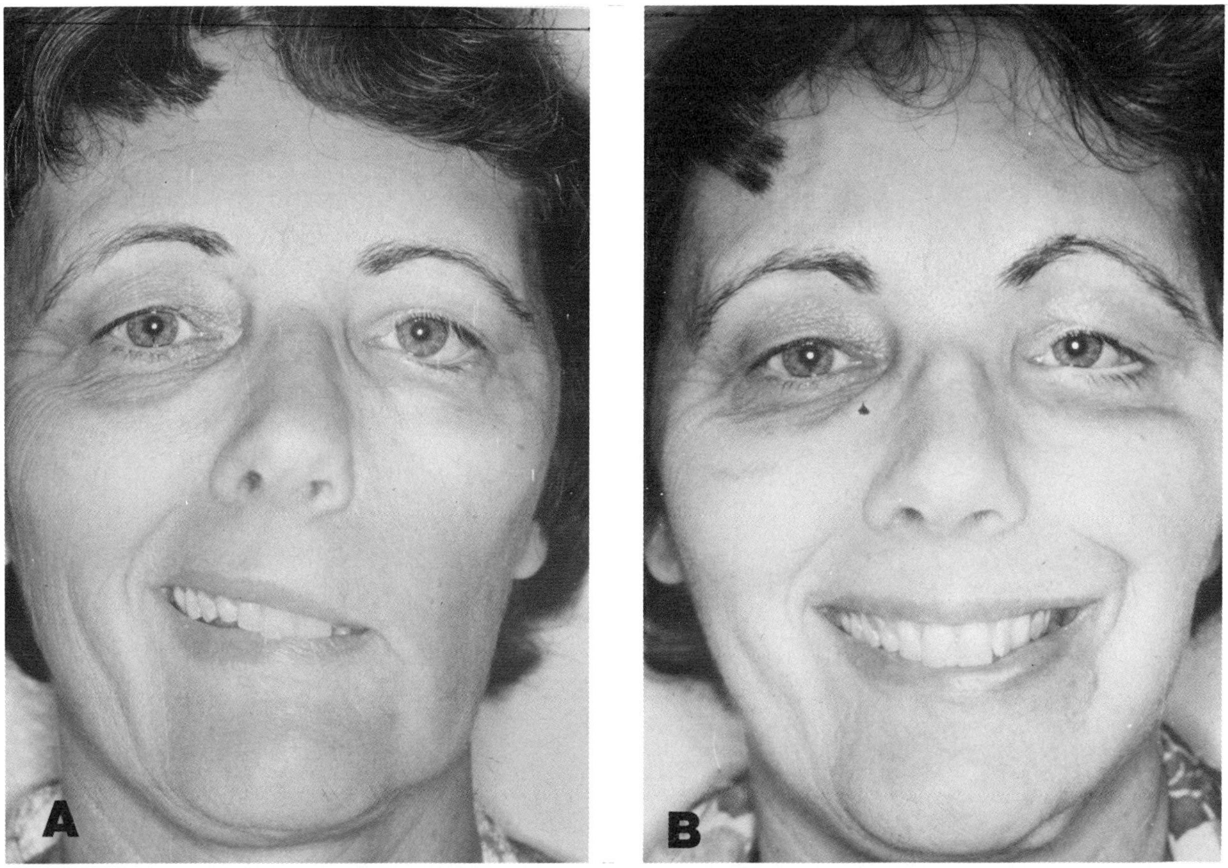

Figure 4 *A*, and *B*, Pre- and postoperative views of a 42-year-old white female who had suffered a complete left-sided facial paralysis after being ill with virus (Bell's palsy). The patient exhibited a zygomatic smile on the normal side. The corrective therapy was the transfer of: (a) the entire temporalis muscle to activate the upper lip, nasolabial fold, and the eyelids; (b) the anterior one-third of the masseter muscle to stabilize the lower lip and corner of the mouth; (c) 1 to 2 cm of the frontalis muscle to activate the medial eyebrow. The postoperative photo is 1 year after the surgery.

pose the teeth and gingiva. As the operation continues, the temporalis muscle stretches and may have to be hiked upward again before closing the wound. The tendon tensions are placed so as to create upper and backward pulls similar to the normal side. Many sutures are used to ensure a firm union. If the patient has a strong canine smile and requires a strong upward pull, a small pulley must be made at the corner of the nose lobule and the upper limits of the new nasolabial fold. This helps redirect the most medial portion of the tendon to simulate the nasal portion of the levator labii superior. At times, with a strong canine smile, this pulley might be used with a separate fascial strip to the temporalis muscle.

Attention is then turned to the lower lip control which is managed with the masseter muscle. The muscle is exposed through an inframandibular upper neck incision. A strip of muscle is tunneled to reach the incision in the lower lip, anterior to and below the corner of the mouth. Since the muscle is just short of reaching its destination, a strip of fascia is needed for attachment. This is brought out through the skin incision and is sutured under great tension to the dermis with 4–0 nylon mattress sutures. This pulls the angle of the mouth and lower lip backward and downward to match the normal opposite side. The nasolabial fold is maintained by suturing the dermis of the inferior side of the wound to the temporalis tendon with 4–0 white nylon.

For brow animation, a segment of frontalis muscle, about 2 cm wide, and of variable length is dissected from its medial edge. Because the frontal nerve enters the muscle laterally, one must be certain that the muscle pedicle is not dissected too high so as to avoid damage to the nerve. A fascia tendon is sutured to the muscle with 4–0 white nylon. This tendon is threaded through the forehead and sutured to the opposite brow with 4–0 polydioxanone (PDS) and 5–0 nylon pullout sutures.

The defect left in the temporal fossa by reflecting the temporalis muscle over the zygomatic arch is filled with a soft Silastic implant, customized at the table. Holes are made in the implant to allow fibrous tissue thin growth to hold the implant in position.

The skin incisions are sutured with 5–0 polydioxanone for subcutaneous tissue and 4–0 black silk subcuticular pullout sutures for the skin edges. A fine suction drain is placed deep in the cheek cavity and a pressure dressing applied.

In the event of bilateral facial paralysis, the procedure is performed on both sides during a single opera-

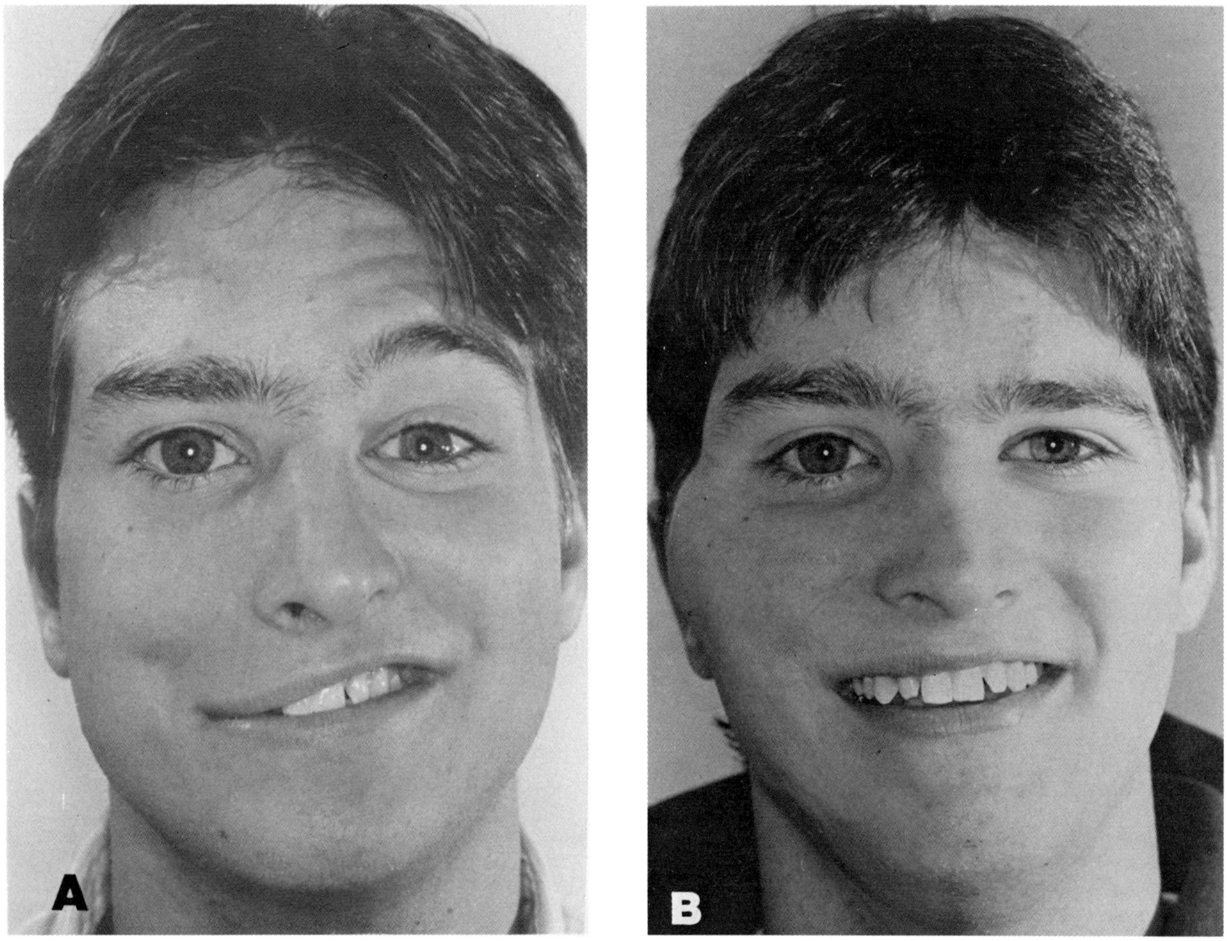

Figure 5 *A* and *B*, Views of a 16-year-old boy with congenital partial right-sided facial paralysis. Electrodiagnostic testing showed 50 percent function of the levator superior muscle and 10 percent function of the zygomatic major. The surgical procedure plicated the levator muscle and a 4 cm strip of temporalis muscle was brought down to substitute for the zygomatic major.

tion. The procedures are the same as for unilateral facial paralysis. However, new nasolabial folds must be made and the temporalis muscle and fascia are brought down at the same procedure. Great care must be exercised to make sure the upward pull is equal on both sides.

The operative treatment of partial facial paralysis requires management of the partially functioning muscles. The levator superior and the zygomatic major muscles are shortened by excisions of about 1 to 2 cm of the muscles, starting at the levels of the nasolabial fold and going superiorly. The exact amount of muscle excision (or plication) can be determined by elevation of the lip up to the desired amount. The cut ends of the muscle are sutured with 4–0 white nylon mattress sutures. At times, the new nasolabial fold requires strips of skin and subcutaneous tissue to be excised on both sides of the new fold. This helps elevation of the lip and takes the burden off weakened levator muscles.

Attention is now paid to the eyelids. A narrow tunnel is made in the lower lid, just below the eyelashes from the outer canthus to the inner canthus, and the inner canthus is exposed and tunneled. A 4 mm temporalis fascia strip is threaded from the outer canthus through the tunnel to the inner canthus and then passed under the latter to emerge about 4 mm above. The fascia is sutured with 4–0 white nylon to the periosteum of the inner orbital wall. In the lateral canthal area, the fascia is pulled tightly and elevates the lower lid as a sling. However, at this movement, the lateral end is relaxed. It will be pulled taut after the upper eyelid spring is placed in position. This spring is formed from stainless steel 0.010 or 0.012 wire. A horizontal incision is made through the skin and orbicularis muscle, 3 mm about the lashes, medially from the lateral canthal area to about 6 mm from the inner canthus. A tunnel is made from the lateral canthus to an incision through skin and orbicularis at the superior orbital rim, midway between the medial and lateral canthi, and a small pocket is developed under the superior orbital rim. The upper limb of the wire spring is inserted. It curves upwards and is sutured to the superior orbital rim periosteum with 4–0 white nylon. The loop of the spring is sutured to the lateral orbital wall periosteum with 4–0 white nylon also. The lower limb of the spring is carefully curved ready for suture to the soft tissue about the orbital cartilage after it has been enveloped with temporalis fascia. The fascia is used to prevent wire breakout through the thin lid skin.

The eyelid closure is tested by gently lifting the lid and allowing it to close. If it does not close readily, the spring tension can be increased by bending the wire at the loop.

The loose end of the lower lid fascial sling is tightened firmly, and the lid margin pulled up as far as it can go. The fascia that covers the wire loop is sutured to the lateral wall periosteum. Thus, the loop is secondarily covered with the lower lid fascia when sutured to the lateral wall. All wounds are closed with 5-0 Vicryl, 5-0 black silk subcuticular pullout suture and Steri-Strips.

POSTOPERATIVE COURSE

Antibiotics are used before, during, and for 2 weeks postsurgery. Drains and pressure dressings are removed in 48 hours. The exaggerated teeth-revealing smile starts to diminish within 24 hours, but may take a month or so to return to normal. The marked facial edema is partially controlled by 8 mg of Decadron given intravenously during surgery, 4 mg that night, and 4 mg the next morning. The edema may last several months. About 25 percent of cases require secondary muscle tightening if the temporalis or masseter relax too much. Hence the need for exaggerated tension at the initial operation.

The end results of the procedure can give a most satisfactory reanimation and enable the patient to smile. However, a long period of learning how to balance the smile is needed and there must be constant exercise and training to make the balanced smile a conditioned reflex. Almost all patients feel greatly pleased by the results.

SUGGESTED READING

Anderl H. Cross nerve transplantation in facial paralysis. In: Marchac D, Hueston JT, eds. Transaction of the Sixth International Congress for Plastic and Reconstructive Surgery, Paris, 1975. Paris: Masson, 1976:337.

Buncke H. Free muscle grafting with cross face nerve grafting for treatment of facial paralysis. Rubin LR, moderator. American Society of Plastic Surgery. Dallas: 1983.

Conley J. Management of facial nerve paresis in malignant tumors of the parotid gland. In: Rubin LR, ed. Reanimation of the paralyzed face. St. Louis: CV Mosby, 1977:224.

Fisch U. Cross-face grafting in facial paralysis. Arch Otolaryngol 1976; 102:453-457.

Rubin LR. Entire temporalis muscle transposition. In: Rubin LR, ed. Reanimation of the paralyzed face. St. Louis: CV Mosby, 1977:194.

Rubin LR. The anatomy of a smile—its importance in the treatment of facial paralysis. Plast Reconstr Surg 1974; 53:384-387.

Rubin LR. Langers lines and facial scars. Plast Reconstr Surg 1948; 3:147-155.

Rubin LR, et al. Reanimation of the long standing partial facial paralysis. Plast Reconstr Surg 1986; 77:41-49.

MICROVASCULAR MANAGEMENT OF FACIAL PALSY

RONALD M. ZUKER, M.D., F.R.C.S.(C), F.A.C.S.

Facial palsy has until recently taken an enormous toll in patient suffering. The effect of facial palsy on self-confidence, professional advancement, and normal social interaction has hindered the enjoyment and productivity of its victims' lives. The challenge of facial paralysis to the reconstructive surgeon has been met with some success. Corneal protection, static suspensions to achieve symmetry, and even a degree of voluntary movement can be achieved by local measures and transfers. However, the key feature of seventh nerve activity is emotional expression and it is here that modern microvascular techniques have made a contribution. The technical advances of microvascular surgery, whereby a muscle may be transplanted to a new site, revascularized, and reinnervated, have allowed a new approach to the facial paralysis problem. Greater muscle excursion can be achieved, more appropriate directional forces can be applied, and activation can be achieved by utilization of the seventh nerve, thus resulting in synchronous and spontaneous activity with emotional expression. In order to achieve this seventh nerve input, a stage-setting transfacial nerve graft may be necessary, as will be outlined herein.

INDICATIONS

The transplantation of a single skeletal muscle cannot be expected to replicate the fine coordinated intricate movements of the facial musculature. Our efforts in muscle transplantation for facial reanimation have been directed toward oral commissure and upper lip activation as we have not, thus far, been satisfied with the results for eyelid function. The lack of commissure and upper lip activation is the most obvious deformity in facial paralysis. It is this problem that muscle transplantation addresses most effectively.

There are three situations in which this occurs. First, there may be unilateral muscle absence due to trauma or surgical excision. In this situation the specific motor nerve supplying these missing muscles is available on the ipsilateral side. Muscle transplantation alone can be of assistance. Second, there may be unilateral absence of both nerve and muscle. This occurs in congenital facial palsy and in acquired paralyses, either through disease, as in Bell's palsy, or through surgery as may follow acoustic neuroma. In these latter situations, the proximal nerve is irreparably damaged and, because of prolonged lack of innervation, the facial musculature served by the damaged nerve loses its ability to recover function. Thus, not only facial musculature is needed, but also additional neural input. To achieve seventh nerve input, a transfacial nerve graft is carried out approximately 1 year prior to the actual muscle transplantation. The third situation, which is much less common, involves bilateral facial paralysis, either congenital, as in Moebius' syndrome, or acquired. In this situation, seventh nerve input is not available, and another motor nerve to power the transplant must be found. Where a normal hypoglossal nerve is available, it is preferable to innervate each muscle transplant via a single fascicle of this nerve. If the hypoglossal nerve is also involved and thus unavailable for use, then the motor nerve to masseter may be used to power each transplant. In these situations, however, synchronous and spontaneous activity can never be fully realized.

PATIENT ASSESSMENT

The severity of the paralysis, as well as the functional and social limitations imposed, must be assessed in each patient. The oral configuration is studied, and measurements are taken of midline deviation at rest and with activation of the normal side. In addition to the extent of excursion, the direction of commissure and upper lip movement is recorded since reconstructive efforts will be directed toward duplicating this on the affected side. The recipient vasculature is assessed by palpation or Doppler, with preference for muscle revascularization given to the facial vessels. If these are not available, then the superficial temporals may be used and, on rare occasions, vein grafting to vessels in the neck may be necessary. The selection of the motor nerve is critical. Ipsilateral, zygomatic, or buccal branches of the facial nerve are preferred, but, if unavailable, a transfacial nerve graft may be utilized. In bilateral facial nerve paralyses it is necessary to plan the use of other facial nerves, e.g., single fascicle hypoglossal or masseter. A thorough discussion of the complexity of the procedures, as well as the potential outcome, must be undertaken. A realistic appraisal of what is possible must coincide with the patient's expectations if success is to be achieved.

STAGE-SETTING TRANSFACIAL NERVE GRAFT

Through a preauricular incision, the facial nerve is identified as it issues forth from the parotid fascia. Muscle relaxants are avoided so that nerve stimulation can be carried out to identify specific responses. After a thorough mapping of the facial nerve, particular attention is directed toward the zygomatic and buccal branches. While sufficient nerve input is left to power the musculature on the normal side, three to five fascicles are selected for transection. The reversed sural nerve graft is tunnelled across the face with the aid of incisions in both nasal vestibules and in the preauricular area of the paralyzed side. Care is taken to place the nerve graft high on the paralyzed side over the body of the zygoma, as this will ease the dissection at the time of muscle transplantation. The fascicular nerve repair with 11–0 nylon sutures is then effected between the selected branches of the facial nerve on the normal side and the sural nerve graft. The nerve graft stump is positioned and anchored in the pretragal region. Regeneration is followed by the Tinel's sign and has generally reached the stump of the graft after 9 months to 1 year. At this time, muscle transplantation can be carried out using this transfacial nerve graft to innervate the muscle.

MUSCLE TRANSPLANTATION

This surgical procedure can be divided into three sections: preparation of the recipient site; elevation of the donor muscle; and muscle transplant with appropriate positioning, revascularization, and reinnervation.

Preparation of the recipient site is via a preauricular incision with a submandibular extension to the approximate midpoint of the mandibular body. A skin flap is elevated, thereby creating a subcutaneous pocket to the oral commissure, the residual musculature of the upper lip, and the inferior border of the zygomatic body and zygomatic arch. The motor nerve to be used is then appropriately identified. This may be the zygomatic or buccal branches of the ipsilateral facial nerve, the previously placed transfacial nerve graft, or—where no facial nerve is available bilaterally—either the single fascicle hypoglossal or motor nerve to masseter. If the hypoglossal nerve is to be used, it is identified in the neck, using the digastric muscle as a guide, then dissected into the tongue musculature itself. A single fascicle is identified, transected, and reflected back laterally. If the motor nerve to masseter is to be used, it is identified as it courses caudad beneath the midportion of the zygomatic arch prior to entering the deep surface of the masseter muscle itself. It is important to evaluate the fascicular pattern of the distal segment of the nerve to be used. Normal-appearing fasciculae must be utilized and, in the case of the transfacial nerve graft, this should be confirmed by quick section. The recipient vessels are then isolated and prepared. Generally, the facial vessels are dissected upward into the cheek, transected, and reflected posteriorly, where they will lie in excellent position to revascularize the transferred muscle.

The donor muscle may be isolated simultaneously by a second team. Although many muscles have been utilized, such as the latissimus dorsi, pectoralis minor, serratus anterior, and extensor digitorum brevis, we have found that a segmental section of the gracilis muscle is preferable. The gracilis has a neurovascular pedicle that is ideal for free tissue transfer. The problem of excess bulk can be avoided by using a small segment of the gracilis; there is no donor functional deficit, and the resultant donor scar in the medial thigh is acceptable. The muscle is easily identified in its superficial position just posterior to the adductor longus, whose tendon of origin is easily palpated with the hip abducted and externally rotated. The dominant pedicle is easily identified 8 to 12 cm from the origin, and consists of a central artery and paired venae comitantes. It can be traced to its origin from the profunda femoris and provides a vascular pedicle of 6 to 7 cm. The motor nerve of the gracilis—a branch of the obturator nerve—enters the muscle just proximal to the vascular pedicle at a 45 degree angle. It is easily traced proximally by retracting the adductor longus. After the neurovascular pedicle is isolated and the entire muscle freed, the fascicular pattern of the motor nerve is noted at the site of predicted nerve repair. The two to four fascicles present at this level are individually stimulated and the segmental contraction effects of the gracilis are noted. Approximately one-third of the width of the muscle is needed to produce the appropriate amount of movement and avoid excessive bulk. The anterior third of the muscle is generally selected, and the fascicle that stimulates this segment is identified. The muscle is then divided longitudinally along the plane of differential contraction, taking care not to separate from its vascular pedicle the muscle that is to be transferred. The length of muscle needed is estimated from the facial dissection. The distance from the commissure to the lower border of the zygoma, matching the direction of the normal side, is noted. Generally, this is about 7 cm on the lower border and 4 cm on the upper border. This segment of muscle is then marked on the gracilis in its stretched position (hip abducted, knee flexed), centered over the neurovascular pedicle. The segment of the gracilis is then removed, along with its vascular pedicle and motor nerve input. The remainder of the gracilis is usually left in situ. The muscle is then transferred to the face (Fig. 1) for final contouring and insertion.

The bulk of muscle at the commissure is reduced by removal of a wedge. The defect is then closed with mattress sutures, which help to anchor the muscle to the commissure and upper lip. The anchoring sutures at the commissure are placed on the deep surface of the residual orbicularis musculature. In this way, the potential for lip eversion upon activation of the muscle is reduced. Three sutures are usually necessary. The most inferior suture is placed at the lateral margin of the lower lip to create a commissural fold, while a second one is placed into the commissure itself. The most superior suture is placed in the upper lip to reproduce the nasolabial fold. The creation of a normal-appearing muscle insertion is a particularly important part of the procedure. With the muscle in its physiologically stretched position, the origin is then secured to the inferior margin of the zygomatic body, or the anterior portion of the zygomatic arch. The muscle position thus corresponds to the normal position of the zygomaticus major, with pains taken to replicate the activity of the normal side.

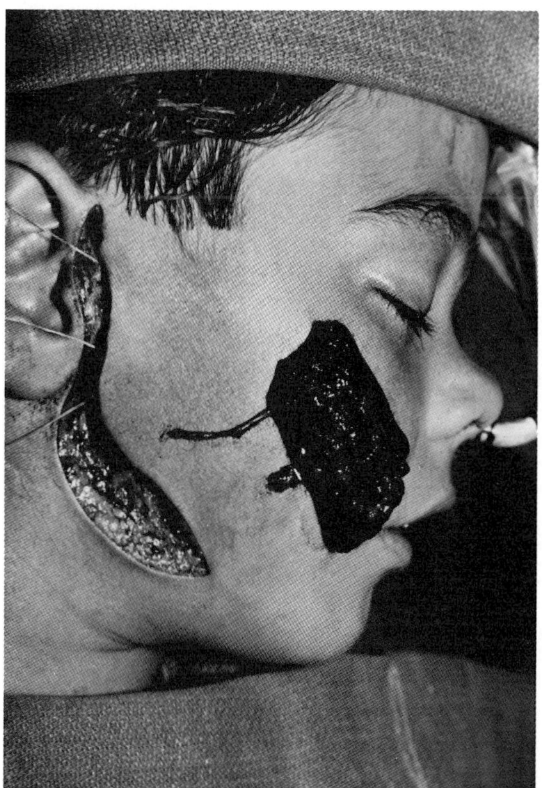

Figure 1 Segmental gracilis free tissue transfer isolated and positioned on face.

Once accurately positioned and secured to the periosteum of the zygoma, the vascular repairs can be carried out. If the facial vessels are used, excellent positioning can generally be achieved. End-to-end microvascular anastomoses of a single artery and single vein are carried out. Finally, the critical nerve repair is done under high magnification. The recipient nerve in the face is anastomosed in a fascicular pattern to the selected fascicles of the motor nerve from the segment of the gracilis being used.

Postoperatively, tension is relieved on both the origin and insertion of the muscle by a hook device that is placed in the commissure and anchored to the scalp. The commissure is thus elevated, and no pressure is placed directly on the muscle (Fig. 2). Although it may be removed for speaking and eating, it remains in place for 10 days.

The time interval between muscle transplantation and muscle reinnervation is generally 3 to 4 months when ipsilateral motor nerves are used. However, this may reach 6 to 9 months when a transfacial nerve graft is used to innervate the muscle. When reinnervation is established, an active exercise program with biofeedback techniques helps to improve strength, excursion, and symmetry of movement.

IMPROVING THE RESULTS

Several factors are important to achieve optimal results from this surgical procedure. The ideal patient is young with excellent potential for nerve regeneration and muscle reinnervation. Unilateral, congenital, facial palsy patients often have lack of commissure and upper lip elevation (Fig. 3A) as their main stigmata. Early surgical treatment by transfacial nerve grafting and muscle transplantation is important in psychosocial development and career guidance (Fig. 3B). Thus, if possible, reconstruction should begin at age 4 to 5 years, as soon as all structures are large enough to be dealt with effectively. Also, muscle transplantation and the rehabilitative stage will be completed by the time the child enters primary school. At the other end of the age scale, the potential for nerve regeneration and muscle reinnervation is reduced. Elderly patients tend not to do well, and are probably best treated by conventional suspension procedures and local muscle transfers.

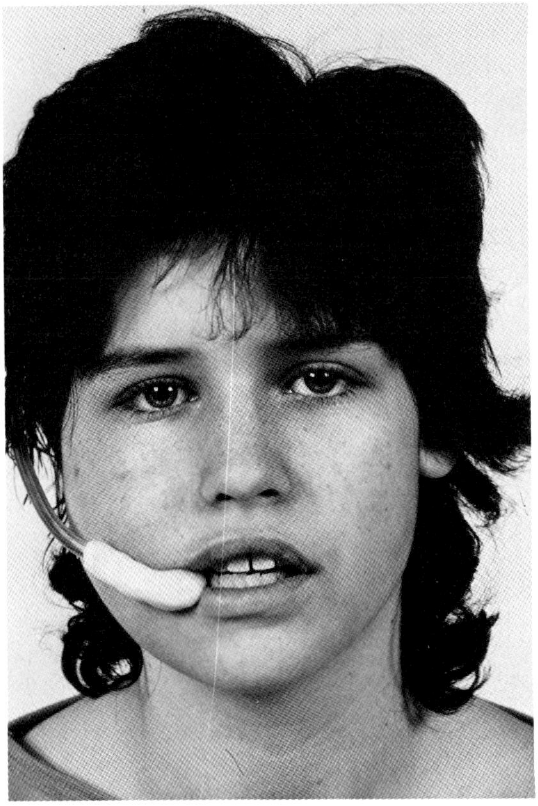

Figure 2 Post segmental gracilis transfer with hook in place to minimize tension at muscle insertion.

The details of these surgical procedures are important. Selection of the appropriate motor nerve for either direct nerve repair, or repair via a transfacial nerve graft, is critical to achievement of the desired spontaneous movement. Meticulous, and exceedingly accurate, neural and vascular repairs are necessary for success. However, in addition to this, great care must be taken in the muscle insertion, muscle origin, and alignment. The muscle origin must be securely anchored to fascia or, preferably, periosteal structures. The muscle insertion in the commissure and upper lip should be to the deep remnants of the orbicularis in order to avoid unsightly lip eversion. Care must be taken to effect a nasolabial crease symmetrical to the normal side. Muscle alignment must also be symmetrical and should simulate the movement of the zygomaticus major. Individual variations will necessitate specific preoperative planning for each patient.

RESULTS

The possibility of transplanting, revascularizing, and reinnervating skeletal muscle for facial paralysis has stimulated a great deal of interest. The procedure is effective and, with the recent refinements in motor nerve selection, muscle orientation, and positioning, it is the procedure of choice for the young and middle-aged patient with longstanding facial paralysis. The previous criticism of excess bulk has now largely been eliminated by use of smaller segments of muscle. After muscle transfer, symmetry at rest is restored as muscle imbalance is eliminated. Muscle

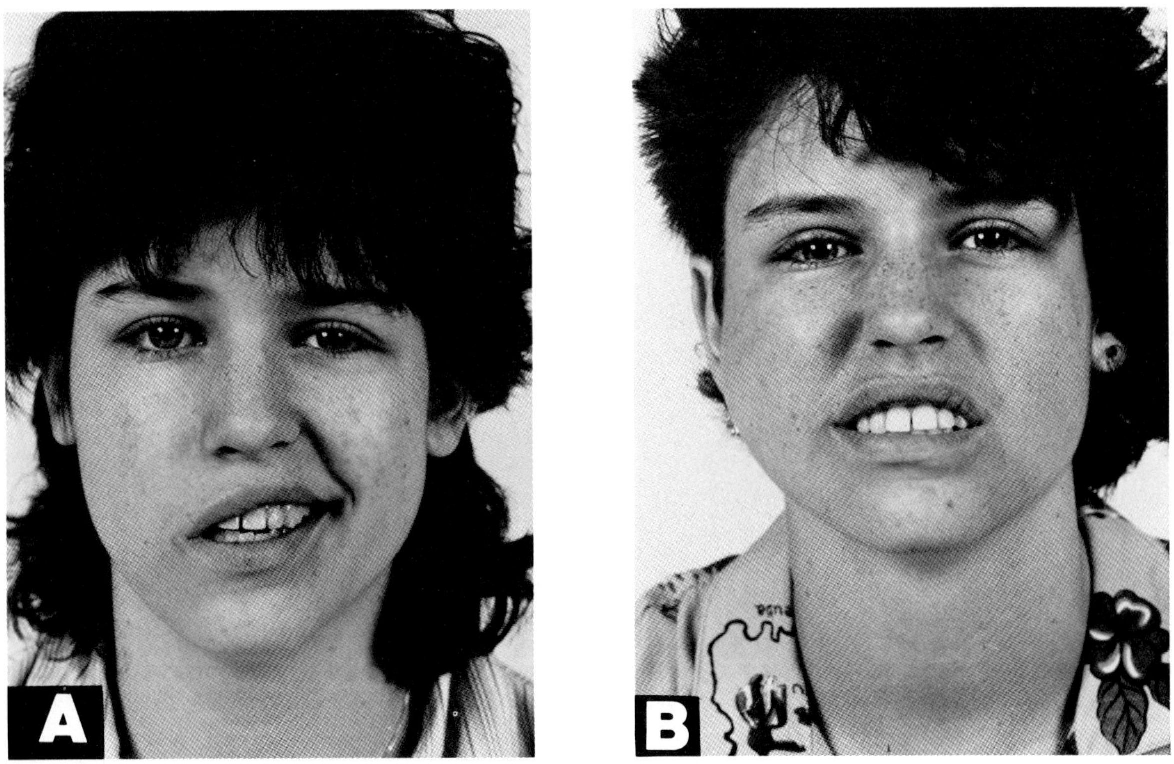

Figure 3 *A*, Congenital unilateral facial paralysis—preoperative view. *B*, Congenital unilateral facial paralysis—post transfacial nerve graft and segmental gracilis free tissue transfer.

excursion is generally just under 1 cm or 15 percent of the length of the utilized muscle. This degree of movement is quite adequate for the production of a symmetrical smile. With the use of the ipsilateral, or the contralateral, seventh nerve via a transfacial nerve graft, spontaneity of contraction with emotional expression has been particularly pleasing. This spontaneous activity is not noted when nerves other than the seventh must be utilized, as in the bilateral congenital seventh nerve paralysis of Moebius' syndrome (Fig. 4A). The expressionless faces of these individuals lead to major problems of interpersonal communication. The degree of facial movement afforded by muscle transplantation is of enormous benefit to these patients (Fig. 4B). If a single fascicle of the hypoglossal nerve is used bilaterally, normal tongue function can be preserved (Fig. 5).

The use of microvascular free muscle transplantation in the field of facial palsy has brought about a major advance in our management of these patients. Further progress will undoubtedly be made through research

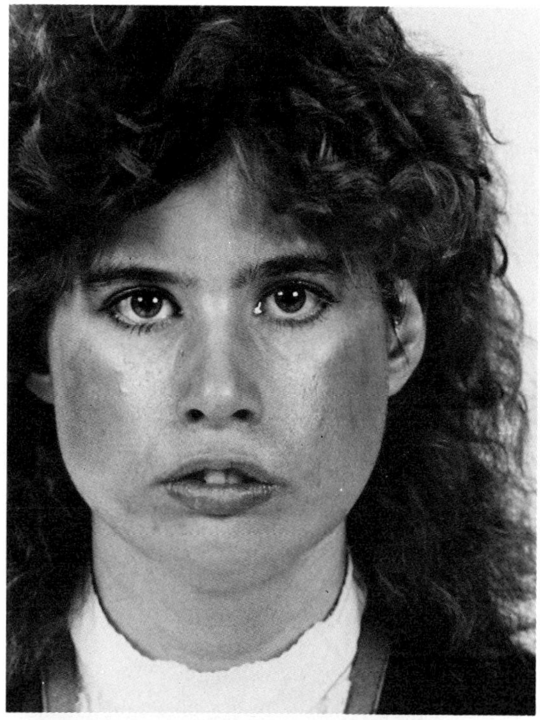

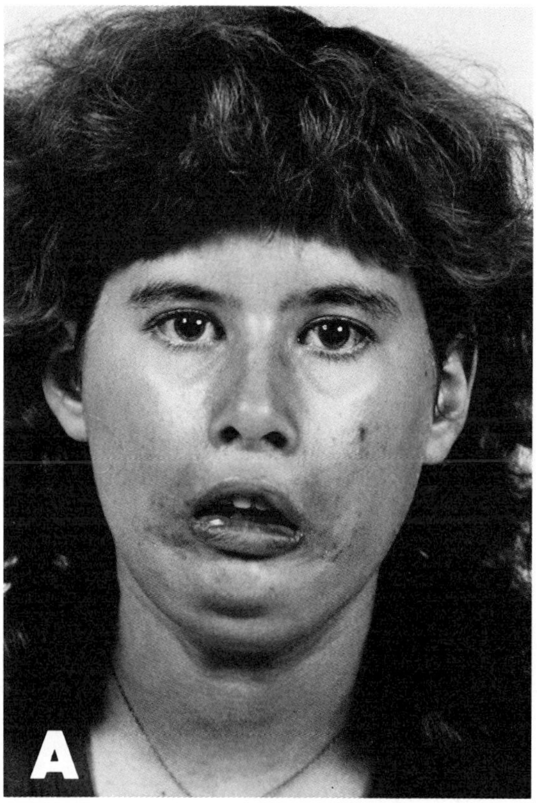

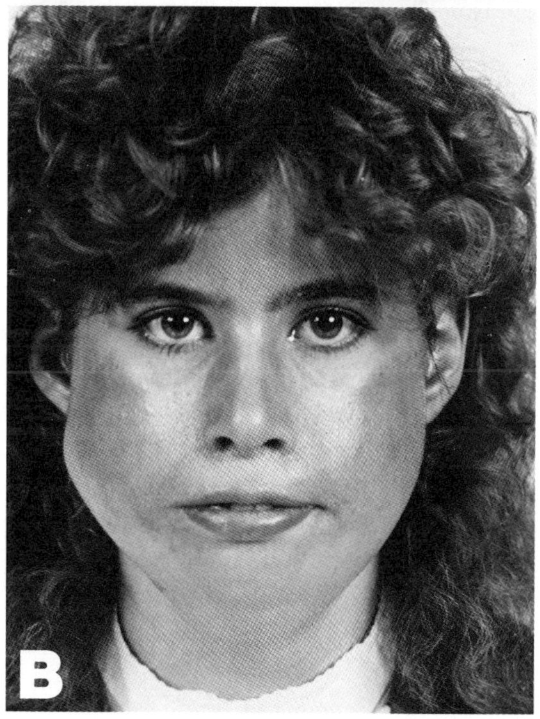

Figure 4 *A*, Bilateral facial paralysis of Moebius' syndrome—preoperative view. *B*, Moebius' syndrome, postoperative view, following bilateral segmental gracilis free tissue transfers: *above*, at rest; *below*, with activation via hypoglossal nerves.

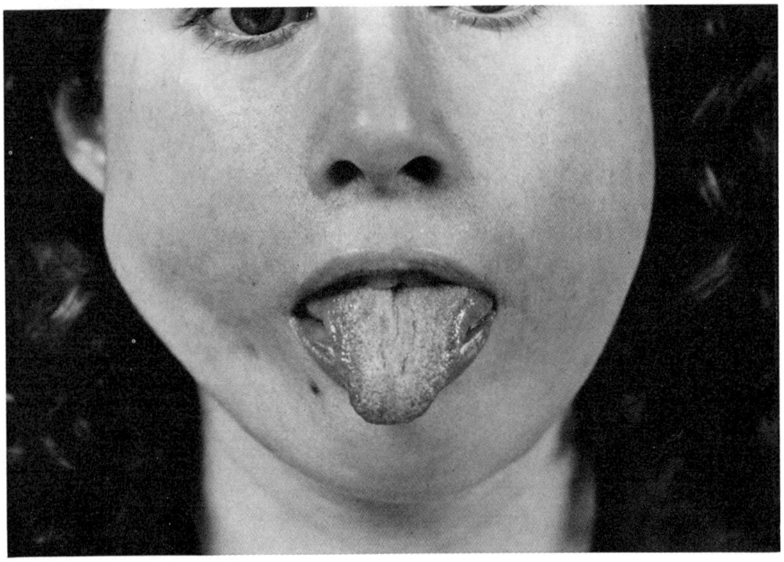

Figure 5 Normal tongue mobility following bilateral use of single fascicle of hypoglossal nerve.

efforts, particularly into eyelid control. We can now be more optimistic that in the future these unfortunate patients can be restored to near normality.

SUGGESTED READING

Harii K, Ohmori K, Torii S. Free gracilis muscle transplantation with microneurovascular anastomosis for the treatment of facial paralysis. Plast Reconstr Surg 1976; 57:133–135.

Manktelow RT. Microvascular reconstruction: anatomy, applications and surgical technique. Facial paralysis reconstruction. Heidelberg:Springer-Verlag, 1986:128.

Manktelow RT, Zuker RM. Muscle transplantation by fascicular territory. Plast Reconstr Surg 1984; 73:751–755.

O'Brien BM, Franklin JD, Morrison WA. Crossfacial nerve grafts and microneurovascular free transfer for long established facial palsy. Br J Plast Surg 1980; 33:202–215.

Tamai S, Komatsu S, Sakamoto H, et al. Free muscle transplants in dogs with microsurgical neurovascular anastomoses. Plast Reconstr Surg 1970; 46:219–222.

Tolhurst DE, Bos KE. Free vascularized muscle grafts in facial paralysis. Plast Reconstr Surg 1982; 69:760–769.

CLEFT LIP AND PALATE

TIMING OF CLEFT LIP REPAIR

R. CHRIS A. WEATHERLEY-WHITE, M.D.

During the past 25 years, a combination of evolving surgical techniques and improved anesthetic management has resulted in significantly higher standards of repair of the cleft lip deformity than previously. Millard's rotation advancement repair of the unilateral cleft and Manchester's simultaneous repair of the bilateral cleft have been significant in this regard. The advent of consistently safe, controlled, endotracheal anesthesia has afforded a degree of security to the surgeon, who can now perform an unhurried repair that was virtually impossible with older and cruder anesthetic methods. In spite of these significant advances, there remain two unresolved and, to some extent, controversial issues that relate to the management of cleft lip. These are the optimum timing of the cleft lip repair and postoperative care. The latter includes feeding techniques and immobilization of both the child and the repaired structures.

TIMING OF THE REPAIR

Currently, the preferred time for cleft lip repair is between 1 and 3 months of age. The most conclusive documentation of this trend is that of Lewin, who published the results of a questionnaire sent to all plastic surgeons in the United States and Canada. He reported that only a small minority repaired the lip in the first week of life, whereas over 90 percent of the respondents performed the surgical procedure between 2 weeks and 6 months of age. He summarized his results by saying that, "A widely acceptable time for the repair of the lip is between 6 and 12 weeks of age." Since this report, the major texts have recommended the delaying of a lip repair until at least 2 months of age. Musgrave urged that surgery not be attempted for at least 10 weeks. In drawing this conclusion, he made reference to his own study that reviewed the results of 500 consecutive cleft lip repairs undertaken over a 15-year period at the University of Pittsburgh. In this carefully documented work, he recommended delaying surgery until the child weighed at least 10 pounds, had a hemoglobin of 10 grams, and a white blood cell count of at least 10,000. He found the postoperative complication rate to be significantly higher when these guidelines were ignored. Both Skoog and Millard were similarly conservative.

All of the above authors quoted three main reasons for delaying surgery. First, anesthetic risks are supposedly lower than in the neonatal period. In addition, allowing some time to elapse between birth and surgery permits the diagnosis of associated anomalies that might increase the hazards of surgery if unrecognized. Second, it was surmised that the larger structures of an older infant would permit a better definitive repair and thus make less likely the chance of a later revision. Finally, it was felt that a period of living with the defect would promote more realistic expectations of the end result and lessen the justified feelings of dissatisfaction attendant upon a less than perfect surgical outcome.

Not all authors, however, adhere to this conservative philosophy. Stark recommended cleft lip repair "as soon as possible after the first day of life." He felt that the neonatal period was the safest from an anesthetic standpoint, and also pointed out that the lip structures grew less than 2 mm of vertical height in the first 3 months of life, thus questioning the concept that enlargement of the lip element permitted a more accurate reconstruction. An editorial by W.B. Cannon recommended surgery in the first 24 hours of life, noting that "with proper anesthesia and adequate supportive treatment, the operation offers no greater risk than one done several weeks later." Bromley reviewed a 15-year series of cleft lip repairs at the New York Hospital and found that there was no greater incidence of operative morbidity when surgery was performed in the first week of life than when it was deferred. Most recently, Desai has strongly advocated neonatal repair of the cleft lip.

Our own study, which involved 100 consecutive lip repairs performed between 1970 and 1978, confirmed both the safety of early repair and the quality of results derived. Half of these patients were operated on during the first 3 weeks of life and the other half later. Subgroups included 26 patients repaired in the first week of life and 17 at an age greater than 3 months. This latter group consisted principally of adopted children from the Far East. An overall complication rate of 16 percent was reported. Predictably, the majority of complications were anesthetic related. This morbidity was, however, unaffected by the age of surgery and occurred with approximately equal frequency whether the repair was undertaken in the first 3 weeks of life or later. Significantly, the subgroup operated upon in the first week of life sustained fewer complications (8 percent) than all other groups.

Long-term follow-up showed that the esthetic results of the procedure were unrelated to the age at which surgery was performed. The necessity for revision—a crude but effective determinant of the adequacy of the original surgery—depended not on the age of the patient at operation but on the type and severity of the cleft. Children born with complete unilateral clefts of the lip and palate were more likely to need revision than those with incomplete isolated cleft lips; and virtually all of the bilateral cleft lips required a subsequent revision. An overall revision rate of slightly less than 50 percent was recorded in this study. No meaningful conclusions could be drawn with respect to the psychological acceptance, or bonding, of the mothers involved, although it was our impression that there was greater satisfaction when repair was accomplished in the first week of life than after a protracted period of living at home with the unrepaired baby.

These objective studies have confirmed our observation that cleft lip repair can be undertaken with safety in the first weeks of life, and that the long-term esthetic result is not jeopardized by early surgical repair. It should be made clear, however, that the safety of an infant undergoing surgery depends far more upon the anesthetic and recovery room staff than on the surgeon! For this reason, unless the anesthesiologist and nursing staff are thoroughly adept at neonatal management, it is probably wiser to defer surgery until the baby is older and thus easier to manage during the postoperative period.

POSTOPERATIVE CARE

The surgically repaired cleft lip, like all other healing wounds, is relatively fragile in the early days after operation. All of the previously quoted authors recommend feeding techniques that are principally designed to avoid undue tension on the repaired structures until an adequate tensile strength has developed in the wound. Most authors utterly condemn the use of a bottle to feed the baby in the first few weeks following lip repair because the activity of sucking imposes undue strain upon the healing wound, and physical trauma inflicted by the hard plastic ring at the base of the nipple may damage the repair.

Two main methods of delivering milk or formula to the baby are widely recommended. One uses a cup and the other a syringe to which is attached a short piece of soft rubber or plastic tubing. In the cup feeding method, a small paper cup is used with part of its circumference pinched into a spout. The baby is held in an upright position to avoid aspiration and milk is poured from the cup into the side of the mouth, away from the cleft. The child will need to be "burped" quite frequently during the feeding as a great deal of air is ingested along with the milk. Most infants adapt to this procedure quite well and obtain, with some patience, adequate nourishment. Alternatively, a syringe with a short piece of soft tubing, often referred to as a "Breck Feeder," may be used. The tip of the tubing is inserted into the mouth and about a teaspoonful of milk deposited on the back of the tongue, at which point the natural swallowing reflex takes over. This method may be necessary for a few days when the infant is initially unwilling to feed from the cup, or it may be preferred by the mother until the child is permitted to return to the bottle. Nasogastric, or gavage, feeding is used only as a last resort, as it inhibits development of the normal sucking and swallowing mechanisms. Both the cup and syringe feeding, as described, are perfectly acceptable methods of ingestion of fluid following lip repair and minimize strain upon the repair structures. However, neither method will appeal to the growing number of mothers anxious to breastfeed.

In this regard, it is noteworthy that none of the authors previously cited mentions breastfeeding, the implication being that it is either extremely difficult to complete satisfactorily, or so obviously hazardous to the repair that it is not worth discussion. It is only in the less developed countries that breastfeeding is widely undertaken following cleft lip repair.

In the pediatric literature, the benefits of breastfeeding are widely accepted, with documentation of the numerous advantages to both mother and child when the mother breastfeeds for at least the first 2 to 4 months. These advantages—nutritional, immunologic, and psychological—are even more important in special situations such as prematurity and prolonged hospitalization. The psychological bond between mother and child that is developed through breastfeeding is widely accepted as a major determinant of the outcome of these higher risk patients.

Until recently, we followed the conventional practice previously described. Cup or syringe feeding was initiated in the hospital and the mother warned against the use of either the bottle or the breast at home. However, it was learned that several mothers had, in fact, breastfed their babies quite soon following surgery without any apparent harm. Accordingly, a study was initiated whereby all mothers of children with cleft lip were offered the option of breastfeeding their infants pre- and postoperatively.

Between 1983 and 1985, 72 infants were operated upon with this option offered. Twenty-two had already been weaned and were, in fact, on a bottle at the time of surgery. This left 50 whose mothers were anxious to attempt breastfeeding through surgery and postoperatively. Of these, 24 completed at least 8 weeks of breastfeeding. The other 26 mothers chose, with approval from the surgeon, to adopt an alternative method within this time period, either because the infants had a very weak suck due to associated cleft palate, or for reasons unrelated to the degree of success attained in breastfeeding, such as a return to work.

No immediate wound problems such as dehiscence occurred in those babies who breastfed from the day of surgery. Although long-term follow-up is not complete, there is no apparent difference in the appearance of the scar when compared with infants who were fed by means of a cup or syringe.

On the other hand, there appear to be significant nutritional benefits to breastfeeding. The weight gain at 1 month postoperative was an average of 28 percent over the operative weight, as opposed to 17 percent for those patients who were fed by cup or syringe. This superior weight gain was maintained through 3 months of age. Those children who breastfed from the day of surgery were discharged from the hospital in a significantly shorter time (median stay 2 days) than those fed by means of cup or syringe (median stay 3 days), with a corresponding reduction in hospital costs. This reduction in morbidity reflected the easier transition from intravenous fluid administration to oral intake when breastfed.

For these reasons, there is encouragement to continue to offer the option of breastfeeding to mothers of patients with cleft lip although it may take more time and patience than feeding with a device, and it may be difficult to the point of impossibility in those patients who have an associated cleft palate.

SUGGESTED READING

Bromley GS, Rothaus KO, Goulian D. Cleft lip: morbidity and mortality in early repair. Ann Plast Surg 1983; 10:214–217.

Cannon B. Current concepts; unilateral cleft lip. N Engl J Med 1967; 277:583–585.

Lewin ML. Management of cleft lip and palate in the United States and Canada. Plast Reconstr Surg 1964; 33:383–394.

Millard DR Jr. Cleft craft. Boston: Little, Brown, 1976:69.

Skoog T. Plastic surgery. Philadelphia: WB Saunders, 1974:97.

Stark RB. Cleft lip and palate. New York: Harper & Row, 1968:427.

Weatherley-White RCA, Kuehn DP, Mirrett P, et al. Early repair and breast feeding for infants with cleft lip. Plast Reconstr Surg 1987; 79:879–887.

Whilhelmsen HR, Musgrave RH. Complications of cleft lip surgery. Cleft Palate J 1966; 3:223–231.

UNILATERAL CLEFT LIP

PETER RANDALL, M.D.

Repair of the unilateral cleft lip continues to challenge and stimulate the plastic surgeon to do better. I use the Millard *rotation advancement* technique for those cases with less displacement of the Cupid's bow (i.e., less than 3 to 4 mm displacement) and the *triangular flap* for those with this amount or more.

OVERALL PLAN

Originally, the incisions were cut perpendicularly through the skin *and* the muscles so that the only part of the muscle that was reoriented was included within the triangular flap. Later, through the work of Fara, it was realized that the muscle fibers roughly parallel the edges of the clefts, so I widely undermined the skin and mucosa, both medially and laterally, cut across the muscle above, and brought the muscles at the alar and columellar bases down in two broad sheets to a horizontal position. The lateral muscle was placed between muscle and mucosa, and the medial muscle was brought more superficially between muscle and skin. Muscle was sutured to muscle. More recently, the studies of Latham have shown that many of the fibers of the orbicularus interdigitate in the midline and insert in the dermis just lateral to the philtrum columns. Duplication of this interdigitation has been tried by dividing each muscle into three slips (sometimes two or four), then interdigitating these slips and suturing them to the dermis. These muscles are quite thin. There are now patients who can whistle and pucker their lips, whereas formerly these patients could not do this symmetrically. There is better positioning of the alar base and a better philtrum ridge on the repaired side, with less "orbicularis bulge," although frequently more fullness is seen in the vermilion on the cleft side compared to the noncleft side. The nasal tip has been an enigma. Progress has gone from doing nothing through various external incisions, to advancing the medial crus and using a Z-plasty laterally, to current use of the McComb technique. The alar cartilage on the affected side is widely undermined without making additional incisions in the nasal vestibule. It is then repositioned in a slightly overcorrected manner and held with through-and-through stitches tied over small boluses of gauze, which are left in place for 7 to 10 days.

LIP ADHESION

Should the lip be very wide, or if there is a great deal of alveolar displacement laterally and anteriorly, a lip adhesion is done at about 3 to 4 months of age, along with closure of the soft palate. Then, 3 to 4 months later, after the lip has become soft, a definitive repair of the lip is carried out and the hard palate is closed using a vomer flap. In addition to being the most gentle and natural way of molding the underlying bone, the lip adhesion repositions the soft tissue—particularly the alar base—and converts a difficult, wide, complete cleft to a much easier, incomplete cleft.

OPERATIVE TECHNIQUE

Markings

The endotracheal tube is placed directly over the center of the lower lip. Midline points are picked at the skin vermilion border and, after straightening the nose, the midline is marked at the base of the columella and the nasal tip. The peak of the Cupid's bow is marked on the noncleft side, then on the cleft side, and the distance from each to the midline is checked. The white roll should still have good definition with the point only 2 to 3 mm lateral to the midline. (Residents in training frequently move these points too far from the midline.) The lateral skin vermilion point is chosen where the white roll has good definition and the vermilion fairly good thickness, although the vermilion is often slightly thin just there. Because this point is usually closer to the commissure on the cleft side than on the noncleft side, it is not selected by measuring commissure to Cupid's bow on the noncleft side and using this distance to mark the cleft side. This almost always puts the marking up into the cleft rather than further laterally (Fig. 1).

Next, the "red line" is marked medially and laterally at the junction of the whitish vermilion skin and the reddish vermilion mucosa. Then a line is drawn on the edge of the nostril laterally, down to the alar base. This helps position the alar base. Finally, the nose is again straightened and symmetrical dots are marked on either side of the columellar base. Measurements are taken from these dots on either side of the columella to the peak of the Cupid's bow on the cleft and noncleft sides. If the Cupid's bow on the cleft side has to be brought down as much as 3 to 4 mm or more, one should preferably use the triangular flap technique and proceed as follows.

A line is drawn from just lateral to the lateral columellar base dot to the peak of the Cupid's bow. A second line, about 3 to 5 mm long, is drawn at right angles from this point towards, but not beyond, the midline of the philtrum. The distance from the lateral columellar dot to the midpoint of the second line is measured and compared with the vertical height on the noncleft side. The difference is the amount that the medial side of the cleft needs to be lengthened by the triangular flap.

A dot is then placed near the alar base so that, when approximated to the medial incision near the columellar base dot, the nostril floor will have the same width as the noncleft side. If there is an appreciable amount of nostril rim flaring, this lateral dot should be placed a little down toward the free border of the lip, so that the lateral nostril base will be moved, not only inward to the nasal spine, but also into the nasal vestibule.

The distance from the columellar base to the peak of the Cupid's bow on the cleft side is now used to determine the distance from the alar base, laterally, to an arc 3 to 4 mm from the skin vermilion border. An isosceles triangle is sketched in, with one limb of the base at the skin vermilion border and one on the arc. The distance across this triangle, between the skin vermilion border and the midpoint of the opposite side, should equal the difference between the vertical height on the noncleft side and the distance from the columellar base on the cleft side to the center of the incision into the philtrum. The triangular flap can be enlarged or decreased in size as needed, but should not be wider than 4 mm.

The points are tattooed into the skin using methylene blue, and the lip is injected with lidocaine 1 percent and epinephrine 1:100,000, in tiny amounts well spread throughout the tissues. It takes 7 minutes for full effect of the epinephrine.

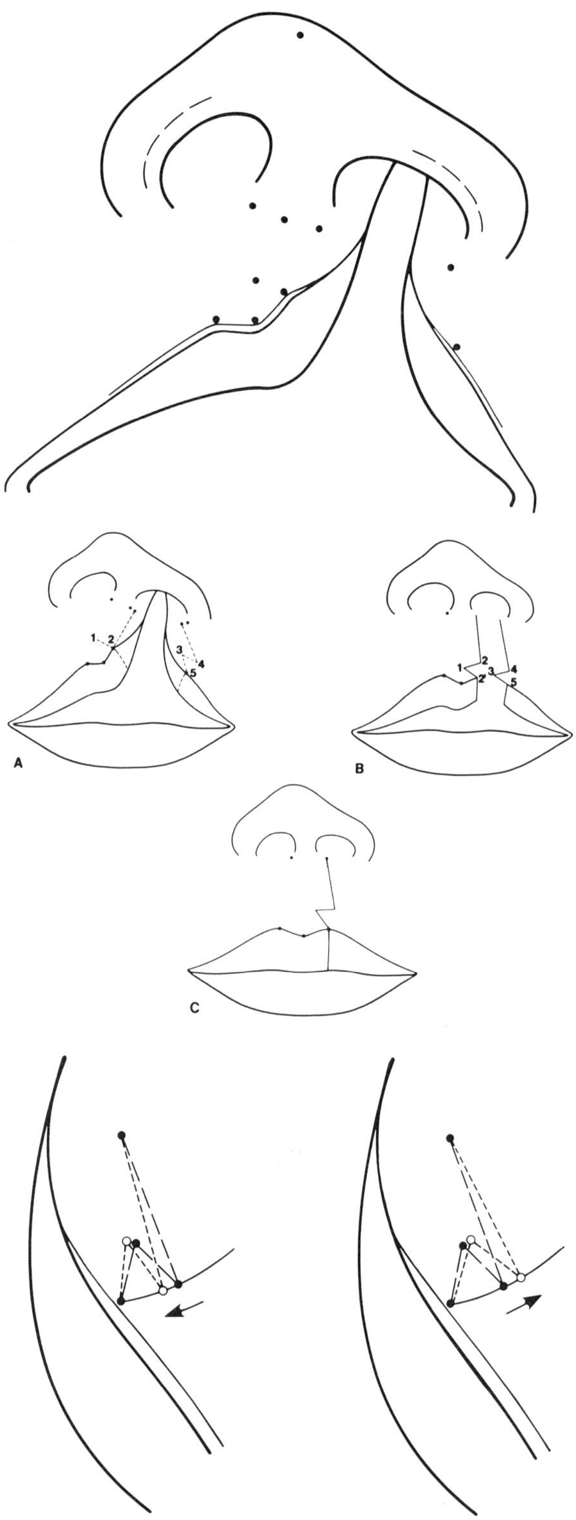

Figure 1 Key markings. The midline points are made first. The peaks of the Cupid's bow should not be too far apart or the lateral skin vermilion point too close to the cleft. The lines on the nostril margin help in selecting the point at the alar base. Point 4 can be moved closer or further away from point 5, depending on the desired width of the triangular flap. (From LaRossa D, Randall P. The unilateral cleft lip. In: Georgiade NG, Georgiade GS, Riefkohl R, Barwick WJ, eds. Essentials of plastic, maxillofacial and reconstructive surgery. Baltimore: Williams & Wilkins, 1987:242.)

Incisions

The skin incisions are carried through to the subcutaneous tissue, following which the vermilion incisions are made in the lip wrinkles. The mucosal edges are continued, roughly paralleling the skin incisions but omitting the triangular flap. The mucosal incision is extended laterally in the buccal sulcus for a shorter or longer distance depending on how much this tissue has to be moved. The incisions in the exposed vermilion are often a little wider apart than one would expect, as this tissue has a tendency to bend up toward the substance of the lip and will leave a whistling defect if too much vermilion is saved. Sponging with a moist sponge is preferred to suctioning, so as to reduce bleeding.

The epithelium on the lip margins is dissected off the underlying muscle. The skin is undermined on top of the muscle, then undermining is continued between muscle and mucosa, sparing the mucous glands. This dissection is taken laterally to the level of the superior part of the nasolabial fold and medially past the midline to the philtral ridge on the noncleft side.

Nasal undermining is now carried out between the skin and the alar cartilages laterally, and between the medial alar crura medially, using the incision at the base of the columella and at the alar base for access so that there are no additional incisions in the vestibule. The closure in the nostril floor is carried posteriorly beyond the alveolus, if possible, and a flap of skin at the alar base is inserted in the base of the medial crus to build up a columella "shoulder" and reconstruct a nostril sill. If the entire nasal tip is *not* undermined (as in the McComb technique), an incision is made just inside the nostril rim in the columella, and a parallel incision is made in the membranous septum so that the medial crus can be dissected completely free and advanced toward the tip for about 3 to 5 mm into a slightly overcorrected position. When this is done, a rectangular flap is taken from the lateral nostril floor to fill in behind this advanced medial crus. In incomplete clefts, these incisions are carried across the nostril floor as two parallel incisions, and a bipedicle flap is used to advance the medial crus superiorly, to move the floor of the nostril into the base of the columella, and to move the alar base toward the nasal spine. To correct the malposition of the lateral alar crus, the dome must be moved cephalad so that the superior margin of the lateral alar cartilage overlaps the inferior margin of the upper lateral cartilage. In addition, a Z-plasty may be needed laterally in the region of the pyriform recess to relieve tightness in this region. With a minimal nasal deformity, the nasal cartilages are not touched at all. During dissection of the flaps from the nostril floor laterally, a good pedicle of fibrous tissue is developed and left attached to the alar base. This flap is sutured to the nasal spine (preferably with 5–0 Vicryl*) to hold the alar base in a corrected position.

* Polyglactin 910, Ethicon, Inc., Somerville, NJ

Muscle

The lateral orbicularis oris muscle is cut across superiorly at the alar base until its fibers can be brought down to the horizontal position. It is then divided into three slips, two long ones superiorly and centrally, and a short one inferiorly. The medial orbicularis muscle is freed from the columellar base and divided similarly. A mucosal flap is developed in the mucosa of the lateral lip element, based laterally. The lateral lip is undermined and dissected off the maxilla only as far as is necessary for easy closure. This lateral flap of mucosa can be divided so that part is used to close the alveolar cleft if it is wide, and part used to reconstruct the gingival buccal sulcus—or all of it can be used in this latter position. If the alveolar cleft is narrow, it can either be left for later closure and bone grafting, or, if the edges are touching, it can be closed with adjacent gingival flaps. Eventually, all alveolar clefts should be closed with gingival mucosa, and most will need bone grafting.

If the labial frenum is tight, it is either cut across and the lateral mucosal flap brought over to the noncleft side, or a Z-plasty can be carried out on the frenum and the mucosal flap taken just to the edge of the "Z". The mucosa is then closed, using 5–0 chromic or 4–0 chromic catgut, to about halfway to the free border of the lip. The nostril floor is closed in the same way and the alar base flap sutured to the nasal spine.

Muscular Interdigitation

The superior lateral muscle flap is also sutured to the nasal spine, using 5–0 Vicryl. The superior medial muscle flap is then sutured to dermis 2 to 3 mm inferior to the alar base, in a position to bring the alar base into a satisfactory orientation (Fig. 2).

The central lateral muscle flap is brought to dermis either just lateral to the philtrum, if it reaches this area easily, or, if it is tight, it is brought to the dermis in the central portion of the philtrum about one-third to one-half of the way between the columella and the lip. The central medial muscle flap is sutured to the dermis laterally in the lip about half to two-thirds of the way from the alar base of the vermilion. The sutures may produce dimples in the skin, but these do not persist.

The inferior two muscle flaps are sutured one on top of the other directly under the skin vermilion border, so as to give additional fullness at this point. This overlap is loose in order not to tighten the free border of the lip. The muscle closure should do a good job of approximating the skin incisions. The mucosa is closed to the free border of the lip. A small V–Y advancement, or a folding of the medial mucosal incision, can be done to produce a small midline tubercle in the vermilion. Occasionally, an ellipse of mucosa needs to be excised laterally if the vermilion is redundant at this point, and a muscle stitch must sometimes be placed lateral to the alar base to replace the attachment of the zygomaticus muscles (Fig. 3).

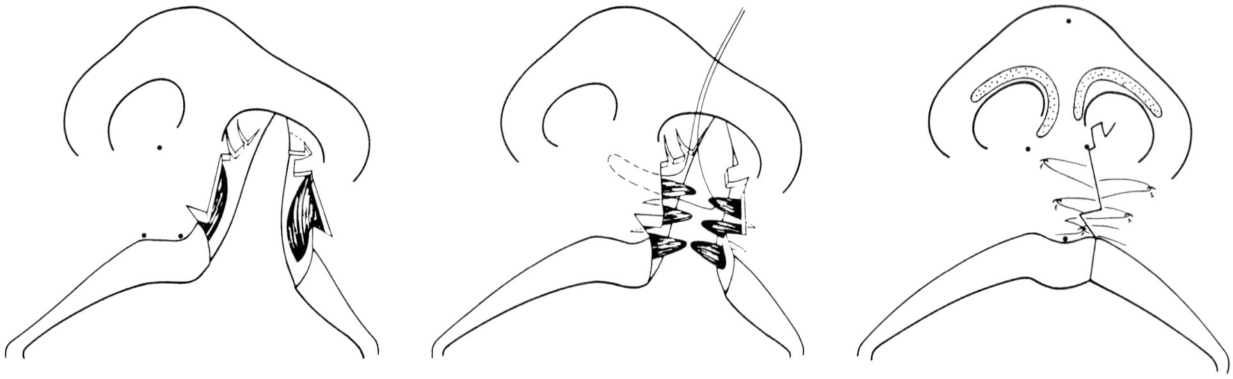

Figure 2 Reorientation, division and interdigitation of orbicularis oris fibers. The top lateral slip is sutured to the nasal spine. The bottom two are sutured to each other, overlapped loosely. The others are sutured to the dermis. (From LaRossa D, Randall P. The unilateral cleft lip. In: Georgiade NG, Georgiade GS, Riefkohl R, Barwick WJ, eds. Essentials of plastic, maxillofacial and reconstructive surgery. Baltimore: Williams & Wilkins, 1987:243.)

Skin Closure

A single, subcutaneous suture of 5–0 chromic catgut is usually needed at the skin vermilion border and another at the base of the columella. The skin is then approximated with interrupted 6–0 nylon or Prolene sutures at the key points. Often a continuous suture is used in the long vertical skin incision to achieve good closure and edge approximation. Magnification is helpful during this part of the operation, and the sutures are tied just tight enough to achieve approximation.

Through-and-through sutures of 4–0 chromic catgut are then placed in the nose, with the medial crus held upward toward the nasal tip in a slightly overcorrected position. Another suture is placed to reproduce the overlap of the superior edge of the lateral crus over the inferior edge of the upper lateral cartilage. Several more are placed laterally in the nasal groove to obliterate the dead space from the undermining. These sutures are tied over small pieces of umbilical tape and are left in for 7 to 10 days (Fig. 4).

Postoperatively

The suture line is covered with a bandaid, which is changed in 2 hours, then every 6 hours for 24 hours. A

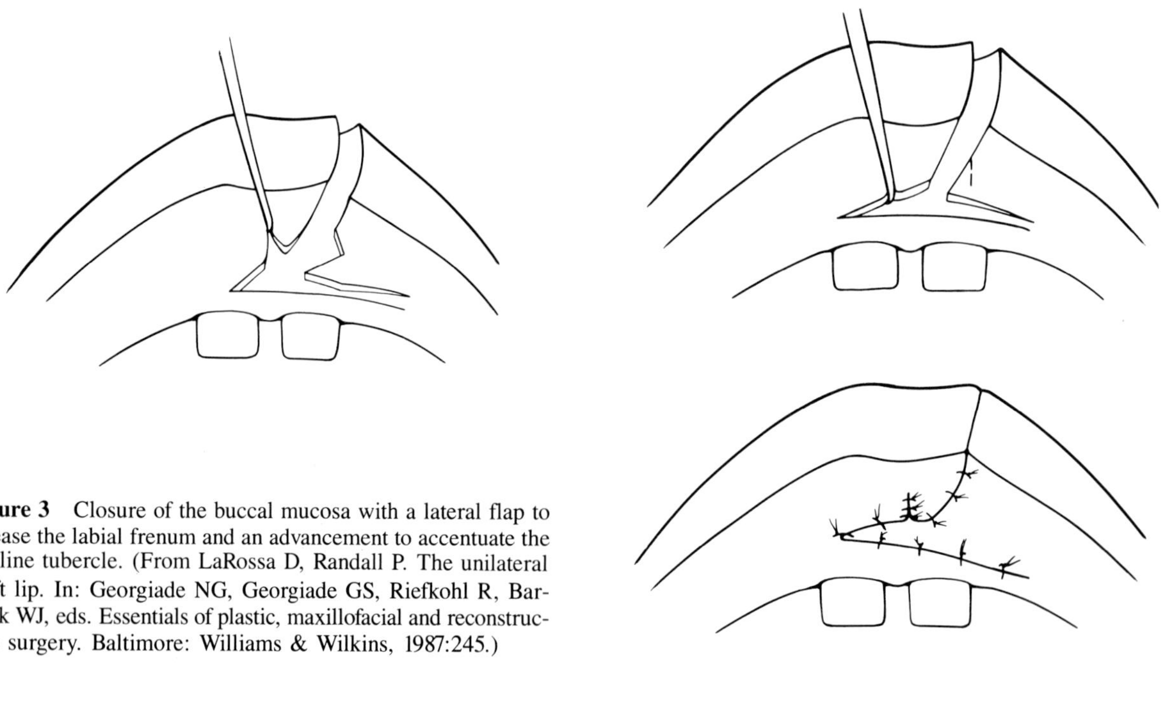

Figure 3 Closure of the buccal mucosa with a lateral flap to release the labial frenum and an advancement to accentuate the midline tubercle. (From LaRossa D, Randall P. The unilateral cleft lip. In: Georgiade NG, Georgiade GS, Riefkohl R, Barwick WJ, eds. Essentials of plastic, maxillofacial and reconstructive surgery. Baltimore: Williams & Wilkins, 1987:245.)

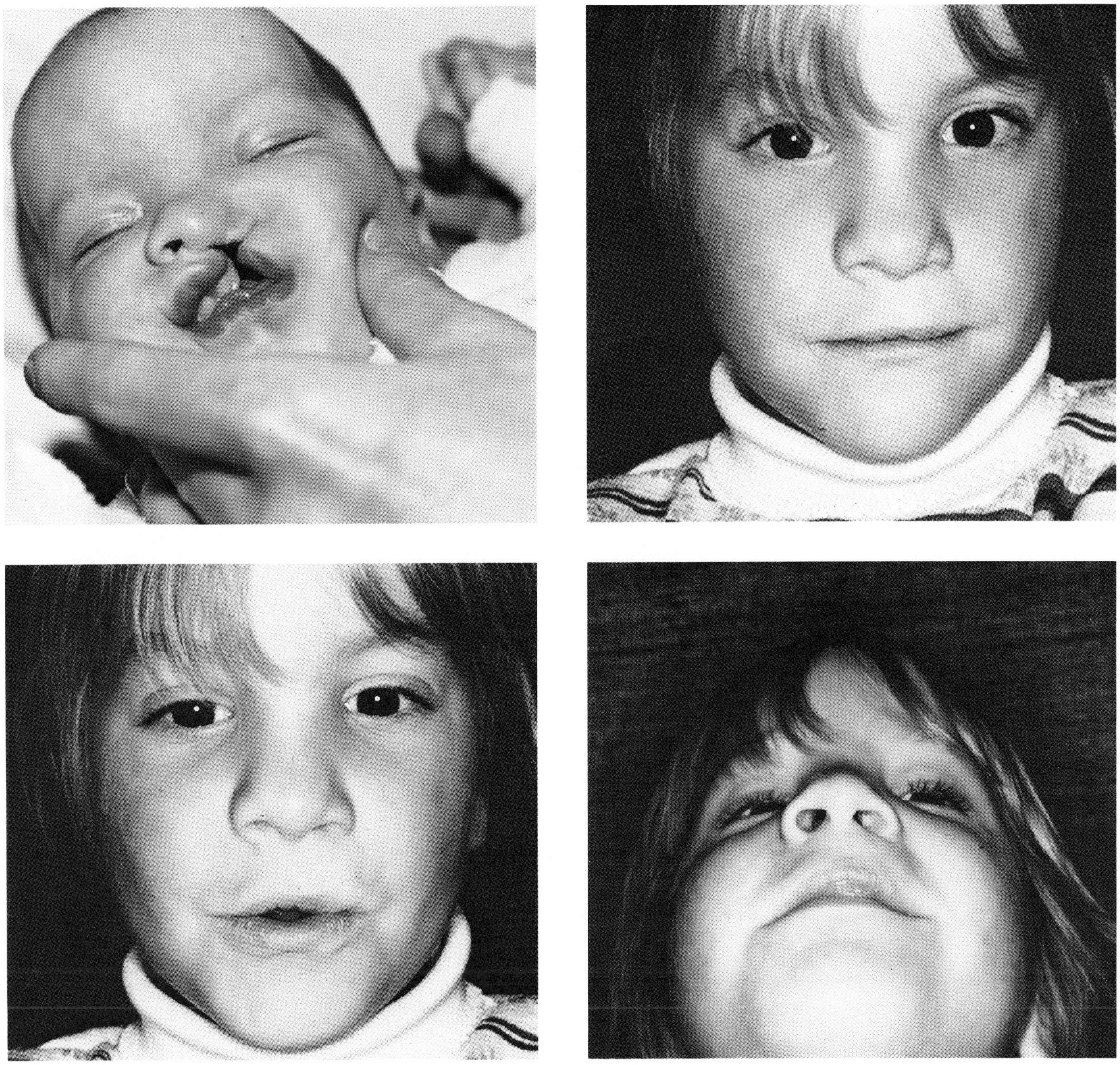

Figure 4 If the edges of the cleft can be approximated with ease (as seen here) a lip adhesion is not used. Postoperatively, there has been fairly good nasal contour, less orbicularis bulge and better symmetrical puckering on whistling.

Logan's bow is not used. At each changing, the old bandaid is removed from the lateral ends toward the center so as not to pull on the suture line, the lip is cleaned with plain soap and water on a piece of sterile gauze, the area is rinsed and dried, and a new bandaid is applied after first removing the paper backing (again to avoid tension). Topical antibiotic ointment is used if desired. Hydrogen peroxide is used only if there are crusts that cannot be removed with soap and water. Systemic antibiotics have been associated with a slight shortening of hospital stay and a reduction of postoperative fever, and are usually used for 3 or 4 days. A full liquid diet or breast feeding is resumed as soon as the patient has recovered from the anesthesia. After the bandaids are discontinued (24 hours), the cleaning routine is continued for a period of about 2 weeks. Sutures are removed in 4 to 6 days with the use of magnification, but not under general anesthesia, after the patient has been given a full feeding. Gentle massage with cocoa butter or cold cream is started in 2 weeks and maintained two or three times a day for 2 to 3 months. Arm restraints are maintained for 2 weeks, and care is taken that the child's lip is not bumped.

The results of the triangular flap repair—used in conjunction with the rotation advancement technique—have so far stood the test of time. The McComb approach to the nasal tip is new to me but seems to be producing good results and avoids incisions in the skin of the vestibule. Reorientation of the orbicularus muscle seems worthwhile, but whether this crude attempt to achieve interdigitation of the muscle will prove to be of value has yet to be determined.

SUGGESTED READING

Fara M. Anatomy and arteriography of cleft lips in stillborn children. Plast Reconstr Surg 1968; 42:29–36.
LaRossa D, Randall P. The unilateral cleft lip. In: Georgiade NG, Georgiade GS, Riefkohl R, Barwick WJ, eds. Essentials of plastic, maxillofacial and reconstructive surgery. Baltimore: Williams & Wilkins, 1987:241.
Latham RA, Deaton TG. The structural basis of the philtrum and the contour of the vermilion border: a study of the musculature of the upper lip. J Anat 1976; 121:151–160.
McComb H. Primary correction of unilateral cleft lip nasal deformity: a 10 year review. Plast Reconstr Surg 1985; 75:791–797.
Noordhoff MS. Reconstruction of vermilion in unilateral and bilateral clefts. Plast Reconstr Surg 1984; 73:52–60.
Randall P. A triangular flap operation for the primary repair of unilateral clefts of the lip. Plast Reconstr Surg 1959; 23:331–347.
Randall P, Whitaker LA, LaRossa D. The importance of muscle reconstruction in primary and secondary cleft lip repair. Plast Reconstr Surg 1974; 54:316–323.
Randall P. A lip adhesion operation in cleft lip surgery. Plast Reconstr Surg 1965; 35:371–376.

BILATERAL COMPLETE CLEFT LIP

JOHN B. MULLIKEN, M.D.

The newborn infant with a bilateral complete cleft lip is a summons to surgical imagination and skill. The surgeon who accepts responsibility for the care of this child must understand the challenge of both the third and fourth dimensions. The operative goal is a normal three-dimensional configuration of the lip and nose, but there is also a temporal dimension. How will the postoperative result be affected by the rapid alterations of the lip and nose that occur with facial animation? The fourth dimension is also expressed by changes in the facial skeletal and soft tissues that take place with growth.

The surgeon who cares for an infant with a bilateral cleft lip cannot wait for the fourth dimension to be revealed. Nor can a child be allowed to grow to adolescence before the surgeon learns from his technical misadventures. One must continually analyze one's own cases, as well as those of predecessors and colleagues, and then inductively determine what operative principles to follow.

The stigmatic look of a repaired bilateral cleft lip is painfully obvious, even at a distance. The nose is flat; the alar bases are widely spaced and malpositioned superiorly. The nasal tip is broad, with splayed and inferiorly-displaced alar genua. The external nares have an abnormal transverse axis. In profile, the columella is short and the nose is snubbed. The prolabial scars are often asymmetrical, bowed, or zigzagged. The prolabium is flat, undimpled, and missing a central cutaneous-vermilion ridge. The distance between the Cupid's bow peaks is usually greater than 15 mm. Bulging of the unconnected orbicularis oris in the lateral lip elements is accentuated by animation. The median tubercle is hypoplastic, and the free margin of the lateral lip elements tends to sag—the so-called "whistling lip" deformity. The central vermilion is thin, with exposed mucosa that is dry and chapped. In profile, the lip is often tight and lacks a pout. There is usually a secondary protuberance of the lower lip; the "cleft lip lower lip deformity."

OPERATIVE PRINCIPLES

Operative *techniques* change constantly and are variably useful in a particular case. Operative *principles*, rather than techniques, are constant guides to the surgeon's craft. Analysis of the residual soft tissue deformities, seen with current methods of bilateral cleft lip repair, suggests that operative principles should be as follows: (1) maintain symmetry, (2) secure primary muscle union, (3) select proper prolabial size and configuration, (4) form the median tubercle and cutaneous-vermilion ridge from the lateral lip elements, and (5) construct the nasal tip and columella by anatomic placement of the alar cartilages.

These operative concepts for bilateral complete cleft lip are still evolving and may need further refinement.

Symmetry

Formation and maintenance of symmetry are the cardinal principles of bilateral lip repair. Symmetry may be the only advantage that a bilateral lip cleft has over its unilateral counterpart. Staged procedures (one side and then the other) portend asymmetry. Even the smallest dissimilarities in the two sides of the lip or nose must be adjusted during the initial repair. Any differences become more obvious with time.

Primary Muscle Continuity

Continuity of the orbicularis oris must be achieved throughout the vertical extent of the lip. Once the lateral lip musculature is fully united, there should be no tension on the prolabial suture lines. Complete repair of the orbicularis oris allows normal muscular forces to act on the underlying premaxilla, maxillae, and nasal cartilages. In addition, a complete dissection of the orbicularis oris bundles rectifies the bulging and festooning of the lateral lip elements.

Proper Prolabial Size and Shape

Many previously described repairs for bilateral cleft lip were conceived on the false notion that the diminutive prolabium has a deficient potential for vertical growth. To compensate for this, various techniques for transposing rectangular and triangular flaps beneath the prolabium were introduced. When observed over time, these patterned repairs usually manifest a long-lip deformity and, often, side-to-side lip tightness. In addition, these techniques result in unnatural geometric lip scars. In fact, the prolabium of a bilateral cleft, once attached to the skin and muscle of the lateral lip, has a remarkable capacity for vertical growth. The expected changes over time must be envisioned in the design of the prolabium, with attention to both size and shape. Inexorably, the prolabium widens, but less so when primary muscle continuity is established. Failure to appreciate this aspect of the fourth dimension results in an excessively bowed and wide prolabium. After the primary repair, the prolabium should measure no more than 4 to 5 mm between the bow peaks, and 2 mm at the columellar-labial juncture. Because of the well-known tendency for hypertrophic scarring in childhood, the lip should not be reincised in an attempt to narrow the prolabium, contrive forked flaps, or revise scars.

Formation of the Median Tubercle from Lateral Lip Vermilion-Mucosa

Older operative techniques usually preserved the tiny central vermilion-mucosal tab, and the result was a dry, fissured, and wrinkled median tubercle. The narrow band of vermilion fails to grow to sufficient height and, in combination with the deficient central mucosa, constitutes the "whistling lip" deformity.

A normal lip has a vertical seam, or raphe, centered on the median tubercle. This anatomic configuration can best be constructed using vermilion-mucosal flaps from the lateral lip elements. The prolabium of a complete bilateral cleft lip lacks a white line roll. Therefore, if possible, this white ridge should also be constructed from the lateral lip, carried atop the vermilion-muscosal flaps.

Early Positioning of the Alar Cartilages to Construct the Nasal Tip and Columella

Current methodology for correction of bilateral cleft lip usually necessitates a secondary columellar lengthening, using either forked flaps or rotation of bipedicled alar base flaps. There are problems with these techniques: scars that disjoin the columellar-labial angle; a tendency to accentuate a long lip; and creation of an abnormally shaped columella.

The most frequently used operations for bilateral complete cleft lip ignore and accentuate the abnormal posture of the alar cartilages. To provide a matrix for normal growth, the alar cartilages and nasal soft tissues must be placed in a normal anatomic relationship as early as possible. The technique described herein is based on this principle. At the first operative stage, the lateral crura are elevated, the alar bases are advanced medially, and forked flaps are turned upward and "banked" beneath the alar flaps. During the second stage, the medial crura are placed into a normal anterosuperior position to elongate the lower columella. The upper columella is lengthened by joining the splayed alar genua. The banked, forked flaps are transposed into the upper nasal vestibules to add lining tissue and accentuate the forward position of the alar cartilages. The columellar-labial angle is not violated by scar, in contrast to other methods for columellar elongation.

CORRECTION

Orthopaedic manipulation sets the stage for symmetrical closure of the bilateral complete cleft lip. A retention appliance with biplane (sagittal and coronal) jackscrews aligns the upper arch by lateral rotation of the palatal shelves and by retrusion and rotation of the premaxilla. This device also restricts vertical growth of the premaxilla. The first stage operative correction is undertaken when the infant is 3 to 5 months of age.

STAGE I

The lip markings are adapted from Millard's descriptions (Fig. 1A). Loupe magnification (2.5X) is used throughout the procedure. With a double hook holding the nares upward in a symmetrical posture, the prolabium is drawn in a biconcave shape. The peaks of the Cupid's bow are set no more than 4 mm apart at the inferior end of the philtral flap. The base of the philtral flap is measured 2 mm wide at the columellar-labial junction. Forked flaps are sketched on each side of the diminutive prolabial flap. The tissue that remains in the prolabium (lateral to the forks) will be rotated into the medial nasal vestibules. The alar base incisions are drawn through the alae, not in the obvious alar-cheek junction, but a little higher so that the scars will lie in the alar crease and not on the cheek.

The lateral point on the lip should be no less than 16 to 18 mm from the oral commissure. The lateral lip flaps are marked exactly on the cutaneous-vermilion junction; however, the most lateral 4 to 5 mm should also include available white roll (see Fig. 1A).

Critical points are tattooed, namely, the base and arrowhead-shaped tip of the prolabial flap, the most lateral points on the cutaneous flaps, and the mucosal-vermilion junctions. The lip segments are infiltrated with 1:200,000 epinephrine solution and, after a suitable waiting period, all lines are carefully scored. The prolabium is cut first and elevated as a trefoil, thereby preserving the tiny vessels from the columella. The two tiny forks are separated from the central prolabial flap. The median vermilion-mucosal flap is turned inferiorly with its blood supply from the premaxilla. The cutaneous-vermilion mucosal flap is cut to the lateral marked point (Fig. 1B). The alar bases are dissociated from the lateral lip elements, and the lateral crura are dissected via an intercartilaginous incision (Fig. 1C). The lateral lip is incised along the gingivolabial sulcus to the maxillary tuberosity. Each lateral lip complex must be completely freed off the anterior maxilla, with the supraperiosteal dissection extended over the malar eminence. The orbicularis oris bundle is carefully dissected to the melolabial crease in the subdermal plane of each lateral lip element (see Fig. 1C). Dissection is also done in the submucosal plane, in order to telescope the muscle from the lip element and minimize mucosal festooning. A small backcut in the superior margin of the muscle bundles may be needed, so that they will lie transversely.

Closure

The intercartilaginous incisions are closed first; in so doing, the lateral crura are advanced superiorly and sutured to the lower edge of the upper lateral cartilages (Fig. 2A). The nostril floor is constructed with a lateral flap from the maxillary alveolus and a medially-based flap from the premaxilla. The next step is crucial—the lateral lip-complex must be transposed medially as the gingivolabial sulcus incision is closed. The premaxillary mucosal flap is folded sagittally and held with a mattress suture to form the frenulum. The translocated lateral lip mucosa is sutured to the premaxillary mucosa, then, for a short distance, it is sutured from one side to the other to form the underside of the lip.

The next step is approximation of the orbicularis oris muscle bundles. The sutures are placed seriatim, inferiorly to superiorly, with progressively wider bites. The uppermost muscle is secured to the anterior nasal spine (Fig. 2B). These maneuvers establish a definitive orbicularis oris closure, promote lip eversion, and diminish the tendency for lingual inclination of the premaxilla.

The closure of the nasal floor is completed by medial transposition of the alar base flaps. Often, the alar bases are sutured to one another in order to adjust their position in relation to the prolabial flap.

Attention must be paid to the construction of the Cupid's bow and completion of the median tubercle. The leading edges of the lateral lip vermilion-mucosal flaps

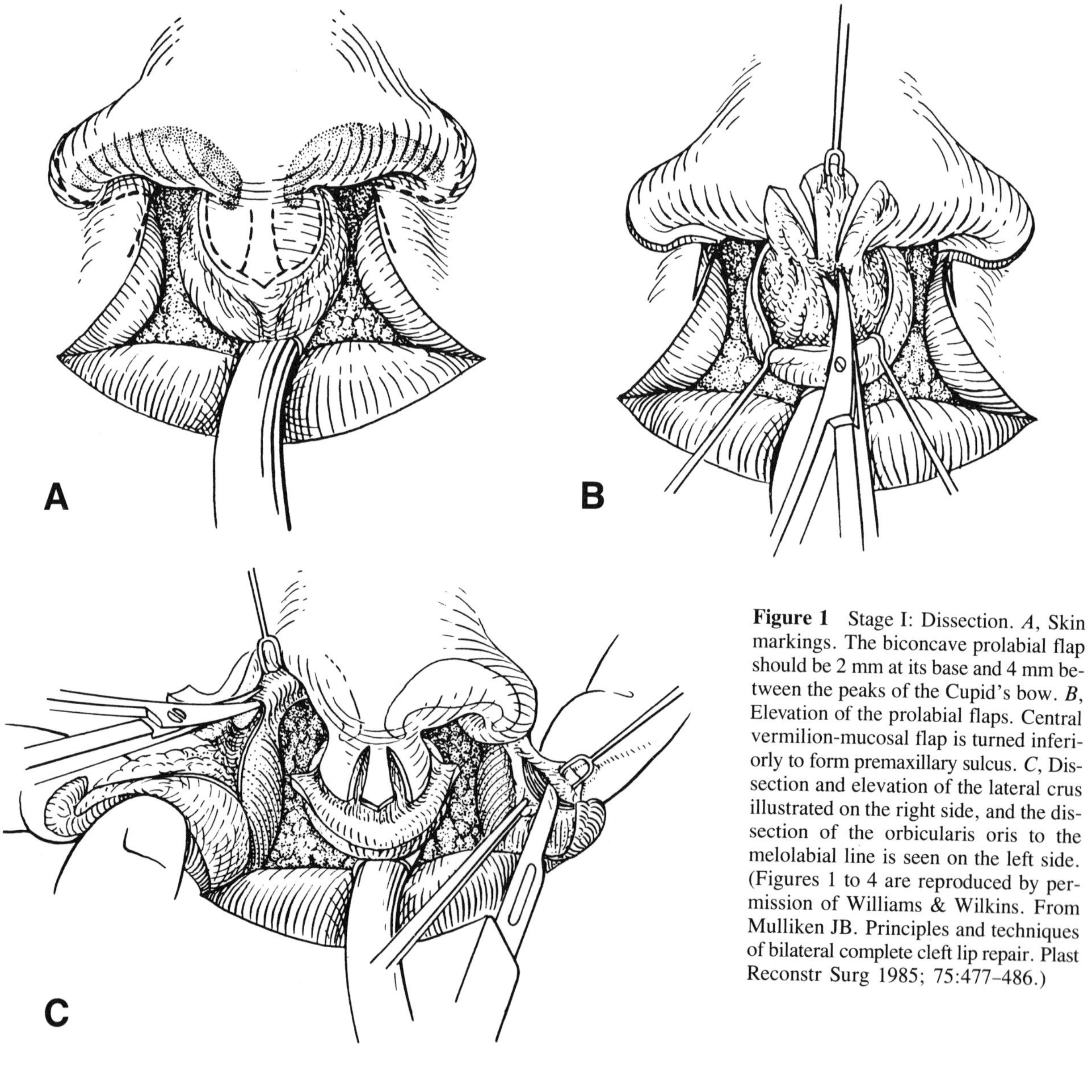

Figure 1 Stage I: Dissection. *A*, Skin markings. The biconcave prolabial flap should be 2 mm at its base and 4 mm between the peaks of the Cupid's bow. *B*, Elevation of the prolabial flaps. Central vermilion-mucosal flap is turned inferiorly to form premaxillary sulcus. *C*, Dissection and elevation of the lateral crus illustrated on the right side, and the dissection of the orbicularis oris to the melolabial line is seen on the left side. (Figures 1 to 4 are reproduced by permission of Williams & Wilkins. From Mulliken JB. Principles and techniques of bilateral complete cleft lip repair. Plast Reconstr Surg 1985; 75:477–486.)

are held downward with single hooks in a "praying hands" fashion. Vertical mattress sutures are used to emphasize eversion of the median tubercle and its central raphe. Rarely should mucosa be trimmed at this stage. If one side of the lateral lip mucosa is excessive, it can be deepithelialized and buried in order to add tissue into the median tubercle. The Cupid's bow is delicately constructed with fine suture that joins the inferior edge of the tiny philtral flap to the apposed lateral white roll–vermilion flaps (Fig. 2C).

The forked flaps are trimmed, if needed, and "banked" in the sill just below the alar base flaps. It is rarely necessary to trim the medial edge of the lateral lip flaps before suturing them to the prolabium. However, it is always necessary to adjust the superior margin of the lateral lip flaps; this is done in a gentle cyma-style curve to fit the vertical dimension of the prolabium and the position of the alar bases. Since there is a tendency for the lateral lip to be vertically long, this excision of the upper margin of skin is critical (see Fig. 2C).

The sill incision should be closed from lateral to medial in order to accentuate the prominence of the central lip. The percutaneous sutures are staggered along the prolabial-lateral lip junctions. There should be absolutely no tension on these suture lines.

A petrolatum-soaked gauze roll placed in each vestibule helps support the alar cartilages and minimize swelling. This completes Stage I.

STAGE II

The cleft of the hard and soft palate is closed as a single procedure when the child is 10 to 12 months of age. Correction of the nasal deformity is undertaken when the child is about 16 to 18 months old. The guiding principles

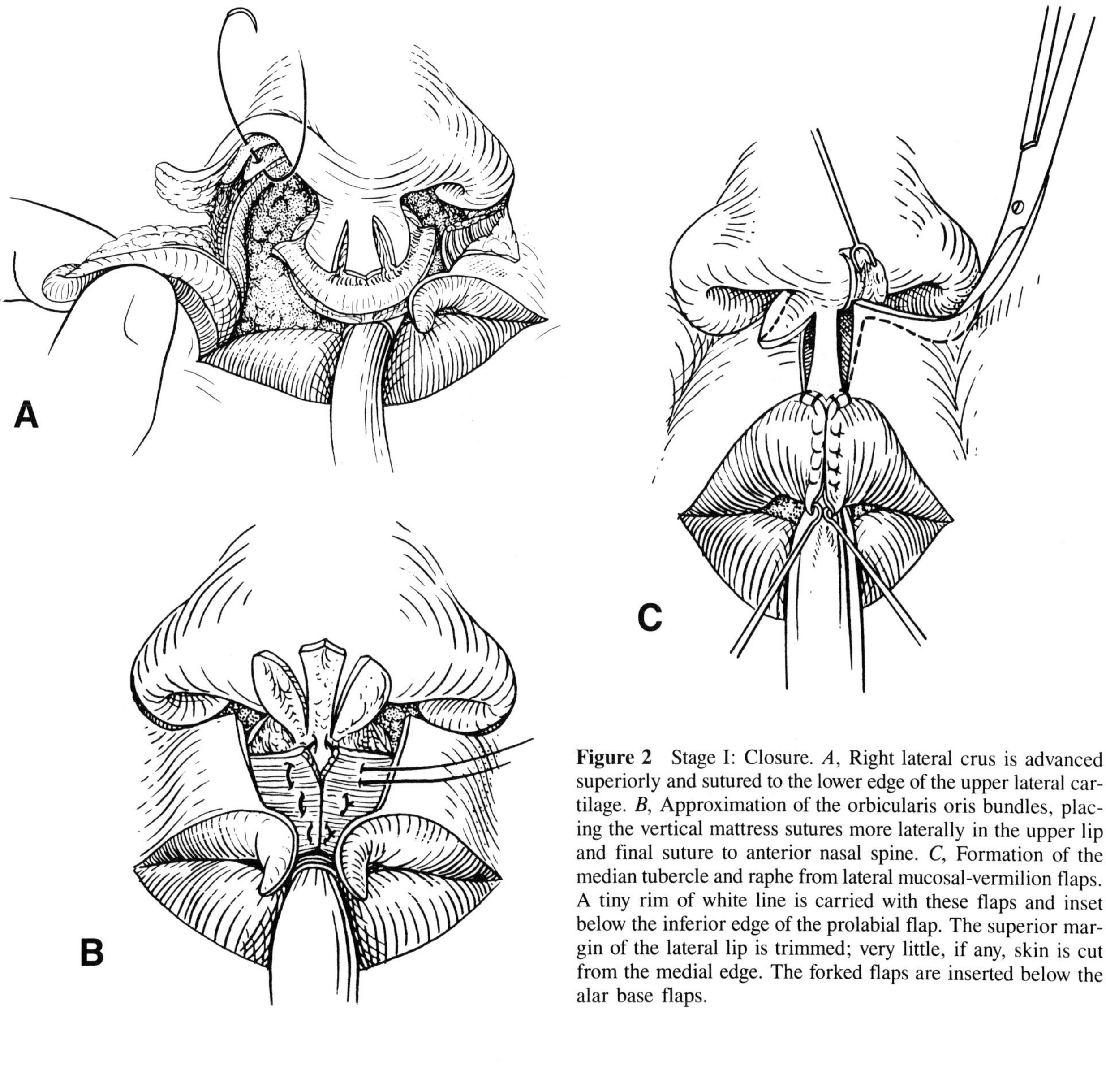

Figure 2 Stage I: Closure. *A*, Right lateral crus is advanced superiorly and sutured to the lower edge of the upper lateral cartilage. *B*, Approximation of the orbicularis oris bundles, placing the vertical mattress sutures more laterally in the upper lip and final suture to anterior nasal spine. *C*, Formation of the median tubercle and raphe from lateral mucosal-vermilion flaps. A tiny rim of white line is carried with these flaps and inset below the inferior edge of the prolabial flap. The superior margin of the lateral lip is trimmed; very little, if any, skin is cut from the medial edge. The forked flaps are inserted below the alar base flaps.

in Stage II are: placement of the alar cartilages in normal anatomic position, and fashioning the draping nasal skin so as to lengthen the columella. The incisions for Stage II are seen in Figure 3A. The alar bases are reincised so that, once again, they can be transposed medially, and the forked flaps are reelevated. A midline nasal tip incision and superomedial rim incisions provide the necessary exposure to the splayed alar domes. The medial crura are located via the tip incision and by extending the sill incision along the intramembranous septum (Fig. 3B). In doing the latter, care must be taken not to transect the crural footplates that are located posteroinferiorly to their normal position. The medial crura are completely exposed and elevated, leaving the lateral crura in place (Fig. 3C).

Once the dissection of the alae is complete, the medial crura are sutured to one another and suspended to the caudal cartilaginous septum. The alar genua are rotated medially and sutured to one another; this corrects the bifid tip deformity and lengthens the upper columella (Fig. 4A). The forked flaps are transposed into the intercartilaginous incisions and secured with fine resorbable sutures (Fig. 4B). The formation of an inverted cone that results from rotation of the forks increases the height of the vestibular domes and brings the nasal tip forward. The alar bases are translocated medially alongside the base of the columella. The undersides of the alar flaps are secured, one to the other, with a nonresorbable mattress suture tunnelled beneath the columellar-labial junction. The lateral genua are suspended to the contralateral septal-upperlateral junction with buried mattress sutures placed through tiny skin incisions (Fig. 4C). The final steps are excision of the redundant skin from the upper edge of the rim incisions, and closure. A petroleum gauze roll is placed in each vestibule.

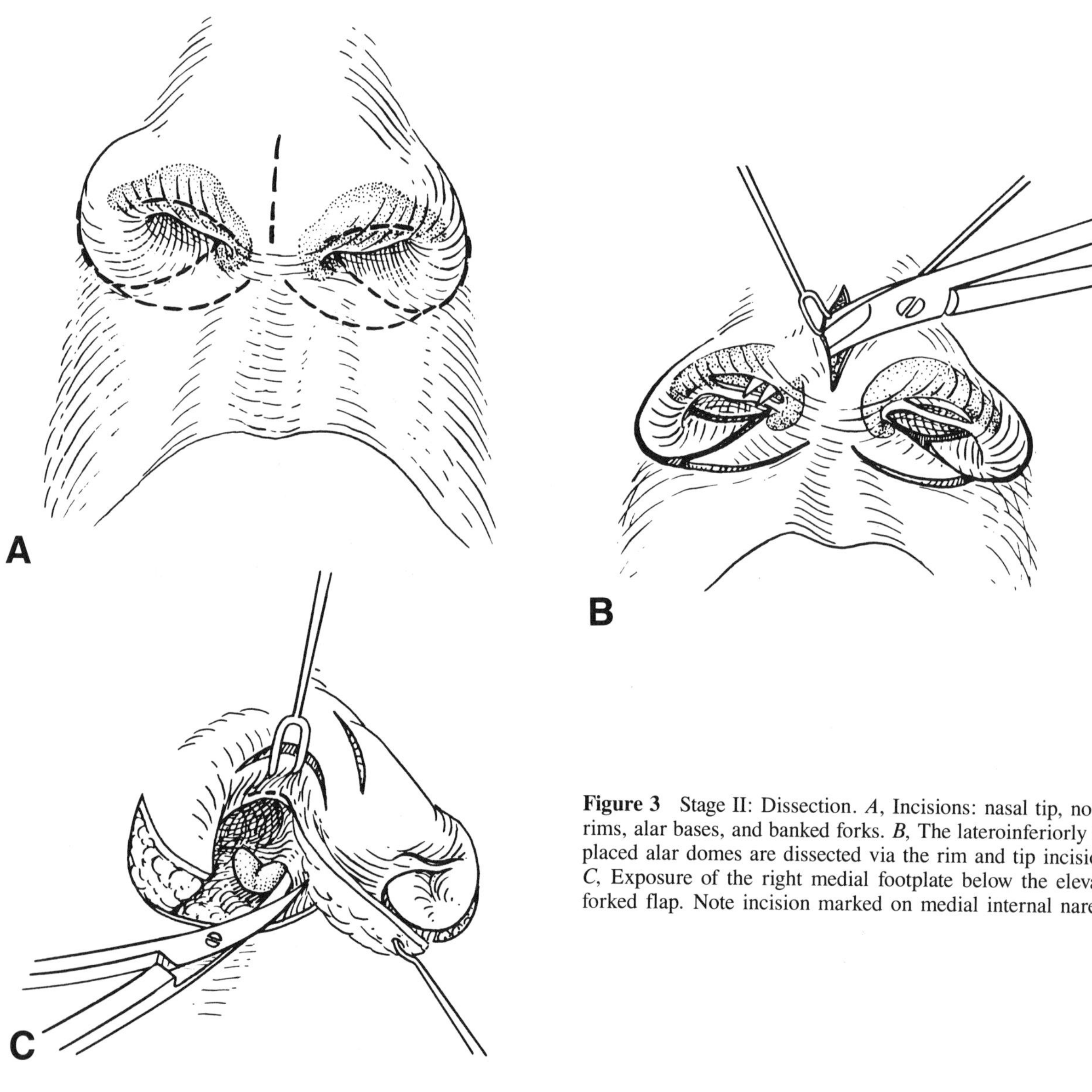

Figure 3 Stage II: Dissection. *A*, Incisions: nasal tip, nostril rims, alar bases, and banked forks. *B*, The lateroinferiorly displaced alar domes are dissected via the rim and tip incisions. *C*, Exposure of the right medial footplate below the elevated forked flap. Note incision marked on medial internal nares.

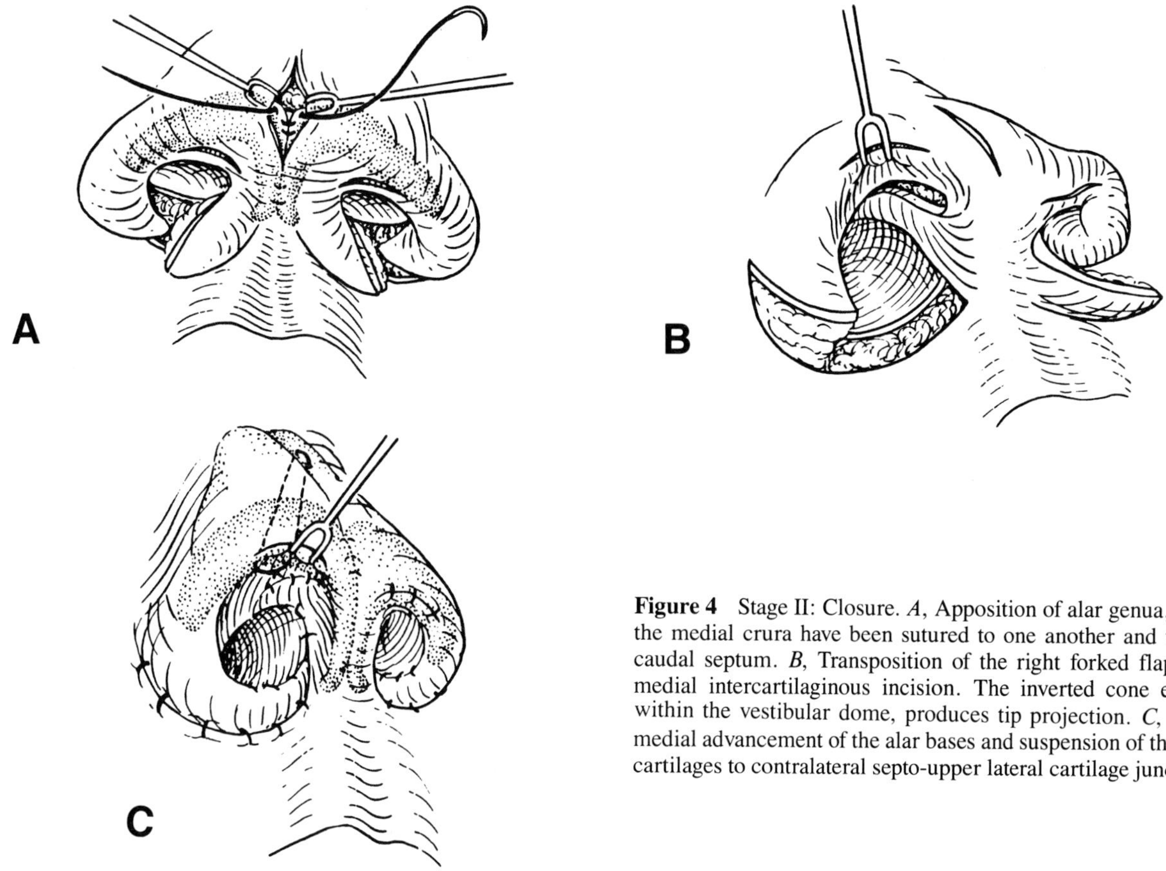

Figure 4 Stage II: Closure. *A*, Apposition of alar genua, after the medial crura have been sutured to one another and to the caudal septum. *B*, Transposition of the right forked flap into medial intercartilaginous incision. The inverted cone effect, within the vestibular dome, produces tip projection. *C*, After medial advancement of the alar bases and suspension of the alar cartilages to contralateral septo-upper lateral cartilage junction.

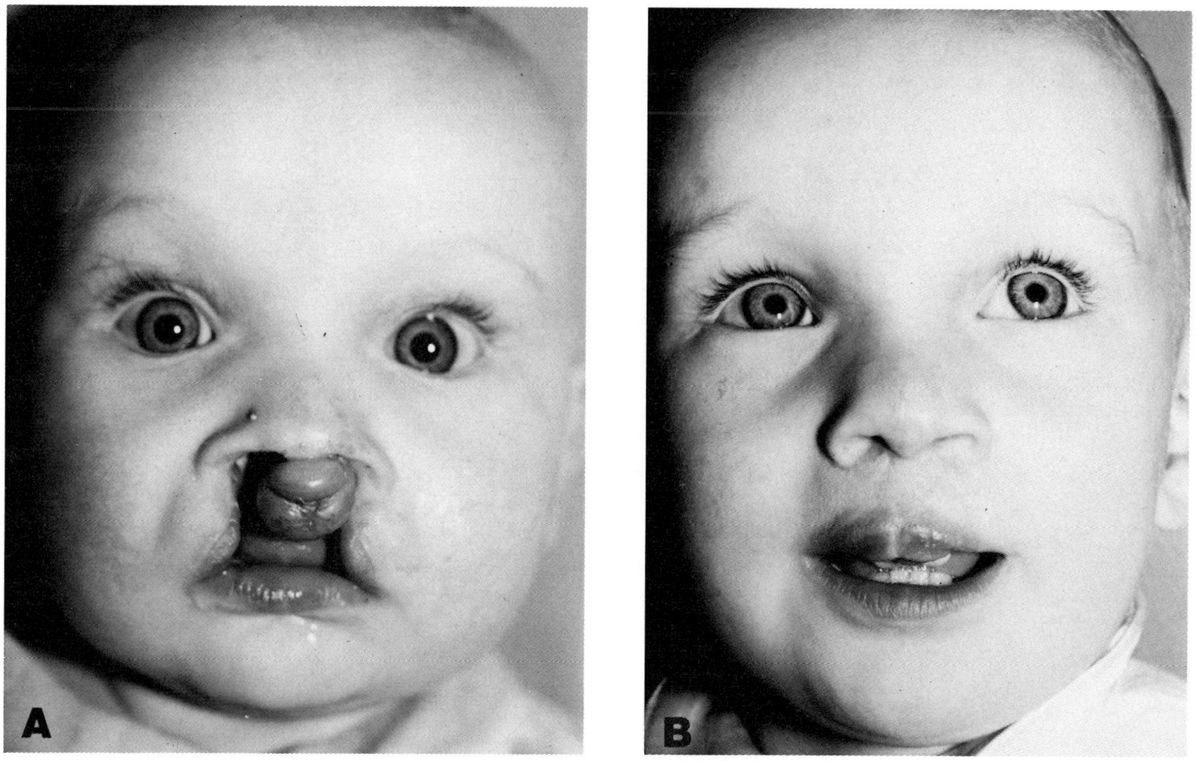

Figure 5 Illustrative case of bilateral complete cleft lip. *A*, Preoperative photograph at 4 months of age. *B*, Postoperative photograph at age 18 months (Stage I at 5 months and Stage II at 15 months).

Figure continues on following page

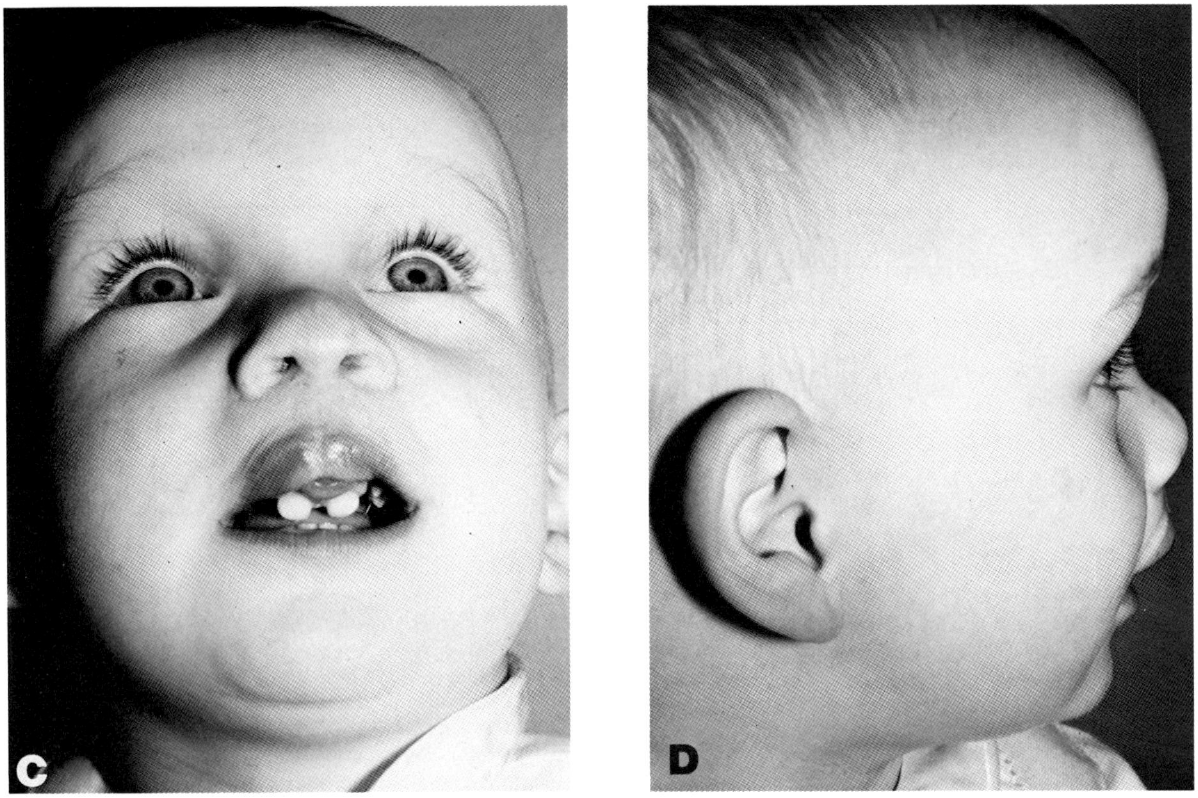

Figure 5 (continued) *C*, Submental photograph, 3 months after alar cartilage positioning and columellar lengthening. *D*, Lateral view, 3 months after Stage II procedure, demonstrates projection of nasal tip and upper lip posture.

RESULTS

This two-stage correction of bilateral cleft lip gives a full central tubercle and a natural posture to the lip. The nasal tip projection and columellar length are maintained with growth; however, there is often a residual transverse axis of the external nares (Fig. 5).

In children over the age of 5, prolabial measurements show a 2.5-fold increase in width at the columellar-labial level and a 2.0-fold widening between the Cupid's bow peaks.

This same approach is used for bilateral incomplete cleft lip deformity. In these cases, if the prolabium has an adequate white ridge and sufficient vertical height of vermilion, then the lateral lip elements are adjusted to the prolabium-vermilion-mucosa. In a minimal bilateral cleft, forked flaps may be unnecessary, although the alar cartilages should be properly positioned. These operative principles also apply to the secondary correction of bilateral cleft lip deformities. The normal anatomic structures that remain elusive are the prolabial dimple and the philtral columns.

SUGGESTED READING

Black PW, Scheflan, M. Bilateral cleft lip repair: "Putting it all together." Ann Plast Surg 1984; 12:118–127.

Broadbent TR, Woolf, RM. Bilateral cleft lip: one-stage primary repair. In: Georgiade NG, Hagerty RF, eds. Symposium on management of cleft lip and palate and associated deformities. St. Louis: CV Mosby, 1974:134.

Millard DR Jr. Cleft craft. The evolution of its surgery. II. Bilateral and rare deformities. Boston: Little, Brown, 1977:359.

Mulliken JB. Principles and techniques of bilateral complete cleft lip repair. Plast Reconstr Surg 1985; 75:477–486.

Noordhoff MS. Bilateral cleft lip reconstruction. Plast Reconstr Surg 1986; 78:45–54.

TIMING AND TECHNIQUE OF CLEFT PALATE REPAIR

MICHAEL B. LEWIS, M.D.

The primary goal of cleft palate surgery is to provide adequate palate function for the development and maintenance of normal speech. Ideally, this should be accomplished without disturbing maxillary growth. This dual objective is not usually attainable and has generated a great deal of discussion.

There are four variables that determine the outcome in cleft palate surgery: (1) the type of cleft, (2) the surgeon, (3) the technique of surgical repair, and (4) timing of the repair. All are important, but only the latter two can be altered to determine the outcome in any particular case. For this reason, they have become the subject of much discussion and controversy.

Eustachian tube-middle ear function and hearing have not been included in this chapter. They are important, but little is known about them as yet vis-à-vis the usual discussion variables.

TIMING

The debate is primarily between the speech pathologist, who favors early repair, and the orthodontist-facial growth specialist who advocates later repair. In the middle of this controversy, but by no means passive, is the plastic surgeon. Because he is performing the surgery, the plastic surgeon has a responsibility for the patient's well-being, speech, and facial growth.

The issues are as follows. Early palate repair provides a better chance for normal speech, but can be detrimental to maxillary growth. Late surgery interferes less with maxillary growth, but provides less chance of normal speech development.

In what appears more and more to be an unsuccessful attempt to compromise, discussion and decisions on the timing of repair have separated the hard palate from the soft palate.

As long ago as 1937, Wardill suggested that the ideal time to repair the palate was before speech developed, thus providing a normal speech mechanism in advance of its use. Because of the limitations of pediatric anesthesia techniques at that time, Wardill was not able to follow his own instincts.

Since then, however, his thoughts on this subject have been confirmed and there is little dissent today. Palate repair before the age of speech development (about 1 year) provides the best opportunity for normal speech. Perhaps the studies by Dorf and Curtin, and Henningsson and Isberg provide some insight into the effectiveness of this common sense approach. If the velopharyngeal valve is not present when speech begins to develop, substitute valving at the pharyngeal and glottal level occurs. Dorf and Curtin found only a 10 percent incidence of pharyngeal and glottal articulation (common compensatory components of cleft palate speech) in children whose palates were completely repaired before 1 year of age, and an 86 percent incidence of these abnormal articulation problems in cases repaired after the age of 1 year—a highly significant difference. Henningsson and Isberg demonstrated that glottal and pharyngeal articulation, as opposed to oral articulation, was associated with poor velopharyngeal closure. Actual paradoxical relaxation of this sphincter can be seen in glottal and pharyngeal articulation. This means the associated cleft palate articulation errors that are more prone to develop if the palate is repaired late will diminish the efficiency of its function, even after it is successfully repaired.

Some of the data available might not withstand scientific scrutiny, but the preponderance of information suggests that the earlier the palate is repaired, (which could be as early as just under 1 year old), the more likely the development of normal speech. It is not clear whether this can be extrapolated to mean that even earlier closure will provide better results. Certainly the ability to do earlier repair exists today, and in some centers it is being done at 6 and even 3 months of age.

There is little doubt that palate surgery has an effect on maxillary growth, and the orthodontists' concerns are well-founded. Two things, however, must be added to the discussion. First, surgery to repair involvement of the primary palate (lip and alveolus) can be equally or even more harmful to maxillary growth than the palate repair. Second, in cleft cases there are varying degrees of inherent maxillary growth deficiency. This is sometimes quite obvious from the initial impression of hypoplasia in the cleft area, but sometimes it is not visible early. This inherent growth deficiency varies not only among cleft types, but also within specific cleft types. Any surgeon who has done a number of cleft cases has noted considerable difference in subsequent maxillary growth, despite having done the same repair in apparently similar cases during the same time period.

There are four general types of spacial maxillary growth: (1) anteroposterior, (2) vertical, (3) transverse, and (4) alveolar arch form. In discussion and conclusions about the effects of surgery on maxillary growth, these are often lumped together, thus suggesting that all are equally important and occur at the same frequency. This is not the case. Most reported maxillary growth problems, especially when one technique, or timing of repair, is compared to another, are either in transverse dimension or arch form. These are less harmful to general facial esthetics than either anteroposterior or vertical growth deficiencies of the maxilla, and are more readily corrected by orthodontic techniques.

These problems make valid conclusions on the issues of maxillary growth and timing difficult to achieve. Undoubtedly, to do no surgery at all would provide the best opportunity for normal maxillary growth. This is, of course, unacceptable and not even a guarantee of normal growth. If the palate *is* to be repaired, it seems to make no significant difference to maxillary growth *when* it is repaired. The exception to this is the timing of hard palate repair, which seems to allow better transverse maxillary growth if delayed past 12 years of age. "Significant" is the keyword because what is significant to the orthodontist may not be so important to the surgeon. It should always be remembered that what is most important is the psychosocial and physical development of the patient.

TECHNIQUE

Although timing is probably more important in determining the speech result, technique cannot be discounted. Variations in technique can also influence the form and degree of maxillary growth disturbance.

For many years, only two techniques for palatal closure were widely used. These were the lengthening procedure of Wardill and Kilner, and the von Langenbeck repair. Both procedures involve submucoperiosteal dissection in the hard palate and leave raw, bony surfaces, which heal by secondary intention, at the completion of the repair. This type of dissection, and especially the raw surfaces, subsequent secondary healing, and scarring, are responsible for most of the observed transverse maxillary and arch form growth disturbances. Because of this, soft palate closure without dissection of the hard palate mucoperiosteum, combined with delayed hard palate closure, has been advocated. This technique causes less deformity of the maxilla but results in very poor speech.

Very few of the many published reports on palate repair that relate speech and maxillary growth to technique are considered highly significant because it is difficult to control all the variables. However, trends or tendencies can be observed. In general, procedures that lengthen the effective soft palate provide better palate function than those that do not. The corollary of this, however, is that they create a somewhat greater maxillary deformity, especially in arch form.

Braithwaite first suggested levator velum palatini muscle retropositioning as an adjunct to palate repair. Although theoretically desirable, no conclusive data are available. More recently, Furlow has described a technique that lengthens the soft palate by a double opposing Z-plasty, without expending hard palate mucoperiosteum. The design of the double opposing Z-plasty also retropositions the effective levator sling. A lot of information is not yet available, but speech results appear comparable to the lengthening procedures. Maxillary growth information is also not yet available.

ESTABLISHING PRIORITIES

After considering the above, it is clear that some compromise must be made. In order to do this, priorities have to be established. Normal speech is the top priority in palate repair. This means acceptance of a potentially greater disturbance in maxillary growth if a better speech result is to be obtained. As regards exact timing and technique of repair, I have been most influenced by Manchester and believe the palate should be completely repaired by 9 months of age, thus allowing sufficient time for softening of the scar tissue before speech begins.

If more than half the length of the hard palate is involved in the cleft deformity, the hard palate should be repaired at an earlier stage, with use of a vomerine mucoperiosteal flap. This repair is usually performed at about 5 months of age and is done in conjunction with the cleft lip repair in cases where there are complete clefts of the primary and secondary palate. This two-staged repair reduces and comes close to eliminating oral-nasal fistulas, even in Manchester's radical lengthening procedure.

The Manchester technique of soft palate repair is an extension of the Wardill-Kilner repair. It uses a preliminary extensive release of the soft palate from the hard palate. Flaps are taken from the nasal surface of the hard palate to line the raw surfaces created on the nasal surface of the lengthened soft palate. I have added levator muscle retropositioning to Manchester's technique.

I have not used the term push-back in this discussion. Even though it is the commonly used descriptive term of the Wardill-Kilner procedure, I feel it is a misnomer. The verb "push" implies movement against force. There should be no feeling of resistance as the palate is lengthened. If an adequate and thorough release is carried out, the soft palate structures will move naturally to a more posterior position (Fig. 1). This thorough release also allows for a tension-free closure. The surgical goal is to keep the retrodisplaced soft palate in this posterior position. This is done by use of the nasal lining flaps to cover the raw nasal surfaces of the lengthened soft palate and by not trying to eliminate all raw bony surfaces on the hard palate, as this would only pull the soft palate back toward its original anterior position.

Briefly, the steps involved in this repair are as follows. The standard V–Ygeometry, first described by Ganzer, is incised on the hard palate (Fig. 2). The position of these incisions is not rigid and depends on the size of the cleft. The incisions can be varied to keep them more posterior and further away from the alveolar area, thus creating less maxillary deformity. Enough tissue should be included to lengthen the palate properly. These oral mucoperiosteal flaps are elevated back to the greater pala-

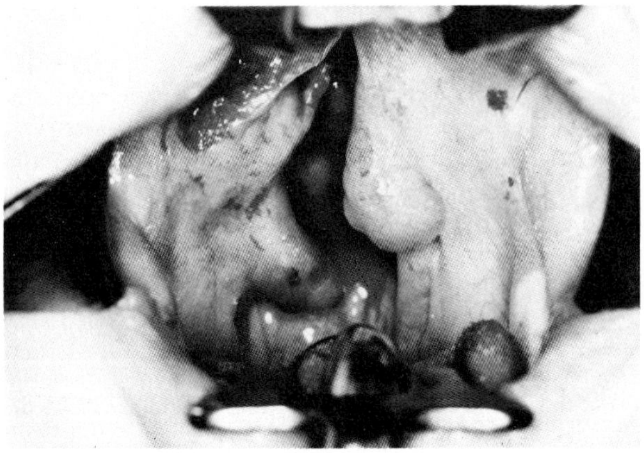

Figure 1 Photograph demonstrates posterior movement of dissected half of palate without "pushing." This movement usually measures 1.5 cm or more.

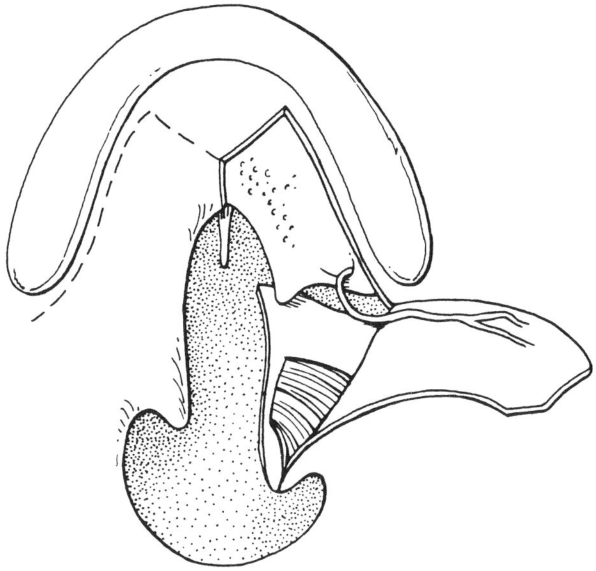

Figure 2 Approximate position of mucoperiosteal incisions on hard palate are shown on left. Right: the appearance of the thoroughly dissected and released soft palate with attached nasal lining flap. Cleft margin has been opened and levator velum palatini muscle dissected and reoriented.

tine neurovascular bundles, which are thoroughly mobilized. At this point the hamular processes are infractured.

Lining flaps from the nasal surface of the hard palate are developed from the oral approach, as described by Manchester, (which differs from the intranasal approach of Cronin). The lateral incisions of this lining flap mobilization are continued vertically up the medial pterygoid bone, completely releasing the soft palate from the hard. The cleft margins are opened, and the levator velum palatini muscle is dissected free from within the substance of the soft palate to allow reorientation, retropositioning, and repair (see Fig. 2).

Repair is started on the nasal surface of the soft palate, by working posteriorly until the uvula is repaired. The levator velum palatini muscle is then retropositioned,

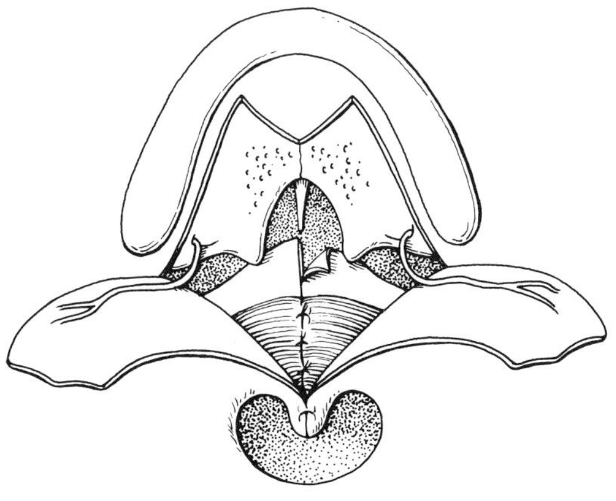

Figure 3 Levator velum palatini muscle reoriented, retropositioned, and repaired. Nasal surface of soft palate and uvula were previously repaired.

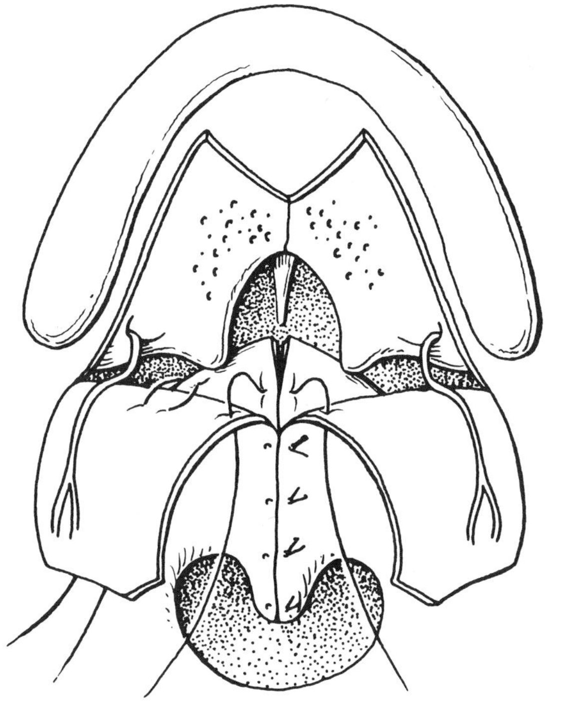

Figure 4 Oral surface of palate is being repaired, with nasal lining flaps incorporated anterior to muscle repair.

reoriented, and repaired with slowly absorbable sutures (Fig. 3). Then the oral surface of the soft and hard palate is repaired with vertical mattress sutures to create a broad area of approximation. Anterior to the muscle repair, the nasal lining flaps are secured to the undersurface of the

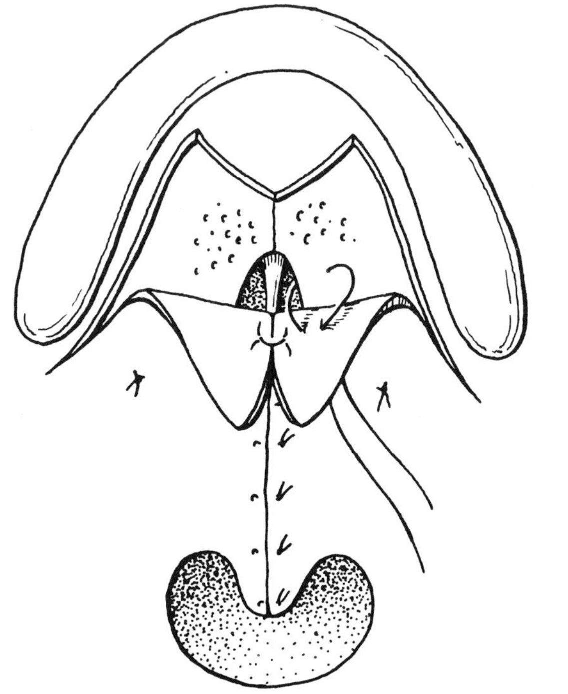

Figure 5 Repaired palate being reattached to hard palate bone in natural retrodisplaced position.

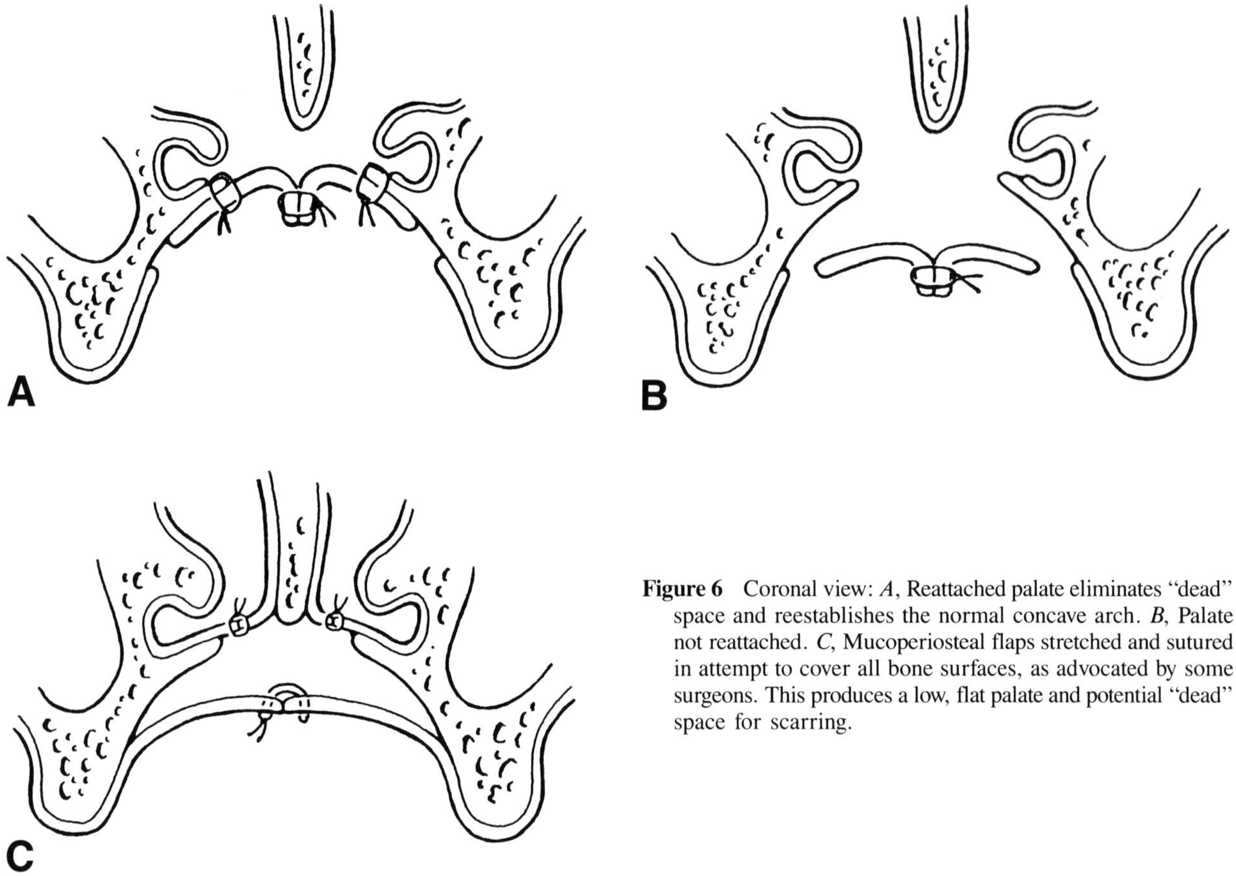

Figure 6 Coronal view: *A*, Reattached palate eliminates "dead" space and reestablishes the normal concave arch. *B*, Palate not reattached. *C*, Mucoperiosteal flaps stretched and sutured in attempt to cover all bone surfaces, as advocated by some surgeons. This produces a low, flat palate and potential "dead" space for scarring.

oral flaps, thereby isolating the muscle within the soft palate (Fig. 4). This prevents any chance of muscle reattachment to the hard palate, which could limit soft palate motion.

Once the repair of the palate is complete, its natural new retrodisplaced position is determined, and it is secured to the hard palate bone with mattress sutures placed through small drill holes (Fig. 5). This usually leaves some uncovered bone surfaces, but does two beneficial things. First, it reconstructs the normal concave palatal arch and, second, it eliminates potential dead space that would be created if the hard palatal mucoperiosteum were stretched in an attempt to cover all raw surfaces. This could be even more harmful than leaving a small area of bone uncovered (Fig. 6).

SUGGESTED READING

Braithwaite F, Maurice DG. The importance of the levator palati muscle in cleft palate closure. Br J Plast Surg 1968; 21:60–62.

Dorf DS, Curtin JW. Early cleft palate repair and speech outcome. Plast Reconstr Surg 1982; 70:74–79.

Furlow LT Jr. Cleft Palate repair by double opposing Z-plasty. Plast Reconst Surg 1986; 78:724–736.

Henningsson GE, Isberg AM. Velopharyngeal movement patterns in patients alternating between oral and glottal articulation: a clinical and cineradiographical study. Cleft Palate J 1986; 23:1–9.

Manchester WM. The repair of double cleft lip as part of an integrated program. Plast Reconst Surg 1970; 45:207–216.

POSTPALATOPLASTY VELOPHARYNGEAL INCOMPETENCY

RAVELO V. ARGAMASO, M.D., F.A.C.S.

Traditionally, nasal hyperresonance following cleft palate repair was believed to be caused solely by failure of the velum to achieve effective approximation with the posterior pharyngeal wall. Based on this hypothesis, corrective measures were directed primarily toward lengthening the soft palate by so-called "push-back" procedures, but results of these operations were rather unpredictable. Further efforts to enhance the range of superoposterior movements of the velum by repair of the levator muscle sling, have also met with limited success. Significant numbers of patients are left postoperatively to contend with varying degrees of hypernasality, despite diverse methods of pharyngeal flap construction.

In recent years, the pathophysiology of the velopharyngeal closure mechanism has been demonstrated through viewing the velopharyngeal port, and the importance of lateral pharyngeal wall movements in the modulation of the velopharyngeal opening has been elucidated. Observations on the functions of the velopharynx, indirectly from multiview videofluoroscopy and directly from nasopharyngoscopy, provided data on the varying patterns of valving during speech. This variability depended on the interplay between the muscles of the velum and pharyngeal walls.

Three patterns of valving have been observed in normal speakers. When the velum assumes the major role in closure, with minimal contributions from the pharyngeal walls, the interaction creates a transverse interface and seals off the nasopharynx from the oropharynx. This pattern of closure is termed "coronal." When lateral pharyngeal wall movements predominate and they meet in the midline, the pattern of closure is referred to as "sagittal." When the velum and lateral pharyngeal walls contribute equally, with little or some additional assistance from the posterior pharyngeal wall (Passavant's ridge), these components are drawn to a point and a circular or true sphincteric pattern of closure is effected. These valving patterns are similarly observed among speakers with velopharyngeal insufficiency, who display gaps of various sizes and shapes from incomplete closure (Fig. 1).

Given the variability in valving patterns among postpalatoplasty patients with velopharyngeal incompetence, the goal of our surgical strategy is the construction of a pharyngeal flap with postoperative width that can be purposely made narrow, wide, or extremely wide, to match the size of the opening in the velopharyngeal closure mechanism. In addition, the pedicle is set to conform with the vertical level and horizontal position of the gap in the velopharyngeal tract. Therefore, in my view, phonation studies in three dimensions with multiview videofluoroscopy and/or fiberoptic nasopharyngoscopy are essential, not only for the surgical indication but also for prognostication of the surgical outcome.

TREATMENT OF VARIATIONS IN VELOPHARYNGEAL INSUFFICIENCY

A superiorly-based pharyngeal flap has been used consistently for over 12 years. Postoperative flap size may be altered by varying flap width at the time of elevation, as well as the site of flap insertion (Fig. 2). Thus, a narrow flap is induced to form from an initially wide, unlined, pharyngeal flap when it is inserted into a pocket created through a transverse incision on the dorsum of the middle third of the soft palate, and its pedicle allowed to heal by tubing itself (Fig. 3).

When the open pedicle is shortened by implanting the distal portion of the flap closer to the posterior third of the soft palate, tubing is hampered and a somewhat wider flap results (Fig. 4). Flap size is further enhanced by increasing the width during elevation. Finally, a flap that almost totally obstructs the velopharyngeal port is created by insertion of the distal end of a very wide, short flap, sandwich fashion, along the free margin of the soft palate, extending to the posterior tonsillar pillars (Fig. 5). Small apertures are left between the base of the flap and the adjacent posterior tonsilliar folds where they merge with the pharyngeal wall.

INDICATIONS AND TIMING OF SURGERY

A team of several investigators and clinicians formulates a treatment plan for any patient who has additional problems other than hypernasal speech. The surgeon should seek the aid of an experienced nasoendoscopist and a radiologist to determine the pathologic mechanics of the valving system and define the nature or extent of the defect in the velopharyngeal port, so that an appropriate flap can be constructed.

The relationship between velopharyngeal insufficiency and articulatory distortion in a given patient is an intricate one, and the judgment of a speech pathologist is invaluable as regards the timing of speech therapy versus pharyngeal flap surgery. Ideally, pharyngeal flap procedures are performed as early as possible, before patterns of articulation disorder are well-established. It is rare that a fistula of the palate alone becomes the dominant cause of hypernasality. However, in an attempt to plug this defect, the tongue often assumes an abnormal position during speech, thereby contributing to errors in articulation. A functional fistula should be closed prior to pharyngoplasty and speech derangements, particularly the glottal stop, corrected to maximize the beneficial effects of surgery.

The prosthodontist may be called on for an alternative solution in special instances where medical intervention is contraindicated. Other colleagues may provide treatment for associated problems that also need attention during the course of therapy. Enlarged tonsils that protrude into and occupy the lateral nasopharyngeal spaces have been known to interfere with velar function and impede lateral pharyngeal wall motion, thus causing nasal

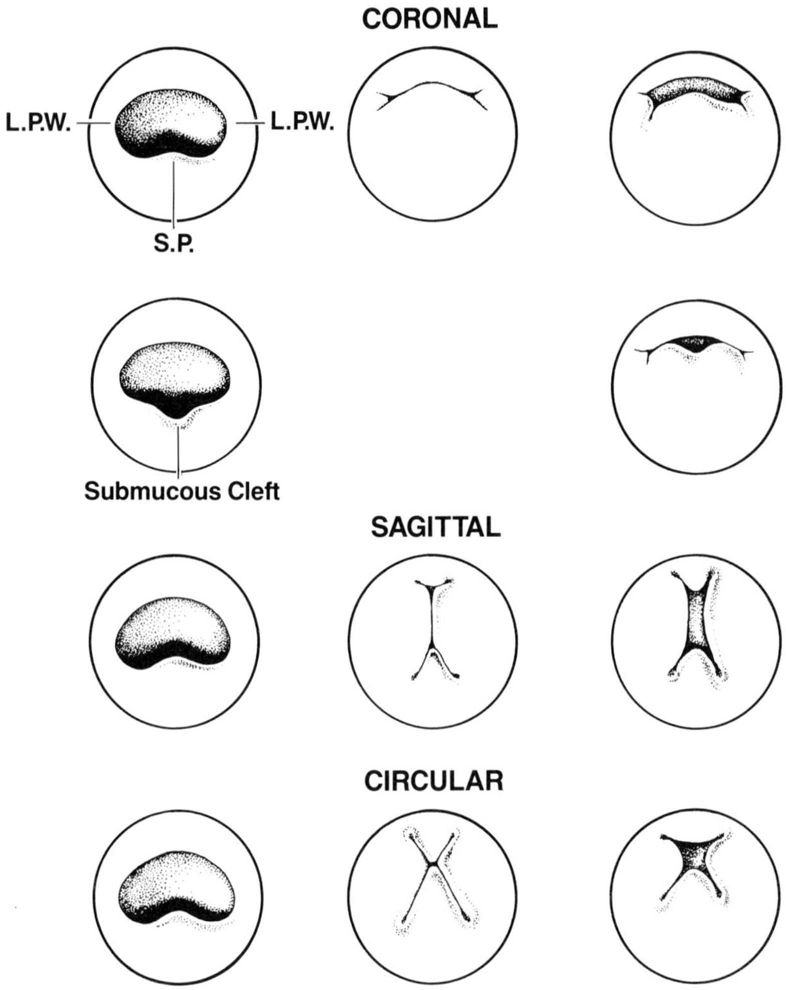

Figure 1 Artist's rendition of velopharyngeal patterns in normal (middle column) and hypernasal (right column) speakers. L.P.W. = lateral pharyngeal wall; S.P. = soft palate. Three patterns of closure are observed: coronal, sagittal, and circular. Note central gap when the central bulge of the musculus uvulae muscle is missing in submucous cleft palate.

air escape. At nasopharyngoscopy, if the tonsils are suspected of interference with velopharyngeal closure, a tonsillectomy without an adenoidectomy is recommended. Reendoscopy may then be performed to assess the competency of velopharyngeal function. An adenoidectomy is contraindicated when the tendency for closure is between the velum and adenoid pad. As a rule, adenoidectomies are avoided for patients who have the stigmata of a submucus cleft.

Mild Hypernasality

Small air leaks, due to a central gap of approximately 4 mm or less, are usually amenable to augmentation of the posterior pharyngeal wall. This defect is commonly present, even with apparently excellent velar movement, when the midline bulge of the musculus uvulae is missing on the dorsum of the soft palate, or when there is a diastasis of the velar musculature. The injection of polytetrafluoroethylene (Teflon paste) at the posterior pharyngeal wall corresponding to the site of insufficiency has had a high rate of success. Unfortunately, this material has been withdrawn from use by the Food and Drug Administration.

My limited experience with collagen as a substitute was promising, but not quite as impressive as Teflon. Until a suitable implant material is available, this degree of insufficiency is managed adequately with a narrow, centralized, pharyngeal flap. A narrow, pharyngeal flap is also indicated for velopharyngeal insufficiencies in the sagittal pattern, where there is excellent movement of the lateral pharyngeal walls. The velopharyngeal port does not have to be maximally obstructed needlessly.

Moderate Hypernasality

A significant amount of air escape results from failure of the velum to reach the posterior pharyngeal wall, with fair movements of the lateral pharyngeal walls. The pattern of insufficiency is usually of the coronal type. Excursions of the lateral pharyngeal walls should be accurately assessed in order to construct a pharyngeal flap with postoperative width that matches the size of the gap. Based on the degree of medial movements of the lateral pharyngeal walls, the flap may be varied from slightly wide to moderately wide. Where there are unequal strengths in wall movements, the flap is skewed to the side of weaker

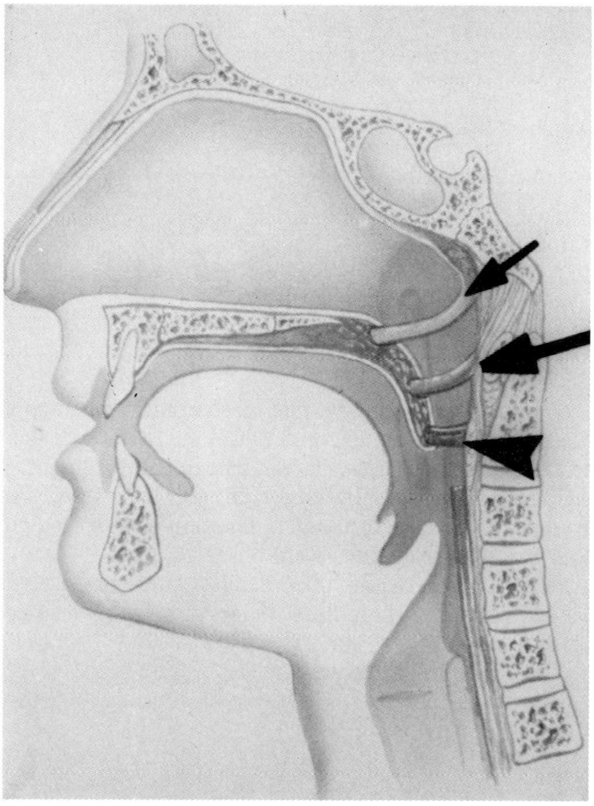

Figure 2 Illustration shows variation in height of the flaps in the nasopharynx and at the site of insertion. Height for narrow (*small arrow*) and wide (*big arrow*) flaps may be altered, depending on vertical level of maximum movement of the lateral pharyngeal wall. Tendency for the pedicle to migrate downward during healing should be taken into consideration. The position of the very wide (subobstructing) flap is low (*arrow head*).

motion. Asymmetrical movements of the lateral pharyngeal walls are commonly encountered among patients with hemifacial microsomia and other syndromic dysmorphology patients with facial asymmetry where the insufficiency is present on the hypoplastic side.

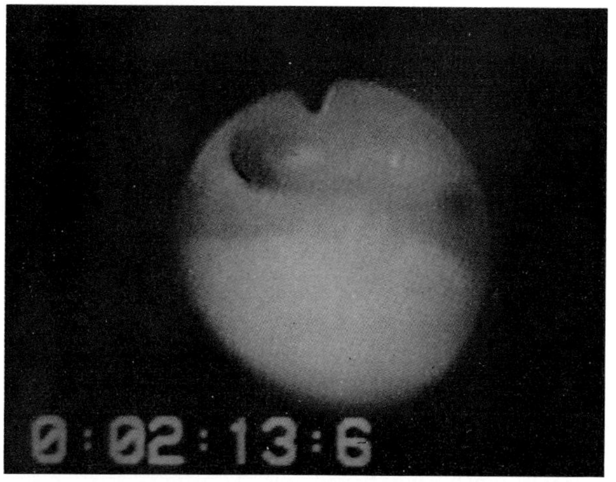

Figure 4 Moderately wide flap, endoscopic view.

Severe Hypernasality

Extreme nasal air emission occurs when velar function is poor in conjunction with weak or absent motion of the lateral pharyngeal walls. In this instance, maximum obturation with a very wide pharyngeal flap is necessary; otherwise, residual hypernasality will persist. Before the procedure is undertaken, patients with a structurally narrow airway (such as Treacher Collins patients) are screened for obstructive sleep apnea, a potentially dangerous condition that could be triggered by subobstruction of the upper airway. Pulsations in the posterior pharyngeal wall, suggestive of aberrant large vessels, should be investigated by angiography, sonography, or magnetic resonance imaging. Although extremely rare, an injury to the internal carotid artery can be a devastating accident.

Candidates for the very wide pharyngeal flap should also be informed of the possible consequences when the nasopharyngeal passage is markedly blocked. These include annoying difficulty in clearing the nose by blowing or sniffling, loud snoring during sleep, occasional noisy breathing during waking hours, and a sense of having a

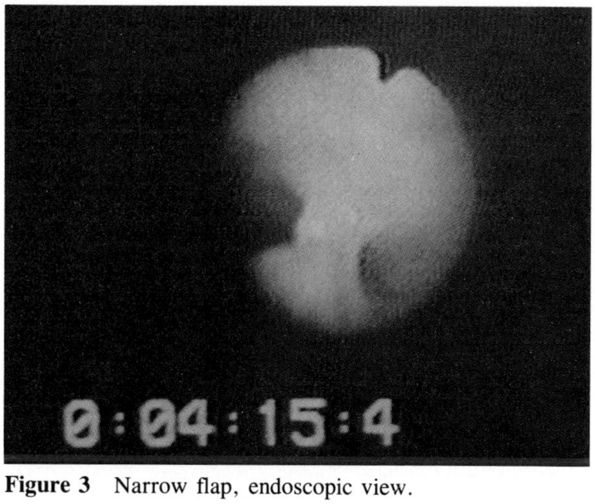

Figure 3 Narrow flap, endoscopic view.

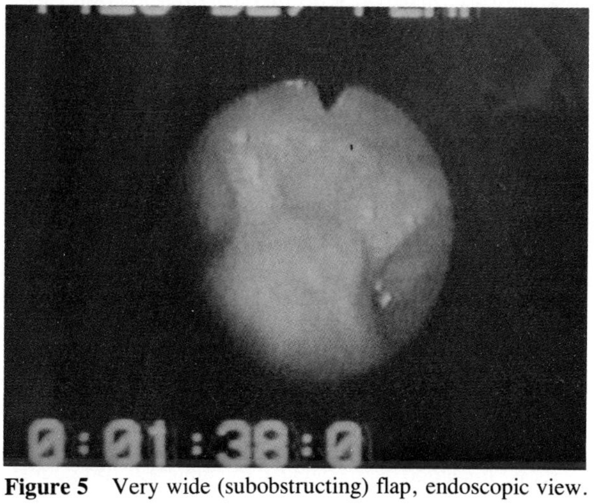

Figure 5 Very wide (subobstructing) flap, endoscopic view.

TABLE 1 Postoperative Results in 180 Patients with Postpalatoplasty Hypernasality

Pharyngeal Flap Type	*No. of Patients*	*Hypernasal*	*Not Hypernasal*	*Hyponasal (intent)*	*Hyponasal (not intent)*
Narrow flaps	37	1	36	0	0
Wide flaps	89	5	84	0	9
Very wide flaps (subobstructing)	54	0	54	11	0
Total	180	6 (3.3%)	174 (96.7%)	11 (6%)	9 (5%)

persistent cold. Hyponasality is common. Young patients seem to tolerate a near total obstruction of the velopharyngeal port much better than adults. As patients grow in stature, their symptoms seem to improve. Among adult patients, the wearing of a well-fitted prosthetic obturator is a tolerable alternative. Such an appliance can be removed at any time including during sleep.

FAILURE OF A PHARYNGEAL FLAP OPERATION

In 20 patients, the two diagnostic modalities mentioned earlier have demonstrated the reasons for failure of the lateral pharyngeal walls to reach the flap and to occlude the lateral portals. In 13 patients, lack of approximation was due to a narrow flap that was well beyond the range of an otherwise good medial movement of the lateral pharyngeal walls. In one patient, the lateral pharyngeal walls moved very poorly. The level of the flap in four patients was at a different height from where the maximum medial movements of the lateral pharyngeal walls occurred. Asymmetrical movements of the lateral pharyngeal walls, or skewing of the flap so that there was a discrepancy in the relationship between the flap and one pharyngeal wall, were observed in three cases.

Since the problems presented were either narrow flaps, wide gaps, or improperly positioned pedicles, another pharyngeal flap was constructed following the principles discussed earlier, i.e., the postoperative width of the new flap was matched with the size and position of the defect in the velopharyngeal tract.

Two additional patients, a singer and a trumpet player, who complained of mild air escape during their musical performances, each had a small flap (superiorly-based, parallel to the original flap) bonded to the first flap on the leaking side.

RESULTS

The speech results of 200 patients with hypernasality, operated on with superiorly-based pharyngeal flaps as described, included a group of 180 consecutive postpalatoplasty patients whose flaps were matched with their velopharyngeal defects, and a group of 20 patients who were postpharyngeal flap failures (unmatched) and had undergone a second pharyngeal flap (matched) procedure.

In the first group, the rate of obturation was highly successful in all flap categories (Table 1). The overall success rate was 97 percent. It should be noted that the high incidence of hyponasality observed with wide flaps was purposely intended in those instances where no lateral pharyngeal wall motions were observed.

In the second group of 20 patients, all hypernasality was eliminated. Of the total number, seven developed denasal speech.

In this series, there were no flap losses, dehiscences, or obstructive episodes. Excessive bleeding occurred in less than 1 percent of cases.

ADVANTAGES

The merit of the procedure lies in its simplicity of execution and its adaptability to variations in the patterns of velopharyngeal insufficiency.

The repaired palate is not reopened for push-back or lengthening procedures, turnover flaps, or other such maneuvers that could risk complications such as fistula formation from wound breakdown or tissue necrosis. There is no strong evidence that any of these additional steps contribute to the improvement in the functional outcome of a pharyngeal flap procedure.

Morbidity is reduced to a minimum. Recovery is rapid, and the hospital stay has been shortened to an average of 3 to 4 days. Results are more predictable, and the success rate is high.

SUGGESTED READING

Argamaso RV. Physical management of velopharyngeal incompetence. J Child Comm Dis 1986; 10:51–57.

Argamaso RV, Shprintzen RJ. Adaptation of a simple single procedure to correct variations in velopharyngeal (VPI) insufficiency: experience in 200 consecutive pharyngeal flaps. Presented at Fifth International Congress on Cleft Palate and Related Craniofacial Anomalies. Monte Carlo, Monaco, Sept. 2–9, 1985.

Argamaso RV, Shprintzen RJ, Strauch B, et al. The role of lateral pharyngeal wall movement in flap surgery. Plast Reconstr Surg 1980; 66:214–219.

Croft CB, Shprintzen RJ, Rakoff SJ. Patterns of velopharyngeal valving in normal and cleft subjects: a multiview videofluoroscopic and nasoendoscopic study. Laryngoscope 1981; XCI:265–271.

Shprintzen RJ, Argamaso RV. Decreasing obstruction with pharyngeal growth following pharyngeal flap surgery. Presented at Second Meeting of the North American Working Group on Cleft Palate and Craniofacial Anomalies. Toronto, Canada, Sept. 1985.

PIERRE ROBIN SEQUENCE

ROBERT W. PARSONS, M.D.

Pierre Robin described respiratory distress in newborns who had a small lower jaw and consequent glossoptosis in 1923. Reports of this clinical picture had previously appeared in the nineteenth century, and a tongue–lip adhesion was proposed as early as 1911. Robin earned his eponym, however, by his insistence on the seriousness of the problem, which might result in death from exhaustion or serious failure to thrive. The Robin sequence may occur as an isolated entity, or as part of other syndromes that also include a small jaw.

The modern terminology of dysmorphology helps us understand this condition, as well as untangle old disputes about whether it results from micrognathia or retrognathia, and whether there is real catch-up growth of the jaw during the early months of life. The cascade of effects from the primary defect of the jaw is referred to as a *sequence*. Thus, we use the term Pierre Robin sequence for this etiologically heterogeneous entity whether the primary defect is a genetic *malformation*, micrognathia, or an intrauterine *deformation,* retrognathia. In either case, the small jaw results in an abnormal posture of the tongue that may prevent the palatal shelves from fusing, if it occurs early enough in fetal development. Thus, a cleft palate is a part of the sequence in about 50 percent of cases. Postnatally, the position of the base of the tongue blocks the airway in the hypopharynx, and extrusion of the tongue is tethered by the retroposed origins of the genioglossus muscles. Deformations tend toward spontaneous improvement when intrauterine influences are eliminated, so that catch-up growth would be expected. However, the child will remain micrognathic in the case of genetic malformation. In either case, the normal vertical growth of the mouth and pharynx tends to provide relief of the respiratory obstruction.

The Robin sequence should be suspected in any baby born with a small lower jaw, especially if there is a cleft palate and if the physical examination shows glossoptosis with a vertical tongue position (Fig. 1). Signs of respiratory obstruction may be noted in the neonatal period, or appear as late as 7 or 8 weeks of age, when it seems there is a period of rapid growth of the tongue. Typically, the child breathes more easily in a prone position, or seated upright. Such babies often have difficulty breathing while eating. When crying and exerting great effort, the baby may be able to keep the tongue forward and ventilate adequately. When tired, the infant falls asleep and the tongue relaxes to produce obstruction. The struggle to breathe then wakes the baby and the effort of crying allows ventilation. Eventually, fatigue makes it impossible to overcome the glossoptosis, and the child may die. Those children who have respiratory distress while eating manifest little or no weight gain and often struggle to maintain their birth weight.

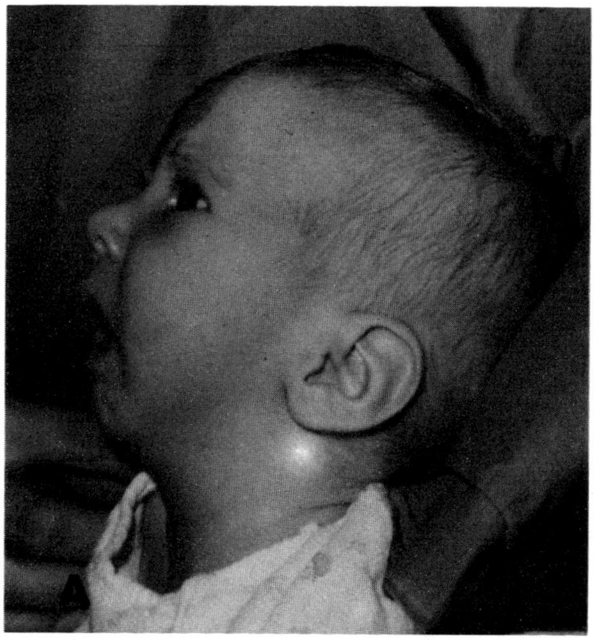

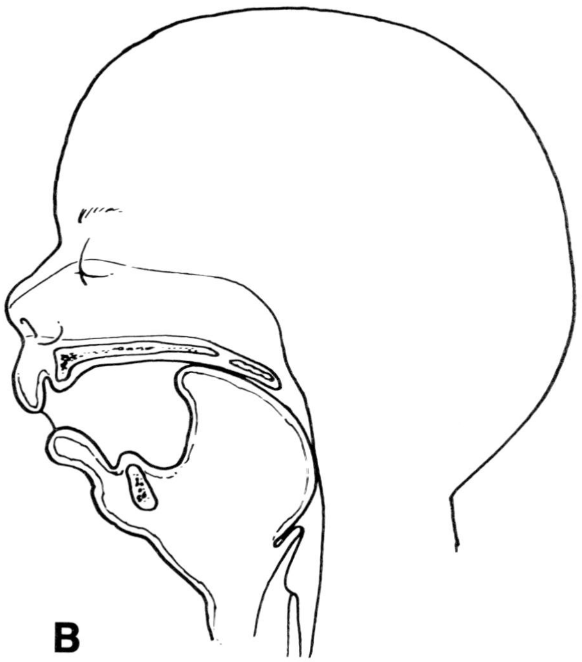

Figure 1 *A,* Infant with typical retrognathia of Robin sequence. *B,* Tracing of lateral x-ray film of head to show retrognathia and glossoptosis with vertical tongue posture. (From Parsons RW, Smith DJ. A modified tongue-lip adhesion for Pierre Robin anomalad. Cleft Palate J 1980; 17:144.

CLINICAL MANAGEMENT

Most babies with a small jaw, with or without a cleft palate, do not have respiratory distress and do not need any special treatment, except observation to be sure that no respiratory or feeding difficulties develop. Most babies with respiratory distress caused by the Robin sequence are successfully managed without surgery by skilled, well-trained neonatologists and nurses in infant intensive care units. Pashayan and Lewis reported 25 consecutive patients who were managed without surgery. The initial step in treatment is to care for the baby in a prone position to allow gravity to assist in keeping the tongue forward. Everything the child needs is done in the prone position, although it may be advantageous for some infants to feed in an upright position while leaning slightly forward. Usually a standard single hole nipple with a crosscut is satisfactory. Various other nipples have been advocated and may be tried if there are problems. Sometimes, it may be useful to use a Breck feeder, which consists of a bulb syringe with a short length of rubber tubing attached. If gavage feedings are necessary, the tube is removed between feedings, provided the airway is patent in the prone position.

When the child has acute obstruction of the airway, it may be necessary to pull the tongue forward mechanically. It has been recommended that a towel clip be used for this purpose, and this is certainly effective. It is important not to grasp the tip of the tongue with the points of the clamp oriented vertically, because the instrument may cut through to produce a bifid tongue. Instead, the dorsum of the tongue should be grasped transversely. Likewise if a heavy suture is placed in the tongue prophylactically for traction in case of obstruction, it should be placed transversely as far back towards the circumvallate papillae as possible (Fig. 2). Traction is then immediately transmitted to the base of the tongue to relieve the obstruction.

In those infants who continue to have respiratory distress or fail to thrive in spite of positioning, the simplest additional step is to place an in-dwelling nasogastric tube. The effect of this is simply to break the seal between the tongue and posterior pharyngeal wall so that the baby can more easily move the tongue to clear the airway. This does increase the risk of aspiration of gastric contents, even with continued prone positioning. Other, usually less effective, measures may include oral and nasal pharyngeal airways to try to bypass the obstructing base of the tongue and prosthetic devices to try to hold the base of the tongue forward. If the airway cannot be controlled by these simpler measures, it is imperative that an endotracheal tube be placed to allow respiration and avoid exhaustion.

It is important to make an accurate diagnosis of the cause of respiratory obstruction, as well as other potential problems that may complicate treatment or be life-threatening in themselves. For example, a baby with a small jaw can also have choanal atresia or laryngotracheal malacia.

SURGICAL MANAGEMENT

Tongue-lip adhesion is the most conservative step available for management of those few infants with Pierre Robin sequence who have persistent respiratory obstruction after an adequate trial of nonsurgical management. There is no precise definition of when a tongue-lip adhesion is indicated, but there are potential complications of

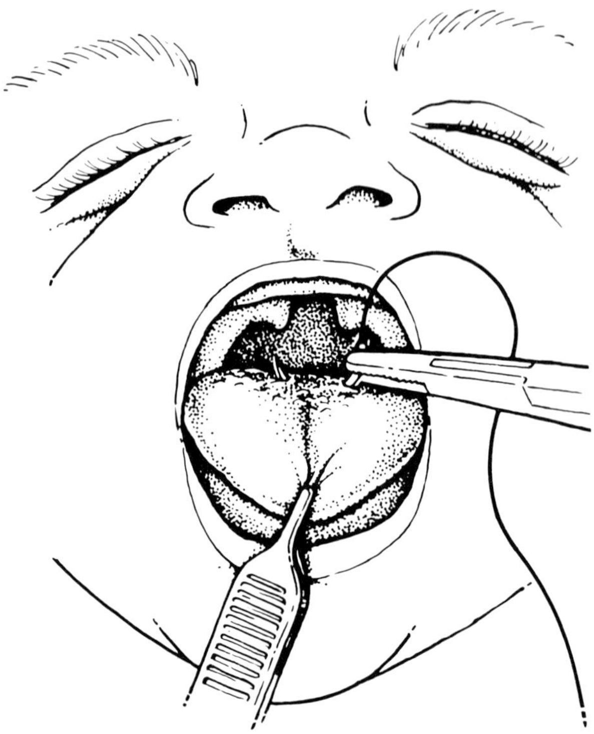

Figure 2 Proper placement of tongue stitch for control of base of tongue in respiratory emergency. (From Parsons RW, Smith DJ. A modified tongue-lip adhesion for Pierre Robin anomalad. Cleft Palate J 1980; 17:144.

long term endotracheal intubation, as well as continuing risks of aspiration and respiratory obstruction. There is also a considerable economic cost for prolonged care in an intensive care unit. We have proposed a rule-of-thumb that a tongue-lip adhesion should be done for babies who do not establish a progressive gain in weight and strength after 7 days of nonoperative intensive care, or those who cannot be successfully extubated after 3 days of endotracheal intubation.

The tongue-lip adhesion was originally proposed by Shukowsky, and was popularized by Douglas with considerable improvement in prognosis for these babies. The modifications of Routledge and Randall reduced the likelihood of injury to the teeth and sublingual ducts and resulted in better control of the base of the tongue. Parsons and Smith further modified Randall's procedure by placing the incisions on the tongue near the floor of the mouth and by freeing the genioglossus muscles from the mandible to allow the obstructing base of the tongue to move further forward.

Tongue-lip adhesions have been tried and abandoned by some surgeons because of dehiscence or failure to relieve the obstruction. These problems should be rare if attention is paid to the technical requirements of a broad area of adhesion, a release of the genioglossus muscles to bring the *base* of the tongue well forward, and a satisfactory glossopexy suture to splint the adhesion during early healing.

Endotracheal anesthesia is used. If the baby has not been intubated already, the pediatric anesthesiologist should be aware of the difficulties and danger of intubation. An experienced surgeon should be present and ready to perform emergency tracheostomy if there is obstruction and the anesthesiologist is unable to place the endotracheal tube. Intubation should be done awake.

Lidocaine 0.25 percent with epinephrine 1:400,000 is infiltrated beneath the mucosa to be incised on the lip and tongue. A transverse incision is made across the mucosa of the tongue just above the floor of the mouth, high enough to avoid injury to the openings of the sublingual glands. The incision is deepened to expose the genioglossus muscles, which are stripped from their origins on the mandible by blunt scissors dissection (Fig. 3*A*). The tongue can then be brought well forward to eliminate the glossoptosis.

A mucosal flap based on the labial sulcus is dissected in the lower lip, long enough to reach the tongue incision and nearly as wide as the lip. This flap is to be turned back over the alveolar ridge and sutured to the inferior margin of the tongue incision (Fig. 3*B*). The flap creates a continuous raw surface for the adhesion that extends from the floor of the mouth onto the lip, but without damage to the alveolus or obstruction of the salivary glands.

The glossopexy suture is passed through one side of the tongue on a reversed Keith needle using a heavy needle holder. The operator's index finger is placed at the base of the tongue, just above the epiglottis, to guide the needle, and one end of this suture is caught with a hook and threaded through a button (Fig. 3*C*). A second Mersilene loop is passed through the other side of the tongue and used to bring the suture back through the tongue (Fig. 3*D*). A length of Mersilene suture is tied to the button before it is put into place so that it can later be retrieved when the glossopexy suture is removed.

The sutures between the lip flap and tongue mucosa are then placed, using 4–0 chromic catgut. Both ends of the glossopexy suture are next passed over the mandible with Keith needles used to bring them out beneath the chin. The muscle of the tongue is sutured to the muscle of the lip on either side of the midline with 4–0 absorbable synthetic suture, and the mucosal suture lines are all closed. The forward position of the tongue is supported by the mucosal sutures at this point.

The ends of the glossopexy sutures are then passed through a submental button and tied (Fig. 3*E*). The tension should hold the base of the tongue forward to maintain relief of glossoptosis, but excessive tension is avoided. The glossopexy suture always tends to cut through the mucosa of the base of the tongue, as well as the skin beneath the chin, because of tension. The glossopexy suture is removed when the buttons are loose, usually between 6 and 10 days postoperatively. The use of a glossopexy suture alone, without the tongue-lip adhesion, is not advisable because of the tendency of the suture to cut through the tissue under tension. On the other hand, the tongue-lip adhesion without an effective glossopexy suture has a high rate of dehiscence.

At the completion of the operation, the tongue protrudes through the lips, but the surgical adhesion is behind the tip of the tongue and below the vermilion border. The tip of the tongue returns to the mouth after several days, thereby allowing the lip to close although the base of the tongue remains forward.

The endotracheal tube is left in place for 24 to 48 hours. Extubation should be done with the patient fully awake and with emergency airway equipment available. Usually, the infant can breathe normally through the nose at this time. Postoperatively, the patient is fed with a Breck feeder. A definite gain in weight and strength should be noted within a few days.

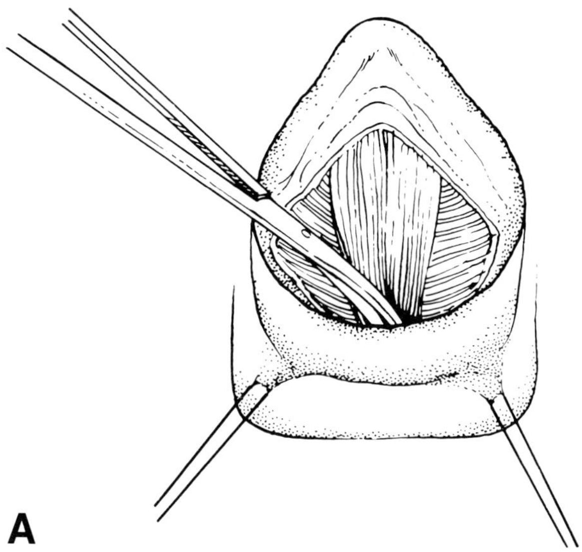

A

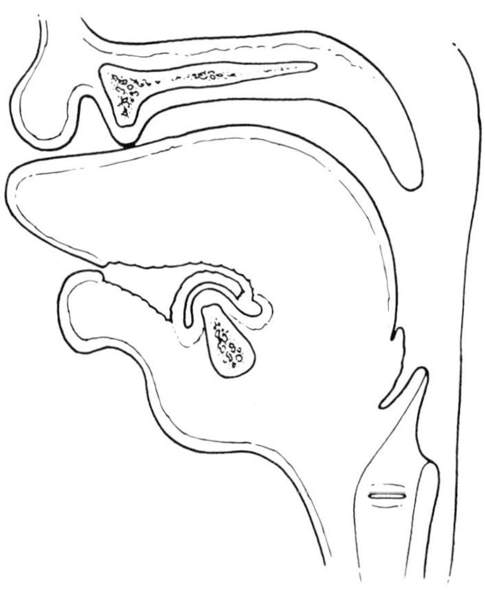

B

Figure 3 *A,* Transverse tongue incision opens widely as genioglossus muscles are released from mandible. *B,* Lip flap is reflected over alveolus to create broad saw surface for adhesion.

Figure continues on following page

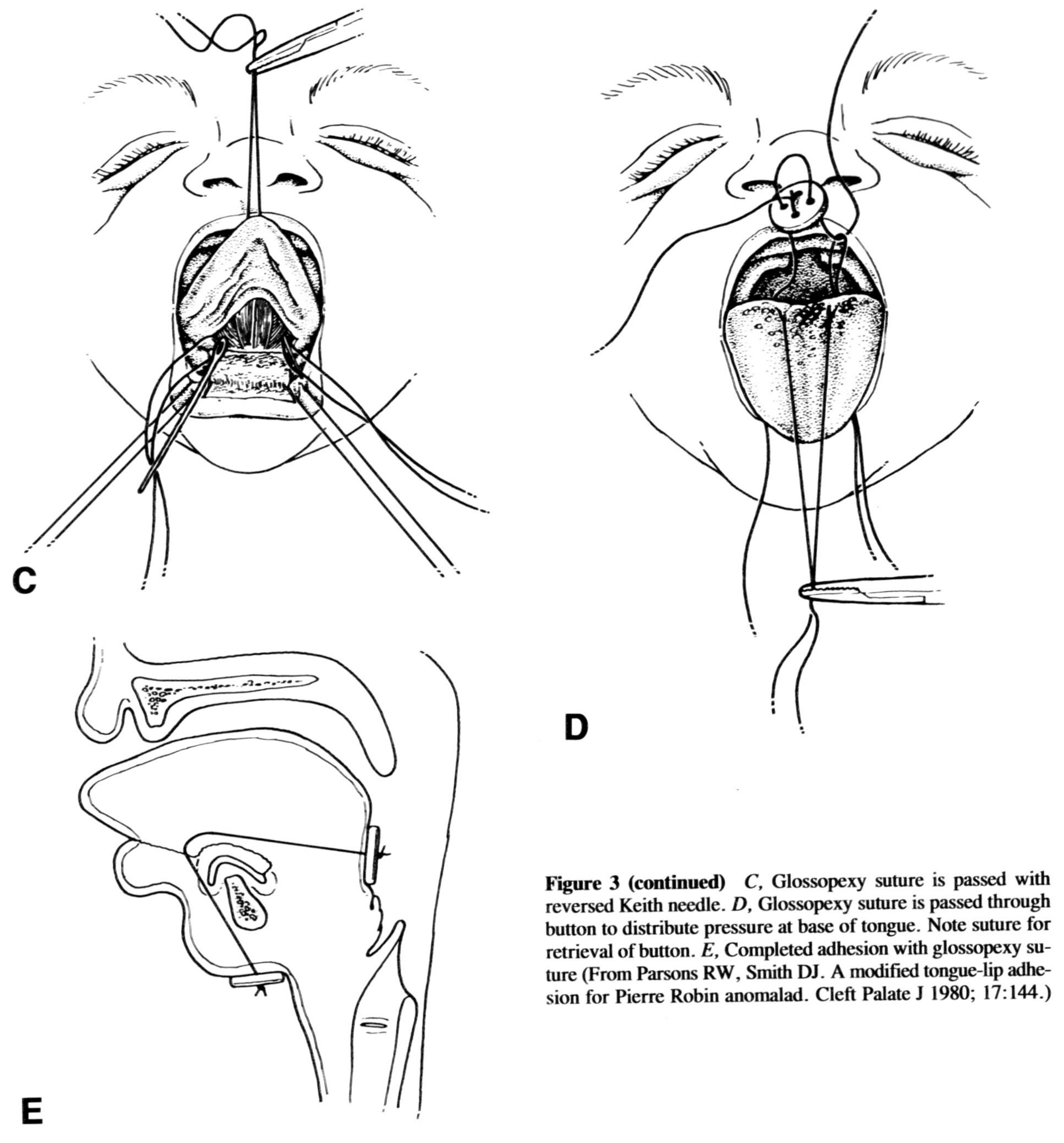

Figure 3 (continued) *C,* Glossopexy suture is passed with reversed Keith needle. *D,* Glossopexy suture is passed through button to distribute pressure at base of tongue. Note suture for retrieval of button. *E,* Completed adhesion with glossopexy suture (From Parsons RW, Smith DJ. A modified tongue-lip adhesion for Pierre Robin anomalad. Cleft Palate J 1980; 17:144.)

There is no great urgency about taking down the tongue-lip adhesion. In a child with a cleft palate, this is usually done at the time of palate repair—at 10 to 12 months of age. In the meantime, the tip of the tongue is mobile enough for eating and sucking motions. Teeth can and do erupt in the tunnel beneath the adhesion, and saliva can drain from the sublingual glands. There is a tendency for tartar to accumulate on the teeth, which should be scaled when the adhesion is lysed.

An alternative procedure has been advocated by Hadley and Johnson and continues to be referenced in current textbooks. It consists of holding the base of the tongue forward while a Kirschner wire is driven across the tissues from one angle of the jaw to the other. The base of the tongue is then skewered in a more anterior position. This operation seems to have the disadvantage of the highly mobile tongue being held forward with a rigid wire. This would be expected to progressively cut through the tissues as the tongue moves, so that it would be useful for a limited time period. However, good experience has been reported with this method.

Tracheostomy is reserved for those rare infants who cannot be intubated endotracheally in an emergency situation; those whose additional diagnoses make tongue-lip adhesion inappropriate; and, of course, those in whom tongue-lip adhesion fails for whatever reason. With careful attention to the basic technical principles, tongue-lip adhesion should be the preferred and eminently satisfactory conservative alternative to tracheostomy in nearly all babies with the Pierre Robin sequence.

Patients with this sequence often have a wide U-shaped palatal defect that is technically difficult to close. In some babies, a progressive narrowing of the cleft can be observed, and surgical closure can be delayed until it is technically easier. In a few patients, the palatal cleft may remain so wide that surgical closure does not become possible and a prosthetic obturator may be necessary.

There have been reports of respiratory problems when pharyngeal flaps were done in children with Pierre Robin sequence, either simultaneously with the palate repair or later. The pharyngeal flap may result in obstruction of an already compromised upper airway, thus causing alveolar hypoventilation, hypoxia and hypocapnia, and pulmonary vasoconstriction. This leads to a reduction in the pulmonary vascular bed and an increased pulmonary artery resistence with pulmonary hypertension, right ventricular hypertrophy, and cor pulmonale. This chain of events may not be clinically obvious and may manifest itself as a late postoperative failure to thrive. In such a situation, it is mandatory to improve the airway by modifying or taking down the pharyngeal flap.

This overall approach to the Robin sequence has the advantage of a graded, conservative series of steps aimed at the specific problem of the glossoptosis and respiratory obstruction. With skilled, intensive neonatal care, surgery of any kind should be reserved for those infants who cannot spontaneously maintain an effective airway after 3 days of rest, or who do not establish a definite weight gain pattern in 7 days. The tongue-lip adhesion described is an effective alternative to tracheostomy in infants who do not have other pathologic reasons for respiratory obstruction.

SUGGESTED READING

Douglas B. The treatment of micrognathia associated with obstruction by a plastic procedure. Plast Reconstr Surg 1946; 1:300–308.

Hadley RC, Johnson JB. Utilization of the Kirschner wire in Pierre Robin syndrome. Plast Reconstr Surg 1963; 31:587–596.

Parsons RW, Smith DJ. Rule of thumb criteria for tongue-lip adhesion in Pierre Robin anomalad. Plast Reconstr Surg 1982; 70:210–212.

Parsons RW, Smith DJ. A modified tongue-lip adhesion for Pierre Robin anomalad. Cleft Palate J 1980; 17:144–147.

Pashayan HM, Lewis MB. Clinical experience with the Robin sequence. Cleft Palate J 1984; 21:270–276.

Randall P. The Robin anomalad: micrognathia and glossoptosis with airway obstruction. In: Converse JM, ed. Reconstructive plastic surgery. 2nd ed. Philadelphia: WB Saunders, 1977:2235.

Robin P. La chute de la base de la langue considérée comme une nouvelle cause du gêne dans la respiration naso-pharyngiene. Bull Acad Med (Paris) 1923; 89:37–42.

Routledge RT. The Pierre Robin syndrome: a surgical emergency in the neonatal period. Br J Plast Surg 1960; 13:204–218.

ALVEOLAR BONE GRAFTING: EARLY

BRUCE S. BAUER, M.D., F.A.C.S.

Considerable controversy exists over whether or not there is a place for primary bone grafting in the treatment of a child with cleft lip and palate. This controversy followed multiple early reports that documented the detrimental effect of this technique on facial growth.

Long-term follow-up of the experience at The Children's Memorial Hospital, Chicago, has demonstrated that primary bone grafting can be used safely and effectively, without significant growth attenuation and with significant long-term benefits. Our approach is described below and clearly demonstrates that the technique differs vastly from those techniques associated with poor results.

Since early bone grafting can be performed safely, the issue is whether early placement provides a benefit. This issue is addressed here with supporting evidence of this benefit.

THERAPEUTIC ALTERNATIVES

As in all other aspects of treatment of cleft palate, there are many approaches to attainment of a particular therapeutic goal. In the present case, the goal is a precise dental alignment with a U-shaped maxillary arch, without collapse of the lesser segment(s) and resultant crossbite.

Alveolar arch molding is directed initially by the use of neonatal orthodontics prior to lip repair and, secondarily, by using the posterior muscle forces against the alveolus following lip repair. This molding is guided by a passive palatal appliance.

Many surgeons feel that an appliance needs regular and repeated adjustments until there is stabilization of arch form at the time of mixed dentition. Others choose initially to ignore the problem and rely on late arch expansion and lengthy orthodontic treatment, in the fear that any early surgical insult to the maxillary segments may result in significant inhibition of growth.

Combined use of neonatal orthodontics and minimal surgical dissection and grafting to stabilize the aligned arch following the use of a single, passive, palatal appliance, offers the benefit of a stable, functional arch that simplifies later orthodontic treatment and avoids significant growth attenuation.

PREFERRED APPROACH

Early, or primary, bone grafting is performed at our institution in all children with complete clefts of both primary and secondary palate (unilateral and bilateral) according to the following standard sequence:

1. An impression is taken and the acrylic palatal appliance (self-retaining) is placed prior to lip repair.
2. Lip repair is routinely carried out at 6 to 8 weeks of age.
3. Arch molding occurs following the lip repair, guided by the external force of lip musculature and internal restraint against collapse of the appliance.
4. The alveolus is bone-grafted when the alveolar segments have aligned and are at maximum 2 to 3 mm apart. (Generally, grafting is not performed earlier than 3 months after lip repair, even if segments abut earlier.)
5. The appliance is retained for at least 8 weeks after the bone graft to maintain stability during healing. Use after that is optional until the time of palate repair (which is at 12 months or less), if it is preferred by the infant during feeding.

In general, the only alterations from this sequence and timing are in cases of bilateral complete cleft lip and palate where the protruding premaxilla is manipulated into more favorable alignment with elastic tape traction before lip repair (thereby delaying the age of lip repair), and in cases where the gap between the alveolar segments remains wide for a prolonged period and the procedure has to be bypassed so as not to delay the palate closure beyond the usual time. In the latter case, the bone grafting is carried out secondarily.

The point that should be emphasized, and is often misunderstood, is that the early bone grafting is carried out only after the arch segments are properly aligned (with maximum 2 to 3 mm gap). Therefore, at no time is extensive dissection needed to place the graft (infra.). This is a key difference between the technique described here and many of the older, abandoned procedures.

SURGICAL TECHNIQUE

The Bone Graft

The bone graft is harvested through an incision that lies at the level of the inframammary crease, positioned so that its medial extent overlies the costochondral junction. In general, the right fifth rib is taken. A 2.5 to 3.5 cm length of rib is taken by subperiosteal dissection from the junction laterally. A slightly longer graft may be taken in bilateral cases. The wound is closed in layers after pleural integrity is assured. Drainage of the wound is not routinely required.

The graft is split with an osteotome and bent to conform to the alveolar curve with cortex outward. The width of the rib is decreased slightly (to approximately 6 mm) and all bone chips are saved.

Dissection of the Alveolus

Flaps are designed along the margin of the alveolar cleft in conjunction with a horizontal incision along the labial sulcus approximately 2 cm on either side of the cleft. As the flaps along the cleft margin are elevated, they fold backward toward one another like the pages of a book. These flaps provide the posterior layer of closure; therefore, dissection is not required posterior to the alveolus. Anterior coverage is obtained by elevation of a mucosal flap through the sulcus incision outward toward the lip margin. This dissection is limited to that required to provide tension-free closure (Figs. 1 to 4).

The anterior dissection proceeds down to the bone with a periosteal elevator along the cleft margin medially and laterally thereby creating a pocket for the graft. The dissection is limited in extent to avoid graft migration and minimize surgical trauma to the maxillary segments. Care is taken not to disrupt the previous nasal floor repair.

Posterior closure is completed before graft placement. The posterior layer is closed with 5–0 chromic catgut. In bilateral cleft cases, the elevation and subsequent closure of the posterior layer is facilitated by side-to-side movement of the premaxilla.

The graft is placed in the pocket so that the main piece of graft spans the cleft, sits snugly within the pocket and rests on the anterior surface of the maxilla. The bone graft does not extend inferiorly into the margin of the alveolus. The remaining extra pieces of bone are converted to chips and packed tightly behind the bridging graft. The labial mucosal flap is then sutured both to the inferior margin of the "book" flaps and to the free edge of the incised alveolar mucosa for completion of the procedure. Closure is facilitated by placement of all of the anterior layer sutures before they are tied down. This provides an accurate edge-to-edge sealed closure and avoids loss of graft chips.

Routine postcleft repair precautions (elbow restraints and syringe feeding for 10 days) are maintained to allow healing. The palatal appliance is left untouched for approximately 2 weeks before routine cleansing procedures

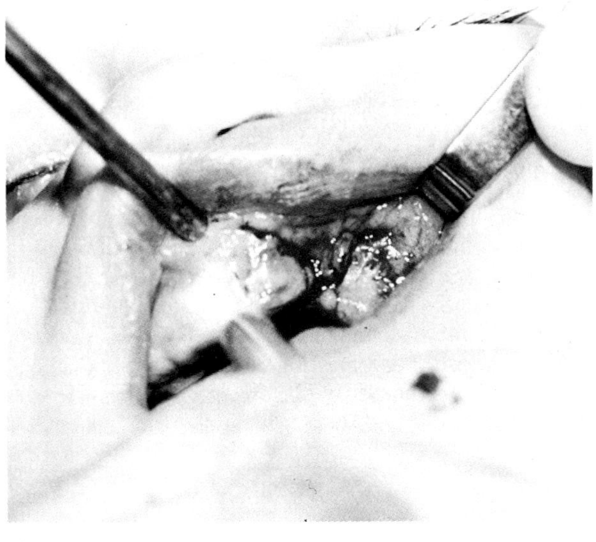

Figure 1 Alveolar segments are in close apposition prior to alveolar bone graft in patient with cleft lip and palate. The incision is marked with methylene blue.

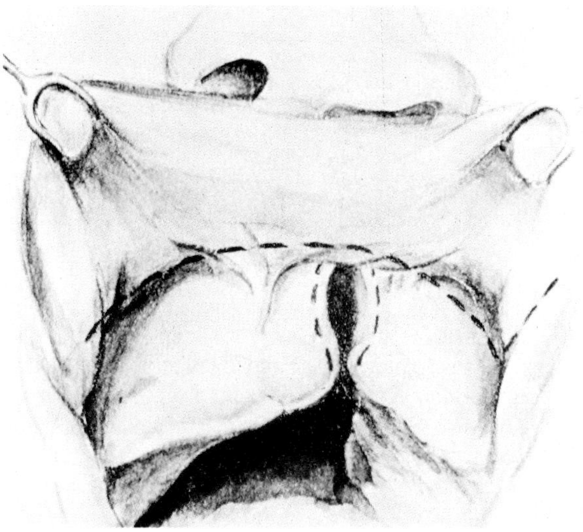

Figure 2 Illustration of incision along cleft margin and in sulcus. Lateral and medial extent of sulcus incision are usually less than illustrated.

are resumed. It is imperative that the palatal appliance be worn for at least 8 weeks following grafting.

Therapeutic Outcome

Following the prescribed technique, the alveolar and maxillary segments are stabilized in the ideal configuration within the first 6 months of life. The single palatal appliance is generally discarded several days before the palate repair but, as noted above, use beyond 8 weeks postgrafting is for the infant's convenience only. The procedure is extremely well tolerated and the complication rate is near zero percent.

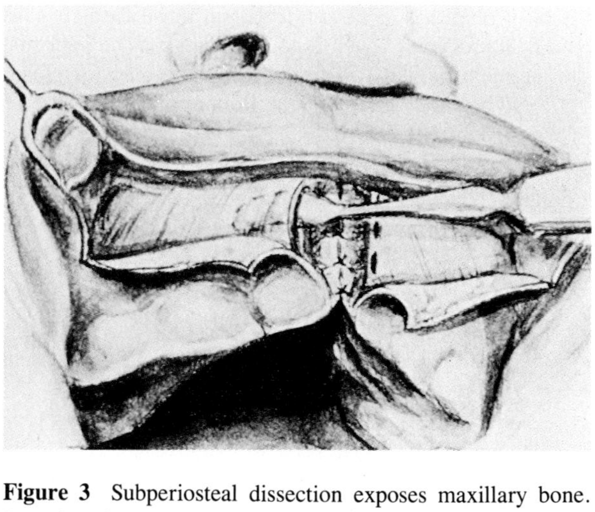

Figure 3 Subperiosteal dissection exposes maxillary bone. Posterior closure with "book" flaps from cleft margin is illustrated.

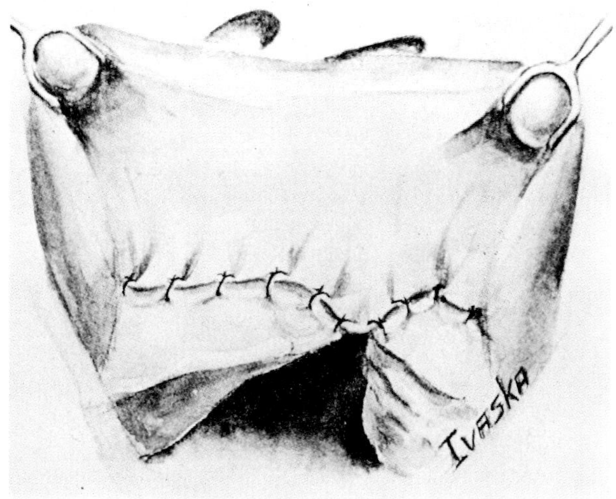

Figure 4 Anterior closure is obtained by advancement of mucosal flap from sulcus. (Figs. 2 to 4 are from Rosenstein SW, Monroe CW, Kernahan DA, et al. The case for early bone grafting in cleft lip and cleft palate. Plast Reconstr Surg 1982; 70:297–307.)

Long-term follow-up by independent observers has demonstrated that the limited dissection described above is not associated with the growth attenuation previously described with those techniques that involved extensive dissection posterior to the alveolus and into the prevomerine and transpalatine suture areas. Further study has shown little difference in maxillary growth between cases of cleft lip and palate that were not grafted and those that were grafted primarily following the above protocol.

The presence of bone in the cleft has facilitated spontaneous eruption of teeth into the area of the previous cleft and/or the orthodontic manipulation of teeth into the grafted bone, thus significantly simplifying later orthodontic treatment.

Two additional benefits of this technique and approach, which have drawn little attention, are: (1) the additional bone present beneath the alar base fills an area of frequent bone deficiency and provides the appropriate foundation for optimal correction of the nasal deformity, and (2) the alveolar dissection and closure facilitates later closure of the anterior hard palate cleft.

SUGGESTED READING

Dahl E, Hanusardotter B, Bergland O. A comparison of occlusions in two groups of children whose clefts were repaired by three different surgical procedures. Cleft Palate J 1981; 18:122.

Hellquist R, Ponten B. The influence of infant periosteoplasty on facial growth and dental occlusion from five to eight years of age in cases of complete unilateral cleft lip and palate. Scand J Plast Reconstr Surg 1979; 13:305.

Nordin KE, Johanson B. Freie Knochentransplantation bei Defekten im

Alveolar-kamm nach kiefer-orthopädischer Einstellung der Maxilla bei Lippen-Kiefer-Gaumenspalten. Fortschr Kiefer Gesichtschir, Bd. 1. Stuttgart: Thieme, 1955.

Rosenstein SW, Monroe CW, Kernahan DA, et al. The case for early bone grafting in cleft lip and cleft palate. Plast Reconstr Surg 1982; 70:297–307.

Ross RB. The clinical implications of facial growth in cleft lip and palate. Cleft Palate J 1970; 7:37.

Ross RB. Treatment variables affecting facial growth in complete unilateral cleft lip and palate. Part 3: Alveolus repair and bone grafting. Cleft Palate J 1987; 24:33–44.

Ross RB. Treatment variables affecting facial growth in complete unilateral cleft lip and palate. Part 7: An overview of treatment and facial growth. Cleft Palate J 1987; 24:71–77.

ALVEOLAR BONE GRAFTING: LATER

A. MICHAEL SADOVE, M.D., F.A.C.S.
CHARLES L. NELSON, D.D.S.
JAMES E. JONES, D.M.D., M.S., M.S.D.

Although considerable controversy still remains concerning the clinical advisability of early alveolar bone grafting, later or secondary osteoplasty is now well accepted. This acceptance stems from the fact that children born with complete clefts have a deficiency in the osseous make-up of their maxilla that leads to several significant functional as well as emotional problems. These problems may include inadequate bony support to the alar base of the nose or to teeth adjacent to the cleft site. This osseous inadequacy also explains the lack of maxillary arch continuity that leads to frequent collapse of the lesser segment (in unilateral clefts) or of the two lateral segments (in bilateral clefts). Further clinical problems associated with secondary alveolar clefts include patent oronasal fistulas that may cause speech or hygiene problems as a result of oronasal reflux.

Patients with bilateral complete clefts have additional problems because of an increased number of at risk teeth adjacent to the cleft sites. If these osseous deficiencies are not dealt with properly, permanent teeth may be lost. This may lead to mucosal-lined periodontal pockets that can increase in size, thus leading to further bony resorption. This unstable osseous condition may limit achievement of even a prosthetic solution to the problem. If the maxillary teeth are not lost into the cleft site, they still may erupt ectopically into the posterior segments or premaxilla; this can cause a problem because of dental crowding. The crowding cannot be dealt with adequately until the segments are aligned and grafted so that teeth may be moved safely into the cleft area with orthodontic treatment.

For all the above reasons, later or secondary bone grafting has been accepted by our cleft team.

THERAPEUTIC ALTERNATIVES

Indications for Bone Grafting

Secondary alveolar bone grafting is indicated in patients with complete clefts (unilateral and bilateral) who have residual osseous deficiency associated with the following: (1) inadequate nasal alar base support; (2) deficient periodontal support; (3) dental arch collapse; or (4) oronasal reflux. Secondary grafts may be indicated in patients who had previous surgeries (primary graft or periosteoplasty) that resulted in osseous inadequacy. Later cleft osteoplasty is also indicated in those patients with unstable prosthetic solutions because of mobile maxillary segments.

Prosthetic Management Alternative

Prosthetic closure of the patent alveolar cleft may at times be an acceptable treatment alternative. This situation could arise in patients who require restoration because of associated congenital dental problems such as ectodermal dysplasia. Prosthetic management may also be indicated in the complex cleft patient with skeletal malocclusion, oronasal fistula, and palatal inadequacy in whom a multidisciplinary, multistaged, treatment plan may be neither financially feasible nor desirable.

Contraindications

The procedure may be contraindicated in those patients with complete clefts who are satisfied and symptom free despite the presence of an osseous defect. Patients with soft tissue inadequacy form another group in which grafting is relatively contraindicated. The procedure is only *relatively* contraindicated in these cases because surgical procedures such as tongue flaps may be performed to augment palatal soft tissue, thus allowing for closure of large palatoalveolar defects. Bone grafting may then be carried out at a later date.

Secondary cleft osteoplasty is absolutely contraindicated in noncompliant patients with poor oral hygiene (gingivitis, caries) in whom the procedure would meet with an unacceptable incidence of failure.

PREFERRED APPROACH

Timing of Therapy

Later or secondary bone grafting is best carried out during the late primary dentition or early mixed dentition stages (5 to 8 years of age). This relative time period is usually selected because of the presence of maxillary molars, which allow placement of expansion devices to correct the dental arch form (Fig. 1, see Fig. 1B). This time period is also desirable because the graft may be placed prior to eruption of the permanent maxillary dentition (see Figs. 1D, 1E and 1F) so that the teeth will not be lost into the cleft site.

Graft Material

Although numerous sources of graft material have been described in the literature, our donor site of choice remains the iliac crest. This donor area allows a two-team approach to be employed, thereby decreasing the total operative time. Donor site problems have been rare (less than 1 percent) and none have been permanent in duration.

Operative Technique

The maxillary labial vestibule adjacent to the alveolar cleft is infiltrated with 3 or 4 cc of 1:200,000 epinephrine solution to aid in hemostasis. Infiltration should also include nasal mucosa accessible through the cleft site and palatal mucosa immediately adjacent to the cleft. We have used several flap designs to accomplish the cleft graft, but our usual and preferred approach is illustrated in Figures 2 and 3 (see Figs. 2A and 3A).

Vertical incisions are made through attached gingiva on the lateral cleft walls superiorly to the level of the nasal floor. These incisions are extended to the proximal surfaces of the adjacent teeth and around these teeth both labially and palatally. Posteriorly, the incision is usually released into the mucolabial fold. Full-thickness mucoperiosteal flaps are developed labially, and the anterior aspect of the nasal floor closure is developed by dissecting the nasal mucosa away from the labial mucosa in a split-thickness fashion. Scissors or a surgical blade are used to free palatal mucosa from nasal mucosa, thereby allowing closure of the nasal floor in the posterior aspect of the palatal cleft (see Figs. 2B and 3B). This dissection is carried posteriorly to include the patent palatal fistula if one exists.

The full-thickness palatal mucosal leaflets are approximated using resorbable simple interrupted or horizontal mattress sutures. The nasal floor closure can be technically difficult while the flaps for this closure are deve-

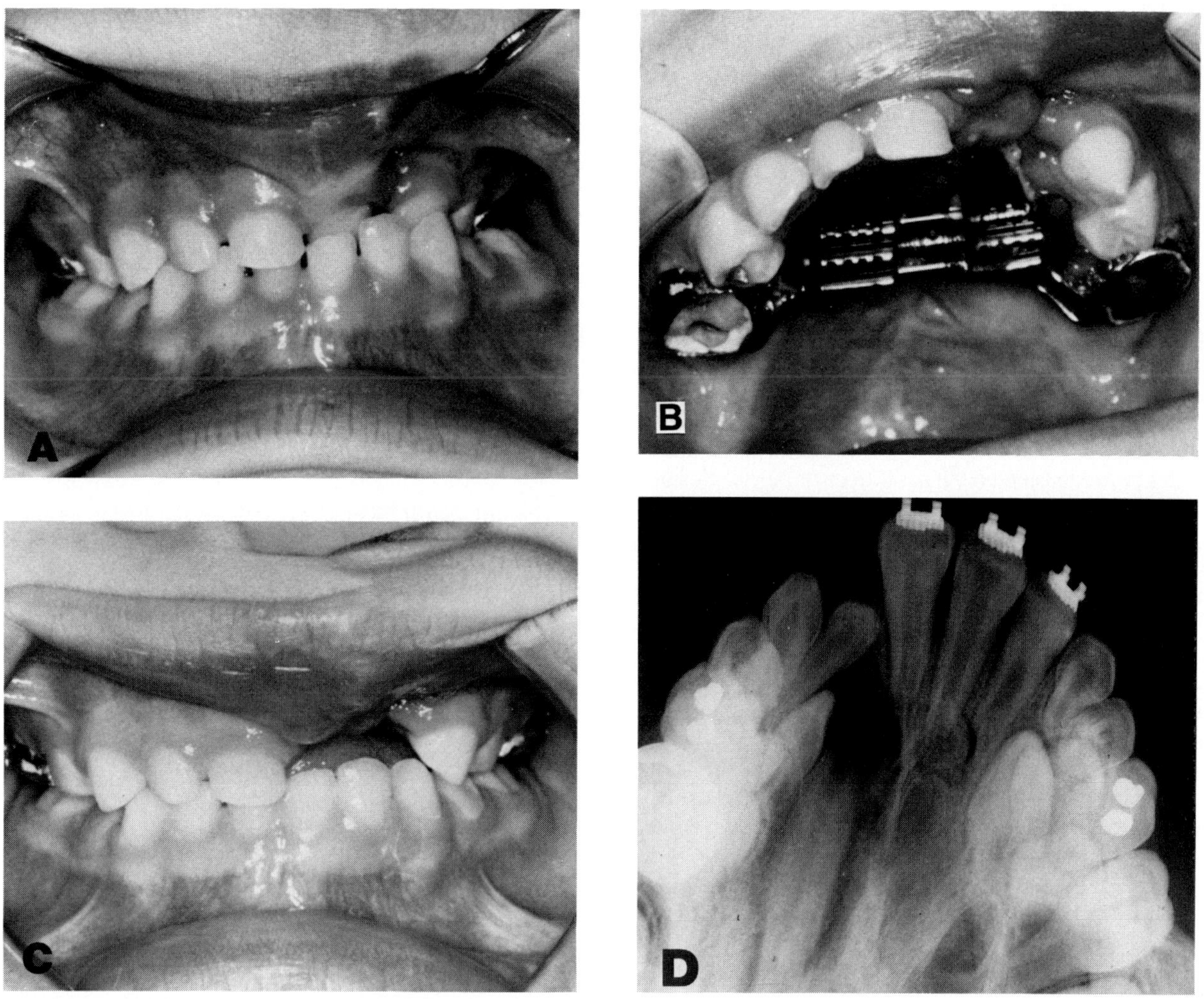

Figure 1 Arch collapse in unilateral complete cleft. *A*, Segmental crossbites requiring correction; *B*, correction is achieved with some form of expansion device; *C*, the desired arch conformation; *D*, grafting of the deficient area may now be carried out.

Figure continues on following page

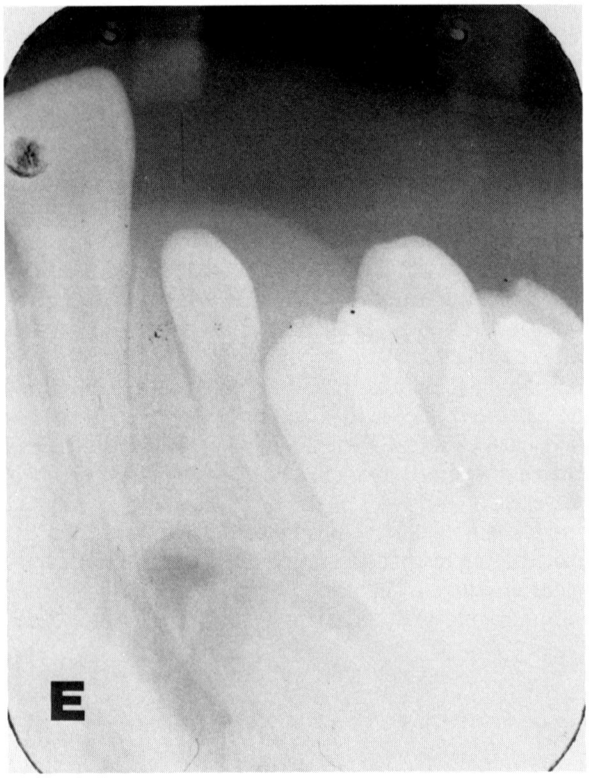

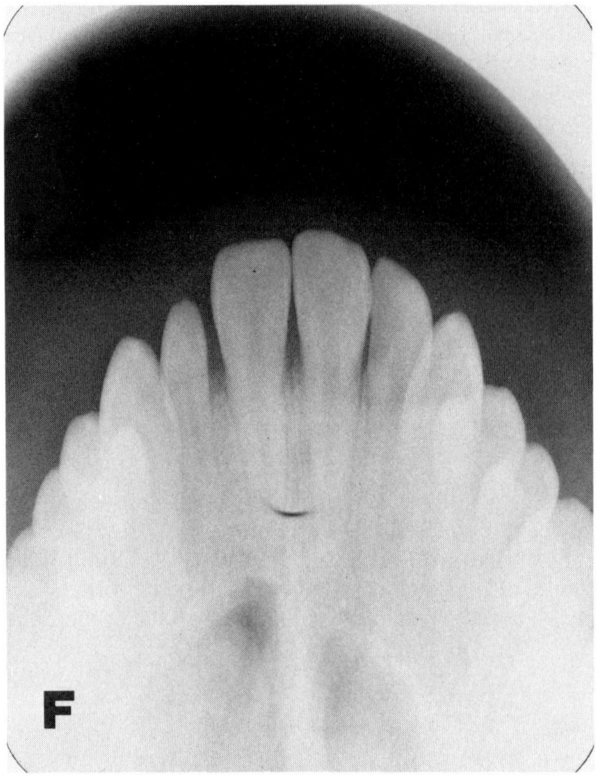

Figure 1 (continued) *E*, the permanent dentition then erupts into the graft; and *F*, this allows later orthodontic alignment.

loped and the posterior aspect is sutured through a narrow cleft site. We use resorbable (usually chromic) gut on a small half-circle needle and a Castroviejo type needle holder. A running suture technique is used to close the nasal floor from anterior to posterior (see Figs. 2C and 3C). This effectively closes the patent oronasal fistula. Cancellous bone harvested from the iliac crest is now packed into the cleft defect to fill the entire alveolus and anterior hard palate (see Figs. 2D and 3D). The bone should be packed densely, but not with such force that it creates undue tension on the nasal floor or palatal closure.

The labial flaps are repositioned and sutured in place with resorbable suture material (see Figs. 2E and 3E). Closure must be without tension; as a result, we often incise underlying periosteum to allow maximum flap mobility.

The technique for secondary grafting in bilateral cleft is not appreciably different. With judicious development of flaps to assure adequate blood supply to the premaxilla, a simultaneous osteotomy and premaxillary setback can be performed at the time of secondary cleft grafting. However, if concomitant Le Fort I osteotomy is necessary, we defer the osteotomy until at least 6 months postgrafting.

Postoperative Care

The patient is usually discharged on the second postoperative day (sooner if donor site drainage is not necessary). Oral hygiene is maintained with frequent mouth rinses. The patient is maintained on a soft diet for 2 to 3 weeks.

An occlusal radiograph is taken at a follow-up appointment approximately 2 weeks postoperatively and again at 2 months to ascertain the integrity of the graft (see Fig. 1E). When the graft has been successful, an orthodontist can begin movement of teeth around and/or into the grafted area.

Therapeutic Outcome

Failures with this technique have not been common (5 percent). Failures usually manifest as loss of the graft and/or reopening of the oronasal fistula. Occasionally, a small fistula reopens even though the bone graft itself has been successful. This seems to happen most often at the apex of the palatal closure in bilateral cleft cases. If the patient is symptomatic, a secondary procedure to close the fistula may be indicated.

Too much tension across flap closure lines leads to wound dehiscence and exposure of the graft. The graft may be lost anytime it becomes exposed. However, if the dehiscence is small, the wound will often heal over with the loss of only a few small spicules of bone. In any event, it is imperative that the flaps for closure be approximated without tension.

Poor tissue quality is another reason for compromised results. Tissue adjacent to the cleft is often chronically inflamed as a result of inherent problems of hygiene. This

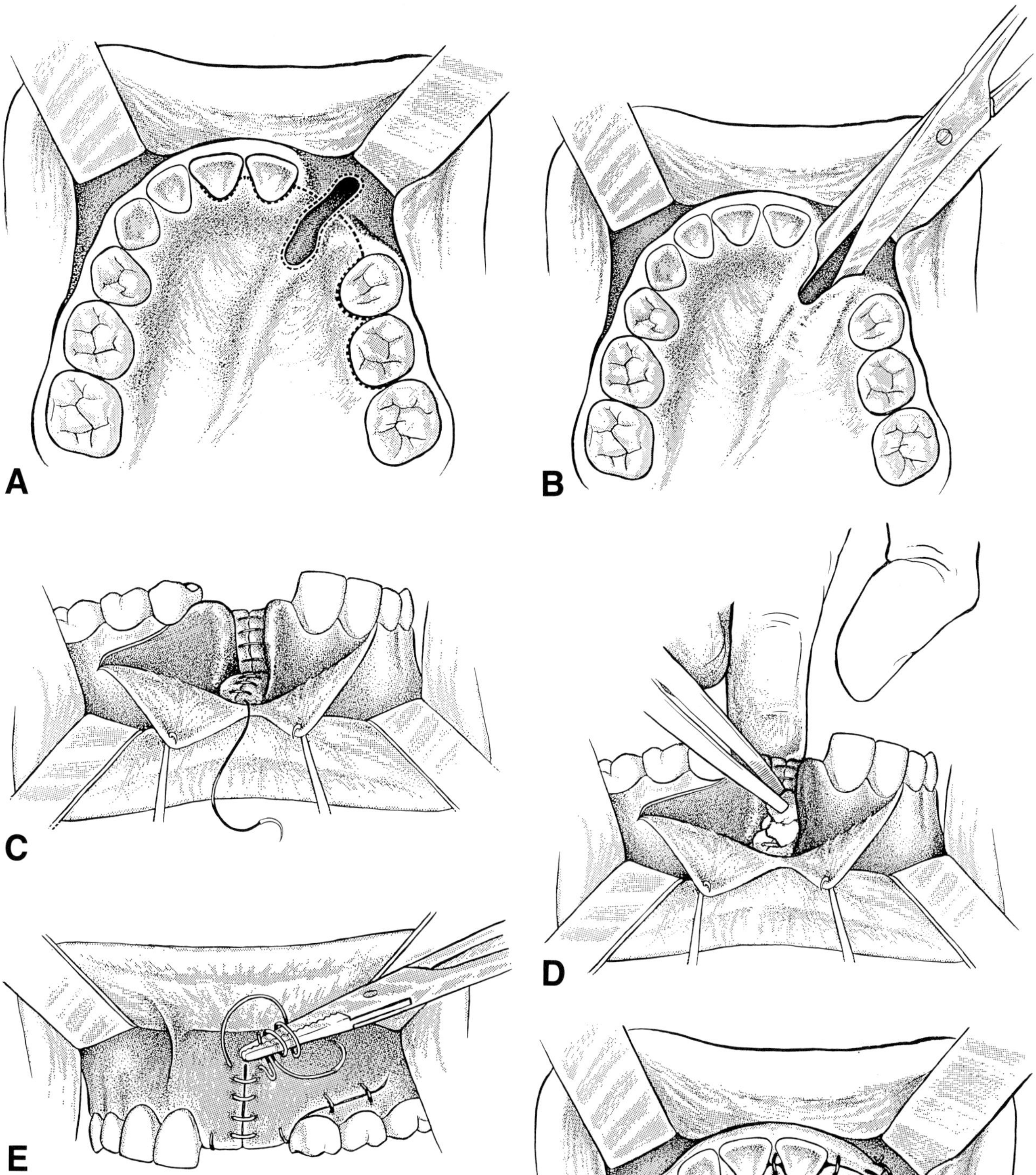

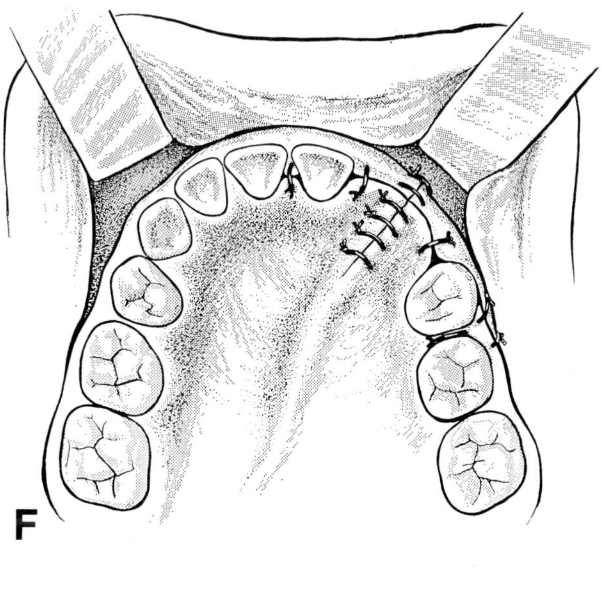

Figure 2 Technique for grafting unilateral complete clefts. *A*, Incisions that allow *B*, dissection of the palatal from nasal mucosa; *C*, after dissection is complete, a running suture technique is used for closure of the palatal and nasal mucosa; *D*, bone graft is then gently packed into the cleft site; *E* and *F*, the alveolus is closed with running and interrupted sutures.

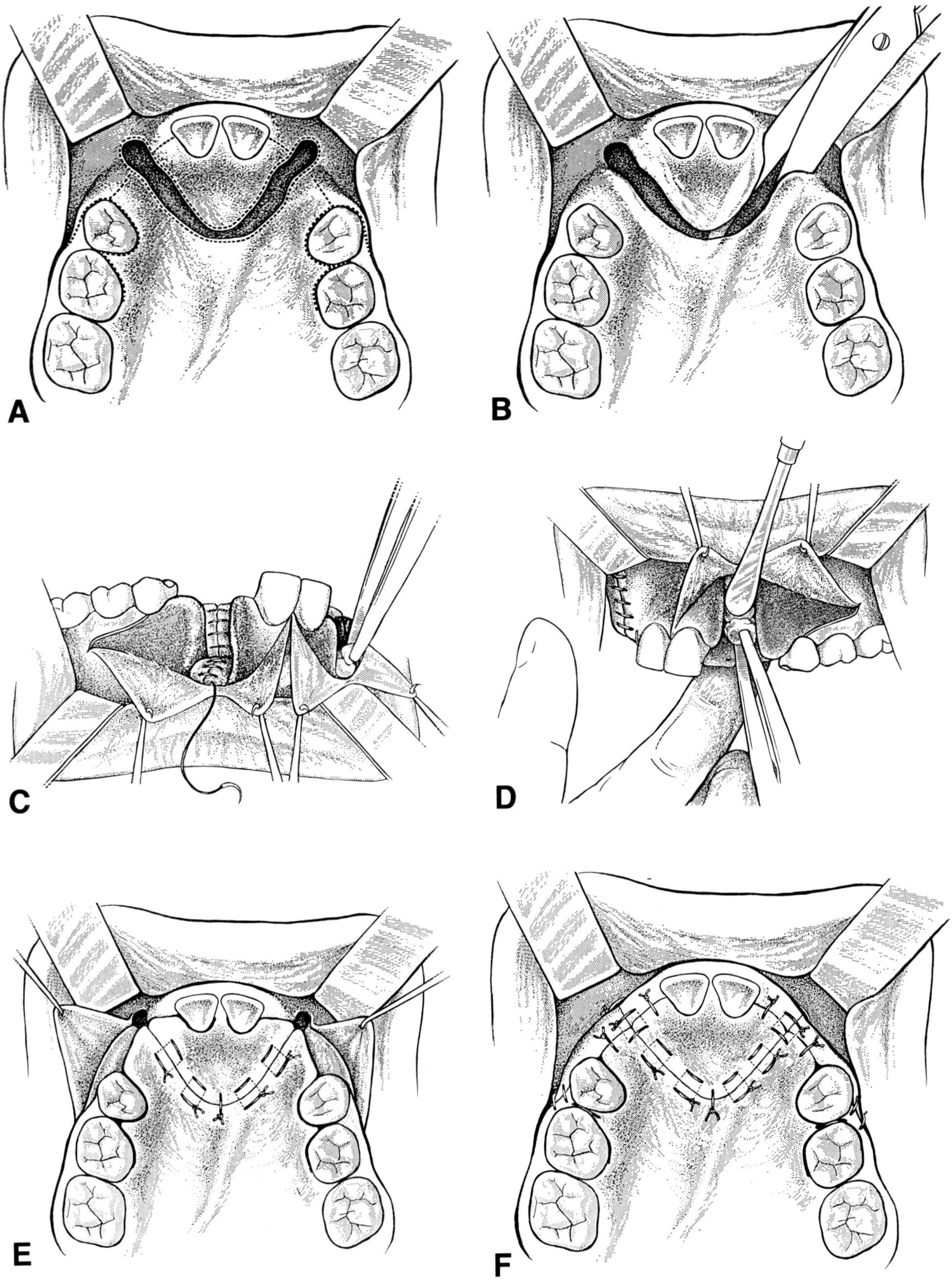

Figure 3 Bilateral cleft grafting technique. *A*, Incision lines; *B*, this allows dissection of the palatal from nasal mucosa; *C*, after dissection is complete, a running suture technique is used for closure of the palatal and nasal mucosa; *D*, bone graft is then gently packed into the cleft site; *E*, mattress sutures are useful to attain approximation of the palatal and premaxillary tissues; *F*, additional sutures are then used to reapproximate the remaining labial flaps.

chronic inflammation often makes the tissue friable and difficult to handle surgically. The tissue may be heavily scarred as a result of previous surgical procedures. Scarring creates problems in gaining closure with proper apposition of the flaps. Compromised healing can be the result.

A "watertight" closure of the nasal floor is necessary for successful grafting. It is often technically difficult to obtain tight closure at the posterior junction of the palate and nasal floor leaflets. Any compromise of closure in this area or in any place along the nasal floor can lead to contamination of the graft by nasal fluids and can result in complete or partial loss of grafted bone.

Perhaps the most serious failure occurs when there is loss of both graft and adjacent teeth. This generally occurs only when one has attempted to graft against root surfaces exposed into the cleft site. Occasionally, bone on the proximal surfaces of teeth adjacent to the cleft has been lost. Bone height on these teeth may be only 50 percent of the total root length. One can graft no higher than the bone height on these teeth. If bone is placed against bare root surfaces, not only will the graft be lost, but external resorption of the teeth occurs; this can result in the loss of these teeth. This is because of the biologic similarity of bone and the cementum of tooth roots. Osteoclasts in this situation cannot differentiate between the two materials, so that resorption of the tooth root surfaces can occur along with resorption and loss of the grafted bone. Therefore, teeth adjacent to the cleft that are devoid of bony support on the proximal surfaces should be extracted prior to grafting. If extraction is deferred, the patient, their family, and the orthodontist should all be reminded of this potential problem. As stated earlier, this pitfall is best avoided by performing the bone graft procedure prior to eruption of the permanent maxillary dentition (5 to 8 years of age).

Risk versus Benefit Analysis

Although this procedure is technically demanding and complications may occur, the benefits of improvement in (1) alar base symmetry, (2) periodontal and dental arch support, and (3) articulation and hygiene far outweigh the potential risks of the procedure. Success rates in excess of 90 percent are expected utilizing this approach for later or secondary cleft grafting. We believe this technique should be considered for the majority of patients with complete clefts of the lip and palate.

SUGGESTED READING

Boyne J. Correction of dentofacial deformities associated with residual alveolar and palatal cleft. In: Bell WH, ed. Surgical correction of dentofacial deformities: new concepts. Philadelphia: WB Saunders, 1985:560.

Epker BN. Bone grafting of alveolar clefts. In: Epker BN, ed. Dentofacial deformities: surgical-orthodontic correction. St. Louis: CV Mosby, 1980:332.

Jackson IT. Use of tongue flaps to resurface lip defects and close palatal fistulae in children. J Plast Reconstr Surg 1972; 49:537–541.

Jones JE, Nelson CL, Sadove AM, Lynch TR. Multidisciplinary team approach to cleft lip and palate management. In: McDonald RE, Avery DR, eds. Dentistry for the child and adolescent. 5th ed. St. Louis: CV Mosby, 1987:806.

Longacre JJ. Transplantation of bone. In: Converse JM, ed. Reconstructive plastic surgery. 2nd ed. Philadelphia: WB Saunders, 1977:329.

CLEFT LIP NASAL DEFORMITY: EARLY CORRECTION

RONALD W. PIGOTT, B.A., M.B., F.R.C.S., F.R.C.S.I.

THE PROBLEM

The simile of visor-like descent of the alar cartilage in the cleft lip nasal deformity suggests that simple lifting of the visor produces a correction. If one wishes to stay with the analogy, one must also say that the helmet was crushed obliquely (the septum deviates to support only the contralateral alar dome), that the rivets on which it hinged were burst, and the visor was squashed almost flat. (The feet of the alar cartilage are displaced and the dome apex opened out.) The helmet was then covered in a dense layer of mud, and, finally, while it was flat, a sheet of leather that united the upper rim of the helmet opening to the upper border of the visor got soaked in water and shrank. The visor cannot be raised until (1) the helmet is straightened (the septum is centralized), (2) the hinge rivets are brought forward (both feet of the alar cartilage are totally freed from the pyriform aperture and nasal spine and advanced to a point where the arc of rotation of the visor is outside the arc of the helmet), (3) the mud is cleared away (the alar visor is totally freed from the covering skin), and (4) the leather sheet is cut (the fascia nasalis is divided, the medial crura are separated and, in extreme cases, the mucosa between the upper and lower lateral cartilages and the mucosa of the membranous septum may also require division to prevent an elastic recoil). These displacements have been described many times. I found the work of Stenstrom and Oberg, 1961, particularly helpful, repeated their work and published the resulting observations (Pigott and Millard, 1971).

This chapter seeks to emphasize the fundamental necessity of primary release of elastic tension in every dimension, as well as straightening of the helmet (septum). To change the simile, the (alar) child may then leapfrog onto the back of his sturdy (septal) friend and sit there securely; his crutch the analogy for the key stitch to be described between medial and lateral crura.

The displacements outlined in this paper were appreciated by Vilray Blair, who described his wide undermining and radical advancement of the lateral crus in his publication of the results of primary surgery in 1930 and the need for medial crus repositioning in a 1923 paper on secondary correction. It is not clear why he did not combine the medial and lateral crus replacements in primary cases. Nor is it clear why those who followed abandoned his techniques. Was the surgery too difficult? Have we the right to assume that there must be a simple solution to a complex three-dimensional problem?

INDICATIONS

The fundamental corrections required to free the alar cartilage are provided by the McComb (1985) and Anderl (1985) extra mucosal dissections, with the exception of mucosal division, which I consider to be essential in order to avoid elastic recoil. Even Anderl admits to an incision up the intercartilaginous line to above the turbinate. It is clear from their publications that substantial, if not perfect, symmetry can be achieved with little or no risk of nostril stenosis.

If it is postulated that there will be some cases so displaced, so hypoplastic, that only the most radical technique could possibly correct them, how are they to be recognized? I do not know, but follow an observation made in bilateral clefts that in cases where there is a shoulder under the skin at the level of the alar dome, then the apex is not pulled out flat and achieves a respectable dome once the alar feet are released. The major deformities occur where, in the bilateral case, the septum is the most anterior point of the nose, no shoulder is visible, and the nose tip skyline forms a tent ridge rather than a dome. This deformity is, of course, visible in the unilateral cleft lip nose of a relatively small proportion of the cases. However, the technique to be described has been applied over-enthusiastically to many incomplete and all complete cases treated since 1972 and, in the light of very good results achieved by less radical procedures, probably unnecessarily.

PREFERRED APPROACH

The alar leapfrog technique (Pigott, 1985) requires a continuous intranasal incision from the tip of the lesser segment, anterior to the turbinate via the intercarilaginous incision, and back down the membranous septum to become continuous with the Millard C flap. This is the V incision of the V–Y alar leapfrog advancement (Fig. 1). A midline incision in the columella extends the C flap into a hemiforked flap (Millard, 1958) and is usually prolonged for 2 to 3 mm anterior to the normal nostril apex. This separates the medial crura. When they are reunited, the apex of the nostrils is carefully leveled (see Fig. 1) and held with transfixion sutures of 6.0 absorbable material. After leveling of the nostril apices, a dogear that must be trimmed may be apparent on the cleft side of the midline incision. Both the midline scar and this 2 to 3 mm-long back cut invariably heal excellently and, because they are below the tip of the nose, they are partly in shadow. If the medial crus is hypoplastic, the dimple at the foot may then be anterior to the normal dimple and a gap of 1 to 3 mm will have opened above the Millard rotation flap. This is eventually filled with the tip of the Millard advancement flap, which may have to be shared with the rotation gap. Excessive rotation to level the Cupid's bow is best avoided because: (1) it lowers the rotation scar inartistically away from the normal philtral column line, (2) excessive length of the rotation flap circumference must be matched by excessive transgression of the natural landmark of the lesser segment mucocutaneous junction and attenuation of the mucosal fullness for lip symmetry, and (3) the Cupid's bow can be leveled with a white roll flap increased from 2 × 1 mm to about 3 × 2 mm.

After preparation of the hemiforked flap, the lateral crus is dissected extraperichondrially (see Fig. 1D) from the covering skin to within 1 mm of the nostril rim, leaving a tongue of fibrofat from the alar base attached to the lip muscle. This is eventually attached to the contralateral nostril floor dermis, deep to the top lip muscle suture, with 4.0 chromic catgut.

The redundant mucosa of the medial lip element (see Fig. 1B) above the Cupid's bow point is dissected off the muscle and kept as a flap on a flap, based on the mucoperiosteum of the premaxilla, which, in turn, comes continuous with the vomer flap that will be used for nostril floor repair. Some or all of this robust little flap is required to break the circular scar of intercartilaginous and membranous septal incisions, thus providing floor to the nose and ending up in the back of the columellar base (see Fig. 1J).

Dissection is completed by wide undermining of nasal skin over both upper lateral cartilages and the anterior surface of the maxilla to the infraorbital foramen. This enables not only the skin and fat of the cheek but also the muscle origins to move medially and removes one of the areas of potential elastic recoil.

LEAPFROG KEY STITCH

The total alar cartilage is lifted upward and forward by a temporary diagonal suture passed through the skin over the contralateral upper lateral cartilage (see Fig. 1F), that picks up the cleft alar dome and goes back through the skin. The weight of an artery forceps clipped to this suture provides the lift to the limit of the tissue dissection. Inspection inside the nose reveals that the lateral crus has moved 3 to 5 mm and the medial crus 2 to 3 mm past the apex of the V where the upper lateral cartilage meets the septum. They are held in this position (see 1F and 1G) by a 6.0 Vicryl suture passed through mucosa of the lateral crus, on through the upper lateral and septal junction, and through mucosa of the medial crus. Once this suture is tied, the alar dome is securely relocated, the traction suture removed, and the intercartilaginous and septal incisions closed from front to back. If the alveolar nostril floor has been closed, premaxillary mucosa is now sutured to the alar mucosa, and the medial lip element mucosal flap-on-a-flap now forms the floor of the nose.

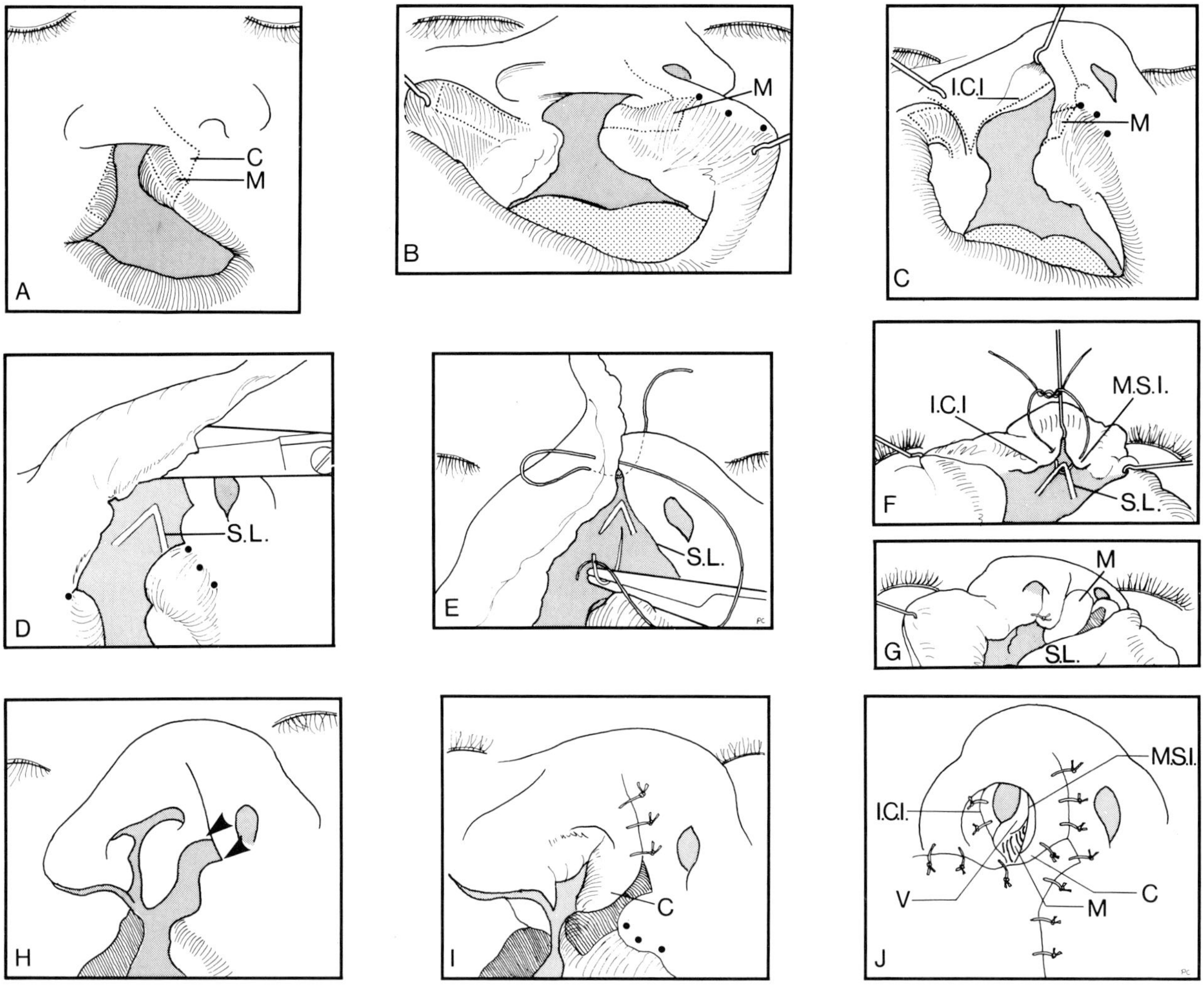

Figure 1 *A* to *J*, Illustrations showing the alar leapfrog technique. M = Medial element mucosal flap based on the vomerine flap; I.C.I. = intercartilaginous incision; M.S.I. = membranous septal incision; V = vomer flap; C = Millard C flap; A = alar base; S.L. = point of fusion of septum with upper lateral cartilage.

A 3 to 4 mm-wide tongue of mucosa is thereby introduced through the otherwise circular scar. The tip of this flap eventually interdigitates with the base of the hemiforked flap until the tail of the C flap turns laterally to tuck under the alar base after completion of the lip repair (see Fig. 1J).

Absorbable mattress sutures are then placed across the membranous septum and from the nostril floor down to the upper buccal sulcus. Finally, mattress sutures are placed over bolsters to pin out the lateral lining to the skin. These are retained for 4 days.

TIMING

The procedure is performed at 3 months of age, general health permitting. This allows the surgeon to take advantage of the considerable hypertrophy of lip muscle that occurs over this period. It also allows the baby's general medical condition to be thoroughly checked out and, as the procedure (vomer flap repair of hard palate, nostril floor repair, alar leapfrog nasal correction, and Millard lip repair) take 1½ to 2 hours of anesthetic time in this nonfatal condition, it is considered safer by the surgical and anesthetic team.

RESULTS

The technique has been performed since 1972 and the oldest children are now 15 (Fig. 2). More than 20 are through puberty.

The advantages of the technique include the following. Growth impairment from this very radical procedure has not been observed and external nasal symmetry has been excellent. Secondary surgery for appearance up to this age has been conspicuously absent. Children are routinely questioned about teasing and almost never attribute it to their noses. Septal correction to improve breathing has usually been performed at some stage between 7 and

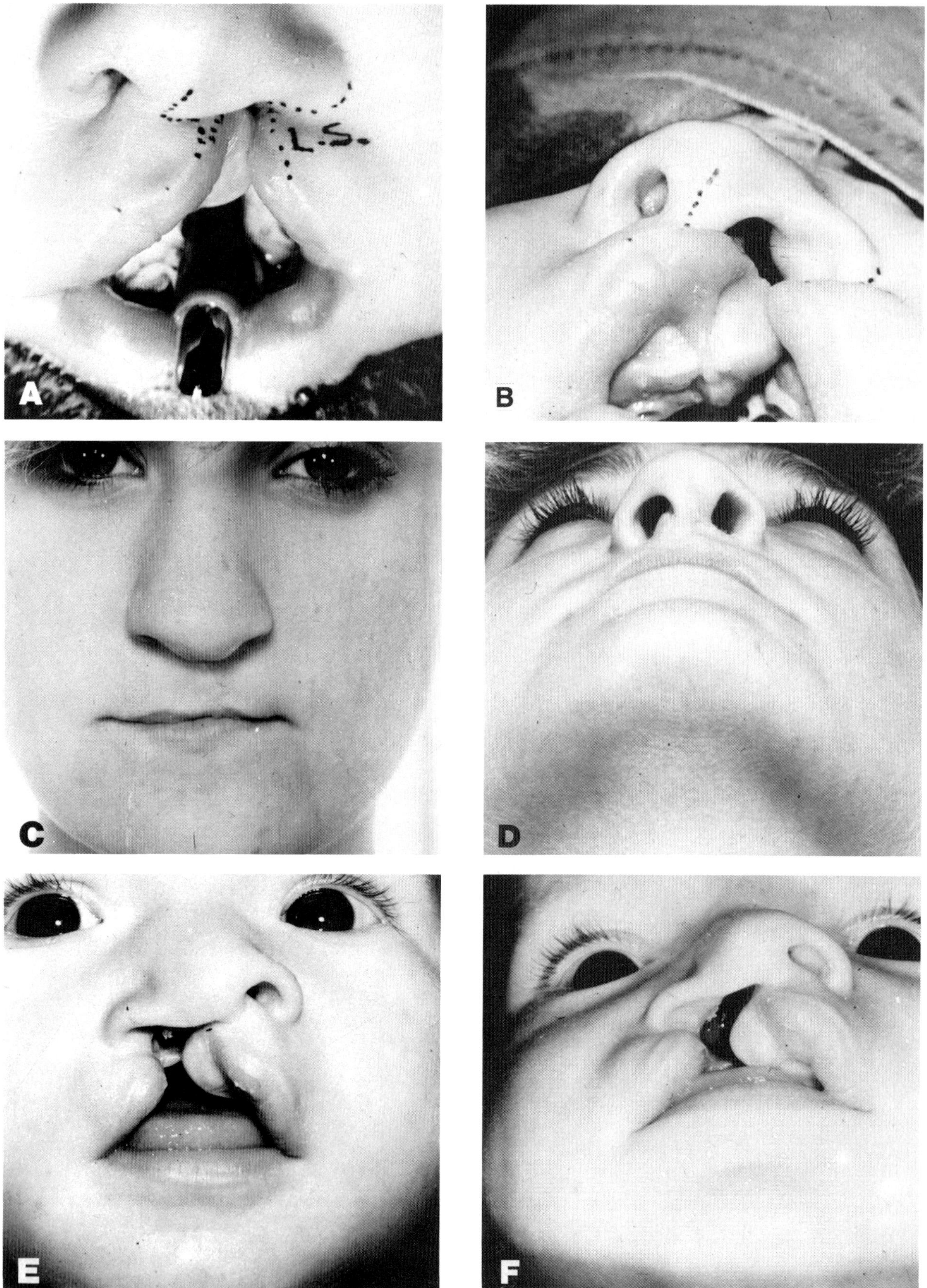

Figure 2 *A* to *H*, 15-year follow-up of two complete clefts that underwent leapfrog. No secondary nasal surgery has been performed.

Figure continues on opposite page

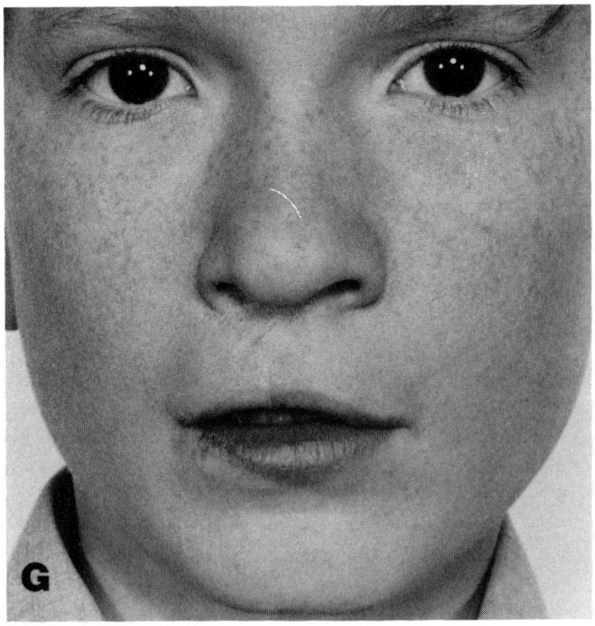

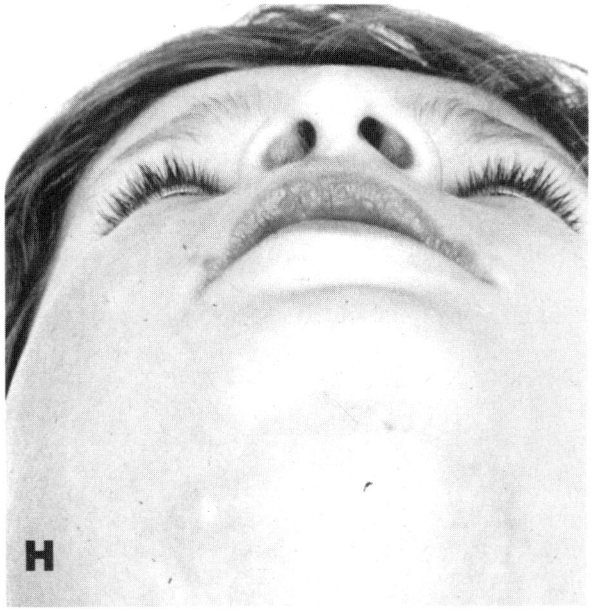

Figure 2 (continued).

14 years in over half the cases, but since adoption of primary septal correction in 1982, the visible septum appears to continue to grow straight (Anderl, 1985).

A disadvantage of the operation is that it is time-consuming. Alar leapfrog, hard palate closure, alveolar nostril floor repair, and Millard's lip repair take 1½ hours operating time. However, the children have tolerated this well. Undoubtedly, the major disadvantage is reduction of intranasal dimensions at the level of the incision. The nares are tested when the infant returns for soft palate repair at 6 months by allowing a forceps to spring open inside the vestibule on each side in turn. The repaired side is usually smaller by 25 percent and occasionally by 50 percent; very occasionally stenosis is almost complete. Because symptoms are very rare in this group, who have never known anything else, it is almost invariably possible to wait until the child comes in for some other procedure between 4 and 5 years of age, before he or she goes to primary school. In other cases, one can wait until 10 or 12 years old and combine the release with alveolar bone grafting. It is possible that more patients will eventually complain of nasal obstruction as their expectations rise in their teens.

CORRECTION OF THE SMALL NASAL AIRWAY

Some or all of the following problems may be found:

1. Anterior synechiae respond well to Z plasty.
2. High nostril floor requires excision of subcutaneous scar tissue and introduction of skin or mucosal graft to the nostril floor. A stent mold is then fashioned and inserted at the end of the operation and converted to acrylic by a dental technician a couple of days later as swelling subsides. It is worn day and night for 3 months and a further 3 months at night only. This has been successful when the family cooperates with the regime. If cooperation is difficult, it is advisable to wait a couple of years before a further attempt is made.
3. Collapse of the pyriform aperture with the maxilla, combined with septal deviation, causes obstruction in cases with no stenosis and must wait until the child is old enough for appropriate treatment.

Since introduction of the medial mucosal flap gusset into the nasal floor, there has been a reduction in cases going to the operating room for treatment of nasal obstruction. It is certainly not the whole answer, but as a good deal of mucosa is advanced to make a normal fornix, a shortage is effectively displayed in the floor, and is filled by this flap.

SUGGESTED READING

Anderl H. Simultaneous repair of lip and nose in the unlilateral cleft (a long term report). In: Jackson IT, Sammerlad BC, eds. Recent advances in plastic surgery. New York: Churchill Livingstone, 1985:1.

Blair VP. Nasal deformities associated with congenital cleft lip. JAMA 1925; 84:185–187.

Blair VP, Brown JB. Mirault operation for single hare lip. Surg Gynecol Obstet 1930; 51:81–98.

McComb H. Primary correction of unilateral cleft lip nasal deformity: a 10 year review. Plast Reconstr Surg 1985; 75:791-797.

Millard DR. Columella lengthening by a forked flap. Plast Reconstr Surg 1958; 22:454-457.

Pigott RW. "Alar leapfrog." A technique for repositioning the total alar cartilage at primary cleft lip repair. Clin Plast Surg 1985; 12: 643-658.

Pigott RW, Millard DR. Correction of the bilateral cleft lip nasal deformity. In: Grabb WC, Rosenstein SW, Bzoch KR, eds. Cleft lip and palate. Boston: Little, Brown, 1971:327.

Stenstrom SJ, Oberg TRH. The nasal deformities in unilateral cleft lip. Plast Reconstr Surg 1961; 28:295–305.

REHABILITATION OF THE CLEFT LIP NOSE

MARK GORNEY, M.D., F.A.C.S.

Despite increased attention to the nasal component of primary cleft lip reconstruction, repair of the secondary cleft lip and nasal deformity is a challenging and often frustrating undertaking. The literature is full of techniques, the success of which is inversely proportional to the severity of the deformity.

The post cleft lip nasal stigma presents a formidable challenge to the nasal surgeon. In this presentation, I define the deformity according to its components, review the groups of procedures available for its correction, and suggest two aggressive approaches that use skeletal support with emphasis upon adequate correction of the nasal tip to obtain better projection.

SURGICAL OBJECTIVES

Regardless of method, the reconstructive surgeon's plan of treatment should aim at the closest approximation to normalcy in the least number of surgical stages with the fewest possible donor site deformities.

In the unilateral deformity, the goal should be the achievement of symmetry relative to the normal side. In the bilateral deformity, the aim should be more tip projection and dorsal height.

In my opinion, it is virtually impossible to achieve an approximation of normality in the significantly deformed nose without the addition of extra structural materials or movement of skeletal segments. The sources of these materials, as well as their relative advantages and disadvantages, are discussed below (Fig. 1).

TIMING OF SURGERY

It is well-known that the nose undergoes growth spurt during puberty. There is a rapid change, not only in size and shape but also in skin thickness. All of these changes are due not so much to the growth of the nasal bones as to the sudden upsurge of the nasal process of the maxilla. This is the route through which the osteotomy chisel must pass in reconstructive rhinoplasty.

During this period of life, a young person undergoes radical emotional and hormonal changes. Thus, it is preferable to postpone reconstructive operations until the nose has achieved its full growth and the patient is emotionally stable. Girls usually achieve physical maturity earlier than boys.

THE LITERATURE OF REPAIR

Unit Rotation Through External Incisions

In this type of repair, the deformed nostril is approached through external skin incisions that extend into the dorsal skin of the nostril, and the deformed portion is rotated cephalad as a unit of skin, cartilage, and, sometimes, mucosa. The principal proponents of this approach do not consider the external scar a drawback and show many excellent results with well-healed, acceptable, but nonetheless visible scars on the columella and dorsal skin of the nasal tip. It is my feeling that if there is any way to achieve the stated goals without an external scar, no matter how unobtrusive, it is preferable to follow it even if it is technically more difficult.

Anatomic Rearrangements Through Internal Incisions

In such procedures, various intranasal or nostril margin incisions are used to expose the abnormal cartilage. This is then rearranged into quasi-normal relationships and held in position with a variety of fixation techniques—either to the upper lateral cartilage directly above, or to the contralateral upper lateral cartilage or normal opposite alar dome. Good results have been achieved by McIndoe, Erich, Potter, Stenstrom, Rees, Spira, Cosman, and Reynolds and Horton. Although these procedures avoid an external scar, and the early results are pleasing, most of them depend on suture fixations

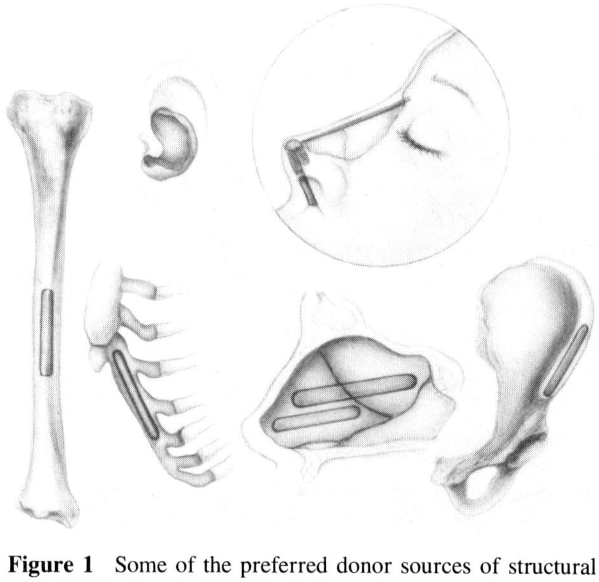

Figure 1 Some of the preferred donor sources of structural material for the significantly deformed nose are shown.

alone, and with the passage of time they tend to show significant loss of improvement.

When this type of repair is done with addition of structural support elements, a combination of incisions is used to reposition or equalize the existing cartilages of the nasal tip and the repair is reinforced with other autogenous structural supports or onlays. Typical of these are those of Millard, Gorney, Musgrave, Cosman, Nishimura, and Dibbell.

Some authors show gratifying results from alloplastic materials. In my experience, alloplastic materials, no matter how well fabricated or innocuous, eventually cause more problem than they are worth. Many eventually extrude.

STATE OF THE ART

It is safe to say that most current thinking about the problem is roughly as follows:

1. If the deformity is minimal, modified tip rhinoplasty techniques, with reduction of the normal side and mobilization of the abnormal one to a more superior medial position, may be sufficient.
2. When the structural elements of the tip of the nose are largely present but malpositioned, they can be rearranged through inconspicuous incisions inside the rim of the nostril. If external support is to be added, it is more easily done through an ''elephant trunk'' exposure, with the skin of the columella lifted up to expose the entire tip anatomy (Fig. 2). It leaves a barely visible scar at the base of the columella.
3. If external scars are to be avoided, and the deformity involves some underdevelopment of the maxillary support on the cleft side, surgical repair must be designed around the addition of adequate structural support for the nasal tip. This support should preferably be autogenous cartilage or bone. When the maxillary support is mildly deficient, an onlay bone graft may suffice. When it is significantly deficient, one should consider a maxillary advancement with or without bone graft.

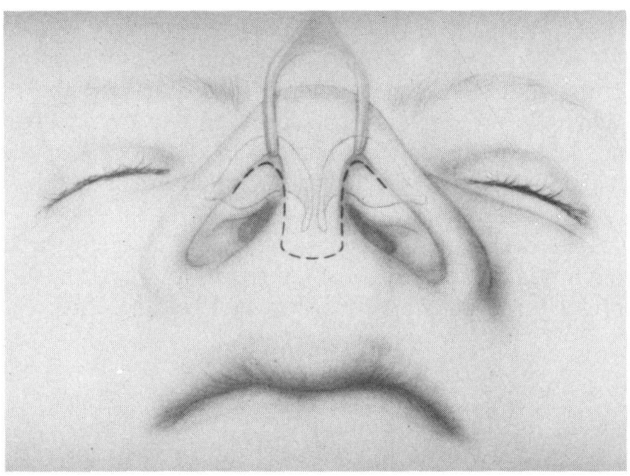

Figure 2 ''Elephant trunk'' incision facilitates addition of external support.

THE UNILATERAL DEFORMITY

For the past 20 years, I have tried various combinations of techniques. In the mid-1980s, I have settled on the following approach, which has stood the test of time.

When the surgical plan calls for structural materials, these are obtained first (except for septal cartilage since the nose is a bacterial zoo anyway). See Figure 1 for the sources of such material. My preferred donor source, whenever possible, is the nose itself. However, the septum is often twisted, inadequate, or insufficient. I then prefer to go to the anterior tibia for bone and the ear for cartilage. (The ear has amazing potential as a donor site with minimal secondary deformity.) I prefer not to invade rib or pelvis if avoidable because of increased morbidity.

The structural anatomy of the nasal tip is easily accessible through incisions just inside the nostril rim. If one extends these incisions down the sides of the columella and joins them across the base, careful dissection of the skin of the columella (the "elephant trunk") reveals with startling clarity the anatomy and the relationship of all the parts (Fig. 3). If there is excess fat on the alar cartilages, it can be easily and accurately removed. The excellence of circulation in the area makes this approach extremely safe, even if one chooses to perform the rest of the rhinoplasty procedure through it (Fig. 4).

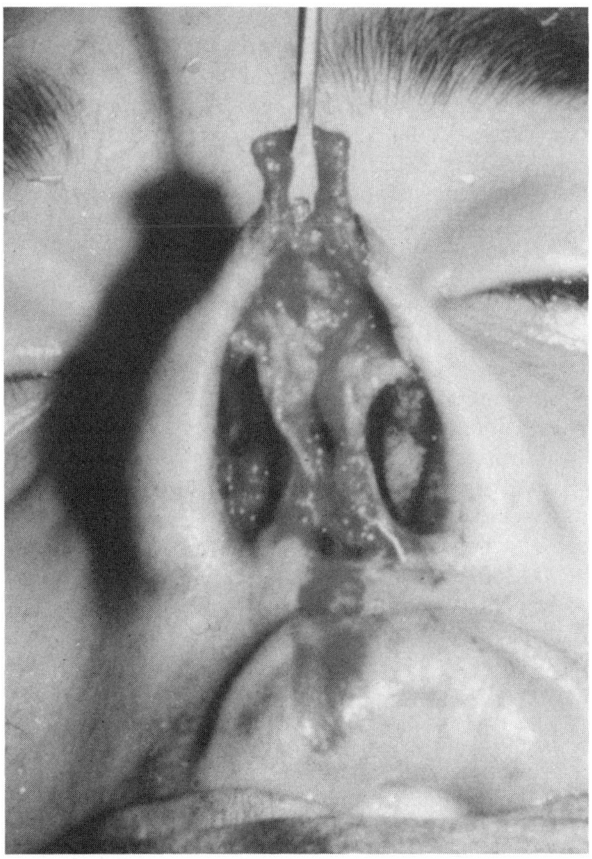

Figure 3 Pathologic anatomy can be clearly seen.

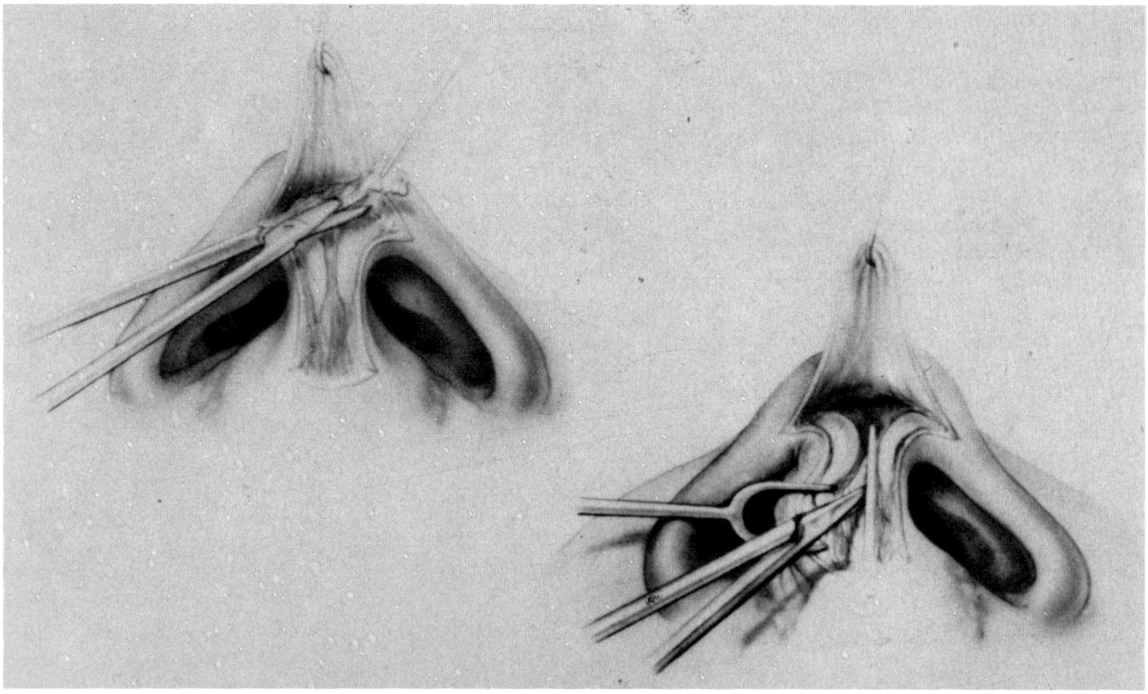

Figure 4 The defatting and harvesting of septum can be performed with great visibility.

When significant asymmetry or disparity exists, this can be addressed directly. In the unilateral deformity, the normal alar cartilage has a lateral crus significantly wider than the opposite side. To correct that asymmetry, the relative excess on the normal side is resected and saved for later use (Fig. 5). Once dimensional parity is achieved, one can assess the degree of positional disparity on the cleft side and correct this in one of several ways. When the end of the lateral crus protrudes into the nostril and the genu is displaced inferiorly, it may have to be dissected out, scored, and reattached in a more normal attitude to the next higher stable point. This may be the dome of the opposite normal side or, more likely, the lowest point of the opposite normal upper lateral cartilage. Either way, such repositioning is much more likely to achieve permanent results and dramatic improvement if a stabilizing strut of cartilage is installed between the medial crura. This strut must sit on the maxillary spine (or what passes for one). It must be thin enough not to make the columella too wide, yet strong enough to act as a support. Stability can be achieved by making it wide enough (in the dorsoventral dimension). If one allows the strut to protrude above the level of both alar domes, it will project under the skin as an abnormal white bump that looks like the top of a tent pole.

The problems of strut camouflage and tip projection can be corrected by fabrication of a cartilage tip graft, preferably of septal cartilage. When this is not available, the most dependent and deeply curved portion of conchal ear cartilage can be used (Fig. 6; see also Fig. 5).

Once the tip of the nose has been balanced, one must then address the problem of the nasal pyramid. If there is adequate structural integrity, standard osteoplastic rhinoplasty with midline osteotomies and lateral infractures will suffice. If the nasal pyramid appears inadequate after the tip deficiency has been corrected, either a dorsal graft or sandwiched septal cartilage or a bone graft must often be used.

THE BILATERAL DEFORMITY

The approach to the bilateral stigma must also vary according to the degree of deformity, but there may be more difficult problems to deal with. Additionally, the surgeon must be prepared to cope with: (1) a short, tight columella, (2) flaring, horizontally-directed nostrils, (3) totally inadequate nostril floor, (4) unstable central maxillary segment (premaxilla), and (5) two vertical scars on an upper lip that may be unsubstantial, too tight, or too long.

When the axis of the nostril is relatively normal, I prefer the same general approach as described above. When the lip is really tight, an Abbe flap transfer into the center of the lip to recreate the philtrum frees up the tethered nasal tip and allows use of lip tissue as additional columella.

In severe cases, when the columella is woefully short, the tip tightly tethered, and the nostril axis horizontal, I prefer the approach I described in 1979 and 1983.

Concept

The basic concept of this procedure is explained by analogy. Let us say the nostril deformity in the double cleft lip is like two pipes, elliptical in cross section, that

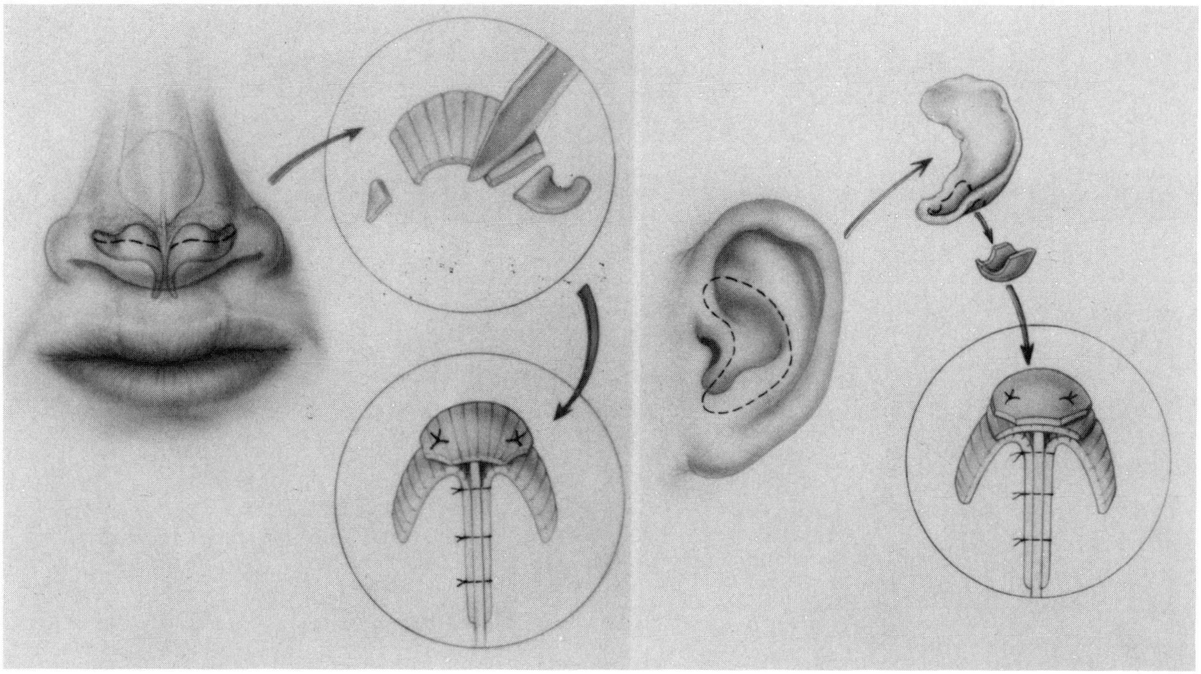

Figure 5 *Left,* If any relative excess material remains from alar cartilage, it should be saved. *Right,* Conchal cartilage will do if nasal cartilage is not available.

are lying on their sides half buried in the ground. The objective is to lift these pipes out of the ground and then rotate them centripetally 90 degrees so that the central axis of the elliptical pipe is turned from a generally horizontal, or oblique plane to a more nearly vertical one. Once this is accomplished the pipes must be held up in the desired position by a vertical support between them. (Fig. 7).

Technique

The addition of tissue to the columella from the nasal floor has proved to be a most satisfactory technique for lengthening the columella. Cronin described this technique in 1958, but noted that others had suggested such an operation. In describing his banked forked flap, Millard notes that this secondary procedure is reminiscent of Cronin's technique, but with more tissue now available.

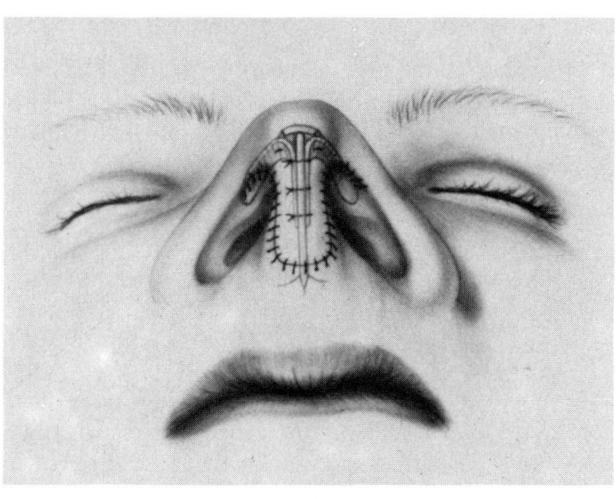

Figure 6 Columellar strut, capped by cartilage, provides needed support for increased projection of nasal tip.

The use of cartilage grafts for nasal support dates back to Von Mangoldt in 1899. In a specific discussion of the bilateral cleft lip nose, Brown and McDowell recommended that an L-shaped, preserved or autogenous, cartilage graft be used for patients with deficient columella and poor septal support. Marcks et al elongated the columella by flap transfer and Z-plasty.

Cronin also suggested a cartilage post; particularly when the soft tissues of the newly lengthened columella do not support the tip.

Meade used auricular cartilage struts in conjunction with a composite auricular graft to augment the columella. Musgrave also recommended additional nasal tip cartilage support as a second stage following composite grafting. Gorney and Falces have devised a gullwing autogenous auricular graft for columellar and alar support.

Dibbell has shown startling results with his "bowie knife" columellar posts.

Millard emphasized the advantages of autogenous septal cartilage for use in the columella. They include its strength, lack of bulk, and availability. Peer observed that septal cartilage grafts transplanted in human tissue maintain their structure.

The incisional design basically follows Cronin's pattern, but the lateral extensions of the incision come around the base of the nostril and well up into the alar crease (Fig. 8). As the dissection of the nostril bases proceeds in depth, maximum traction should be exerted on the tip of the nose

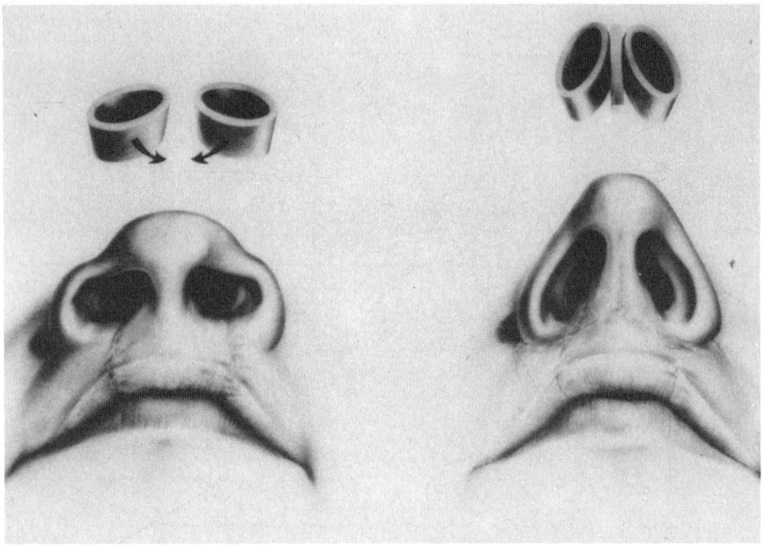

Figure 7 The "pipes" are released and turned centripetally to support them on a post.

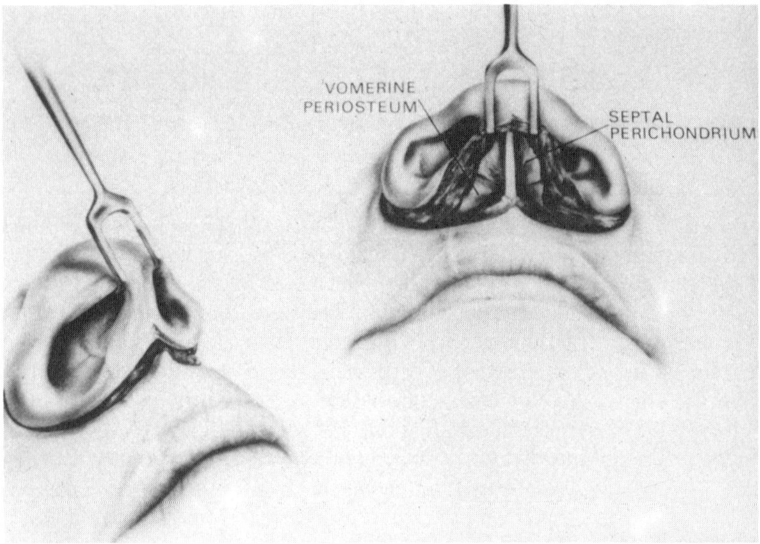

Figure 8 *Left*, The tip is released, and dissection of the subperichondrial flaps is advanced. *Right*, The lower half of the nose is being degloved.

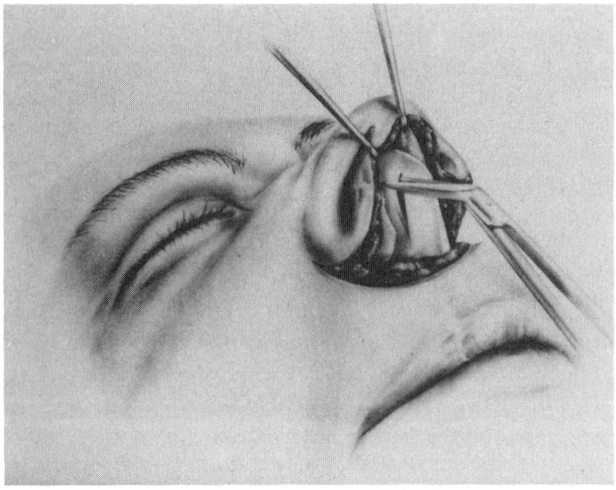

Figure 9 Septal cartilage is divided and installed where needed—thickest and longest segment should be used for vertical strut.

with a hook. After the initial skin and subcutaneous incision, the dissection should proceed obliquely downward so as to include not only the nostril bases but as much of the floor of the nose as possible. Unlike the classic Cronin procedure, there is no separation of the cutaneous columella from the septal mucosa immediately contiguous. As the dissection proceeds medially toward the septum, one should insinuate a small, sharp, submucous elevator under the periosteum of the vomer and the perichondrium of the cartilaginous septum and continue the elevation in the plane as far back as is normally done in the septoplasty. In addition, it should continue superiorly all the way to the skin of the dorsum of the nose.

After this maneuver is completed, and with continuing traction on the tip of the nose, the soft tissue of the entire tip, which includes the alar cartilages, should be literally degloved from the cartilaginous septum (Fig. 9).

It is now possible to obtain from the septum enough cartilaginous material for both the tip strut and the dor-

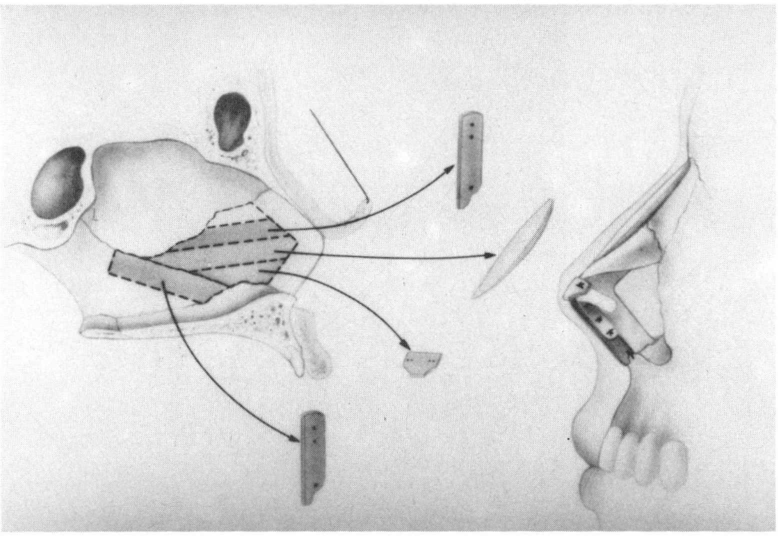

Figure 10 The cartilage is easily harvested through the degloving approach. Enough should be left behind to assure structural support.

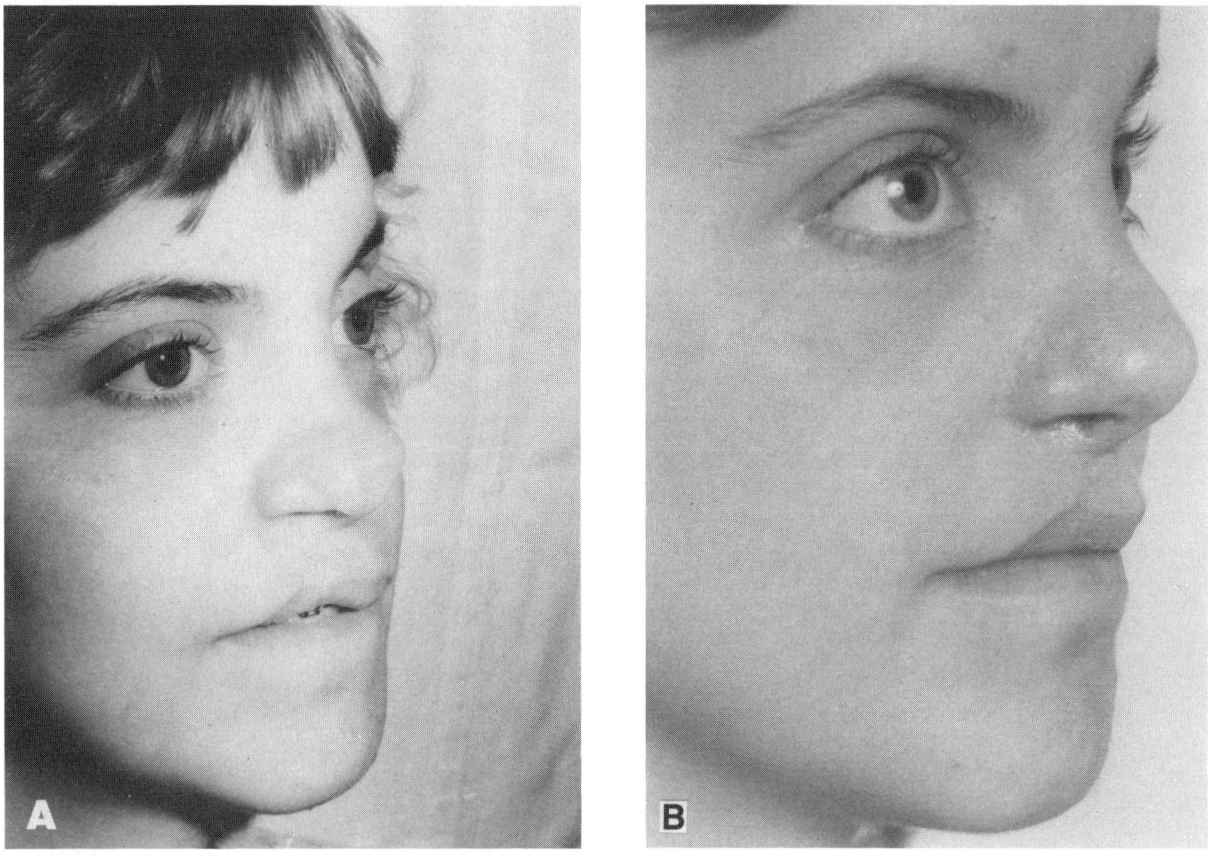

Figure 11 *A*, Preoperative and, *B*, postoperative appearance.

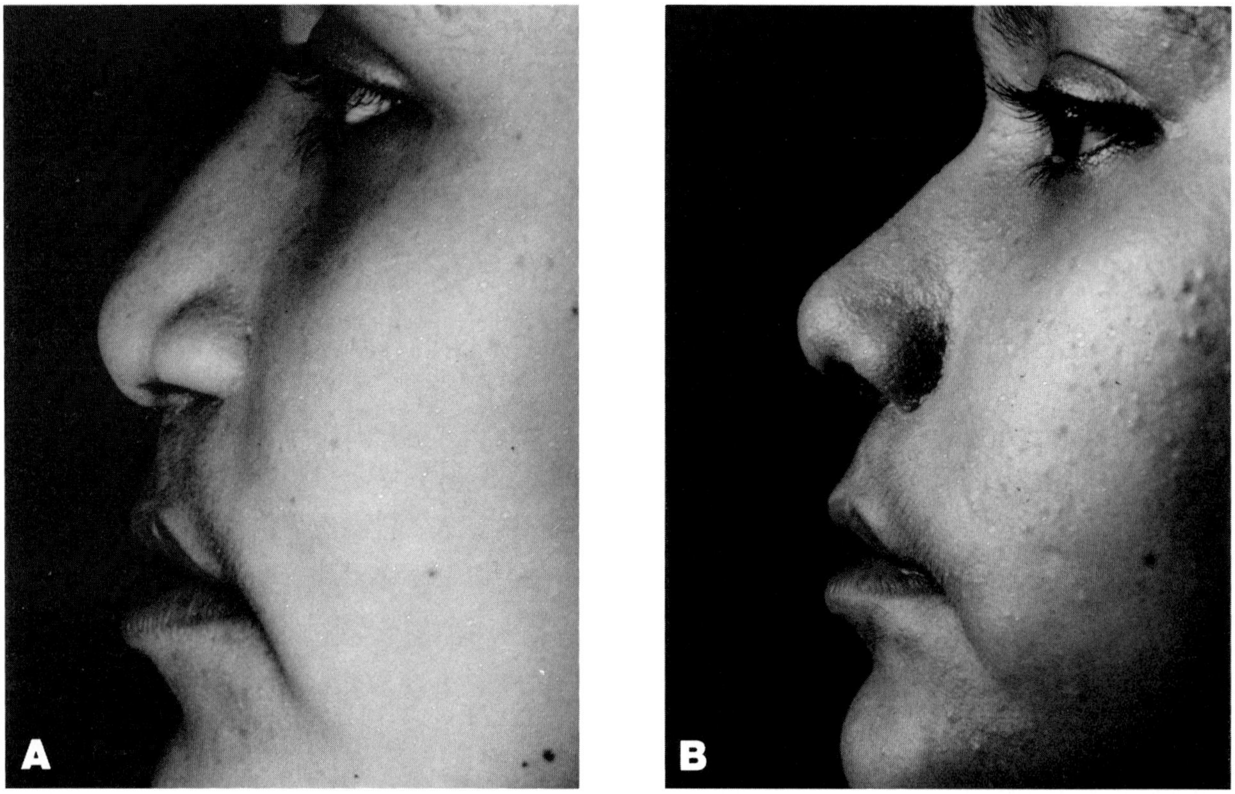

Figure 12 *A*, Preoperative appearance and *B*, Postoperative appearance. Patient's ethnic look has been preserved.

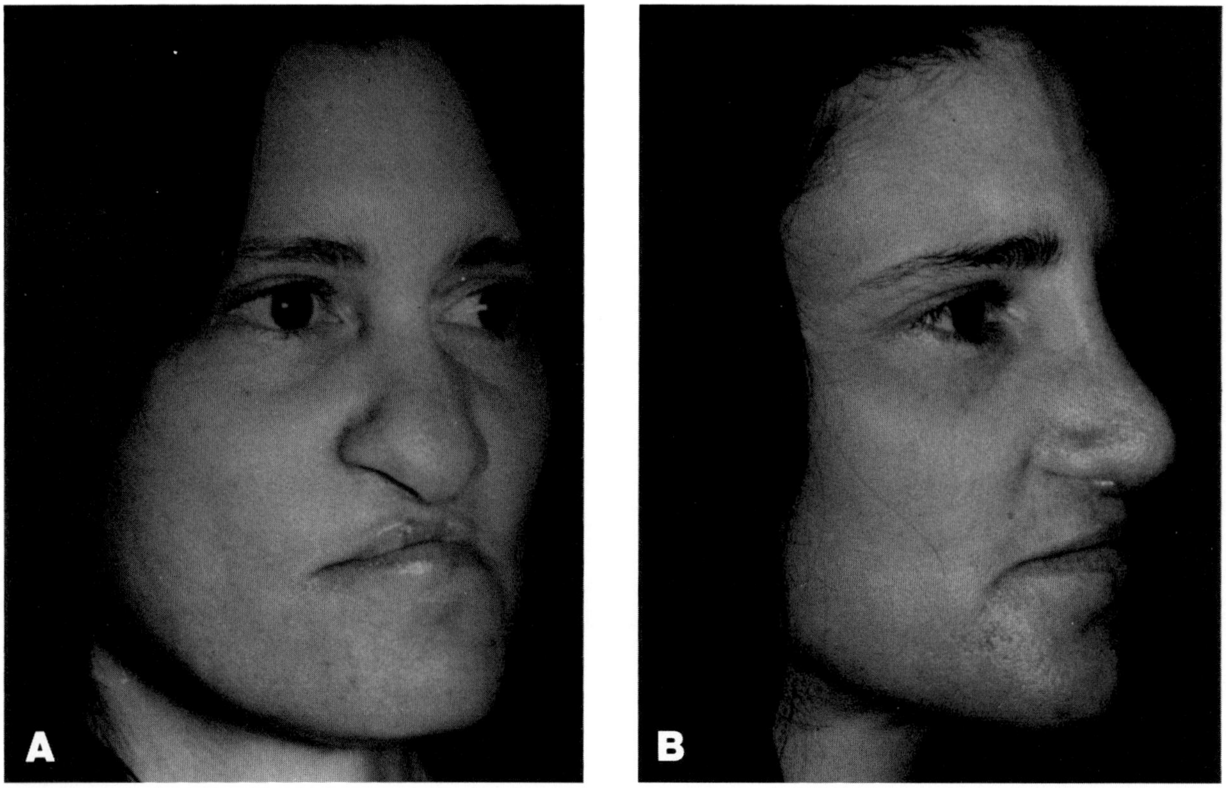

Figure 13 *A*, Multiple attempts at revision had failed in thick-skinned nose with no support. *B*, Appearance 6 months after reconstruction is shown.

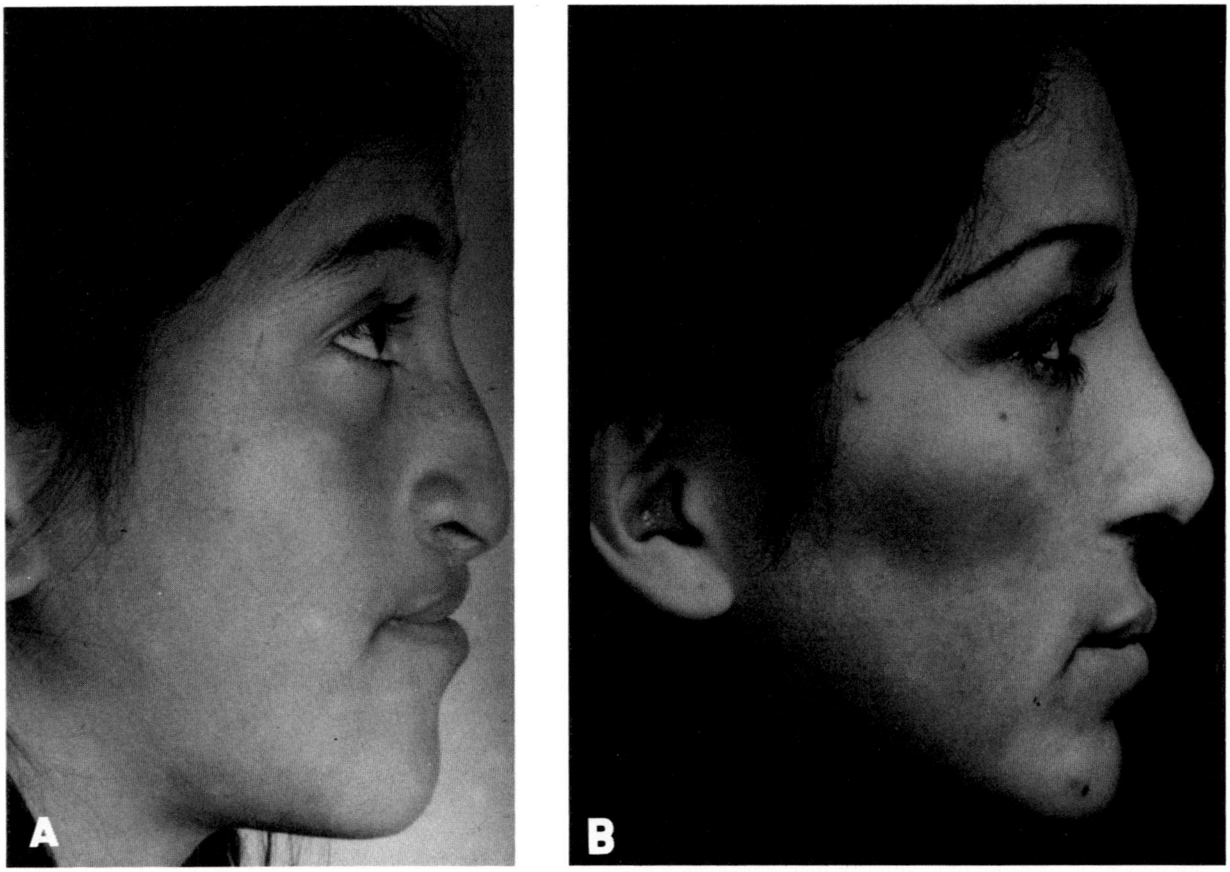

Figure 14 *A*, Appearance preoperatively and *B*, 12 years postoperatively. (Courtesy of Interplast and D. Laub, M.D.)

sum, if necessary. As much septal material as is compatible with continuing adequate dorsal support should be removed (Fig. 10). The material obtained from the septum must now be divided into either two or three segments, depending on the requirements.

When no osteoplastic rhinoplasty is contemplated, a much greater illusion of narrowing can be obtained by addition of dorsal height. This is achieved by the trimming and tailoring of a section of the material obtained to insert under the dorsal skin of the nose, either as a single "spear" or as a "sandwich" graft.

The best segment of the septal material must be saved for use as a strut between the medial crura of the liberated alar cartilages. The bottom of this strut should fit into the nasal spine by either a notch or a mortise and tenon arrangement. Any suitable nonabsorbable suturing material can now be used to fix the medial crura of the ala to the cartilage strut. The base of the supporting strut may be fixed to the spine if desired (see Fig. 8).

Any remaining material can now be used as a separate subcutaneous tip graft to give the blunted tip more definition and projection and improve the profile.

Figures 11 through 14 show the results that can be achieved by careful tailoring of the procedure to meet the patient's needs.

SUGGESTED READING

Berkeley WT. The cleft lip nose. Plast Reconstr Surg 1959; 23:567-575.

Cronin TD. Lengthening columella by use of skin from nasal floor and alae. Plast Reconstr Surg 1958; 21:417-426.

Dibbell DG. A cartilaginous columella strut in cleft lip rhinoplasty. Br J Plast Surg 1976; 29:247–253.

Gorney M, Falces E. Use of ear cartilage grafts for nasal tip reconstructions. Plast Reconstr Surg 1972; 50:147

Gorney M. Centripetal rotation-advancement for bilateral cleft lip nasal deformities. Ann Plast Surg 1979; 2(5):374-380.

Millard DR Jr. The unilateral cleft nose. Plast Reconstr Surg 1964; 34:169–175.

Nishimura Y. Autogenous septal cartilage graft in the correction of cleft lip nasal deformities. Br J Plast Surg 1978; 31:222–226.

Reynolds JR, Horton CF. An alar lift procedure in cleft lip rhinoplasty. Plast Reconstr Surg 1965; 35:377–385.

Stenstrom SF. The alar cartilage and the nasal deformity in unilateral cleft lip. Plast Reconstr Surg 1966; 38:223-231.

MAXILLARY AND MANDIBULAR SURGERY FOR CLEFT LIP AND PALATE

RICHARD E. ALBIN, M.D., Ph.D., F.A.C.S., F.A.A.P.

What is the role of maxillary and mandibular surgery in the patient with a cleft lip and palate? What can it accomplish, who needs it, at what age should it be performed, should one or both jaws be operated on? How does orthodontia relate to this type of surgery? None of these questions has universally accepted answers. This chapter attempts to provide both background information and specific facts for a better understanding of this particular area of plastic surgery in which several fields of expertise come together.

ORTHODONTIA AND ORTHOGNATHIC SURGERY

To determine whether or not a particular patient would benefit from jaw realignment surgery, it is necessary to consider two factors: dental occlusion and facial profile. Do the teeth occlude normally in the anteroposterior direction, i.e., do the maxillary incisors overlap the mandibular incisors without either of them protruding at an abnormal angle from the underlying bone? Normally, the mandibular teeth come out of the bone essentially vertically, whereas the maxillary teeth come out of the bone slightly inclined anteriorly. In many patients with cleft lip and palate, the mandible is anterior to the maxilla, and either the orthodontist or the teeth themselves try to occlude the teeth normally by tilting the mandibular teeth backwards and the maxillary teeth forward. If this exaggerated tilt causes the maxillary teeth to overlap the mandibular incisors, it is not normal occlusion and surgery should be considered.

Orthodontia can move teeth within the bone but cannot change the position of the bone. Surgery can move the bone so that the teeth can be moved within it to achieve normal occlusion. One might consider the role of jaw surgery as the rough tuning and orthodontia as the fine tuning control. Therefore, when the jaw discrepancy is small and the teeth can be moved by orthodontic appliance so as to occlude normally, surgery is not indicated. Conversely, when the jaw discrepancy is large, then surgery is needed in order to reduce the bone discrepancy sufficiently to allow orthodontics to restore a normal occlusion.

Jaw surgery can do more than provide a foundation for normal occlusion; it also can provide a more normal facial profile. In many cleft palate patients, the maxilla does not project forward sufficiently, thereby giving the mandible the appearance of prognathism and the patient a dishface appearance. This situation cannot be remedied by orthodontia alone but rather in combination with surgery to move the midface forward, and possibly also the mandible backward.

Therefore, jaw surgery can be used to accomplish two goals: movement of the jaws into a close enough relationship to enable orthodontics to restore normal occlusion, and creation of a more normal facial profile.

TIMING OF SURGERY

As a basic rule, maxillary and mandibular surgery should be performed when facial growth has ceased. Ordinarily, facial growth is complete in women by 18 years of age and in men by about 20 years. However, as with all rules, there are legitimate exceptions. These are average ages for normal patients. A cleft maxilla is not a normal maxilla and may not have normal growth potential. Therefore, when serial examinations have documented cessation of growth prior to 18 or 20 years of age, surgery can be performed at an earlier age when indicated.

The mandible is another consideration. When there is no normal occlusion and the maxillary teeth do not overlap the mandibular teeth, the mandible encounters less growth-restraining force and can continue to become more prognathic. When this is the situation, it is better to operate on the jaws prior to complete mandibular growth so that restoration of a normal occlusion can help minimize the problem of further mandibular growth.

Another valid consideration as regards timing is whether or not the patient is suffering significant psychological harm from the deformity. If so, then earlier surgery should be considered as a possible therapeutic alternative. However, if the patient is undergoing relatively normal psychological problems of growth and development, there is no reason to perform surgery 5 years sooner. Jaw surgery can and should be moved up if the patient is suffering unusual psychological trauma, and if it seems likely that a successful surgical outcome would be of significant psychological help.

ONE JAW OR TWO?

At first glance, most patients with clefts appear to have mandibular prognathism. Upon closer examination, one usually finds that the maxilla is not sufficiently anterior, i.e., the middle third of the face is recessed or hypoplastic. If the maxilla were repositioned anteriorly, then the mandible would, in fact, be normal. Another possibility is that the maxilla is recessed and the mandible is too far forward. If the second situation is the case, then the surgical decision is easy—move the maxilla forward and the mandible backward. However, even in the first situation it is sometimes advisable to operate on both jaws, not on a theoretic basis but on a purely pragmatic level. If one attempts to move a cleft maxilla forward a large distance, e.g., about 1 cm or more, relapse often occurs due to the inexorable backward pull of the soft tissue. The amount of relapse increases as the forward movement increases. In all published series, the cleft maxilla relapses more than the noncleft maxilla, when advanced. Therefore, it is thought to be prudent to split the difference. Rather than advance the maxilla 1 cm, why not, for example, advance the maxilla 6 mm and set back the mandible 4 mm. In this way there is less relapse and, while the ideal profile might not be achieved, a stable, significant improvement can more readily be obtained and maintained (Fig. 1).

ROLE OF THE ORTHODONTIST

Orthognathic surgery requires much cooperation between surgeon and orthodontist. It is only by discussion of a case at regular intervals that the best possible care can be rendered. The orthodontist can provide the surgeon with growth and development data, as well as recommendations for the type of surgery and the amount to move each jaw. However, the surgeon must take an active role so that he is not forced into an attempt to perform technically difficult or hazardous procedures in order to attain a normal profile when this theoretically desirable goal may not be practical.

Once the surgeon and the orthodontist agree on the surgical procedures and their timing, the orthodontist begins brace therapy designed to get the teeth into proper

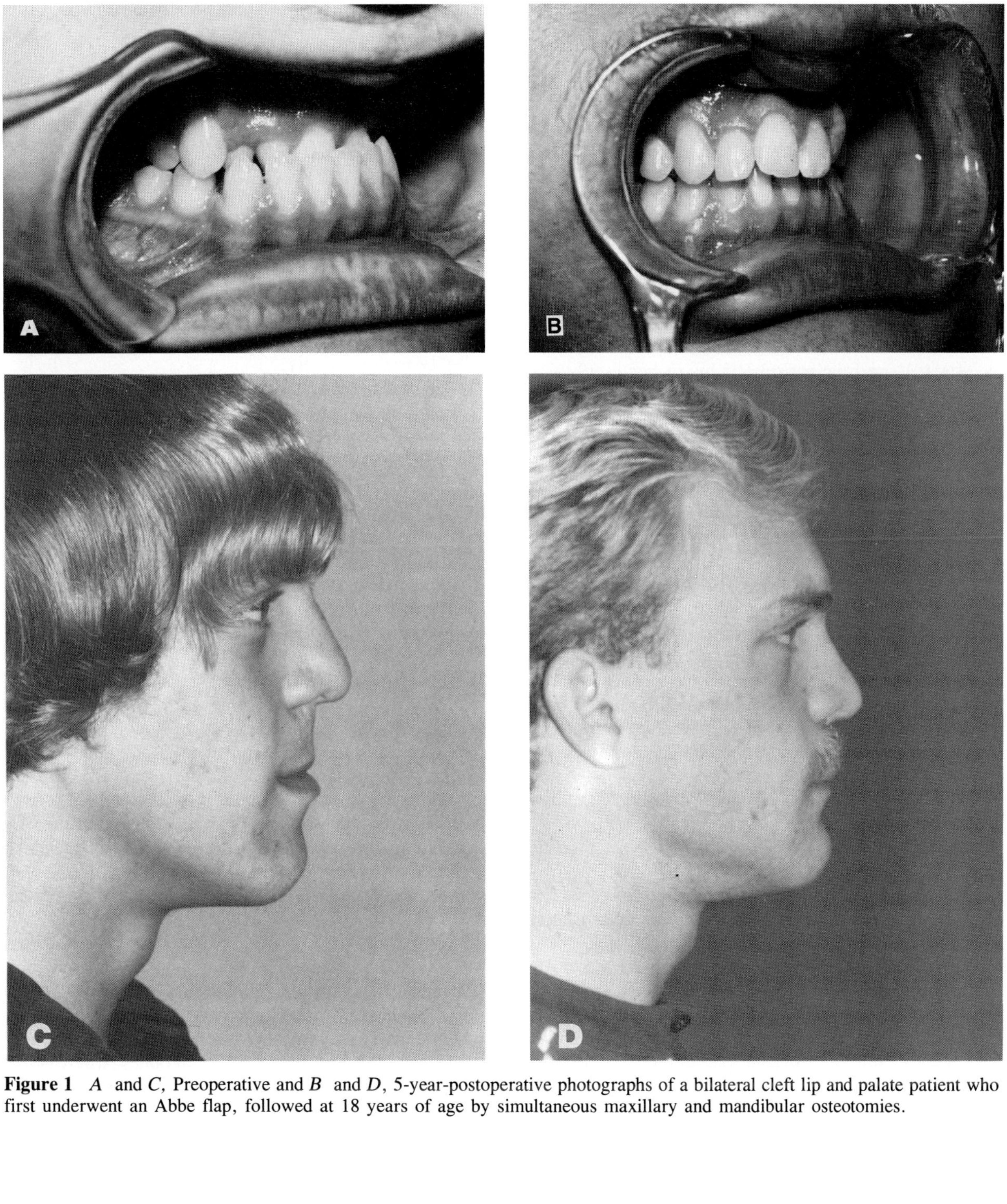

Figure 1 *A* and *C*, Preoperative and *B* and *D*, 5-year-postoperative photographs of a bilateral cleft lip and palate patient who first underwent an Abbe flap, followed at 18 years of age by simultaneous maxillary and mandibular osteotomies.

position for surgery. It is important to have the teeth positioned so that immediately after surgery they are in occlusion. Relapse is then less likely to occur. Just prior to surgery, the orthodontist may make the splints that will be used during surgery and also applies any wires or appliances that are necessary for the operation.

Postoperatively, the orthodontist follows the patient and documents the early and late effects of the surgery with x-ray films and dental models. He assesses healing and, when the bones are stable, proceeds with brace therapy to fine tune the occlusion. When this is completed, he fits the patient with a retainer. The reason for a retainer is to allow the bone to solidify or heal around the tooth once it has been moved into its proper position. Tooth movement within bone is accomplished by inducing a small amount of bone resorption at the leading surface of the moving tooth. As a result of tooth movement, a bone gap results at the trailing surface. If the teeth are held with a retainer, bone is allowed to fill in the gap and solidify the tooth in its new position. This entire process takes many years to complete. It is not unusual for the orthodontist to work with an individual cleft palate patient for 15 years or more to achieve a satisfactory outcome.

ANCILLARY PROBLEMS

Once the surgeon and orthodontist agree that surgery is indicated, and the patient and his or her family wish to proceed, several other factors need to be addressed. These involve dental soft tissue and nasal configuration issues.

Prior to surgery, dental hygiene must be satisfactory with all cavities filled and periodontal disease resolved. Other surgical procedures, such as palatal fistula closure or bone grafting of an alveolar ridge defect, may also be required. Transverse maxillary expansion and placement of a stabilizing bone graft may be necessary to achieve better symmetry, eliminate crossbite, and allow the maxillary arch to fit over the mandibular arch, thereby providing stable occlusion. These procedures can be done at the same time as the maxillary surgery, and sometimes should be done at the same time if, for example, the exposure would be better. However, it is generally advisable for the neophyte surgeon to keep things as simple as possible for the first few times by closing fistulas before maxillary surgery or by bone grafting a bilateral cleft maxilla before maxillary advancement.

When the cleft lip repair has resulted in a tight lip, or when there is significant upper to lower lip disparity, an Abbe flap should precede the maxillary advancement in order to decrease the soft tissue forces that promote relapse.

Most teenage and adult cleft palate patients who are about to undergo maxillary and mandibular surgery have significant nasal deformities, which can, in theory, be corrected at the same time as the jaw surgery. I do not think this is either safe or desirable, particularly for someone who is a novice at this type of surgery. The nasal correction should be performed after the maxillary surgery. Typically, nasal tracheal intubation is used for jaw surgery, which precludes adequate nasal correction. If first the jaws are operated with nasal intubation and then the tube is moved intraorally to perform the nasal surgery, it would then be very hazardous to put the patient into intermaxillary fixation. If the patient were left out of fixation until the next day, then the jaw fixation might be compromised. The recent advent of compression plate usage may make this option more feasible but for the present I believe the patient gets a better result if the nasal surgery is deferred until after the maxillary surgery. Since maxillary surgery changes the nasal foundation, it is usually contraindicated to do a reconstructive rhinoplasty before maxillary surgery. This is not to be confused with primary repair of the cleft lip nose, which I feel should be performed at the same time as the original cleft lip repair.

CAN MAXILLARY SURGERY AFFECT VELOPHARYNGEAL INSUFFICIENCY?

In a word-Yes! Maxillary advancement can make preexisting velopharyngeal insufficiency (VPI) worse and it can make an individual with no clinical VPI symptomatic. The frequency of either of these unfortunate events varies widely in the literature but they can and do occur. The patient and his family must be warned about this possibility preoperatively.

When a patient has an apparently functional pharyngeal flap in place, it should be lengthened at the time of maxillary surgery. When the flap has contracted into a narrow band, then it probably can be transected safely.

SELECTION OF PROCEDURE

Mandibular setback can be achieved by several methods. One of the most commonly used methods today is an intraoral, sagittal split. Maxillary advancement can be achieved with a Le Fort I, II or III maxillary osteotomy with bone grafting. The most common procedure for cleft lip and palate patients is a high Le Fort I. Occasionally another procedure is preferable and this, of course, depends on whether and by how much other facial structures need to be advanced differentially relative to the tooth movement. A deficient nasal projection can be improved either by a Le Fort II or III maxillary osteotomy or a Le Fort I followed by nasal bone grafting. The latter option is preferable if the amount of advancement in the two areas is very disparate. Similarly, deficient inferior orbital rims and malar eminences can be advanced with either a Le Fort III or a Le Fort I and onlay bone grafts placed on the orbital rims and malar eminences.

Bone grafts have traditionally been harvested either from iliac crest or ribs, but these sites have been supplanted in recent years by outer table cranial bone. This is now the preferred site for several reasons. Cranial bone is membranous bone, as are the facial bones, whereas iliac and rib bones are cortical bone. The scar for cranial bone harvesting is not visible, whereas the scars for the other sites are. Donor site pain is far less for cranial bone harvesting. Experimental data and empiric observations indicate that cranial bone undergoes less resorption in the face than either rib or ilium. Demineralized cadaver bone powder can be used as an aid to stimulate faster bone union at osteotomy sites. This has been observed empirically, but not documented.

CAVEATS

As with any type of surgery, experience is an excellent teacher and the surgeon's results in the first ten cases usually will not be as good as in later cases. Therefore, case selection is particularly critical when someone is first performing this type of surgery.

A Le Fort I osteotomy and advancement is not a particularly difficult procedure in a normal jaw. However, the same operation on a cleft maxilla is a difficult and tedious procedure that should not be undertaken by the inexperienced surgeon.

The proper instruments are important for any type of surgery, but are particularly critical for jaw surgery in order to provide adequate, safe exposure, make precise osteotomies, and stabilize the fragments securely. If the surgeon does not have access to all the necessary instruments, he should not perform the surgery.

The blood supply to the lower maxilla is primarily via the greater palatine vessels, but also through the vestibular and nasal floor mucosa. During a Le Fort I maxillary osteotomy, the nasal floor and vestibular blood supply is almost completely eliminated. Therefore, if the greater palatine vessels have been interrupted during earlier surgery, then a Le Fort I is contraindicated and a Le Fort III is necessary, but still somewhat hazardous. If there is any doubt as to the patency of the greater palatine vessels, arteriography is indicated. There have been isolated reports in the literature of maxillary necrosis following Le Fort I maxillary advancement in the cleft palate patient.

SUGGESTED READING

Drommer R. Selective angiographic studies prior to Le Fort I osteotomy in patients with cleft lip and palate. J Maxillofac Surg 1979; 7:264–270.

Drommer R, Luhr H. The stabilization of osteotomized maxillary segments with Luhr miniplates in secondary cleft surgery. J Maxillofac Surg 1981; 9:166–169.

Henderson D, Jackson I. Combined cleft lip revision, anterior fistula closure and maxillary osteotomy; a one stage procedure. Br J Oral Maxillofac Surg 1975; 13:33–39.

Moser K, Freihofer H. Long-term experience with simultaneous movement of the upper and lower jaw. J Maxillofac Surg 1980; 8:271–277.

Poole M, Robinson P, Nunn M. Maxillary advancement in cleft palate patients. A modification of the Le Fort I osteotomy and preliminary results. J Maxillofac Surg 1986; 4:123–127.

Schendel S, Oeschlaeger M, Wolford L, Epker B. Velopharyngeal anatomy and maxillary advancement. J Maxillofac Surg 1979; 7:116–124.

Schendel S, Delaire J. Functional musculoskeletal correction of secondary unilateral cleft lip deformities: combined lip-nose correction and Le Fort I osteotomy. J Maxillofac Surg 1981; 9:108–116.

CRANIOFACIAL DEFORMITIES

FREE FLAPS IN CRANIOFACIAL SURGERY

WILBUR L. BAIRD, M.D.
FOAD NAHAI, M.D., F.A.C.S.

Craniofacial deformities result from disturbance in the normal growth and development of the face and cranium. A wide variety of syndromes are seen, with varying degrees of expression. Both hard and soft tissues exhibit abnormalities in the craniofacial deformities. However, in the majority of syndromes, the skeletal deformities are of much more consequence than those of the soft tissues. Major advances have been made in the past two decades in the treatment of these skeletal abnormalities. Soft tissue aspects of the syndromes have also been addressed, but the procedures have often been cumbersome and the results unpredictable.

Several soft tissue problems require attention: (1) contour deficits, (2) unsuitable beds or severe deficiency of tissue that does not permit underlying skeletal work, and (3) muscular deficits. With the perfection of microvascular techniques, various free tissue transfers are available that are capable of addressing these soft tissue problems. This chapter discusses our experience with free tissue transfer in the treatment of two craniofacial deformities: hemifacial microsomia and hemifacial atrophy. Our major emphasis has been on soft tissue augmentation to alleviate contour deficits.

HEMIFACIAL MICROSOMIA

Hemifacial microsomia is a congenital deformity. It consists of deficiencies in bone and soft tissue of considerable phenotypic variability among affected individuals. Minor deformities may be corrected by minimal skeletal surgery. However, severe deformities may require extensive skeletal surgery in addition to soft tissue augmentation. While there is no universal agreement on the timing of surgery for these patients, the overall surgical plan, which includes ear reconstruction, must be considered in the timing of the microvascular procedure.

Skeletal problems are addressed first. Soft tissue reconstruction is considered early only when the soft tissue is inadequate to support underlying skeletal procedures. After skeletal correction, soft tissue augmentation is considered when significant contour deficits remain. Historically, the soft tissue problems have been addressed with various pedicled or tubed flaps, fat grafts, and dermis grafts. Various free flaps have also been utilized for soft tissue augmentation of the face; however, we feel that omentum and lower abdominal flaps are best suited for this purpose. The omentum provides a significant amount of tissue that may be fashioned into separate fingers of tissue for placement into different areas of the face. However, the omentum suffers from lack of structural integrity and is victim to gravitational sag. Lower abdominal flaps provide more structural support but cannot be sculptured as easily as the omentum. Free muscle flaps have been used, but because they atrophy with time their volume is not as predictable as omentum flaps.

Preoperatively, the degree of soft tissue contour deficiency and its distribution are determined by clinical exam. When the area is large and requires several separate sub-areas of augmentation, omentum is chosen. Less severe deformities can be corrected with de-epithelialized lower abdominal flaps. When skin is required, the omentum can be skin-grafted, or the skin may be left intact on an abdominal flap. The areas of the face that require augmentation are undermined via a preauricular facelift-type incision. The pockets are dissected in a very superficial plane, similar to the facelift. In certain cases, depending on the degree of soft tissue deficit, it may be prudent to expose the facial nerve directly to avoid injury. Once adequate pockets have been dissected, acceptable recipient vessels are located in the upper neck.

Future, or previous, ear reconstruction incisions must be kept in mind when incisions are planned. In addition, great care must be taken to preserve the superficial temporal vessels, because damage to them, or to their use as recipient vessels, would negate future use of the temporoparietal fascial flap, which may, at times, be needed for ear reconstruction. The flap of choice is then harvested. The omentum is harvested through an upper midline incision and is based preferably on the right gastroepiploic vessels. The superficial inferior epigastric artery (SIEA) flap is our skin–dermis flap of choice. The vessels are exposed through a transverse incision along the inguinal crease. If adequate vessels are identified, then the flap design is outlined and the flap elevated. In the absence of the SIEA vessels, a standard groin flap may be utilized. A two-team approach for synchronous facial and flap dissections significantly decreases operative time.

The flap is then transferred to the face and anastomoses are performed in the upper neck with standard microvascular techniques. The vascular supply is reestablished prior to any flap alteration. This is particularly important with the omentum so that devascularization and resultant fat necrosis of a portion of the flap does not occur with trimming. Similarly, the SIEA flap may be split along the plane of Scarpa's fascia to distribute bulk, but this should be done only after revascularization. The flaps are secured into position with mattress sutures through flap and skin and are tied over bolsters. Postoperative wound care consists of Polysporin ointment over the suture lines without any compressive head dressings. The flaps are monitored by clinical examination via a small opening in the incision and also by Doppler.

HEMIFACIAL ATROPHY

Hemifacial atrophy, or Romberg's disease, is a form of craniofacial deformity, although it is not congenital in nature. It is an idiopathic progressive wasting of the subcutaneous fat, followed in some patients by atrophy of the skin, cartilage, bone, and muscle. The usual age of onset is in the first or second decade, and the end result may be very similar to that of hemifacial microsomia. The timing of treatment in this deformity is more certain and is begun when the wasting has progressed fully and is stable.

In contrast to hemifacial microsomia, skeletal surgery is rarely necessary in Romberg's disease. The primary surgical problem is that of soft tissue augmentation. In the past, this problem has been addressed using fat grafts, dermis grafts, various pedicled grafts, and liquid silicone injections. More recently, free tissue transfer has become the accepted procedure for significant contour deficits. As in hemifacial microsomia, omentum and lower abdominal flaps have been our flaps of choice depending on the degree and distribution of the deficits.

The preoperative evaluation and operative techniques are very similar to those described for hemifacial microsomia. It should be noted that additional skin is often required in Romberg's disease, particularly when patients have been previously treated with liquid silicone injections. The indications and the relative advantages and disadvantages of the various flaps are the same as described for hemifacial microsomia.

CLINICAL EXPERIENCE

Four patients with hemifacial microsomia underwent free tissue transfer for correction of contour deficits. The omentum was used in three patients and a lower abdominal flap in one. A representative case is shown in Figure 1. Nineteen patients with hemifacial atrophy underwent similar therapy; the omentum was used in 14 patients and lower abdominal flaps in the remaining five. Representative cases of each flap type are seen in Figures 2 and 3.

The follow-up period ranges from 15 months to 10 years. There has been no total flap loss but two partial losses have occurred: one partial loss of omentum with fat liquefaction, and partial loss of a skin–dermis flap. All patients have required at least one further operation for contour adjustments. In addition, resuspension has been necessary in all the patients with omental transfers in order to correct the sagging that occurs over time. This gravitational sag has not been a problem with the lower abdominal flaps. There has been no clinically apparent resorption of the transferred free flap after the initial operative swelling subsides. Finally, there have been no significant complications from the donor site.

For many surgeons. free flaps are now the procedure of choice for soft tissue restoration in the craniofacial region, and there will likely be greater use of free flaps in the future. As expertise in this field grows, the esthet-

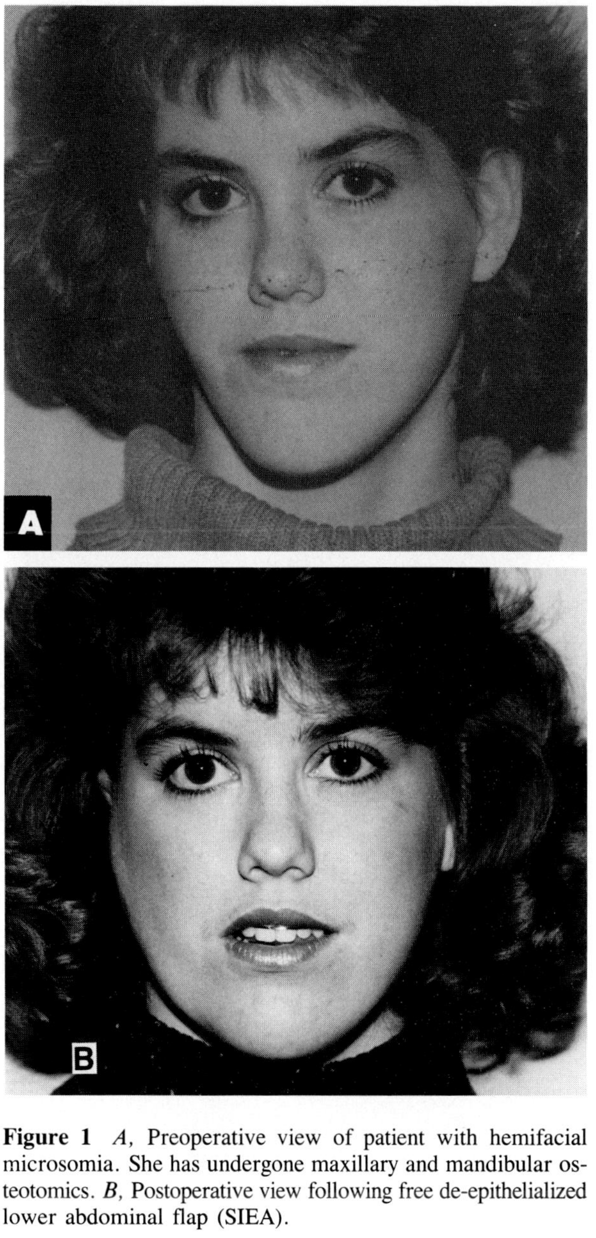

Figure 1 *A*, Preoperative view of patient with hemifacial microsomia. She has undergone maxillary and mandibular osteotomics. *B*, Postoperative view following free de-epithelialized lower abdominal flap (SIEA).

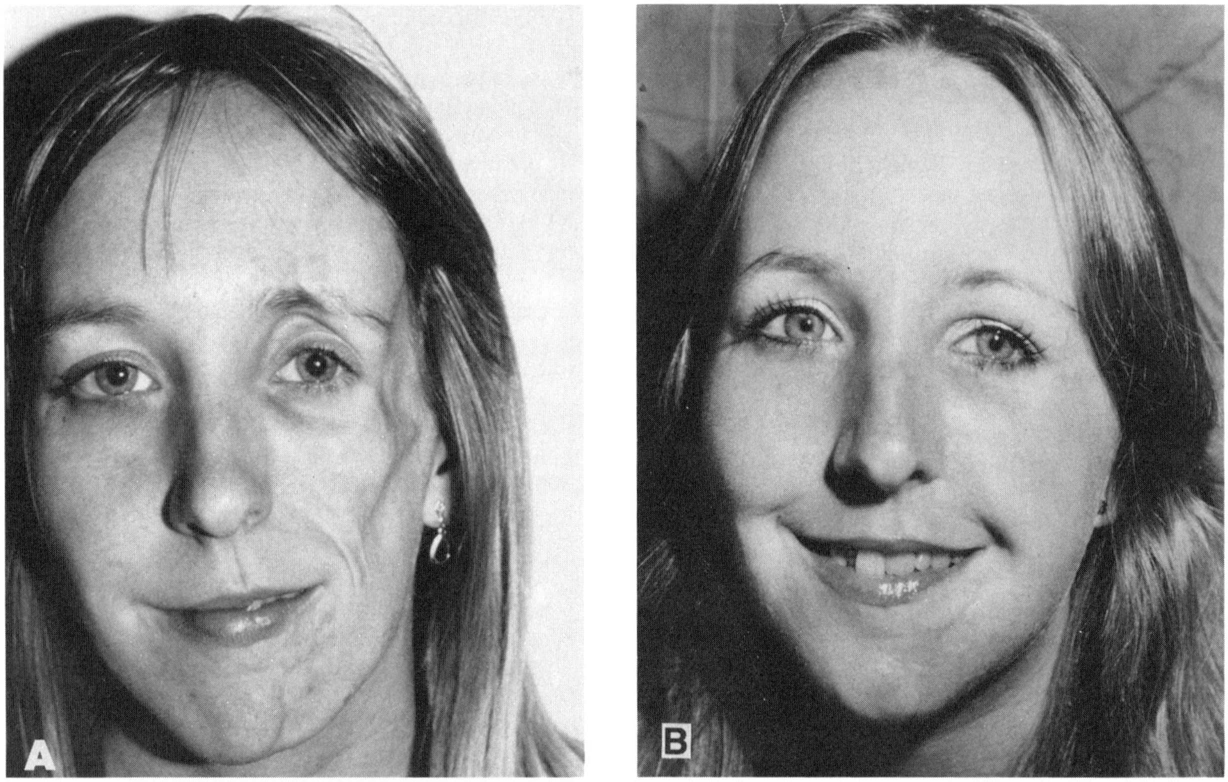

Figure 2 *A,* Preoperative view of woman with stable hemifacial atrophy, and *B,* Postoperative view following free omental transfer and one debulking procedure. (From Wallace JG, et al. Reconstruction of hemifacial atrophy with a free flap of omentum. Br J Plast Surg 1979; 32:15–18.)

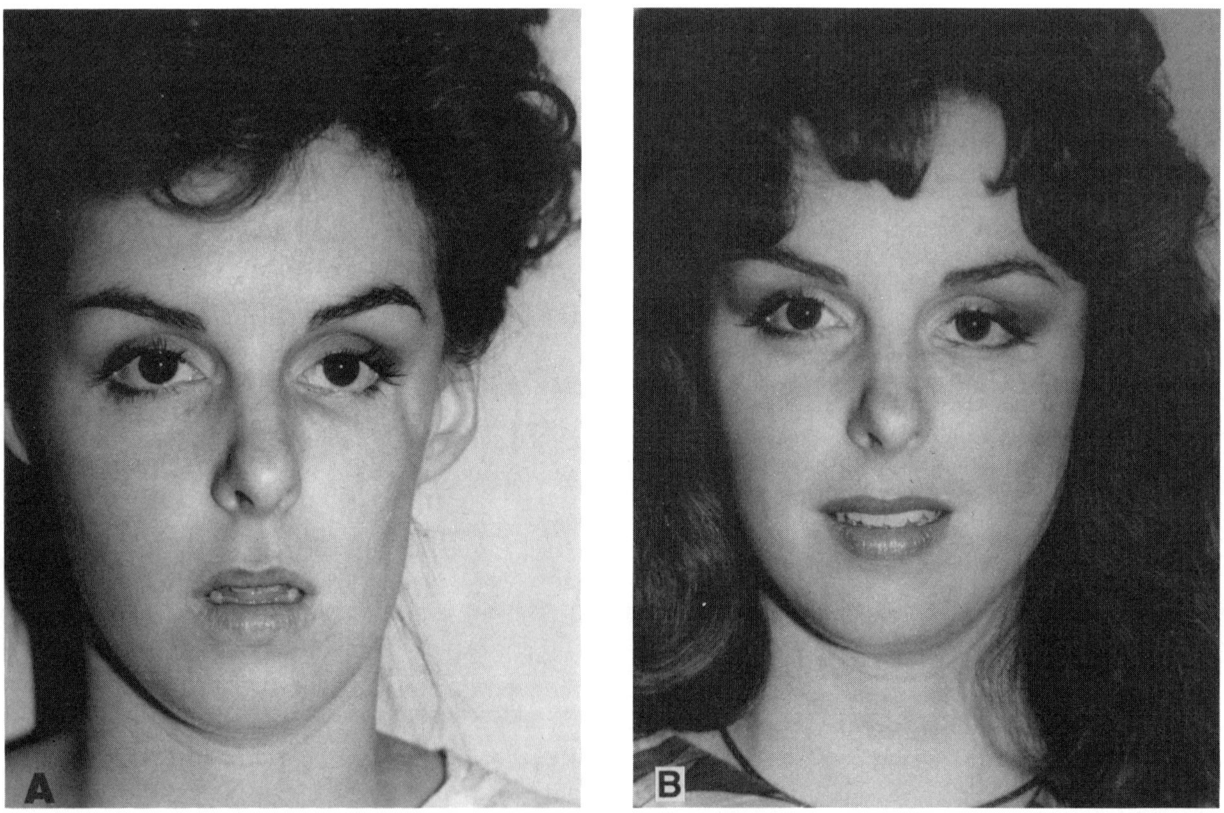

Figure 3 *A,* Preoperative view of patient with stable hemifacial atrophy, and *B,* the same patient postoperatively following free de-epithelialized lower abdominal flap (SIEA) and flap debulking in which suction lipectomy was used.

ic demands will increase and other possibilities of free tissue transfers may be considered in the treatment of craniofacial deformities, e.g., vascularized bone flaps, innervated and functional muscle transfers, and possibly even free tissue allografts.

A final comment should be made regarding the use of craniofacial techniques in areas other than congenital deformities. The techniques developed have enabled tumor resections in the craniofacial area that were not previously possible. In addition, the techniques have greatly influenced our early and late treatment of craniomaxillofacial trauma. Free tissue transfer will obviously be required for closure and various cavity isolations in many instances of tumor resection. Free flap use in the treatment of trauma, early and late, has obvious appeal and may be more widely used in the future.

SUGGESTED READING

Hester TR, Nahai F, Beegle PE, Bostwick J. Blood supply of the abdomen revisited, with emphasis on the superficial inferior epigastric artery. Plast Reconstr Surg 1984; 74:657–666.

Jurkiewicz MJ, Nahai F. The omentum: its use as a free vascularized graft for reconstruction of the head and neck. Ann Surg 1982; 196:756–765.

Jurkiewicz MJ, Nahai F. The use of revascularized grafts in the Amelioration of hemifacial atrophy. Plast Reconstr Surg 1985; 76:44–54.

Rossa DL, Whitaker L, Dubb R, Millissinos E. The use of microvascular free flaps for soft tissue augmentation of the face in children with hemifacial microsomia. Cleft Palate J 1980; 17:138–143.

Wells JH, Edgerton MT. Correction of source hemifacial atrophy with a free dermis-fat flap from the lower abdomen. Plast Reconstr Surg 1977; 59:223–229.

FREE FLAP CONTOURING OF FACIAL ASYMMETRIES

BERNARD S. ALPERT, M.D., F.A.C.S.
HARRY J. BUNCKE, M.D., F.A.C.S.

The facial contouring problems discussed in this chapter are those that result from hemifacial atrophy (Romberg's disease), hemifacial microsomia and its variants, surgical ablation, radiation, and overwhelming infection. These problems present with varying reconstruction requirements, and an individual analysis of each case with its functional (if any), and esthetic deficits is required. Specific deformities to be considered in each case are in the bony skeleton, facial skin, soft tissue fill (fat and muscle), and lining of facial cavities. The approach to reconstruction of facial nerve paralysis is not discussed. The methods utilized represent our own individual approaches to complex facial contouring problems, using vascularized tissues.

THERAPEUTIC ALTERNATIVES

Many alternative methods have been and are currently used in the treatment of facial contouring. These include vascularized local flaps, composite grafts or nonvascularized tissue (e.g., dermis-fat, fascia), alloplastic materials, and injectables (collagen, fat, silicone).

The use of vascularized local flaps in the contouring of major deformities may have the disadvantage of producing a significant secondary facial contour problem because of the parasitization of local tissue. Examples include use of the temporalis and sternocleidomastoid muscles. In addition, because of the many specialized tissues of the face, the number of acceptable local flaps is limited. Examples of vascularized regional attached flaps with acceptable donor sites that may be used for significant deformities are the calvarial osseofascial flap and the pectoralis major musculocutaneous flap after being tunneled and de-epithelialized.

Nonvascularized grafts of bone, dermis-fat, and fascia have unpredictable volume preservations and require an intact, richly vascularized bed for survival. Given an excellent local environment, all of these may be used with varying degrees of success. They may be useful adjuncts to free flaps in the treatment of extensive deformities. They, obviously, are not useful in a poorly vascularized environment that has been radiated, has extensive scarring, or contains a full-thickness tissue defect.

Alloplastic materials, of all kinds, have been used for a long time to treat facial contour problems. Success is more frequent when small implants are placed in areas where they can be covered by significant amounts of soft tissue. The use of such implants in the chin, malar region, and premaxillary area is currently quite common. Extrusion and infection may be problems, particularly in areas where the overlying soft tissue cover is thin. Malposition, implant perimeter visibility, and palpability are recognized potential disadvantages. Underlying bony erosion has been seen in some cases. Small implants that are well covered with vascularized tissue may be an adjunct in the refinement phase of treating extensive facial asymmetries.

The use of injectable fat and silicone remains experimental at this time. The unpredictability of the injection of significant volumes of fat over a long term has become apparent. Similarly, the use of commercially available forms of injectable collagen provides only temporary correction, particularly for larger defects.

PREFERRED APPROACH

Each patient is evaluated with regard to the specific requirements of reconstruction. The ultimate goal in every case is to achieve as normal a result as possible, both functionally and esthetically. We attempt to achieve this by leaving as little evidence of surgery behind as possible. In so doing, two basic tenets are observed: (1) great care is taken to design incisions so that they are as acceptable and disguised as possible, and (2) since a flap in the face is a patch in the face, we attempt to make all flaps used in reconstruction disappear in the eyes of the beholder: the disappearing flap.

In order to accomplish the above goals, we do not always adhere to one basic principle of reconstruction; namely, the ideal of always replacing like tissue with like. Specifically, bone is not always replaced with bone, and subcutaneous fat not always with fat. The reasons for this are given later during the discussion of the principles of the therapeutic approach.

Very few patients are rejected as candidates for microvascular facial contouring surgery. Acceptable vasculature in the recipient region of the head and neck is an obvious prerequisite for reconstruction. Most patients undergo preoperative angiography; certainly if there is any question as to the status of the external carotid artery system. Many of these patients have had either congenital or acquired alterations of the vessels, and knowledge of their preoperative status is essential. It is quite unusual, however, to find a patient without at least a single artery and vein suitable for recipient vasculature in reconstruction; although interposition vein grafts may be required.

As regards timing of surgery, it is advisable to have all local tissues in the recipient area stable and not evolving, either with regard to scar formation or progression of a disease process. An example of the latter would be in cases of progressive hemifacial atrophy. There is always a fear that the tissues used in reconstruction will become subject to the same disease process, particularly if the procedure is performed as the disease manifestations are evolving.

It is usually beneficial to perform the facial contouring procedures subsequent to other operations on the face for major functional deficiencies. Examples of this would be craniofacial, Le Fort, and mandibular osteotomies to reposition major bony segments. Orthodontia and orthognathic surgical procedures are best concluded prior to the microsurgical facial contouring.

Obviously there are cases, such as loss of mandibular segments, where the restoration of function, as well as facial contour, is accomplished in and by the same procedure. Appropriate examples are discussed later in this chapter.

PRINCIPLES OF THERAPEUTIC APPROACH

As previously stated, the basic principles of treatment are to produce the best functional and esthetic results while minimizing incisions and "flap tracks." When we plan incisions, we commonly use those employed in esthetic procedures such as rhytidectomy or coronal browlift. Natural skin lines (e.g., nasolabial folds), blepharoplasty, and intraoral incisions are also used when necessary. In previous years, extended incisions on the face and neck such as for parotidectomy, or a radical neck dissection, were used for exposure when performing free flap facial contouring. Currently, we are more likely to use, for example, a rhytidectomy incision combined with a small submandibular incision in order to expose the facial vessels. This may require tunneling of a vascular pedicle in order to reach its recipient vasculature, thereby violating a previously adhered to rule of microvascular surgery. As long as attention is paid to detail in the creation of tunnel width and direction of the vascular axis, flap survival is not sacrificed by these modifications.

Since a flap in the face always appears as a patch, great efforts should be made to have all such flaps ultimately covered by facial skin. A bulky flap beneath normal facial skin is also conspicuous by its size, however, and attempts should be made to reduce evidence of the flap's presence by appropriate secondary trimming and debulking procedures. A flap in the face that is both bulky and not covered by facial skin is often as conspicuous in its own way as the original deformity. (See case example below).

There should essentially be no outward evidence of the existence of a flap of appropriate bulk, placed through well-designed incisions and positioned totally beneath facial skin, as anything but a normal, integrated part of the face. The flap essentially disappears as an identifiable entity. If facial skin is deficient and flap skin must be placed externally, efforts should be made secondarily to reduce and, one hopes, eliminate the size of the added external skin. Fortunately, in many such cases the flap itself acts as an autogenous tissue expander, thereby allowing the adjacent normal facial skin to relax and stretch, often aided by the excess weight of the flap and gravity. Facial skin edges that have been indurated and tight with contracture often soften up nicely when sewn to well-vascularized bulky flap edges. This aids the ability of the normal facial skin to expand on its own. If additional expansion with alloplastic tissue expanders is required, this may be utilized. In our experience, however, this is not often required. The flaps themselves are excellent autogenous expanders. Subsequent secondary procedures of de-epithelialization and burying of the skin paddle portions of the flap, accompanied by appropriate debulking such as with suction lipectomy, allow such patches in the face subsequently to "disappear" and leave no "flap tracks."

CASE EXAMPLES

Specific Flaps

The advantages and disadvantages of commonly used flaps are listed in Tables 1 and 2.

Romberg's Disease

In advanced cases, the defects that require soft tissue fill are classically serpentine in nature. (Figs. 1 and 2) The serratus anterior muscle, with its own slip-like serpentine shape, is ideal to match the defects with a custom-fitted flap. One, two, or three slips of the serratus anterior may be used, depending on the requirements of the defect.

TABLE 1 Commonly Used Flaps

Muscles
Serratus anterior
Gracilis
Rectus abdominis
Latissimus dorsi
Skin flaps (usually de-epithelialized)
Scapular
Groin
Superficial inferior epigastric artery (SIEA)
Osteocutaneous flaps
Deep groin (DCIA)
Scapula

Good quality facial skin is almost never deficient in these patients, and the entire flap is placed beneath the skin, thus allowing the flap to "disappear." Seventh nerve function is normal and continues to be so postoperatively, without interference from the intervening flap. There is usually no associated bony defect and, certainly, no functional bony deficit. The muscle is placed in the subcutaneous plane and is sewn precisely beneath the flap to the exact margins of the defect. The muscle is not innervated, because obviously no undesirable muscle function is sought. The disadvantage of the use of the muscle in these cases is an unpredictable amount of atrophy, up to 30 or 40 percent. However, the most prominent feature of these patients' deformity is the skeletal appearance of the affected part of the face. The bone edges are not blunted, because of the lack of subcutaneous tissue. Even with muscle atrophy, the blunting of bony prominences is maintained by the remaining muscle, thus producing a much softer appearance to the face, which is within the normal range of facial asymmetry postoperatively. It is common for the bulk of the serratus anterior muscle to overcorrect a Romberg's defect by approximately 25 percent at the time of surgery. The resultant atrophy usually places the final result within 15 percent of undercorrection, thereby maintaining the soft blunting of the skeletal edges. Smaller isolated defects may be corrected with small pieces of muscle, again placed through esthetically acceptable incisions.

In keeping with the principles outlined previously, the serratus anterior muscle is placed through a rhytidectomy incision, combined with a small submandibular incision to dissect the facial vessels. By turning the lowest three slips of the serratus anterior upside down, the vascular pedicle is placed ideally for anastomosis to the facial artery and vein as recipient vasculature. This also places the flap vascular pedicle in an ideal position for venous drainage. The quality of these vessels is far superior to the temporal vessels which, if necessary, may also be used.

Hemifacial Microsomia

In patients with hemifacial microsomia (Fig. 3), the maxillofacial surgery is performed prior to any microsurgical facial contouring. The remaining deficit usually does not have a bony requirement because the functional bony deficit has been corrected by the maxillofacial surgery. The shape of the deformity in hemifacial microsomia is usually ovoid, and lends itself to reconstruction with a de-epithelialized skin flap. If desired, muscle may also be used. Facial skin cover may or may not be adequate. Ideally, all of the flap is covered by facial skin, as noted previously. If not, efforts should be made secondarily to resect serially any skin-grafted portions of the de-epithelialized skin flap or cutaneous portions of such flaps, and ultimately cover them with normal facial skin that has relaxed secondary to the autogenous expanding nature of the skin flap reconstruction.

Deformities Secondary to Surgical Ablation for Cancer

When radiation is not involved, it is often possible to place all of the reconstruction beneath normal facial skin. This is one of the ideal settings for reconstruction (Figs. 4 to 6). When a bony deficit exists, a distinction must be made as to whether or not it is a functional bony problem. If it is, then appropriate osseous reconstruction

TABLE 2 Advantages–Disadvantages of Flaps by Type

Type	*Advantages*	*Disadvantages*
Muscle	Serpentine defects Easily harvested Good donor sites (serratus, gracilis)	Atrophy Involuntary contractions
De-epithelialized skin flaps	Predictable bulk Easily harvested (Scapular only) Ovoid defects Good donor sites (groin, SIEA)	Less adaptable
Osteocutaneous flaps	Good functional bony substitute Versatile (Scapular)	Bulky (DCIA) Bone-skin relationship may be restrictive (DCIA)

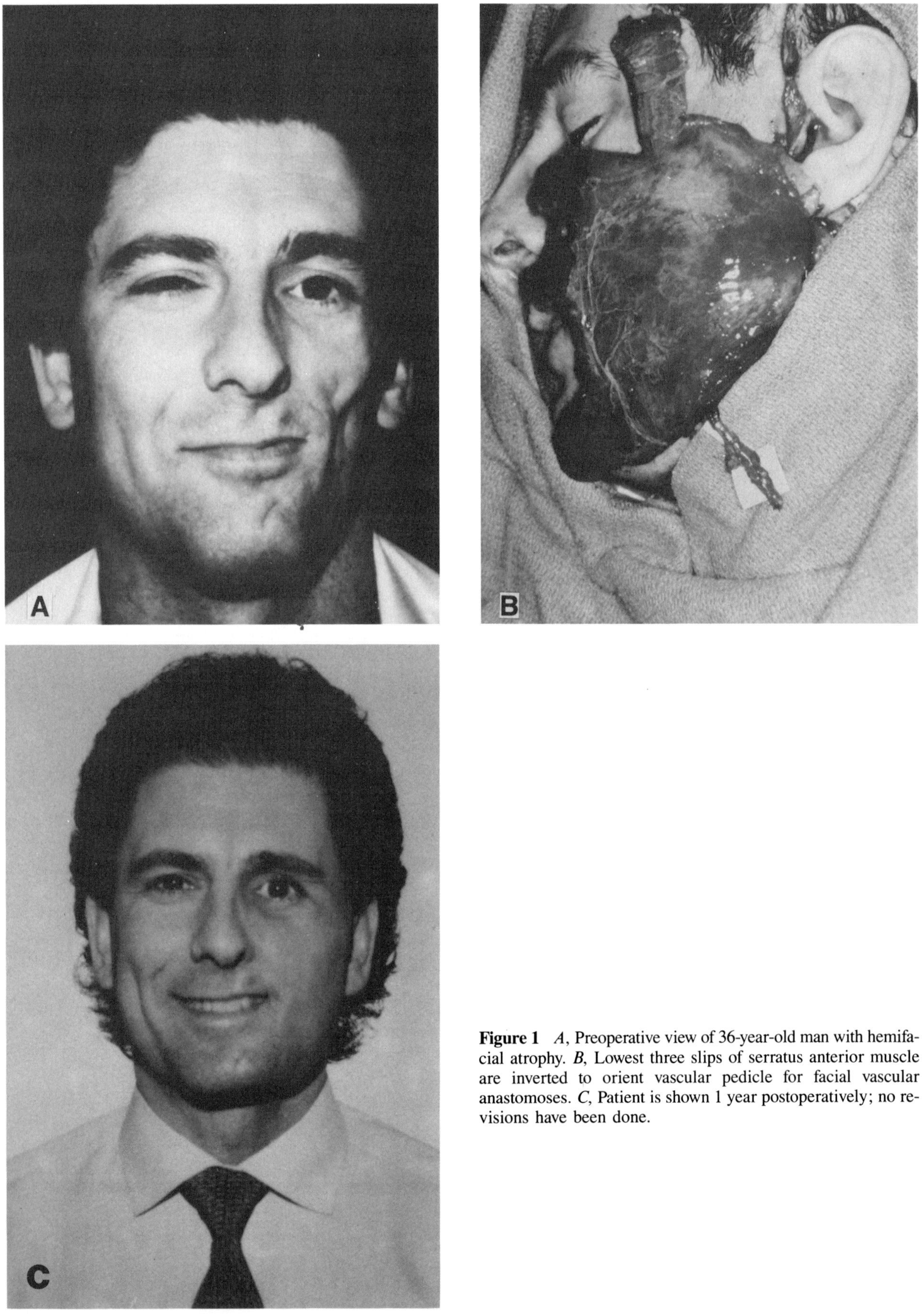

Figure 1 *A*, Preoperative view of 36-year-old man with hemifacial atrophy. *B*, Lowest three slips of serratus anterior muscle are inverted to orient vascular pedicle for facial vascular anastomoses. *C*, Patient is shown 1 year postoperatively; no revisions have been done.

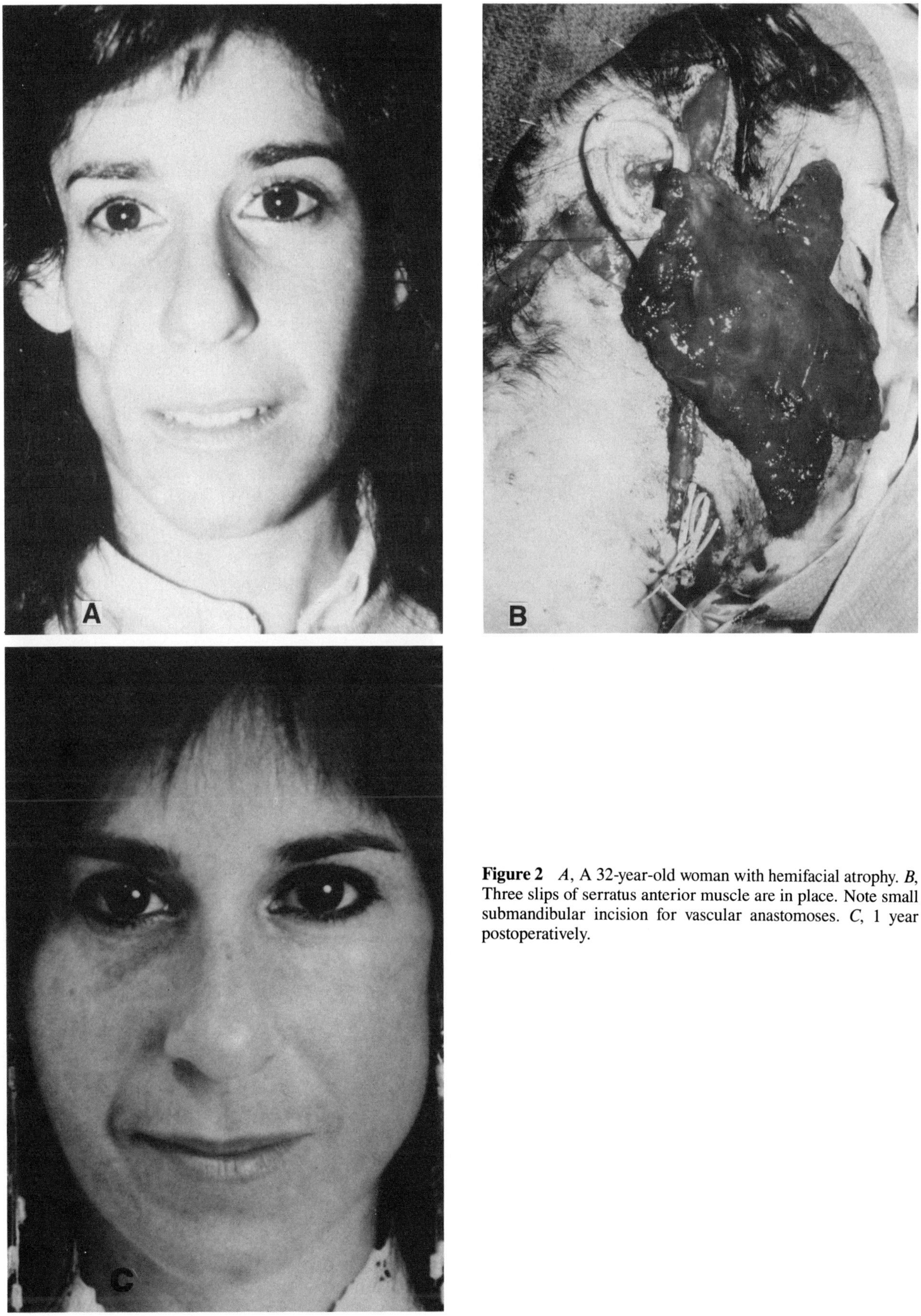

Figure 2 *A*, A 32-year-old woman with hemifacial atrophy. *B*, Three slips of serratus anterior muscle are in place. Note small submandibular incision for vascular anastomoses. *C*, 1 year postoperatively.

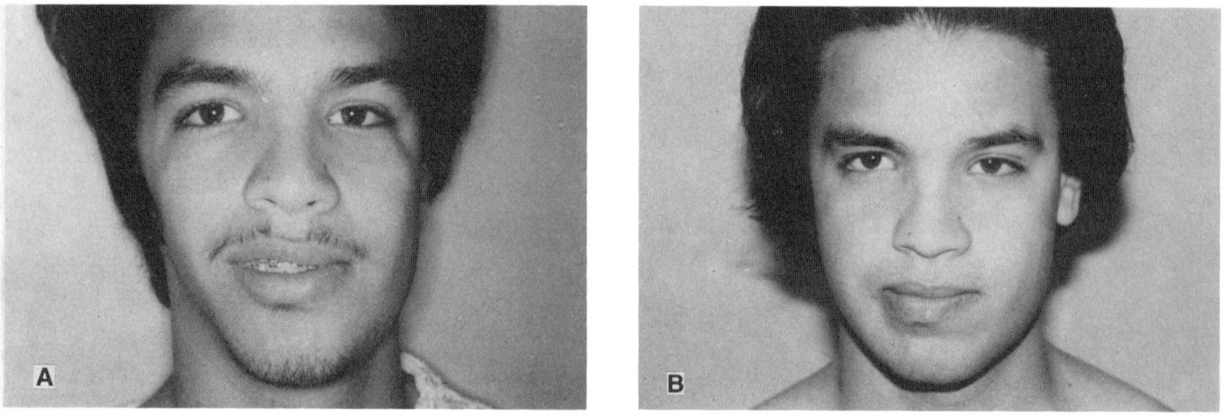

Figure 3 *A*, A 19-year-old male with hemifacial microsomia; skeletal osteotomies, orthodontic and ear reconstruction were completed prior to the soft tissue contouring. *B*, One year postoperatively. A serratus anterior muscle was used in this case. De-epithelialized skin flaps are also applicable here as the defect is ovoid in shape.

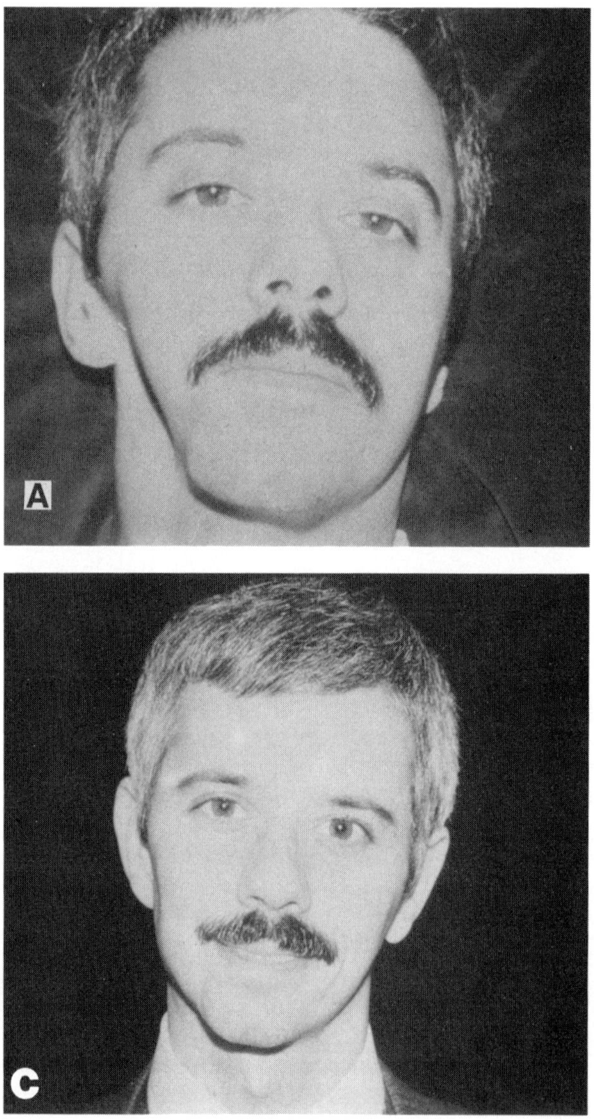

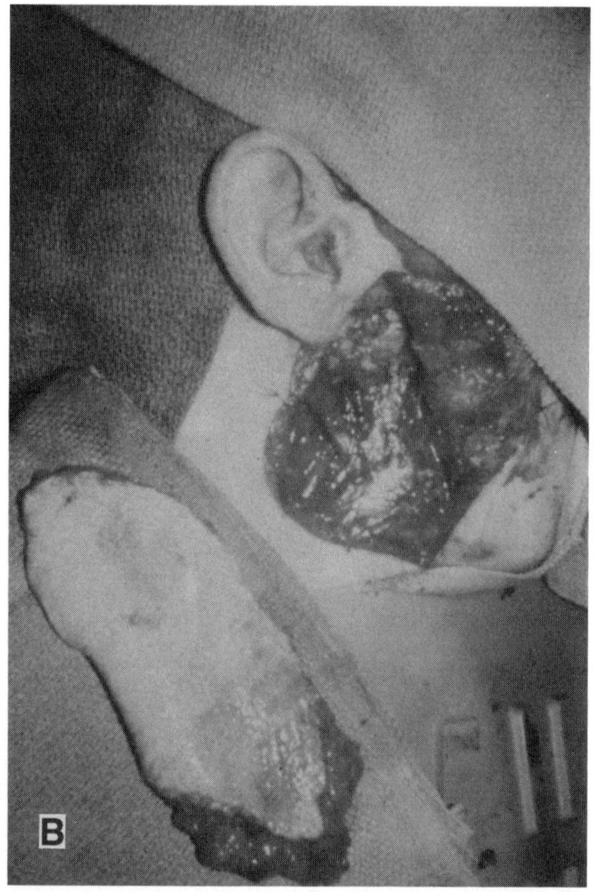

Figure 4 *A*, Young man is shown post segmental mandibulectomy for carcinoma. Mastication is normal. *B*, De-epithelialized groin flap is used. *C*, The patient is shown 2 years postoperatively.

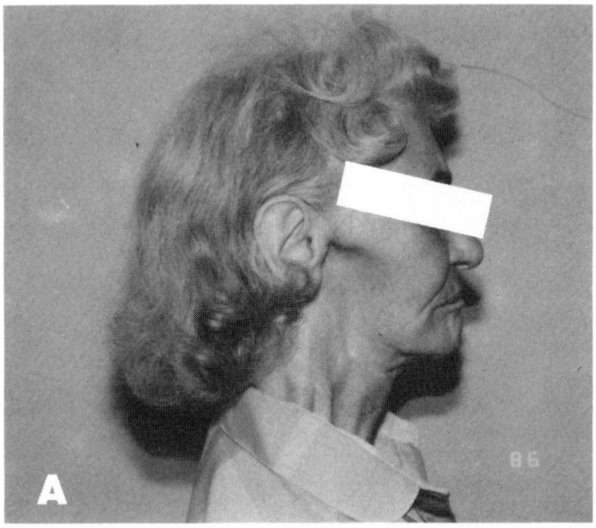

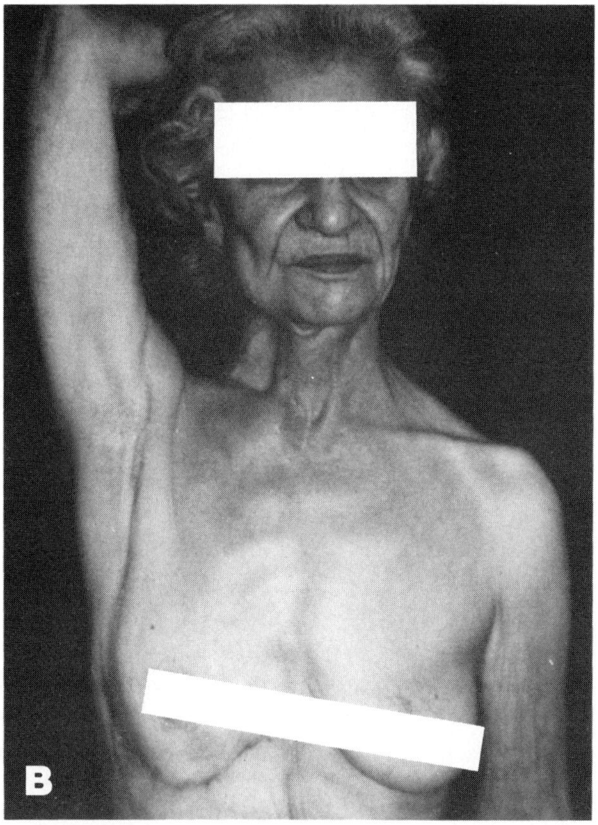

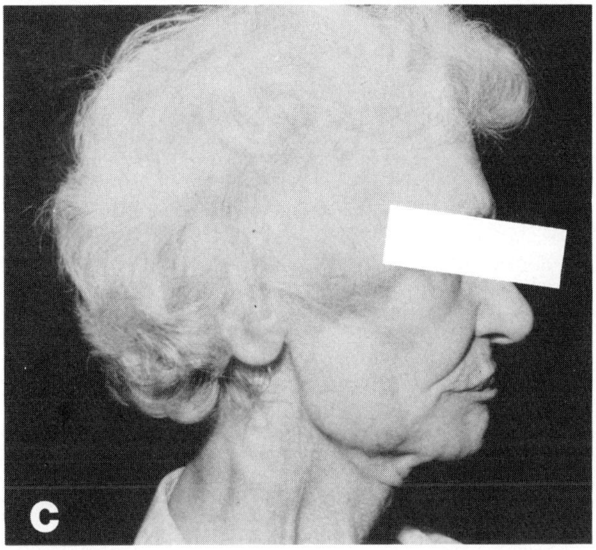

Figure 5 *A*, Photograph of a 67-year-old woman after mandibulectomy, parotidectomy, and radial neck dissection for ameloblastoma. *B*, Postoperative results. The mandible was reconstructed with vascularized iliac bone through the deep circumflex iliac vessels to the external carotid using vein grafts. A pectoralis musculocutaneous flap with de-epithelialized skin island was used for neck and cheek fill beneath the patient's normal face and neck skin. *C*, Face and neck contour are good with acceptable donor incisions. Mandible has no deficit, mastication is good, and vestibuloplasty and denture fitting are planned (or osteointegrated dental implants).

has to be a part of the reconstructive procedure. This bone may be part of an osteocutaneous flap; or the bony and soft tissue corrections may be done independently. This approach offers increased versatility in the reconstruction, without any constraints upon positioning because of the intimate attachments between the bone and skin portions of an osteocutaneous composite flap (see Fig. 5). When the bony deficit is not a functional one, and no radiation has been involved, it may be possible to use only soft tissue for facial contouring. This goes against the basic principle of replacing like with like; however, predictable and precise facial contour may be achieved with esthetically pleasing incisions without disturbing the facial skeleton (see Fig. 4).

When radiation has been involved in the treatment of the patient's malignancy, it is most likely that external facial cover will have to be provided at the initial reconstruction. When a functional bony deficiency also exists, it is likely that a composite miscrovascular osteocutaneous flap will be used (see Fig. 6). If this is the case, all useful facial skin should be preserved. The cutaneous portion of the composite flap is used as an autogenous expander. The epidermis of the cutaneous island is ultimately removed and the dermis covered by facial skin.

The Autogenous Flap as Tissue Expander

The patient in this case example (Fig. 7) is a brittle diabetic with an extensive facial defect secondary to mucormycosis infection. The patient is extremely short of tissue, i.e., lining, bone, muscle, fat, and skin. The use of a large latissimus musculocutaneous flap allows the marginal facial skin to soften and stretch under the weight of the flap along with gravity. There is a bony defect, but it is not a functional one. Therefore, bone is not an absolute requirement of reconstruction. In this particular case, the autogenous expander nature of the flap allows subsequent advancement of normal facial skin over a de-

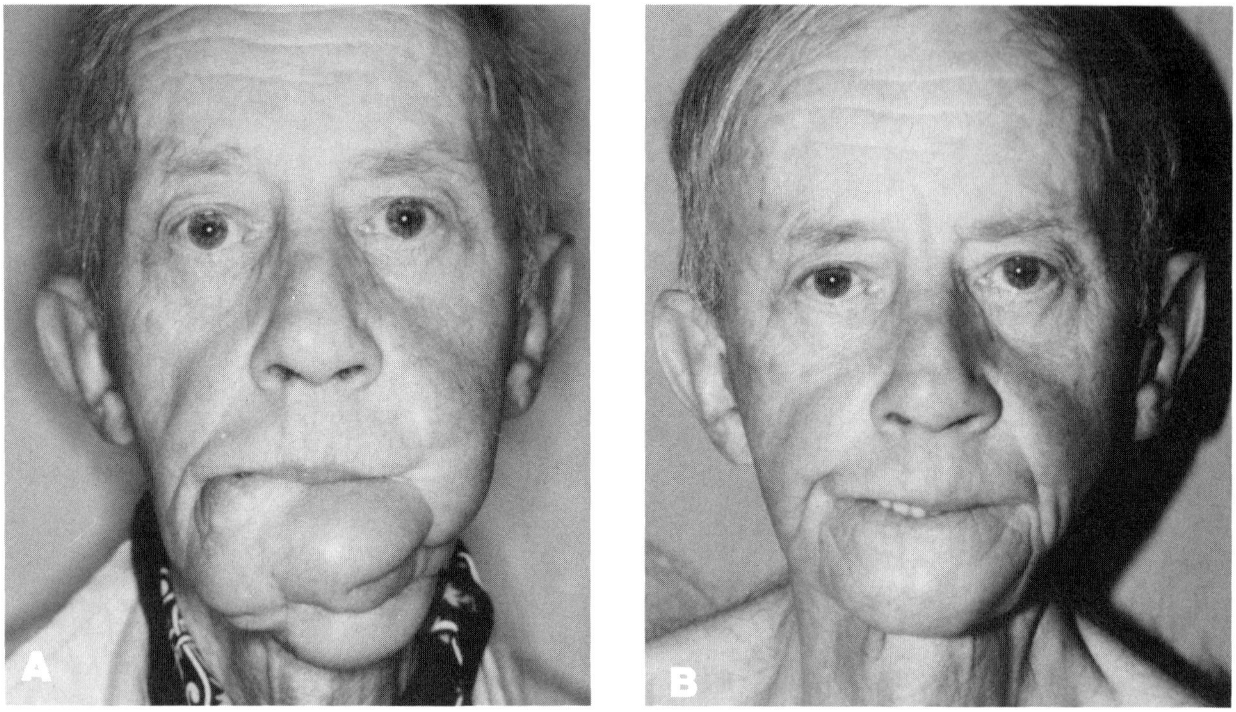

Figure 6 *A*, A 56-year-old patient had osteoradionecrosis of the mandible shown here after scapular osteocutaneous flap reconstruction. The flap is bulky, deforming, and appears as a patch. *B*, After 1 year, the adjacent facial and neck skin had relaxed. The cutaneous portion of the osteocutaneous flap was debulked by suction lipectomy, de-epithelialized, and buried beneath good quality adjacent facial and cervical skin. Photograph shows appearance 2 years postoperatively after vestibuloplasty and denture fitting.

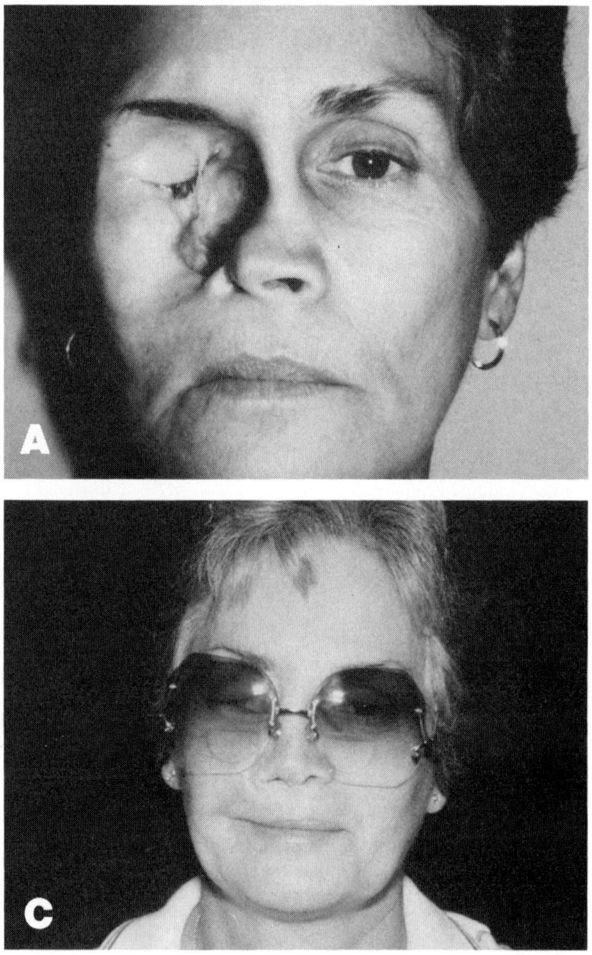

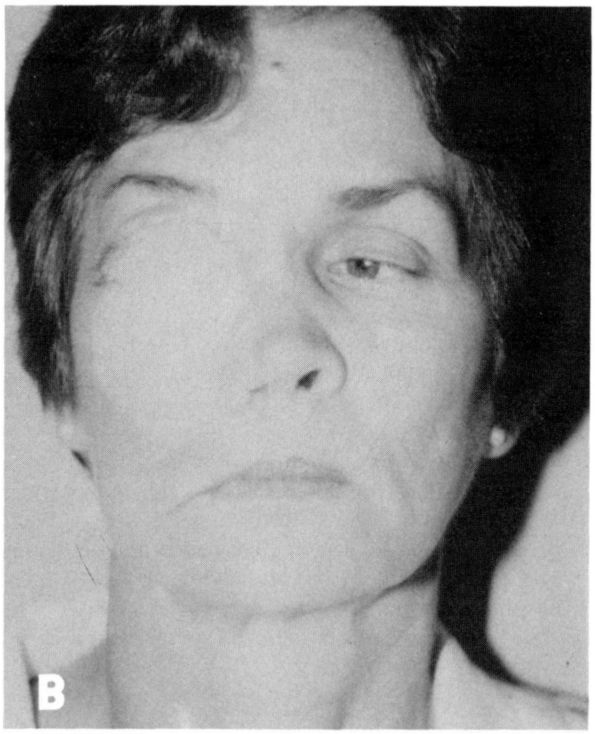

Figure 7 *A*, A 50-year-old brittle insulin-dependent diabetic with extensive deformity following mucormycosis infection. *B*, She is shown after first stage with large latissimus musculocutaneous flap filling the defect. Adjacent facial skin then softens and relaxes, allowing staged debulking, de-epithelialization, and advancement. *C*, The patient 18 months postoperatively. The only remaining portion of skin island is in the orbit. Ocular prosthetic fitting is planned.

epithelialized cutaneous portion of the flap, so that the only remaining flap patch is that in the orbital socket. Incisions were designed at the nasomaxillary junction and orbital rim to maximize the esthetic potential of the result. The flap was easily contoured and no bone was used in the reconstruction. After orbital prosthetic fitting, the patient, who had an extensive deformity now essentially has a flap that has totally disappeared, with minimal signs of reconstruction.

CRANIOSYNOSTOSIS

LINTON A. WHITAKER, M.D.

Craniosynostosis leads to craniostenosis with restriction of growth of associated calvarial and facial structures. As a result, problems may occur related to inhibition of calvarial growth with increased intracranial pressure and abnormality of cranial and facial contour. The treatment of craniosynostosis and its secondary problems is a balancing act that attempts to take advantage of the generally positive effects of: rapid brain expansion in the first 3 years of life; the malleability and capacity for regeneration of calvarial bone, especially in the first 18 months of life; and the lack of advance psychological effects with early surgery. Opposing the positive influences are: the uncertain growth patterns inherent in some of the syndromes; the fact that previous surgery on bone, when not totally corrective, makes subsequent surgery more difficult; the inherent risks of any operative procedure, especially when it is certain that one cannot fully correct the problem; and the compromising of calvarial bone graft donor sites as a result of early surgery.

Thus, the timing of surgery for treatment of patients with craniosynostosis is exceptionally important. If it can be expected that one operative procedure will correct the structural and functional problems, it should be done as early as possible. If, on the other hand, the initial operation only partially corrects the problem and makes subsequent procedures more difficult, then the value of the earlier procedure becomes questionable. In our experience, based on the treatment of 195 patients, aged 1 month to 40 years, since 1972, those patients with fundamentally asymmetrical problems treated within the first 18 months of life have a greater than 90 percent chance that this surgery, excepting a minor revision, will be the only operation required. In contrast, in patients with generally symmetrical problems, including most of those with hereditary disorders and with named syndromes, the chances of complete or almost complete correction of the problem with one operation in the first 18 months of life is reduced to less than 50 percent. Consequently, one must more carefully consider alternative timing of treatment for these patients until better understanding of the outcome of surgery and subsequent growth is known. In the more severe problems, such as Apert's syndrome, the need for further surgery that is at least as great as the original procedure is nearly 100 percent. This makes it essential that we continue to evaluate current techniques, attempt to improve them, and strive to understand the pathophysiology of the problems involved. Once the timing of surgery is determined, the calvaria and face are considered architecturally and one of several operative procedures is done to establish normal relations.

THERAPEUTIC ALTERNATIVES

The initial overriding concern with craniosynostosis is whether or not brain function is being compromised, as manifested by increasing intracranial pressure, by the pathologic process. A second and generally lesser concern is corneal exposure related to exophthalmus. Rarely, nasal airway function may be motivation to perform a procedure early in life. Jaw function is generally not a primary consideration until well into the mixed dentition stage. Finally, while appearance and the psychological effect of the contour deformities are dominant concerns, they must be secondary to functional considerations at least until age 4 years—and perhaps much later.

Neurosurgical intervention may be important within the first few weeks of life for severe problems associated with craniosynostosis. In these instances, the neurosurgeon should proceed with whatever basic procedure is considered advisable for release of the growing brain. Neonates who require perinatal intervention almost invariably have the named syndromal and symmetrical manifestations of craniosynostosis. It should be emphasized to the parents that multiple operations will be necessary. A second operation for reshaping the calvaria and orbits can be considered at 6 to 12 months of age. Even then, it is likely that subsequent, often major, revisions, as well as midface reconstruction, will be necessary between ages 4 and 12 years.

Because of the compromise in results that may occur in patients with severe synostoses, deferral of subsequent surgery, other than the basic neurosurgical procedures, should be considered. While it is psychologically trying for a family and for a child to wait, it may be advisable physically for growth to be nearly complete in some instances. An intermediate stage that consists of repositioning of the orbits, reshaping of the forehead, and augmentation of the midfacial skeleton may be done in these patients. Midface osteotomies are generally reserved, except in the most extreme cases, until past 8 years of age. In those patients where it is possible to defer the surgery until the teenage years, primarily those with moderate to severe problems, the likelihood of having one major craniofacial reconstructive procedure is much higher.

Patients with plagiocephaly have fundamentally normal growth potential. The chances of full correction of the problem with one-time surgery, are sufficiently great (more than 90 percent), that the presence of a clinically important asymmetrical synostosis is sufficient indication for surgery. As demonstrated in comparative studies, the unilateral treatment of asymmetrical synostosis is as effective as bilateral treatment, and the ideal age is 6 to 9 months. While the surgery can be done earlier, it is more difficult because of the delicate nature of the bones and no structural advantage is gained. In the milder forms of symmetrical synostosis, the same statements are generally true, although the possibility of increased intracranial pressure must be watched carefully.

The only absolute contraindications to cranial osseous surgery are uncorrected hydrocephalus, extreme mental retardation, and at the opposite end of the scale, problems that are so minor they are difficult to detect. The latter most often occur in patients with plagiocephaly. They also may occur in the extremely mild symmetric forms of craniosynostosis where consideration should be given to delaying surgery until the teenage years.

PREFERRED APPROACH

The calvaria and face must be assessed in detail prior to surgery by a comprehensive physical examination, adequate radiographic examination (generally computerized tomography [CT] scan with 3-dimensional imaging), and examinations by the ophthalmologist, neurosurgeon, and orthodontist, when the jaws are involved. Symmetry of the calvaria, orbit to eye, and midface to upper and lower face relations must be considered along with known esthetic standards of facial norm, which includes physical anthropologic assessment. Based on these findings, and on x-ray studies, photographs, and consultants' reports, the surgery is planned.

All surgical approaches involve a coronal incision, with exposure of the frontal bones, orbits, base of the nose, and part of the midface. Soft tissue is mobilized adequately for comparative purposes in the unilateral problems, and for osteotomies in the bilateral problems. In asymmetrical problems, a unilateral frontal craniotomy and a shift of approximately two-thirds the circumference of the orbit is our procedure of choice. The osteotomy enters the orbit from the frontal craniotomy at the juncture of the superior and medial orbits, goes across the anterior cranial base immediately behind the posterior table of the frontal bone, and extends as a tongue-in-groove into the temporal region. The tongue-in-groove is cut, including the pterion, and the cut is extended down the posterior lateral orbit a variable distance. If the deformity stops at the zygomaticofrontal suture, a half Z-plasty may be done. If, however, as is more often the case, it extends to the zygoma, the osteotomy is carried to just lateral to the infraorbital nerve. The segment is shifted anteriorly after it has been freed entirely, it is wired superiorly and medially as a hinge, advanced the appropriate amount laterally and superiorly, with the tongue-in-groove used for fixation, and a bone graft is placed behind the advanced lateral orbit to reconstruct its continuity as well as provide fixation. Where advisable, craniectomy bone is used as an onlay to the anterior surface of the zygoma. When a tendency to enophthalmus is noted, bone grafts are placed in the orbit to shift the eye forward. In rare instances, both sides are operated on in patients with asymmetrical synostoses (Figs. 1 and 2).

In the symmetrical (bilateral) problems, an osteotomy of the superior and lateral orbit is done with a tongue-in-groove extension into the temporal bone laterally. It is carried across the anterior cranial base and into the nose at the nasofrontal suture, or down to the inferior border of the nasal bone so that it can be advanced in its entirety. Laterally, a half Z-plasty at the zygomaticofrontal suture is done in most instances, but, occasionally, the osteotomy is carried into the infraorbital area. After the orbits are freed in approximately two-thirds of their circumference, they are advanced and rigidly fixed by wires or miniplates to the facial skeleton and temporal calvaria.

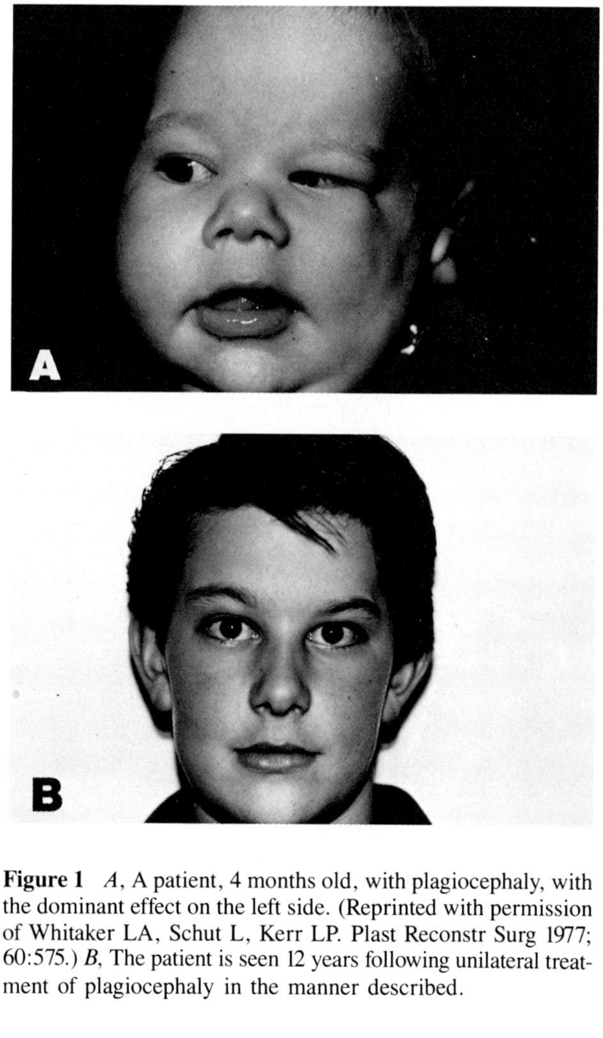

Figure 1 *A*, A patient, 4 months old, with plagiocephaly, with the dominant effect on the left side. (Reprinted with permission of Whitaker LA, Schut L, Kerr LP. Plast Reconstr Surg 1977; 60:575.) *B*, The patient is seen 12 years following unilateral treatment of plagiocephaly in the manner described.

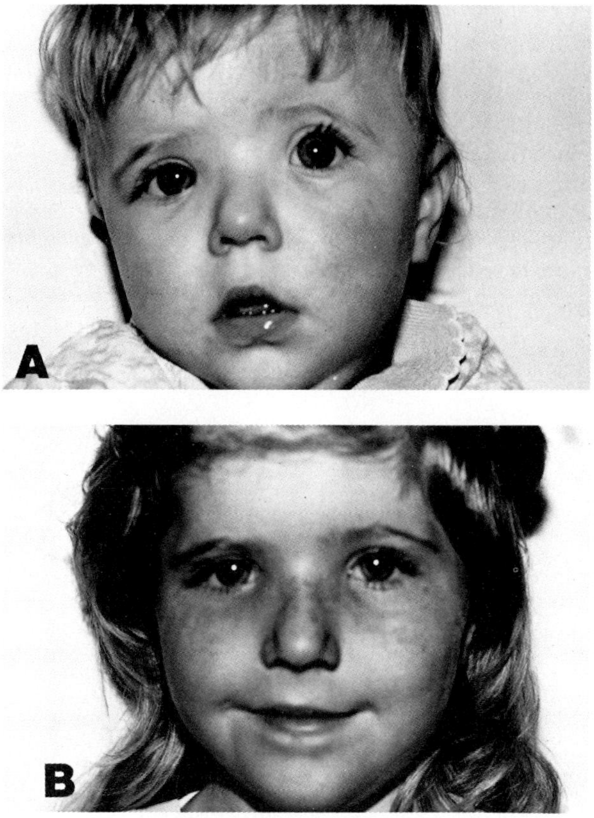

Figure 2 *A*, A 6-month-old patient with plagiocephaly, with bilateral involvement. *B*, The patient is seen 4 years after right unilateral orbital repositioning, bilateral frontal bone repositioning, and bilateral medial canthopexies.

These procedures are done with the assistance of a bifrontal craniotomy. The frontal bone is shaped with either reorientation or contouring, following the orbital advancement, to achieve the proper slope, symmetry, and contour desired. Bone grafts are used to fill in some of the calvarial defects, although these are generally left open in infants to close spontaneously. In patients more than 4 years of age, variations of craniofacial disjunctions are done. Monoblock supraorbital, orbital, and midface advancement have been the most frequent procedures (Fig. 3).

Treatment of trigonocephaly or metopic synostosis with orbital hypotelorism is extremely effective and should ideally be carried out at 4 to 6 months of age if the patient is otherwise healthy. The procedure involves a bifrontal craniotomy and an osteotomy of the midportion of the nasal bone, plus a lateral shift of the medial, superior, and lateral orbital walls, with a compensatory bowing out of the supraorbital ridge and temporal bones. A bone graft is placed in the interorbital space, and the medial canthal ligaments are not detached.

Patient Selection or Rejection

All patients with plagiocephaly, and those with mild to moderate symmetrical synostosis, are candidates for sur-

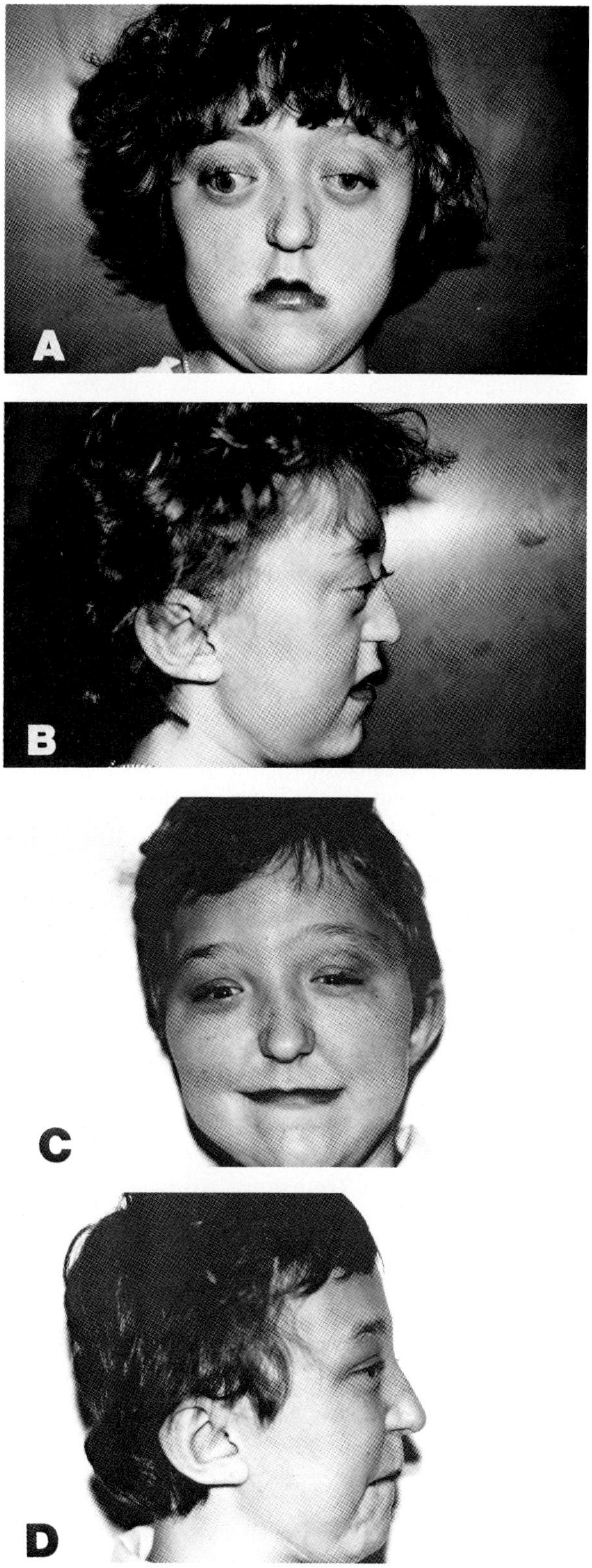

Figure 3 *A*, A patient with Crouzon's syndrome, whose only previous operative procedure was a craniectomy. She is seen at age 8 years. *B*, The same patient is shown in profile. *C*, The patient is seen 2 years following monobloc frontal bone, orbital, and midface advancement. *D*, The same patient again in profile.

gery if the deformity is sufficiently severe to warrant operation and there are no contraindications. These would include severe mental retardation or other severe physical problems. When the deformity is mild, the decision for surgery can be difficult. In general, the deformity should be sufficiently obvious that a beneficial change would be noticeable to virtually all observers. Realistic expectations of what the corrective procedures can achieve should be analyzed. This is best based on the surgeon's own experience, or lacking that, on the published and stated experience of others. For patients with severe problems, the same realistic expectations are essential. Severe problems almost always mandate surgery, but future reconstructive procedures will also almost always be necessary. The moderately severe deformities are more difficult to judge. In some instances, future major procedures will not be necessary, although revisions will be advisable in virtually all cases.

Timing

In plagiocephaly, the optimum time for treatment is 6 to 9 months of age. At that time, the bones are sufficiently well-formed that they can be fixed securely into position. Brain and eye function are protected and structural outcome is assured. Even up to 18 months of age, similar statements can probably be made, but surgery becomes more difficult as the bones develop.

In the symmetrical synostoses, which include most of the named syndromes, neurosurgical considerations must be given first priority. When, for purposes of brain growth, a craniectomy must be done, it should be carried out by the neurosurgeon as early in life as thought advisable. However, orbital and cranial advancement or reshaping procedures should not be done at less than 3 months of age, and the ideal time is 6 to 9 months. Final osteotomies on the upper- and midface would ideally be done well into the mixed dentition stage (age 8 to 9 years), or if possible, later (age 13 to 16 years) for optimum stability.

Principles of Treatment Approaches

In plagiocephaly, the object is to establish symmetry at surgery, with expectation of subsequent normal growth. The normal side is used as reference, and the structures shifted so as to achieve symmetry. In the mild to moderate symmetrical synostoses, the same concepts apply, except that bilateral operative procedures are carried out. The problem occurs when growth potential is not normal. In severe symmetrical synostosis, orbital and frontal bone advancement are carried out to near maximum. The limitations of soft tissue and severely compromised growth potential make overcorrection impossible. In addition, brain growth may not be symmetrical or normal, and distortions of surface contour and growth patterns appear. If normal orbital and frontal bone relations are maintained, a Le Fort III or I osteotomy, or on rare occasions a Le Fort II osteotomy, may be considered once the patient is in the mixed dentition stage. The older the patient and the more complete the growth, the better. Age 16 years might be ideal, but it is rarely possible to wait that long because of psychological concerns. In patients with metopic synostosis, trigononcephaly and orbital hypotelorism, the surgery should be carried out at age 4 to 9 months since treatment is highly predictable and growth potential seems much like that for mild coronal synostoses. It should be emphasized to all parents and patients that more than one operation will probably be necessary except in cases of mild symmetrical and asymmetrical synostosis. In the more severe synostoses, several major osteotomies will usually be necessary (Fig. 4).

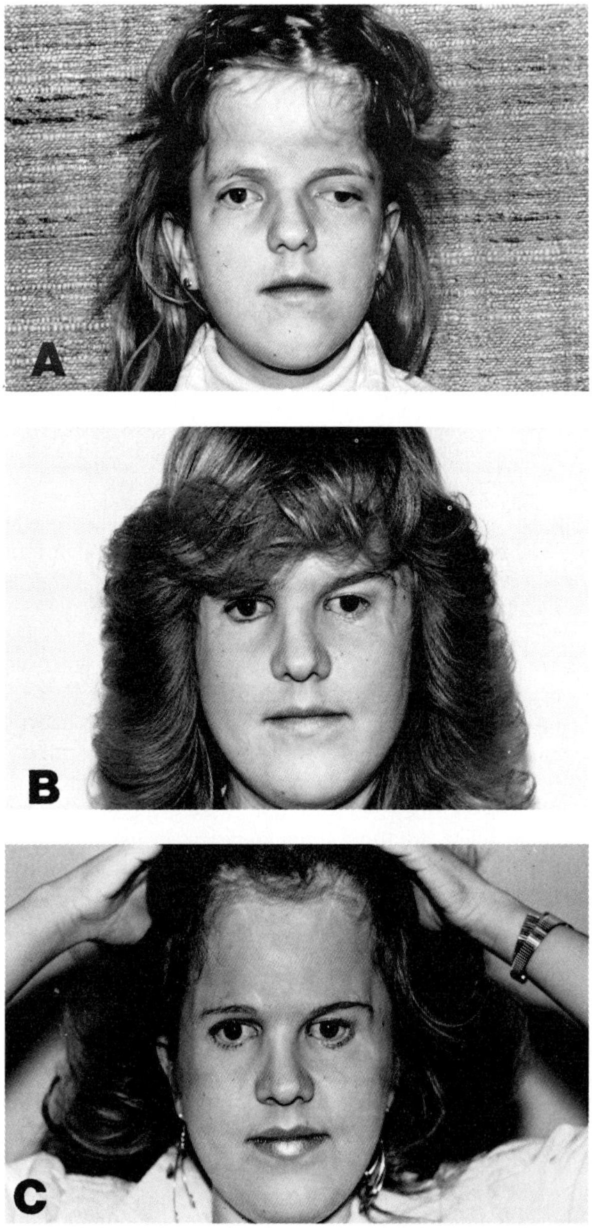

Figure 4 *A*, A 12-year-old patient who had had multiple operative procedures done elsewhere for craniosynostosis. *B*, and *C*, The patient is shown following extensive fronto-orbital reconstruction, that included bilateral orbital advancement, forehead advancement and reshaping, and canthopexies. The result is now stable at age 18 years.

Tricks and Traps

In the asymmetrical synostoses, cranial bone can be used as an onlay on the anterior surface of the zygoma to establish symmetry or it can be placed in a grooved surface of the lateral orbit and temporal bone to reconstruct the lateral orbital wall. This is held by tension of pull of the tongue-in-groove fixation laterally, and the wires medially. When the deformity stops at the zygomaticofrontal suture, a half Z-plasty transposition allows greater stability, without adding fixation to the calvaria. The lateral canthus should be reattached, otherwise there is a tendency for it to drift downward. In addition, cranial bone can be placed behind the eye to shift it outward if there is a tendency to enophthalmus. There is a high incidence of ocular adnexal problems with plagiocephaly. Strabismus is especially frequent.

In patients with bilateral forms of asymmetry, the growth pattern behaves more like that of the symmetrical synostoses and thus there is a higher chance of need for subsequent surgery.

A maximal advancement is often necessary, and miniplate fixation is advisable to overcome the counterpull of soft tissues when the coronal flap is sutured back into position. It is unnecessary to close all of the calvarial defects, even in older patients. One should avoid doing too much in the younger patient with a severe symmetrical problem, since future operations will be necessary. It is important also to avoid consumption of bone graft donor sites in the posterior calvaria so that these sites will be available for grafts at a later date.

In infants, midface along with orbital and frontal bone advancement has been reported, with some evidence of success. The concern is the extremely major nature of the operation and its safety. Long-term effect on growth remains to be seen. Because it may make subsequent operative procedures more difficult, it becomes an even greater concern as to whether or not this is an advisable operation.

Therapeutic Outcome

In our experience, patients with asymmetric synostosis have a greater than 90 percent chance of a successful outcome of surgery, with, at most, only a minor revision necessary if operated on at less than 18 months old. If surgery is done after 18 months, approximately two-thirds of patients will have similar benefits and one-third will require subsequent osteotomies.

In symmetrical problems, metopic synostosis has a highly predictable outcome. There seems to be normal growth potential in more than 90 percent of patients who are sufficiently corrected by the initial operative procedure (done at 4 to 6 months of age) to need no subsequent revisions, or only minor ones. The symmetrical coronal and syndromal problems are much different, however. In patients less than 18 months old, with mild to moderate symmetrical problems, approximately 50 percent have sufficiently complete corrections that only a minor operative procedure that does not require an osteotomy will be necessary. The other 50 percent require major repeat osteotomies for treatment of recurrent patterns of facial deformity. The likelihood of this occurring is similar in patients older than 18 months up to approximately 13 years of age. After 13 years of age, the need for repeat osteotomies is much less, and the results and long-term stability are highly predictable. In the severe problems, represented by Apert's syndrome and some other synostoses, the likelihood of major repeat osteotomies after the initial one is near 100 percent. Generally, these involve procedures at least as complicated as the original one.

RISK: BENEFIT RATIO

In our entire series, there has been no mortality or blindness. There is a substantial incidence of strabismus, sixth nerve palsy, ocular adnexal problems, nasolacrimal obstruction, and minor contour defects following the surgery described. For the procedures carried out in infancy, the risk:benefit ratio is highly favorable. The main risk is that in addition to the problems just described, further, usually minor, revisions may be necessary. A carefully planned approach to timing and procedures should be made to try and minimize the number of operations each child will require. Orbital, supraorbital, and forehead advancement have major beneficial effects on intracranial hypertension. Surgery done in infancy may have an extremely positive psychological benefit if the child has no awareness of ever having been different. When multiple operations are necessary, that benefit is lost. In addition, when full correction cannot be achieved, the distortions of bone and the greater difficulty of subsequent operations make limited surgery more advisable. In older patients, the possibility of infection becomes greater. Surgery on the midface involves open sinuses and nasal cavity, and communication with the oral cavity becomes more likely. In the infant procedures, where these communications do not exist, infections are unlikely. However, when a monobloc procedure is done in infancy, the chances of infection approach 25 percent. Consequently, consideration should be given to the Anderl approach, or to staged or modified procedures.

SUGGESTED READING

Anderl H, Muhlbauer W, Twerdy I, Marchac D. Frontofacial advancement with bony separation in craniofacial dysostosis. Plast Reconstr Surg 1983; 71:303–306.

Jackson I, Munro I, Salyer K, Whitaker L. Atlas of craniomaxillofacial surgery. St. Louis: CV Mosby, 1982.

Marchac D, Renier D. Craniofacial surgery for craniosynostosis. Boston: Little, Brown, 1982.

Mühlbauer W, Anderl H, Heeckt P, Ramatschi P, Vertesy E. Early facial advancement in craniofacial stenosis. In: Marchac D, ed. Craniofacial surgery. Berlin: Springer-Verlag, 1987:123.

Ortiz-Monasterio F, Fuente del Campo A, Carrillo A. Advancement of the orbits and midface in one piece, combined with frontal repositioning for the correction of Crouzon's deformities. Plast Reconstr Surg 1978; 61:507–516.

Tessier P. The definitive plastic surgical treatment of the severe facial deformities of craniofacial synostoses. Crouzon's and Apert's disease. Plast Reconstr Surg 1971; 48:419–442.

Whitaker LA, Bartlett S, Schut L, Bruce D. Craniosynostosis: an analysis of the timing, treatment, and complications in 164 consecutive patients. Plast Reconstr Surg 1987; 80:195–206.

Whitaker LA, Bartlett S. The craniofacial dysostoses: guidelines for management of the symmetric and asymmetric deformities. Clin Plast Surg 1987; 14:73–81.

CRANIOSYNOSTOSIS SYNDROMES: SURGERY IN INFANCY

WOLFGANG MÜHLBAUER, M.D.
HANS ANDERL, M.D.
ANDREAS SCHMIDT, M.D.
PETER HEECKT, Cand. Med.
JÖRG ZENKER, M.D.
BERND SCHAARSCHMIDT, M.D.
FRANK HÖPNER, M.D.
ESTHER VERTESY, M.D.

We believe that craniofacial dysostosis results basically from premature synostosis of skull sutures, with unknown degrees of growth deficiency. Such congenital deformities progressively worsen without treatment. Retardation of growth becomes more pronounced and, as a consequence, so also do the degree of disfigurement and the functional problems, as the child ages.

The logical treatment of craniofacial stenosis syndromes is, therefore, the complete disjunction of all involved suture lines in the cranium and the face, with appropriate remodeling and repositioning to a more normal anatomic situation as early in life as possible.

With modern techniques, expert pediatric anesthesia, and intensive care available, complex one-stage corrections may be safely carried out during infancy with a number of benefits to the little patient, the family, and even the therapeutic team.

PROBLEMS AND SOLUTIONS

Table 1 lists the major problems and their appropriate solutions at the various craniofacial levels, such as the cranium, the orbits, and face. These well-established techniques utilize osteotomy, disjunction, mobilization, advancement, repositioning, and remodeling. The goals of early complete craniofacial mobilization are to restore normal anatomy, appearance, and development as early as possible (Table 2).

INDICATIONS AND TIMING

In the course of our experience since 1980, a number of sound medical, psychosocial, and technical reasons have convinced us that the ideal time for treatment is the first year of life, preferably the first 6 months. Emergency situations necessitate immediate surgical intervention when they arise any time after birth. In order to prevent progressive functional and developmental retardation, we feel justified in operating prophylactically within the first year even in less severe cases (Table 3).

DYNAMIC REMODELING IN INFANCY

The mobilized skeletal components in adolescents and adults with craniofacial dysostosis are rigidly fixed in a permanent position with use of bone grafts to bridge eventual gaps and prevent relapses (Table 4).

In infancy, we approach craniofacial stenosis syndromes with a different concept. The stenosing sutures of the cranial vault and anterior base are widely resected and the gaps left open. The constricting sutures of the facial skeleton are disjuncted and mobilized as far as possible, then stabilized with miniplates for only a very short period to prevent relapse through the traction of soft tissues. Screws and plates are then removed to make full use of the reshaping powers of the no-longer constricted, rapidly-expanding brain. For this purpose, we create a sort of floating cranio-orbito-facial complex that can readily be pushed forward, downward, and even sideways during this critical period with the help of the rapidly-growing brain.

OPERATIVE TECHNIQUES

We approach the skeleton through a single coronal incision. An additional subciliary incision in the lower eyelid rarely is necessary. This is an intracranial, extranasal, and extraoral approach with dissection in the epiperiosteal and submucosal planes. Much of the bone-cutting can be performed with scissors when the operation is performed at this early age. The ethmoid bone is still cartilaginous and the paranasal sinuses have not yet been pneumatized; a fact that markedly decreases the chance of infection. An infant's cranium is characteristically larger than its face. This allows easy surgical access to the pterygopalatine fissures through the temporal fossae from above (Fig. 1).

The stenosed sutures are widely resected and the neurocranium is mobilized, remodeled, and/or advanced as desired.

The orbits and facial skeleton are mobilized either as a monoblock, or in two, three, or multiple fragments. The circular orbital osteotomy is done through the anterior cranial and temporal fossae with an oscillating saw and fine curved osteotomes. The zygomatic arches are transsected, and the pterygopalatine fissures are gently separated via the temporal fossae.

The interfrontal suture and nasal bones are separated in the midline, thereby exposing the still-cartilaginous ethmoid, the septum, and the nasal mucoperichondrium. A submucosal tunnel is dissected in front of the cribriform plate down to the nasal pharynx under digital control using a small periosteal elevator. A fine guarded osteotome separates the septum from the base of the skull. Fibrin glue is injected into the tunnel to reattach the mucoperichondrium and occlude the opening to the nasal pharynx.

The facial skeleton can now be repositioned by gentle traction with the Rowe forceps over a period of 3 to 5 minutes in order to stretch the soft tissues without major laceration or tearing of blood vessels. One or two malleable miniplates are attached in the temporal fossa and/or on the zygomatic arch to fix the mobilized bones into the ideal position. The average advancement is between 15 and 20 mm. No bone grafts are interposed, in keeping with the concept of the dynamic procedure.

TABLE 1 Craniofacial Stenoses

Problems	*Solutions*
Cranium	
Elevated pressure	Craniotomy, resection of sutures
Skull deformity	Mobilization, remodeling
Orbits (threatened vision through)	
Atrophy of optic nerve, exorbitism, exposure, keratitis-ulceration, or proptosis	Expansion, elongation, repositioning
Face (midfacial hypoplasia and retrusion)	
Nasopharyngeal obstruction	Facial osteotomy, mobilization, repositioning
Breathing, sleeping, eating, speech, or weight-gaining difficulties	Remodeling
Malocclusion	Advancement
Disfigurement	Esthetic correction
Restricted skeletal growth	Release of skeletal stenoses

TABLE 2 Indications for Early, Complete Craniofacial Mobilization

Medical
Decompression of intracranial pressure; preservation of mental capacity; decompression of optic nerve; protection of eyes; restoration of nasopharyngeal airway; restoration of normal occlusion; release of skeletal stenoses; maximum cerebral growth within 0 to 2 years.

Psychosocial
Disfigurement is obstacle to psychosocial acceptance and development

Technical
Dissection in virginal planes; malleable bones facilitate remodeling; brain is plastic and compensative; paranasal sinuses are not yet developed; extramucosal dissection is possible; risk of infection is minimal; extraoral skeletal fixation with miniplates is possible; excellent healing capacity; complete reossification; minimal absorption.

TABLE 3 Timing of Early, Complete Craniofacial Mobilization

Emergency operation
Threat to life, brain, vision, airway, or nutrition—after birth anytime.

Elective operation
Slowly rising intracranial pressure, moderate functional deficits—months 3 to 6.

Prophylactic operation
Slowly progressive functional deficits and disfigurement—months 6 to 12.

TABLE 4 Craniofacial Surgery Procedures

Dynamic (Infants)	*Static (Adolescents and Adults)*
Release and mobilization temporary fixation to keep position and bony gaps (removal of plates after 2 to 6 months); reshaping through progressive growth.	Osteotomy and advancement into permanent position; stable skeletal fixation; prevention of relapse with bone grafts.

The ease and variability of miniplate fixation permits division of the orbits and face into several fragments. Indications for fragmentation include a midline split and resection to correct orbital dystopia in hypertelorism and plagiocephaly and to widen the narrow and high, gothic palate of Apert's syndrome, as recently advocated by Tessier.

At the end of the procedure, the remodeled frontal bone plates, or a suitable piece of cranium, are fixed with wire sutures to the advanced supraorbital rim via

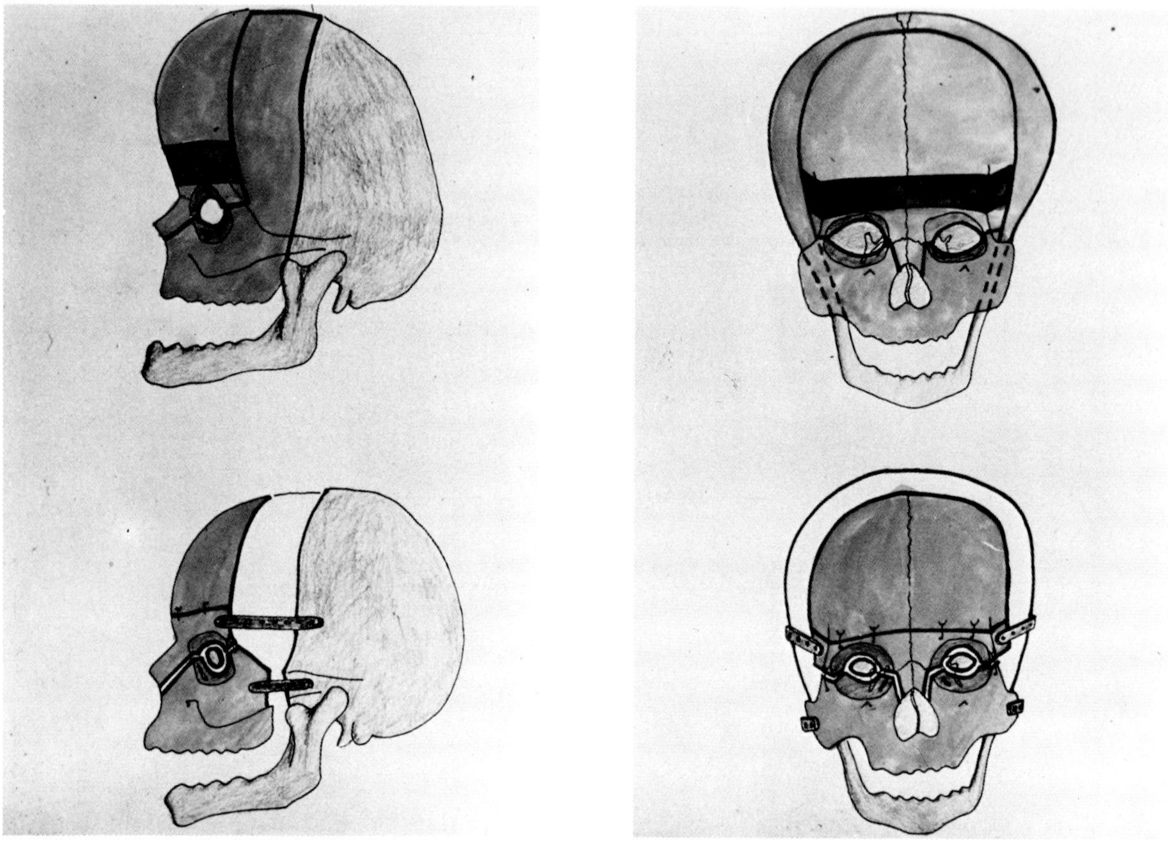

Figure 1 Schematic drawings of operative procedure: stripping of the synostosed coronosphenotemporal sutures plus resection of a supraorbital strip of bone; caudal displacement and advancement of frontal bone plate by 25 mm; transorbitonasal osteotomy and advancement of the hemiorbitonasal segment by 15 mm; facial osteotomy and disjunction (without nasal bones) and advancement by 10 mm; fixation with two miniplates in the temporal fossa and the zygomatic arch on either side.

Marchac's floating forehead principle: Bony irregularities may be filled with bone paste made of crushed bone and fibrin adhesive. The soft tissues are then redraped over the remodeled craniofacial skeleton. The miniplates resist any adverse traction forces from the soft tissue envelope.

RESULTS

Thirty-two infants with various forms of craniofacial stenosis, such as pansynostosis (Kleeblattschädel), Crouzon's disease, Apert's syndrome, and craniofacial scoliosis, who were operated on during the first year of life, were carefully followed over a maximum period of 6 years (1980–86) with clinical examinations, x-ray films of the skull, computed tomography (CT) scans, and cephalometry (Figs. 2 and 3). In 21 infants, we performed a one-stage, complete, craniofacial mobilization. Eight infants underwent various forms of multisegmental mobilization on the cranio-orbito-facial skeleton. Three cases were done in two stages.

In 29 cases, all cranial and orbital problems such as increased intracranial pressure, skull deformities, and exorbitism were relieved. In 25 cases, the facial problems (nasopharyngeal obstruction and malocclusion) were markedly improved. All but one patient rapidly gained weight and developed satisfactorily, including the degree of disfigurement. In the majority, the postoperative skeletal growth was amazingly good and in many instances compared favorably with the growth pattern of normal children. In four patients, only an insufficient advancement could be achieved during the operation. It was interesting to note how even these patients improved continuously over the follow-up period. However, four infants later developed dysproportional growth of the maxilla and mandible.

COMPLICATIONS

Analysis of our series of 32 infants operated on within the first year of life revealed a surprisingly low incidence of complications; much lower than in a series of children upon whom we operated later in life.

Early in the series, we lost more than one circulating blood volume during the operation on three patients. The blood was replaced without any sign of coagulopathy. No events of brain damage, epidural or subdural hematoma, injury to the eyes or effects on vision, or bone absorption were encountered.

One infant developed bacterial meningitis as a consequence of cerebrospinal fluid leak. It was controlled by conservative treatment.

One patient with an extreme case of pansynostosis of the Kleeblattschädel type, with associated hydrocephalus,

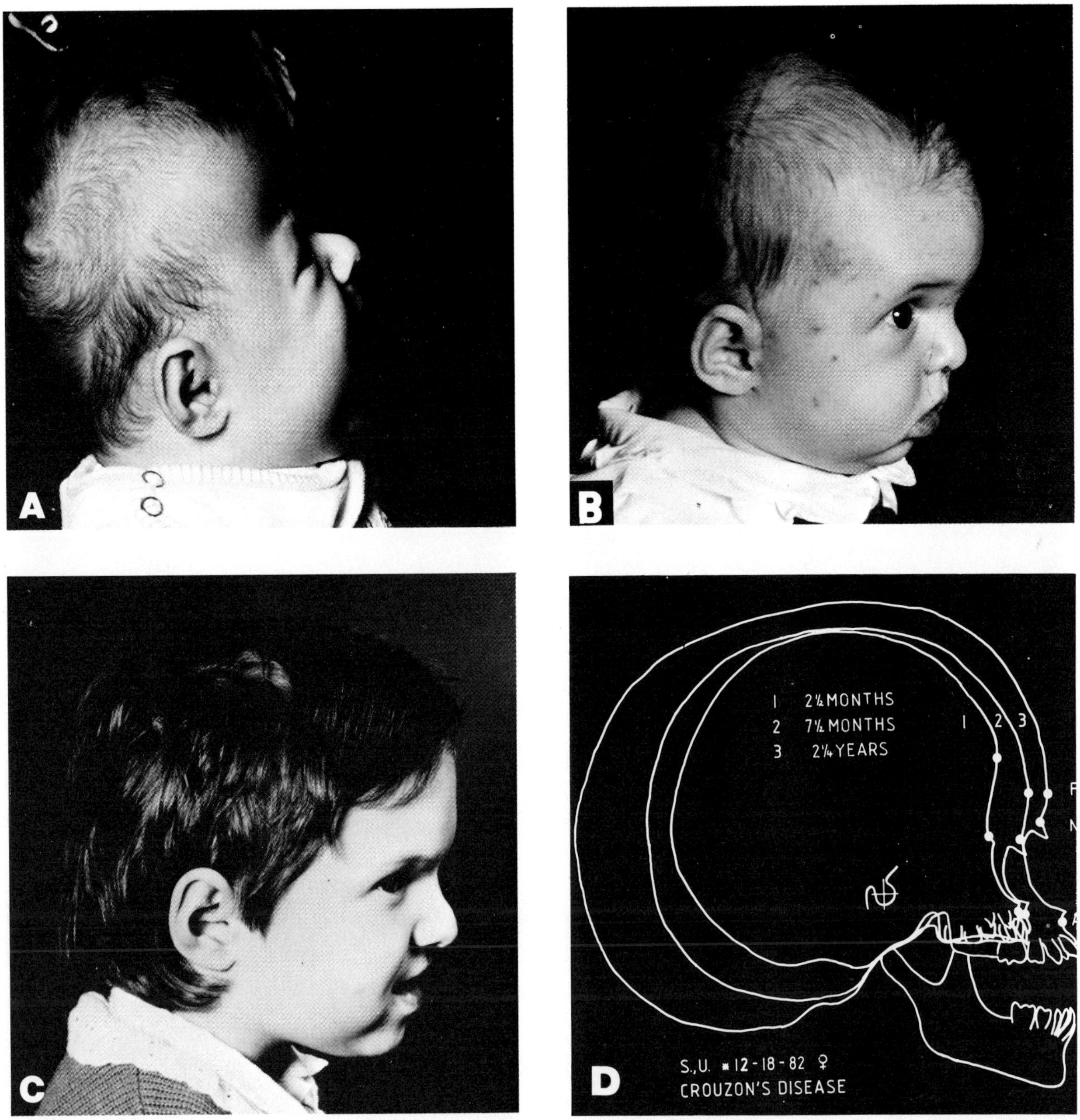

Figure 2 *A*, A 2-month-old infant with craniofacial dysostosis (Crouzon's disease) shows brachycephaly, moderate exorbitism, and midfacial hypoplasia. *B*, The same child at 6 months, shortly after the one-stage, three-segment cranio-orbito-facial mobilization and advancement (see schematic drawings of Fig. 1). *C*, The child is shown again at 5½ years of age. *D*, Cephalometric tracings before and at various intervals after the operation.

died from cardiopulmonary complications 2 weeks after an emergency operation at 6 weeks old. We were obliged to save at least one eye after spontaneous bilateral proptosis. It was an extreme case with grave prognosis from the start.

DISCUSSION

Many infants with craniofacial dysostosis must be operated on during the first year of life for medical reasons, such as decompression of a rising intracranial pressure and preservation of vision. The exorbitism can be corrected satisfactorily when both the orbital roof and the orbital floor are advanced. Since an operation is already in progress, it seems logical also to disjunct the facial stenoses and advance the midface to open the blocked nasopharyngeal airway at the same time. This one-stage procedure is superior to a two-stage approach, which entails a much higher risk due to the need to dissect through scar tissue. In our experience, the first time is

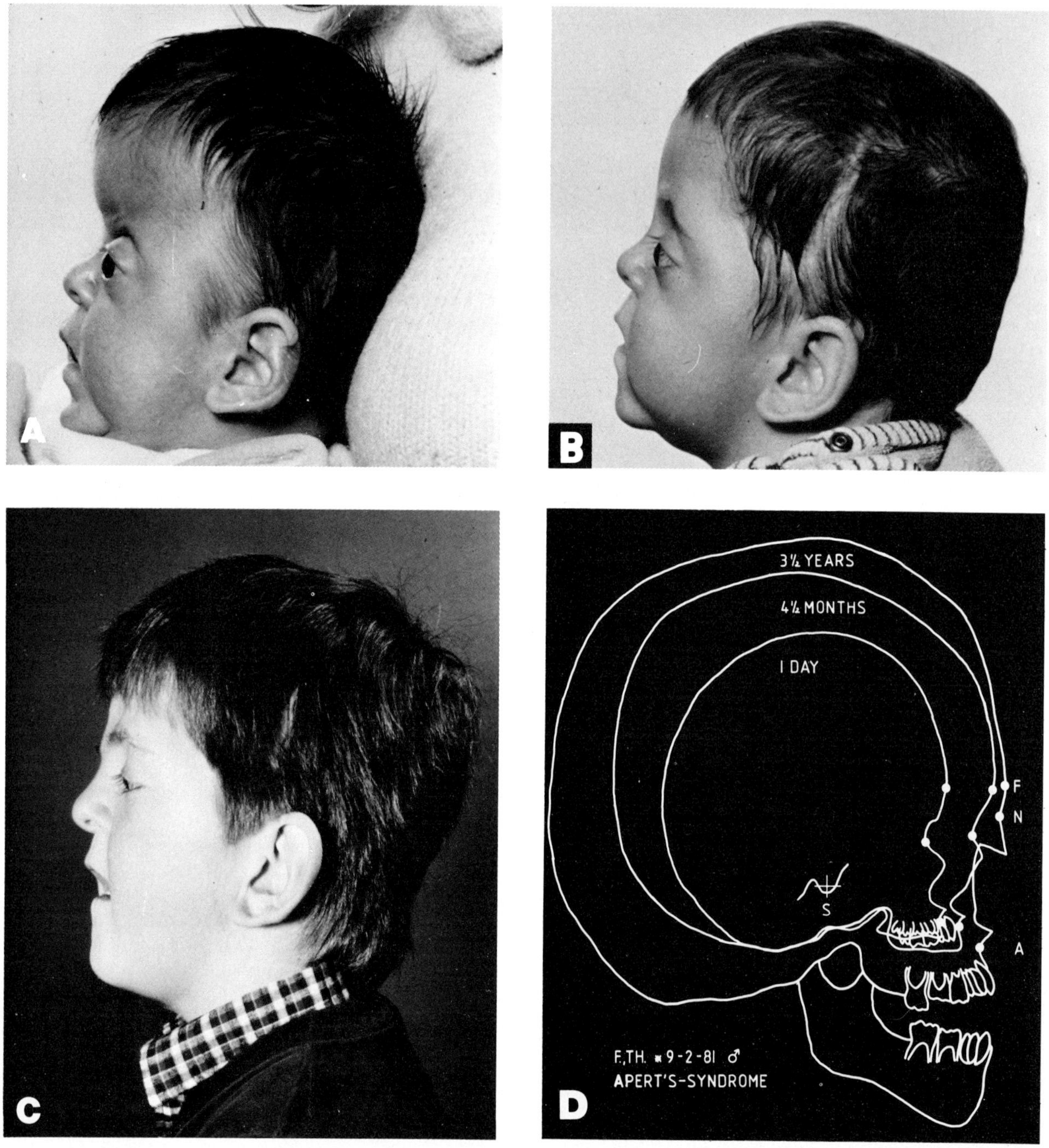

Figure 3 *A*, Three-month-old infant with craniofacial dysostosis (Apert's syndrome) shows acrobrachycephaly, exorbitism, midfacial hypoplasia, and retrusion with nasopharyngeal obstruction. *B*, The same child at 9 months (operation was performed at 3 months of age) after one-stage complete resection of stenosed sutures, craniofacial disjunction, and two-segment cranio-orbito-facial advancement of 20 mm. *C*, The same child is shown at 6 years of age. *D*, Cephalometric tracings before and at various intervals after the operation.

the best time to do all the necessary corrective surgery. There are also technical advantages to one-stage surgery in infancy, namely: (1) dissection in virginal planes is rapid and nearly bloodless, (2) much of the skeletal separation and disjunction can be done with scissors, or even bluntly, (3) the bones are malleable and easily remodeled without any tendency to absorption (we leave the periosteum attached), (4) the neurocranium in infants is much larger than the face, which permits the dissection and disjunction to be completed from above through a single coronal incision without additional incisions in the nasal or oral cavities, and (5) after the skeletal disjunction, the restrictive soft tissues can be expanded much easier than in older children or adults.

The use of miniplate skeletal fixation, which we began in 1980, has been a major breakthrough for us and has made this type of infant surgery possible. Miniplates greatly help otherwise difficult stabilizations, especially in multisegmental surgery. The plates and screws are generally removed after 3 months through small stab incisions in order to create the floating fronto-orbito-facial complex that is further advanced and reshaped by the rapidly-growing brain of the infant.

When expert anesthesia and intensive care are provided, the risk of complications is much lower in infants than in later life. The healing capacity of infants is striking, which means minimal morbidity. The low rate of infection may be explained also by the fact that the paranasal sinuses are not yet developed.

We use a synthetic vasopressor (POR 8, Sandoz) to diminish blood loss. Fibrin glue (Immuno) is used to seal off any communication between the cranial fossae and the pharynx or nasal cavity. Osseous irregularities may be smoothed by bone paste made of bone dust and fibrin glue.

The infant's brain is plastic; capable of compensating for an eventual operative trauma. In our opinion, the postoperative growth pattern has proved our hypothesis of the dynamic nature of the very early disjunction and mobilization at all levels of the craniofacial skeleton. In craniofacial stenoses, disjunction appears more important than initial advancement, which, in very favorable cases, may reach 20 to 25 mm. So far, the maximum follow-up is 6 years. Although we cannot predict the skeletal growth in the years to come, we believe that minor corrective procedures and orthodontic treatments later in life are no contraindication to this early approach.

The earliest possible correction of the congenital malformation is also of great psychosocial importance. Many studies show that a normal parent-child relationship is established within the first year of life. The disfigured infant runs a higher risk of being rejected despite a satisfactory corrective operation later in childhood or adolescence. Even a fatal outcome of the operation is more easily accepted by the parents earlier rather than later. Ideally, the child born with a congenital anomaly should never become aware of the disfigurement.

SUGGESTED READING

Anderl H, Mühlbauer W, Marchac D. Moulding the craniofacial skeleton with a paste of concentrated fibrin and bone dust. In: Marchac D, ed. Craniofacial surgery. Berlin: Springer-Verlag, 1987:274.

Marchac D, Renier D. Early monoblock frontofacial advancement. In: Marchac D, ed. Craniofacial surgery. Berlin: Springer-Verlag, 1987:334.

McCarthy JG, Coccaro PJ, Epstein F, Converse JM. Early skeletal release in the infant with craniofacial dysostosis. Plast Reconstr Surg 1978; 62:335–346.

McNamara JA, Carlson DS, Ribbens KA. The effect of surgical intervention on craniofacial growth. Ann Arbor: Center for Human Growth and Development, The University of Michigan, 1982.

Mühlbauer W, Anderl H, Heeckt P, Ramatschi P, Vertesy E. Early facial advancement in craniofacial stenosis. In: Marchac D, ed. Craniofacial surgery. Berlin: Springer-Verlag, 1987:121.

Mühlbauer W, Anderl H. Use of miniplates in craniofacial surgery. In: Marchac D, ed. Craniofacial surgery. Berlin: Springer-Verlag, 1987: 334.

Ortiz-Monasterio F, Fuente del Campo A, Carillo A. Advancement of the orbits and the midface in one piece, combined with frontal repositioning, for the correction of Crouzon's deformity. Plast Reconstr Surg 1978; 61:507–516.

CRANIOSYNOSTOSIS SYNDROMES: SURGERY IN INFANCY AND CHILDHOOD

JOSEPH G. McCARTHY, M.D.

The goals of surgery of the infant (early surgery*) with a craniosynostosis are two-fold: (1) decompression of the intracranial space (to reduce intracranial pressure, to prevent visual problems and to permit normal mental development); and (2) achievement of satisfactory craniofacial form.

CRANIOFACIAL GROWTH

Before I embark on a description of the various treatment regimens employed in the infant with craniofacial synostosis, a discussion of craniofacial skeletal growth is indicated.

The head and neck region is no longer viewed as a composite consisting of isolated bones, muscles, and glands; rather, it is considered as a number of relatively independent, yet interrelated, units of function. The original concepts of functional craniology of Van der Klaaw began with the recognition that the functions of the head and neck are subserved by "functional cranial components." The latter are formed by all of the soft tissues (viscera, such as muscles and glands and visceral spaces, such as the mouth and pharynx, which are related to specific function) and those related skeletal tissues that serve to protect or support the soft tissues. Moss popularized the concept of the functional matrix in which any given bone grows in response to functional relationships, which represent the sum of all of the soft tissues operating in association with that bone.

STRIP CRANIECTOMIES

Prior to the turn of the century, several case reports of strip craniectomies were recorded in the literature. By the 1920's, the technique had found wide clinical acceptance in the United States for the treatment of craniosynostosis.

* Early surgery is defined as surgery performed before the patient is 12 months of age.

Neurosurgical strip craniectomies have traditionally been advocated before the age of 3 months. While adequate cranial decompression was obtained, the techniques generally failed to yield satisfactory results in terms of craniofacial form. Shillito and Matson reviewed 519 patients with craniosynostosis who had undergone strip craniectomies and noted that only 52 percent of the patients had a satisfactory appearance after surgery; the best results in terms of craniofacial appearance were observed in infants with isolated sagittal sutural synostosis.

In isolated sagittal synostosis either sagittal or parasagittal strip craniectomy is the treatment of choice. In bilateral coronal synostosis strip craniectomy (bilateral coronal) has been replaced in recent years by frontal bone advancement and cranial vault remodeling. However, in infants with a *mild* degree of bilateral coronal synostosis with no evidence of exophthalmus an extended coronal-sphenozygomatic strip craniectomy may occasionally be indicated.

The author has abandoned simple strip craniectomy techniques in the treatment of plagiocephaly, trigonocephaly or the craniofacial synostosis syndromes (Crouzon, Apert and Pfeiffer).

FRONTAL BONE ADVANCEMENT WITH OR WITHOUT STRIP CRANIECTOMIES

In the infant with bilateral coronal synostosis and a moderate degree of exophthalmus and in the infant with one of the craniofacial synostosis syndromes, the Tessier type of frontal bone advancement is preferred with additional extension of the osteotomy along the lateral orbital wall to encompass wide bony resection in the region of the sphenozygomatic suture (Fig. 1). This procedure, which is performed with more facility in the infant than in the adult, is usually performed at approximately 6 months of age. Osteotomies are made across the nasofrontal junction, across the roof of the orbit, and along the lateral orbital wall. Extensions are made into the temporal fossa to provide a tongue-in-groove arrangement, a maneuver that obviates the need for bone grafts for fixation purposes. The frontal bone flap is wired to the advanced supraorbital bar, or the forehead is reconstructed by a parieto-occipital calvarial bone graft of suitable size and contour. The frontal bone has been advanced as far as 20 mm, with significant expansion of orbital volume (Fig. 2). Closure of the bicoronal scalp incision, although difficult following a large degree of frontal bone advancement, can be facilitated by incisions in the galea.

For unilateral coronal synostosis, Hoffman and Mohr described a type of frontal bone advancement which, with modification, is my preferred procedure. A supraorbital osteotomy (Fig. 3) is made approximately 1.5 cm above the roof of the orbit and carried into the temporal region; burr holes in the middle cranial fossa are usually required to prevent injury to the temporal lobe. A counter osteotomy is made halfway up the medial orbital wall, across the roof, and through the lateral wall in a full-thickness fashion. It is essential that the osteotomies extend across the midline to the less affected side so that, when the greenstick fracture is accomplished, there is no resulting depression in the midline. Plagiocephaly should be regarded as a bilateral deformity. In recent years, a bilateral frontal bone advancement has become customary and a single-piece calvarial bone graft used to restore the forehead contour (Fig. 4).

The affected supraorbital arch is usually flat and lacks the desired convexity. Restoration of contour can be ac-

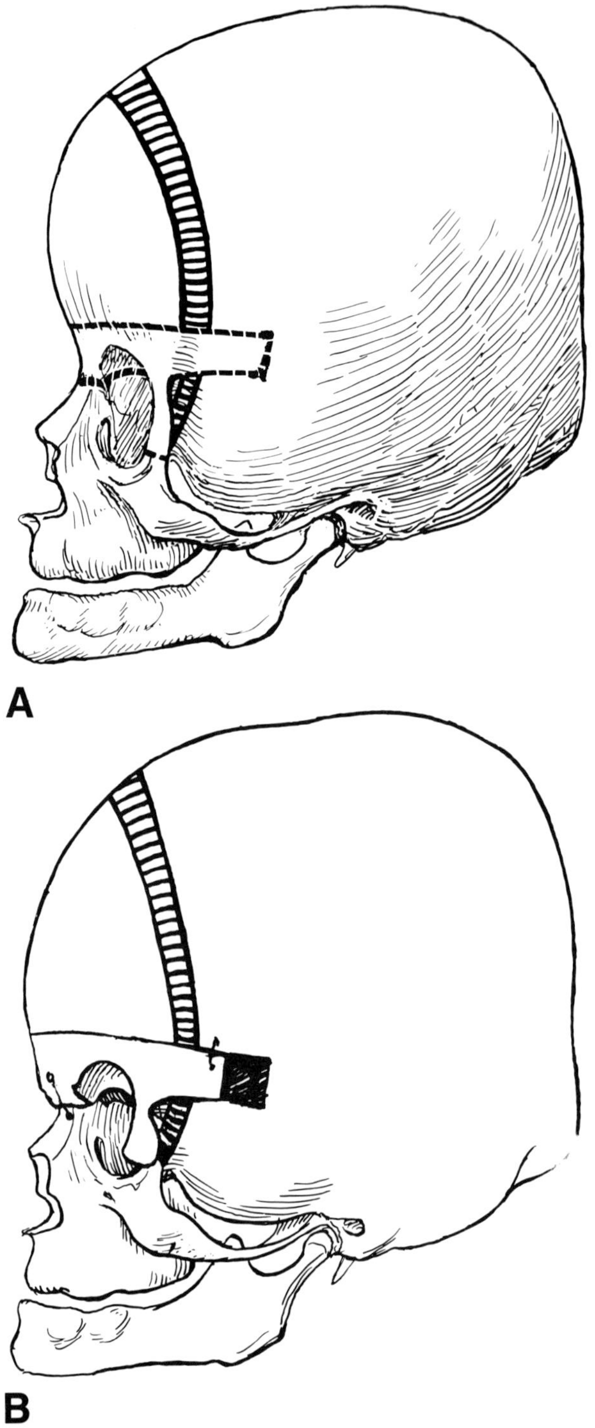

Figure 1 Frontal bone advancement or fronto-orbital remodeling. *A*, Lines of osteotomy/ostectomy; *B*, Following advancement and recontouring.

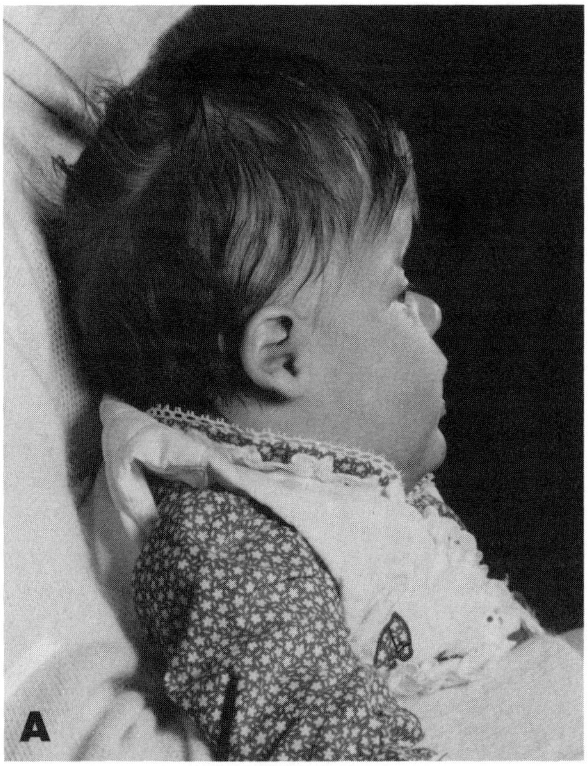

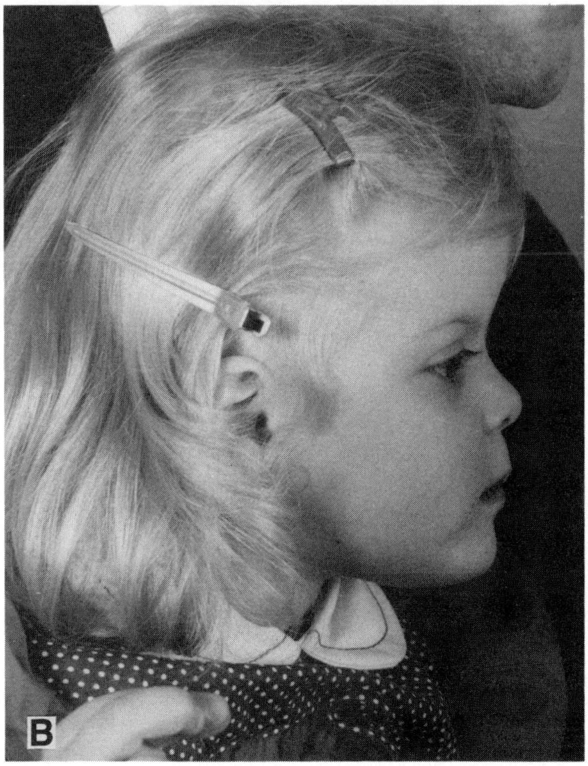

Figure 2 Infant with bilateral coronal synostosis, retrusion of the brow and exophthalmus. *A*, Preoperative appearance; *B*, Eighteen months following the technique illustrated in Figure 1.

complished by bending the mobilized bony segment after making posterior cuts or by placing onlay bone grafts (removed from the frontal bone plate) on the anterior aspect of the supraorbital arch. The osteotomized segment is wired in a slightly overcorrected position by placing stainless steel wires between the "tongue" extension and the temporal bone. The resulting gap in the orbital roof does not require bone grafting.

Metopic synostosis (trigonocephaly) is usually associated with a supraorbital rim, which is recessed in the sagittal dimension. The procedure of Marchac is used. A supraorbital bar with a greenstick fracture at the midline is advanced as needed, and the forehead is reconstructed by 2 remodeled frontal bones or by a single-piece calvarial bone graft removed from the parieto-occipital portion of the calvaria.

It has been my observation that residual frontal bone defects that remain at the conclusion of surgery in the infant are usually replaced by new bone in the following months.

OTHER TECHNIQUES

Cranial Vault Remodeling

Additional cranial vault remodeling may be indicated when there is an associated turricephaly. Munro described a technique in which a frontal bone advancement (Tessier tongue-in-groove), as described above, is initially done. A radical calvariectomy is performed bilaterally, but a central strip of bone is preserved over the sagittal sinus. A segment of the strip is resected, and the strip is advanced in an anterior and inferior direction and secured with wire to the previously advanced frontal bone segment. Consequently there has been a two-dimensional remodeling of the cranial vault: sagittal advancement and vertical reduction.

An alternative technique for reducing the vertical height of the cranial vault is the "barrel stave" osteotomy reported by Persing and associates. The prone position with the patient's neck hyperextended allows circumferential lowering of the cranial vault.

A patient who underwent cranial vault remodeling is illustrated in Figure 5.

Monobloc or Craniofacial Advancement

For infants with a severe variant of a craniofacial synostosis syndrome characterized by midface retrusion, respiratory distress and exophthalmus with corneal exposure, Mühlbauer and associates have recommended a monobloc advancement ("Le Fort IV") or simultaneous advancement of the forehead, orbits, and midface. This is a potentially dangerous procedure in an infant and should be reserved for the child with combined corneal and respiratory threats. It has been my experience that all cases of craniofacial synostosis and corneal exposure can be successfully managed by frontal bone advancement alone (see

Fig. 1). A tracheotomy can relieve the respiratory distress of the newborn with a craniosynostosis syndrome. I am not a proponent of the monobloc advancement in the infant.

Shunt Surgery

The presence or absence of hydrocephalus and ventricular enlargement can be easily assessed by computed tomography (CT). It is preferable that shunt surgery is done prior to the craniectomy and cranial vault remodeling.

LATE SURGERY

Late surgery is defined as surgical procedures performed on the patient with craniofacial synostosis after 1 year of age.

Despite the aggressive surgical treatment plan advocated for the infant with a craniosynostosis syndrome, many patients develop a significant midface hypoplasia as they grow, which is apparent by age 4 years.

Le Fort III Advancement Osteotomy

Gillies and Harrison reported the first high maxillary (a modified Le Fort III) osteotomy in a patient with craniofacial dysostosis (Fig. 6). The technique was popularized by Tessier who employed it mainly in the adult and the adolescent. McCarthy and associates reported a series of patients with craniosynostosis who underwent Le Fort III advancement under 6 years of age (Fig. 7). The study demonstrated a remarkable degree of skeletal stability (minimal relapse of the advanced segment), and some patients showed evidence of postoperative maxillary growth, albeit minimal. With the period of mandibular growth observed in puberty and adolescence, some

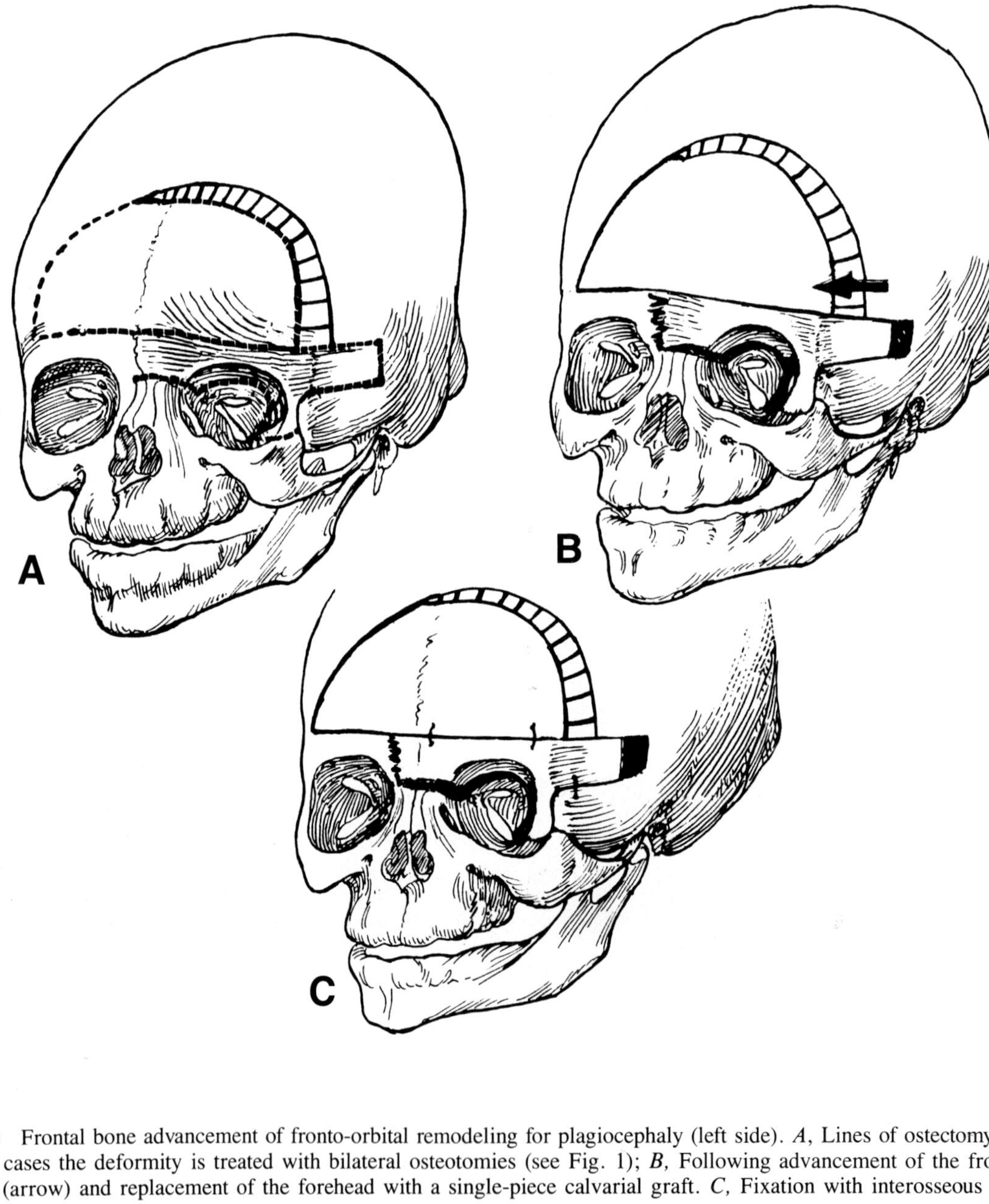

Figure 3 Frontal bone advancement of fronto-orbital remodeling for plagiocephaly (left side). *A*, Lines of ostectomy/osteotomy In many cases the deformity is treated with bilateral osteotomies (see Fig. 1); *B*, Following advancement of the fronto-orbital segment (arrow) and replacement of the forehead with a single-piece calvarial graft. *C*, Fixation with interosseous wires.

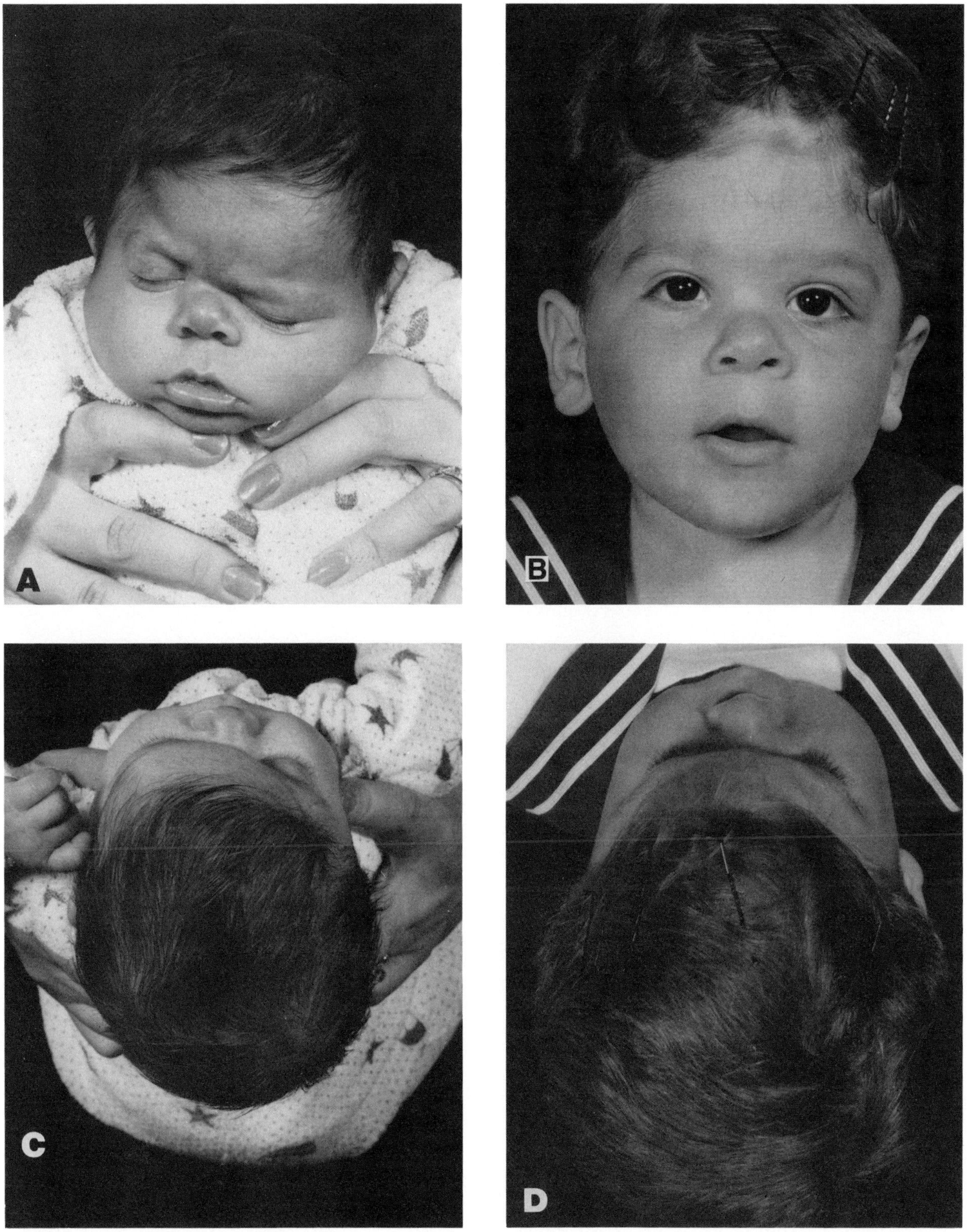

Figure 4 Newborn male with plagiocephaly/unilateral coronal synostosis. *A*, Preoperative frontal view. Note rightsided plagiocephaly and recession of the brow. There is frontal bossing on the opposite side. *B*, Appearance following the technique illustrated in Figure 3. *C*, Preoperative superior view. *D*, Postoperative superior view.

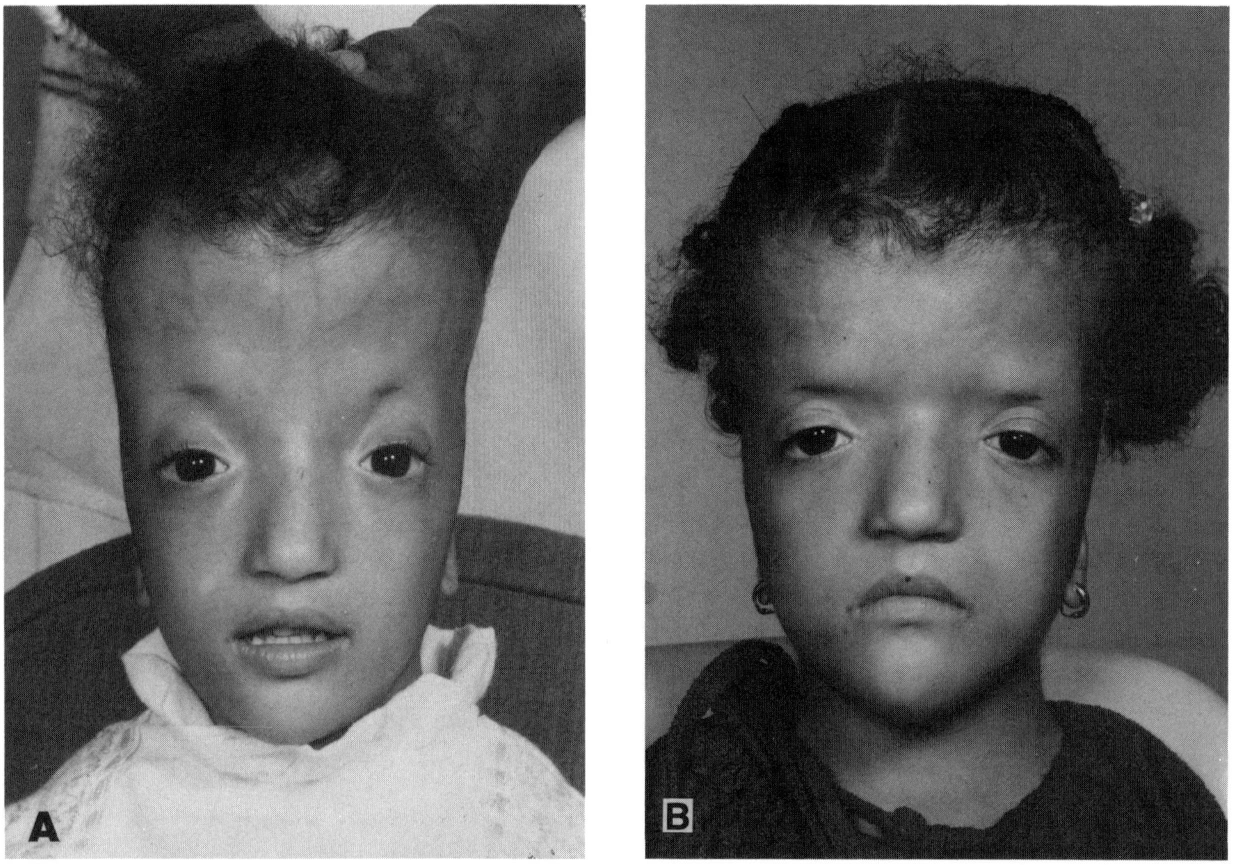

Figure 5 A 3-year-old girl with craniosynostosis (pansynostosis): *A*, Preoperative appearance; *B*, After cranial vault remodeling.

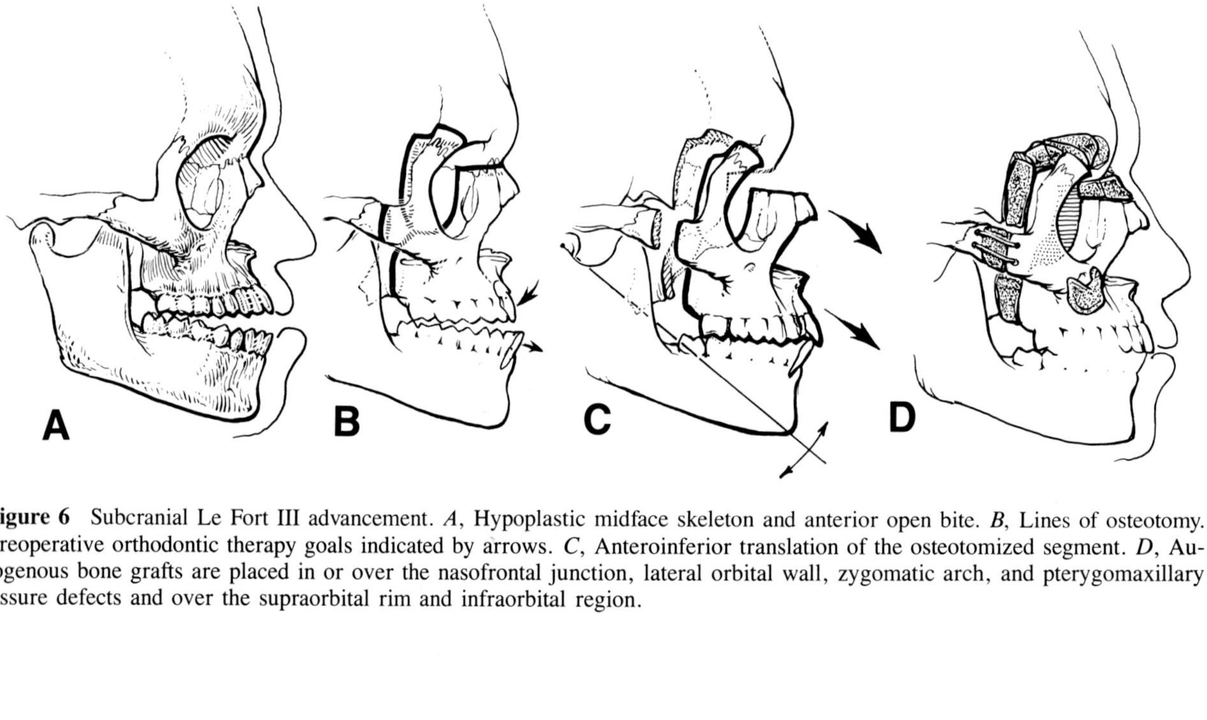

Figure 6 Subcranial Le Fort III advancement. *A*, Hypoplastic midface skeleton and anterior open bite. *B*, Lines of osteotomy. Preoperative orthodontic therapy goals indicated by arrows. *C*, Anteroinferior translation of the osteotomized segment. *D*, Autogenous bone grafts are placed in or over the nasofrontal junction, lateral orbital wall, zygomatic arch, and pterygomaxillary fissure defects and over the supraorbital rim and infraorbital region.

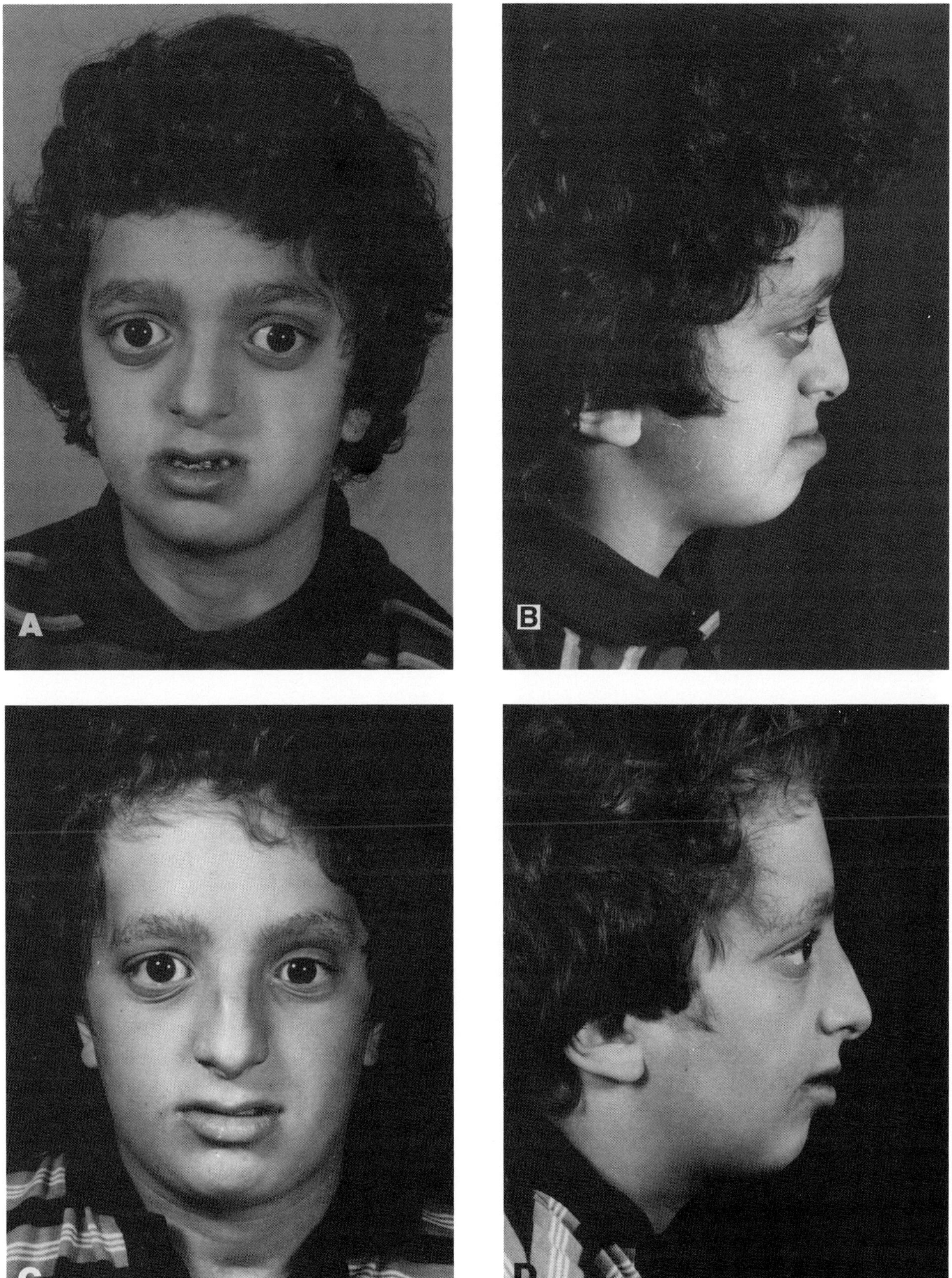

Figure 7 Le Fort III advancement in a younger boy. *A* and *B*, Preoperative views. Note the midface hypoplasia, exophthalmus and lip relationships. *C* and *D*, Appearance after Le Fort III advancement.

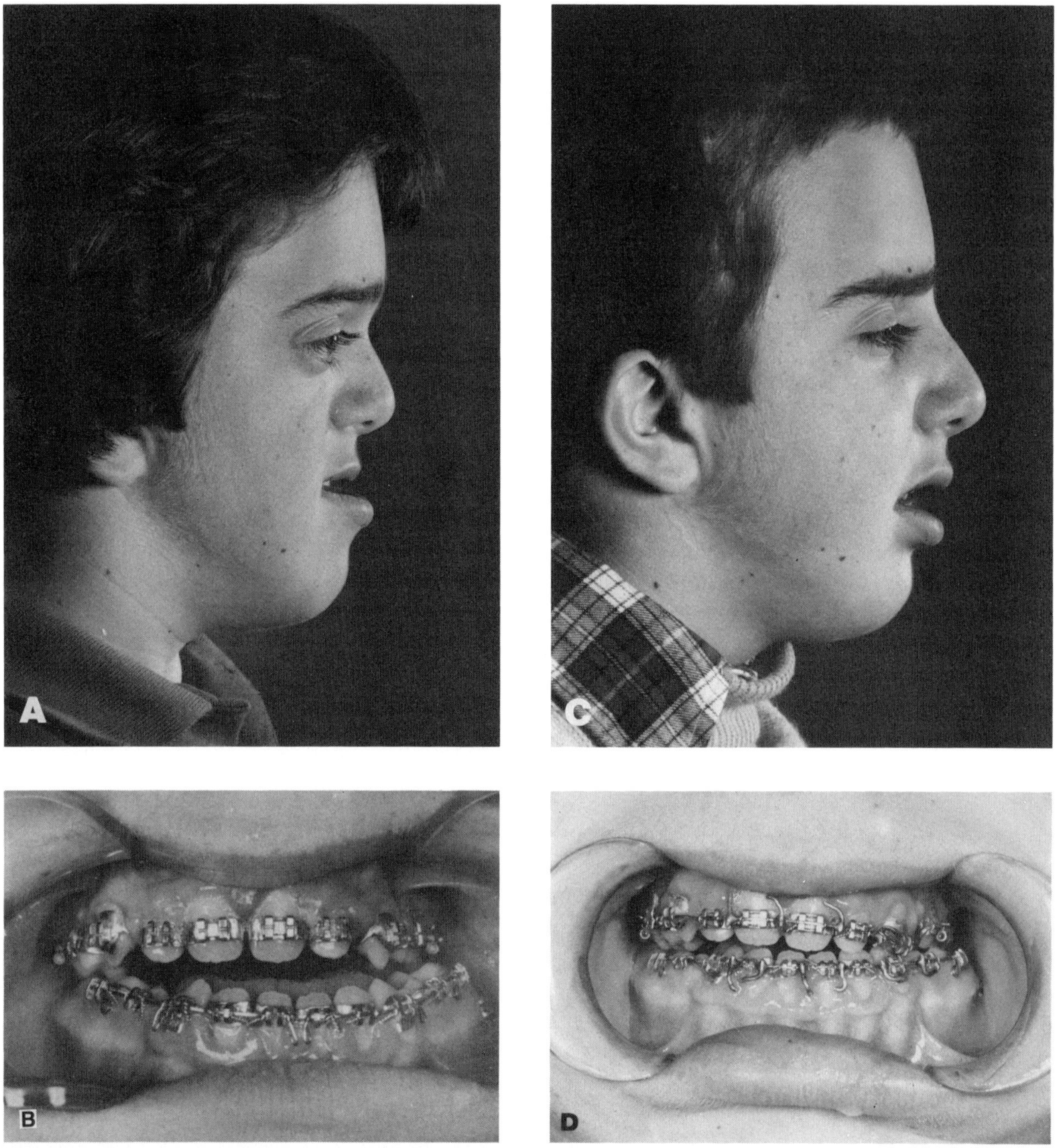

Figure 8 Longitudinal study of a male with Pfeiffer syndrome. *A* and *B*, Age 14: note the midface hypoplasia and anterior crossbite. *C* and *D*, Age 15 following Le Fort III advancement. There has been improvement in facial form and the malocclusion has been corrected.

Figure continues on opposite page

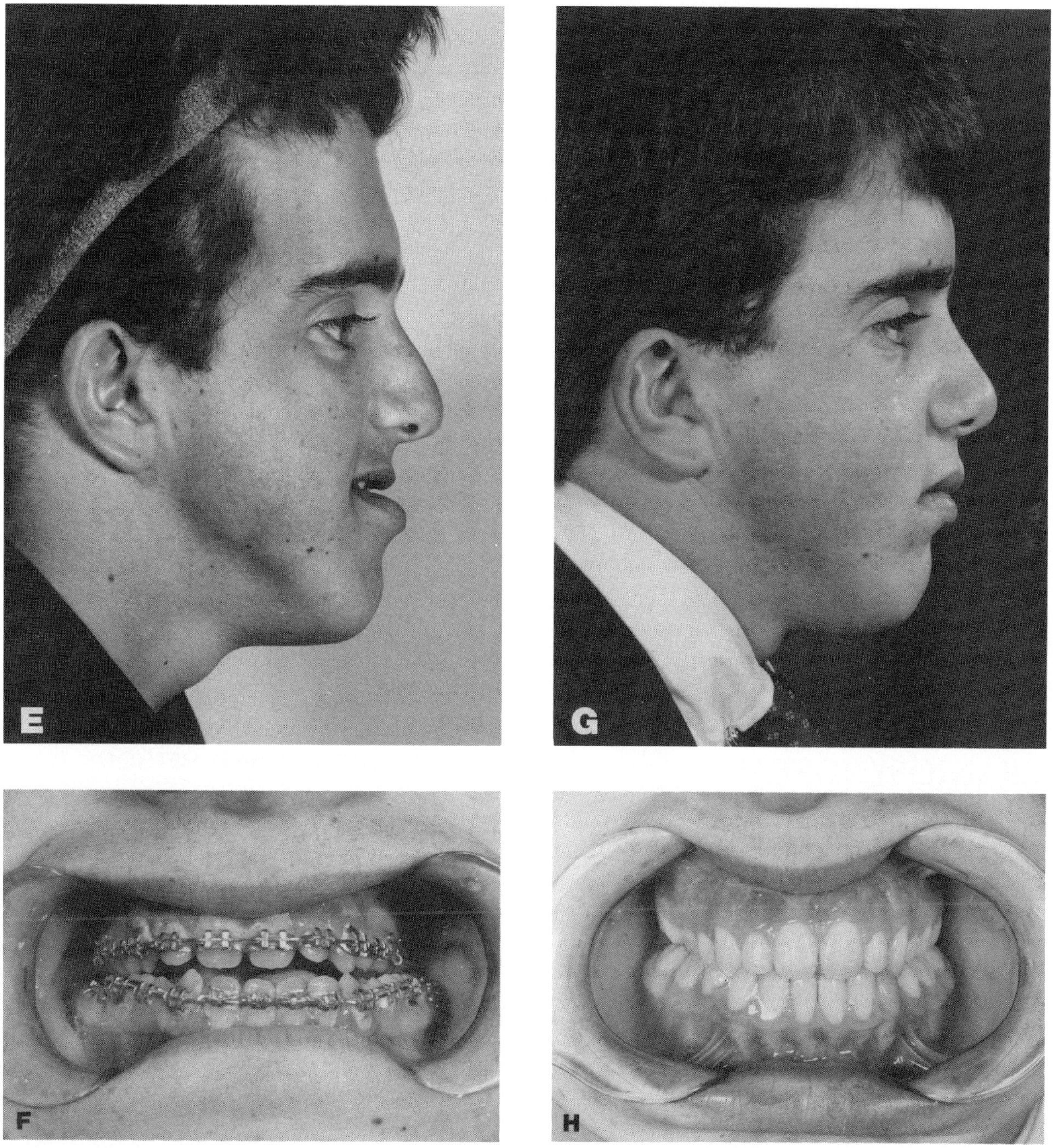

Figure 8 (continued) *E* and *F*, Age 17: with expected mandibular growth there is an anterior crossbite and jaw-lip disharmony. *G* and *H*, Age 18: after a Le Fort I advancement there is satisfactory jaw-lip relationship and the occlusion is class I.

TABLE 1 New York University Protocol

Age	*Treatment*
Neonate	Tracheotomy if there is severe respiratory distress
Six months	Strip craniectomy and/or frontal bone advancement and/or cranial vault remodeling and/or shunt surgery (shunt surgery should precede skeletal remodeling)
Three to four years	Le Fort III advancement (if necessary)
Early adolescent	Jaw surgery (if indicated)

patients develop an anterior crossbite, which was corrected by a Le Fort I maxillary advancement (Fig. 8).

NEW YORK UNIVERSITY PROTOCOL

The current New York University surgical protocol for the patient with a craniosynostosis is listed in Table 1.

SUGGESTED READING

Hoffman HJ, Mohr G. Lateral canthal advancement of the supraorbital margin. J Neurosurg 1976; 45:376–381.

Marchac D. Radical forehead remodeling for craniostenosis. Plast Reconstr Surg 1978; 61:823–835.

McCarthy JG, Epstein F, Sadove AM, Grayson B, Zide B. Early surgery for craniofacial synostosis: an eight-year experience. Plast Reconstr Surg 1984, 73:521–530.

McCarthy JG, Grayson B, Bookstein F, Vickery C, Zide B. Le Fort III advancement osteotomy in the growing child. Plast Reconstr Surg 1984; 74:343–354.

Munro IR. Reshaping the cranial vault. In: Converse JM, ed. Reconstructive plastic surgery. 2nd ed. Philadelphia: WB Saunders, 1977:2492.

Persing JA, Edgerton MT, Park TS, Jane JA. Barrel stave osteotomy for correction of turribrachycephaly craniosynostosis deformities. Ann Plast Surg 1987; 18:488–493.

Reid CA, McCarthy JG, Kolber AB. A study of regeneration in parietal bone defects in rabbits. Plast Reconstr Surg 1981; 67:591–596.

CRANIOSYNOSTOSIS SYNDROMES: SURGERY IN ADOLESCENCE

DOUGLAS K. OUSTERHOUT, D.D.S., M.D.
KARIN VARGERVIK, D.D.S.

Surgical advancement and lengthening of the midface is the accepted form of treatment for the hypoplastic midfacial structures that are usually present in individuals with conditions such as Crouzon, Pfeiffer, and Apert syndromes. The credit for the widespread acceptance and use of these procedures goes to Tessier, who improved upon and popularized the techniques first described by Gilles. The Le Fort III advancement procedures are now performed on a regular basis at major centers for craniofacial anomalies around the world.

The functional and aesthetic benefits to be obtained by such surgery are now well-established. The improved maxillary-mandibular relationship, the opening of the nasopharyngeal airway, protection of the globe by correcting the exorbitism, and an overall facial aesthetic improvement are all well-accepted.

Although the Le Fort III procedures were originally completed on adolescents or older individuals, the age at which these major facial reconstructive procedures are being done has been lowered to include patients as young as 3 years. Under certain circumstances, such operations have even been completed on neonates. There is still controversy as regards the optimal timing.

MATERIALS AND METHODS

All patients in the series presented here were treated by our team at the Center for Craniofacial Anomalies at the University of California, San Francisco. A sample that consisted of 21 consecutive patients with craniosynostosis syndromes (seven with Apert, ten with Crouzon, and four with Pfeiffer) aged from 12 to 24 years (mean age 17) was analyzed. Only three of these patients showed mandibular growth after the Le Fort III facial advancement.

Preoperative orthodontic coordination of the dental arches is desirable and was completed in most cases. Preoperative dental casts and lateral head films in conjunction with the clinical examination were utilized to determine the amount of anteroinferior movement of the midface. In six cases where the lower, dental portion of the maxilla had to be advanced more or less than the upper portion, where intrusion was required, or where there was asymmetry between the upper and lower maxillary portions, a combination of Le Fort III and Le Fort I was completed. All of the Le Fort III procedures completed in this series were subcranial (Tessier modification); no self-retaining Le Fort III (Tessier V) procedures were utilized. All advancements were maintained with intermaxillary fixation, iliac crest bone grafts to the glabellar and lateral orbital rim areas, and split rib grafts secured to the infraorbital rims, which extended around onto the zygomatic arches. Metal plate fixation was not utilized.

In all cases a prefabricated registration bite-block was made from the dental casts. This splint was utilized to hold the maxillary dental arch in the most desirable location.

The splint was made high with a large anterior hole that facilitated postoperative suctioning, augmented the airway (especially in the immediate postsurgery period when edema was greatest), and allowed for easier food ingestion. In each case, custom-made, well-fitting, round wire arch bars were also made on the dental casts and were placed on the teeth with wire ligatures the day before surgery.

Shortly after surgery, a lateral head film was obtained. Postoperatively, the patients were maintained in intermaxillary fixation for 8 weeks, after which a thinner bite-block was fabricated and stabilized to the maxillary dental arch with elastics, thus allowing easy removal and cleaning. This splint provided even occlusal forces during mastication as well as maintenance of the occlusal relationships. Each patient maintained this splint for 3 to 4 months postsurgery, by which time bone graft ossification was completed. Final orthodontic detailing was then completed. Lateral head films were again obtained, at least 1 year postoperatively and again at a later date, if possible. Six patients were followed between 1 and 2 years postsurgery: nine between 2 and 5 years; and six between 6 and 9 years. Standard techniques for obtaining the head films were utilized.

It was felt that lateral head films would be most useful in our long-term evaluation of midfacial advancement results. Previously described landmarks for head film analysis (Kaban et al and Coccaro et al) were not reliable in our series. Nasion could not be utilized in these measurements as it was destroyed during the Le Fort III procedure by the transglabellar osteotomy. Orbitale is very difficult to reproduce on cephalometric tracings, partly because it is a bilateral structure but also because the infraorbital rim was thin in all of these syndrome patients and was augmented in each case with split rib grafts. Since all the patients in our series were adolescents or older, and growth changes were minimal, we were able to compare lateral cephalometric tracings by superimposing the sella, the anterior cranial base structures, the posterior tubercle of the atlas, and the contours of the occipital bone. All of these areas were unaffected by the surgery. Comparative measurements could thus be obtained. The landmarks, superimposition, and measurements used are shown in Figure 1.

Additionally, the majority of these patients underwent further reconstructive surgery to maximize the aesthetic result once the Le Fort III advancement was stable. Thirteen patients also underwent a nasoseptal reconstruction, four underwent a sliding genioplasty, and fourteen had a forehead reconstruction. The sliding genioplasty was utilized to advance the retruded chin but also to reduce its vertical height, which is frequently excessive in these individuals. In all cases, the forehead reconstruction was the last procedure completed. This augmentation was designed to obtain a more normal supraorbital rim, with protection of the globes from above, and to improve the basic forehead contour (Figure 2). This was accomplished by performing a methyl methacrylate cranioplasty. We do not complete forehead advancements in this age group for fear of resulting infection, with possible bone loss and

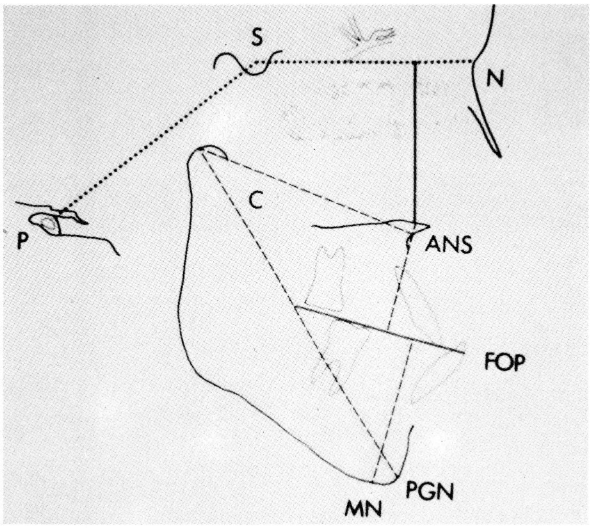

Figure 1 An example of the cephalometric tracing shows the position of the various points and lines utilized to evaluate the patients in this series. (From Ousterhout DK, Clarks S, Vargervik K. Midface position after Le Fort III procedures. Cleft Palate J 1986; 23[Suppl]:91–101.)

meningitis. A recent report confirms our longstanding impression. The implant model was sculptured in wax, either on a forehead plaster cast obtained from a facial moulage or from a CAD–CAM (computer aided designed-computer aided machined) model obtained from computed tomography (CT scans); the latter being the newer and preferred procedure. The resulting precast implant was gas-sterilized, then placed directly on the frontal bone and stabilized with cold-curing methyl methacrylate. None of the patients required additional or repeated procedures, except for an occasional secondary rhinoplasty. Some of the patients declined these additional procedures.

The same 21 consecutive patients were also evaluated for aesthetic result. The purpose of the study was to compare patients with these syndromes to faces of normal size and shape. We could determine from pre- and postoperative evaluation and comparison to normal standards whether these patients were approaching norms from a control group. The evaluation was accomplished by comparison of specific measurements, lengths, and angles from both the preoperative and final (long-term postoperative) lateral tracings (bony and soft tissue) with the same lengths and angles for normal individuals of similar age and sex. These measurements are shown in Figure 3. The normal standards were obtained from accepted anthropologic soft-tissue data (Farkas and Behrents) and bony measurements (Burlington study—Harvold).

Results

The results of these studies indicated a mean forward advancement (CO-ANSii) of 8.6 mm (with a range of 2 to 17 mm) and a mean downward movement (SN-ANSi) of 11.7 mm (the range being 5 to 21 mm). During the long-

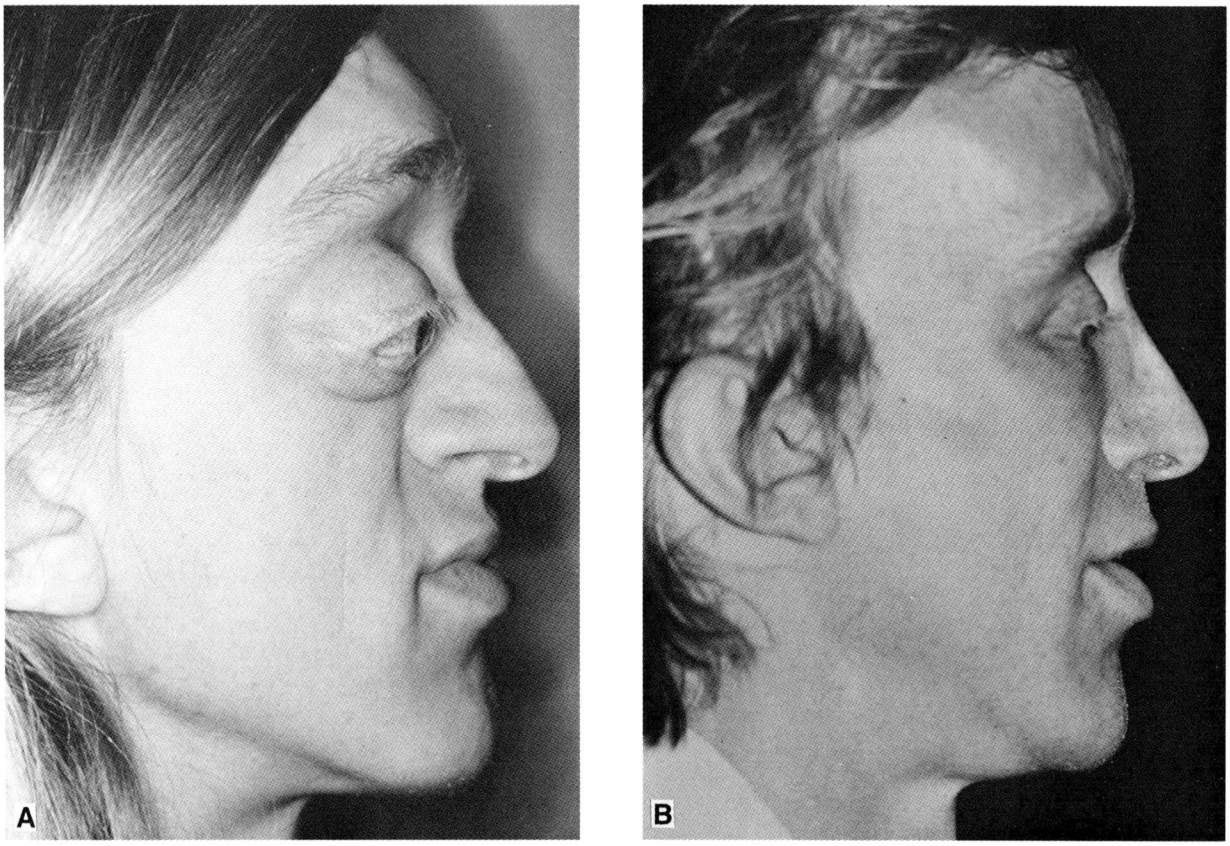

ure 2 Twenty-three-year-old patient with Crouzon syndrome. Operations performed were Le Fort III and I, nasoseptal reconstruction and cranioplasty. *A*, Preoperative view and *B*, 3 years postoperative.

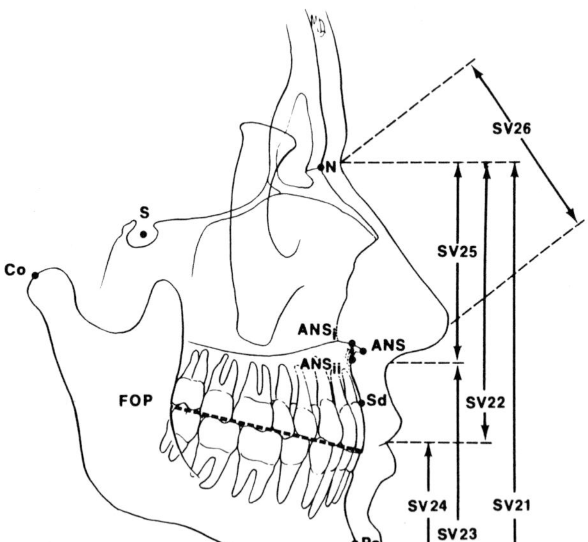

Figure 3 The cephalometric bony distances and planes and the soft tissue distances evaluated were: Nasion—anterior nasal spine (N-ANS); Anterior nasal spine—menton (ANSi-M); Sella—supradentale (S-Sd); Condylion—anterior nasal spine (Co-ANSii); Condylion—pogonion (Co-Po); Angle of the functional occlusal plane as it relates to the line sella—nasion (FOP-SN); SV–21 morphologic height of the face (nasion—menton); SV–22 physiognomic height of the upper face (nasion—stomion); SV–23 height of the lower face (subnasale—menton); SV–24 height of the lower third of the face (stomion—menton); SV–25 length of the nose (nasion—subnasale); and SV–26 length of the nasal bridge (nasion—pronasale). (From Ousterhout DK, Vargervik K. Aesthetic improvement resulting from craniofacial surgery in craniosynostosis syndrome. J Craniomaxillofac Surg 1987; 15:189–197.)

term follow-up, the average change in vertical height was 0.33 mm (2.8 percent) and the average change in advancement was 1.0 mm (11 percent). These changes were not statistically significant. Therefore, it can be concluded that our technique shows consistent and stable results for midfacial advancement in adolescents and adults treated for midfacial hypoplasia secondary to craniofacial synostosis syndromes.

The findings from the aesthetic evaluation indicated that a significant change from the preoperative deformity towards a more normal facial appearance occurred with the operative procedures previously described (Figs. 4 and 5, see also Fig. 2). It was clear, however, that these faces and skulls were very abnormal preoperatively and, even with marked improvement towards normal, truly normal proportions were obtained in only a few cases. The deformities vary considerably in patients with these syndromes and surgery must be individualized, based on both objective and subjective evaluation. The best results were obtained when the patient allowed us to complete *all* the surgical procedures we had proposed for that individual, thereby developing the most harmonious relationship between the facial areas in conjunction with the overall size of the craniofacial skeleton and soft tissue drape. Interestingly, some of our best results occured when the Le Fort III was completed with a Le Fort I osteotomy (see Figs. 2 and 4).

COMPLICATIONS OF SURGERY

There were major complications in four subjects in our long-term follow-up series of Le Fort III surgical procedures, which includes the 21 patients previously described. No additional surgical procedures were necessary as a result of these complications.

There was one patient with a major infection, which responded to antibiotics without loss of position or bone grafts. Two patients had a temporary seventh nerve paralysis that, in neither case, seemed to be present in the first couple of days following surgery, but in both cases it responded without treatment or sequelae. One patient lost vision in one eye following the Le Fort III advancement. Hemorrhage was never a major problem in any of the cases, although they all required blood replacement during surgery. There were no permanent complications in any of the patients following the nasoseptal reconstructions or the sliding genioplasties. The forehead augmentations with the methyl methacrylate implant have also been without complications. There has been no evidence of bone resorption with subsequent migration of the methyl methacrylate prosthesis into the skull, nor has there been any case of infection. In two patients, a temporary collection of serous fluid developed over the implant but responded rapidly to aspiration. There were no other significant complications in this series from any of the procedures completed.

DISCUSSION

It has been established that the results of the described procedures are stable and there was aesthetic improvement. The operations were completed in a minimum of pro-

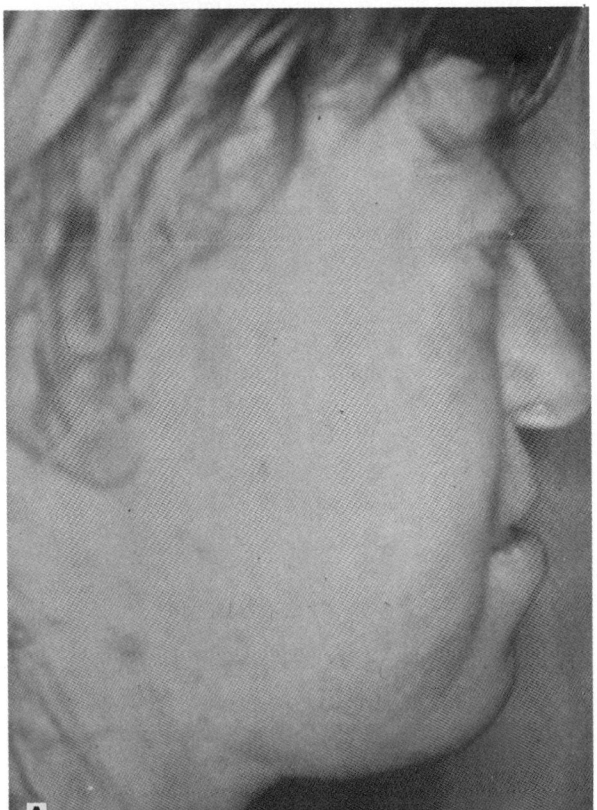

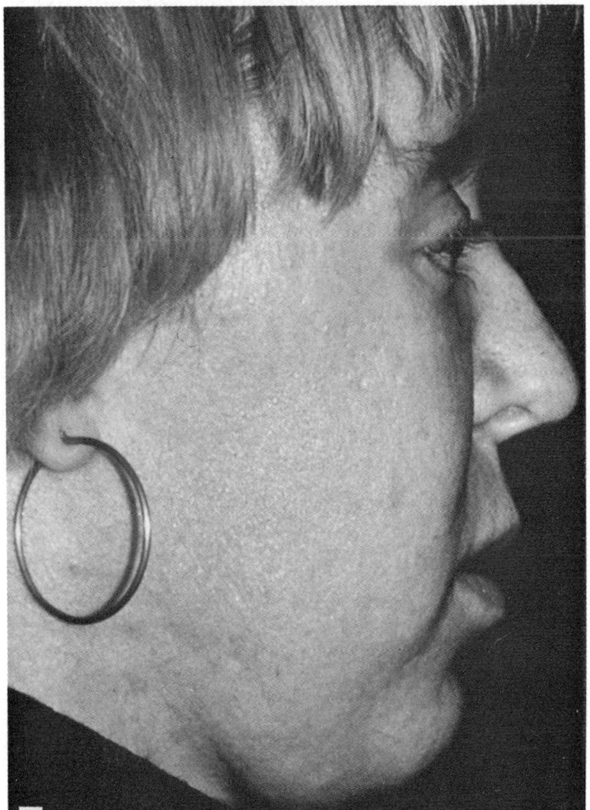

Figure 4 Views of a 20-year-old woman with Apert syndrome. Operations performed were Le Fort III and I, nasoseptal reconstruction and cranioplasty. *A* and *B*, Preoperative views.

Figure continues on following page

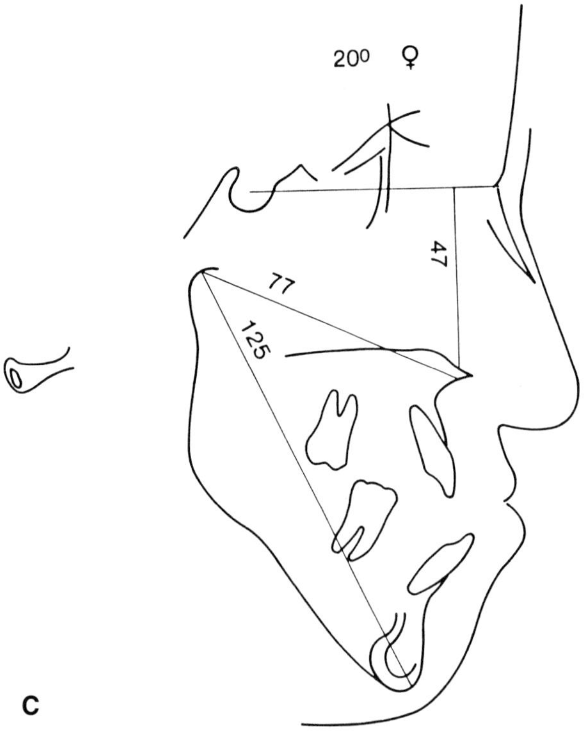

C

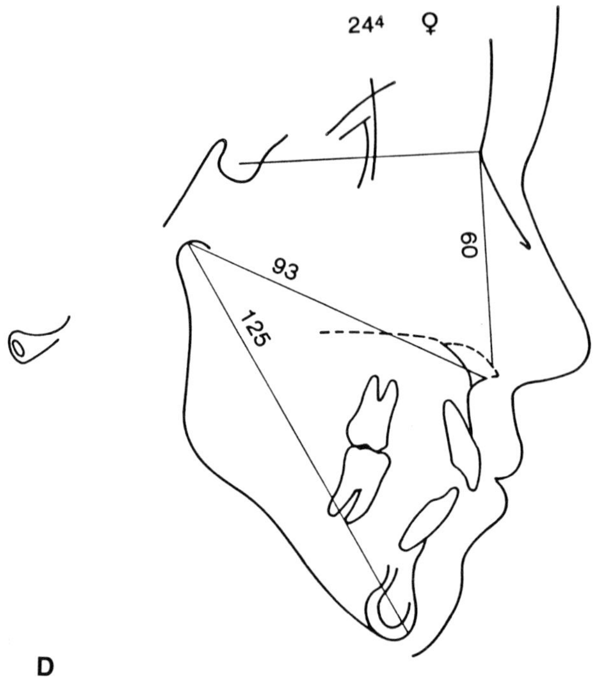

D

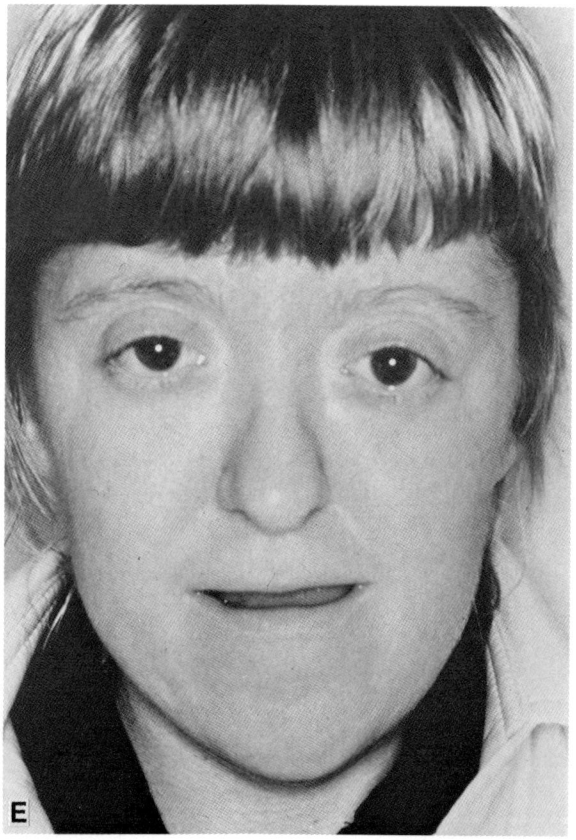

E

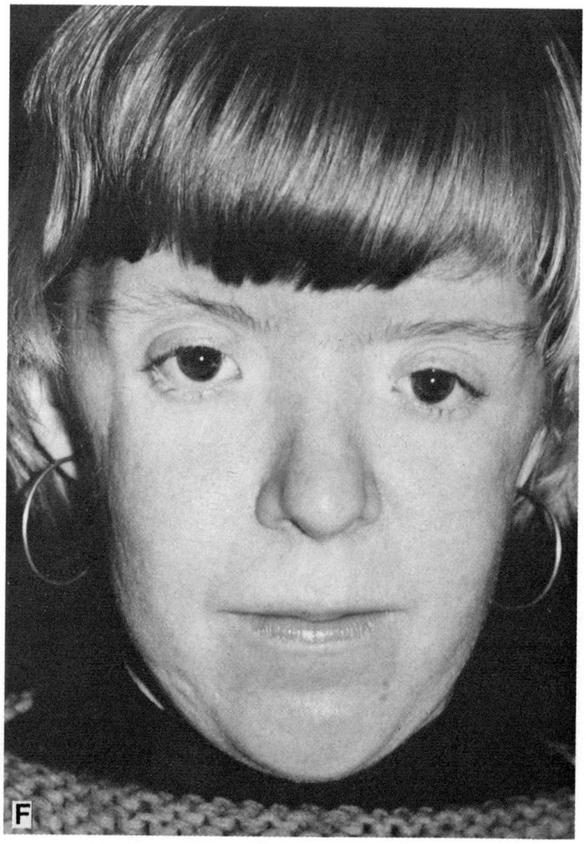

F

Figure 4 (continued) *C*, Preoperative cephalogram tracing. *D*, Postoperative cephalogram tracing and, *E*, view 4 years postoperatively. *F*, Another postoperative view.

dures. There has been only one long-term significant complication in all of the surgeries.

Our position is that it is important to complete the total reconstruction, and achieve the best functional and aesthetic goals, in as few surgical procedures as possible because each procedure must be considered to cause both physical and psychological trauma.

There is major interest in the completion of midfacial advancements in early childhood, e.g., ages 3 to 10. Proponents of this philosophy are willing to accept that additional surgical procedures, (often a Le Fort I and cheek augmentation, but usually a repeat of the Le Fort III) may be necessary in adolescence, but they consider that the psychological benefits outweigh the disadvantages.

It is our opinion, endorsed by the pediatric psychiatrist who sees our patients, that it is more difficult to have a young child undergo repeated operations, with varying degrees of residual (and recurring) deformity between the operations, than it is to give the child psychological support until adolescence and then complete the reconstruction in a minimum number of procedures. Bachmayer et al stated in the conclusion of their recent article that surgery in early childhood "is a justifiable and often necessary procedure because it leads to improved psychological adjustment." There is no discussion nor reference within their article to support this hypothesis. Kreiborg and Aduss have made the same statement, also without supportive evidence. While it is probably true that psychological adjustment does occur in those conditions that can be permanently corrected at an early age, e.g., prominent ears, we question whether it is generally true in conditions where there is a recurring deformity that requires additional major surgery.

Bachmayer et al have shown that children who undergo Le Fort III advancement for midfacial hypoplasia secondary to craniosynostosis syndromes, have had little, if any, additional forward growth following their surgery. It is primarily vertical growth that occurs as a result of alveolar bone growth with development of the permanent dentition. This clinical finding has recently been confirmed experimentally by Nanda et al, who have demonstrated midfacial growth impairment following midfacial surgery in adolescent monkeys. These studies confirm those completed by Shapiro et al and Wade et al. We have also described three patients who, following midfacial trauma in childhood, developed midfacial hypoplasia that required a Le Fort III advancement to correct the resulting facial deformity. In the above two clinical series, not only was the lower maxillary bone deficient but, additionally, the cheeks were also hypoplastic. If Le Fort III surgeries are done in childhood and result in growth impairment, secondary advancement procedures will be necessary. Subse-

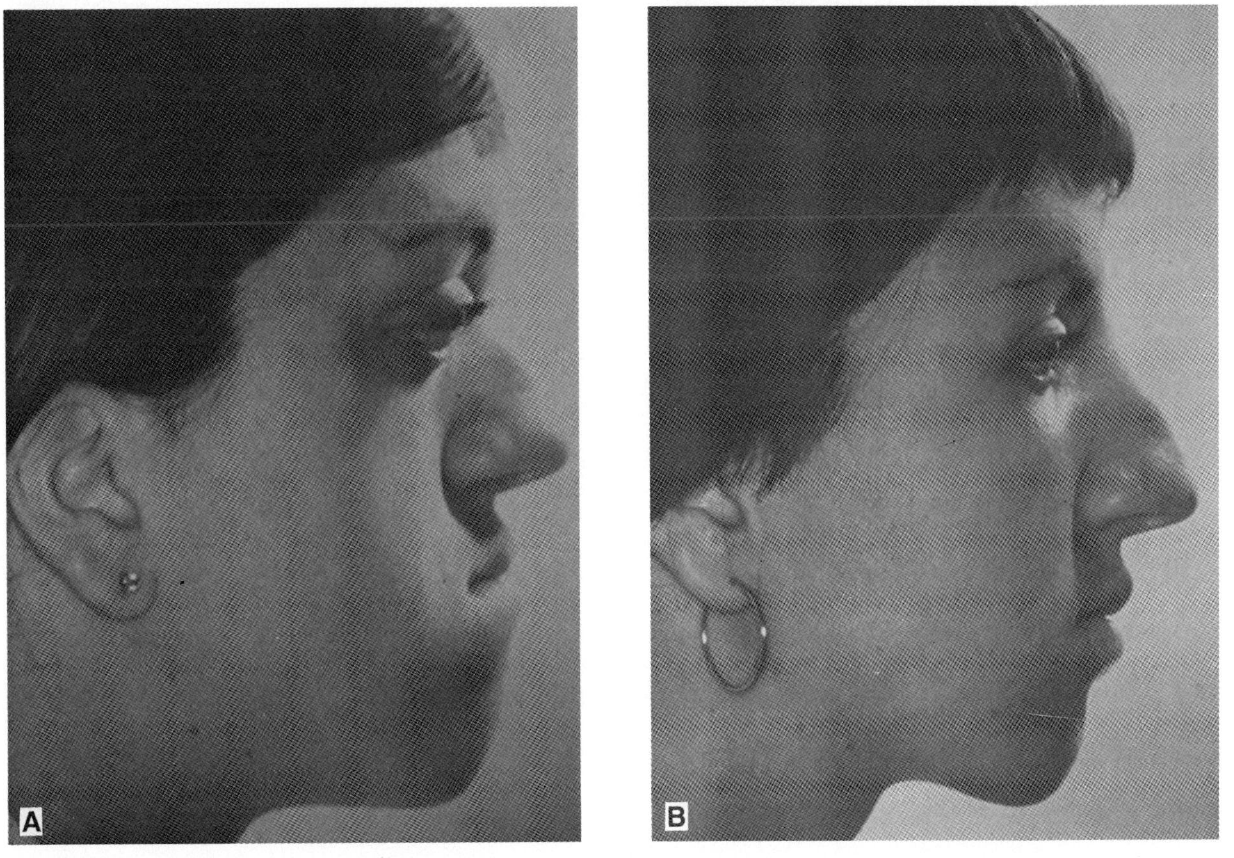

Figure 5 Seventeen-year-old patient with Crouzon syndrome. A Le Fort III operation was performed. *A*, Preoperative view; *B*, postoperative view.

Figure continues on following page

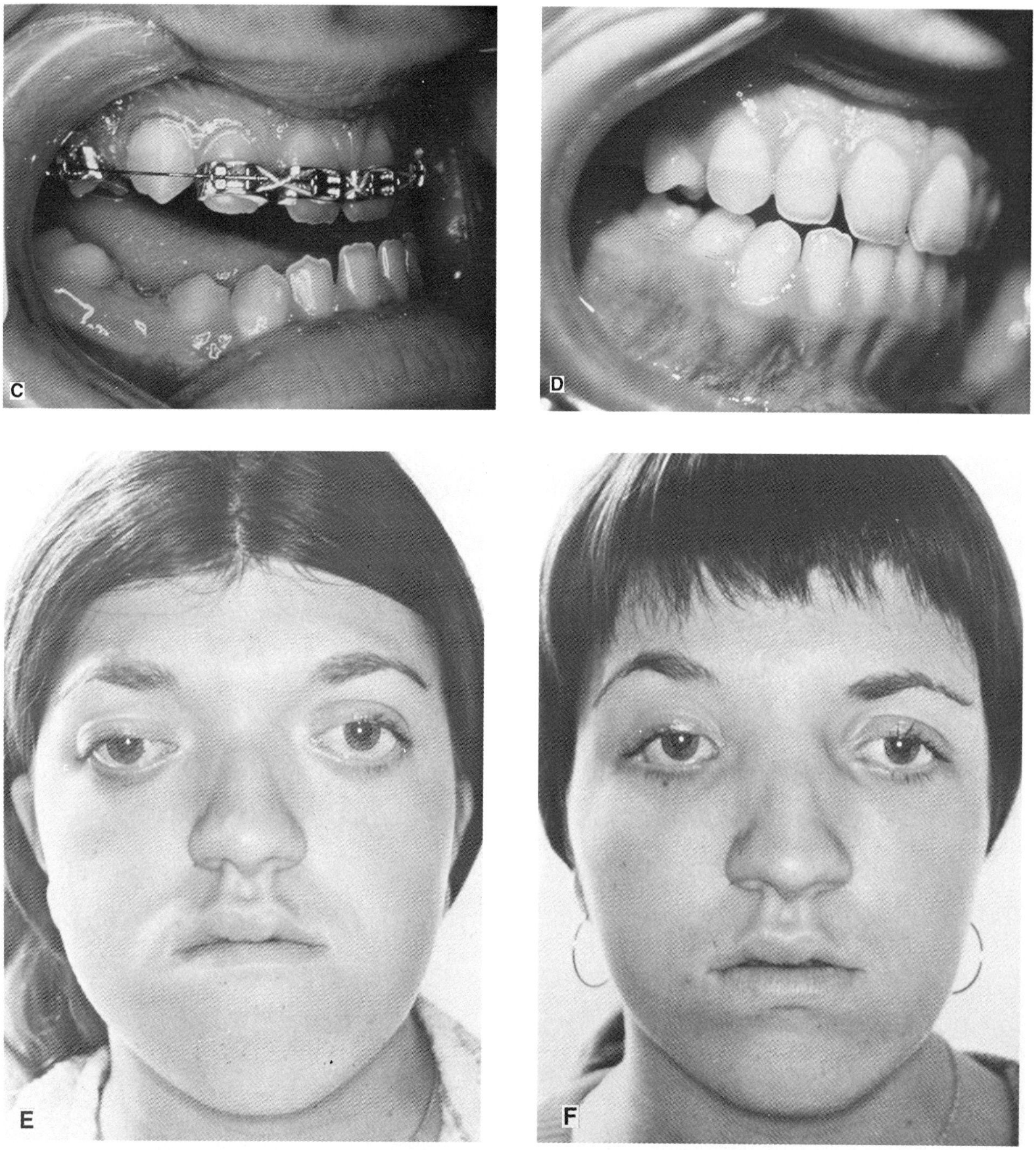

Figure 5 (continued) *C,* Postoperative occlusion; *D,* postoperative occlusion; *E,* preoperative front view; *F,* frontal view of patient 6 years postoperatively.

quent completion of the reconstruction will require not just a Le Fort I and cheek augmentation but also a secondary Le Fort III, as indicated in our post-trauma mid facial hypoplasia cases. A secondary Le Fort III procedure could certainly be completed, but it is our opinion that this will be associated with a higher complication rate—physically and, possibly, also psychologically.

SUGGESTED READING

Bachmayer DI, Ross RB, Munro IR. Maxillary growth following Le Fort III advnacement surgery in Crouzon, Apert, and Pfeiffer syndromes. Am J Orthod 1986; 90:420–430.

Behrents RG. An atlas of growth in the aging craniofacial skeleton. Monograph 18. Ann Arbor: Center for Human Growth and Development, 1985:1960.

Kaban LB, Conover M, Muliken JB. Midface position after Le Fort III advancement: a long-term study. Cleft Palate J 1986; 23(Suppl): 75–77.

Kreiborg S, Aduss H. Pre- and postsurgical facial growth in patients with Crouzon's and Apert's syndromes. Cleft Palate J 1986; 23(Suppl):78–90.

Nanda R, Bouayad O, Topozian RG. Facial growth subsequent to Le Fort I osteotomies in adolescent monkeys. J Oral Maxillofac Surg 1987; 45:123–136.

Ousterhout DK, Baker S, Zlotolow I. Methylmethacrylate onlay implants in the treatment of forehead deformities secondary to craniosynostosis. J Maxillofac Surg 1980; 8:228–233.

Ousterhout DK, Vargervik K. Maxillary hypoplasia secondary to midfacial trauma in childhood. Plast Reconstr Surg 1987; 80:491–497.

Ousterhout DK, Vargervik K, Clark S. Stability of the maxilla after Le Fort III advnacement in craniosynostosis syndromes. Cleft Palate J 1986; 23(Suppl):91–101.

Shapiro PA, Kokich VG, Hohl TH, Low C. The effects of early Le Fort I osteotomies in craniofacial growth of juvenile macaca nemestrea monkeys. Am J Orthod 1981; 79:492–499.

Tulasne JF, Tessier PL. Long-term results of Le Fort III advancement in Crouzon's syndrome. Cleft Palate J 1986; 23(Suppl):102–109.

Wade T, Kremenak CP, Miyazaki T. Midfacial growth effects of surgical trauma to the area of the vomer in beagles. J Osaka Univ Dent School 1980; 20:241–276.

Whitaker LA, Bartlett SP, Schut L, Bruce D. Craniosynostosis: an analysis of the timing, treatment and complications in 164 consecutive patients. Plast Reconstr Surg 1987; 80:195–206.

ORBITAL DYSTOPIAS

S. ANTHONY WOLFE, M.D., F.A.C.S.

Since the original description of transcranial correction of orbital hypertelorism by Tessier in 1967, little has changed in the basic approach to the correction of orbital dystopias.

The normal interorbital distance, measured between the dacryons, ranges from 18.5 to 29 mm in the adult female and 19.5 to 30.7 mm in the adult male. Interorbital distance increases from a mean of 18.5 mm at 1 year of age to 26 mm at 12 years. The two orbital cavities, of course, normally lie on the same transverse axis.

Tessier introduced the concept of the "effective orbit," and showed that the globe can be safely moved in any of the four directions in the coronal plane by performing circumferential osteotomies both inside and outside the pyramid of the orbital cavity. A displacement of the effective orbit is thus possible in a superior, inferior, lateral, or medial direction. Anterior or posterior movement of the orbital framework is also possible to prevent exorbitism or enophthalmos.

Of the four possible movements in the coronal plane, superior repositioning and movement away from the midline are accomplished with ease. Inferior displacement of the orbital framework requires removal of bone from the anterior maxilla and is somewhat more difficult than superior repositioning. Medial movement of the orbital cavity, or cavities, requires removal of interorbital bone and almost always, therefore, requires some sort of nasal reconstruction at the same time. It is, in fact, the nasal reconstruction, rather than the displacement of the orbital cavities, that makes the correction of orbital hypertelorism a challenging procedure. Since orbital hypertelorism is only a symptom and not a diagnosis per se, many of the patients with this deformity have concomitant deformities of the nose, or congenitally short noses, that require nasal bone grafting and, in some cases, total nasal reconstruction.

Correction of orbital hypertelorism may be accomplished without difficulty at age 2 years or older, but subsequent nasal surgery may be necessary if the nasal bone graft does not keep pace with facial growth (Fig. 1). There is no evidence that early correction of orbital dystopias in any plane interferes with subsequent maxillary growth in the sagittal direction. However, Tessier has reported some cases where early surgery was performed and the maxilla was subsequently shorter than the anticipated normal vertical dimension.

In most instances, a transcranial procedure is safer because it allows direct visualization and protection of the contents of the anterior cranial fossa. In experienced hands, however, extracranial correction may be carried out, in which the roof of the orbit is left intact and both medial and lateral walls and floor are moved en bloc. In these instances, careful radiologic evaluation should be carried out beforehand to establish the position of the cribriform plate, which will indicate how low the dura can be expected to descend into the interorbital space. In some instances, vertical malposition of a globe, associated with enophthalmos, can be corrected by bone grafting of either the orbital roof or floor. In some other circumstances, the orbit can be opened into either the frontal or the maxillary sinuses to create more orbital capacity, so that a bone graft can be placed to bring the globe down or up without causing exorbitism.

Usually, unless there is significant malformation of the cribriform plate and anterior cranial base, correction of orbital hypertelorism can be performed with preservation of olfaction. None of the other movements of the orbital cavity should cause damage to the sense of smell. In milder cases, correction of the orbital deformity can be performed entirely through intraoral and coronal incisions, with no visible incisions on the face whatsoever (Fig. 2).

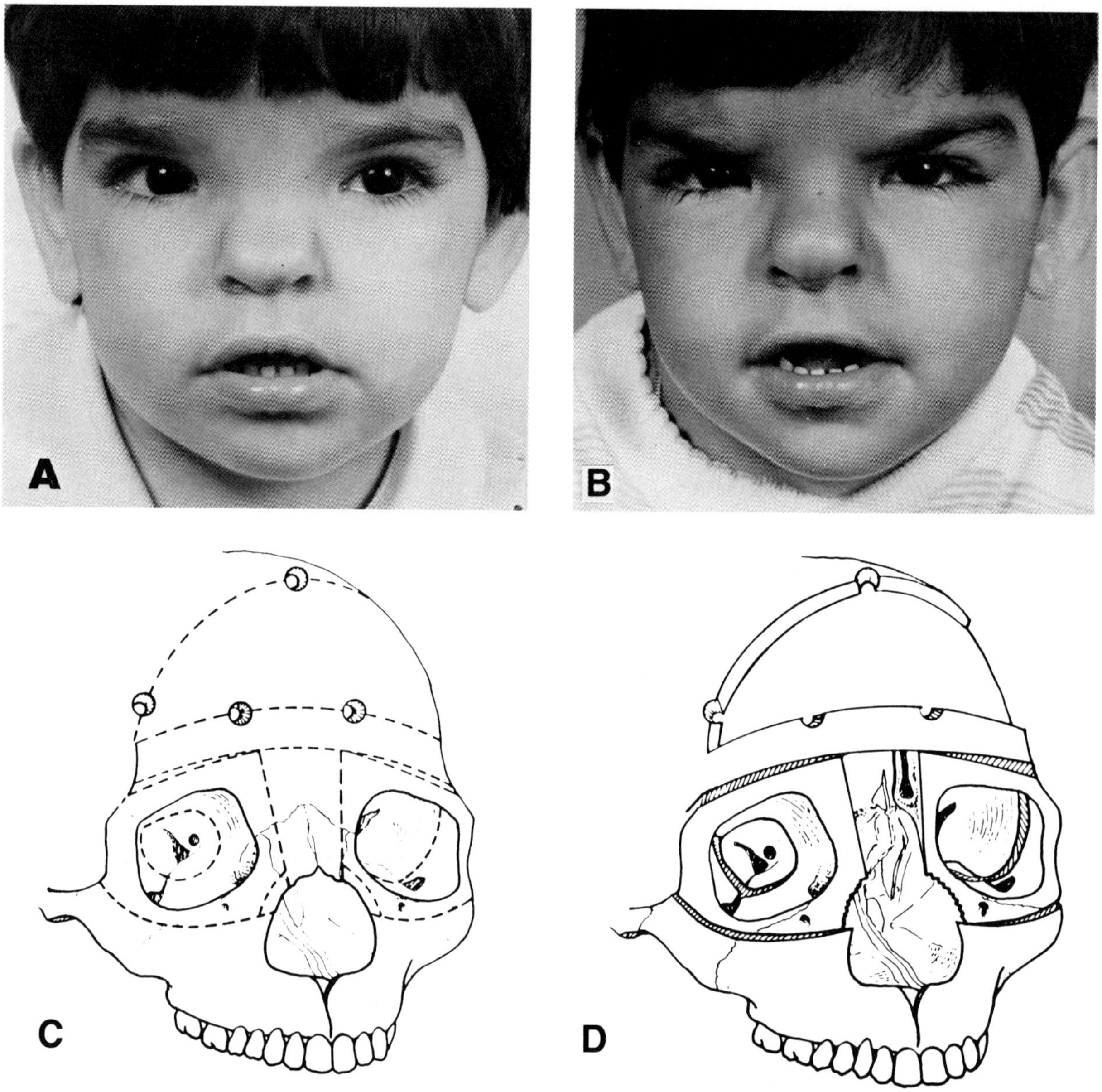

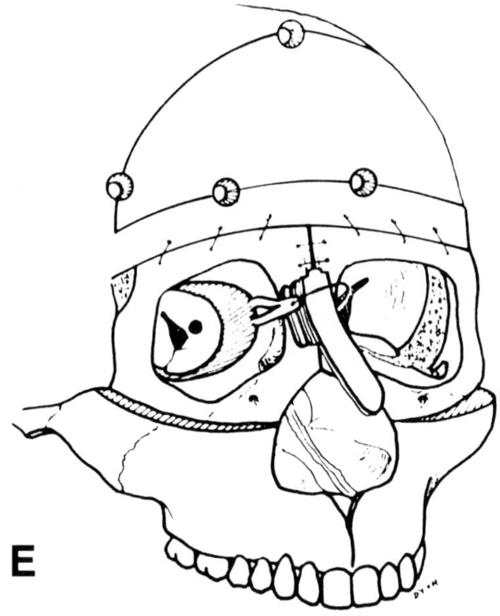

Figure 1 *A*, A 2-year-old child is shown before transcranial correction of orbital hypertelorism. *B*, The postoperative result at 3 months. Coronal and intraoral incisions were used to provide access for orbital osteotomies, and a Rethe incision was used for exposure of the nasal tip. *C*, *D*, and *E*, Osteotomy lines for transcranial correction of orbital hypertelorism. In the young child, the infraorbital osteotomy should be very close to, or through, the infraorbital foramen to avoid damage to permanent teeth roots. Some bone may need to be removed from the piriform rim area to prevent impingement on the nasal airway.

Figure continues on opposite page

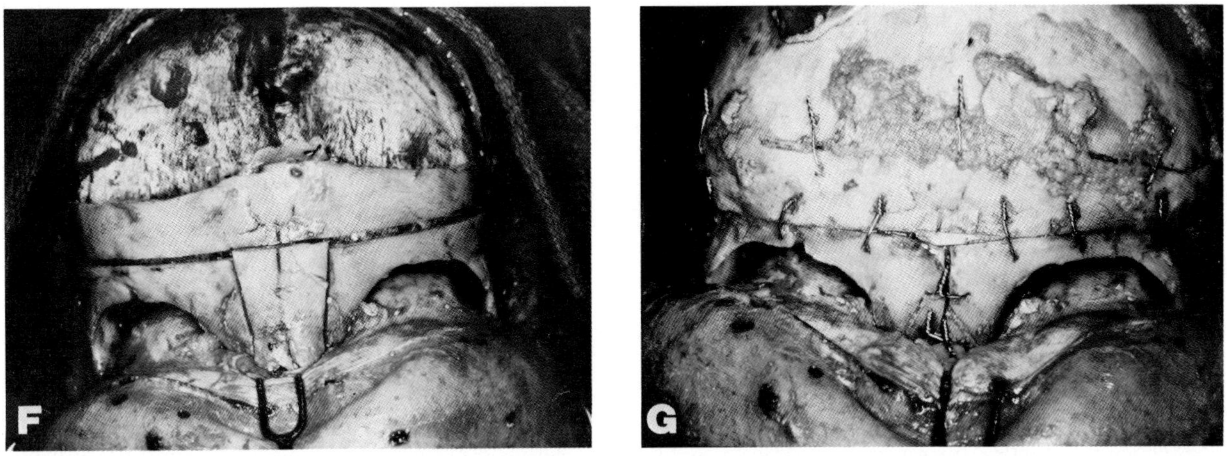

Figure 1 (continued) Operative photographs show the same patient before *F*, and after, *G*, medial displacement of the orbital cavities. The frontal bandeau is useful both to provide orbital fixation and to prevent enophthalmos or exophthalmos by inadvertent sagittal displacement of the orbital framework. The interorbital distance in this case was 38 mm preoperatively and 17 mm postoperatively.

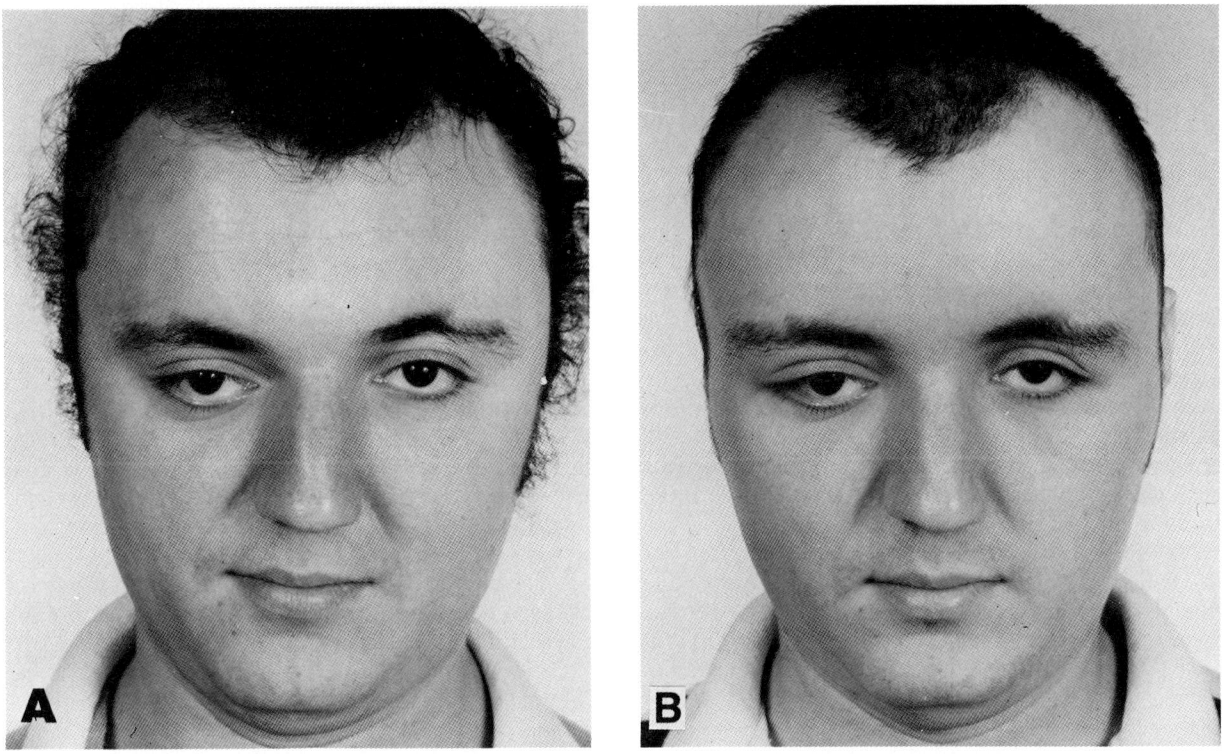

Figure 2 *A* and *B* show a 28-year-old patient with a vertical, orbital dystopia caused by a giant hyperpneumatization of the right frontal sinus. Transcranial correction of the right orbital dystopia was performed, which elevated the right orbit 8 mm. This was performed through a combined coronal and intraoral approach. Other causes of vertical, orbital dystopia include torticollis and hemifacial microsomia, and other types of facial clefts.

It has been found that some overcorrection of hypertelorism beyond the anticipated normal values for age provide a better result. Also, whenever possible, the medial canthal tendons should be kept attached to the medial orbital wall, thus preventing the need for later revision of medial canthal relapse.

SUGGESTED READING

Günter H. Konstitutionelle Anomalien des Augenabstandes und der Interorbitalbreite. Virchows Arch 1933; 290:373.

Lejoyeux E, Tulasne JF, Tessier PL. Maxillary growth following total septal resection in correction of orbital hypertelorism. Cleft Palate J 1986; 23(Suppl):27–39.

Tessier P. Experiences in the treatment of orbital hypertelorism. Plast Reconstr Surg 1974; 53:1–4.

Tessier P, Guiot G, Rougerie J, Delbet JP, Pastoriza J. Osteotomies cranio-naso-orbitales. Hypertelorism. Ann Chir Plast Esthet 1967; 12:103.

HEMIFACIAL MICROSOMIA

IAN R. MUNRO, M.D., M.A., M.B., B.CHIR, F.R.C.S.(C)

The term hemifacial microsomia (HFM) is now the most widely accepted term for unilateral facial asymmetry of congenital origin. It has displaced terms such as first and second branchial arch syndrome or lateral facial dysplasia. A common variant of HFM is Goldenhar's syndrome. The additional features that permit this latter diagnosis are the presence of an epibulbar dermoid and cervical spine anomalies.

A rare variant is bilateral HFM, which must be differentiated from Treacher Collins syndrome. In the latter case there may be a family history of a similarly involved member. Clinically, HFM does not have a preauricular tongue of hair or absence of eyelashes in the medial two-thirds of the lower eyelids. Treacher Collins patients may have an absence of the zygomatic arch, but never an absence of the mandibular condyle. In Treacher Collins syndrome there is usually an antigonial notching of the lower border of the mandible. The mandibular gonial angle is usually more obtuse and the chin point is more posterior and closer to the hyoid. The Treacher Collins patient typically has a very high-bridged nose, often with absence of the glabellar notch. The lower anterior maxilla is frequently protrusive and there is no occlusal tilt upwards to one side. In bilateral HFM there is usually a marked degree of asymmetry between the two sides and an occlusal tilt is not uncommon. It is important to differentiate bilateral HFM and Treacher Collins syndrome because of the genetic implications. Treacher Collins syndrome is an autosomal dominant inherited condition, whereas HFM is always a spontaneous mutation and not inherited.

The only other diagnoses that may be considered, but which are easily rejected by the history, are Romberg's hemifacial atrophy and acquired deformities such as those secondary to temporomandibular ankylosis or torticollis. Hemifacial hypertrophy can be differentiated because other parts of the body may be enlarged and the dentition is enlarged on the involved side. For pragmatic reasons it is useful to separate HFM from the more involved form that affects the orbit and skull on the same side, to which the term craniofacial microsomia (CFM) is applied. This pragmatism will influence decision-making with regard to treatment.

FACTORS IN TREATMENT DECISIONS

Although there is a wide spectrum of treatments available, the decision as to which treatment should be used cannot be based solely on the anatomic problem or the patient's age.

The order of importance for making a decision is: (1) severity of deformity, (2) age of patient, (3) psychosocial concern of patient and/or parents, and (4) presence or absence of skeletal parts. In considering the severity of the deformity, the most important factor is what the patient looks like, rather than the actual anatomic problems. A mild-appearing deformity may have severe anatomic deficiencies and vice versa.

EXAMINATION OF THE PATIENT

The detailed physical examination is the most important factor in deciding what needs to be corrected—and by how much. All other investigations, such as diagnostic radiology and anthropology, should be considered conjunctive and do not override the clinical physical examination.

It is the external appearance that must be changed. Good skeletal correction is only secondary to the need of the external appearance. Sometimes, extensive correction is needed for relatively mild deformities and is justified if there is sufficient parent and/or patient concern. However, the corollary is also true. Sometimes, a mild external deformity may mask a severe skeletal problem, yet it may not be necessary to correct the skeleton completely.

The physical examination should be from the top of the head downward, looking for asymmetry in position and size. The forehead may be recessed; the eyebrow, orbit, and also the lateral canthus may be lower. The ear is frequently microtic or displaced. The zygomatic arch, glenoid fossa, mandibular condyle, or ascending ramus may be dysplastic or absent. If there is an occlusal plane tilt, there will be a labial fissure tilt and displacement of the chin to the involved side—and usually backwards as well. The muscles of mastication and the parotid gland may be hypoplastic or absent. Branches of the facial nerve may not be working. Sometimes, the ipsilateral side of the palate may be paralyzed. Intraorally, the dental arches may show narrowing on the involved side with a lingual tilt to the teeth and a posterior rotation of the entire arch.

Diagnostic radiology should include cephalometric and panorex studies, computed tomography (CT) and three-dimensional reconstruction, and it is of primary importance to note the asymmetry and tilting, and what bone is missing. If the condyle and part of the ascending ramus are absent, then the residual ascending ramus will be displaced medially. If a line is drawn upwards along the outside of the ascending ramus on the normal side, it points to the side of the head (Fig. 1), whereas a line drawn on the involved side points to the orbit. This is the main cause of the facial flatness on that side.

When the CT scan in the coronal view is examined, it will be seen that the distance between the lateral surface of the mandible and the skin on the normal side is not very thick, and the distance on the involved side may be equally thick. This is the whole premise for treatment: *first the bone then the soft tissues*. Indeed, in most cases, once the skeleton is aligned and size corrected, there is no need to add soft tissue.

TREATMENT PLANNING

For ease of planning, a surgical–anatomic classification of five types has been devised. In Type I the skeleton is intact but hypoplastic whereas the other types have increasing degrees of absent bone and displacement. Type I is further divided into Type Ia, with a horizontal occlusal plane and labial fissure, and Type Ib, with an occlusal tilt.

In principle, it is easier to augment bone than soft tissue. Thus, it becomes easier in many cases to overcorrect the hypoplasia of bone rather than add a free flap of tissue. Types I to IV can be corrected skeletally in one operation. Type V, with orbital displacement (that constitutes craniofacial microsomia), requires a two-stage correction.

In planning the actual skeletal movement, it is important to realize that this is a three-dimensional deformity; not two-dimensional as often portrayed. The skeleton is tipped upwards on the involved side; it is displaced posteriorly and medially contracted or positioned. Thus, it is important to level the occlusion, advance the skeleton forward, and rotate it laterally. Although the opposite side of the patient may appear normal, the mandible is usually retrognathic on that side as well as on the involved side and, therefore, the mandible, and usually also the chin, must be advanced.

The planning of the leveling and rotation of the skeleton must be done around the facial midline. If the maxilla is positioned correctly, then the mandible is simply placed in relationship to the level maxilla. The positioning of the maxillary occlusal plane therefore becomes the basis of correction of Types Ib to IV. The dental arch must be lowered on the involved side, but the hinge point must be the facial midline and not the opposite zygomatic buttress, otherwise the incisors and canines on the normal side are lengthened and have an abnormal relation to the lip line. Thus, a wedge of bone is removed on the normal side while the involved side is lengthened, advanced, and rotated out laterally. These measurements can be calculated precisely from cephalometric radiologic studies, dental models on the articulator, and direct patient examination. The mandible position is just calculated to fit the maxilla.

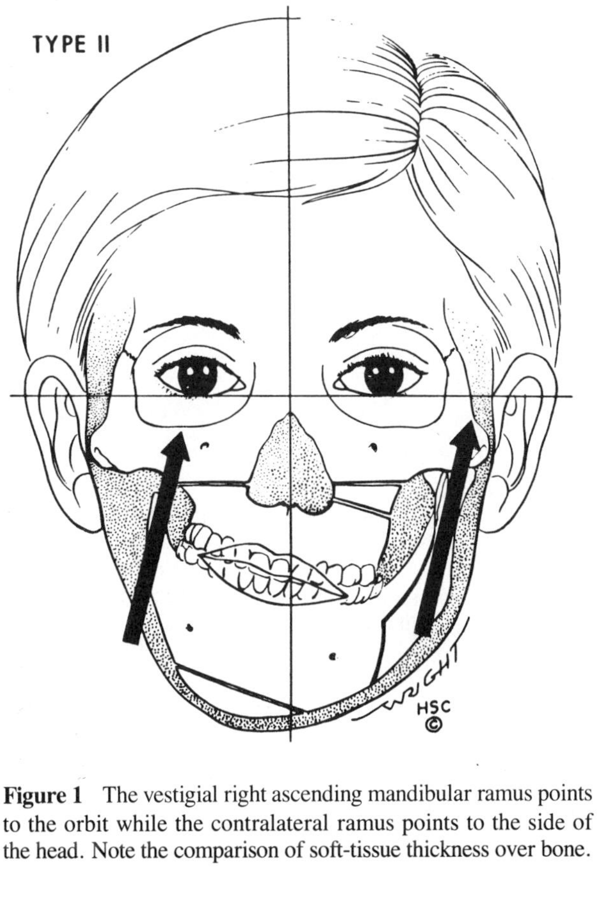

Figure 1 The vestigial right ascending mandibular ramus points to the orbit while the contralateral ramus points to the side of the head. Note the comparison of soft-tissue thickness over bone.

TECHNIQUES OF SKELETAL TREATMENT

Bone Harvesting and Augmentation

Originally, split rib grafts were used for augmentation. They were easy to contour but had a high resorption rate and caused chest morbidity. Split cranial grafts cause no local morbidity (provided they are removed by someone familiar with the technique). They have little resorption, but are difficult to contour. A hemicoronal incision is used to expose the parietal bone. No hair shaving at all is necessary. The bone must always be removed at least 1½ to 2 cm lateral to the sagittal suture. The squamous temporal area can be augmented from this approach, if necessary. If the zygomatic arch or zygoma are to be enlarged, a full coronal incision is necessary. The zygoma (without the arch), maxilla, mandible body, and ascending ramus can all be reached intraorally. The quickest way to attach the onlay bone is with a lag screw. Layers of bone can be used to provide the necessary soft tissue external contour (Fig. 2).

Osteotomies

In Type Ib with an intact skeleton, an intraoral exposure is used for the Le Fort I maxillary osteotomy, sagittal split mandibular osteotomies (on both sides), and the genioplasty. The mandible almost always needs lengthen-

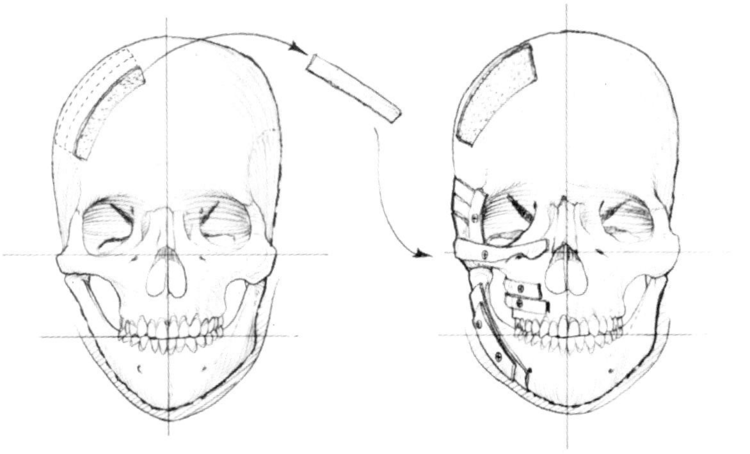

Figure 2 Type 1A, deformity shows the various areas that can be augmented with split cranial grafts attached by lag screws.

ing on the normal side. A sagittal split is used for all mandibular osteotomies. In order to simplify the surgery, it is best to expose the chin first, perform the mandibular sagittal splits and then carry out the Le Fort I maxillary osteotomy. The wedge of maxilla to be removed should have been precisely calculated preoperatively as should the lengthening, advancement, and lateral rotation of the involved side. The fitting and holding of a wedge of bone into the gap on the involved side is technically very difficult. The self-retained Le Fort I osteotomy principle can be used to make fixation easier, quicker, and more stable (Fig. 3). Although the various maxillary movements can be calculated theoretically with a good degree of accuracy, the level and rotation of the occlusal plane should be checked visually with a tongue depressor or flat rule held against the teeth, to see if the occlusal plane is parallel to the orbits. Verification should also be made by direct measurements from the teeth to the lateral and medial canthi on either side. The maxilla is fixed with miniplates and screws and predesigned occlusal acrylic wafer is inserted. The mandible is adjusted to the occlusal wafer as well as to the maxilla. The sagittal split is fixed with screws or a miniplate. Finally, the osteotomy of the chin is performed with advancement and movement into the midline as needed. A three-dimensional rotation of the genioplasty segment is usual, thereby following the principles of the Le Fort I maxillary osteotomy.

In types II and III with absent bone, a costochondral graft is first taken from the contralateral chest (about the sixth rib). This provides the correct convexity to the face. Prior to the intraoral exposure, a preauricular incision is made and the glenoid fossa, when present, is exposed. When there is no zygomatic arch, then the correct location for the glenoid fossa on the side of the skull is identified. Once the intraoral exposures are complete, a tunnel is made from the body of the mandible to the preauricular region, kept deep to the facial nerve. The osteotomies of the maxilla, mandible, and chin are performed and secured as in the Type Ib deformity.

When a glenoid fossa is present, the cartilage of the costochondral graft is carved to fit it. The rib is brought through the tunnel and along the body of the mandible

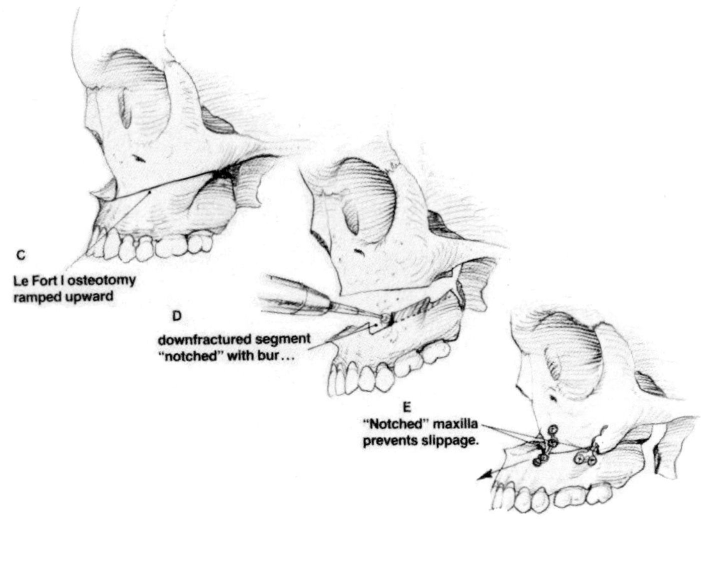

Figure 3 Self-retained Le Fort I osteotomy shows how the bone is cut horizontally at the front of the maxilla but ramped upwards as it passes posteriorly thus allowing advancement, vertical lengthening, and self-retention without necessity of bone grafts. Miniplate bone fixation is used.

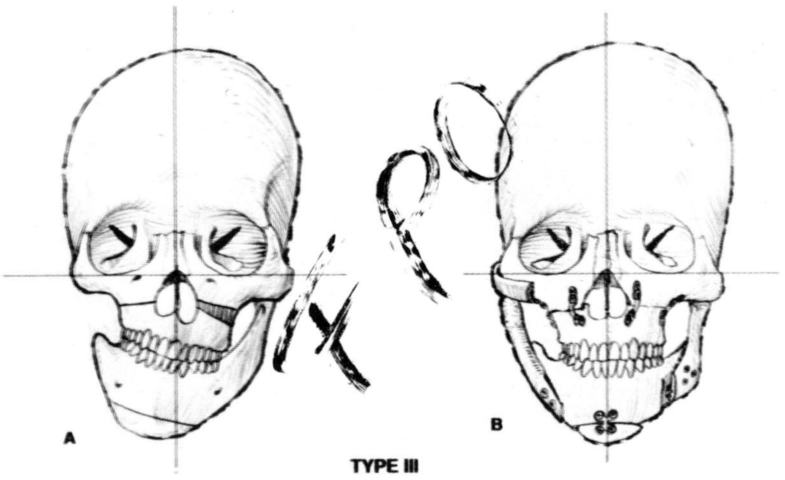

Figure 4 *A*, Type III skeletal deformity shows the three-dimensional deformity and rotation. *B*, The zygomatic arch and glenoid fossa are constructed with rib and cartilage. A Le Fort I osteotomy is used to level and rotate the maxilla using self-retained technique (see Fig. 3). The mandible is advanced with sagittal split, centralizing genioplasty, and costochondral graft construction of the temporomandibular joint.

to the lateral margin of the genioplasty segment. Over the distal 2 cm of this rib the medial cortex is removed, thus allowing attachment of rib cancellous bone to the cortex of the mandible—which is best done with two screws. In Type III cases with absence of the zygomatic arch and glenoid fossa, a new arch is built from full-thickness rib to pass from the inferior orbital rim to the side of the skull. A glenoid fossa is carved from the rib and lined with costal cartilage (Fig. 4).

In young patients before eruption of the secondary dentition, screws and plate fixation are not possible. Wires must be used to prevent damage to the permanent teeth.

For Type IV cases, hemi-Le Fort III and contralateral Le Fort I osteotomies have been described. The periorbital osteotomy repositioned the hypoplastic and displaced lateral orbital wall and inferior orbital rim wall. However, the orbital floor was also lowered. Thus, bone grafts had to be inserted on the orbital floor to prevent lowering of the eye. Because split skull grafts are readily obtainable and do not resorb, it may be easier to do a Type III skeletal correction and merely augment the periorbital bones with split cranium (Fig. 5).

CRANIOFACIAL MICROSOMIA (TYPE V)

When the eye is displaced downward by only 2 to 3 mm, it is possible to raise it by upward contouring of the anterior orbital roof and superior orbital rim and placement of split cranial grafts into the floor. This can be done at the same operation as the other osteotomies. When the eye displacement is greater, however, a full osteotomy of the entire orbit via the intracranial route is necessary. In such patients, the forehead is frequently also displaced backwards and can be advanced simultaneously. At the same operation, the zygomatic arch and glenoid fossa can be constructed.

In severe cases of HFM or CFM, it is necessary to build or push the skeleton a long distance laterally and, usually, lengthen it at the same time. The bone reconstruction of the temporomandibular joint and insertion of the long costochondral graft is deep to the facial nerve, which is thus pushed laterally and must curve over a much longer arc. It is not unusual for the patient to have a facial neuropraxia for a time after surgery as a result of this stretching. In CFM, at the first operation of orbital repositioning, a tissue expander can be inserted against the squamous temporal bone and done to the region of the ascending ramus, deep to the facial nerve. Progressive expansion over several weeks prevents the development of a facial neuropraxia at the second operation.

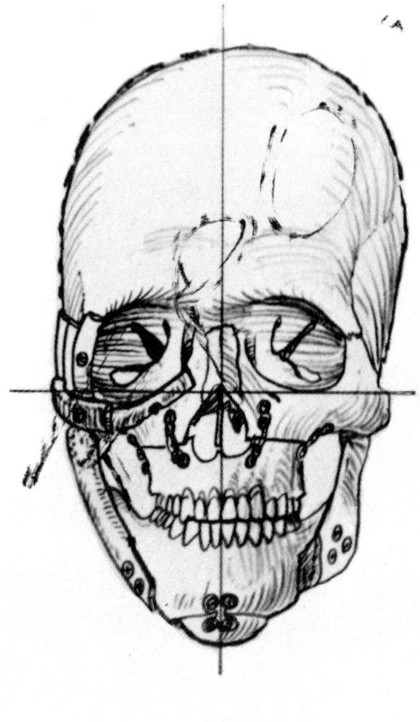

Figure 5 The lower and midface osteotomies of Type IV are the same as for Type III. In addition split cranium augments the lateral orbital wall, inferior orbital rim, and temporal fossa.

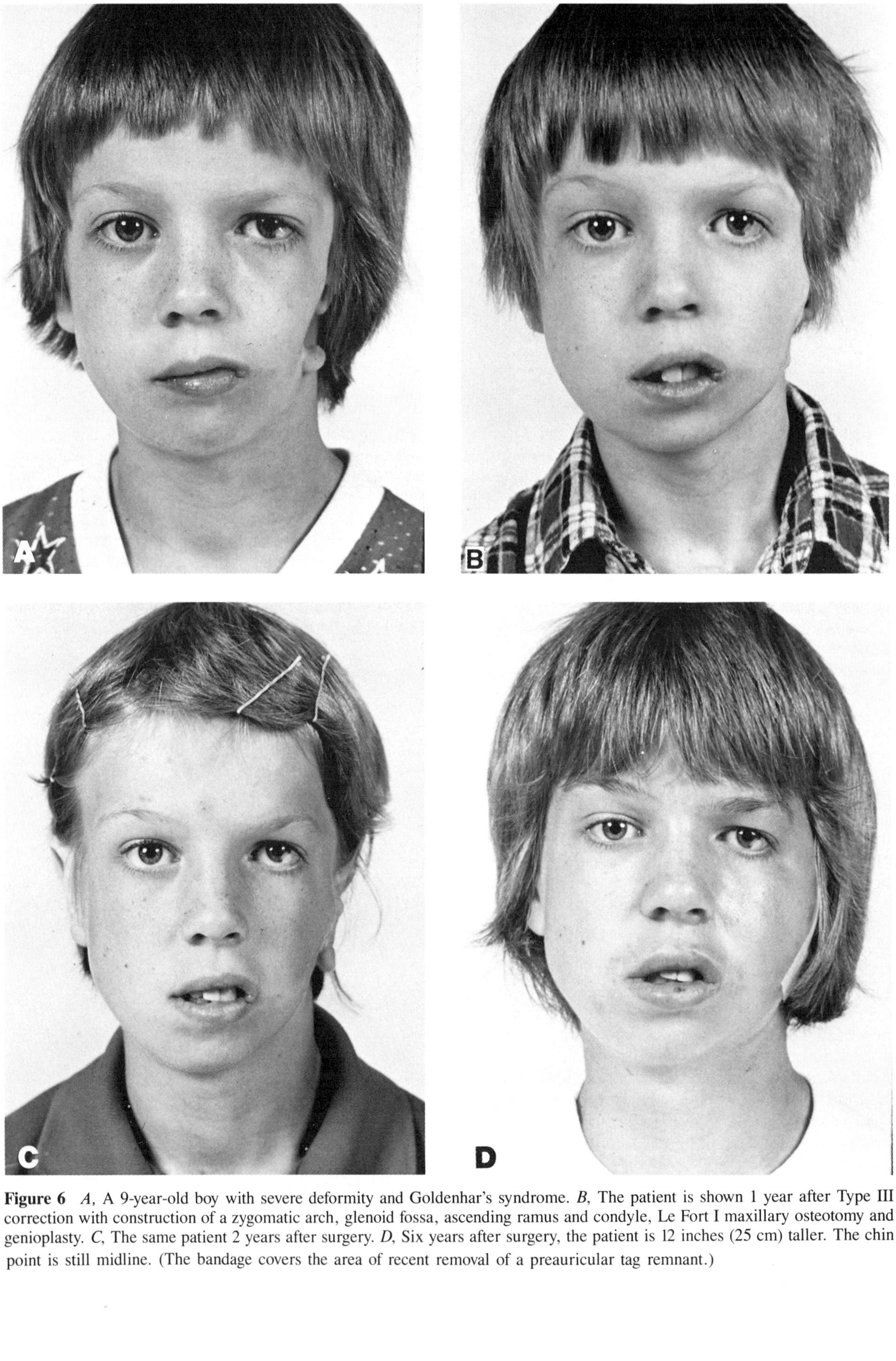

Figure 6 *A,* A 9-year-old boy with severe deformity and Goldenhar's syndrome. *B,* The patient is shown 1 year after Type III correction with construction of a zygomatic arch, glenoid fossa, ascending ramus and condyle, Le Fort I maxillary osteotomy and genioplasty. *C,* The same patient 2 years after surgery. *D,* Six years after surgery, the patient is 12 inches (25 cm) taller. The chin point is still midline. (The bandage covers the area of recent removal of a preauricular tag remnant.)

The key feature in skeletal correction is not just to level the skeleton but to build it out laterally far enough to produce the correct width to the face. This puts the maximum stretch on the facial nerve and diminishes or eliminates the need for additional secondary soft-tissue augmentation. The labial fissure tilt follows the occlusal tilt and is corrected with leveling of the occlusion.

ADDITIONAL PROCEDURES

When the patient has microtia, it ideally should be corrected after the skeleton has been aligned. In severe cases, with complete absence of masseter and parotid gland, correction or even overcorrection of the skeleton will still leave asymmetry. An extra 2 to 4 mm of soft-tissue thickness can be gained by rotating down a large pericranial flap. However, for the small percentage of cases in which this is not enough, a free flap is necessary. The disadvantages of free flaps are (a) donor site scar, (b) size of scar on face or neck, and (c) the fact that it is usually necessary to perform a second operation to "trim the flap." Flaps that contain fat also retain the growth pattern of the donor site. Thus, as body habitus changes, further trimming will be necessary. In general, patients prefer to look a little bit too thin rather than too fat on one side. Thus, free flaps should be used with reluctance and caution.

The ideal time for surgery is to have the patient look as normal as possible before entering Grade 1. Originally, it was unknown what the effect of growth would be on the osteotomized segments—especially the free nonvascularized costochondral graft. Recently, it has been found that these grafts do, infact, grow and further surgery may not be necessary (Fig. 6).

The standard operations may be varied according to the severity of the problem and the age and geographic location of the patient. This last factor can be used if the patient can be closely followed orthodontically. In patients with an absent condyle, the mandible is tilted up on that side. This has a secondary adverse effect on alveolar bone growth of the maxilla. When the secondary dentition is not fully erupted and the patient lives locally, the mandible can be leveled and centralized but no osteotomy of the maxilla is performed. This causes an open bite on the involved side. During fixation an acrylic splint is made to maintain this open bite. The most posterior tooth on each jaw on the involved side can be left uncovered and will erupt during the fixation period. Subsequent to removal of fixation, an orthodontic splint is made to uncover the teeth progressively and allow them to erupt and gradually close the bite. This produces alveolar bone growth and can avoid the necessity of a maxillary osteotomy.

SUGGESTED READING

Beals SP, Munro IR. The use of miniplates in craniomaxillofacial surgery. Plast Reconst Surg 1987; 79:33–38.

Munro IR. The self-retained Lefort I osteotomy. Craniofacial surgery. Marchac D, ed. Proceedings, First International Congress, International Society of Cranio-Maxillo-Facial Surgery. Berlin: Springer-Verlag, 1987; 326.

Munro IR. One-stage reconstruction of the temporomandibular joint in hemifacial microsomia. Plast Reconstr Surg 1980; 66:699–710.

Munro IR, Lauritzen CD. Classification and treatment of hemifacial microsomia. In: Caronni EP, ed. Craniofacial surgery. Boston: Little, Brown, 1985:391.

Phillips JH, Munro IR, Ross RB, Griffen G. Growth after reconstruction of the temporomandibular joint. Paper presented at the Canadian Society of Plastic Surgeons annual meeting, Toronto, May 1986.

MANDIBULOFACIAL DYSOSTOSIS

JEAN-FRANCOIS TULASNE, M.D.
PAUL TESSIER, M.D.

The facial anomalies of mandibulofacial dysostosis result mainly from hypoplasia of the zygoma and mandible. In the orbital region, even an absence of the malar bone is compatible with normal ocular function and binocular vision. The problem is different in case of extreme mandibular hypoplasia that results in nasopharyngeal obstruction and, therefore, breathing difficulties. The current treatment of mandibulofacial dysostosis takes into account these functional anomalies that are an integral part of the facial dysmorphia, at least in the lower face.

MALFORMATIONS AND FUNCTIONS INVOLVED

In the orbital complex, all the deformities proceed from a basic defect that consists of an absence, or marked hypoplasia, of the zygoma and overlying superficial musculoaponeurotic system. The malar eminence does not exist and there is lateral canthal looseness and dystopia, upper eyelid pseudoptosis, and antimongoloid slant of the palpebral fissure. There is also a coloboma or marginal hypoplasia of the lower eyelid. Mechanical upper eyelid ptosis and, sometimes, ocular deviation are associated with the syndrome.

In the jaws, there are two basic defects. The first is posterior shortness of the maxilla, narrowness of the palate and choanal atresia. The second is shortness of the ramus and body of the mandible. As a result, there is micrognathia, a foreshortened floor of the mouth and suprahyoid region, obstruction of a small hypopharynx by the base of the tongue, anterior open bite, and retrogenia (Fig. 1). These anatomic findings often produce breath-

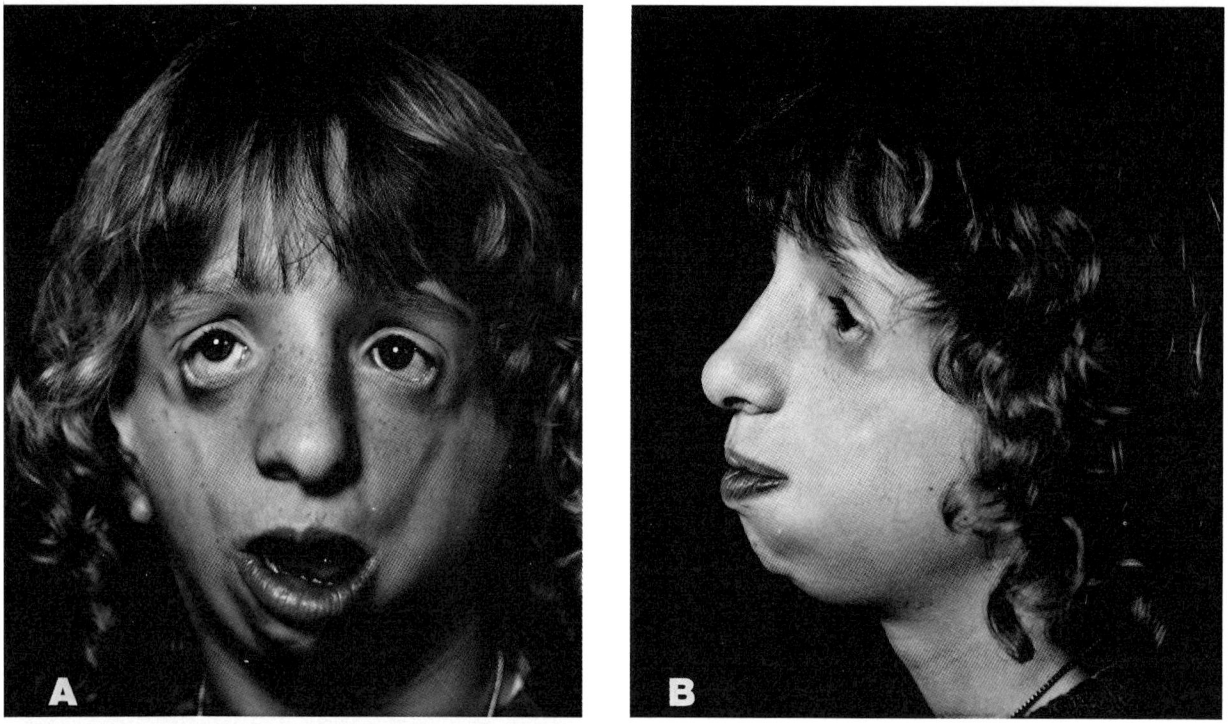

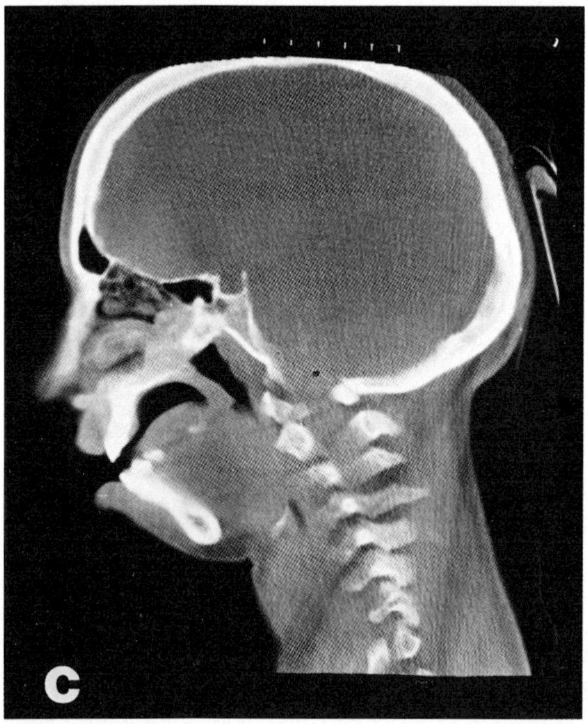

Figure 1 *A*, and *B*, Complete form of Treacher Collins syndrome in a patient with severe breathing difficulties. *C*, Sagittal section on computed tomography scan demonstrates choanal atresia and obstruction of the hypopharynx by the tongue.

ing impairment secondary to obstruction of the nasopharynx and hypopharynx.

Microtia and middle ear anomalies may cause hearing loss and subsequent impairment of speech and intellectual development. Speech problems are common in these patients as the result of hearing loss, choanal atresia, pharyngeal obstruction, soft palate or pharyngeal incompetence, and incomplete dental and labial occlusion. Lip occlusion is incompetent because of the macrostomia, weakness of the levators of the upper lip, and retrogenia, which pulls away the lower lip.

Finally, there is underdevelopment of the body, presumably related to chronic respiratory deficiency.

The objectives of treatment are: (1) to restore normal nasal and oral breathing, (2) to develop the pharyngeal space for the tongue and breathing, (3) to give projection to the mandible and chin, (4) to normalize the dental occlusion, (5) to restore the orbital contours, the malar eminences, and a normal level of the lateral canthi, (6) to construct the auricles, and (7) to improve hearing function.

PRINCIPLES OF SURGICAL TREATMENT

The basic therapeutic principle developed by Tessier in 1982 is to restore normal nasal and oral breathing by enlargement of the choanae and the pharyngeal space through a combined rotation of the midfacial segment and mandibular lengthening. The counter-clockwise rotation of the lower face also adds to the projection of the receding chin, which is advanced by a genioplasty.

Using the Le Fort III-type osteotomy as a model, the midfacial element is not advanced, but rotated around a transverse axis with the frontonasal angle acting as a fulcrum.

This midfacial rotation involves the orbital complex, nasopharynx, maxilla, ramus, mandibular body, and floor of the mouth. In practice, the procedure requires only one osteotomy at the frontonasomaxillary junction and a disjunction between the maxillary tuberosity and the pterygoid process.

Combined Midfacial Rotation and Mandibular Lengthening

Technique for Rotation of Midfacial Segment

Dissection of the midface is made through coronal and infraorbital incisions. A contour resection is made along the overhanging supraorbital ridge, from the supratrochlear notch to the temporal crest. This fragment can be used as a graft for the contralateral inferior orbital rim. At the frontonasomaxillary junction, a reverse V-shape osteotomy is made. It enters the frontal sinus. Laterally, the osteotomy cuts the medial orbital wall down to the floor and is completed via the infraorbital approach. A curved chisel is used to disjoin the hypoplastic maxillary tuberosity and the pterygoid process. The midfacial segment is disimpacted with a Rowe-Epker forceps by a downward movement. A burr is used to remove bone from the frontal bone and to allow a deeper impaction at the frontonasal angle.

The rotation has the following effects: (1) shortening of the anterior face, (2) forward movement of the anterior teeth, (3) downward movement of the posterior maxilla, which also enlarges the nasopharynx, and (4) downward displacement of the zygomatic remnant, which slightly enlarges the vertical diameter of the orbit. As a result, the maxilla becomes more horizontal and is given more anterior projection. This also allows lengthening of the mandible, both vertically and sagittally. However, intermaxillary fixation of an overlengthened mandible with a shortness of soft tissue submits the midfacial segment to considerable backward force. In consequence, the midface must be stabilized and the orbital deficits closed with bone grafts.

Stabilization of the Midface and Orbital Construction

Stability is provided by bone grafts taken from the calvaria in the parietal region. Depending on the patient's age, the grafts can be either half thickness, taken discontinuously, or harvested as a single full-thickness fragment that is cut in several bands and split.

The frontonasal angle is stabilized with two interosseous wires. The key point for sagittal stability is the bone graft interposed between the temporal bone and the maxilla. Fixation must take into account the backward stress caused by the mandible.

The parietal area gives the proper curvature to the temporomaxillary bone graft. The posterior end of this graft is fixed to the cranium through a hole that enters the middle cranial fossa anteriorly, or above the mastoid process. The anterior end is fixed under the malar stump

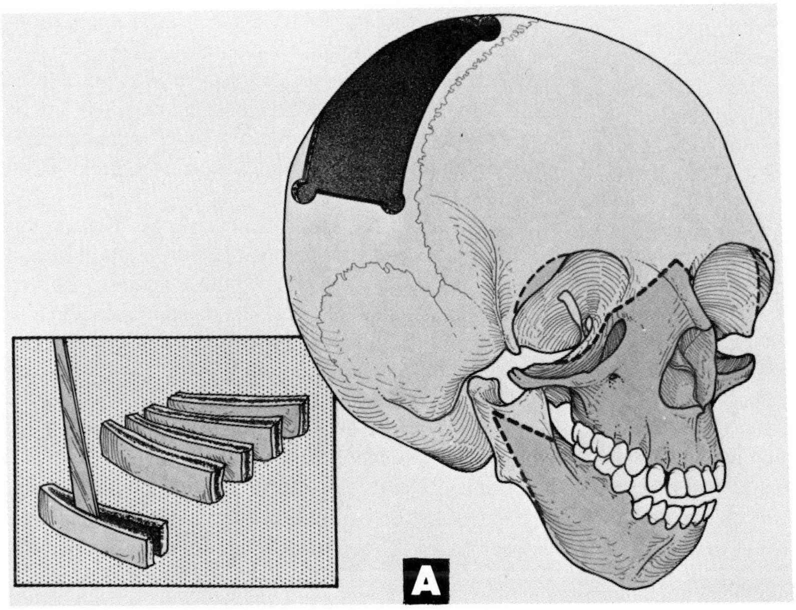

Figure 2 Combined rotation of the midfacial segment and mandibular lengthening. *A*, Outlines of the midfacial segment osteotomy and V-shaped osteotomy of the ramus. Five calvarial strips of bone are split for use in the orbital region, zygoma, and, if appropriate, ramus.

Figure continues on following page

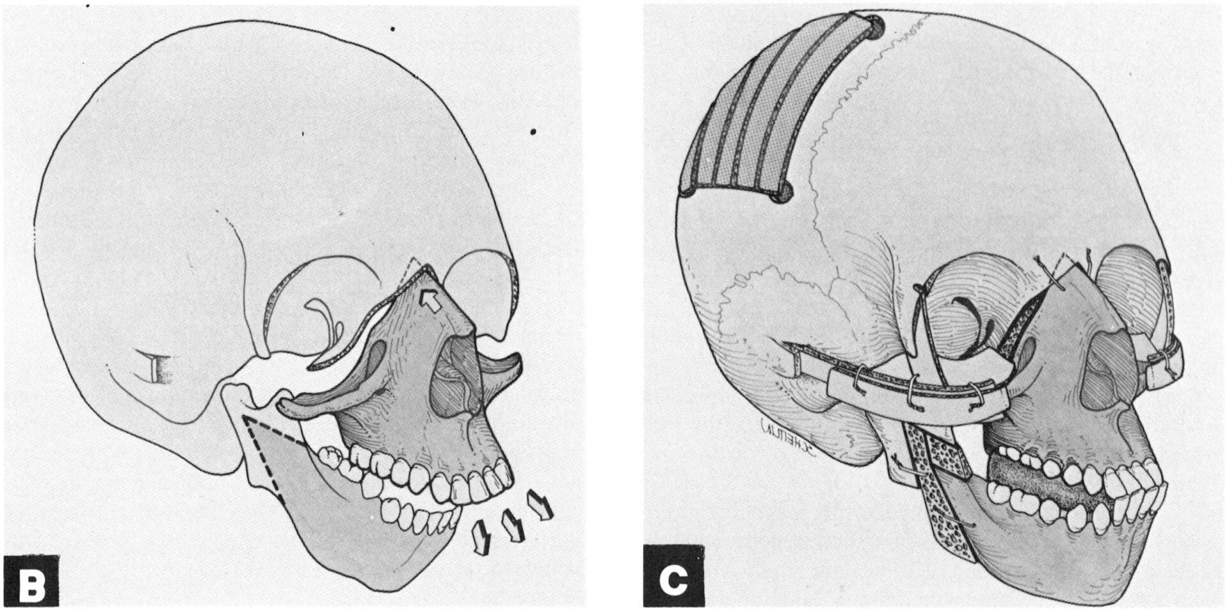

Figure 2 (continued) *B*, Rotation of the midfacial segment. The inverted V at the frontonasal angle is deeply impacted into the frontal sinus. *C*, Lengthening of the ramus and mandibular body by a V-shaped osteotomy and, eventually, by a bone graft between the fragments. The mandible is advanced on a splint in an anterior cross bite position and a posterior open bite. Construction of the orbital region and zygoma is completed with calvarial grafts. Tibial or iliac cancellous grafts fill up the dead spaces between the main supporting grafts. The calvarial donor site is covered by the other part of the split of the parietal bone.

against the maxilla. A graft placed between the tuberosity is displaced below the small pterygoid plate.

The orbital complex is also constructed with calvarial bone grafts to the lateral orbital wall, inferior lateral angle, floor, and inferior orbital rim. The latter graft is reinforced by the resection made at the superior orbital ridge. Cancellous grafts from the tibia can also be used to fill in the dead space between the major grafts.

Lengthening of the Mandible

Mandibular lengthening can be performed in two different ways, depending on the patient's age and the degree of ramus hypoplasia. In a young child where the ramus is almost nonexistent, the initial construction is made with the cranial graft interposed from the glenoid fossa to the angle. When a ramus exists in older children, it can be lengthened by a V- or S-shaped osteotomy. The defect is also filled with calvarial grafts. There is almost no limitation to mandibular lengthening.

The mandible is fixed to the maxilla with a splint in an anterior cross bite and posterior open bite position.

One- or Two-Step Procedure

The stability of the midfacial segment is important. Therefore, it may be best to separate the midface rotation and the mandibular procedures (Fig. 3).

In theory, the midfacial segment ought to be rotated first. However, this results in a severe anterior open bite until the mandibular lengthening is carried out. When the mandible is lengthened first, a splint is needed to maintain the posterior open bite, which will be changed to the appropriate size at the time of the midface rotation.

OTHER PROCEDURES

1. Hearing aids are preferred to procedures on the middle ear, which are often unsuccessful and carry the risk of possible damage to the facial nerve.
2. Auricle construction is done according to Brent's method. It is generally performed in three or four stages, depending on the severity of the malformation. It includes implantation of a costal cartilage framework with later lobule transposition, tragus construction, and conchal excavation.
3. Lowering of the posterior part of the maxilla is achieved by a Le Fort I maxillotomy or a Le Fort II-type midfacial rotation. It can also be accompanied by a disjunction of the palate in order to enlarge the maxilla.
4. Lengthening of the ramus and angle by V-shape osteotomy and bone graft advances the mandible and thus expands the floor of the mouth and the pharyngeal space. It also corrects the dental malocclusion and gives more normal projection to the lower face.
5. A segmental anterior mandibular osteotomy may be required to correct the anterior open bite, either simultaneously or secondary to mandibular lengthening, according to the age of the patient.
6. Genioplasty and elongation of suprahyoid tissues achieve a better contour to the chin and the whole lower face. If necessary, another advancement

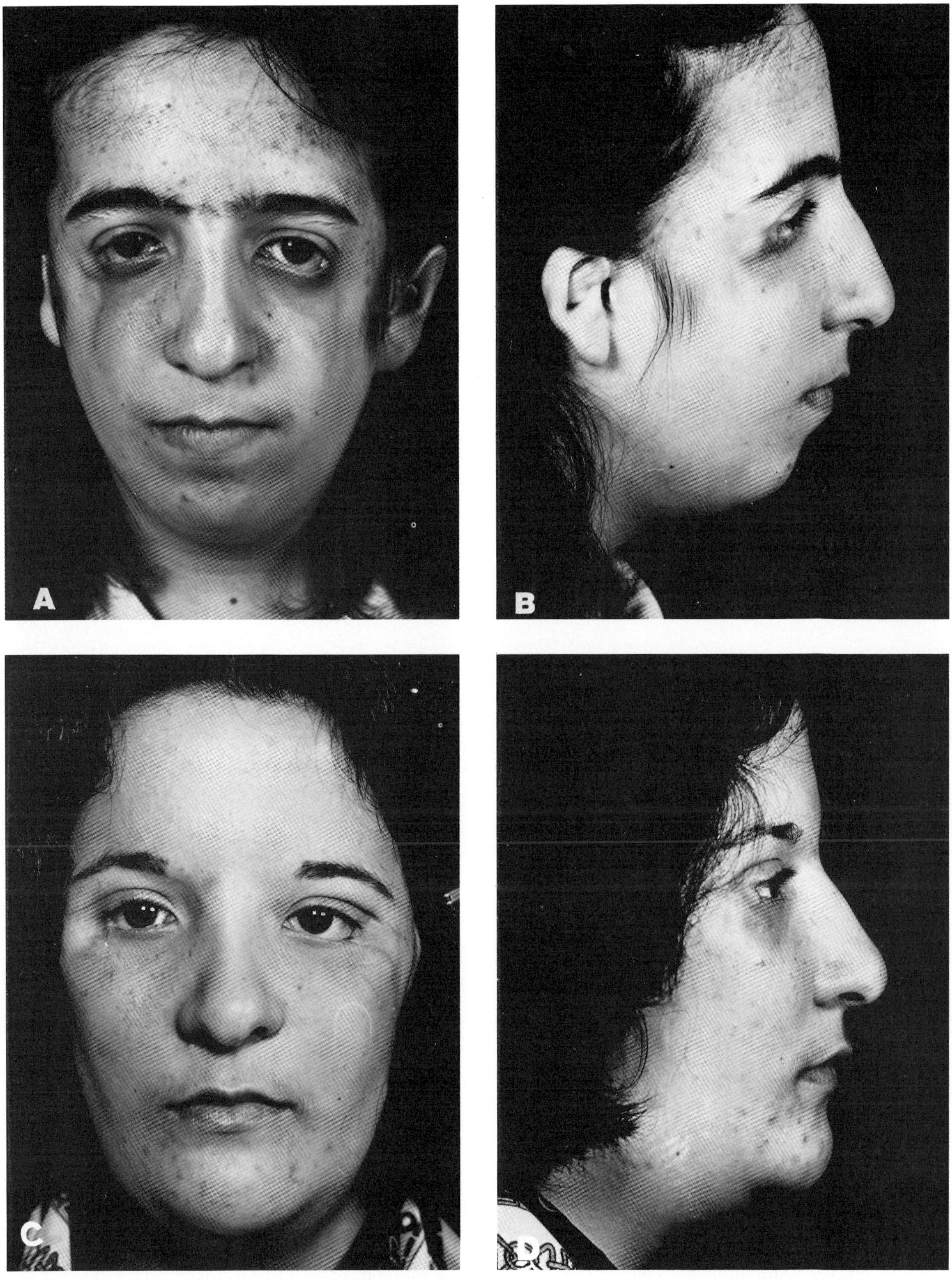

Figure 3 Patient operated on for Treacher Collins syndrome. *A* and *B*, Appearance at 16 years (before treatment). *C* and *D*, at 20 years following a two-stage radical procedure (with genioplasty) and two additional operations on the orbits and eyelids.

genioplasty can be done again after 2 years through the transplanted inframandibular segment.

7. The orbital complex and zygomatic arch are constructed and reshaped in two or three stages with bone grafts from the calvaria, ilium, tibia, or ribs and, in the final stage, with rib cartilage.
8. Eyelid coloboma is corrected by dissection of the edges of the cleft and careful approximation of the conjunctiva, orbicularis oculi muscle and skin (Tessier's procedure). Chondromucosal grafts from the upper lateral cartilage are useful in cases of severe hypoplasia of the lower eyelid.
9. A lateral canthopexy must be done each time the orbital complex is constructed or reinforced.
10. Vertical shortness of the lower eyelids and infraorbital regions is corrected at a final stage with supraclavicular full-thickness skin graft.

Orthodontic treatment is always necessary to align the teeth preoperatively and after surgical correction.

The Timing

1. Hearing aids should be used as early as possible.
2. Eyelid colobomata can be corrected in the first years of life.
3. Ear construction can begin after 8 years of age, when there is substantial rib cartilage available.
4. Surgery of the jaws should be performed between 6 and 10 years only when the child has major breathing problems.
5. Orbital surgery can begin within the same age range.

Based on the distribution of the deformities, priority is given to the orbital complex or to the jaws. In cases with severe breathing problems, the correction of the maxilla and nasopharynx, lengthening of the mandible, and the primary construction of the orbits are performed simultaneously according to the rotation of the midfacial segment pattern.

SUGGESTED READING

Tessier P, Rougier J, Hervouet F, Woillez M, Lekieffre M, Derome P. The Franceschetti syndrome. In: Plastic surgery of the orbit and eyelids. Report of the French Society of Ophthalmology. New York:Masson, 1981: 165.

Tessier P, Tulasne JF. Treacher Collins syndrome. Combined rotation of the midfacial segment and mandibular lengthening. In: Marchac D, ed. Craniofacial surgery. Berlin: Springer-Verlag, 1987.

Raulo Y, Tessier P. Mandibulofacial dysostosis. Analysis, principles of surgery. Scand J Plast Reconstr Surg 1981; 15:251–256.

Raulo Y. Treacher Collins syndrome: analysis and principles of surgery. In: Caronni P, ed. Craniofacial surgery. Boston: Little, Brown, 1985: 371.

NEUROFIBROMATOSIS

VICTOR L. LEWIS Jr., M.D.

Neurofibromatosis is a progressive, incurable, autosomal-dominant, congenital disease that affects approximately 1 in 3,000 individuals. Progression may be slow, as with the development and enlargement of cutaneous neurofibromas, or rapid, as with the appearance of the disease at puberty, or the detection of a sarcoma. Current therapy is symptomatic as there is no cure or palliative medical treatment known. Surgical therapy is either aggressive or staged.

The most common surgical treatment is removal of cutaneous and subcutaneous neurofibromas for appearance, size, and location. Major operations are indicated for extensive plexiform neurofibromas and pachydermatoceles that distort features and impair function.

THERAPEUTIC ALTERNATIVES

The forms of neurofibromatosis that may be treated by the plastic surgeon include: (1) dermal and subcutaneous neurofibromas, (2) plexiform neurofibromas, (3) pachydermatoceles (molluscum pendulum), (4) cutaneous pigmentations, including café au lait spots, axillary freckles, hairy nevus, and melanomas that arise in pigmented areas, and (5) neurofibrosarcoma and malignant schwannomas that arise from preexisting neurofibromas.

The decision to operate upon or observe the benign lesions is based upon: (1) the possibility to preserve function, (2) the opportunity to prevent further deformity or restore form, (3) the potential to improve appearance, (4) the wishes of the patient, and (5) consideration of the observation that children of mothers with neurofibromatosis may have a more severe disease course. Treatment of malignant disease by debulking for palliation or resection for cure depends on resectability and systemic spread.

PREFERRED APPROACH

The preferred approach for the manifestations of neurofibromatosis varies for each case, because of the great differences in time of presentation, potential for deformity, associated manifestations, and potential for benefit to the patient.

In patient selection, the surgeon must consider the neural crest origin and generalized manifestations of neurofibromatosis. The associated central nervous system (CNS) manifestation of low intelligence, seizure disorders, hydrocephalus, acoustic neuromas, and macrocephaly may limit the benefit of aggressive therapy for some patients. Elevated blood pressure or hypercalcemia dictate evaluation for pheochromocytoma or parathyroid adenoma before elective operation.

The treating surgeon should remember that the lifespan of many individuals with neurofibromatosis is shortened. In one series, 41 of 110 patients died of complications of the condition.

Operation for large plexiform neurofibromas or pachydermatoceles may be associated with poor wound healing, extensive blood loss or both. The wound-healing problems may be due to tissue compromise from extensive debulking or to the chronically denervated nature of the tissue. Blood loss is due to the large number of dilated, friable vessels found in these lesions. When the patient's overall condition will not tolerate hemorrhage or secondary operation for tissue loss, observation may be indicated.

Alternatively, spontaneous hemorrhage may be an indication for emergency operation for neurofibroma. Shock and death have been reported after spontaneous hemorrhage from large neglected neurofibromas. Emergency operation is also required for sudden paralysis from plexiform neurofibromas that involve the spinal canal or cranial fossae. A clue to the involvement of the axial nervous system by plexiform neurofibroma is the extension of the darkly pigmented skin overlying the tumor to the dorsal midline.

OPERATIVE THERAPY OF SPECIFIC MANIFESTATIONS

Cutaneous Pigmentation

Café au lait spots appear by 1 year of age in neurofibromatosis (Fig. 1). They are a hallmark of the condition, but not by themselves diagnostic. There is a condition of multiple café au lait spots along with neurofibromas. Their surgical significance lies in the cases of melanoma that have been described as arising in café au lait spots.

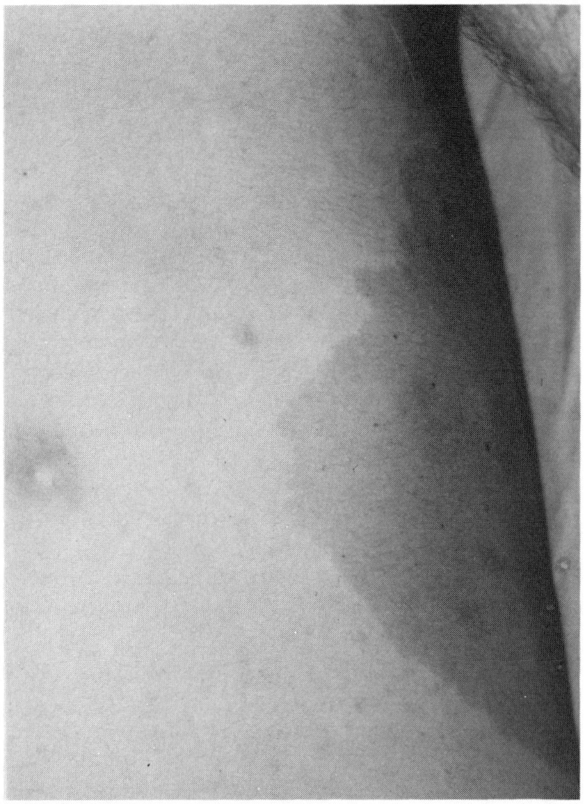

Figure 1 Café au lait spot with characteristic margins and pigmentation.

Axillary freckles are pathognomonic of neurofibromatosis. They are found at the apex of the axilla, and have no surgical significance.

There is an increased incidence of hairy nevi in neurofibromatosis. There is no difference in their surgical significance from their occurrence alone.

Cutaneous and Subcutaneous Neurofibromas

These, the most common lesions of the condition, usually appear in large numbers at puberty (Fig. 2). In women, the numbers may increase rapidly with pregnancy, and a characteristic location is the areola. Though called "cutaneous," these lesions also may be found in deep, soft tissues and visceral cavities. Indications for removal include size, location, interference with function, irritation, itching, and esthetics. There is indication for operative removal, usually under local anesthesia, when the above symptoms exist. The trade-offs are a scar and the possibility of recurrence. Excision is performed with

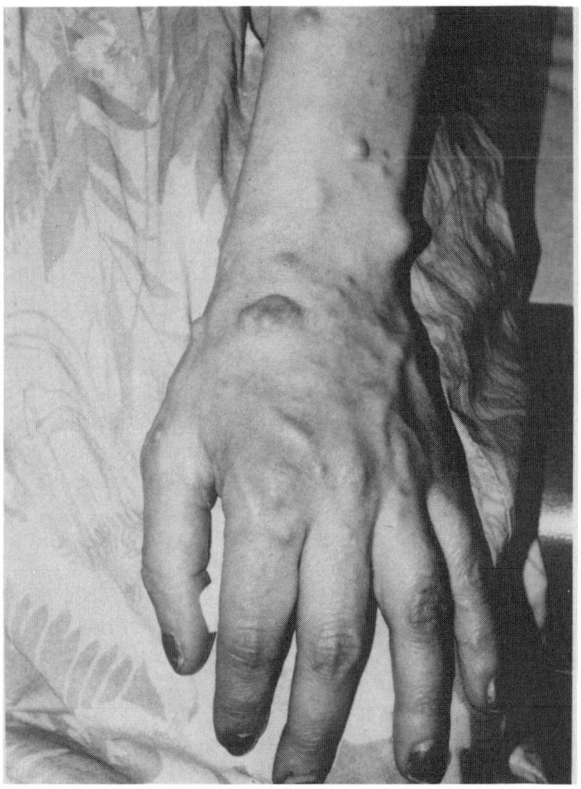

Figure 2 The appearance of subcutaneous neurofibromas as they develop in the young adult.

the realization by both the patient and the surgeon that new lesions will occur, and the patient cannot be freed of tumors. One unusual location of neurofibroma, the tongue, can also be managed by local excision.

Pachydermatoceles

These large masses of loose, corrugated skin develop over time, frequently in areas where plexiform neurofibromas occur. They contain skin and fibrous tissue, with very large blood vessels. Operation is indicated for control of bleeding, to debulk the mass, and to improve function. Complete removal is not mandatory. In the face, an extended rhytidectomy incision frequently permits removal of the mass and redraping of the skin. Depending upon location, other incisions may be placed along lines of facial expression or skin folds, as appropriate to excise the mass. Usually, the remaining skin redraped, albeit hyperpigmented and wrinkled, looks better esthetically than a split-skin graft that covers the debulked facial tissues.

Plexiform Neurofibroma

This manifestation of neurofibromatosis is characteristic of the head and neck, especially the orbit (Fig. 3). The tumors involve sensory and motor nerves (fifth and seventh). Due to their bulk, they displace and distort normal structures. Tumors of the orbit and maxilla may interfere with vision, breathing, and mastication. The tumor may be present in the orbit by the sixteenth week of intrauterine life, be apparent at birth, or appear in infancy.

The plexiform neurofibroma of the orbit has a characteristic constellation of deformities that include proptosis, with or without pulsation, absence of the greater wing of the sphenoid, deformity of the bony orbit, and herniation of the temporal lobe of the brain through the sphenoid defect. For the orbital neurofibroma, especially for the young individual with an amblyopic or blind eye, aggressive resection and reconstruction are indicated. The reconstruction requires orbital osteotomies and split rib grafts.

Epiphora is improved by removal of the eyelid adnexal structures, with the remaining lid skin used to line the reconstructed orbit. This technique also resolves the problem of shortening the overlong eyelid, which was stretched by the tumor. Facial paralysis and distortion of the oral commissure can be improved after debulking by static fascial suspension.

For the older patient, or for the patient with plexiform neurofibroma of other areas of the face, when function can be preserved, debulking operations, (staged when the tumor interferes with function) can preserve facial features and expression. There is no evidence that debulking causes malignant degeneration. Some have suggested that debulking slows tumor growth. Some individuals, especially older people with multiple stigmata of neurofibromatosis, may be benefited by debulking, to the point that they decline craniofacial extirpation of their lesions, even when technically possible. As with the cutaneous lesions, complete excision of most plexiform neurofibromas for cure is not possible. Those with extension of tumor or pigmented skin to the dorsal midline require close follow-up for intramedullary CNS involvement.

Sarcoma

Neurofibrosarcoma and malignant schwannoma arise from preexisting neurofibromas. Eighty-five to 90 percent occur in association with the most common form of cutaneous and subcutaneous neurofibromas, many in deep tissue spaces. The overall risk in common neurofibromatosis is about 5 percent. In one series of childhood sarcoma, 12 of 28 were neurofibrosarcomas of the head and neck associated with neurofibromatosis. Unexplained pain, or recent growth of neurofibromas, should lead to a search for a malignant tumor and appropriate biopsy.

Principles of treatment do not differ from those for sarcomas unassociated with neurofibromatosis. Biopsy confirmation and evaluation for systemic disease, precede wide excision of the malignancy. All potentially involved structures are sacrificed. Reconstruction is with regional or distant flaps. Prognosis is unfavorable; tumors of the proximal neural axis have a worse prognosis than the more peripheral ones. The biology of these tumors is not extensively documented.

UNDOCUMENTED POTENTIAL TREATMENTS

The possibility of debulking neurofibromas with liposuction cannula has been mentioned by one author, without specification of the type of cannula used.

Elevated levels of nerve growth factor have been documented in patients with central neurofibromatosis (acoustic neuromas). The possibility exists that nerve growth factor, or a similar substance, contributes to the growth of peripheral neurofibromas. If so, at some point, a blocker for nerve growth factor may be available and might control growth of the tumors.

Itching as a symptom of neurofibromatosis, and the presence of mast cells in neurofibromas, have been combined with research on two murine models that link mast cell abilities to change local cellular environments. These studies suggest that mast cell antagonists might be used to block the development of neurofibromas. There are no clinical data to support these suggestions.

RISK–BENEFIT ANALYSIS

Patients with neurofibromatosis are similar to burn patients in that most will submit to any operation in the hope of a little improvement. Even more important, parents are willing to submit their children to extensive procedures in the hope of preventing deformity. Timely craniofacial resection of orbital neurofibromatosis can halt the progression of deformity and give the patient a defect that can be covered by a prosthesis. Repeated resections can lessen the most unpleasant features of myriad cutaneous neurofibromata. Vigilance may save those whose

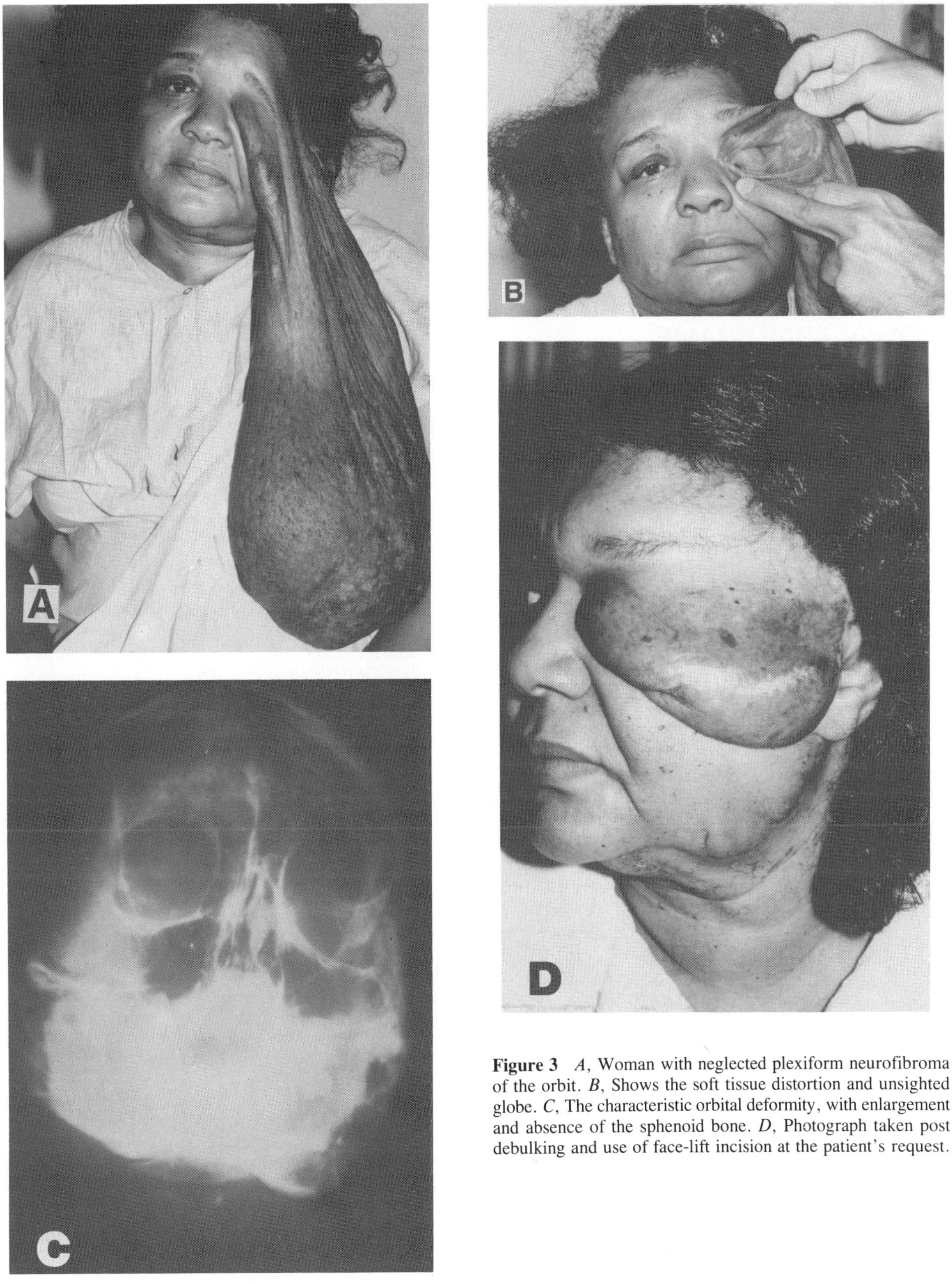

Figure 3 *A*, Woman with neglected plexiform neurofibroma of the orbit. *B*, Shows the soft tissue distortion and unsighted globe. *C*, The characteristic orbital deformity, with enlargement and absence of the sphenoid bone. *D*, Photograph taken post debulking and use of face-lift incision at the patient's request.

tumors have undergone malignant degeneration. The goal — to erase the deformity of the Elephant Man — is yet before plastic surgery.

SUGGESTED READING

Griffith BH, Lewis VL Jr, McKinney P. Neurofibromas of the head and neck. Surg Gynecol Obstet 1985; 160:534–538.
Jackson IT, Laws ER Jr, Martin RD. The surgical management of orbital neurofibromatosis. Plast Reconstr Surg 1983; 71:751–758.
Martin G, Kleinsasser O. Neurogenic sarcomas of the neck in neurofibromatosis. Arch Otorhinolaryngol 1981; 232:273–283.
Rasi HB, Herr BS, Sperer AV. Neurofibromatosis of the tongue. Plast Reconstr Surg 1964; 35:657–665.
Riccardi VM. Von Recklinghausen's neurofibromatosis. N Engl J Med 1981; 305:1617–1627.
Riccardi VM. Neurofibromatosis: clinical heterogeneity. Curr Prob Cancer 1982; 7:1–34.
Van der Meulen JC, Moscona AR, Vandrachen M, Hirshowitz B. The management or orbitofacial neurofibromatosis. Ann Plast Surg 1982; 8:213–220.

DOWN SYNDROME FACE RECONSTRUCTION

MENACHEM R. WEXLER, M.D.

The most expressed deficiency of Down syndrome is mental retardation, characterized by an incapacity for abstract thought, especially in mathematics. Mental retardation in the Down syndrome patient (DSP) is, however, of varying degrees, and many of them suffer, on top of their inborn retardation, from environmental retardation due to their rejection by society.

Appearance, speech, and eating behaviors are important components of interhuman relationships and the aim of surgery is to improve these abnormal components in the DSP. In pursuit of this aim, several plastic surgeons have attempted to change Down syndrome facial characteristics (Hohler, Lemperle and Radu, Olbrisch, Rosner, Wexler and Peled). It is estimated that more than 700 patients have undergone surgery: more than 500 have been operated upon in Germany; more than 100 in Israel; close to 40 each in Australia and Canada, and several in the United States. Detailed follow-up studies have documented the merits and limitation of the operative procedures and results (Tables 1 to 7).

FACIAL REHABILITATION

The facial stigmata in Down syndrome and their possible surgical corrections are:

1. Oblique eye axis—slanting: correction by detachment of the lateral canthal tendon and its insertion in a lower location.
2. Epicanthal folds: correction by augmentation of the nose is generally advised. This eliminates the epicanthal folds. In a few cases, five-flap technique is used.
3. Receding cheeks: correction by insertion of silicone prosthesis over the malar eminence.
4. Flat dorsum of the nose: correction by insertion of silicone prosthesis.
5. Receding chin: correction either by insertion of silicone prosthesis, or by subcutaneous flip flap from the submental area over the chin, or by mandibular advancement.
6. Macroglossia: correction by wedge excision of the anteriorly-projected tip of the tongue and primary suture (partial glossectomy).
7. Submental fat deposit: excision and suture; it could be used as a filling material to augment the chin.
8. Dysplastic external ears: correction by otoplasty.
9. Redundant lower lip (hypotonia): correction by wedge excision of the lower lip (vertical or horizontal).
10. Forward inclination of lower incisors (mandibular incisor overjet): we did not attempt correction in our series. In some cases, it is spontaneously corrected following partial glossectomy.
11. Drooling: this improves spontaneously following partial glossectomy in most cases. We did not attempt correction in our series.
12. Occipital heaviness: we did not attempt correction.
13. Strabismus: we did not attempt correction.
14. Round cheeks: correction by removal of the buccal pad of fat.

TABLE 1 Population of Down Syndrome Patients

Age	*Frequency (%)* Male	Female	Total (%)
1–6	7 (11.9)	8 (13.5)	15 (25.4)
7–10	7 (11.9)	10 (16.9)	17 (28.8)
11–14	5 (8.5)	8 (13.5)	13 (22.2)
15+	10 (16.9)	4 (6.9)	14 (23.8)
Total	29 (49.2)	30 (50.8)	59 (100)

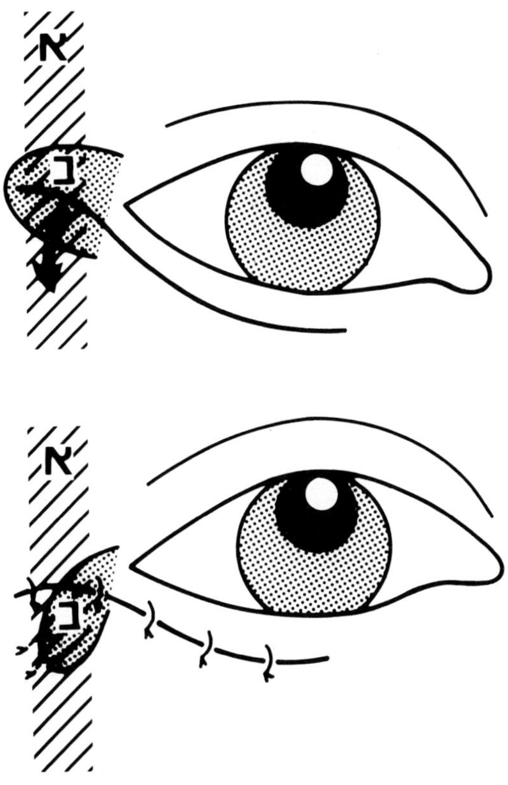

Figure 1 Schematic drawing of a lateral canthoplasty. The subcutaneous lateral canthal flap is lowered and fixed in this lower location, thereby changing the typical slanting.

Slanting Eyes

A lower blepharoplasty incision extends almost 1 cm laterally from the end of the palpebral fissure (Fig. 1). The skin is elevated carefully as it is adherent to the orbicularis oculi. The lateral canthal tendon, which is not always a defined structure, is released from the lateral orbital wall. This actually includes a flap of orbicularis muscle attached to the lateral palpebral fissure. The periorbita is elevated with a Joseph periosteum elevator. Care should be taken not to pull the lateral canthal tendon laterally but to lower it in a caudal direction only. The best reinsertion is by drilling a hole through the lateral orbital wall almost 1 cm below the original insertion, with a delicate stainless steel wire used for fixation and another nylon 4–0 suture added for reinforcement. The wound is not closed before both sides are compared to make sure that the new locations are symmetric. The skin is sutured with a running intracuticular 5–0 suture. It is advisable not to use interrupted sutures in Down syndrome patients as they may present obstinate resentment to stitch removal, and a sharp instrument brought near the globe may prove harmful.

Epicanthal Folds

In most cases in our series, the epicanthal folds were eliminated by augmentation of the root of the nose with a silicone prosthesis. In two patients only, we eliminated the epicanthus by direct approach and used the five-flap technique, composed of double opposed Z-plasty and Y–V advancement, which is a modification of Mustardé operation for telecanthus.

Receding Cheeks

Correction is achieved by augmentation with a silicone prosthesis. The expected location of the prosthesis is marked over the skin. The muscles are stripped from the malar eminence through a lower eyelid blepharoplasty incision, and a pocket is created. The separation is done in such a way that the periosteum remains adherent to the bone. The prefabricated silicone prosthesis is inserted into the pocket and is anchored to its place with two 4–0 nylon stitches. Most prefabricated malar silicone prostheses have an oval shape; this makes it difficult to obtain identical results on both sides. Because of unfavorable results, we changed the shape into a round one in several cases (as happened in the past with breast prostheses). Lately, we have used miniscrew fixation of the prosthesis. The screw is introduced through a small incision, and its outside 4 mm are left projecting from the bone. The prosthesis is attached to the bone by pressing the screw head into the prosthesis. The muscles are then sutured above it with two 5–0 nylon sutures and the lower eyelid incision is sutured with a running intracuticular 5–0 nylon stitch. Two-year follow-up has disclosed no bony resorption in the malar region.

Flat Root of The Nose

Elevation of the root of the nose is achieved by a silicone prosthesis inserted through an intercartilaginous intranasal incision. A pocket is created of sufficient size to accommodate the prosthesis. There was no fixation of the prosthesis in most of our cases. The intranasal incision is sutured with 5–0 absorbable material. Some of the complications that have occurred, for instance, migration of the prosthesis in a cephalad direction toward the glabella in several cases, and rotation of the prosthesis on itself, could be attributed to the fact that the prosthesis was not fixed, and this was corrected by external manipulation. To avoid these complications, a circumferential suture has been introduced. From the side of the nose, through a small hole, a straight needle is inserted from right to left through the cartilage. If the needle is resisted, a delicate drill is used to create a passage for the needle. Then the needle is passed through the same hole in the skin, this time above the prosthesis. One knot is tied adjacent to the incision, again through the same skin incision. A nerve hook is then introduced through the intercartilaginous incision to fish out the two tails and they are then tied with the aid of a needle holder. The intercartilaginous incision is sutured. Steristrips are glued to the skin over a thin layer of tincture of benzoin.

Receding Chin

The correction of this by insertion of a silicone prosthesis should be carried out in adult Down syndrome patients only. Insertion of a silicone prosthesis in children

TABLE 2 Parents' Evaluation of Postoperative Changes in Various Facial Compoments*

	Deterioration		*No Change*		*Improvement*	
	F[†]	*%*	*F*[†]	*%*	*F*[†]	*%*
Tongue	1	2.1	2	4.3	44	93.6
Eyes	3	7.7	2	5.1	34	87.2
Cheeks	3	11.5	3	11.5	20	77.0
Nose	4	17.4		–	19	82.6

* n=59.
[†] F=Frequency.

TABLE 3 Parents' Evaluation of Postoperative Changes in Oral Functions

	Deterioration		*No Change*		*Improvement*		
	F[†]	*%*	*F*[†]	*%*	*F*[†]	*%*	*Total*
Drooling	3	8.4	7	19.4	26	72.2	36
Opened mouth	1	2.0	14	28.0	35	70.0	50
Protruding tongue	1	2.2	4	8.7	41	89.1	46
Sores around the mouth	1	4.5	6	27.3	15	68.2	22

* n=59.
[†] F=Frequency.

resulted in bone resorption in most cases. It seems, however, that if the periosteum is left intact, and the prosthesis is inserted on top of a thin soft tissue padding, the resorption does not take place, although the prosthesis is then not firmly fixed and may be moved slightly from side to side. The prosthesis is inserted through an intraoral transverse incision 1 cm beyond the gingivolabial sulcus. The bone is reached and the prefabricated PDMS prosthesis is inserted and fixed in place with 4–0 nylon sutures. In several cases, it was fixed with stainless steel miniscrews. The wound is washed with gentamicin (80 mg in 5 to 10 cc) prior to closure. This is used for all the locations in which prostheses are inserted. The muscles are sutured over the prosthesis with 4–0 chromic catgut, and the mucosa is sutured with a running over-and-over 4–0 chromic stitch.

Horizontal mandibular osteotomy and advancement was not done in our patients. Another method for augmentation of the receding chin, done recently in four patients with encouraging results, consists of elevation of a submental dermis flip flap, turned over subcutaneously and fixed over the chin. This allows removal of the submental fat accumulation and augmentation of the chin in the same operation. This procedure does not cause any bone growth disorder. The follow-up of the four patients who underwent this procedure is, however, less than 1 year.

Macroglossia

Not every Down syndrome patient has macroglossia and needs his or her tongue reduced. This section refers to those DSP who need improvement by partial glossectomy. The correction consists of a wedge excision of a rhomboid-shaped form from the anterior tongue. The patient is anesthetized through an oral intubation with the endotracheal tube fixed sideways by a stitch around one of the molar teeth. A 3–0 silk suture is introduced vertically into the tongue and held with a hemostat (Fig. 2). The tongue is pulled forward from the oral cavity, and the maximal protrusion point corresponding to the lower lip vermilion is marked with methylene blue. Then, the tongue is slightly released back into the oral cavity and another point is marked on either side of the tongue. These points correspond to the tips of the two tails that are created following wedge excision of the tongue. Care should be taken to leave the tails long enough for the patient to be able to wet the vermilion and avoid crusting. The wedge is not a straight line, but rather has a bell shape so the future new tip will not be too pointed. On the other hand, the wedge should not be too short or the tongue will be too round. One can go further posteriorly since the DSP tongue is also too wide. By following the markings on top of the tongue, a wedge is marked below. This wedge is, however, shorter and should not reach the base of the tongue. Still following the marking, we infiltrate the tongue with 5 to 10 cc of 0.5 percent Marcaine with 1:200,000

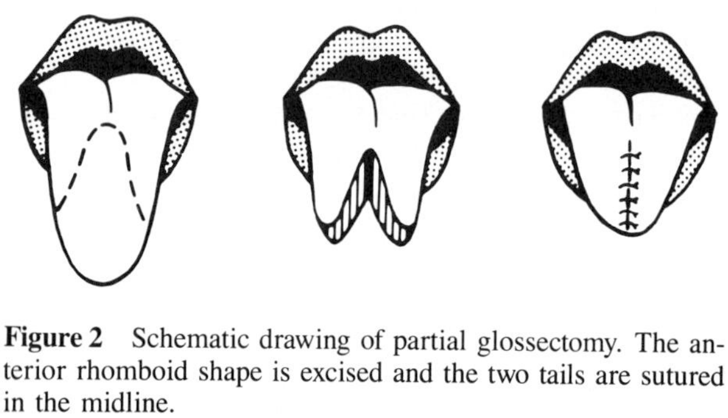

Figure 2 Schematic drawing of partial glossectomy. The anterior rhomboid shape is excised and the two tails are sutured in the midline.

TABLE 4 Parents' Evaluation of Postoperative Changes in Respiratory Function*

	Deterioration		*No Change*		*Improvement*		
	F†	*%*	*F*†	*%*	*F*†	*%*	*Total*
Mouth breathing	1	3.1	8	25.0	23	71.9	32
Snoring	5	10.4	22	45.8	21	43.8	48
Running nose	5	10.0	26	52.0	19	38.0	50

* n=59.
† F=Frequency.

Adrenalin solution. This eliminates postoperative pain and reduces bleeding. The anesthetized tongue could have been the reason one patient bit the tip of his own tongue. Two sutures are then introduced vertically into the tongue, each on one future tail. The tongue is held between the surgeon's fingers while the three sutures pull the tongue, and the wedge is cut. The section starts on the dorsal aspect, continues on the ventral aspect, and terminates through the muscles between the two incisions. Bleeding is minimal; the cut arteries are clamped and cauterized.

While the two tails are displaced medially and are being held together, 4–0 Vicryl sutures are used to approximate the muscles, generally in two layers. Then the mucosal layer is sutured, starting from inside so that the tie remains buried within the tongue and the patient does not open it by rubbing the tongue toward the hard palate. After the suturing of the upper suture line, suture of the undersurface of the tongue takes place in the same manner. There has been occasional small wound dehiscence among our patients. Then, a through-and-through 1-0 silk suture, used in abdominal surgery, is introduced transversely through the anterior part of the tongue and tied to a loop hung out of the tongue. This suture serves as a pulley to correct postoperative acute airway obstruction by pulling the tongue forward. This suture is taken out the next day provided there have been no respiratory problems.

There was no need for blood transfusion in any of our patients. The patient has intravenous infusion for 24 to 48 hours and oral, clear liquid intake is started from the first day.

The initial swelling, which reaches its peak on the second postoperative day, gradually reduces and reaches its final size 4 to 6 weeks postoperatively (Fig. 3).

Submental Fat Deposit

The correction of the heavy chin by submental liposuction and excision has recently been done on six patients and we do not have a long follow-up.

Skin undermining is accomplished through a transverse incision in the submental crease, similar to a face-lifting dissection. The submental fat is then dissected off the platysma muscles. If augmentation of the chin is desired, it should be lifted as an anteriorly-based flap. Following hemostasis, the wound is sutured. We added liposuction towards the angle of the mandible, but the yield of this liposuction in our cases was poor.

Dysplastic External Ears

Some of the DSP operated upon had small prominent ears. Various methods of otoplasty were used.

Redundant Lower Lip (Hypotonia)

This is corrected by wedge excision. A midline wedge is excised and sutured in three layers, with 4–0 Vicryl used for the muscle and 5–0 chromic for mucosa and skin so that stitch removal is not needed. In DSP capable of higher performance, nonabsorbable 5–0 nylon stiches are used for the skin. Occasionally, fusiform-shaped protrusive mucosa is excised horizontally, thus hiding the suture line intraorally.

We have not attempted to correct forward inclination of the lower incisors, drooling, occipital heaviness, or strabismus.

TABLE 5 Parents' Evaluation of Postoperative Changes in Eating Behavior*

While Eating & Drinking	*Deterioration*		*No Change*		*Improvement*		
	F†	*%*	*F*†	*%*†	F†	*%*	*Total*
Cleanliness around mouth	2	4.3	17	36.2	28	59.6	47
Protruding tongue	1	2.3	7	16.3	35	81.4	43
Open mouth	1	2.0	14	28.0	35	70.0	50

* n=59.
† F=Frequency.
* This represents the number of the subjects whose parents defined their state in each area as less than satisfactory prior to the surgery.

TABLE 6 Parents' Evaluation of Postoperative Changes in Various Aspects of Speech*

Speech Aspect	*Deterioration*		*No Change*		*Improvement*		
	F†	*%*	*F*†	*%*	*F*†	*%*	*Total*
Intelligibility	1	1.8	18	32.7	36	65.5	55
Articulation	4	7.3	21	38.2	30	54.5	55
Hoarseness	2	4.9	27	65.8	12	29.3	31
Stuttering	2	6.1	18	54.5	13	39.4	33
Self confidence in speech	1	2.3	19	44.2	23	53.5	43

* n=59.
† F=Frequency.

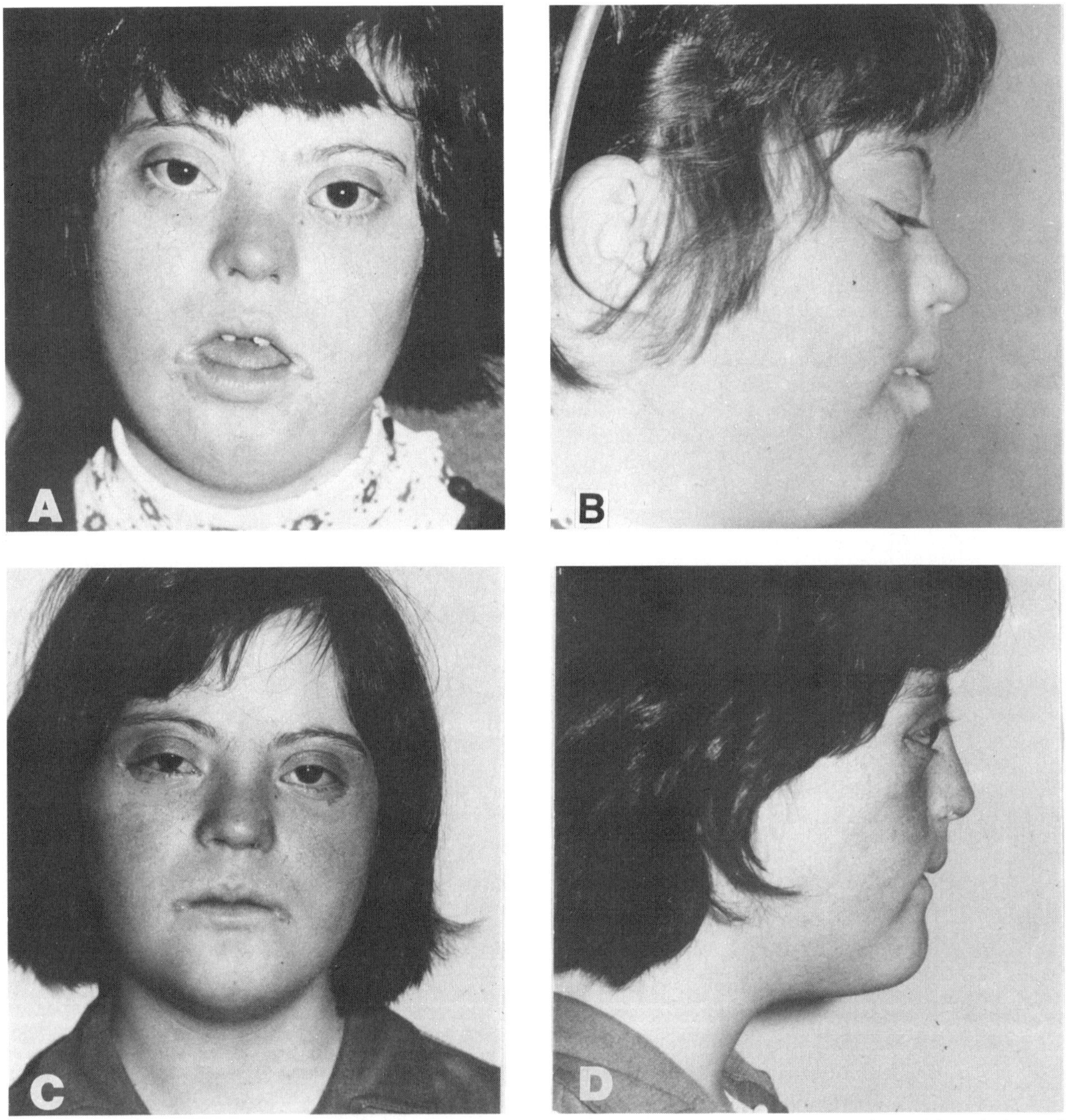

Figure 3 *A* and *B*, Preoperative anterior and lateral views of a Down syndrome patient. *C* and *D*, Anterior and lateral views of the patient after she underwent partial glossectomy, lateral canthoplasty, and augmentation of the nose, cheeks, and chin with silicone prostheses. (From Wexler MR, Peled IJ, Rand Y, Mintzker Y, Feuerstein R. Rehabilitation of the face in patient with Down syndrome. Plast Reconstr Surg 1986; 77(3):387.)

TABLE 7 Parents' Ranking Order of Down's Syndrome Characteristics Based on Weighted Scores*

Characteristic	*Preoperative*	*Postoperative*
Protruding tongue	1	6
Open mouth	2	3
Speech	3	1
Running nose	4	2
Slanted eyes	5.5	7.5
Drooling	5.5	7.5
Eating behavior	7	5
Gait	8	8

* n=59.

Round Cheeks

This procedure, suggested by Salyer, entails removal of the buccal pad of fat and was successfully used in four patients. Blunt tipped scissors are introduced and opened through an intraoral horizontal incision in the cheek mucosa anterior to Stensen's duct papilla. The buccal pad of fat is then fished out, cauterized, and excised. A milking maneuver on the cheek facilitates its removal.

PATIENT SELECTION

Indication and Contraindication

Almost all our patients underwent psychological evaluation and family interview through the Hadassah Wizo Canada Research Institute, which specialized in education of retarded children. The decisions concerning surgery were made collaboratively by parents, the institute, and the surgeons. The only exceptions were very young patients. In these, the protruding tongue was the major indication and was the only operation done.

According to our postoperative follow-up studies, the patients performing at high level benefited from the surgery more than low-performers, and we now try to do fewer procedures on a Down syndrome patient when his or her level is low. It has been found that if the parents have specific expectations, e.g., "I am bothered by the big protruding tongue of my son," the results are better appreciated than when there are vague general expectations, such as, "I want my son to look normal", without specifying how.

From the age of 7 years, a youngster has to participate in the decision-making process. This is applicable to Down syndrome patients. Many times, they are aware of the fact that they are different from their friends, yet they know they resemble other DSP. Following surgery, it was noticed that they resembled their relatives to a higher degree.

TIMING OF SURGERY

Tongue reduction can be done as young as 6 months of age, although most of our patients were at least 3 years old. Lateral canthopexy can be done on patients of three years of age. Silicone prostheses were not inserted before 5 years of age, and the family was notified that this prosthesis should be changed to a bigger one in the future, if necessary. We have stopped using a chin prosthesis on the growing face.

To our surprise we have had no instance of infected prosthesis in all our cases—and only a few extrusions. We have used our hospital-fabricated PDMS prosthesis.

SUGGESTED READING

Hohler H. Changes in the facial expression as a result of plastic surgery in mongoloid children. Aesthetic Plast Surg 1977; 1:245

Lemperle G, Radu D. Facial plastic surgery in children with Down's syndrome. Plast Reconstr Surg 1980; 66:337

Olbrisch RR. Plastic surgical management of children with Down's syndrome. Indications and results. Br J Plast Surg 1982; 35:195

Rosner L. Facial plastic surgery for Down syndrome. Lancet 1983; 1320.

Wexler MR, Peled IJ, Rand Y, Mintzker Y, Feuerstein R. Rehabilitation of the face in patients with Down's syndrome. Plast Reconstr Surg 1986; 77:383

MICROTIA: AUTOGENOUS FRAMEWORK

DAVID C. LEBER, M.D., F.A.C.S.

Reconstruction of the external ear for correction of microtia or traumatic loss of the external ear presents one of the greatest challenges in plastic and reconstructive surgery. This chapter presents the use of rib cartilage as the framework, with detail of the harvesting, carving and implanting of the cartilage framework. Emphasis is placed on total ear reconstruction for the classic microtia deformity, with additional suggestions for partial absence of the external ear.

THERAPEUTIC ALTERNATIVES

One alternative to ear reconstruction is the use of an external ear prosthesis. Problems associated with this method include possible embarrassment from dislodgment of the prosthesis and color changes as the prosthesis ages.

Silicone framework implants are an alternative to the use of costocartilage for ear reconstruction. This method is discussed in the following chapter. A criticism of this method is the frequency of infection and exposure that results in removal of the implant.

PREFERRED APPROACH TO EAR RECONSTRUCTION

Analysis of the Deformity

The microtic ear, which can present in a variety of forms, should be compared with the patient's normal ear. In the classic microtia deformity, it is obvious that the entire ear requires reconstruction. The soft tissue present is used to form the lobule of the new ear. In some patients there is considerably more soft tissue present, which may represent as much as one-half of the external ear. Careful judgment is needed to determine how the tissue can best be utilized. Formation of the lobule should have priority, while the remaining soft tissue can be used for the upper one-third of the ear or can be simply left in place and excised after insertion of the framework, if it is not needed.

Preoperative Planning

Any method that helps to determine the correct size and position of the reconstructed ear, as compared with the normal ear, should be utilized. It should include measurements of height and width of the normal ear and distance from the lateral canthus. Clear x-ray film can be used to draw the outline of the normal ear and its relationship to the lateral canthus, midforehead, and tip of the nose. The film can then be flipped to the opposite side of the face to determine the position of the new ear. Guides can be made to sight the superior and inferior poles of the normal ear from the frontal view as a placement aid for the new ear. The latter should be in the same relative position on the head as the normal ear whenever possible. Patients with hemifacial microsomia, or those with an existing external canal in an abnormal location, sometimes make this ideal positioning impossible.

Acrylic models made from alginate impressions of the normal ear are a helpful guide in the operating room when the cartilage framework is being carved.

A working pattern of the normal ear, drawn on clear x-ray film, is the most important step in carving a framework that resembles the normal ear (Fig. 1). This pattern represents the outline that the rib cartilage graft is to assume.

Staging of Reconstruction

Stage I—Harvesting, Carving, and Implantation of Cartilage Framework with Lobule Rotation

The sixth, seventh, and eighth costal cartilages from the contralateral chest wall are used for construction of the framework. Exposure is through an 8 cm transverse incision in the sixth intercostal space (Fig. 2). The perichondrium is dissected free and preserved to allow regrowth of fibrocartilage, thus preventing chest wall deformities. There is also reduced risk of creating a pneumothorax.

With the ear framework pattern and acrylic models of the normal ear used as guides, the cartilage is carved

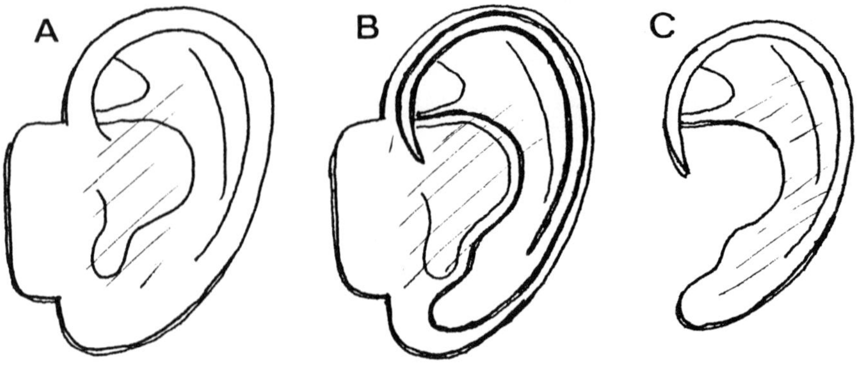

Figure 1 *A*, An outline of the normal ear is drawn on clear x-ray film and cut out. *B*, The pattern of the cartilage framework is drawn from the pattern of the normal ear. Note the allowance for thickness of the overlying skin along the helical rim and concha. *C*, Pattern to be used intraoperatively during harvesting and carving of the cartilage framework.

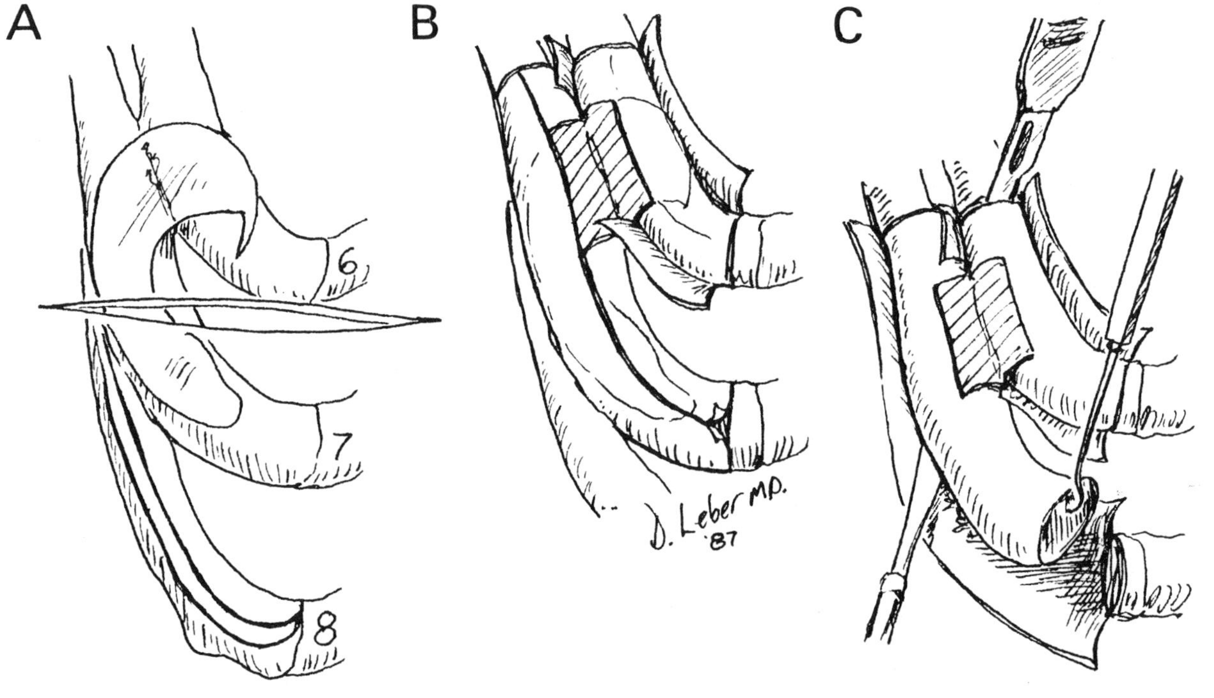

Figure 2 Harvesting costocartilage. *A*, Transverse skin incision is made midway between sixth and seventh ribs. *B*, The perichondrium is incised along the longitudinal axis of the ribs. The synchondrosis of the sixth and seventh ribs is left intact. The perichondrium is carefully dissected with use of a Freer elevator. *C*, The cartilage is transected with a knife and completed with a Freer elevator. The perichondrium is separated from the underside of the ribs, with care taken not to create a pneumothorax.

in a stepwise manner, which accurately and efficiently achieves the desired shape (Fig. 3). Instruments for carving include No. 15 and No. 10 surgical blades, 3/8 inch and 3/32 inch U X-ACTO* gouges and a No. 6 aluminum handle. The handle can be sterilized and the gouges replaced when they become dull.

The lobule is rotated into position by means of a Z-plasty (Fig. 4). I prefer to rotate the lobule at the same time as implantation of the cartilage framework so that the tail of the framework can be fitted into the lobular skin. It is unnecessary to rotate the lobule as a separate first stage. Any residual deformed microtic cartilage is carefully removed during dissection of the pocket. The thin skin that remains can be used to advantage for lining the recesses of the cartilage framework. A combination of petrolatum gauze stents and suction is used to coapt the skin to the cartilage framework. The stents remain in place for 3 weeks.

Stage II—Elevation of Ear and Creation of Postauricular Sulcus

Four to 6 months after Stage I, the ear is lifted away from the side of the head through a periauricular incision (Fig. 5). The posterior scalp skin is undermined and advanced anteriorly to reduce the size of the defect and to hide the skin graft behind the ear.

* Registered trademark of Hunt Manufacturing Co.

Stage III—Concha and Tragus Formation

If there is inadequate conchal depth, an anteriorly based skin flap can be raised from the conchal floor and the floor further excavated, with care taken not to injure the facial nerve, which could be in an abnormal location. The flap is tucked under its base to form the tragus, and the conchal floor is covered with a full-thickness skin graft taken from the opposite postauricular sulcus (Fig. 6).

Where there is adequate conchal depth, the tragus can be created from a composite ellipse of cartilage and skin taken from the opposite ear when the latter is being set back to improve symmetry.

Patient Selection

Virtually any patient with microtia is a candidate for reconstruction. There are patients with atypical deformities where the lower half of a normal ear exists, but the upper half is absent or severely deformed. When the upper half is absent, the rib cartilage framework is placed under the scalp skin and fashioned to fit into the lower normal portion in such a way that the upper position of the ear will be supported. When there is deformity of the upper half, it is usually difficult or impossible to place the framework into the existing external ear skin. It is best to place the framework under the scalp skin and excise the abnormal skin at a later time (Fig. 7).

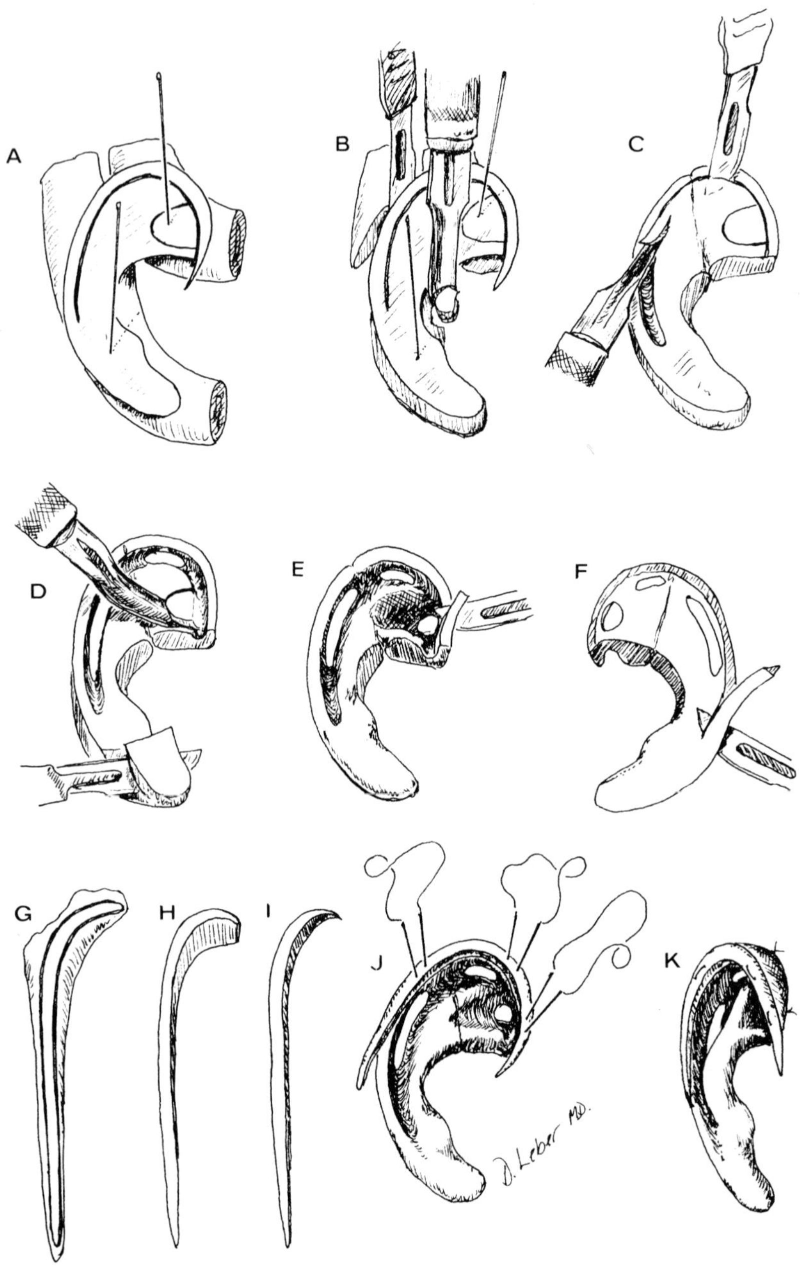

Figure 3 Carving cartilage framework. *A*, The x-ray film pattern of the framework is pinned to the sixth and seventh ribs. *B*, The outline of the framework is cut with a No. 10 blade, taking care to keep the cuts perpendicular to the surface. The concha is easily cut with 3/8 inch U X-ACTO gouge. *C*, The 3/8 pattern is removed and a checking cut is made 2 to 3 mm into the cartilage along the helical rim with a No. 10 blade, followed by carving out the recessed area of the scapha with a 3/32 inch U X-ACTO gouge. *D*, The triangular fossa is excavated with the larger gouge. The tail of the framework is thinned out on the dorsal side, which also permits the tail to warp in a posterior direction. Note that the excavation of the scapha is carried through to the posterior surface, which enhances skin coaptation to the cartilage graft. *E*, Finishing touches to the framework include a slight beveling cut to the root of the helical rim and all edges of the cartilage are rounded off with fine knife strokes. *F*, The framework is turned over and the leading edges are rounded, thus providing a more realistic appearance when the ear is lifted away from the side of the head and grafted. *G*, The eighth costal cartilage is used to carve an additional piece for the helical rim so as to provide greater projection. *H*, The rim piece is cut in the shape of a hockey club. It is important to remove equal amounts of cartilage from each side so that warpage will not occur. *I*, The rim piece is completed by thinning out the anterior and posterior aspects of the rib then, *J*, It is fixed to the main framework with clear nonabsorbable suture, double armed with taper-point needles. Four or five sutures are required. *K*, Shows a three-quarter view of the completed framework.

Timing of Surgery

I prefer to perform the rib cartilage framework surgery at age 8 years or older. This provides a larger block of cartilage to work with and much improved patient cooperation during postoperative care. However, many surgeons prefer to begin ear reconstruction at a much earlier age to avoid psychological trauma to the patient. In my experience, it is usually the parents who are overanxious to have the surgery completed at an early age.

The second stage of creation of the postauricular sulcus can be done 4 months after the first stage, or any time thereafter. Concha and tragus formation and minor soft tissue revisions can be done 4 to 6 months after the second stage.

Tricks and Traps

At times, one must be ready to deal with ossified rib cartilage. This condition has been encountered in one 16-year-old patient. When this occurs, the dental drill can be used to shape the framework satisfactorily.

One must be aware of tremendous variations in the shape and relationship of the sixth, seventh, and eighth costal cartilages. The eighth rib may be firmly fused to the seventh rib. It may be difficult to identify the sixth and seventh ribs due to their shape.

If one makes use of the fifth costal cartilage, great care must be taken not to create a pneumothorax. The pleura seems to be much more easily penetrated in that location.

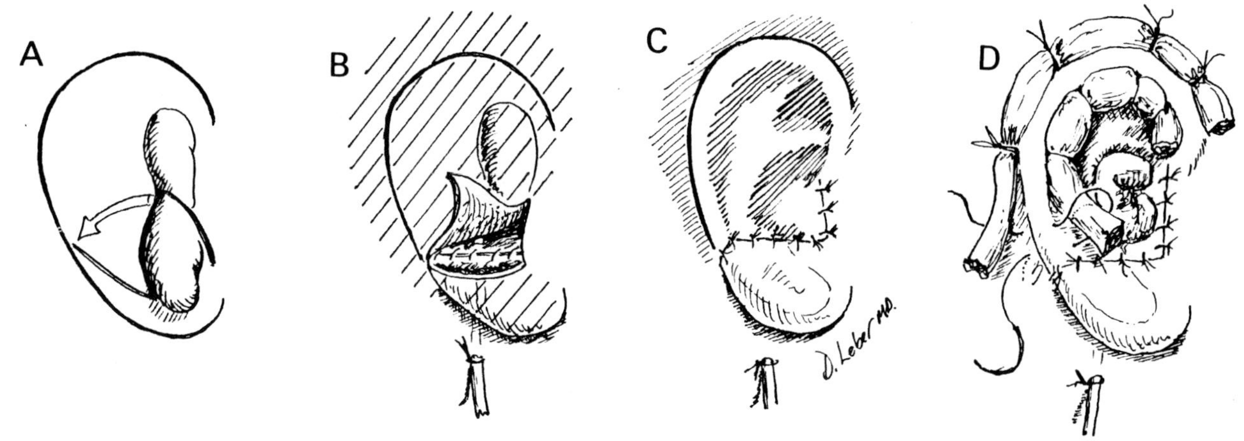

Figure 4 Rotation of lobule and implantation of framework. *A*, The proper position of the reconstructed ear is marked on the skin. The lower half of the existing deformed microtic ear is rotated into position by means of a Z-plasty. *B*, The scalp skin is carefully undermined with scissors, to extend at least 1 cm beyond the outline of the ear. All remaining deformed cartilage is removed from the microtic tissue. A pocket is created in the lobular tissue to receive the tail of the cartilage framework. The posterior skin edges are sutured with absorbable sutures, and a silicone suction drain is placed in the wound and brought out below the lobule. *C*, The carved cartilage framework is then inserted in the space created by rotation of the superior portion, followed by insertion of the tail of the helix into the lobule. The skin is closed with fine sutures. At times, a skin graft is needed to complete closure of the concha. Suction is applied in order to reveal the contour of the framework beneath the overlying skin. *D*, Rolled bolsters of petrolatum gauze are placed inside and outside the helical rim and held in place with 0000 nylon mattress sutures. These bolsters assure coaptation of the skin to the framework and are left in place for 3 weeks. Care should be taken not to tie these too tightly so as not to compromise the skin circulation.

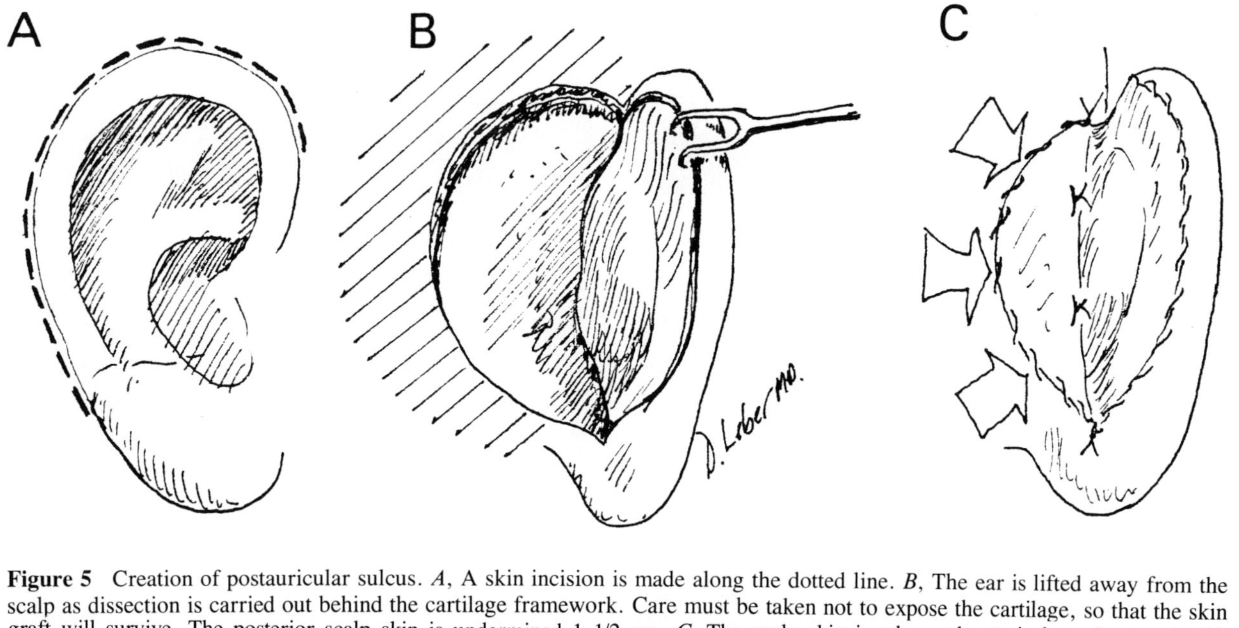

Figure 5 Creation of postauricular sulcus. *A*, A skin incision is made along the dotted line. *B*, The ear is lifted away from the scalp as dissection is carried out behind the cartilage framework. Care must be taken not to expose the cartilage, so that the skin graft will survive. The posterior scalp skin is undermined 1 1/2 cm. *C*, The scalp skin is advanced anteriorly and sutured with 0000 absorbable sutures. This helps to hide the grafted area behind the ear and also helps to give the ear more anterior projection. A full-thickness skin graft, taken from the lower abdomen, is used to cover the remaining defect.

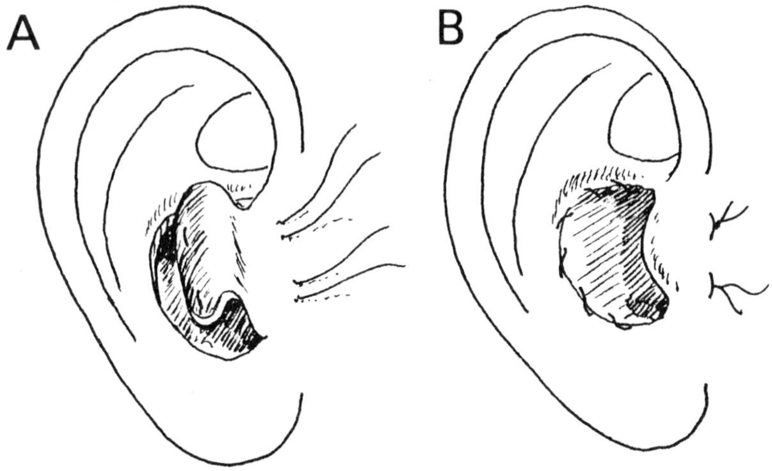

Figure 6 Formation of tragus and concha. *A*, The tragus can be constructed and the concha deepened at the same time. An anteriorly based flap is elevated out of the existing concha and folded upon itself. The flap is held with two or three mattress sutures. *B*, Before the sutures are tied, the concha is deepened, with care taken not to injure the facial nerve, which can be in an abnormal position. A full-thickness skin graft, taken from the postauricular sulcus of the opposite ear, is attached to the free edge of the flap and the mattress sutures are then tied.

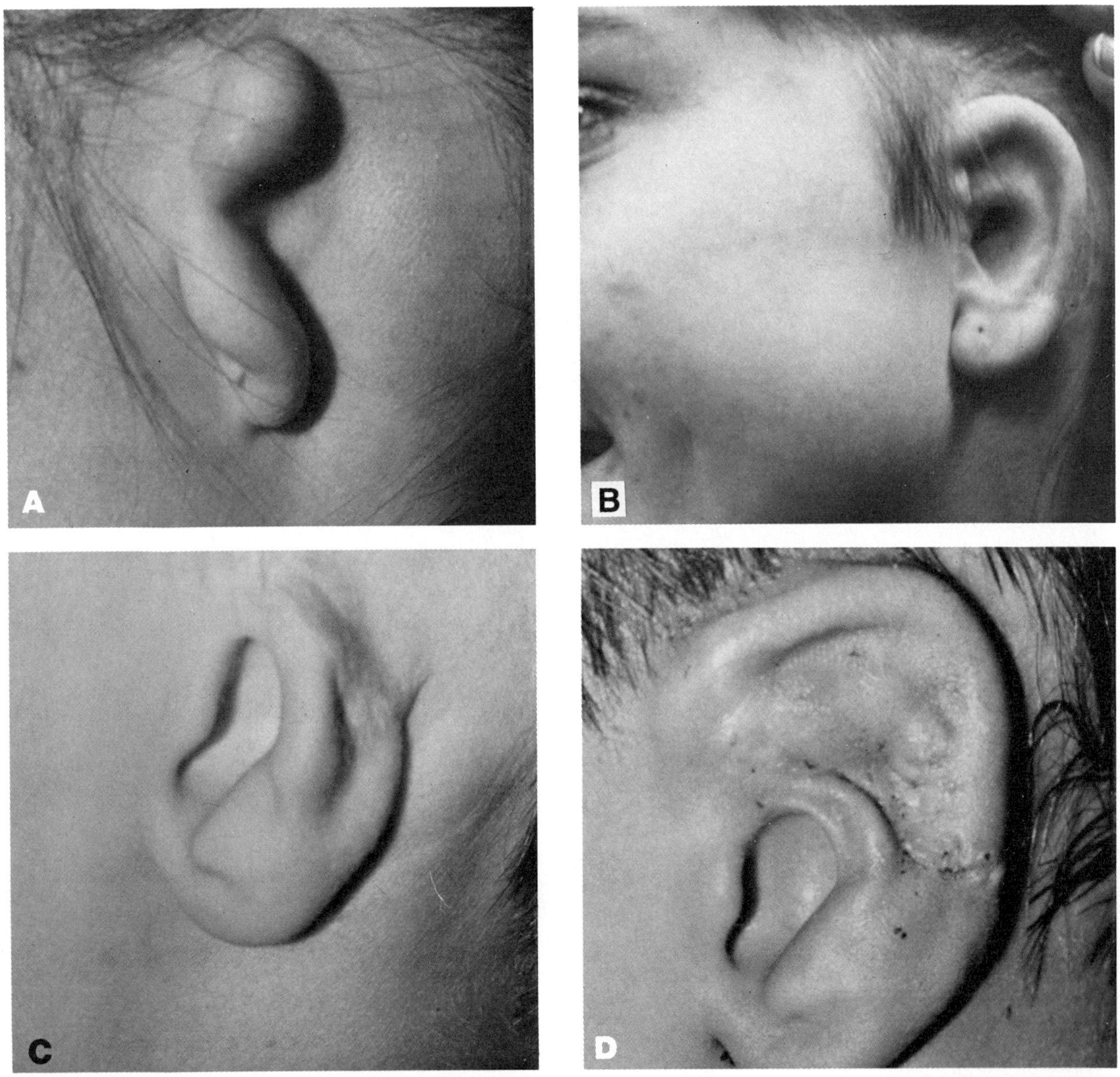

Figure 7 *A*, Preoperative findings of classic microtia deformity. *B*, Postoperative results after use of the techniques described. *C*, Congenital absence of superior half of external ear. A full concha and external canal are present. *D*, Results after placement of rib cartilage graft. The cartilage graft extends into the lobule just as in a complete ear reconstruction. Formation of the postauricular sulcus has not yet been completed.

There may be times when a very small area of skin becomes necrotic, with minimal exposure of the cartilage framework. These ears usually heal without difficulty if a little of the exposed cartilage is cut back and the skin edges are permitted to granulate across the framework.

When there are problems with insufficient skin, as in burn patients or those where the framework becomes exposed due to infection or necrosis of the overlying skin, adequate coverage can be achieved with the use of a temporalis fascia "fan flap" and skin graft, or a temporoparietalis fascia flap and skin graft.

Therapeutic Outcome

Ear reconstruction is difficult and often frustrating because the final shape and details do not always fulfill expectations. Fortunately, most patients are grateful for any attempt made at ear reconstruction, provided the new ear is the proper size, well-shaped and properly located.

BENEFIT-RISK ANALYSIS OF PREFERRED APPROACH

The benefits for a patient with microtia of having an ear constructed of his own body tissues are much greater than with the use of alloplastic materials. The final results, however, depend heavily on the surgeon's ability to harvest the rib cartilage with ease and efficiency and to carve the cartilage into a well-planned framework, based on the size and shape of the patient's normal ear. Care is required in handling the soft tissue coverage of the framework to prevent necrosis of the skin. This is not a procedure that should be undertaken if one performs only one ear reconstruction per year.

SUGGESTED READING

Brent B. A personal approach to total auricular construction. Clin Plast Surg 1981; 8:211–221.

Brent B. The correction of microtia with autogenous cartilage grafts: I. The classic deformity. Plast Reconstr Surg 1980; 66:1–12.

Fox JW, Edgerton MT. The fan flap: an adjunct to ear reconstruction. Plast Reconstr Surg 1976; 58:663–667.

Leber DC. Ear Reconstruction. In: Georgiade NG, Georgiade GS, Riefkohl R, Barwick WJ, eds. Essentials of plastic, maxillofacial and reconstructive surgery. Baltimore: Williams & Wilkins, 1987:493.

Tanzer RC. Total reconstruction of the external ear. Plast Reconstr Surg 1959; 23:1–15.

Tegtmeier RE, Gooding RA. The use of a fascial flap in ear reconstruction. Plast Reconstr Surg 1977; 60:406–411.

MICROTIA: SILASTIC FRAMEWORK

SEIICHI OHMORI, M.D.

Since Radford Tanzer published his idea to reconstruct microtia by using an ear frame made of rib cartilage, this method has been accepted as the most reliable method in the world. As far as the technique of arranging or carving the frame is concerned, some different methods have been described by Brent, Davis, and Matsumoto among others. However, these authors all accept the premise that autogenous cartilage should be used for the framework.

On the other hand, Cronin reported another method of microtia reconstruction in which a Silastic frame was used instead of autogenous cartilage. In 1968, soon after I personally examined that patient's result in Houston, I started to apply this method in Tokyo. I repeated trial and error to find the most reliable method for utilization of a Silastic frame microtia reconstruction and arrived at the safest method around 12 years ago.

I classify microtia into two types (Fig. 1) with respect to the planning of the treatment. Type 1 microtia, has no concha; type 2 microtia has a concha with underdevelopment of the upper part of the auricle. It is somewhat difficult to classify the type of microtia in which the formation of the concha is too small, and the classification is made according to the experience of the surgeon.

TREATMENT PLAN

The treatment plans for types 1 and 2 microtia are different, as will be described.

Treatment of Type 1 Microtia

A Silastic frame edged with a bonded Dacron mesh is used (Fig. 2). At the first operation, switchback of the lobule is carried out. The expected axis of the reconstructive auricle is planned parallel to the nasal axis. The rudimentary cartilage mass is excised. The second-stage procedure is performed 3 months later. An L-shaped incision is made bordering on the lobule (Fig. 3) and the superior flap is undermined sufficiently to accommodate the Silastic frame. Hemostasis should be meticulously maintained. The soft tissue of the conchal area, including a part of the parotid gland, is excavated to the periosteum of the mastoid (Fig. 4). This excavated area accommodates the conchal part of the frame, thereby avoiding any pressure on the overlying flap. Then soft tissue of the lobule is separated with scissors, thus making a pocket into which the tail of the frame is placed (Fig. 5). A T-shaped incision is marked on the temporal region of the skull, about 8 cm superior to the mastoid hairline. The superficial tem-

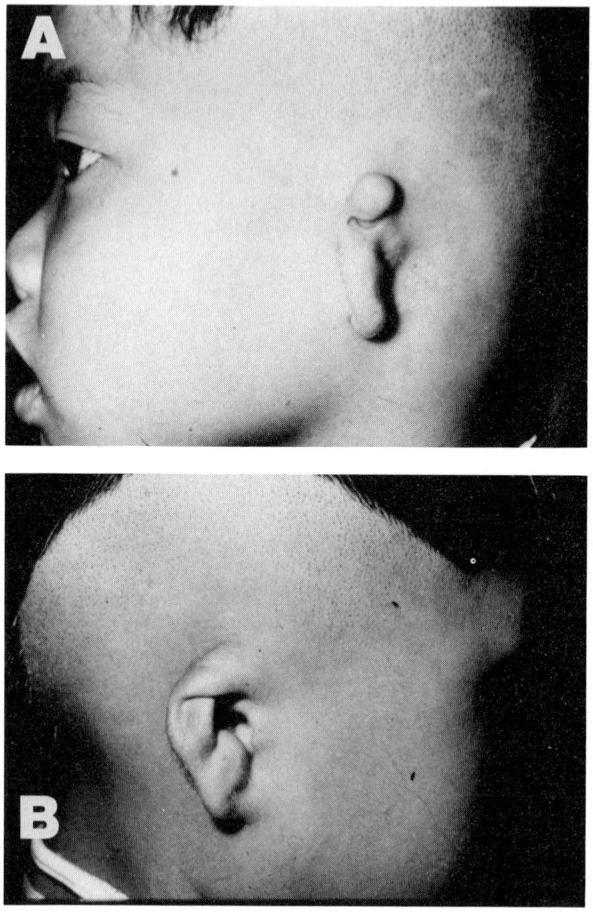

Figure 1 *A*, Shows type 1 microtia. *B*, Shows type 2 microtia.

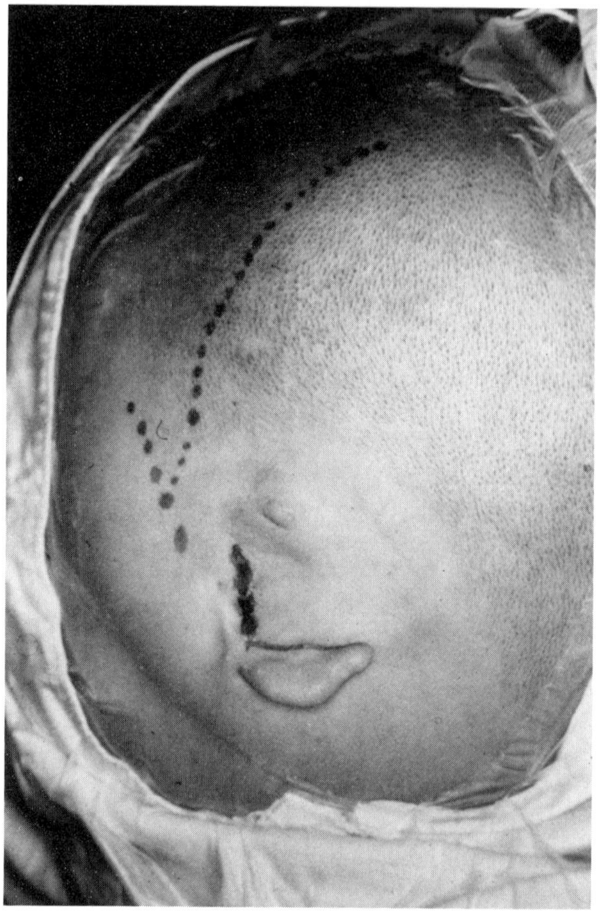

Figure 3 After switchback of the lobule, 3 months should elapse before the second-stage operation. An L-shaped incision is performed and the flap undermined. Then the superficial temporal artery's path is marked.

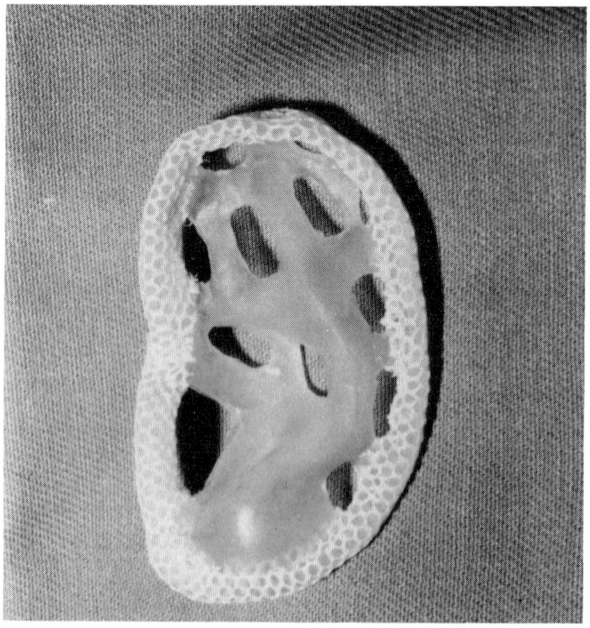

Figure 2 The rim of the Silastic frame is edged with bonded Dacron mesh.

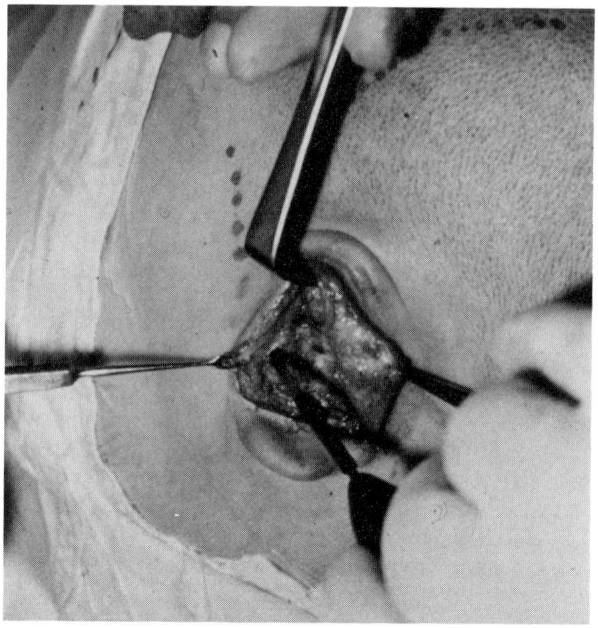

Figure 4 Soft tissue of the conchal area is excavated by electrocautery to the periosteum of the mastoid.

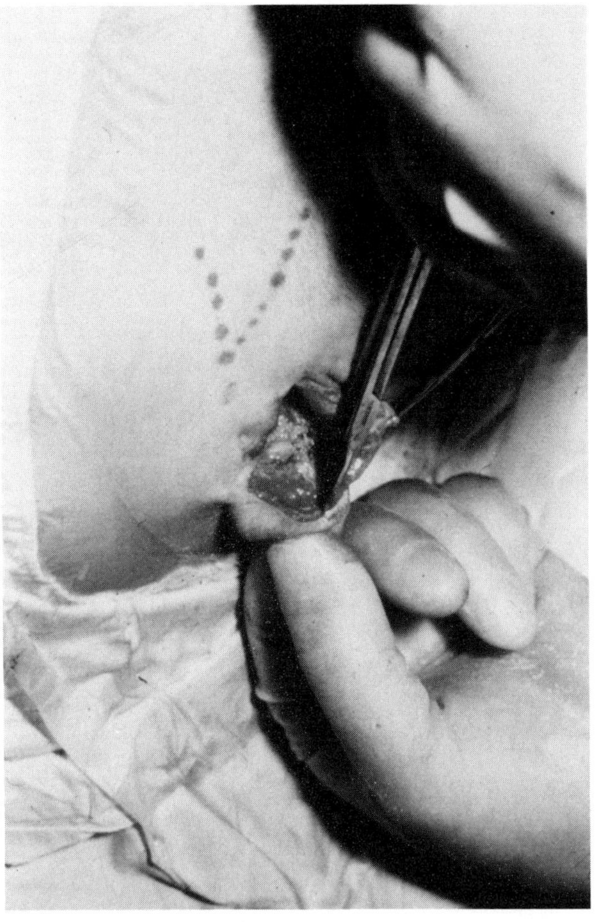

Figure 5 The lobule is separated into two flaps and the tail of the frame is inserted into the pocket created.

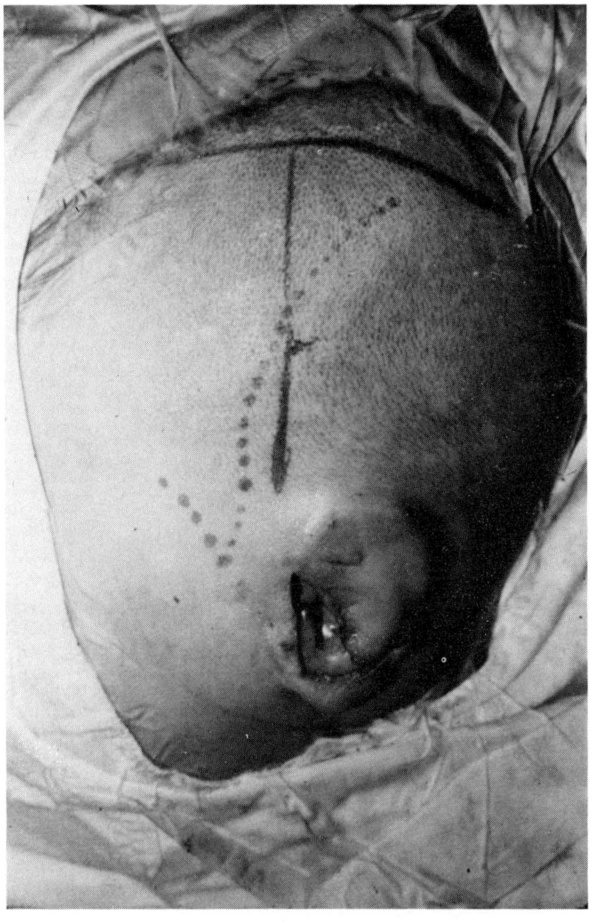

Figure 6 The flap is undermined enough to keep the frame safely, and a T-shaped mark is drawn on the temporal area.

poral artery is marked along its path prior to making the T incision (Fig. 6).

After injection of saline solution with epinephrine (1/200,000) subcutaneously, the T incision is carried out and the temporoparietal muscle fascia is exposed (Fig. 7). This muscle fascia is separated carefully from the temporalis muscle to avoid damaging the superficial temporal artery.

Then, the Silastic frame is inserted into the dissected area. A silicone drainage tube, with five to six small holes at its end, is inserted beneath the antihelix of the frame and suction is applied.

The temporoparietal muscle fascia is passed beneath a skin tunnel in front of the auricle and used to cover the conchal part of the frame (Fig. 8). This muscle fascia flap is anchored to the surrounding area of the concha with 5–0 Dexon suture. As suction is applied, the depth of the concha appears. The tip of the flap is sutured to the concha of the frame with 5–0 Nylon. Upon this deep concha, a full-thickness skin graft, taken from the inguinal region, is secured with a tieover dressing (Fig. 9).

The third stage is performed 3 months later. The reconstructed auricle is raised from the skull and the auriculocephalic sulcus is lined with a full-thickness skin graft (Fig. 10).

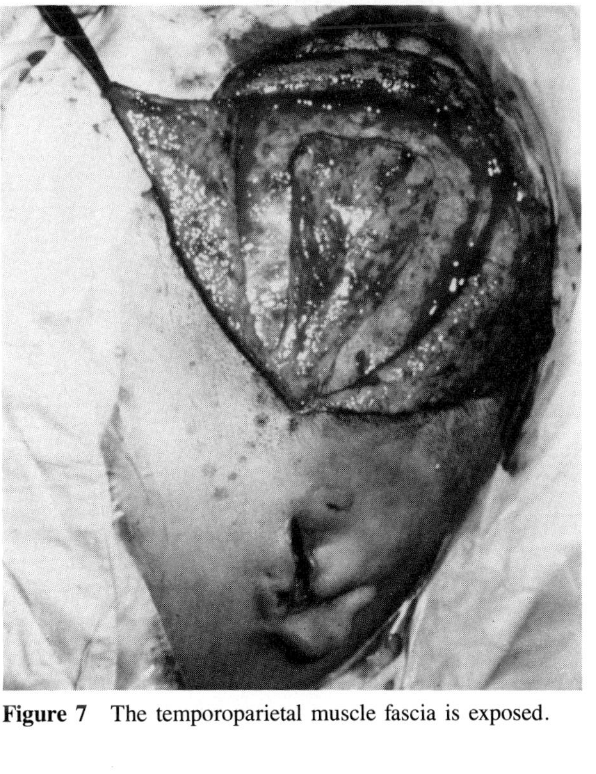

Figure 7 The temporoparietal muscle fascia is exposed.

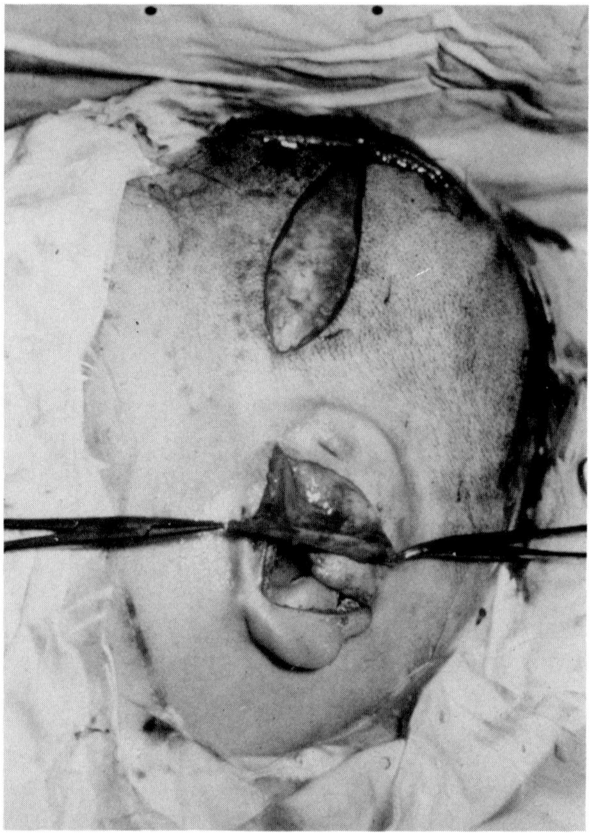

Figure 8 The temporoparietal muscle fascia is introduced beneath the skin to the conchal part of the frame. Under suction, this muscle fascia flap is anchored to the surrounding skin. The deep concha appears.

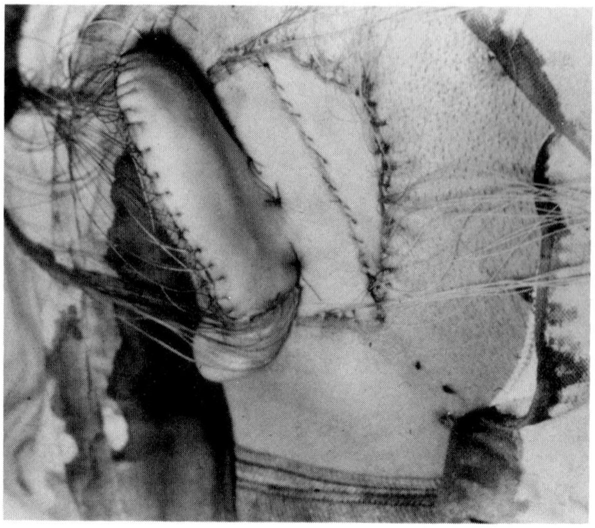

Figure 10 The reconstructed auricle is separated from the skull by skin grafting.

Treatment of Type 2 Microtia

In the case of type 2 microtia, the rim of the Silastic frame is not bordered completely by Dacron mesh. The part of the rim facing the tragus is freed of the mesh covering and this part is cut horizontally. The concha of the frame is excised (Fig. 11).

The rudimentary helical cartilage is excised, preserving the concha (Figs. 12 and 13). It is most important in type 2 cases that the size of the concha be trimmed or enlarged so as to be the same size as the concha of the Silastic frame.

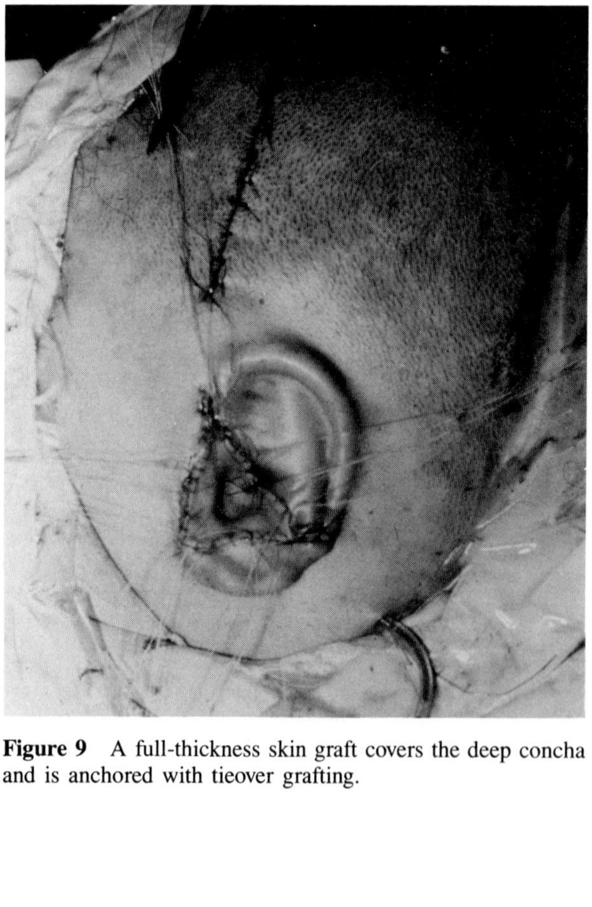

Figure 9 A full-thickness skin graft covers the deep concha and is anchored with tieover grafting.

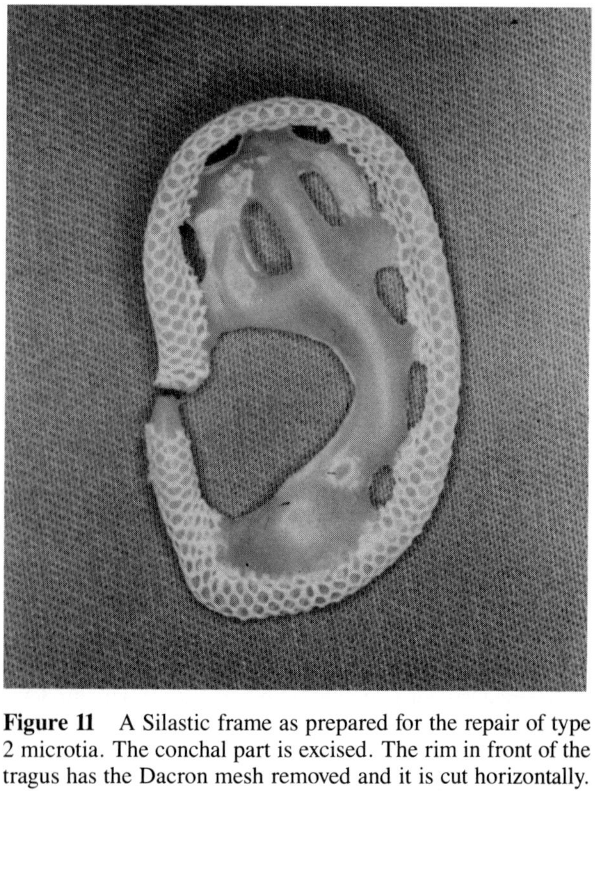

Figure 11 A Silastic frame as prepared for the repair of type 2 microtia. The conchal part is excised. The rim in front of the tragus has the Dacron mesh removed and it is cut horizontally.

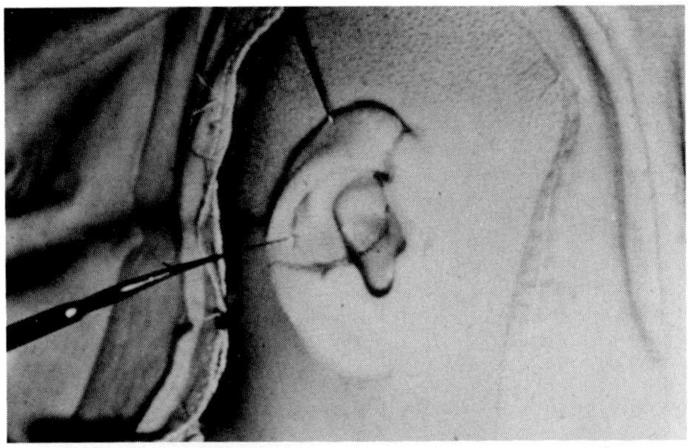

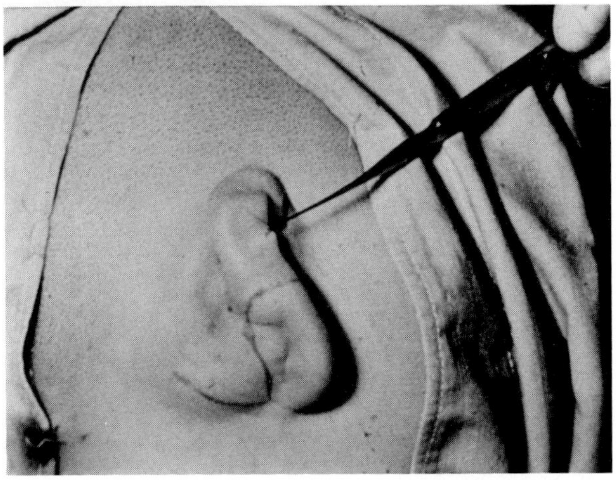

Figure 12 Incision line for repairing type 2 microtia.

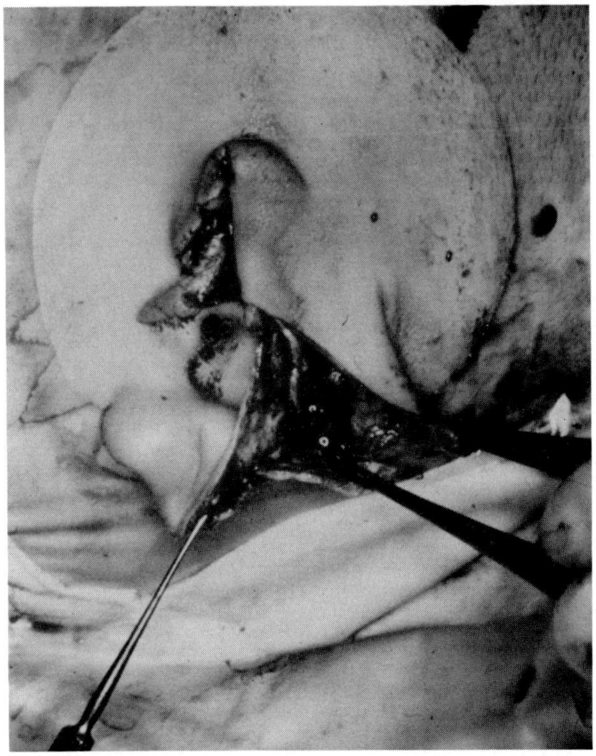

Figure 13 Rudimentary cartilage, except the conchal part, is excised.

An incision is made in front of the tragus and subcutaneous pockets are formed. The upper and lower rims of the frame are inserted and the cut ends are then pulled into the incised area and tied together with nonabsorbable suture. A piece of cartilage is placed on this and the skin is closed (Fig. 14). Suction is applied as in type 1 microtia reconstruction (Fig. 15).

Three months later, the reconstructed auricle is freed in the same manner as for type 1 microtia.

FOLLOW-UP STUDY

I published a follow-up study of Silastic frame microtia reconstruction in *Aesthetic Plastic Surgery* (1984; 8:1).

Another follow-up study was made in 1986. All patients were between 3 and 12 years postreconstruction. There were 169 cases of type 1 microtia (Table 1) and 56 cases of type 2 (Table 2). Of the 169 type 1 reconstructions, 87 ears were in good condition: 82 ears were not evaluated. Of the 56 type 2 microtia reconstructions, 28 ears were in good condition; 28 ears were not evaluated.

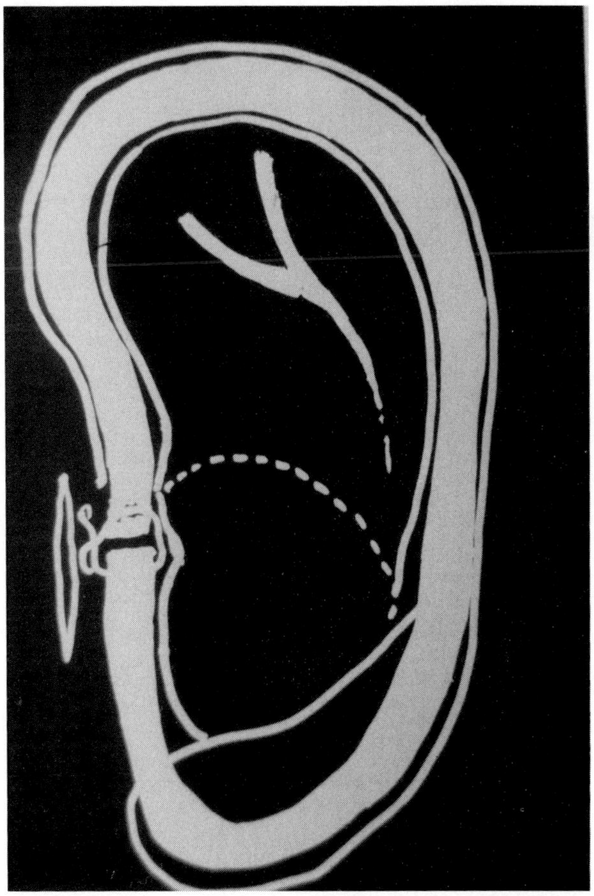

Figure 14 This shows frame utilization for the repair of type 2 microtia.

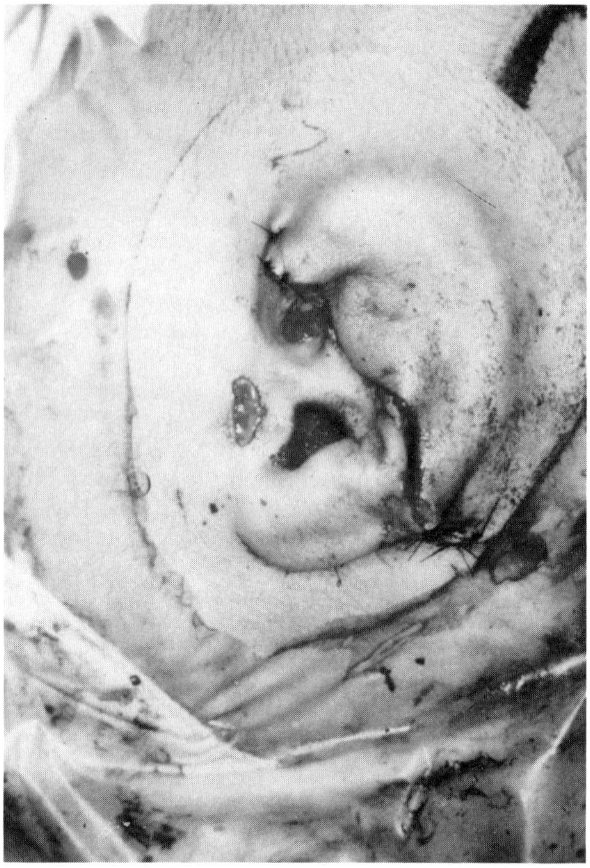

Figure 15 Postoperative view just after the completion of the first stage procedure for type 2 microtia.

TABLE 1 Time Elapsed and Patients' Response in a Follow-Up Study of Modified Reconstruction of Typical (Type 1) Microtia

Time Elapsed Since Surgery (in years)	*Number of Patients*	*Follow-Up* Direct Observation	Questionnaire	No Response	Lost
12	5	0	1	0	4
11	11	1	5	1	4
10	25	3	11	5	6
9	28	3	4	12	9
8	22	6	11	3	2
7	22	4	5	10	3
6	14	2	3	7	2
5	14	3	10	1	0
4	15	3	4	6	2
3	13	1	7	4	1
Total	169	26	61	49	33

Patients' Attitudes and Feelings Toward the Reconstructed Auricle

Approximately two-thirds of the patients do not pay any extra attention to the reconstructed auricle. Of those who do, cleansing and protection against trauma were reported most frequently (Table 3).

While patients report more satisfaction and confidence with their reconstructed auricle, they still seem to have an inferiority complex concerning the deformity. Three-fourths of the patients used a long hairstyle to conceal their reconstructed ear (Table 4).

Sports Engaged In

Approximately half of the patients participate in contact sports including judo, rugby, and soccer (Table 5), any of which could result in trauma to the reconstructed auricle.

Clinical Examples

Figures 16 to 25 as part of the follow-up study show the results of modified reconstruction of microtia.

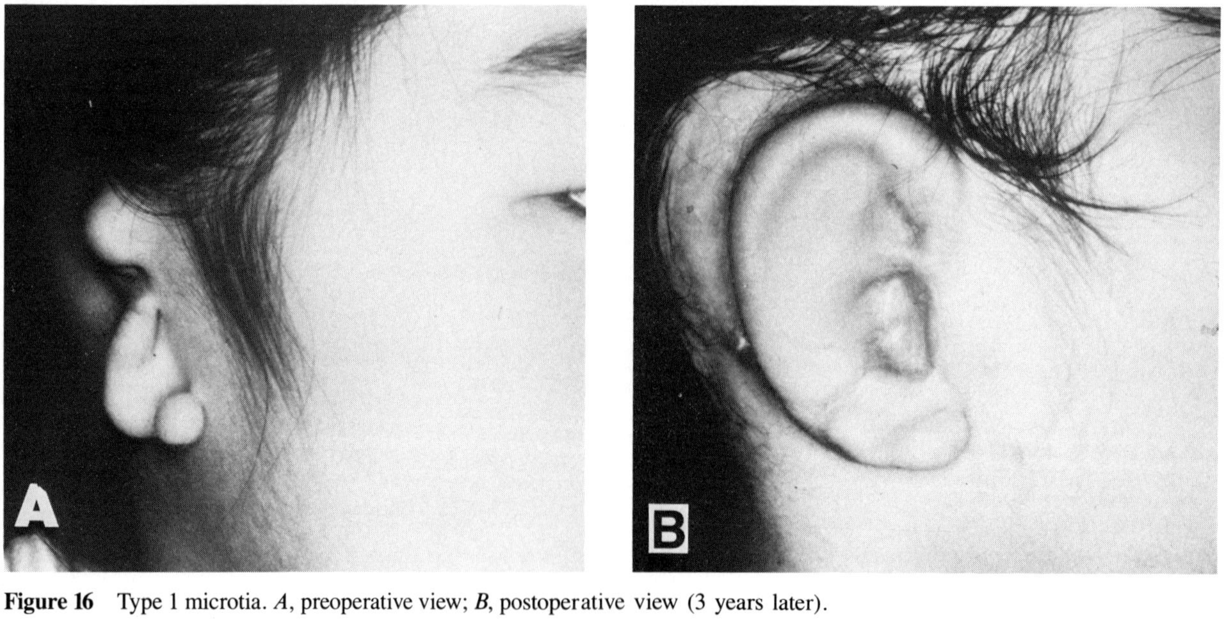

Figure 16 Type 1 microtia. *A*, preoperative view; *B*, postoperative view (3 years later).

TABLE 2 Time Elapsed and Patients' Response in a Follow-Up Study of Modified Reconstruction of Minor-Grade (Type 2) Microtia

Time Elapsed Since Surgery (in years)	*Number of Patients*	*Follow-up*			
		Direct Observation	*Questionnaire*	*No Response*	*Lost*
12	2	0	1	1	0
11	7	0	2	2	3
10	8	1	2	3	2
9	12	2	3	3	4
8	8	2	3	0	3
7	4	2	2	0	0
6	6	1	2	3	0
5	4	2	0	1	1
4	4	1	2	0	1
3	1	0	0	1	0
Total	56	11	17	14	14

TABLE 3 Patient Attention Paid to Reconstructed Ear

Type of Extra Attention	*Typical Microtia*	*Minor-Grade Microtia*
None	54	16
Some	25	7
Clean up	11	3
Protection against trauma	9	0
Protection against frostbite	3	4
Epilation	2	0

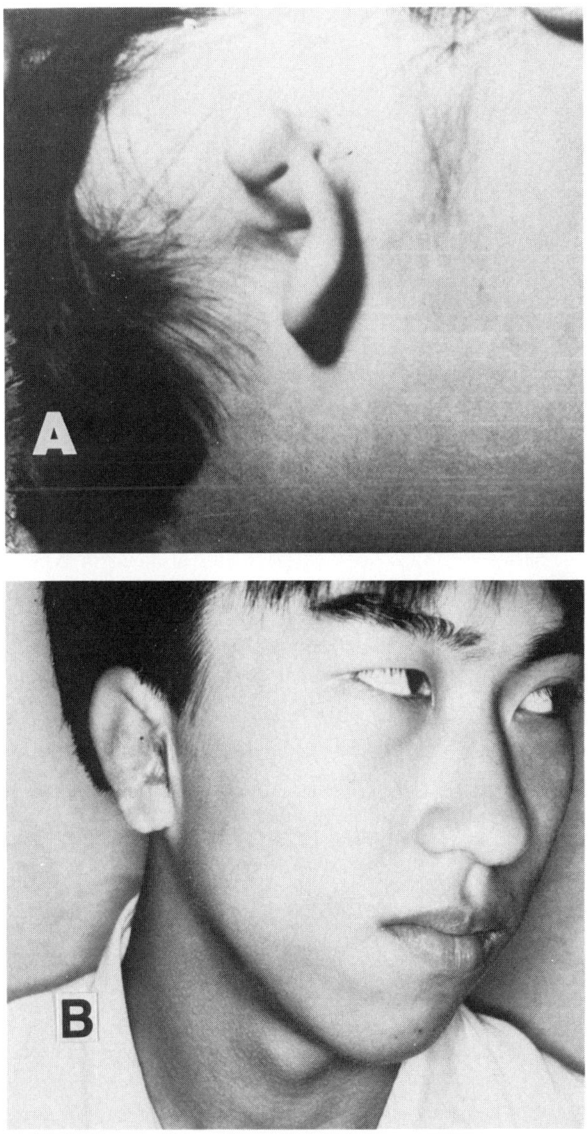

Figure 17 Type 1 microtia. *A*, Preoperative view; *B*, Postoperative view (10 years later).

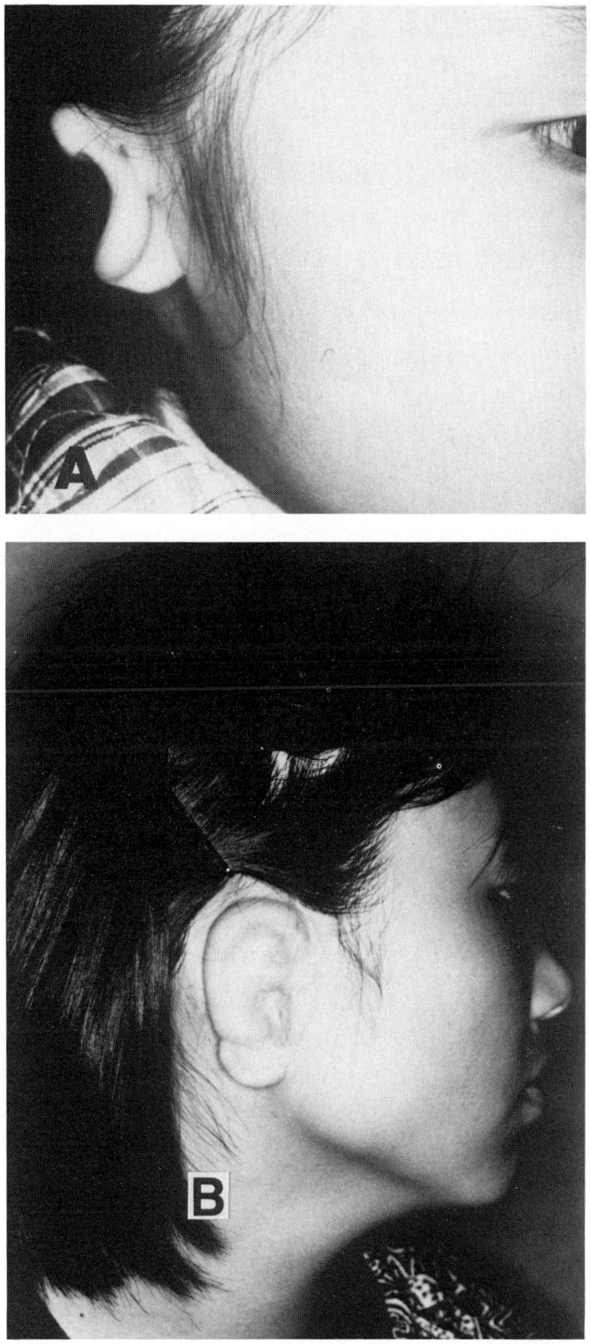

Figure 18 Type 1 microtia. *A*, Preoperative view; *B*, Postoperative view (10 years later).

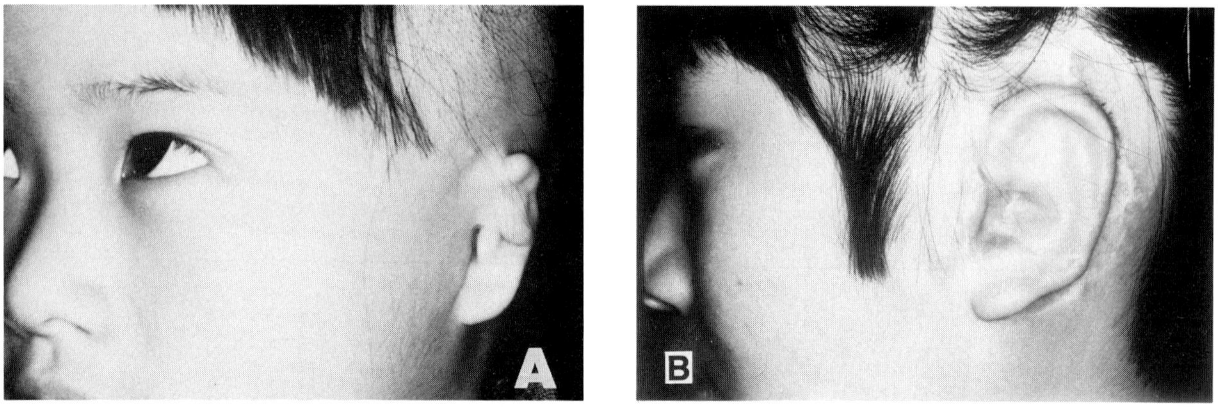

Figure 19 Type 2 microtia. *A*, Preoperative view; *B*, Postoperative view (8 years later).

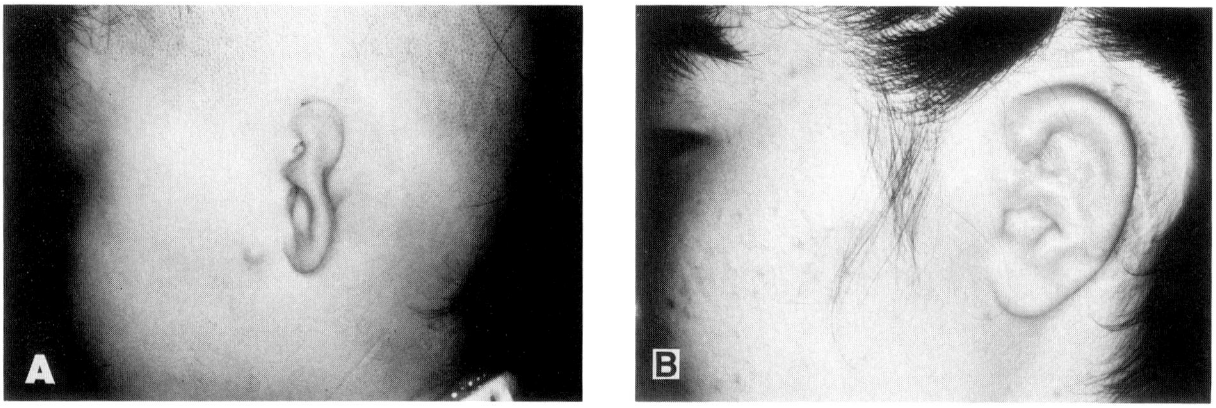

Figure 20 Type 2 microtia. *A*, Preoperative view; *B*, Postoperative view (9 years later).

TABLE 4 Patients' Hairstyle After Microtia Reconstruction

Type of Hairstyle	*Typical Microtia*	*Minor-Microtia*
Long (for concealment)	60	13
Exposed Ear	22	10
No Answer	1	5

TABLE 5 Sports Activities of Patients After Microtia Reconstruction

Sport	*Typical Microtia*	*Minor-Grade Microtia*
Soccer	10	1
Rugby	1	0
Judo	2	0
Fencing, Chinese judo	1	1
Basketball	3	3
Baseball	10	2
Softball	2	0
Volleyball	1	1
Athletics	7	0
Swimming	4	4
Tennis	5	4
Ping-Pong	4	0
Badminton	1	0
Total	51	16

COMPLICATIONS

Among 136 cases of type 1 microtia, at least 3 years after completion of reconstruction, two Silastic frames have been removed: one because of infection and one because of unknown cause. Among 44 cases of type 2 microtia, no frame removal was necessary.

However, 33 cases of type 1 and 14 cases of type 2 microtia were lost to follow-up. In my experience, the patients who did not respond to the questionnaire had no complications in connection with the reconstruction, since we are usually contacted promptly whenever something goes wrong with the auricle.

SUGGESTED READING

Cronin TD. Use of Silastic frame for construction of the auricle. In: Tanzer RC, Edgerton MT, eds. Symposium on reconstruction of the auricle. St. Louis: CV Mosby, 1974:33.

Davis DKB, Jones SM. The complications of Silastic implants. Br J Plast Surg 1971; 24:405–411.

Davis J. Aesthetic and reconstructive otoplasty. New York: Springer-Verlag 1987:319.

Edgerton MT, Bachetta CA. Principles in the use and salvage of implants in ear reconstruction. In: Tanzer RC, Edgerton MT, eds. Symposium on reconstruction of the auricle. St. Louis: CV Mosby, 1974:58.

Ohmori S. Follow-up study of the reconstruction of microtia using Silastic frame. Aesth Plast Surg 1984; 8:1–6.

Ohmori S. Reconstruction of microtia using the Silastic frame. Clin Plast Surg 1978; 5:379–387.

Ohmori S, Matusmoto K, Nakai H. Followup study on reconstruction of microtia with a silicone framework. Plast Reconstr Surg 1974; 53:555–562.

PROTRUDING EARS

RAY A. ELLIOTT Jr., M.D., F.A.C.S.

The correction of excessive protrusion of the ears has been a popular topic in the surgical literature for many decades. However, the variable nature of the deformity escaped many of the earlier writers. The resulting plethora of authoritative techniques often disappointed and confused the surgeon in search of predictable esthetic results.

Some protrusion of the ears is normal; excessive protrusion results most commonly from a failure of antihelix folding, hypertrophy of the concha, malposition of the concha, or a combination of these three. Malposition of the earlobe may also contribute to the deformity.

Perhaps stimulated by the inevitable failures from use of a single technique, individualized correction of specific deformities gradually evolved. The current therapy for protruding ears utilizes refined techniques selected for reliability in correction of a specific deformity. These are used in combinations when dictated by a diagnosis of combined deformities.

After 25 years of experience, refinement, and teaching of the composite approach to the treatment of protruding ears, I remain convinced that the concept is sound, esthetic results are easy to predict and duplicate, and complications are unusual.

PATIENT SELECTION

The primary goal of aesthetic surgery is patient satisfaction. Not everyone can be satisfied completely, but astute patient selection certainly improves the odds.

Given a truly protruding ear, the single most compelling indication for correction is the patient's personal motivation to have it corrected. Peer pressure and parental suggestion to the young patient are most important; self-image and personal interest should be evaluated at any age.

The motivation of an adult who seeks correction of protruding ears requires particular scrutiny. Latent hostility and unreasonable expectations are more common in older adult patients, particularly males. Thorough preoperative counseling may help borderline patients enjoy a good result; psychotic patients should be identified and surgery avoided.

Medical contraindications do exist, as for any surgery, but this surgery should be relatively atraumatic; blood loss is not a concern, infections are rare, and most patients beyond age 10 are candidates for local anesthesia. This is an ideal operation for outpatient surgery, in a relaxed office setting if available.

Growth of the ear is essentially complete in the preschool age group, but today we seldom see a patient younger than age 8; the average age at the initial consultation is, at present, 11 years. There is no upper age limit if general health, motivation, and expectations are favorable. Otoplasty patients tend to be very pleased, if properly selected and well treated.

SURGICAL PRINCIPLES

The ideal procedures selected for correction of ear protrusion should be reliable, safe, and reproducible. They should also be reversible during surgery. Patients undergoing elective cosmetic surgery often experience guilt, and sometimes even a temporary depression; as a group they do not tolerate complications well. Easy adjustment of the surgical correction permits refinement of the result.

Careful tissue handling and hemostasis are important. Today, cartilage is seldom thinned or incised. The result is a softer antihelix roll. Once the cartilage spring has been lessened by scoring the perichondrium, the cartilage can be positioned readily with multiple sutures. White, nonabsorbable sutures are preferred. If the concha is retropositioned, removal of the muscle and fibrofatty tissue behind the ear is routine. This important step eliminates tension on the conchal-mastoid sutures and avoids recurrence.

Skin excision is not recommended for positioning the ear. It is used only for decreasing redundancy in the sulcus. Absorbable sutures are feasible for the postauricular skin closure. Dressings are used to protect the ear in the early postoperative period. They do not prevent hematomas, but may decrease edema and bruising.

EVALUATION OF THE DEFORMITY

The esthetic ear tends to protrude less than 2.0 cm from the head, as measured from the lateral plane of the helix to the mastoid prominence at the midpoint of the ear's length.

The scapha should have a soft antihelix fold that does not obscure the helical rim on the anterior view. Failure of the antihelix fold permits lateral protrusion of the helix. This is often associated with lateral displacement of the tail of the helix on the posterior surface of the concha, thus resulting in prominence of the lobule as well.

A very large, deep concha thrusts the entire ear laterally. Anterior rotation of the concha causes protrusion because of the associated rotation of the entire ear.

Each of these can occur alone. More commonly, two or more deformities combine to create the excessive protrusion.

PREFERRED SURGICAL APPROACH

The composite of otoplasty techniques that I prefer has been detailed in numerous publications since 1965. I remain indebted to those authors whose teachings and writings have influenced the evolution and refinement of the composite approach. My personal contributions are also a matter of record.

I always approach a failure of scaphal folding with a combination of anterior perichondrial scoring and horizontal mattress sutures (Fig. 1). This virtually eliminates the 8 percent recurrence seen with sutures alone.

If there is protrusion of the lobule, the first suture lowers the tail of the helix on the posterior surface of the concha. Then the remaining scaphal sutures are placed in radial fashion to form a curved antihelix. In a reconstruction of the entire antihelix, five or six mattress sutures are placed, tested individually, and then serially tied from inferior to superior with the progressive laxity that creates a normal fold. The technique is completely reversible at this point; sutures can be added or replaced until the desired appearance is achieved. It is important to avoid separation of the lobule from the tail of the helix, as this adherence is the key to control of the lobule. Where combined techniques are used for scaphal and conchal deformities, folding of the scapha is done first.

The most common problem with the concha is malposition. Excision of the postauricular muscle and fibrofatty tissue in the sulcus, to create a pocket for the concha, diminishes the importance of the conchal-mastoid suture since it eliminates the potential for a fulcrum. This modification of the popular suture technique permits many mild to moderate cases of conchal hypertrophy to be nicely masked in most views without resorting to conchal reduction. Today, some degree of conchal setback is used in almost every case of protruding ear (Fig. 2).

Conchal reduction can be accomplished from an anterior or posterior approach. The anterior approach is much easier to judge, as the excision is limited to cartilage that overlaps when the ear is manually positioned. The scars have been uniformly good, and the procedure is compatible with the described techniques for scaphal folding and conchal repositioning (Fig. 3). Today, conchal reduction is reserved for patients with severe conchal hypertrophy. When combined with scaphal folding, the excision is placed a few millimeters lower on the posterior conchal wall.

Most cases of protruding lobule are corrected by controlling the tail of the helix, but, occasionally, a dermal-mastoid suture is required. I avoid skin excision for control of the lobule; a skin excision that obliterates the sulcus behind the lobule is never esthetic.

RESULTS AND COMPLICATIONS

The described procedures, alone or in combination, provide the flexibility required to correct most protruding ears. The steps are easily learned, and the techniques

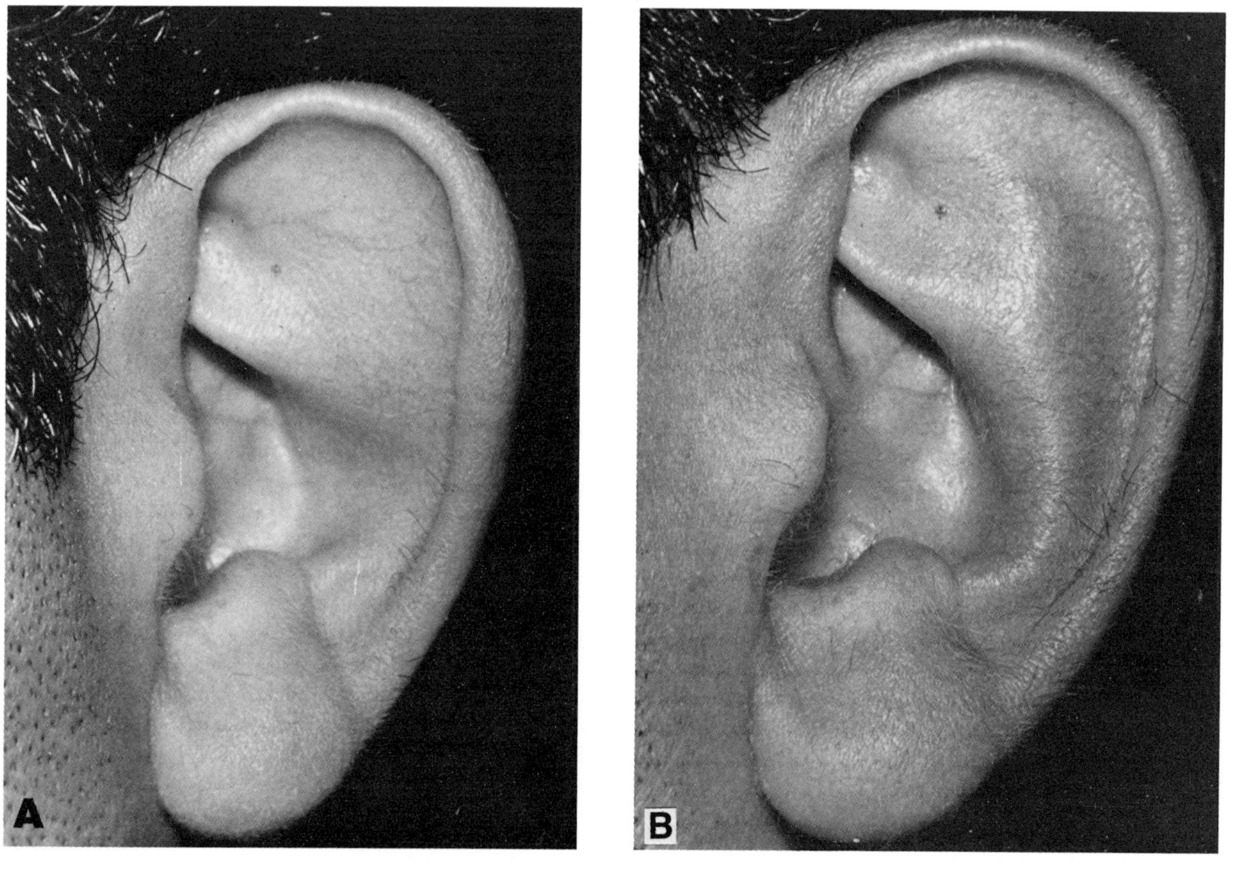

Figure 1 *A*, Failure of antihelix. *B*, Soft reconstructed antihelix roll.

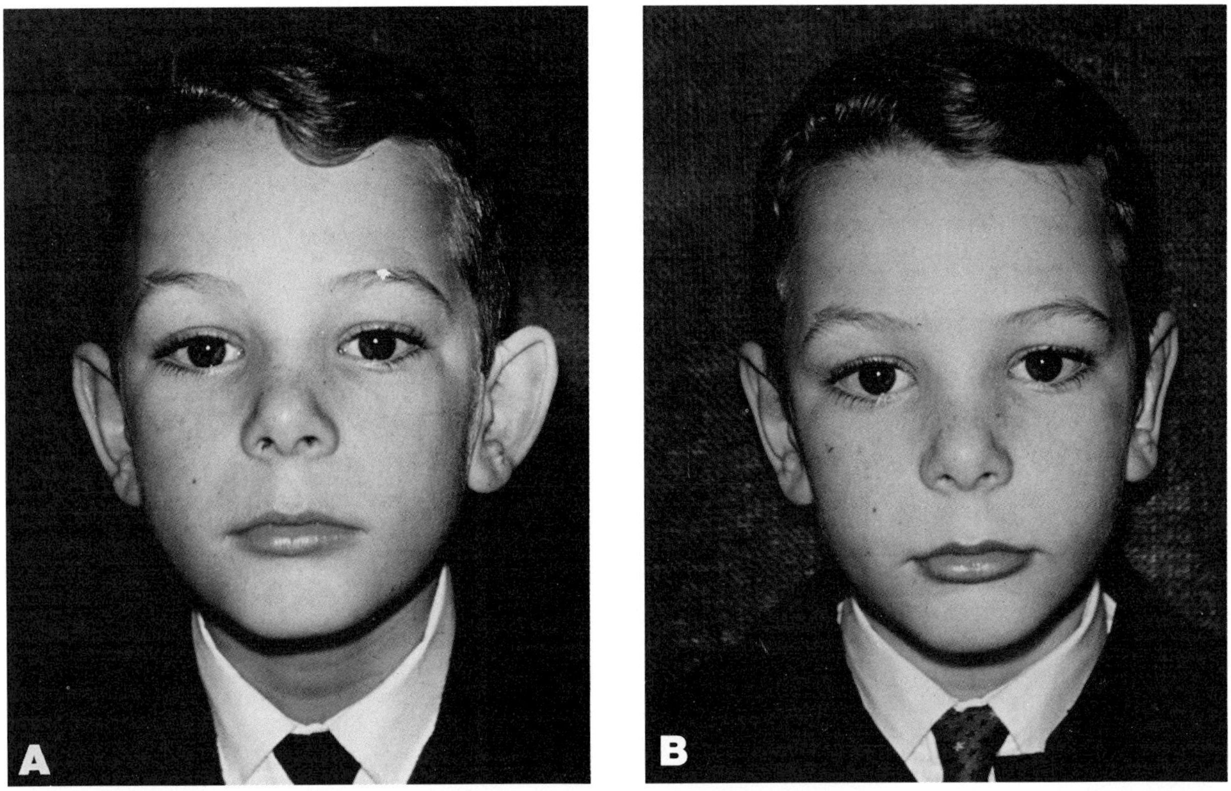

Figure 2 *A*, Unilateral failure of antihelix folding. *B*, Antihelix reconstruction, unilateral.

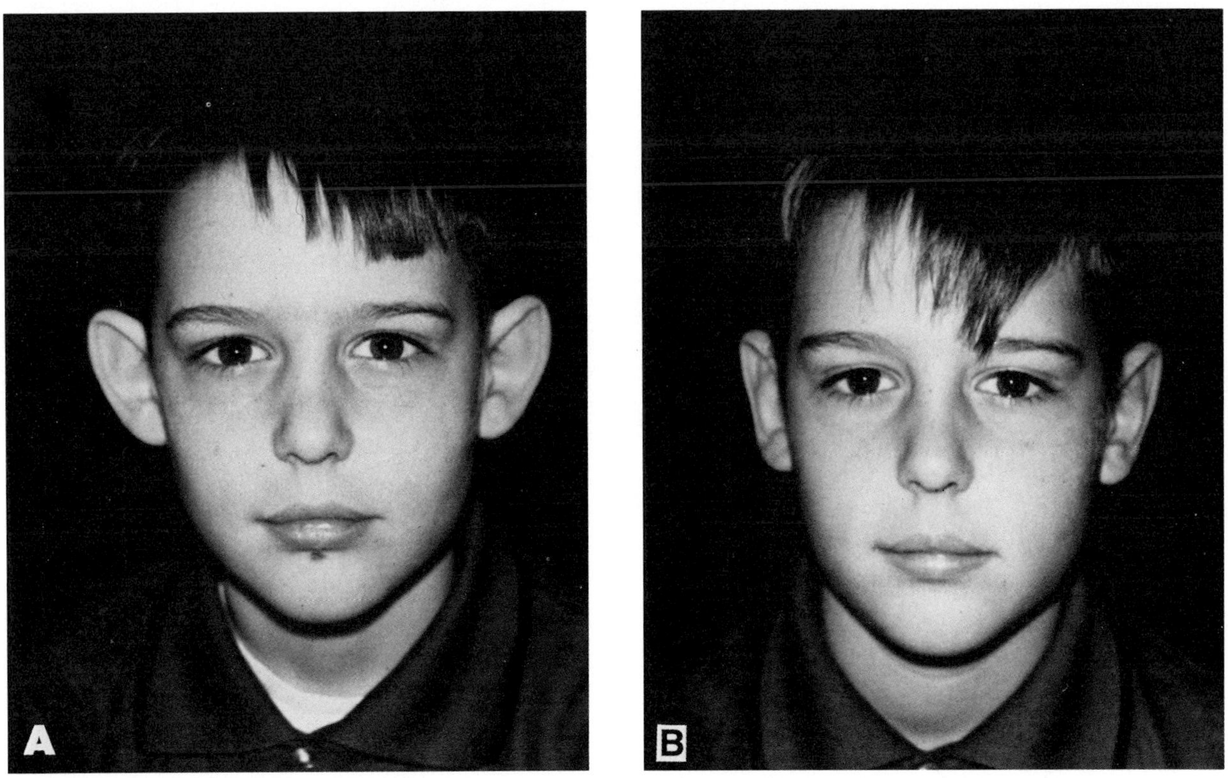

Figure 3 *A*, Failure of antihelix folding, deep concha, and malrotation of concha, asymmetrical. *B*, Bilateral antihelix reconstruction and conchal setback; left conchal reduction.

are reliable and adjustable. Sharp edges, deformed scapha, hidden helix, uncontrolled lobule prominence, asymmetry, and recurrent protrusion can become historical; they give way to ears with a natural appearance and an esthetic degree of protrusion.

SUGGESTED READING

Elliott RA. Aesthetic otoplasty. In: Regnault P, Daniel R, eds. Aesthetic plastic surgery. Boston: Little, Brown, 1985.

Elliott RA. Aesthetic surgery of the ears. In: Georgiade N, ed. Essentials of plastic, maxillofacial and reconstructive surgery. Baltimore: Williams & Wilkins, 1984.

Elliott RA. Complications in the treatment of prominent ears. Clin Plast Surg 1978; 5:479–490.

Elliott RA. Composite otoplasty. In: Stark RB, ed. Plastic surgery of the head and neck. New York: Churchill Livingstone, 1986.

Elliott RA. Otoplasty. In: Courtiss E, ed. Trouble—how to avoid it and how to treat it. St. Louis: CV Mosby, 1978.

Elliott RA. Otoplasty for prominent ears. Surg World News 1965; 1.

Elliott RA, Hoehn JG. Otoplasty for prominent ears: a composite approach. JAMA 1974; 227:992–994.

CONSTRICTED EARS

DAVID C. LEBER, M.D., F.A.C.S.

Constricted ears include a variety of deformities that range from simple hooding of the helical rim to the severely constricted cockleshell ear and the miniature ear. This chapter attempts to sort the deformities into groups and suggest ways each group can be corrected.

PREFERRED CORRECTION APPROACH

Analysis of the Problem

When one ear is deformed and the opposite ear is normal, comparisons should be made as to how the two ears differ. If both ears are involved, they should be compared to some normal standard.

When a deformed ear is compared with a normal or near-normal ear, the vertical height, the shape of the helical rim, and the overall shape of the scapha and lobule should be noted. When dealing with a miniature ear, or a markedly deformed ear, one should think of the ear in terms of upper, middle, and lower thirds (Fig. 1). What parts are present and what parts are absent? In this way, one can determine whether repositioning of the parts and reconstruction with cartilage grafts, flaps, and skin grafts will be necessary. It should be remembered that minor differences in size and shape can go untreated since both ears are not usually visualized at the same time.

Treatment

Deformities of Helical Rim

The most common deformities of the helical rim involve hooding of skin and cartilage, often associated with some rumpling of the rim cartilage.

If the outer rim contour is smooth and does not create a marked reduction in the vertical height of the ear, then simple excision of skin and cartilage is indicated (Fig. 2). This can be done through an incision within the helical rim sulcus (Fig.3).

If the outer rim is not smooth, or if there is insufficient vertical height, then a skin incision can be made in the postauricular sulcus, and the skin degloved over the helical rim, thereby exposing the entire helical rim cartilage (Fig. 4). Overhanging cartilage can then be excised, and residual indentations corrected by scoring the cartilage with a knife over the concave surface where depressions

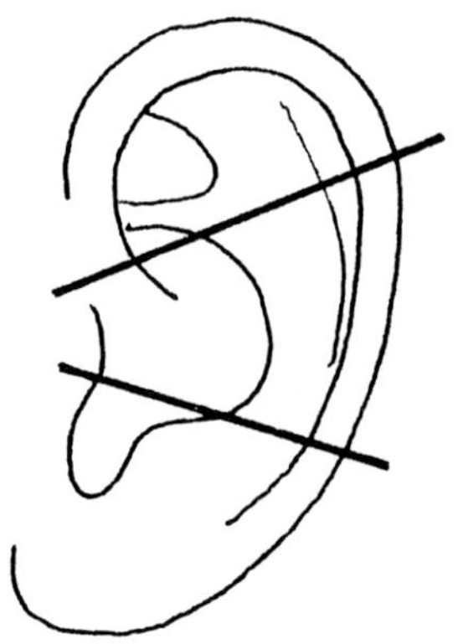

Figure 1 The ear is divided into thirds for purposes of evaluating deficiencies.

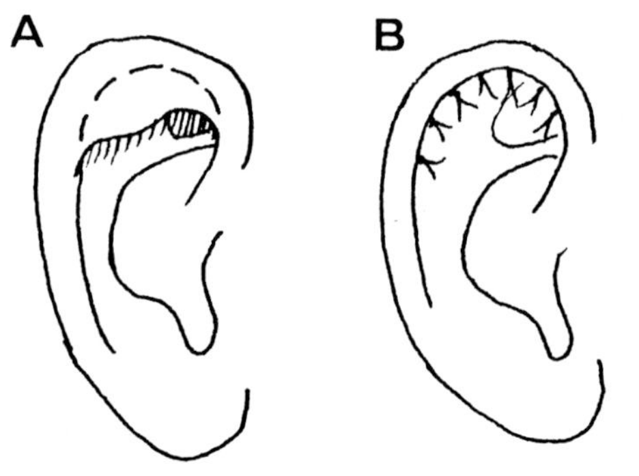

Figure 2 *A*, Constricted ear with minor skin defect only. *B*, Correction made by excision of hooded, redundant skin at inner margin of helical rim.

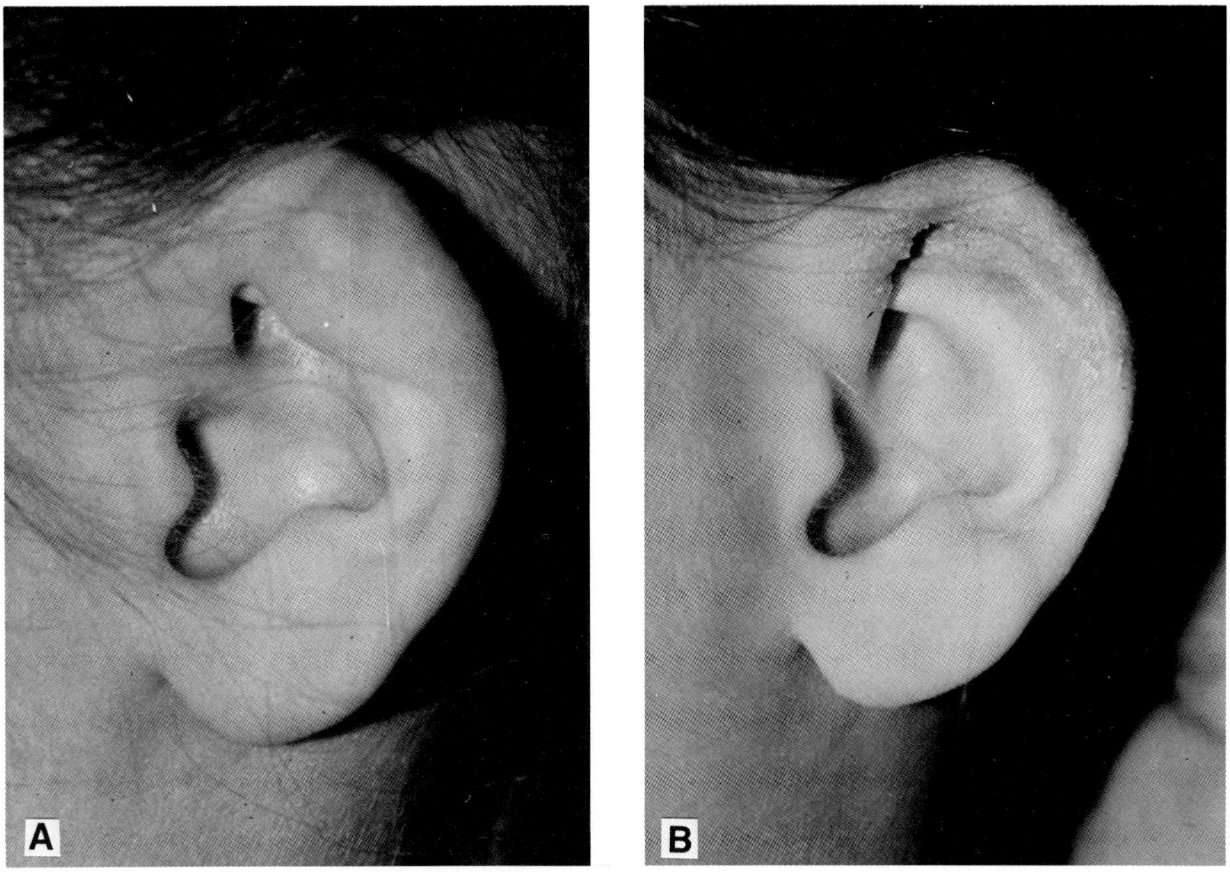

Figure 3 *A*, Preoperative findings of ear with hooding of helical rim and minimal distortion of cartilage. *B*, Postoperative results after removal of excess skin and cartilage through helical rim incision.

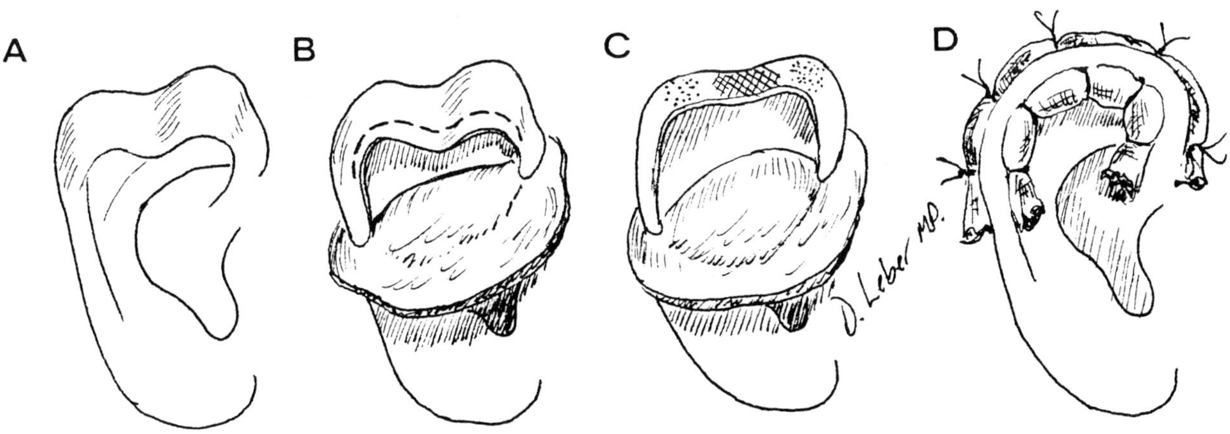

Figure 4 *A*, Constricted ear with cartilage and skin defect. *B*, Cartilage is exposed through postauricular incision. The skin is carefully degloved and excess cartilage is marked. *C*, Excess cartilage is excised and the cartilage is reshaped by scoring with a knife blade. Scoring should be on the concave side or constricted side. Scoring of the cross-hatched area on the outer surface and the stippled area on the inner surface should correct this contour deformity. *D*, The skin is reapplied to the cartilage and held in place with rolled petrolatum gauze stents and 4–0 nylon mattress sutures.

exist. If additional vertical height is needed, then a cartilage graft taken from the opposite ear can be added to the superior aspect. The skin is then redraped and held in place with through-and-through mattress sutures tied over rolled bolsters of petrolatum gauze. Sometimes it is necessary to thin out the skin where it folds over the previous helical rim margin to permit better draping, but one must be careful not to injure the blood supply to the skin.

A set-back otoplasty may be indicated to correct abnormal projection of the deformed ear due to absence of the antihelix or conchal abnormalities.

Complex Deformities

Miniature Ear. A miniature ear can look very much like a normal ear except it may be only one-half the size of the normal ear. The best treatment is to divide the ear in half, reposition the upper and lower parts, and place a postauricular and scalp flap in the defect (Fig. 5). A rib cartilage graft is then harvested and carved to the shape of the scapha and helical rim of the middle third of the ear (see Fig. 2 in the chapter *Microtia: Autogenous Framework* for technique of harvesting rib cartilage grafts). Extensions of the carved cartilage graft are necessary to maintain the support of the upper and lower thirds. After 4 months, the ear is lifted away from the side of the head and a full-thickness skin graft applied to the postauricular sulcus (Fig. 6).

There are times when a compensatory revision of the normal ear is indicated in order to obtain better symmetry. A set-back otoplasty, or a reduction in the size of the normal ear by wedge excision of cartilage and skin, or wedge excision of the lobule, may be required.

Cockleshell Ear. The cockleshell ear is the most difficult of the constricted ear deformities to correct. Such ears usually have a normal concha, with an external auditory canal, and a normal lobule. The upper third of the ear, however, is curled over the concha and inserted in an abnormal location. The entire ear is usually low-set on the side of the face, and is often associated with hemifacial microsomia. There appears to be ample thin skin available for reconstruction, but when the ear is released and unfolded surgically, it becomes evident that the anterior upper third of the ear is absent.

Treatment of the cockleshell ear is directed at unfolding the existing parts, inserting them into the side of the

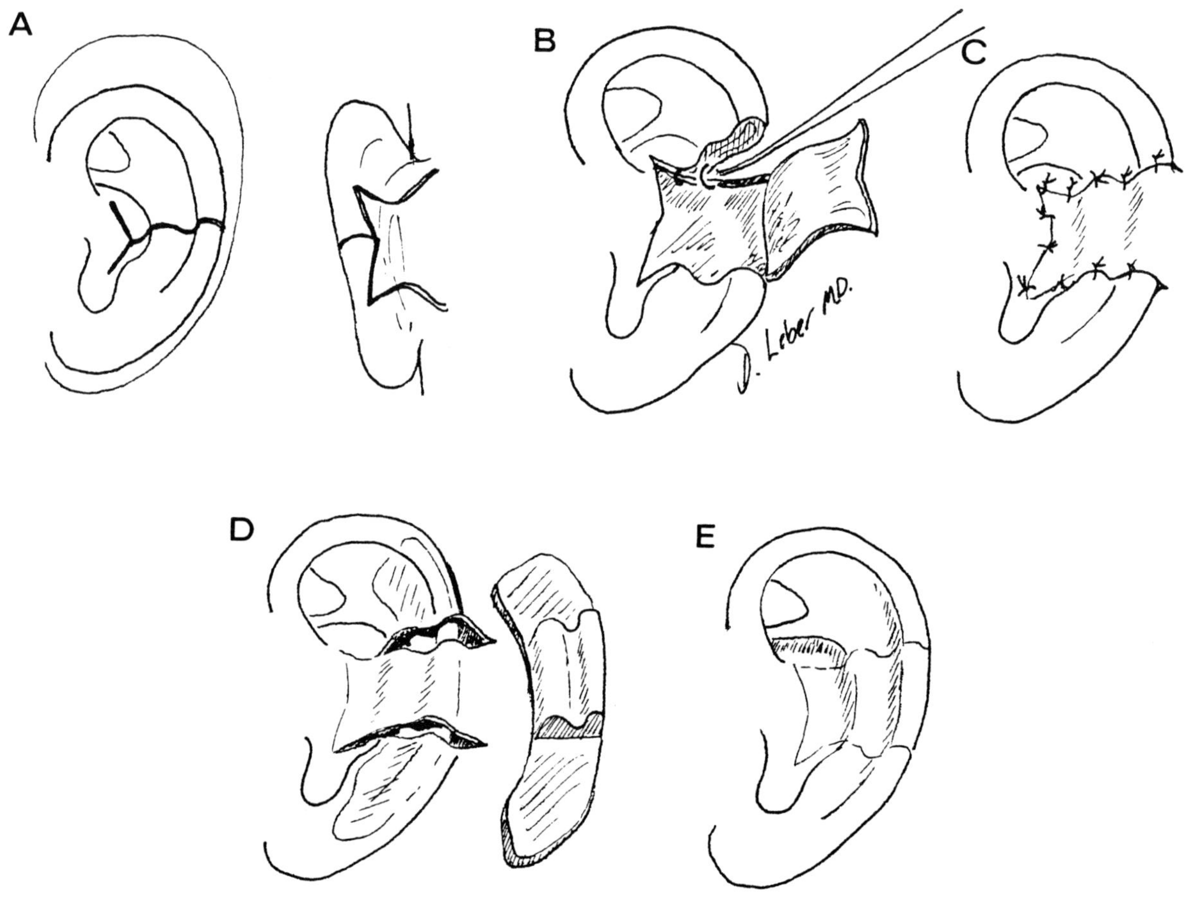

Figure 5 *A*, The miniature ear is expanded by dividing the ear as shown. *B*, The posterior ear skin is sutured to the scalp skin with absorbable sutures. *C*, The postauricular and scalp flap is sutured into the anterior defect. *D*, A costocartilage graft is carved in the shape of the defect. Support struts are carved into the graft to fit behind the existing ear cartilage and the graft is inserted through the tunneled incisions. *E*, The postauricular space is recreated after 4 months with a full-thickness skin graft.

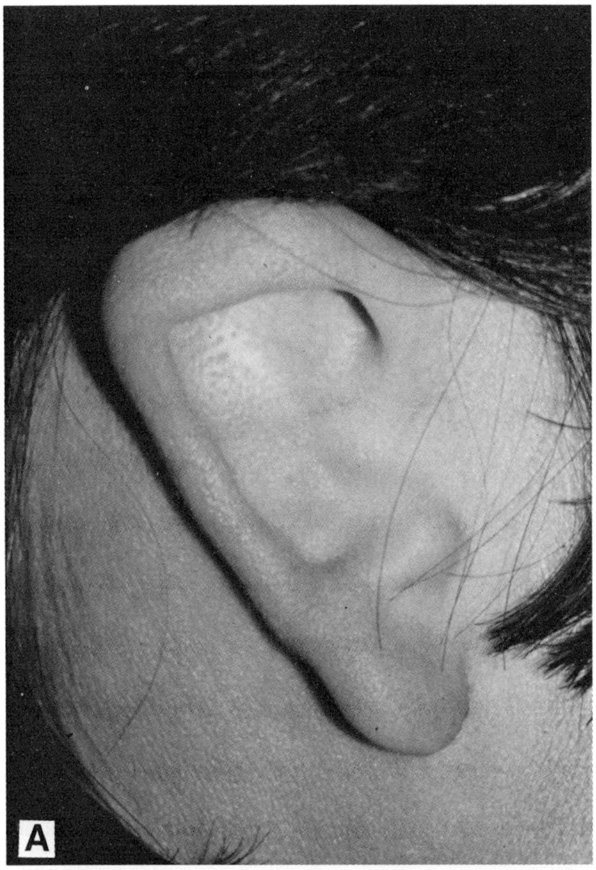

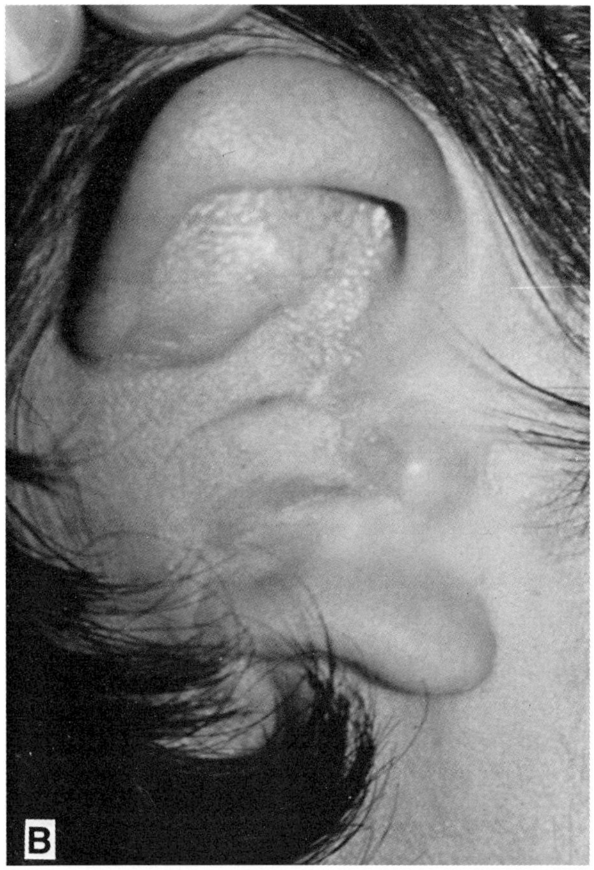

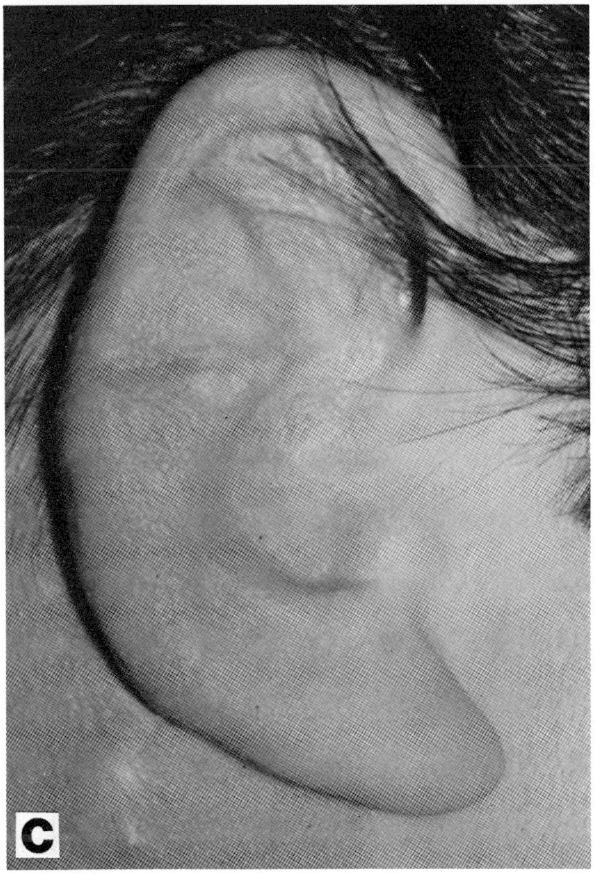

Figure 6 *A*, Preoperative findings of a miniature ear without an external auditory canal. *B*, The ear has been divided, expanded to the size of the normal ear, and sutured to the scalp. *C*, Final result after insertion of cartilage graft, creation of postauricular sulcus, and correction of hooded helical rim. Formation of tragus and deepening of the concha are planned.

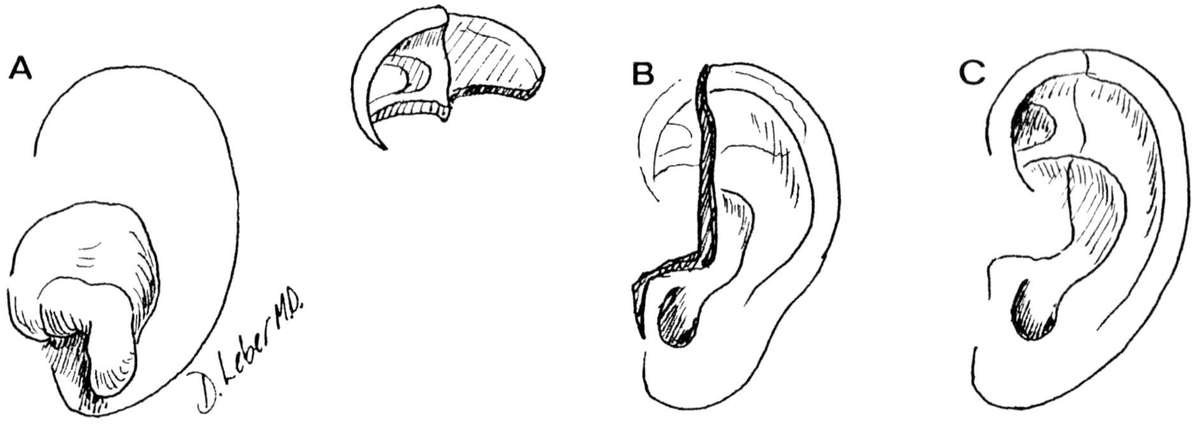

Figure 7 *A*, Cockleshell ear deformity, showing normal size and position of the opposite ear. *B*, The ear is reconstructed by incision of its superior attachment, unfurling of the ear, and its insertion into the hairless scalp skin. The missing cartilage of the anterosuperior aspect of the ear is carved from costocartilage and can be inserted at the same time, or as a second procedure. Note the strut used to support the graft attachment to the remaining normal ear cartilage. *C*, The ear is completed by creating a postauricular sulcus with a full-thickness skin graft.

scalp in proper position, and then reconstructing the anterior upper third of the ear with a rib cartilage graft and postauricular skin graft (Fig. 7).

Since there is an external auditory canal present in an abnormally low position, it is impossible to relocate this ear to its normal anatomic position as compared with the opposite ear (Fig. 8).

Timing of Surgery

Minor corrections that involve the helical rim can be performed anytime after 4 years of age.

Major procedures that require repositioning of tissue, and subsequent rib cartilage grafts, can be done in two stages. The repositioning surgery can be done at an age

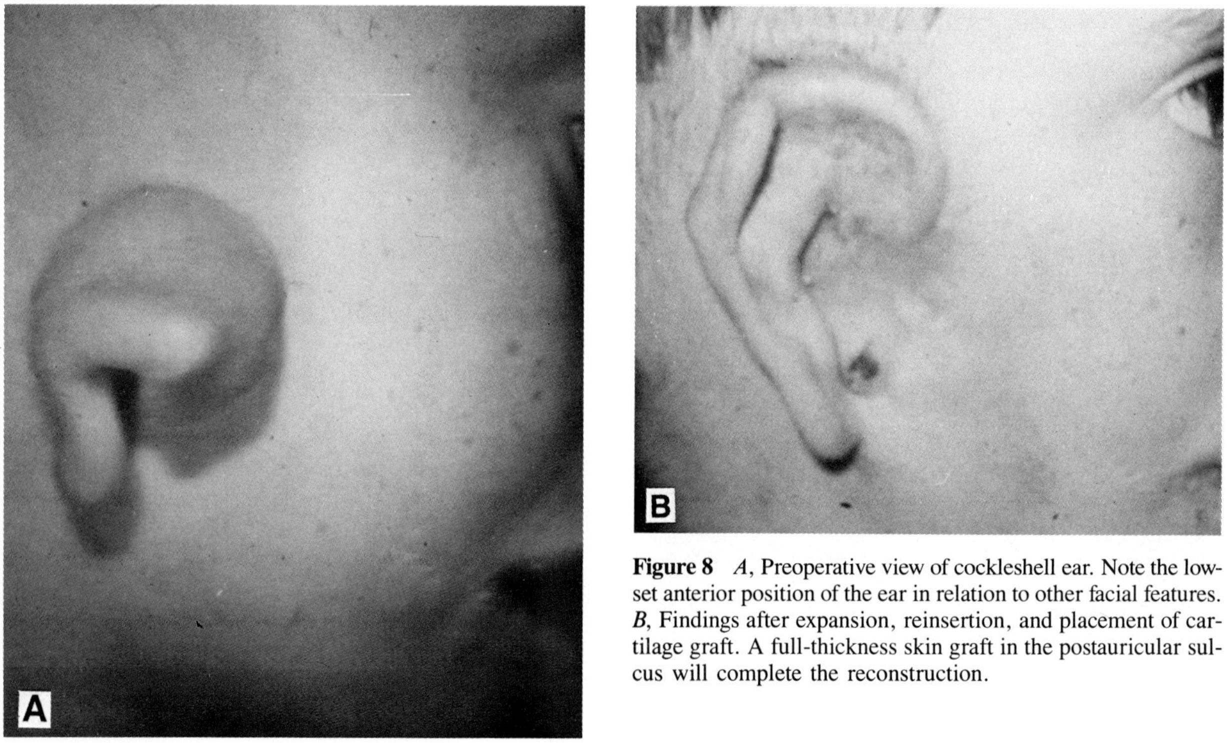

Figure 8 *A*, Preoperative view of cockleshell ear. Note the low-set anterior position of the ear in relation to other facial features. *B*, Findings after expansion, reinsertion, and placement of cartilage graft. A full-thickness skin graft in the postauricular sulcus will complete the reconstruction.

when proper position can be determined accurately and this is usually any time after 5 or 6 years of age. It is important to wait until the child has developed enough to have sufficient rib cartilage for the second stage. If a small graft is needed, the surgery can be done as early as 6 years of age. If a large framework is required, it is best to wait until the child is 8 to 10 years of age.

Complications and Problems

Possible complications that can occur in correction of constricted ears include hematomas, infection, and skin necrosis, although these are quite rare.

When working with one abnormal and one normal ear, it is important to inform the patient and family that the two ears will never look exactly alike.

The difficulty for most surgeons who undertake ear reconstruction is their ability to carve cartilage implants to the precise size and shape required and to accomplish this efficiently. This requires frequent practice.

Benefit-Risk Analysis of Preferred Approach

There have been many operative procedures suggested for correction of a large variety of constricted ear deformities. The benefit of the approach presented here is that the deformities are divided into two major groups; those with simple helical rim deformities, and those that require repositioning of ear segments with the use of local flaps and rib cartilage grafts. Accurate preoperative assessment of the deformity is necessary if proper treatment is to be expected. When properly analyzed through comparison with the opposite normal ear, or when compared to a standard normal ear in bilateral deformities, good results can be anticipated with little risk of disappointment—on the assumption that the surgeon has experience and confidence in working with cartilage and the carving of cartilage grafts.

SUGGESTED READING

Brent B. The correction of microtia with autogenous cartilage grafts: II. Atypical and complex deformities. Plast Reconstr Surg 1980; 66:13–21.

Converse JM. Reconstruction of the auricle. Plast Reconstr Surg 1958; 22:150–163.

Leber DC. Ear reconstruction. In: Georgiade NG, Georgiade GS, Riefkohl R, Barwick WJ, eds. Essentials of plastic, maxillofacial and reconstructive surgery. Baltimore: Williams & Wilkins, 1987:501.

Tanzer RC, Edgerton MT, Eds. Symposium on reconstruction of the auricle. St. Louis: CV Mosby, 1974.

Tanzer RC. The constricted (cup and lop) ear. Plast Reconstr Surg 1975; 55:406–415.

ANOPHTHALMIC ORBIT

LARS M. VISTNES, M.D., F.R.C.S.(C)

An anophthalmic orbit may be either congenital or acquired. The scope of this chapter does not allow discussion of the congenital anophthalmic orbit. Furthermore, since removal of the globe before the age of 2 years interferes with bony orbital growth later in life, and because such removal is usually secondary to tumor (retinoblastoma) and is followed by irradiation (which in itself tends to further interfere with bony growth), this very difficult problem also has to be excluded.

Accordingly, the discussion will be confined to those orbits where the anophthalmic state is secondary to removal of the globe beyond the age of 2 years, and where there has been no trauma to the bony orbit itself.

The result of such surgery is the production, either immediately or over time, of a series of distinct physical findings known as the *anophthalmic orbit syndrome*. These are: (1) superior sulcus (supratarsal) depression, (2) enophthalmos of the artificial eye, (3) ptosis of the lower eyelid, and (4) ptosis of the upper eyelid (Fig. 1).

If trauma was associated with the event that necessitated removal of the globe, as well as extensive soft tissue damage, scarring and deficit of conjunctiva frequently cause problems related to the socket designed to contain the prosthesis. Inadequate and, often, contracted sockets create a further problem that should be discussed under the topic of the anophthalmic orbit, but this must be omitted from this chapter.

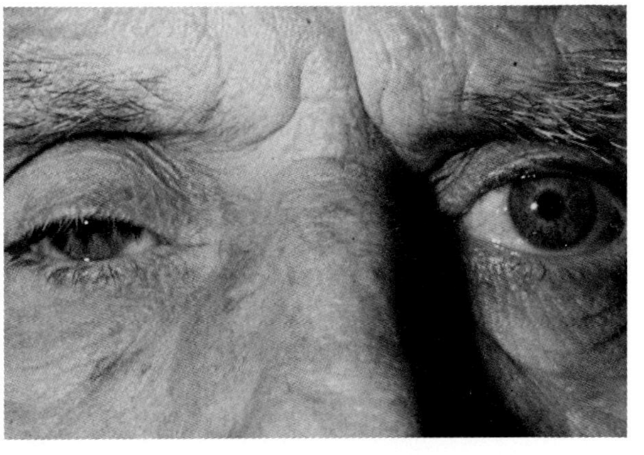

Figure 1 Patient shows all features of the anophthalmic orbit syndrome: supratarsal depression, enophthalmos of the artificial eye, lower lid ptosis, and upper lid ptosis. (From Vistnes LM. Surgical reconstruction in the anophthalmic orbit. New York: Aesculapius Publishers, 1987.)

THERAPEUTIC ALTERNATIVES

For a variety of reasons, some patients who have had surgical removal of the globe have a result that does not call for surgical intervention, at least not immediately. Some of these patients have a truly remarkable result. Even the most critical surgeon, patient, or ocularist cannot find need for improvement in such fortunate situations.

The first line of defence for these patients is usually the ocularist or the anaplastologist depending on the medical care delivery system. The ophthalmologist, by virtue of his training and orientation, is more concerned with the remaining eye than the one that has been removed. Since it was the ocularist who made the artificial eye (prosthesis), he or she is contacted first if the appearance becomes unsatisfactory. The ocularist can often achieve significant improvements in appearance by alterations in shape and size of the prosthesis. Such changes in the size of the prosthesis often make good sense, since the most significant and the earliest changes in appearance after enucleation are due to a discrepancy in volume between the enucleated globe and the material that replaces it in the orbit (the implant buried in the muscle cone and the prosthesis seated in the socket). Eventually, however, the prosthesis may become so large that it is difficult to get it through the palpebral fissure into the socket, and its weight will eventually produce lower lid ptosis. Upper lid ptosis, when present, may be partly corrected by a change in the prosthesis through addition of bulk in the upper sulcus. Such an addition may, however, eventually lead to so much physical obstruction in the upper sulcus that it interferes with lid closure. A well-trained ocularist knows when the limits of his ability have been reached and he should refer further problems in appearance or function to an ophthalmic or plastic surgeon who is familiar with the problems involved.

As stated above, the main problem is lack of adequate volume in the contents of the bony orbit, and many materials have been used over the years to augment orbital volume, with greater or lesser success, i.e., bone, cartilage, fat, dermis, fascia, precarved silicone blocks, and glass or silicone beads. I have for the past 15 years used room temperature vulcanizing (RTV) silicone,* which technique will be described presently. Ophthalmic surgeons have recently revived the use of dermis fat grafts for volume augmentation in these patients. Plastic surgeons have not found dermis fat grafts, when used elsewhere in the body, to be reliable in their behavior as regards take and eventual volume. I have no reason to believe that they will behave any differently when placed in the orbit.

If the pathomechanics of the anophthalmic orbit syndrome are not fully understood by the treating surgeon, there is a temptation to treat individual components according to one's training and inclinations. This is a mistake, because it may preclude ideal treatment of another component of the syndrome later. Thus, if a fascial sling is placed in the lower lid to support sagging, it would be an effective physical barrier to a later attempt to move an enophthalmic prosthesis to a more anterior position.

* Dow Corning Corp.

PREFERRED APPROACH

Correction of Enophthalmos and Supratarsal Depression

As already indicated, there is a basic discrepancy in the volume of orbital contents if one compares the volume of the average eye globe (7.5 ml) with the volume of its replacement following enucleation. The combined volume of prosthesis and implant is typically around 5.0 ml. My approach to correction of this deficit has been to use RTV silicone.

With the patient supine and asleep under general anesthesia, a 1 cm incision is made in the upper eyelid over the lateral orbital margin just superior to the lateral canthal tendon. The periosteum is incised for the same length and, with a Freer elevator, the periosteum (periorbita) is separated from the bony orbital wall laterally and along the floor of the orbit so as to create a pocket that will push the orbital contents superiorly and anteriorly when filled with RTV silicone (Fig. 2). After hemostasis has been obtained by packing the pocket thus created with half-inch gauze stripping for 5 minutes, the RTV silicone is put into the pocket via a piece of intravenous connector tubing attached to a 5 ml syringe. This contains the RTV silicone mixed with the appropriate amount of catalyst. (Five drops of stannous octoate mixed with 5 ml of the silicone monomer produces a rubbery polymer in about 5 minutes.) Prior to surgery, a competent ocularist should have fabricated an ideal prosthesis for the patient's socket and this sterilized prosthesis (soaked in Betadine solution for 10 minutes) is placed in the socket before the silicone mixture is pushed into the predissected pocket. Enough

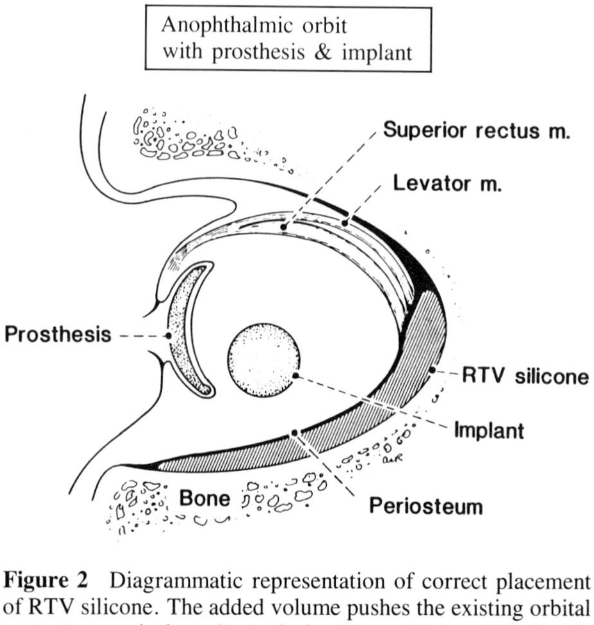

Figure 2 Diagrammatic representation of correct placement of RTV silicone. The added volume pushes the existing orbital contents superiorly and anteriorly. (From Vistnes LM. Surgical reconstruction in the anophthalmic orbit. New York: Aesculapius Publishers, 1987.)

RTV silicone to produce a satisfactory appearance is pushed into the predissected pocket in the orbit, with any perioperative edema taken into account. On average, 2.5 to 3.0 ml is needed. After vulcanization has taken place (the mixture left in the syringe is a good indicator), the tubing is gently dislodged and pulled out, and the polymer is cut at the orbital margin. The incision is closed in layers, and an eyepad is placed as a dressing, with care taken to keep the prosthesis in the socket at all times. Prophylactic antibiotics (1.0 gm cephalosporin), started intravenously before surgery, are continued for 72 hours.

Correction of Lower Lid Ptosis

Various approaches to adding support to the sagging lower lid have been tried over the years by different surgeons. Shortening of the lid by various methods has been tried with immediate good results, but with disappointing long-term results as the lid continues to stretch due to the continued and relentless weight placed on it by the otherwise unsupported prosthesis. Similarly, the lid has been propped up by cartilage, either from the ear or the nasal septum. It has been my practice to support the lid by creation of a sling that holds the lid in the desired position with absolutely firm anatomic anchors. Long-term follow-up of this method has shown it to be reliable.

Small incisions over the lateral orbital rim and the medial canthal tendon make it possible to drill a hole in the orbital rim and clearly identify the external portion of the medial canthal tendon. With a Crawford fascial stripper, a 2.5 to 3.0 mm wide piece of fascia lata is obtained, which, after placement in the lid margin (using a Wright's fascial passer), is passed around the canthal tendon and through the hole in the orbital rim. After suturing the strip of fascia to itself medially, the tension is adjusted laterally with the prosthesis in place in the socket, and similarly sutured to itself with interrupted sutures of fine nonabsorbable suture material (Fig. 3). The prosthesis which has been sterilized by soaking in Betadine solution, is placed in the socket for the critical adjustment of sling tension, and remains in the socket thereafter. Prophylactic antibiotics (cephalosporin), started intravenously at the beginning of surgery, are continued for 72 hours. When a fascial sling is used in this manner, it is not necessary to overcorrect in the expectation that there will be later relaxation, as is done, for instance, in the correction of facial nerve paralysis. Because each end of the fascial strip is connected to a rigid anatomic structure, there is no change.

Upper Lid Ptosis

Of the manifestations that make up the anophthalmic orbit syndrome, upper lid ptosis is usually the last to show itself. For reasons outside the scope of this discussion, it occurred in only approximately 20 percent of a series of 200 patients. Minor degrees of ptosis can be corrected by the ocularist by the addition of a small ledge on the superi-

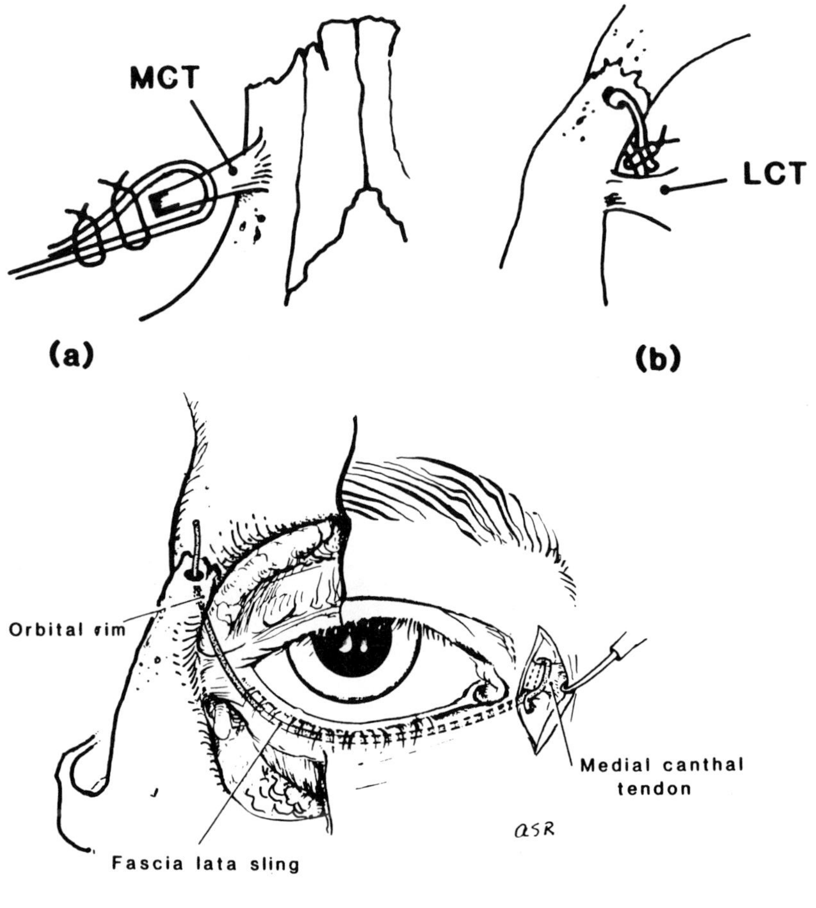

Figure 3 *Above*, diagrammatic representation of detail of inset of fascial strip medially and laterally. *Below*, position of the sling in the lower lid. (From Nolan WB, Vistnes LM. Correction of lower lid ptosis in the anophthalmic orbit—a long-term follow-up. Plast Reconstr Surg 1983; 72:289.)

or aspect of the prosthesis. This is, in fact, so commonly done that the surgeon never sees many of these patients. When ptosis is sufficiently severe that surgical intervention is necessary, it is corrected in much the same manner as the conventional treatment.

A mild degree of ptosis (1 to 2 mm) is most easily corrected by a lid-shortening operation such as that described by Fasanella and Servat. In the rare patient who has a marginal socket with a poor upper sulcus, such an operation may produce a totally inadequate socket, since twice the amount of conjunctiva is removed when the lid is everted and turned on itself. The procedure may correct the ptosis, but the lid cannot close since there is a physical barrier to closure in the upper sulcus. In such patients, correction of the upper lid ptosis is best achieved by the judicious removal of a wedge of conjunctiva and tarsal plate only (i.e., an intratarsal lid shortening).

More severe ptosis is most easily corrected by direct exploration of the levator apparatus via an external lid excision in the classic manner described by Berke. Occasional patients who have had a large prosthesis with a large ledge superiorly will be found to have a levator disinsertion. The more common finding is a relatively normal-looking levator apparatus that is lax and needs tightening. In these patients, correction is easily obtained by a conventional levator shortening procedure as described in standard texts.

TIMING OF SURGERY

Correct timing, or sequencing, of the procedures described above is essential. The operations should be performed in the sequence in which they have been described, even if all the components of the anophthalmic orbit syndrome are present. Adjustment of both lower lid and upper lid ptosis is so critical that it is essential to do both these operations in tissues that are not edematous. The operation for the correction of deficit in the orbital contents' volume produces a great deal of edema at times, even intraoperatively. To follow such a procedure immediately, or in conjunction, with ptosis correction would produce a less than satisfactory result. I, therefore, plan these operations at least 6 weeks apart. It is rare to find a patient who needs only one of these procedures. Most commonly, the patient presents with enophthalmos of the artificial eye along with supratarsal depression. After the correction, with a new prosthesis in a more anterior position, the laxity or ptosis of the lower lid becomes apparent. This is corrected next and the adjustment of the upper lid, if needed, is the "frosting on the cake."

THERAPEUTIC OUTCOME

The described approach to the anophthalmic orbit syndrome has yielded a satisfactory result over the past 15 years. Critical long-term analysis, of both the use of RTV silicone and fascial strips for support of the lower lid, has stood up to time. There has been no migration of the silicone, which has conformed well to the compound curvature of the orbit (in contrast to silicone and glass beads, which migrate with relative ease). Similarly, the unyielding anatomic structures to which the fascial strip is attached (a hole in the lateral bony orbital rim and the medial canthal tendon), do not allow for further stretching of the lower lid over a period of time (Fig. 4).

BENEFIT-RISK ANALYSIS

In the ongoing analysis of the stated approach, benefits continue to outweigh the risks. Since adoption of prophylactic antibiotics more than 10 years ago, whenever either a foreign body (RTV silicone) or autogenous fascia is used in the region of a potentially contaminated surgical field (the socket), no problem with infection has been

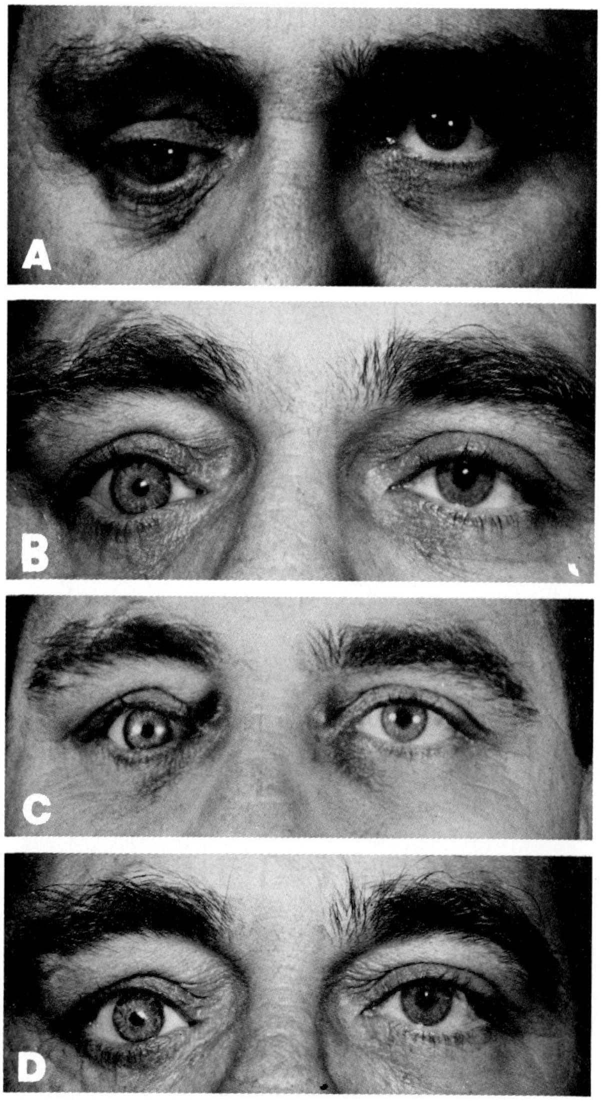

Figure 4 Therapeutic outcome of described operative approach. *A*, Preoperative appearance. *B*, After placement of RTV silicone, but prior to correction of lower lid ptosis. *C*, Appearance 2 years after both operations. *D*, Appearance 8 years after original surgery. Good correction is maintained. (From Vistnes LM. Surgical reconstruction in the anophthalmic orbit. New York: Aesculapius Publishers, 1987.)

experienced. Migration of the implant has not been a problem and, when the pocket for the silicone is correctly dissected, the material achieves the purpose for which it is intended. I am aware of complications that have arisen when inexperienced operators have placed the materials in the incorrect anatomic location, or in incorrect amounts (usually by overcorrection). This is failure on the part of the surgeon rather than failure of the method. If the described philosophy of treatment is followed, the final result should yield a satisfied patient every time provided the patient's expectations are realistic. One should aim for the improvement that is always possible rather than for the perfect result, which is not attainable because the missing eye can never be truly replaced.

SUGGESTED READING

Nolan WB, Vistnes LM. Correction of lower lid ptosis in the anophthalmic orbit—a long-term follow-up. Plast Reconstr Surg 1983; 72:289–292.

Sergott T, Vistnes LM. Long-term follow-up of the use of RTV silicone in the augmentation of volume of orbital contents. Plast Reconstr Surg 1987; 79:331–338.

Vistnes LM. Surgical reconstruction in the anophthalmic orbit. New York: Aesculapius Publishers, 1987.

SURGICAL CORRECTION OF DROOL

ROBERT M. FAGGELLA Jr., M.D., M.S.S., F.A.C.S.
JOHN M. OSBORN, M.D., F.A.C.S.

The care and management of chronic drool problems have been long neglected. Drugs, radiation, and transtympanic resection have been ineffectual treatments due to the lack of prolonged clinical success. The surgical correction of drool was first reported by Theodore Wilke in 1964. Garry Brody joined with Dr. Wilke and they perfected the technique. Today, surgical correction is an acceptable treatment of sialorrhea.

The classic Wilke-Brody operation consists of bilateral submaxillary gland resection and intraoral repositioning of the parotid duct to the tonsillar fossa. Subsequently, other authors have reported series of complete ligation of parotid ducts, rather than transpositions, in conjunction with submaxillary gland resection. A review of our long-term case follow-ups, using the Wilke-Brody technique, suggested recurrence of a little excess saliva with that technique, versus too dry a mouth with complete ligation. We, therefore, started a new series that included bilateral submaxillary gland resection, ligation of one parotid duct, and the transposition of the other. After long-term evaluation of this technique in over 90 patients, we feel that it results in a desired amount of residual saliva.

Evaluation of the patient with chronic drool is important. Close attention must be paid to the number and type of medications the patient may be taking. Most patients will be on anticonvulsive and muscle-relaxant drugs. Age does not seem to be a factor in surgical success. We have performed the procedure in age groups 4 to 48 years. We find the surgery is easier in the 8 to 16 year age group. Most of these patients are noncommunicative. Those who are, fully realize their drool problem and express their desire for improvement. Surgery is warranted also in the noncommunicative, nonambulatory, or the noncomprehending patient. The nursing care problems that chronic drool produces will be relieved. The results facilitate better care for the patient. Two classes of patients should be approached cautiously for drool surgery: athetoid patients and those with small mandibles. The athetoid patient will place great stress on the flap postoperatively. The patient with a small mandible makes the technical aspects of tunneling and flap formation more difficult.

SURGICAL PROCEDURE

The submaxillary glands are resected through an external approach. Once the patient's head is turned to the side, the musculature and contents of the neck pull the gland more posterior towards the angle of the mandible. One generally finds the gland through a small incision, one finger breadth below the rim of the mandible at the junction point of the proximal and middle third of the mandible. Invariably, there are very large lymph nodes present on top of the cervical fascia, which must be moved. The platysma muscle is split in the direction of its fibers. Beneath the muscle, there is a walnut-size tan-gray racemose gland in a filmy capsule. The gland is tucked under the rim of the mandible. A subcapsular dissection of the submaxillary gland is desirable and, with care, is virtually bloodless.

The anatomic compartment of the submaxillary gland is important. The gland is beneath the mandible, resting on the glossopharyngeal muscle. Care is necessary in the deep dissection to preserve the lingual nerve. The lingual nerve can be tented up with the traction on the submaxillary gland due to its connections with the otic ganglion. Frequently, it must be dissected free. The hypoglossal nerve lies more inferiorly, below the digastric tendon and rarely is seen. The dissection of Wharton's duct does not need to extend anteriorly under the mylohyoid muscle. Frequently, one will see small glandular attachments to Wharton's duct that appear like grape clusters. Suture ligation of the divided duct is all that is necessary. A small drain is brought out through the wound. Only subcuticular skin closure is carried out to coapt the wound because suture removal is difficult in these patients. The drain is removed in 2 to 4 days. On one occasion, we were unable to find submaxillary glands on either side. Subsequently, radioactive uptake confirmed the congenital absence of these glands.

Ligated Stensen's Duct

Finding the papilla of Stensen's duct is sometimes difficult. The duct surface is not always in the described anatomic position opposite the second upper molar tooth. External massage of the parotid gland may emit a localizing drop of saliva at the papilla. Gentle probing with a number 0 or 1 lacrimal duct probe will suddenly enter the orifice. In our series there was one case of congenital absence of Stensen's duct. This duct makes a sharp bend in the midportion of the cheek and it is easy to trace it surgically through the cheek with the probe in place. After freeing up the papilla, a suture ligature helps to keep the duct taut. On the side for suture ligation, the ligature should be placed as close to the gland parenchyma as possible.

Transposition Site

This portion of the procedure necessitates planning. The flap is designed to run parallel to the buccal sulcus from the papilla to the approximate area of the mandibular incisor. The flaps should be drawn an ample distance above the sulcus in order to ensure adequate mucosa adjacent to the gingiva for ease of closing the defect. The incision around the papilla should leave a cuff of mucosa so as to maintain circulation and stability to the head of Stensen's duct. This diversion is based on the Dennis Brown principle of buried epithelium tending to tube itself. The flap is harvested moderately thick, with a layer of fibroareolar tissue attached to the mucosa. Gentle freeing-up of the bulk of tissue surrounding the cuff and Stensen's duct is necessary for a short distance so that this area can eventually be folded.

The crucial aspect of this operation is the creation of the submucosal tunnel. The tunnel extends from the inferior incision site, down the cheek, and over the pterygomandibular ligament into the tonsillar fossa area. Most problems of breakdown with subsequent fistula are caused by a tear in the mucosa overlying the tunnel, particularly where it is thin overlying the ligament. Injection of the mucosa with saline solution of Xylocaine is helpful; however, do not puncture the mucosa directly over the area of undermining. A puncture acts as a weak point, and the mucosa may perforate easily at that site. A flatnose scissor facilitates the tunnel dissection. At the pterygomandibular ligament, extreme care and caution is necessary. The tunnel should be wide enough to accommodate the flap. We use a 2–0 silk ligature at the distal tip of the flap for traction, and thread this silk through the tunnel. We then grasp the base of the flap with a fine tooth pick-up and turn the flap 90 degrees over. Gentle traction on the ligature delivers the flap into the tunnel without corkscrewing. The mucosal surface is turned down in the tunnel. The head of the papilla (opening of Stensen's duct) is then buried deep into the tunnel. There is a tendency for the head and cuff to ride up and suture fixation sometimes helps to keep the head in place. As much length of flap should be maintained as possible. When the patient is awake, considerable stretch will result from mouth movements. The distal stoma is simply sutured in place with three interrupted 4–0 Vicryl sutures. No other treatment is necessary.

POSTOPERATIVE EXPECTATIONS

The sialorrhea is noticeably reduced immediately. All of the patients will have moderate to marked swelling for which ice bags are recommended. Good cheek hemostasis helps to minimize the swelling. The major swelling lasts 3 to 5 days. Intraoral discomfort and swelling usually prevent the patient from taking oral fluids so intravenous replacement is needed during this period. Pain is not a major factor in most cases.

Hospitalization depends on the patient's progress and usually lasts 3 to 6 days. Patient comfort and ability to take oral fluids are the key factors. As the swelling subsides, the patient returns to a more normal state and is discharged. Antibiotic administration has been optional and infection, early or late, is uncommon.

Good preoperative counseling to parents, nurses, or others will alleviate many anxieties over the patient's initial swollen appearance.

LONG–TERM CARE

Residual swelling subsides in approximately 4 to 8 weeks. Mouth care must become an important daily routine for those taking care of the patient. There can theoretically be an increase in caries due to the decrease in saliva. This reduced saliva can cause crusting of mucus on the exposed teeth, with associated bad odor. Many patients experience transitory swellings of the cheek, similar to the appearance of mumps. Onset is generally rapid and painless. Usually there is fever, tenderness, or malaise. We have treated the event symptomatically with warm compresses, mouth care, anticholinergic drugs, and, occasionally, antibiotics. The swelling disappears as quietly as it appeared and its etiology is not clear.

Frequently, a small nodule about the size of a marble can be palpated in midportion on either side of the cheeks. Such nodules represent dilatations of the duct or development of a cyst. Generally, they present no problems. On occasion, we have seen the mass point into the external cheek and have incised and drained it intraorally. If the mass presents with no appreciable symptoms, watchful waiting is the best treatment. Long-term infection is rare and we have seen it occur in only two cases over the past 18 years.

Surgical correction of drool is an emotionally rewarding procedure for doctor, patient, parents, and nursing personnel.

SUGGESTED READING

Faggella RM, Osborn J. Surgical correction of drool. A comparison of three groups. Plast Reconstr Surg 1983; 72:478–482.

Glass LW, Nobel GL, Vecchione TR. Treatment of uncontrolled drooling by bilateral excision of submaxillary glands and parotid duct ligation. Plast Reconstr Surg 1978; 62:523–526.

Guerin RL. Surgical management of drooling. Arch Otolaryngol 1979; 105:535–537.
Wilke T, Brody G. The surgical treatment of drooling. A ten year review. Plast Recostr Surg 1977; 59:791–798.
Zohn H. Corda tympanic neurectomy. A new approach to submaxillary gland sialolithiasis. J Laryngol Otol 1968; 82:835–837.

MANDIBULAR OSTEOTOMIES

JAMES A. LEHMAN Jr., M.D.

Surgery for the correction of dentofacial deformities, and more specifically for mandibular deformities, should be simple and straightforward, as this chapter will show. The difficult aspect is the diagnosis and presurgical planning. This will not be discussed in the text, but I refer the reader to the "Suggested Reading" at the end of the chapter.

The aims of any surgical procedure on the mandible are to obtain a stable, functional occlusion and good facial esthetics. Various types of osteotomies or, occasionally, bone grafts can be performed on either the body or the ramus to correct mandibular deformities. These procedures require adequate exposure, which can be obtained by either extraoral or intraoral approaches. Procedures that do not alter the dental arch are usually preferred and have less tendency to relapse. Rather than attempt to describe all the techniques available, this paper focuses only upon those that have been found to be reliable, safe, and technically simple. These techniques are all within the capabilities of any plastic surgeon doing maxillofacial surgery.

Mandibular body osteotomies are of historical interest and will not be discussed. The most reliable procedures are those performed on the ramus. Presurgical orthodontics, to produce two well-aligned dental arches that can be fitted together accurately at surgery without tooth interference, improves the stability of the operation.

There are two preferred ramus procedures: (1) subcondylar osteotomy, and (2) sagittal osteotomy.

SUBCONDYLAR OSTEOTOMY

Subcondylar osteotomy is a procedure designed for mandibular setback, although occasionally it can be used to level the occlusal plane. It can be performed with either an extraoral or intraoral approach. It has the advantage of avoiding injury to the mandibular nerve so there is no potential for loss of lower lip sensation.

The external approach has the advantages of better visualization and complete access to the pterygoid muscle. It is indicated for setbacks greater than 10 mm and in patients having a repeat setback. In addition, it is easier to position the proximal segment, especially if rigid fixation is planned. The disadvantage is the cutaneous scar.

Extraoral

A 2 cm curved incision is marked approximately 0.5 cm below the angle of the mandible. The incision is carried through the platysma. The superficial layer of the deep cervical fascia is inspected for the mandibular branch of the facial nerve. The nerve is retracted superiorly and the exposure is extended through the pterygomasseteric sling. A periosteal elevator is then used to elevate the tissues from the ascending ramus up to the sigmoid notch. The fiberoptic lighted channel retractor* is then inserted into the sigmoid notch and the line of the osteotomy marked with a sterile pencil. The osteotomy line is marked from the sigmoid notch to the angle staying posterior to the bony protuberance that corresponds to the lingula medially. Using the Midas-Rex power burr, the osteotomy is completed. In setbacks greater than 10 mm, the coronoid may need to be divided to allow for complete setback. The pterygoid muscle is stripped from the proximal segment sufficiently to allow the proximal segment to overlap the distal segment laterally. On completion of the osteotomies on both sides, the occlusal splint is inserted, and the teeth placed in intermaxillary fixation. The proximal segments are then positioned laterally and held with a wire or rigid fixation. With rigid fixation, the intermaxillary fixation can be removed after the incision is closed. When the segments are held with a single wire, intermaxillary fixation is maintained for 6 weeks (Fig. 1).

Intraoral

The intraoral approach is designed for setbacks of less than 10 mm. It has the advantage of no external scar, but the disadvantage of being technically more difficult.

The incision line is marked from a point 1 cm below the coronoid process down the ascending ramus, staying far enough lateral to facilitate wound closure. The incision line is carried forward to the second bicuspid. After the incision is made through the mucosa, a periosteal elevator is used to expose the lateral, posterior, and inferior borders of the mandible. Blunt dissection avoids exposure of the buccal fat pad. The Bauer sigmoid notch retractor is inserted in the sigmoid notch, and the L & M retractor is inserted inferiorly. The osteotomy cut is made with the sagittal saw from the sigmoid notch to the angle, as in the external approach. It is technically more difficult to make

* All instruments mentioned are available from Walter Lorenz Co.

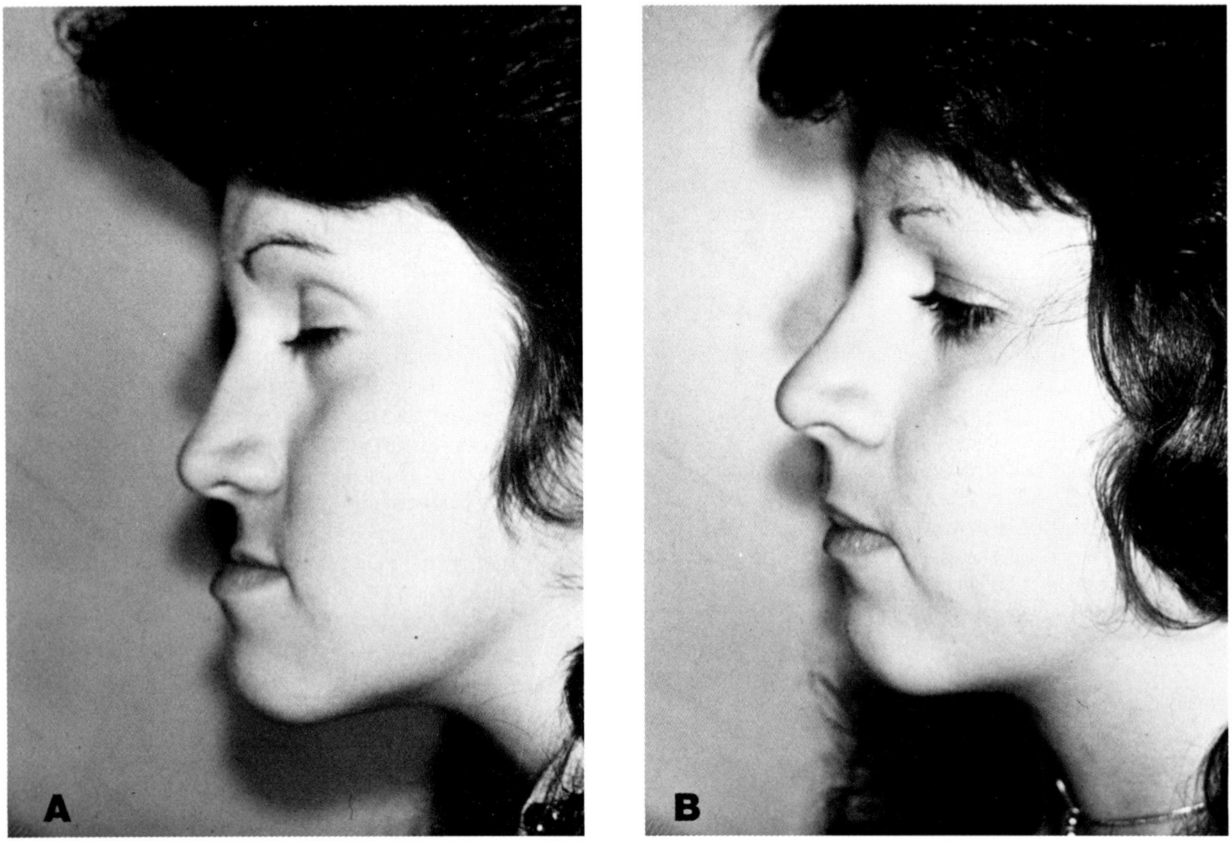

Figure 1 *A*, An 18-year-old female with mandibular prognathism is shown. *B*, The result 1 year after an external subcondylar osteotomy and setback.

the cut because visualization is poor. There is also a greater risk of injury to the vessel, and bleeding can be difficult to stop.

Upon completion of the osteotomy, the medial pterygoid muscle is stripped from the proximal segment to allow lateral positioning of that segment. After completion of both osteotomies, the teeth are placed in intermaxillary fixation using the occlusal splint. The proximal segment is positioned laterally, and the drill holes are marked. Intermaxillary fixation is then removed, the drill holes made, and a wire passed. The intermaxillary fixation is then restored with the splint in place, and the wire is tightened as the condyle is seated in the fossa. Lag screw fixation also can be used to obtain rigid skeletal fixation and avoid intermaxillary fixation. However, it is more difficult because of the narrow area of overlap. The mucosal incision is then closed (Fig. 2).

SAGITTAL OSTEOTOMY

This procedure has undergone numerous modifications since its original description and has evolved into the technique used today. It is currently the most popular mandibular osteotomy. It can be used for mandibular advancement, mandibular setback, or vertical lengthening of the ramus. It is the preferred procedure for mandibular advancement.

Sagittal osteotomy, however, has some serious risks that are not associated with the subcondylar osteotomy. These include injury to the inferior alveolar nerve, with permanent sensory loss to the lower lip and avascular necrosis of the proximal bony segment. These risks can be avoided by careful adherence to the technical details of the procedure.

Sagittal ramus osteotomy is a transoral procedure. The mucosal incision extends from 2 cm below the coronoid down the lateral retromolar area and then forward to the second bicuspid. The subperiosteal dissection is started anteriorly and continued cephalad toward the coronoid. Laterally, the periosteum is elevated to the inferior border of the mandible and, posteriorly, to and around the angle. There should be no lateral dissection cephalad to an imaginary line from the retromolar area to the angle in order to maintain the vascular integrity of the proximal segment and, thereby, prevent avascular necrosis and skeletal relapse. The buccal fat pad can be avoided by not extending the incision too cephalad on the ascending ramus and by using blunt dissection when exposing the bone along the ascending ramus. Medially, the soft tissues are elevated, exposing the lingula and the inferior alveolar neurovascular bundle. The channel retractor is inserted medially and the L & M retractor laterally. The osteotomy line is marked horizontally on the lingual cortex about 3 to 5 mm above the lingula. Then it extends down the anterior border of the ascending ramus to the second molar and

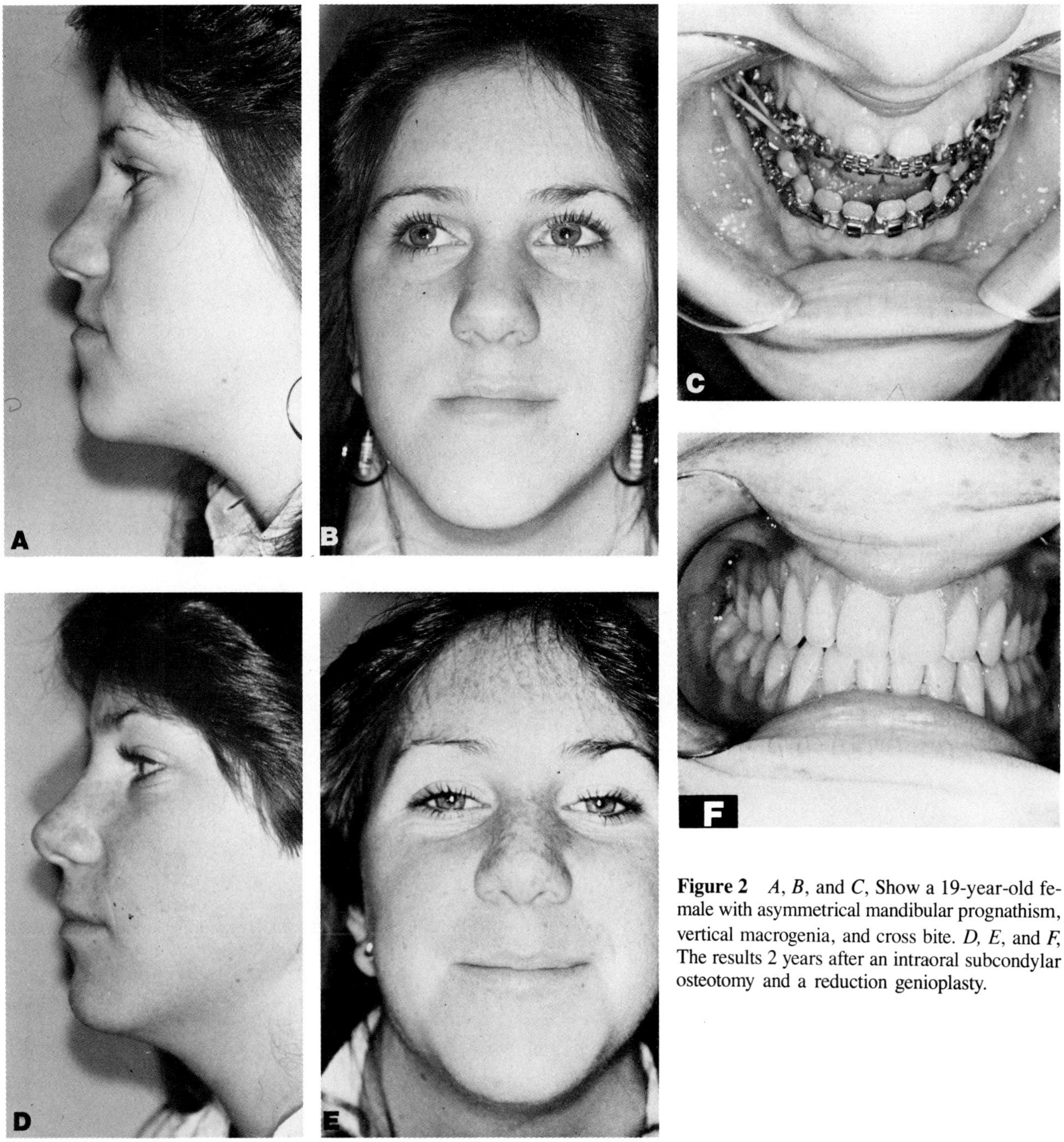

Figure 2 *A*, *B*, and *C*, Show a 19-year-old female with asymmetrical mandibular prognathism, vertical macrogenia, and cross bite. *D*, *E*, and *F*, The results 2 years after an intraoral subcondylar osteotomy and a reduction genioplasty.

curves along the oblique line to the inferior border. The medial cut is made and extended posteriorly, approximately 2 cm from the anterior border. The osteotomy is then carried down the ascending ramus. The lateral osteotomy is completed through the lateral cortex and should extend through both cortical plates of the inferior border of the mandible to avoid splitting off the outer cortex when the chisel is inserted. After completion of the bone cuts with the power burr, a curved chisel is used to start the separation of the lateral cortex. A wedge osteotome is then levered to increase the separation until the neurovascular pedicle is visualized. A straight osteotome then can be passed over the bundle and the sagittal split completed. Care is taken to free the soft tissue attachments from the distal segment. After completion of both osteotomies, the occlusal splint is inserted and intermaxillary fixation applied. The proximal segment is positioned with the condyle in the fossa, and drill holes are placed so that the wire seats the condyle in the fossa as it is tightened. Presently we use lag screw fixation and remove the intermaxillary fixation at the completion of the procedure (Fig. 3).

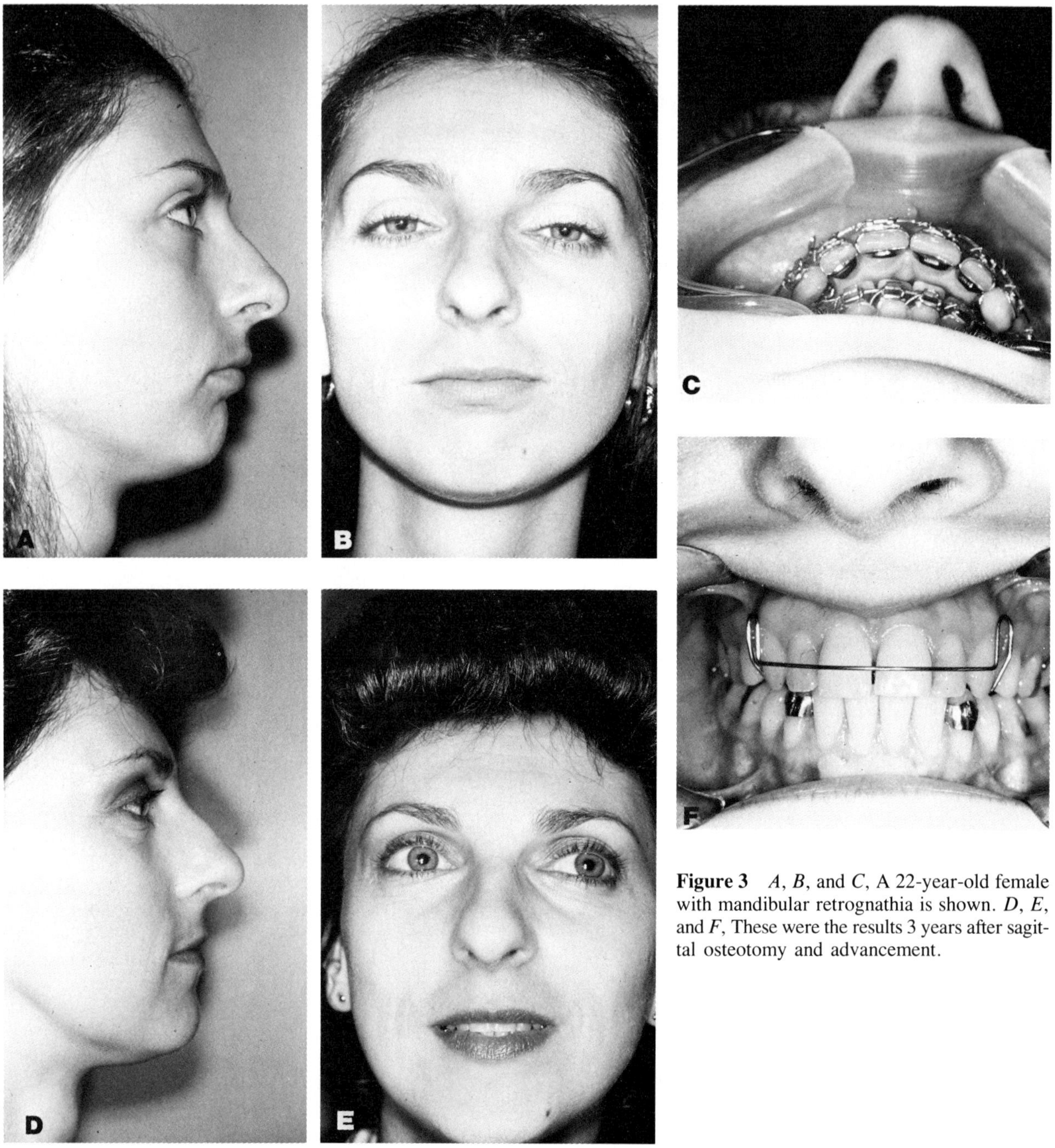

Figure 3 *A*, *B*, and *C*, A 22-year-old female with mandibular retrognathia is shown. *D*, *E*, and *F*, These were the results 3 years after sagittal osteotomy and advancement.

COSTOCHONDRAL GRAFTS

Costochondral grafts to the mandible are indicated for the congenitally absent condyle, as in hemifacial microsomia, acquired condylar destruction resulting from trauma, ankylosis, or rheumatoid arthritis, and ablative removal of the condyle for tumor resection. Loss of the condyle in the young patient usually results in a high mandibular plane angle class II malocclusion, which is frequently associated with an anterior open bite. Reconstruction of the condyle with a costochondral graft provides horizontal as well as vertical lengthening of the mandible.

The costochondral graft is obtained from the fifth rib on the contralateral side. There should be approximately 1 cm of cartilage on the bone. The contralateral rib is preferred because the curve of the rib follows the contour of a normal mandible. The fifth rib is utilized so that the synchondrosis of the sixth and seventh rib is not disturbed. This may be required for subsequent ear reconstruction in patients with hemifacial microsomia.

The surgical approach is the same as that used for an external subcondylar osteotomy. The incision, however, is extended proximally and distally about 1 cm to provide access to the angle and ramus. An extensive subperiosteal dissection is done to allow for horizontal and vertical lengthening. Care must be taken to preserve the neurovascular bundle which might be abnormally located, especially in hemifacial microsomia. The glenoid fossa can usually be exposed through the neck incision because of the short ascending ramus. In some patients, a second preauricular incision must be made to facilitate exposure and avoid injury to the facial nerve. In severe cases of hemifacial microsomia, the entire glenoid fossa must also be reconstructed. After mobilization, the mandible is positioned by using the occlusal splint, and intermaxillary fixation is obtained. The deformed condyle can be removed or partially resected. The cartilage cap is carved to the appropriate shape and inserted into the fossa. The cortical plate is removed from the lateral border of the ascending ramus and the medial border of the bone graft, and the graft is secured with two lag screws. The soft tissue is closed, and intermaxillary fixation maintained for 6 weeks. In some cases of unilateral grafting, a contralateral subcondylar osteotomy may be required to position the mandible properly (Fig. 4).

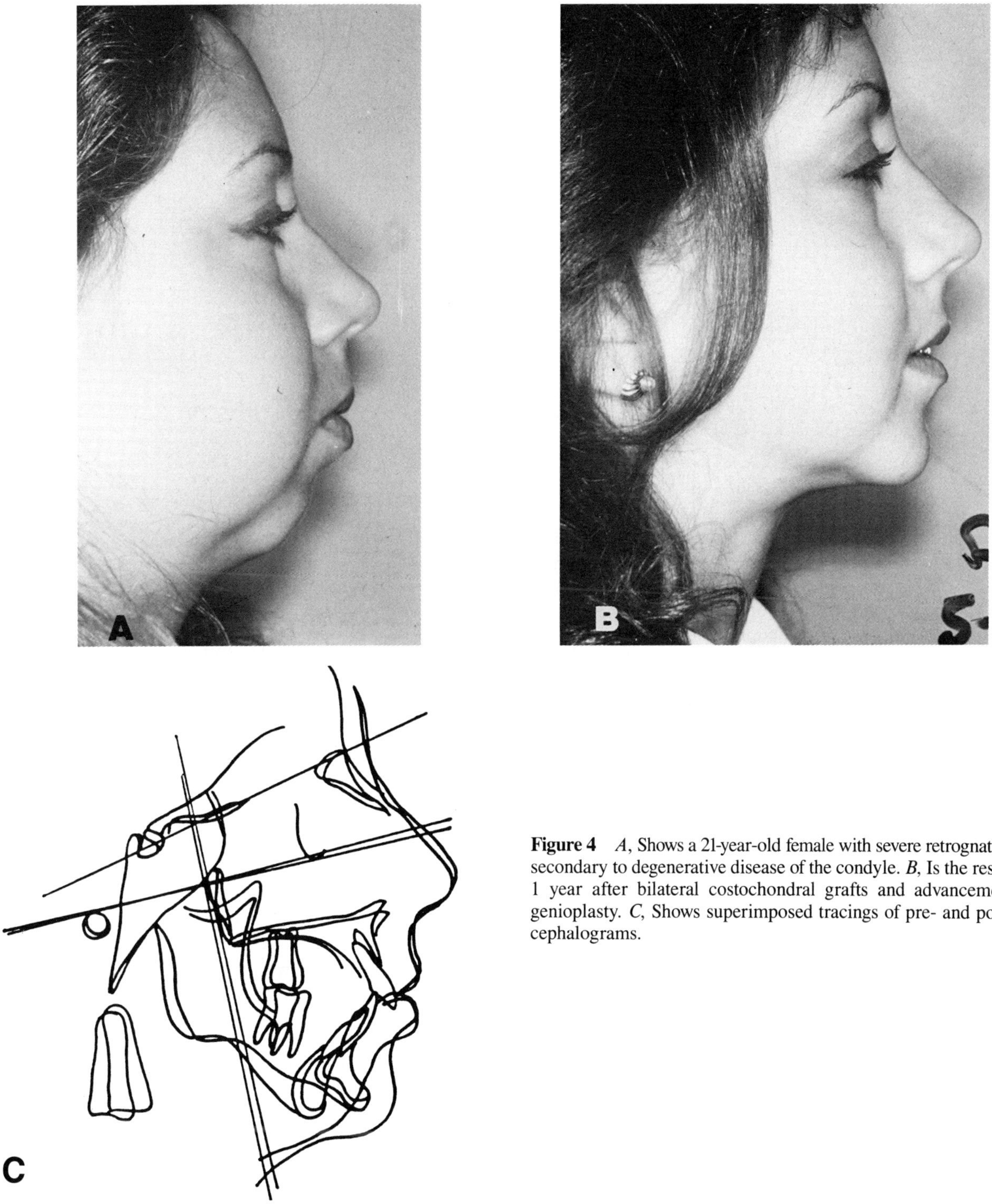

Figure 4 *A*, Shows a 21-year-old female with severe retrognathia secondary to degenerative disease of the condyle. *B*, Is the result 1 year after bilateral costochondral grafts and advancement genioplasty. *C*, Shows superimposed tracings of pre- and post-cephalograms.

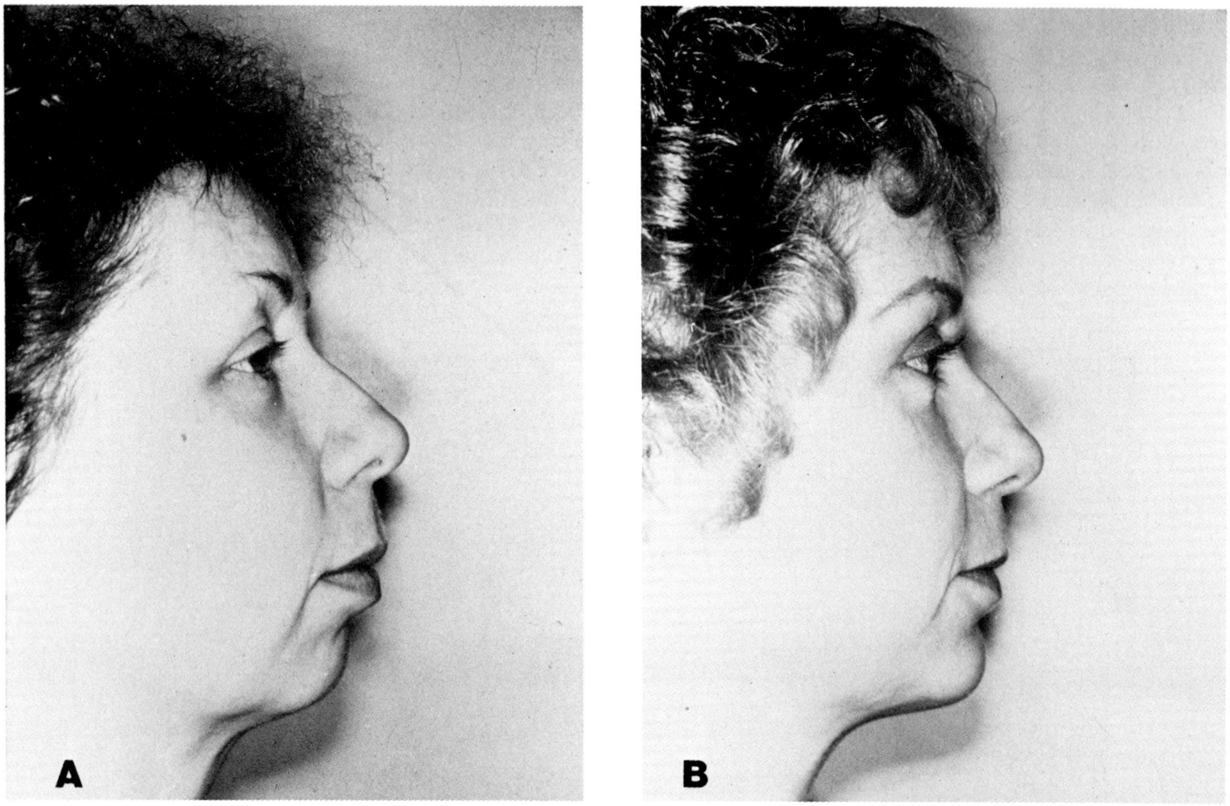

Figure 5 *A*, A 35-year-old female with microgenia. *B*, Postoperative result after a 10 mm augmentation (osseous advancement) genioplasty performed under local anesthesia on an outpatient basis.

GENIOPLASTY

The chin must also be considered in the overall planning of mandibular surgery to achieve ideal facial esthetics. In treatment planning, the lateral cephalogram with the soft tissue profile is important. The two most common procedures are augmentation and reduction genioplasty. Correction of asymmetry and vertical deficiency can also be performed. The majority of genioplasties can be performed on an outpatient basis through intraoral approach under local anesthesia.

Augmentation Genioplasty

An anterior lower buccal sulcus incision is made from cuspid to cuspid, leaving a 5 mm cuff of mucosa beyond the gingiva. The incision is carried into the muscle and then downward to the periosteum. This leaves a flap of mucosa and muscle attached to the dentoalveolus to facilitate wound closure. The periosteum is then elevated to deglove the symphysis. Laterally, the elevation is extended to expose the neurovascular bundle as it exits the foramen. The geniohyoid muscles are left attached to the bone. The osteotomy line is marked 3 to 4 mm below the apices of the cuspids and extends laterally below the mental foramen. The horizontal osteotomy is completed through both the labial and lingual cortices. By varying the angle of the cut it is possible either to increase or decrease the lower third facial height as well as advance the pogonion. The bone is then advanced the desired distance and stabilized with wires or rigid fixation plates. The incision is closed in two layers (Fig. 5).

Reduction Genioplasty

A reduction genioplasty can be designed to reduce the chin in either the vertical or anteroposterior direction, or a combination of both. The operation is determined by the soft tissue profile analysis. To reduce the chin in an anteroposterior direction, an osteotomy similar to that for augmentation is made, and the bone is moved posteriorly the desired distance and fixed with lag screw technique. To reduce the chin in a vertical direction, the transverse osteotomy is made, and the inferior segment left attached to the geniohyoid muscles. The amount of bone to be removed is measured along the intact symphysis and then removed. The inferior segment is then moved superiorly and fixed with screws. The symphysis should not be degloved and bone removed inferiorly, as this leads to distortion and malposition of the overlying soft tissue.

SUGGESTED READING

Holdaway RA. A soft tissue cephalometric analysis and its use in orthodontic treatment planning. Part I. Am J Orthod 1983; 84:1–28.

Legan HL, Burstone CJ. Soft tissue cephalometric analysis for orthognathic surgery. J Oral Maxillofac Surg 1980 38:744–751.

Lehman JA. Soft-tissue manifestations of aesthetic defects of the jaws: diagnosis and treatment. Clin Plast Surg 1987; 14:767–783.
Lehman JA, Tabbal N, Haas DG, Haas AJ. The combined surgical and orthodontic treatment of mandibular prognathism. Ann Plast Surg 1981; 7:458–463.
Park YC, Burstone CJ. Soft tissue profile—fallacies of hard tissue standards in treatment planning. Am J Orthod 1986; 90:52–62.
Worms FW, Isaacson RJ, Speidel TM. Surgical orthodontic treatment planning: profile analysis and mandibular surgery. Angle Orthod 1976; 46:1–25.

MAXILLARY OSTEOTOMIES

GREGORY S. LA TRENTA, M.D.
BARRY ZIDE, M.D., D.M.D.

Maxillary (Le Fort) osteotomies are the cornerstones for treatment of skeletal maxillary excess and deficiency states. These osteotomies differ in their treatment and effect on the nose, zygomas, orbits, and teeth (Fig. 1, A to C). The lower maxillary osteotomy (Le Fort I) extends transversely from the piriform apertures. The cuts occur at least 5 mm above the level of the dental roots, backward to the pterygomaxillary groove, thereby separating the maxillary tuberosity from the pterygoid plates. The "pyramidal" naso-orbital maxillary osteotomy (Le Fort II) begins at the nasofrontal angle and extends to the posterior lacrimal crest down the medial wall of the orbit to the orbital floor, through the orbital rim medial to the infraorbital foramen, obliquely below the zygomatic process of the maxilla toward the pterygomaxillary junction. The craniofacial disjunction, or Le Fort III *subcranial* osteotomy, also begins at the nasofrontal angle and extends behind the posterior lacrimal crest on the medial wall of the orbit, then through the orbital floor into the inferior orbital fissure. The osteotomy then extends across the fissure, thus encompassing the entire zygomatic complex at the sphenozygomatic interface to the frontozygomatic junction, transversely above the frontozygomatic suture, then vertically through the arch anterior to the temporozygomatic suture. The osteotomy is completed by connecting the inferior orbital fissure to the pterygomaxillary disjunction osteotomy. As in the Le Fort II, an osteotome must sever the posterior portion of the nasal septum for completion.

In general, the Le Fort III osteotomy tends to advance and downwardly displace the nose, the lower orbits, and the maxilla, in addition to correcting any class III malocclusion (with or without open bite). It can be combined, albeit rarely, with a Le Fort I osteotomy, if a class I occlusion exists. The Le Fort II osteotomy advances and downwardly displaces the nose and maxilla, in addition to correcting any class III malocclusion. A Le Fort I osteotomy, the most versatile and commonly performed osteotomy, is capable of advancing, recessing, downwardly or upwardly displacing, and rotating the tooth bearing segment of the maxilla. As with other Le Fort osteotomies, the Le Fort I may be combined with surgical procedures on the mandible. Unlike the Le Fort II and III osteotomies however, the Le Fort I osseous unit may be segmented as necessary to correct transverse or protrusive problems.

Le Fort I

The Le Fort I unit may be impacted, retruded, downfractured, advanced or rotated depending on the problem (Fig. 2). Segmentation of the lower maxilla may correct transverse or protrusive problems as well. The stability of each type of movement varies. Maxillary excess, or "long face syndrome" is characterized by a gummy smile with or without an anterior open bite. Associated stigmata include lip incompetence, narrow alar bases, prominent nose, and recessed chin. The chin muscles tend to overwork in compensating for the excessive labial gap by chronically trying to close the lips. Excessive incisor show at rest (greater than 3.5 mm in males, greater than 5.0 in females), although always present, does not necessarily occur with a gummy smile. The surgeon must be cautious to treat only the latter or an apparently "edentulous" postoperative result may ensue. Superior maxillary repositioning impaction is the preferred correction of this syndrome. The indication for simultaneous augmentation genioplasty depends upon the degree of rotory movement of the mandible in correcting chin recession (Fig. 3). When a marked class II malocclusion exists, simultaneous mandibular advancement may also be necessary (with or without chin work). In addition, the surgeon must assess the nasal passages preoperatively as maxillary elevations may reduce the airways. We frequently reduce turbinate bulk as part of this procedure.

Vertical maxillary deficiency, or "short face syndrome," in the absence of associated nasal, zygomatic, and orbital deformities occurs infrequently. In the absence of cleft lip and palate deformities, patients are usually noted to have a square, protruding jaw with an everted lower lip. The patient commonly displays a deep labiomental fold and accentuated nasolabial folds. There is minimal or no incisor showing, even with smiling. Le Fort I osteotomy with inferior displacement and interpositional bone grafting with or without lower jaw surgery is the preferred correction. As this procedure tends to be unstable due to bone graft resorption, adjunctive methods of fixation are required. Plate fixation with screws or pinning, which spans from splint to zygomatic buttress, is used to reduce mandibular pounding on the graft. Some surgeons have mixed *nonresorbing* material, namely, hydroxyapatite, with the bone to reduce this tendency toward graft resorption.

Setback of the anterior or entire Le Fort I segment

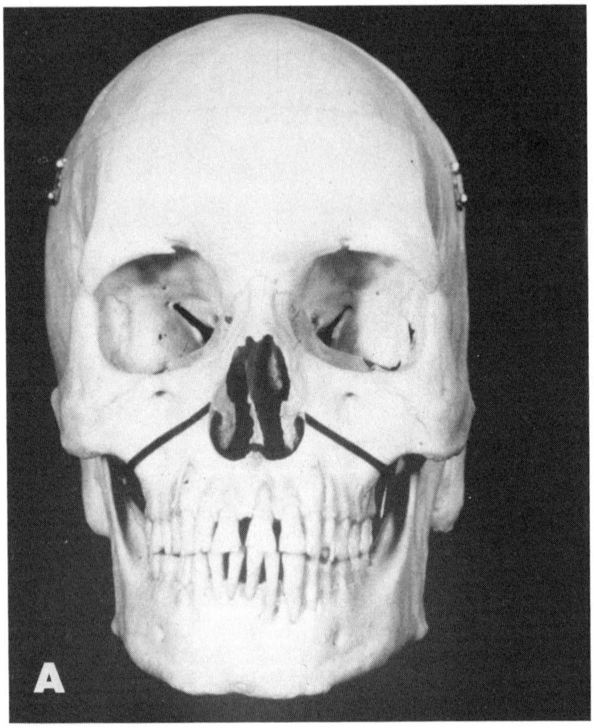

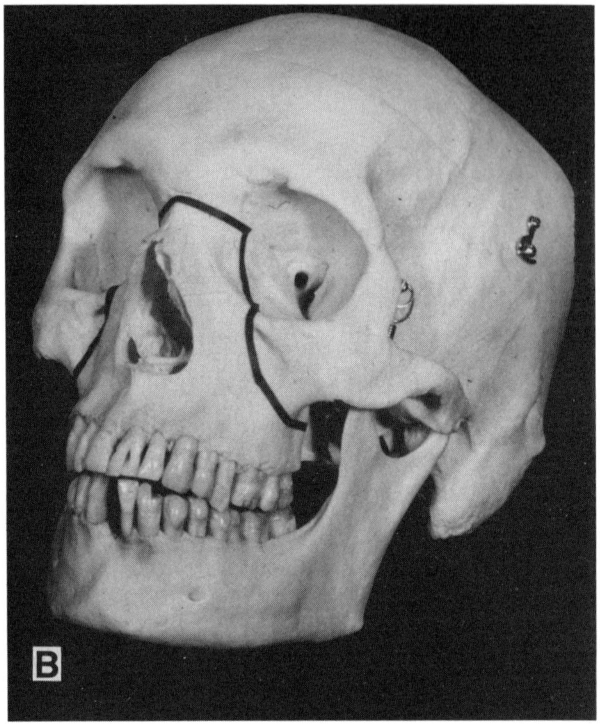

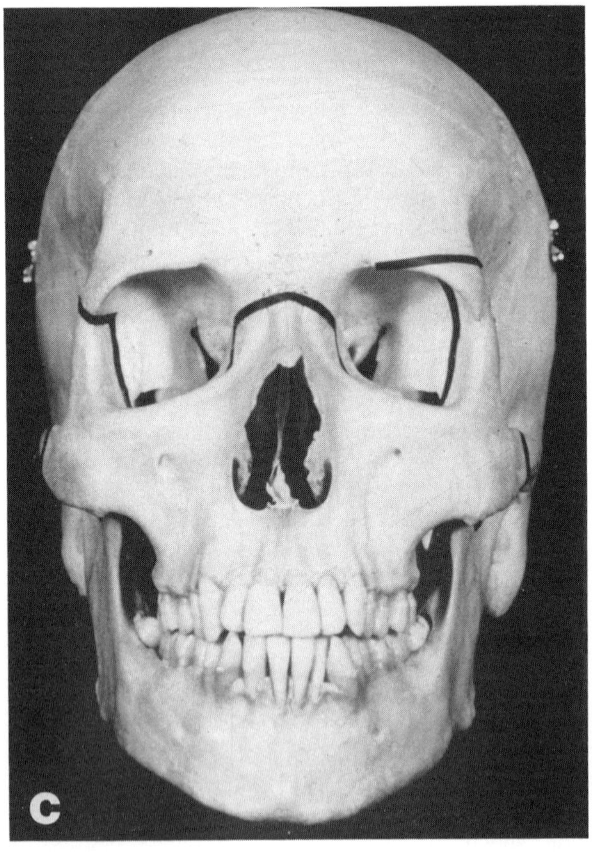

Figure 1 *A*, Le Fort I osteotomy. The osteotomies course across the maxillary face. This lower segment is freed from the pterygoid plates and mobilized as required. *B*, Le Fort II osteotomy. This "pyramidal" osteotomy is always advanced without or with downrotation to lengthen the nose or close an anterior open bite. The cheek bones are left alone. *C*, Le Fort III osteotomy. This total maxillary disjunction is used primarily to correct syndromal midface deficiency. As noted, the upper lateral orbital rim cuts may vary to advance (left) or not advance (right) the upper lateral brow.

is used primarily for situations when marked dental procumbency is present. Occasionally, the occlusal plane may require leveling. This opens the nasolabial angle.

Surgical advancement of the Le Fort I segment corrects certain class III malocclusions when maxillary hypoplasia is present. This procedure is less stable with the greater advancements. It tends to flare the alar bases, fill out the piriform areas, and thin the upper lip slightly.

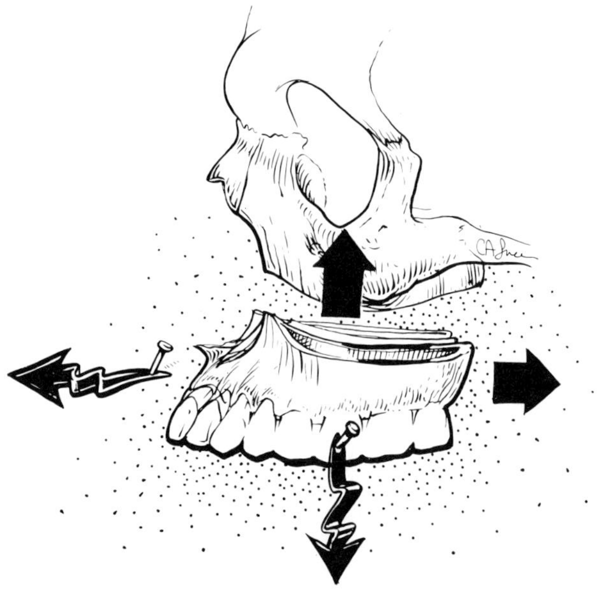

Figure 2 Le Fort I stability. Movements upward or backward tend to be stable (solid arrows) while movements downward and forward may require special treatment to reduce relapse. Of course, the amount of postoperative regression depends on many factors, e.g., clefting, amount of movement, prior surgery, etc.

Le Fort II

Le Fort II maxillary osteotomy is not discussed in depth due to its infrequent application. Suffice it to say, however, the Le Fort II advances the occlusal plane, midface, and nose, while leaving the malar bones in situ. It is used when the midface is retruded, but the cheekbones are sufficiently prominent. Certain syndromes, e.g., Binder's syndrome or nasomaxillary hypoplasia, may benefit from this procedure.

Le Fort III

The usual patient who would have this procedure suffers such craniofacial syndromes as Apert's, Pfeiffer's, or Crouzon's disease (Fig. 4). Certain atypical Tessier facial clefts or severe post-traumatic deformities might also receive this procedure. These syndromes are associated with severe maxillary micropathies as well as naso-orbital and zygomatic retrusion. Nasofrontal flatness, exorbitism, and malar flatness are the presenting facial complaints.

Preferred Approach to Maxillary Dentofacial Deformities

All patients receive cephalograms, photographs, dental study models, and clinical evaluations by the plastic surgeon and the orthodontist. The diagnostic cephalometric analysis is used only to assist formulation of the treatment plan; it does not dictate the procedure or the orthodontic therapy, which usually precedes maxillary osteotomy. Elimination of active peridontal disease and caries control are performed preoperatively to reduce postoperative tooth movement and infection. Professional preoperative photographs are taken by protocol including occlusal and smiling views. The surgeon and orthodontist confer after complete data are obtained. Occlusal splint fabrication occurs according to the preoperative mock surgery. When two-jaw surgery is required, in which both the maxilla and mandible are cut, an intermediate splint is required after the first jaw is mobilized. The final splint is then provided following stabilization of the maxilla.

Le Fort I

After nasotracheal intubation, the maxillary vestibule is infiltrated with an appropriate amount of 0.5 percent Xylocaine with 1:200,000 epinephrine. A transverse incision is made through the alveolar mucosa in the labial sulcus. The incision should not go much beyond the distal first molars to reduce the fat pad herniation into the field. The entire anterolateral face of the maxilla is exposed from the piriform aperture to the infraorbital rim, and posteriorly to the pterygomaxillary groove. A Lempert square-ended mastoid periosteal elevator works well for this part of the procedure. The infraorbital nerves are preserved. Nasalis muscles and mucoperiosteum are then dissected off the anterior nasal spine and anterior alveolus. The vomer and septum are isolated anteriorly. Using a round ended periosteal elevator, the nasal floor is cleared along with the lower lateral walls of both sides of the nose. The septum is dislocated from the vomer along its full length. Vertical scoring lines are made on the maxillary face with a fine saw or drill. These lines should be long enough as not to be removed with the osteotomy.

The Le Fort I transverse osteotomy is then begun with the sagittal or reciprocating saw at least 5 mm above the canine roots (as approximately measured on Panorex). With the aid of calipers, the exact height of the osteotomy is determined. The osteotomy, if necessary, is marked as determined from the preoperative surgical prediction tracing, beginning at the piriform aperture medially. The saw is used to cut the osteotomies from the piriform rims to the lower buttress areas.

To complete the anterolateral osteotomy, two techniques work well. The reciprocating saw may be placed within the maxillary sinus to complete the procedure from inside out, or the osteotome may be used to complete the bony cut from the buccal aspect toward the pterygoid plates. The mucoperiosteum is undermined below the inferior turbinates along the lateral nasal walls. A small osteotome is then tapped along this route for a distance of about 3 cm. This distance is chosen because haphazard osteotomy beyond this point may cause bleeding from the greater palatine vessels. It is much easier to clamp these under direct vision after the down fracture.

Bilateral greater palatine vessel transsection with cauterization does not reduce the segment's viability if the palatal mucosa is intact. Vertical pterygomaxillary dis-

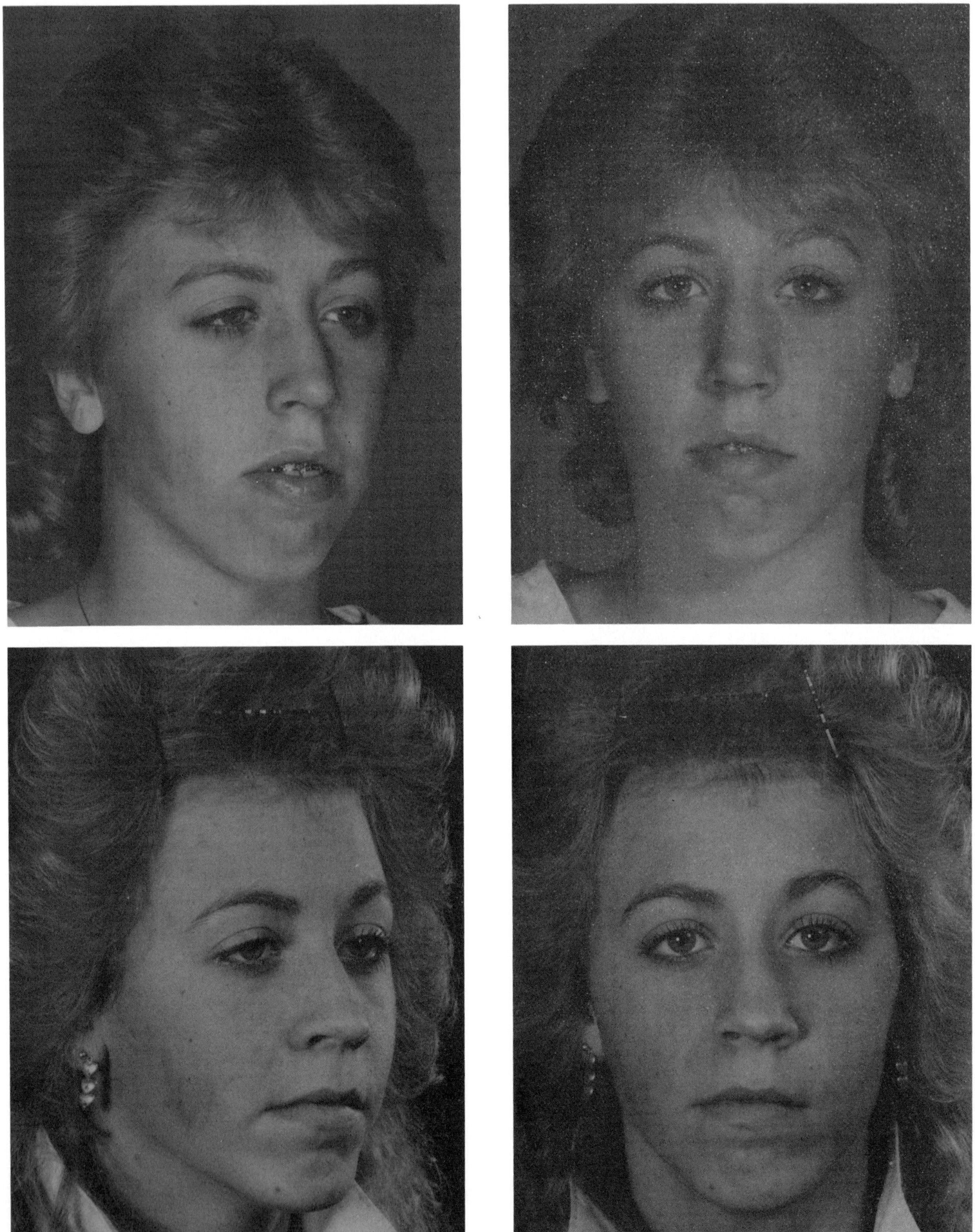

Figure 3 Le Fort I maxillary impaction. This patient had long face syndrome. The procedure consisted of elevation of the lower maxilla with simultaneous advancement osteotomy at the symphysis.

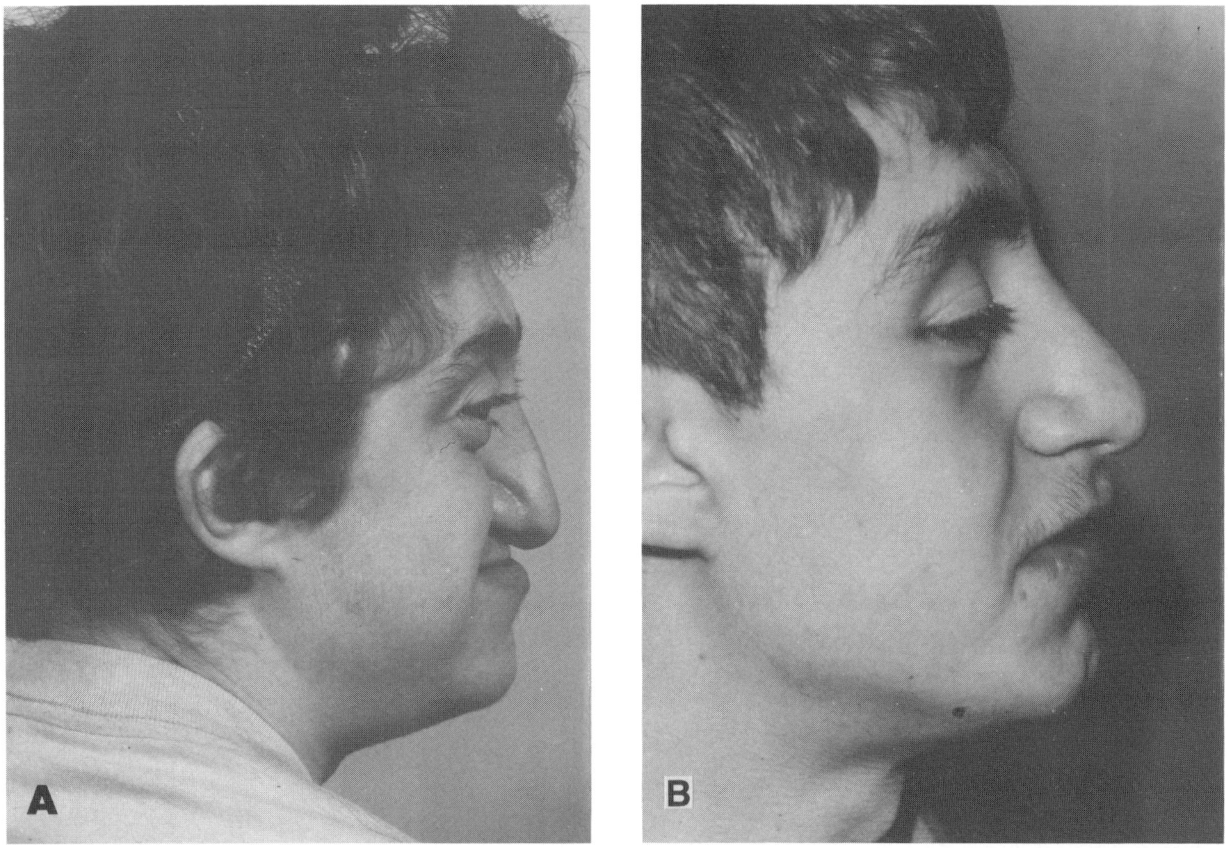

Figure 4 Le Fort III. This patient with Crouzon's disease underwent Le Fort III osteotomy in his teens. At age 19, his facial appearance is stable and greatly improved.

junction is performed bilaterally with a curved Kawamoto osteotome at the pterygomaxillary junction. The position of the osteotomy should be on the lower 8 to 15 mm of the pterygomaxillary groove (Fig. 5). Prior to down fracture, all osteotomies are checked. Down fracture may then be performed manually with inferiorly directed force using the thumbs placed at the incisor edge. If down fracture is difficult, the pterygomaxillary osteotomy is usually incomplete and the curved osteotome is reinserted and applied. If bleeding is encountered posteriorly at this time, the greater palatine vessels can usually be clamped in their canals with a tonsil clamp and either electrocoagulated or hemoclipped. The maxilla is rocked and loosened so that easy mobility is achieved.

The above discussion pertains to the simple Le Fort I procedure used for advancement or retrusion. For retrusion, the third molars and associated bone may be removed. Some surgeons favor the third molar area for the posterior osteotomy sites. In certain cases, segmental osteotomies are done to allow transverse widening or anterior segment setback. When the maxilla is elevated, however, attention is directed to the overall lower maxillary shape. If the lower maxilla is narrow and must be moved superiorly more than 5 to 6 mm, the surgeon should be wary of telescoping the lower segment into the upper maxilla. For this reason, osteotomy is only performed 2 ½ cm from the piriform aperture and not from

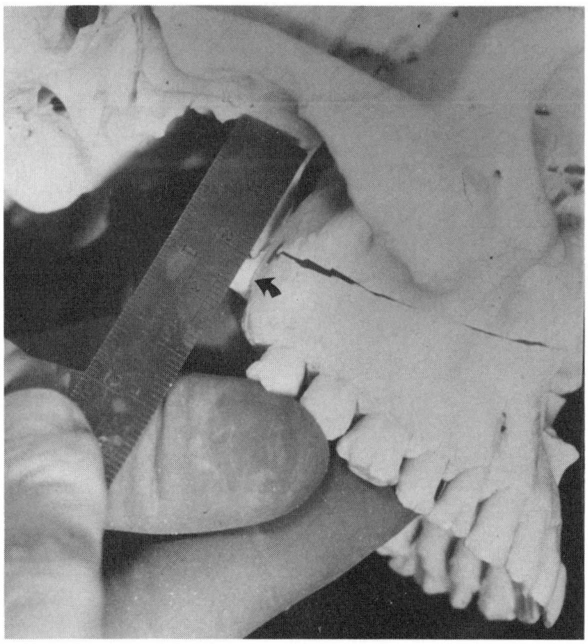

Figure 5 Pterygopalatine disjunction. Separation of the palate from the pterygoid plates is best done in the lower 10 cm of the pterygomaxillary groove (arrow). Osteotomies at this level are at least 15 mm below the region of the internal maxillary artery.

the buttress prior to down fracture. Any additional bone removal is done piecemeal to avoid telescoping, which can occur at the buttresses. Only grooves may be required at the buttresses.

Further ostectomy, if needed, is then carried out manually with a rongeur or air-driven burr. The vomer is easily taken down with a large burr to prevent septal deviation with elevation. Septal cartilage may be trimmed with a Foman's scissors. The lateral nasal walls, i.e., medial maxillary sinus walls, are resected by rongeur as required. The anterior nasal spine and some of the piriform aperture may require removal to enlarge the airway. Inferior turbinate removal may also be indicated. A longitudinal cut in the nasal mucosa will expose the offending turbinates. As much turbinate as required (often two-thirds) may be removed. The mucosa is closed with a 4–0 running chromic gut suture. The occlusal splint is then secured to the maxillary teeth and the mandible is autorotated into the splint, with care taken not to dislocate the condyles. If necessary, the previously started sagittal split osteotomy of the mandible may be completed after setting maxillary position firmly. If a symphyseal genioplasty is required, it should be completed prior to intermaxillary fixation (IMF) to prevent wire loosening, which occurs with sawing while in IMF. Interosseous wires or rigid internal fixation plates may be placed depending on the amount of movement and the tendency to relapse.

A nasogastric tube is always inserted prior to IMF, which is performed with No. 26 surgical steel wire.

Fixation

Superior approximating wires (circumzygomatic or from the infraorbital rims) are utilized in cases where internal fixation plates have not been chosen. Plates are used primarily in cases of high relapse potential, although they may be used in all cases. When wires are used, they are secured to loops on the occlusal splint. Anterior suspension from the infraorbital rim tends not to displace maxillary advancement posteriorly as the pull is primarily vertical. Twenty-four to twenty-six gauge steel wires are tightened after twisting down the interosseous wires. The interosseous wires may in some cases encompass bone grafts and/or alloplast if down fracture for short face has been performed. As previously stated, down fracture with interposition bone grafting may result in significant relapse unless plate fixation is applied. All wires are manually stretched prior to their use to minimize postoperative loosening. Elastics may be used adjunctively with wires to hold the IMF and continued for physiotherapy after IMF is removed. In general, IMF is continued for 5 to 6 weeks for stable procedures and longer (6 to 10 weeks) if the stability is more risky.

Alternate fixation with rigid internal fixation miniplates, especially with inferior maxillary positioning, has several advantages. In addition to compression osteosynthesis and enhanced three-dimensional precision fixation, IMF can usually be released very early postoperatively. Our orthodontist feels more comfortable with at least 2 weeks of intermaxillary fixation to allow for postoperative settling, although it may be unnecessary.

The disadvantages of plates are that they require a good bone stock for placement, excellent passive fit prior to fixation, and removal is recommended at 1 year. In general, with the Le Fort I osteotomy, two inverted 45 degree miniplates are applied at each anterior and posterior buttress bilaterally, making certain not to enter the tooth roots, especially anteriorly.

Relapse

Anteroposterior. Anteroposterior relapse may be reduced with two-jaw surgery if the overall amount of movement exceeds 12 mm. Lesser movements tend to relapse less. In contrast, patients with maxillary hypoplasia, e.g., cleft patients, requiring more than 7 mm anterior movement for a class III malocclusion tend to be unstable. When the anterior or entire lower maxilla is set back, relapse tends to be minimal as long as the surgical cuts are exact and the splint fits well. The maxilla should heal with a bony union.

Vertical. Inadequate elevation of the tooth-bearing segment occurs with improper planning or insufficient ostectomy. Excessive superior repositioning of the anterior maxilla, i.e., telescoping, may happen with injudicious planning or ostectomy with catastrophic results. The teeth may not show during smiling. The surgeon should always err on the conservative side, especially in older patients whose lips tend to sag. Although the time for fixation may be reduced to zero with plates, we tend to adhere to short fixation times when plates are used. When wires alone are used after elevation, the patient may be taken out of IMF at 4 weeks. With the splint left in, the patient's occlusion is then cautiously directed by the orthodontist for the next few weeks.

Down fracture cases with inferior maxillary repositioning and bone grafts are usually left in intermaxillary

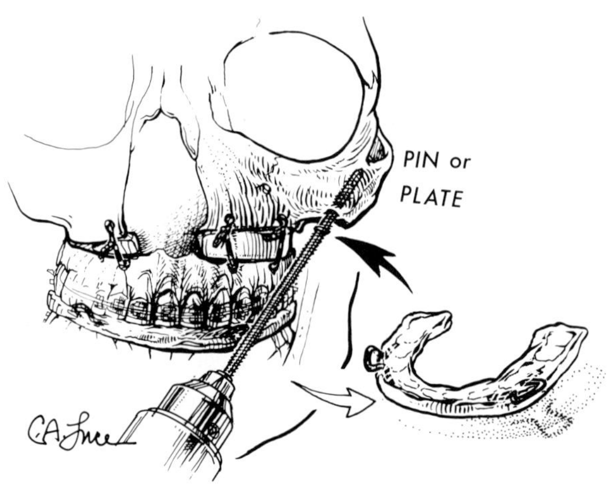

Figure 6 Down fracture cases are best secured by pinning or plating. A Steinmann pin burred into the buttress and "acrylic-wired" to the splint reduces the relentless pounding from the mandible. Alternatively, Luhr or Champy plates may be similarly used.

fixation for 8 to 12 weeks to reduce the tendency for bony resorption. Two methods of fixation have been used. Steinman pins may be driven into the buttresses and secured to the splint (Fig. 6), or internal plate fixation. Down fracture with bone graft interposition is commonly used for hemifacial microsomia and short face cases.

Effects

Risk–Benefit of Le Fort I. Risk-benefit ratio can be analyzed according to anatomy. In the nose, vertical impaction widens the alar base and raises the tip slightly, thus giving more supratip break. The nasolabial angle may be opened slightly but the amount varies. The effect of removing or leaving the anterior nasal spine has never been determined exactly. These changes would obviously benefit the patient with a narrow nose, minimal hump, and plunging tip, but would be "hazardous" to patients with a broadbased nose. When the maxilla is advanced, the lip tends to move forward slightly less, as some thinning is noted. Impactions and retrusive maxillary movements tend to allow the lip to look fuller in contrast. For each posterior 1 mm movement, the lip tends to drop 0.5 mm. Midline mucosal V-Y advancement may be helpful in situations where more central lip tubercle is desired.

SUGGESTED READING

Bell WH, Proffitt WR, White RP. Surgical correction of dentofacial deformities. Philadelphia: WB Saunders, 1980.

Epker BN, Fish LC. Dentofacial deformities. St. Louis: CV Mosby, 1986.

Epker BN, Turvey TA, Fish LC. Indications for simultaneous mobilization of the maxilla and mandible for correction of dentofacial deformities. Oral Surg 1982; 54:369.

MALIGNANT DISEASE

EVALUATION OF THE PATIENT WITH HEAD AND NECK CANCER

THOMAS A. MUSTOE, M.D.

The evaluation of a patient with head and neck malignancy has evolved over the last 10 years with new additions in technology; but the basic principle of a thorough, careful physical examination of the head and neck remains as the cornerstone. This chapter discusses what is involved in the initial careful head and neck exam; the value of office biopsies, both direct and skinny needle; the cost-effective approach to radiologic work-up; and, finally, the approach to endoscopy in the proper evaluation of the patient prior to surgical treatment.

Most of the discussion centers on the patient with squamous cell carcinoma of the upper aerodigestive tract. Statistically, these are by far the most common malignancies of the head and neck excluding skin tumors. The unknown primary lesion that presents as a mass in the neck is considered in some detail. Skin tumors are excluded from this discussion.

SALIVARY GLAND TUMORS

In the patient who presents with a parotid swelling, the first consideration is whether the swelling is most consistent with tumor, an obstructed gland secondary to sialolithiasis, an inflammatory process, or diffuse swelling secondary to Sjögren's syndrome. Examination and history usually delineate quite easily the differences between these etiologies. An obstructed gland should fluctuate in size in relation to meals, with post prandial swelling. Diffuse swelling of the gland is evident on physical examination and is almost certainly not due to tumor. Sjögren's syndrome is the most common cause of diffuse parotid swelling.

If an obstructed gland is suspected, palpation of the gland, with visualization of Stensen's duct simultaneously, should reveal whether or not saliva is being produced and if so, whether it is clear or not. If there is significant suspicion of obstruction, a sialogram is the next diagnostic step. However, in the absence of suspected obstruction or inflammatory disease of the parotid gland, a sialogram is generally unnecessary.

In a patient with a discrete mass in the parotid gland with the mass presenting externally in the cheek, the next appropriate diagnostic step in the healthy individual is excisional biopsy, i.e., a superficial parotidectomy. Diagnostic roentgenography is not useful in the evaluation of a typical benign parotid mass that is clearly intraparotid because it can not differentiate between a superficial and a deep lobe tumor. The facial nerve divides the parotid into superficial and deep lobes, but this is an arbitrary rather than an anatomic segmentation: there is no fascial plane that can be demonstrated radiologically between the superficial and deep lobes. Therefore, it is impossible to tell whether a mass that is near the facial nerve is just underneath it, and thus pushing the nerve superficially, or is just over it, pushing the nerve deeply.

If there is a suspicion of malignancy, concern of parapharyngeal extension, or a mass in the tail which is difficult to distinguish from a cervical lymph node, then computed tomography (CT) scan is helpful. A CT scan with contrast can clearly differentiate whether a mass is intra- or extraparotid, which differentiation governs therapy. CT scan also helps confirm the suspicion of malignancy if the tumor is quite infiltrative, and defines extension for deep lobe tumor into the peripharyngeal space. At this time CT scans have largely supplanted the need for a sialogram. In an occasional patient a sialogram is performed to further delineate the parotid gland; however, I believe its role is limited.

The skinny needle biopsy is a consideration in an office diagnosis of parotid tumor. Although there have been multiple studies in the last several years that suggest relative accuracy of skinny needle biopsy, parotid salivary gland tumors remain difficult to read pathologically, even on permanent section, and cytology does not have sufficient accuracy. Furthermore, there is significant variation in histology from point to point in a tumor, such that a random sample that discloses pleomorphic adenoma can not rule out a focus of malignancy elsewhere in the mass. Therefore, I believe that skinny needle biopsy for the salivary glands is not yet useful in the average patient. Such biopsies do have a potential role in the very ill patient in whom it would be desirable to avoid an operative procedure. In a tumor with a benign clinical course, a skinny needle biopsy that showed a benign tumor would reassure me to defer an operation on such a patient.

In physical examination of patients with submandibular masses, it is very difficult to distinguish a submandibular tumor from a submandibular lymph node. In addition, sialolithiasis is much more common in the submandibular than the parotid gland, probably as a factor of anatomy. The submandibular gland lies below its orifice in the mouth, and, therefore, inspissation of salivary material is more likely. In patients with submandibular swelling, a sialogram is more useful than in those with parotid swelling and may delineate a submandibular mass from an extraglandular mass. A CT scan may also do this, but it can be quite difficult on CT scan to distinguish between a node adherent to the gland and the gland itself. Again, negative or benign skinny needle biopsies for submandibular gland tumors should not be relied upon in evaluation.

MALIGNANCY OF THE UPPER AERODIGESTIVE TRACT

In evaluation of the patient with malignancy of the upper aerodigestive tract, it is worthwhile to note that the overwhelming predisposing factors are a combination of smoking with the synergistic effects of alcohol intake. This results in a field cancerization defect such that a patient with malignancy in one site in the head and neck is at high risk for a second primary, either synchronously or asynchronously. For this reason, it is vital for a patient with a small tongue carcinoma, for example, to have a thorough examination of the entire head and neck, including the nasopharynx, hypopharynx, and larynx, as well as the remainder of the oral cavity and neck. Currently, the risk of a synchronous second primary at the time of presentation of the regional tumor is as high as 3 to 7 percent and this rises to 20 to 25 percent asynchronous primaries in patients followed over several years. These statistics include tumors of the esophagus and lung and, therefore, these areas need to be evaluated as well.

To return to the patient with a small early carcinoma of the tongue, my approach in the office would be to do a thorough inspection of the oral cavity including buccal sulci, entire jaw and teeth, the floor of mouth, tongue, retromolar trigone, and oropharynx. I generally find a head mirror or headlight useful to free up both hands and I use two throat sticks to examine the region thoroughly. The region behind the anterior tonsillar pillar is searched with special care, particularly in a patient with an unknown primary, because early carcinomas can present in this area and be easily missed.

I then use a head mirror (or headlight) and laryngeal and nasopharyngeal mirrors to examine the nasopharynx, hypopharynx, and larynx. If the patient has a strong gag reflex and I cannot get an adequate view, I use a fiberoptic laryngoscope. These are now available with external diameter as small as 2.3 mm and can easily be passed through the nose without any anesthesia, except perhaps some topical spray. They give even the novice an extremely good view of the nasopharynx and larynx and obviate somewhat the need for a skillful indirect examination. I also routinely use a nasal speculum to examine both nares in order to rule out sinus tumor, particularly in a patient with an unknown primary. I also examine the ears to rule out serous otitis as a potential complication of nasopharyngeal carcinoma in particular.

If the patient with tongue cancer has not had a tissue diagnosis, a biopsy can be easily obtained in the office with a small amount of local anesthesia and small forceps. Alternatively, if the patient has a mass that is less suitable for office biopsy, or if there is any question at all of staging, I usually schedule panendoscopy to include direct laryngoscopy, esophagoscopy, and, where appropriate, fiberoptic bronchoscopy.

Most patients on whom we plan to operate for malignancy of the aeordigestive tract receive a staging panendoscopy prior to surgery. Direct laryngoscopy provides an optimal view of the larynx. Examination of the tongue and neck by manual palpation is facilitated with maximum relaxation under anesthesia. This examination is useful for staging purposes because the patient can be examined without pain and the tumor mapped meticulously. In addition, if I believe the patient has stage III or IV disease and is a candidate for preoperative chemotherapy, I routinely tattoo the planned surgical margins with India ink. Therefore, if the tumor responds well to chemotherapy, I do not compromise on my margins but go back later and resect the tumor precisely as I would have done before. In addition, rigid esophagoscopy, which is very sensitive, is performed in order to rule out cervical esophageal tumor. While barium swallows are also useful, even good examinations can miss small cervical esophageal tumors. Rigid esophagoscopy, therefore, supplants the need for routine barium swallow in ruling out a second primary and, in addition, is more accurate for examination of the upper cervical esophagus. Bronchoscopy is not necessary in the face of a negative or clear routine chest x-ray study. However, with a potential mass revealed on the chest x-ray film, I perform fiberoptic bronchoscopy with bronchial washings of the appropriate areas. If a bronchial lesion is seen, a brushing of the lesion can be performed as well. Coordination with a thoracic surgeon should be done in a patient with a possible lung carcinoma, pulmonary metastasis, or when the head and neck surgeon lacks significant bronchoscopy experience.

The foremost reason for endoscopy is to stage the lesion accurately. Although CT scan can be very helpful in documenting soft tissue spread, direct palpation of a tongue carcinoma, to define its extent and approximate invasion, is critical. It also finds the extent of a tumor in the posterior oral cavity and its invasion of the neck. Accurate examinations cannot generally be carried out in a conscious patient because of the pain involved. Finally, any additional masses can be biopsied at the time of the panendoscopy.

NECK MASS WITHOUT OBVIOUS PRIMARY LESION

A special situation is the evaluation of a patient found, on thorough head and neck examination, to have a neck mass without an obvious primary (Fig. 1). In a patient with a mass in the supraclavicular triangle, the tumor is most likely a metastasis from a primary malignancy be-

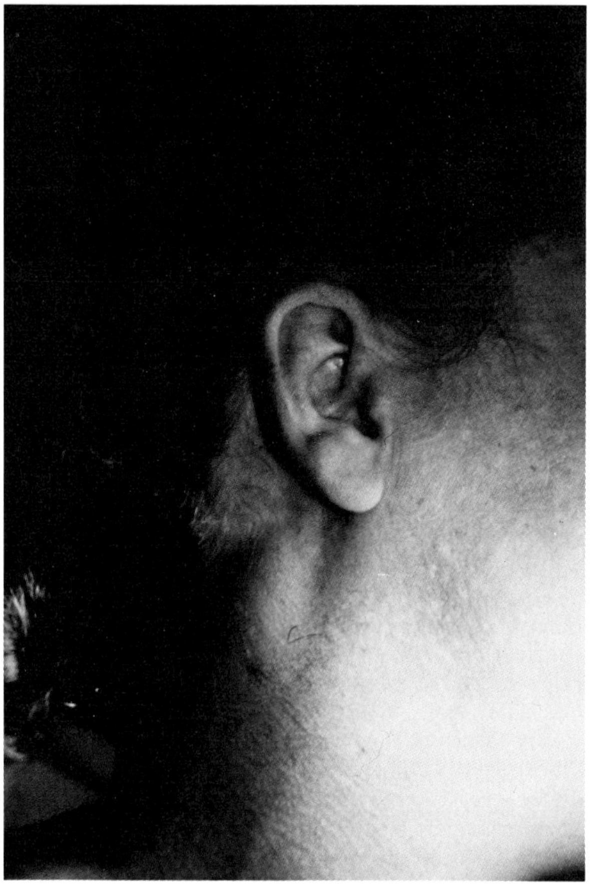

Figure 1 Patient with neck mass of 3 months' duration without visible primary on thorough examination. Location in posterior triangle raises suspicion of nasopharyngeal carcinoma.

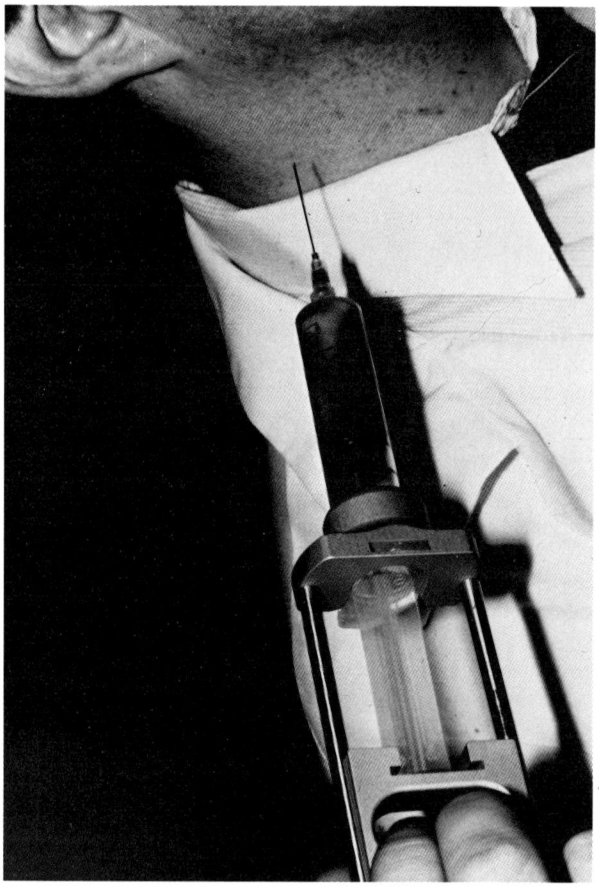

Figure 2 Needle aspiration cytology performed in the office on initial examination.

low the clavicles. Such a patient already has systemic disease, and therefore the foremost consideration should be to obtain a diagnosis. In these patients, I proceed directly to an open lymph node biopsy. In a patient with masses in the upper portion of the neck, in a nonsmoker under the age of 40, or in a patient with lymphadenopathy persistent beyond 2 to 3 months, I believe the most appropriate measure is to do an open neck biopsy. There is a significant chance that if the tumor is malignant, it would represent a lymphoma, and needle biopsies are not helpful in this situation. If the mass is in the region of the thyroid, it should be treated presumptively as a thyroid tumor and should be worked up accordingly with needle biopsy, scan, and thyroid functions.

When the patient is over the age of 40, or younger with a significant smoking history, and has a persistent neck mass that appears to be noninflammatory in origin, skinny needle biopsies can be quite helpful. These are performed with a 20-cc syringe and a 22-gauge needle (Figs. 2 and 3). A pistol grip holder for the syringe to allow one to hold the syringe with one hand and palpate and fix the mass with the other, makes this somewhat easier. The needle is passed into the mass, and suction is placed on the syringe. Several passes are made through the tumor, keeping the vacuum in the syringe. Before the needle is removed from the skin, the vacuum is released that keeps the aspirated material in the needle itself. This material is then spread onto a slide, fixed with alcohol, and sent for cytology. The results can often be obtained the same day from an experienced cytology laboratory. Squamous cell carcinoma can usually be read quite well from aspiration cytology; and this may be the most cost-effective way to obtain a rapid diagnosis of a neck mass.

If the tumor is squamous cell carcinoma, then a very careful work-up needs to be carried out for a primary in the head and neck. Panendoscopy would be performed to include selected "random" biopsies of the nasopharynx because of the well-known incidence of submucosal nasopharyngeal tumors with mucosal abnormalities that can first present as neck node metastases. Other areas to be examined carefully are the tonsillar fossa, the base of the tongue, and the piriform sinuses. Any even mildly suspicious lesions in these areas should be biopsied. Finally, when neither panendoscopy nor skinny needle biopsy have disclosed a diagnosis, it is appropriate to do an open neck biopsy. Prior to panendoscopy, a CT scan of the en-

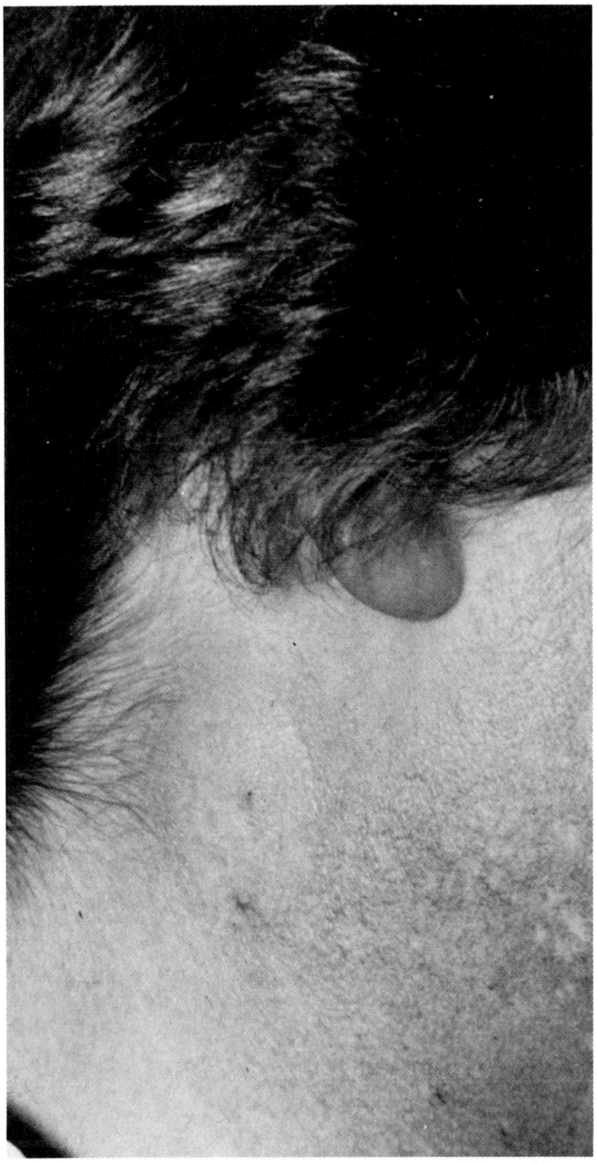

Figure 3 Needle puncture site from needle biopsy. There are no recorded cases of tumor tracking with the use of a skinny needle (22 gauge). The diagnosis of malignancy was obtained that day.

tire head and neck, from the nasopharynx to the clavicle, should be carried out. Particular attention should be paid to the nasopharynx and, of course, the sinuses also are displayed on this examination. I believe that a CT scan in this situation is the most cost-effective test, and essentially obviates the need for other radiologic diagnostic methods. If there is suspicion that the mass may be thyroid in origin, a thyroid scan is helpful. In general, for head and neck masses, I believe that CT scan has largely supplanted all other radiologic maneuvers. There is occasional need for a barium swallow, and a straight lateral of the neck can be helpful in some situations. If a CT scan is obtained, it should disclose all the information necessary to rule out a sinus tumor; and, in general, tomograms or laryngeal fluoroscopy do not add additional information. In a tumor where there is suspicion of jaw involvement, a panorex is useful to define dental relationships.

The role of magnetic resonance imaging (MRI) is still being defined for head and neck tumors. MRI can help differentiate soft tissue densities that can not be distinguished on a CT scan, but MRI resolution is still significantly less than that of CT scans. A potential use for MRI would be evaluation of a mass that was felt to be intraparotid but was not well-defined on CT scan.

SUGGESTED READING

Chretien PB, Johns ME, Shedd DP, Strong EW, Ward PH, eds. Head and neck cancer. Vol 1. Toronto: BC Decker, 1985: 87, 130, 214, 279.

Jesse RH. General considerations. In: Suen JY, Myers EN, eds. Cancer of the head and neck. New York: Churchill Livingstone, 1981:1.

Lingemann RE, Singer MI. Evaluation of the patient with head and neck cancer. In: Suen JY, Myers EN, eds. Cancer of the head and neck. New York: Churchill Livingstone, 1981:12.

McGregor I. Cancer of the face and mouth. New York: Churchill Livingstone, 1986:382.

Million RR, Cassissi NJ. Management of head and neck cancer. A multidisciplinary approach. Philadelphia: JB Lippincott, 1984.

Montgomery WW. Surgery of the upper respiratory system. Vol 2. Philadelphia: Lea & Febiger, 1973.

Pernkopf E. Atlas of topographical and applied human anatomy. Vol 1. Ferner H, ed. Baltimore: Urban & Schwarzenberg, 1980.

SURGICAL TREATMENT OF CANCER IN THE NECK

DAVID L. LARSON, M.D.

The most common surgical disease of the neck is metastatic squamous carcinoma from the oral cavity or upper aerodigestive tract. When a regional deposit of tumor presents itself as a neck mass, the patient's survival is reduced by one-half. Therefore, it is vital that the surgeon have a clear, logical understanding of the treatment of cancer in the neck. This will necessarily include answers to the following questions: When should I do an elective neck dissection? What type of neck dissection is appropriate—radical, modified, or functional? How should radiation therapy be incorporated into the treatment plan, if at all? These and other questions will be addressed in this chapter.

MASS IN THE NECK

When confronted with a mass in the neck, it is important to do a thorough examination of the oral cavity, larynx, hypopharynx, and the remainder of the neck to search for a primary tumor and any other neck disease. If the mass is low in the neck (near the clavicle), a workup should include diagnostic studies of the gastrointestinal and urinary tracts. Most masses are in the anterior and lateral areas of the neck. Following a good history and physical examination, diagnostic studies should include a chest roentgenogram (looking for a primary tumor), esophagram, thyroid scan, soft tissue lateral of the neck, and routine blood studies (including liver function and the human immunodeficiency virus [HIV] tests). Following review of these results, a fine needle aspiration is appropriate, providing no primary tumor has been seen. If the aspirate is positive for squamous cancer, a direct laryngoscopy is performed; this should be negative before proceeding to the neck dissection. If the aspirate suggests lymphoma or some other uncommon tumor, an open biopsy to remove the mass and some associated lymph nodes is performed to obtain the additional information necessary to proceed with appropriate treatment.

LYMPHATIC ANATOMY OF THE NECK

Although there are over 300 lymph nodes in the neck, only a few are of clinical significance to the surgeon. These can be grouped on either side of the neck according to their location (Fig. 1). These groups are chosen because they represent echelons of nodal drainage of primary tumors of the oral cavity, oropharynx, and hypopharynx. Knowledge of these lymphatic drainage echelons has been acquired by both clinical and pathologic evaluation of large numbers of patients who had previously untreated squamous carcinoma of the upper aerodigestive tract. It is vital that this information be kept in mind when viewing metastatic cancer in the neck as a surgical disease. This knowledge will allow the surgeon to make logical decisions when deciding on the type of neck dissection to use in a given clinical setting.

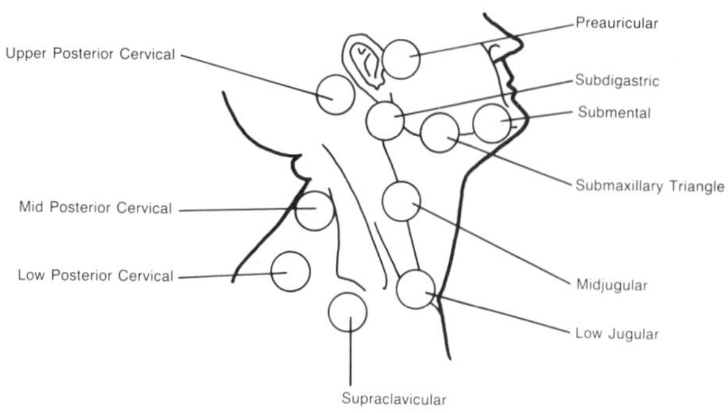

Figure 1 The names and locations of nodal groups that constitute the echelons of lymphatic drainage of squamous carcinoma of the upper aerodigestive tract.

The patient with oral cancer can be classified according to the TNM (Tumor, Node, Metastasis) schema of the American Joint Committee on Cancer (Table 1).

ELECTIVE NECK DISSECTION

As its name implies, elective neck dissection (END) is an option of the surgeon. The following examples of lip and tongue cancer demonstrate clinical application of END. Unless there are clinically positive nodes in the neck, there is no indication for elective neck dissection in lip cancer. This is primarily because the incidence of subclinical metastasis is so low (less than 10 percent) that, regardless of the size of the primary tumor, the yield from surgery does not justify the procedure. This clinical setting is in complete contradistinction to the small T_1 (up to 2 cm) or T_2 (2 to 4 cm) lesion of the floor of the mouth and mobile (anterior two-thirds) of the tongue. As

TABLE 1 TNM Clinical Staging of Oral Cancer

Tumor size
T_1–up to 2 cm
T_2–between 2 and 4 cm
T_3–greater than 4 cm
T_4–massive involvement of adjacent structures (bone, muscle, nerve)
Node status
N_0–clinically negative
N_1–one clinically positive node up to 3 cm
N_{2a}–clinically positive node greater than 3 cm, but less than 6 cm
N_{2b}–clinically positive nodes at multiple levels
N_{3a}–clinically positive node greater than 6 cm in size (usually a confluency of nodes)
N_{3b}–clinically positive nodes bilaterally, these are usually staged separately (e.g., N_{3b}, CN_1, N_{2b})
N_{3c}–clinically positive contralateral node **only** (extremely unusual)

the size of the primary lesion increases in size, the probability of microscopic foci of disease in the lymph nodes increases from 18 percent for a T_1 lesion to 35 percent for a T_2 lesion. Over half of all patients with larger lesions, T_3 and T_4, have these microscopic deposits even if they do not already have clinically positive neck nodes. Although the grade of the tumor does not have significant influence on nodal involvement, higher-grade tumors are less differentiated and usually should be viewed more aggressively. I feel that lymphadenectomy is in order when a tumor has greater than 20 percent chance of harboring microscopic disease in the regional lymph nodes. By removing the first and second echelon of nodal drainage of the primary tumor, the surgeon performs both a therapeutic and a diagnostic service and obtains valuable information regarding prognosis. If the nodes are all negative and a good margin is obtained around the primary tumor, the patient has received maximal treatment and carries a good prognosis. If the first echelon of nodes is positive and particularly if extracapsulary extension is present, adjunctive radiation is indicated. If there are multiple levels (first and second) of nodes involved, then postoperative radiation is essential.

The concept of extracapsular extension has only recently come to light. Though most frequently present in large nodes (greater than 3 cm), extracapsular extension may also be present in a clinically negative neck and is not necessarily related to the size of the node. When the tumor extends beyond the capsule of the node, the cure rate is reduced by almost 50 percent if radiation therapy is not given postoperatively. It is important to alert your pathologist to the clinical significance of extracapsular extension so that it will be included in his written report when present.

It is not a good idea to depend upon the clinical exam to make the final decision regarding need for an END. Recent unpublished data from M.D. Anderson Hospital, Houston, Texas and from Sloan-Kettering Hospital, New York City, suggest that *experienced* head and neck surgeons underestimate the staging of the neck in over 20 percent of patients and overestimate the incidence of positive neck disease more than 30 percent of the time, based on their clinical exam. The smaller the tumor burden in the neck, the greater the probability of misreading the neck nodes.

It should now be obvious that there are a number of risk factors related to the patient, the tumor, and the surgeon that must be taken into account before deciding on the correct treatment of cancer in the neck. Generally speaking, when the primary tumor is small (less than 4 cm) and will be treated surgically, serious consideration should be given to an END if the chance of subclinical nodal disease is greater than one in five. Adjunctive radiation should be given for a specific reason, e.g., questionable margins of the primary tumor, multiple echelon involvement, and/or extracapsular extension. It is usually inappropriate to treat T_1 and T_2 lesions with more than one modality. I prefer surgery as the only reasonable treatment of these lesions because of its ease, pathologic availability of the specimen, and lack of both short- and long-term morbidity.

MODIFIED RADICAL NECK DISSECTION?

In my mind, there is no indication for a classic radical neck dissection in the treatment of the N_0 neck (a neck that has no clinically positive nodes). This procedure should be reserved for the presence of clinically positive nodes at multiple levels when there is no question that surgery must be performed.

Although all surgeons know that the classic radical neck dissection removes the sternomastoid muscle, the XI cranial nerve, and the internal jugular vein, the "modified" neck dissection remains a mystery to most. As the name implies, each surgeon has the potential to modify the procedure to his or her own liking, and many do. I generally describe the modified neck dissection as a procedure that removes the first and second echelon of nodes at risk while preserving the muscle, nerve, and vein that are usually taken in the classic procedure. In most oral cavity tumors, this procedure removes the submaxillary, upper cervical (or subdigastric), and midjugular nodes. This is also called a supraomohyoid neck dissection because it removes all the nodes above the omohyoid muscle. It has also been called a functional neck dissection because it preserves function and results in little morbidity. For insurance purposes, it should be called a functional radical neck dissection so that reimbursement is commensurate with the difficulty of the procedure (CPT #38724), since it takes longer and is technically more difficult than a classic radical neck dissection.

The reader can understand the confusion arising from the term modified neck dissection. I feel the safest thing to do is to label the operation with the anatomic structures removed, e.g., lymphadenectomy removing the ipsilateral submental, submaxillary, subdigastric, and midjugular nodes. This approach leaves little to the imagination and is essential for retrospective review of your cancer treatment. The surgeon must orient the surgical specimen from such cases for the pathologist, since there are no normal anatomic structures for reference within the specimen, e.g., muscle, jugular vein.

Bilateral modified neck dissections are indicated when a primary lesion is in the midline. This occurs most commonly in a floor-of-mouth lesion. Midline tongue lesions are distinctly uncommon. Larger tongue lesions that cross the midline frequently have clinical nodal disease on the ipsilateral side; this dictates a neck dissection. The opposite side of the neck can be treated with a modified neck dissection or radiation therapy (5,500 cGy in 5½ weeks).

Since we know that therapeutic radiation can sterilize an N_0 neck of microscopic disease, it is most appropriate to apply that modality as the only treatment of choice when the primary tumor is being radiated. I feel that it is unwise to use both radiation and surgery on a small (T_1 or T_2) cancer of the oral cavity. When given the choice, I prefer surgery, for the reasons previously stated.

One may ask, why not wait for a metastatic node to evolve and then operate on the neck? Unless a patient is extremely dependable and their tumor is equally predictable, the concept of "watchful waiting" may result in an N_0 neck becoming an N_2 or an N_3 neck before surgical follow-up is sought. Studies have shown a survival rate of only 56 percent in "waiting" for neck to evolve into palpable regional disease.

SURGERY FOR THE NECK WITH CLINICALLY POSITIVE NODES

There is no decision apart from surgery when there are clinically palpable neck nodes. There is little indication for initial radiation in an N_1, N_{2a}, N_{2b}, or N_{3b} neck. In these cases, radiation is an adjunct to an appropriate neck dissection, usually a radical neck dissection with optional preservation of the XI nerve. The classification N_{3a} (node greater than 6 cm) implies an extremely grave prognosis. With a survival rate of less than 10 percent, this patient deserves extraordinary measures that go beyond the usual capabilities of most surgeons. I feel the patient should be referred to a tertiary care facility or at the very least should be placed in one of the experimental protocols addressing this problem.

By application of basic lymphatic anatomy and knowledge of the primary tumor and its most probable paths of lymphatic spread, the surgeon can make a rational treatment decision related to the nodal groups to be removed and the need for adjunctive radiation therapy. Using the information presented above, a cure rate of between 80 and 90 percent can be attained for T_1 and T_2 oral cavity lesions and better than 50 percent for most larger lesions.

SUGGESTED READING

Byers RM. Modified neck dissection: a study of 967 cases from 1970 to 1980. Am J Surg 1985; 150:414–421.

Byers RM, Wolf PF, Ballantyne AJ. Rationale for elective modified neck dissection. Head Neck Surg 1988; 10:160–166.

Johnson JT, Cunningham MJ, Myers EN, et al. Cervical lymph node metastasis after local excision of early squamous cell carcinoma of the oral cavity. Am J Surg 1986; 152:361–365.

Larson DL, Ballantyne AJ, Guillamondegui DM, eds. Evaluation and treatment of cancer in the neck. New York: Macmillan, 1986.

Lindberg RD. Distribution of cervical lymph node metastases from squamous carcinoma of the upper respiratory tract and digestive tract. Cancer 1972; 29:1446–1449.

FUNCTIONAL NECK DISSECTION

STEPHAN ARIYAN, M.D., F.A.C.S.

Any operation designed for the treatment of cancer should have as its purpose the removal of all cancer-bearing tissue and any tissue suspected of harboring cancer cells that surrounds the malignancy. There are two other instances in which cancer operations may be considered; one of these is a cancer so extensive that cure cannot be achieved, but that, without surgical removal, could grow through the skin and result in deformity, bleeding, or malodor and, thereby, prevent the patient from staying with friends or loved ones. The other circumstance might be an operation to remove tissue suspected of harboring cancer—even though this may not be clinically detectable. These general statements on the principles of cancer surgery are most applicable to a cancer that either exists in the neck or that may have spread to related structures.

At the turn of this century, Crile proposed the operation we have come to know as the *radical neck dissection* for the removal of cancers that have spread to the neck from primaries in the oropharyngeal area. Crile felt that distant metastases were rare and that spread of cancer was from the primary site to the regional neck nodes. Although advocating the radical removal of all the neck contents for squamous cell carcinomas, Crile was much more conservative in his treatment of papillary carcinoma of the thyroid. This was because he felt that removal of the thyroid decreased the chances of metastases to the neck nodes. In modifications of neck operations for removal of lymph nodes in thyroid cancer, great variability exists in techniques; these range from "node picking" to "partial" neck dissection in which only the palpable nodes are removed with the internal jugular vein (as has been advocated by Lahey et al).

On the other hand, Crile was very aggressive in the management of metastatic nodes in squamous cell carcinoma of the head and neck, and advocated removal of the internal jugular vein because he believed the lymphatic structures immediately surrounded it and he felt that the removal of the sternocleidomastoid muscle would provide easier access to the internal jugular vein. Interestingly, he did not report removal of the spinal accessory nerve as part of the operation. Hayes Martin felt that the only operation for metastatic carcinoma of the neck was a standard radical neck dissection with removal of all the structures, including the spinal accessory nerve. Because of Martin's influence on head and neck cancer surgery, and his many trainees who believed in his principles, this more aggressive neck dissection became the standard procedure to which all other techniques had to be compared. However, one must keep in mind that with other cancers that metastasize to the axillary, inguinal, or iliac nodes, lymphadenectomy is performed with preservation of the nerves and veins, yet still achieves cure and control rates comparable to those with the radical neck dissection

Bocca and Pignataro advocated a conservative neck dissection in patients who required prophylactic lymphadenectomies for laryngeal cancers. They cited the work of Suarez, who demonstrated that the lymph nodes in the neck lie within a closed space surrounded by the two layers of the cervical fascia (Fig 1). Although lymph nodes lie close to muscular structures and vascular aponeuroses, they are not found within vessel walls or the overlying muscles.

Few surgeons would try to preserve these structures if there is a tumor growing through the lymph node capsule, adherent to the adjacent muscle or jugular vein. On the other hand, unless there is such extension outside the lymph node capsules, there appears to be no justification for the routine removal of the jugular vein from within the carotid sheath while the carotid artery, vagus nerve, and sympathetic chain are spared. Similarly, there appears to be no reason for routine removal of the spinal accessory nerve while the hypoglossal nerve and the lingual nerve in the neck contents are spared.

Bocca reported a series of 500 neck dissections performed for N_0 necks in patients with cancer of the larynx, in which he spared the jugular vein and the sternocleidomastoid muscle (SCM) without alteration of the overall disease-free rates. Skolnik et al demonstrated that there were no metastatic lymph nodes in the posterior triangle in either therapeutic or prophylactic neck dissections in patients with cancer of the larynx, pharynx, and oral cavity. Additional reports have demonstrated the low probability of metastases to lymph nodes in the posterior triangle from primaries in the oropharyngeal area unless there is also extensive involvement of lymph nodes in the anterior triangle.

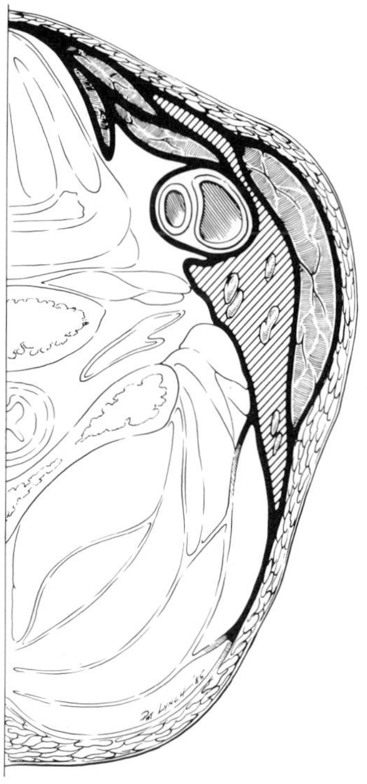

Figure 1 The lymphatic contents of the neck are enveloped within the superficial and deeper layers of the cervical fascia, which lie under the sternocleidomastoid and over the carotid sheath and its contents. The superficial layer of the cervical fascia divides in two to envelope the sternocleidomastoid and then reforms into one layer along the anterior triangle.

The purpose of this chapter is to demonstrate my preference for a radical neck dissection that still preserves the function of the structures of the neck because the internal jugular vein, the sternocleidomastoid muscle, and the spinal accessory nerve are kept intact.

SURGICAL TECHNIQUE

Although a number of acceptable neck incisions have been described in the past, I most often prefer an L-shaped incision that extends from the mastoid region down to the shoulder and lies about 2 cm behind the anterior border of the trapezius muscle. At the shoulder, the incision extends medially below the clavicle (Fig. 2). If this incision is made in front of the border of the trapezius muscle, there is risk of injury to the spinal accessory nerve that lies very superficial to, and just beneath the cervical fascia under the platysma muscle. Also, scar contraction after incision wound healing can cause a webbed neck, whereas when the incision overlies the muscle fascia, the wound scar heals to the muscle without any webbing due to scar contraction.

The neck flap is elevated deep to the platysma muscle and superficial to the underlying cervical fascia. Care must be taken to incorporate the platysma muscle with this skin flap in order to prevent ischemic necrosis of the tip of the flap over the shoulder. This technique has resulted in safe elevation of the entire neck skin, even in previously-irradiated necks. With the skin flap elevated, together with the platysma muscle, the entire contents of the neck can be seen intact with the cervical fascia.

As mentioned earlier, the lymphatic contents of the neck are incorporated within the two layers of the cervical fascia deep to the sternocleidomastoid muscle. As such, the superficial layer of the cervical fascia comes along the posterior triangle, divides in two to pass superficially and deep to the sternocleidomastoid muscle (see Fig. 1), and then reforms to one layer to cover the anterior cervical triangle. Therefore, the sternocleidomastoid muscle (SCM) can be elevated by incision along its anterior and posterior borders and by dissection away from the deeper half of this split cervical fascia. The origins of both the sternal and clavicular heads of this muscle are then transected, and the muscle is elevated up and away from the cervical fascia (see Fig. 2B). I developed this technique of elevation of the SCM muscle from my experience with the use of this muscle to transport paddles of skin for reconstructions of defects in the oropharyngeal area. As previously reported, cadaver dissections demonstrated that the sternocleidomastoid muscle has three blood supplies, which provide circulation through the upper, middle, and lower portions of the muscle (Fig. 3). Therefore, preservation of the superior blood supply and the eleventh nerve to the muscle result in a functional preservation of this muscle.

During the elevation of the SCM muscle from the deeper layer of the enveloping cervical fascia, care must be taken to prevent damage to the spinal accessory nerve in the upper portion of the muscle (Fig. 4). One approach would be to identify the spinal accessory nerve (SAN)

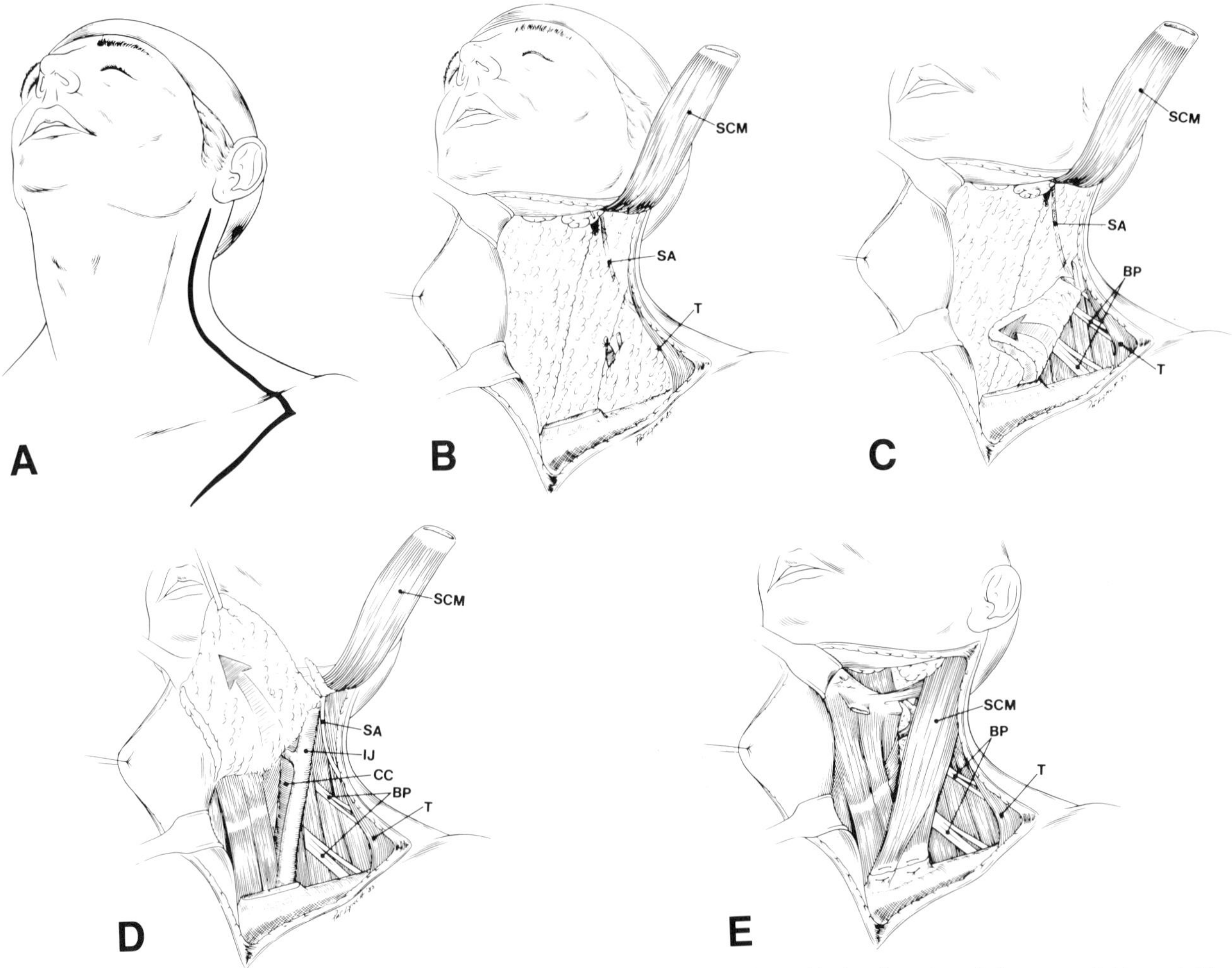

Figure 2 Artist's depiction of the neck incision *(A)*, and the dissection, beginning with the elevation of the sternocleidomastoid *(B)*, and the removal of the neck contents (*C* to *E*), while vessels and nerves are preserved. The muscle is sutured back in place at the end of the procedure. (SCM = sternocleidomastoid muscle; SA = spinal accessory nerve; IJ = internal jugular vein; CC = common carotid artery; BP = brachial plexus; and T = anterior border of trapezius muscle). (From Ariyan S. Functional neck dissection. Plast Reconstr Surg 1980; 65:768.)

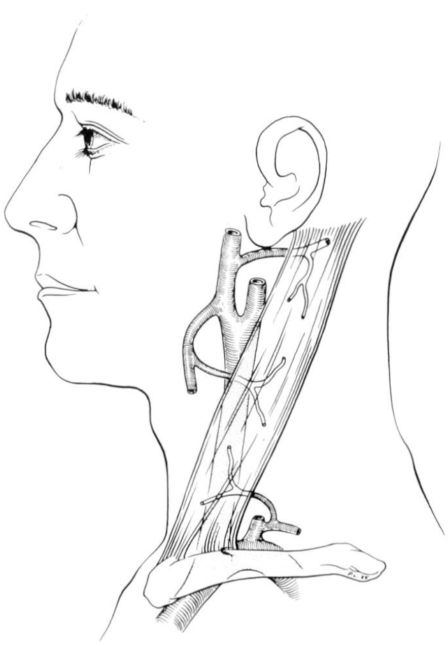

Figure 3 There are three blood supplies to the sternocleidomastoid muscle. Superiorly, there is a branch from the occipital artery; in the midportion, a branch from the superior thyroid artery, and, below, a branch from the thyrocervical trunk.

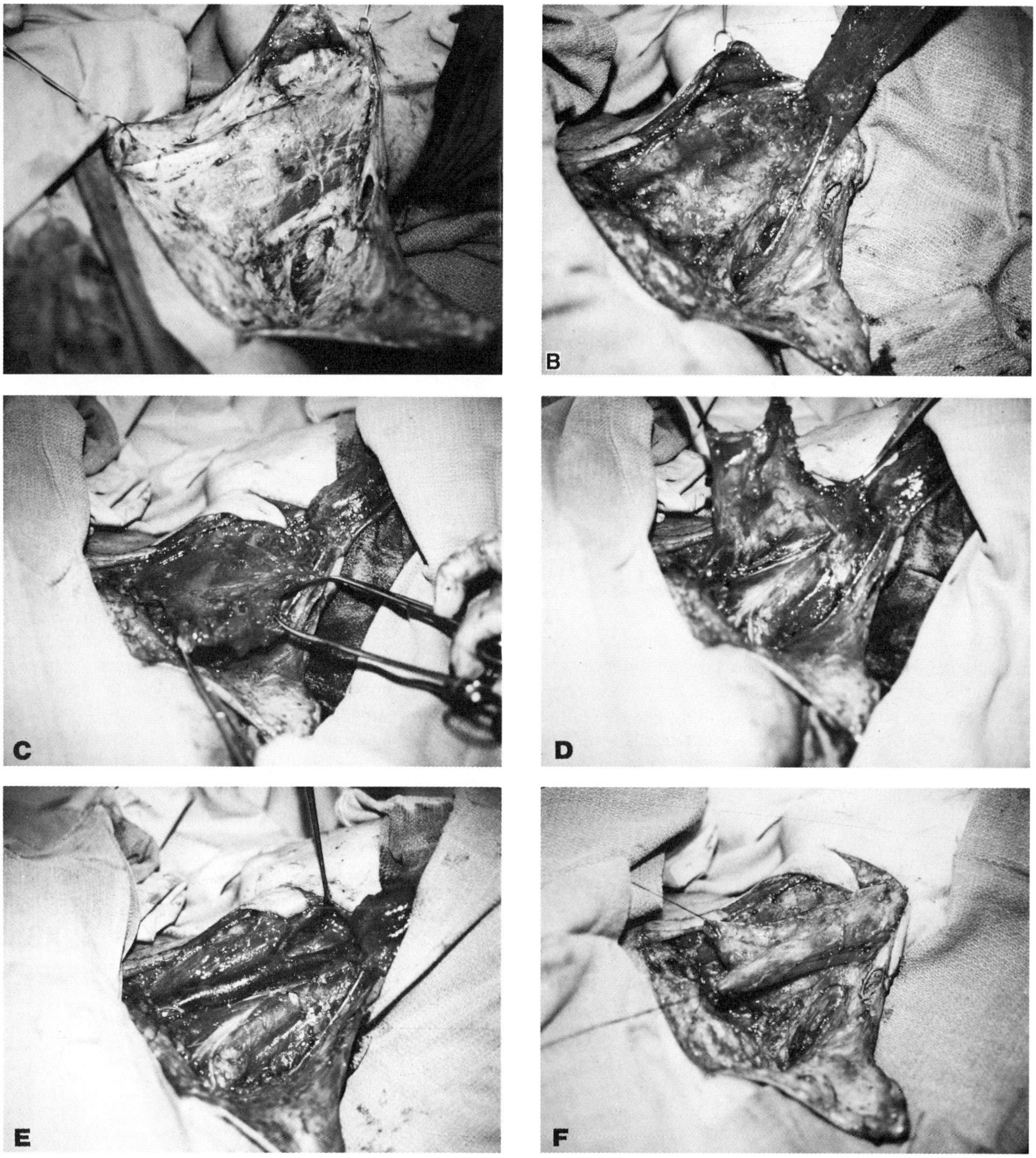

Figure 4 *A*, The elevation of the skin flap shows the cervical contents together with the cervical fascia that envelopes the sternocleidomastoid muscle. *B*, With the fascia incised along the anteroposterior borders of the SCM, the muscle can be elevated away from the deeper half of the cervical fascia. The spinal accessory nerve has been dissected along the posterior triangle up to the sternocleidomastoid muscle to prevent damage to the nerve. *C*, The dissection of the neck contents begins along the posterior triangle as they are elevated with a deep layer of the cervical fascia from the neck musculature and the branchial plexus. *D*, As the dissection is carried up to the carotid sheath, it is then incised to remove this sheath together with the specimen, while the major vessels and nerves are preserved. *E*, Following completion of the neck dissection, the jugular vein, brachial plexus, carotid artery, vagus nerve, and spinal accessory nerve can be seen preserved. *F*, The sternoclavicular origins of the SCM are then brought down to their points of attachment and sutured with several heavy absorbable sutures.

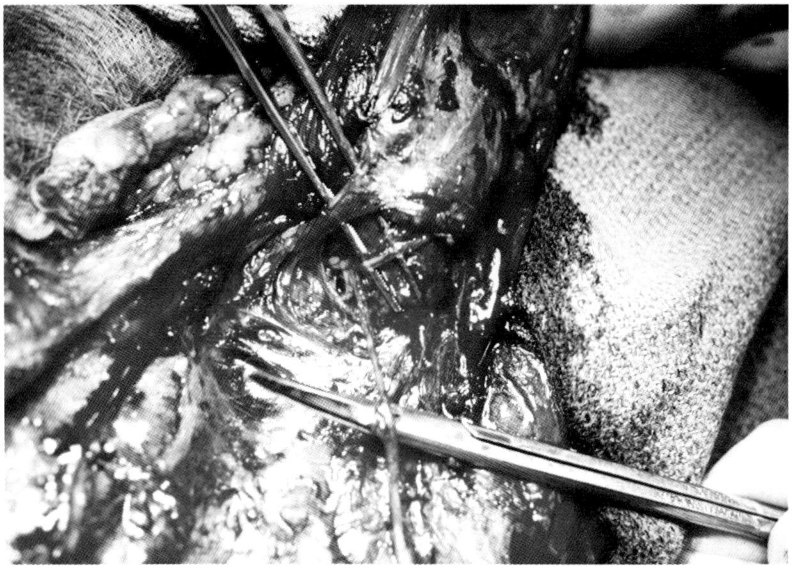

Figure 5 In the dissection of the upper portion of the sternocleidomastoid muscle, the spinal accessory nerve can frequently be seen to travel under the muscle, giving a motor branch to it rather than traveling through the muscle itself.

along the anterior border of the trapezius muscle and dissect it up to the posterior border of the SCM muscle prior to elevation of the latter (see Fig. 4B).

Dissection of the lymphatic contents of the neck is begun from the posterior triangle along the border of the trapezius muscle anteriorly towards the carotid sheath. The latter is incised anteriorly to expose and identify the internal jugular vein, the carotid artery, the vagus nerve, and the sympathetic chain (see Fig. 4D). The dissection continues cephalad and the sensory cutaneous branches of the cervical plexus are then transected in the midportion of the neck above the phrenic nerve. With the dissection carried more cephalad, care must be taken to dissect out the spinal accessory nerve meticulously to the sternocleidomastoid base. At this point, it can be determined whether the spinal accessory nerve travels through the sternocleidomastoid muscle on its way through the trapezius, or travels under the SCM giving it a motor branch (Fig. 5). The upper portion of the neck contents are now dissected from the hypoglossal nerve, and dissection is continued to the mylohyoid muscle in the same way as in a standard radical neck dissection.

Following removal of the cervical lymphatics, the SCM is returned to its former position, and the two tendinous heads of the muscle are sutured to their sites of origin with interrupted 3–0 Vicryl sutures (see Fig. 4F).

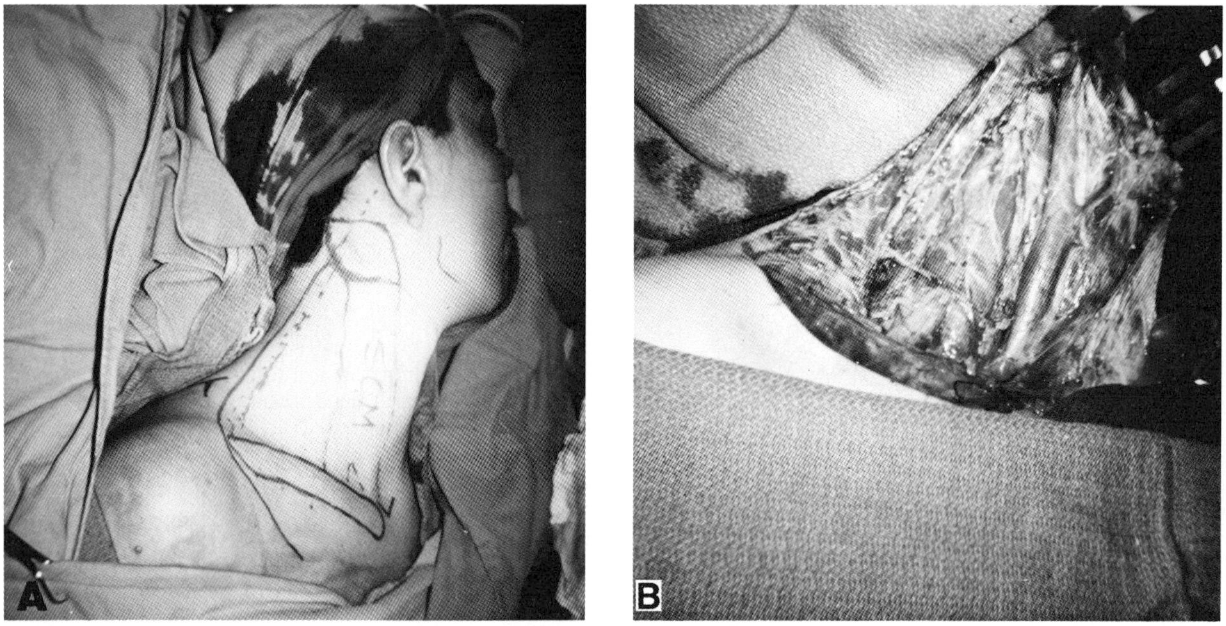

Figure 6 *A*, A patient with a high-risk melanoma of the neck required a wide excision and lymphadenectomy. *B*, Following completion of the neck dissection, it can be seen that the main structures of the neck are preserved while at the same time a complete excision of the lymphatic contents has been performed.

Figure continues on opposite page

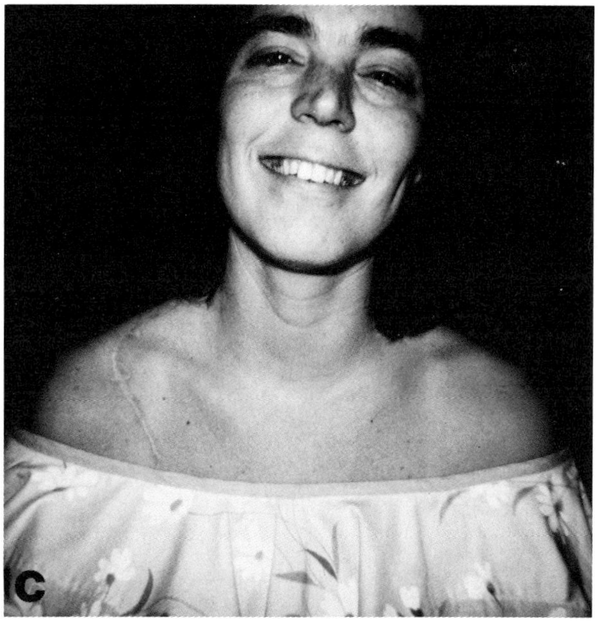

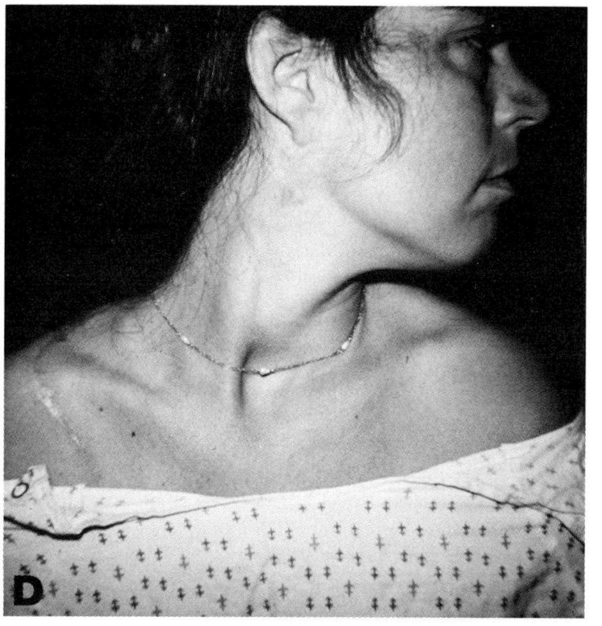

Figure 6 (continued) *C*, The scars are quite acceptable and pleasing when the shoulders are exposed in a summer dress, while the muscle provides symmetry to the neck. *D*, There is normal functioning to this muscle through the intact nerve and blood supply.

It helps to have some silk sutures placed as marks at the site of the origins of the muscle on the sternum and the clavicle in order to identify the proper location when one has reached this point near the end of the operation. The silk sutures can be removed when the origins have been sutured in their proper position. Several sutures are required for each tendinous origin because, if the patient becomes combative while awakening from anesthesia, the muscle could be pulled away. Large suction catheters are then placed in the neck contents from the direction of the shoulder, and the neck flap is repositioned and sutured in two layers. The first is the platysma-fascial layer and the second is the skin layer.

If the patient requires bilateral neck dissections, both can be readily performed at the same operation since the jugular veins can be preserved. In the postoperative period, the suction catheters are removed when the daily recordings of the volume of drainage demonstrate that it is significantly decreased, rather than when any particular numerical volume is reached. In general, the patient

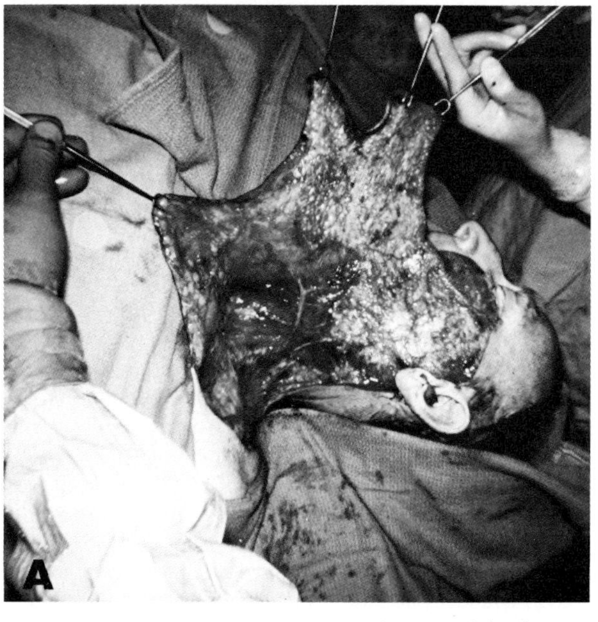

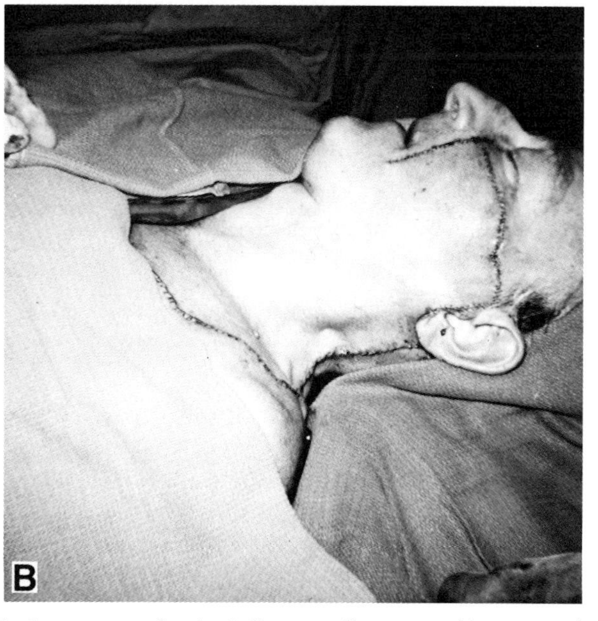

Figure 7 *A*, A wide resection of a melanoma of the face required advancement of a cheek flap as well as a parotidectomy and neck dissection. *B*, This flap was then advanced for the closure of the defect as well as the neck contents.

Figure continues on following page

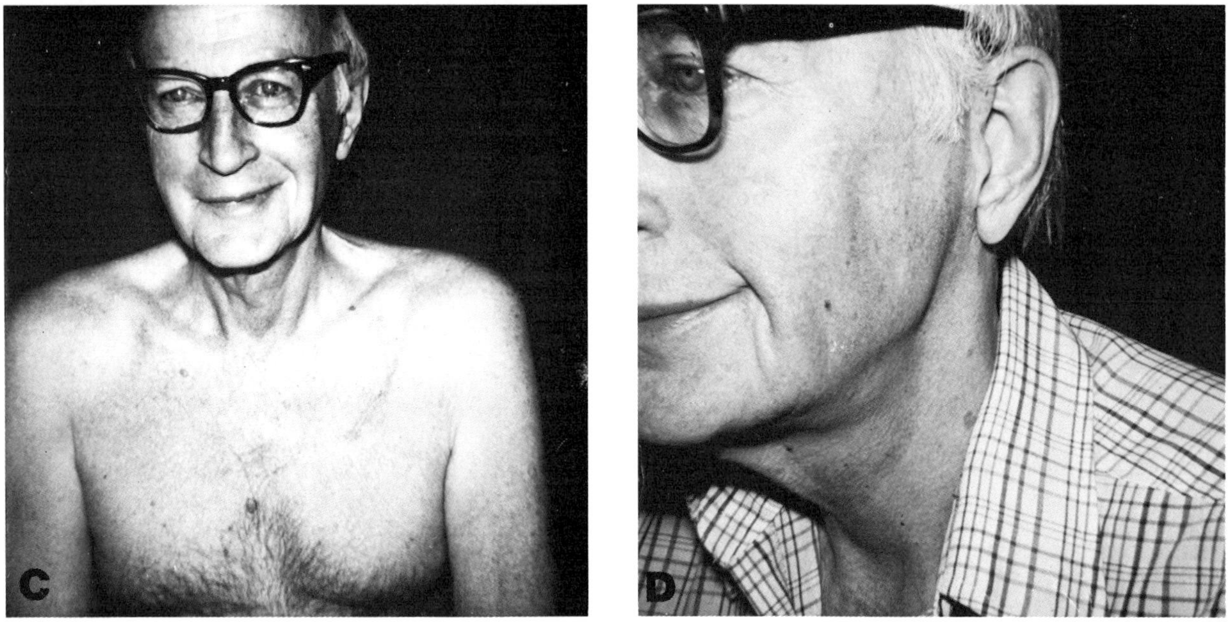

Figure 7 (continued) *C*, This provided symmetry to the neck, an acceptable incision scar, and functional sternocleidomastoid muscle. *D*, The advancement of the cervical flap provided a very good match for coverage of the facial defect.

is discharged from the hospital in 5 to 7 days. At two weeks after the operation, I recommend that patients begin to swim in a pool in order to increase the range of motion. Swimming has been the most successful way to return full function to the shoulders (most commonly within a period of 1 week)—much more so than any other exercises that we tried with patients.

The functional results of this technique are quite rewarding (Figs. 6 and 7). The patients are pleased with the relatively symmetrical result and the good function of the muscles of the neck and shoulder. In addition, the incision wounds heal frequently with a pleasing result. The scar location permits patients to wear wide-open shirts and V-neck sweaters, yet still conceal the scars.

SUGGESTED READING

Ariyan S. One-stage reconstruction for defects of the mouth using a sternomastoid myocutaneous flap. Plast Reconstr Surg 1979; 63:618–625.

Ariyan S. Functional neck dissection. Plast Reconstr Surg 1980; 65:768–776.

Bocca E. Conservation neck dissection. Laryngoscope 1975; 85:1511–1515.

Drile G. Excision of cancer of the head and neck. JAMA 1906; 47: 1780–1786.

47:1780–1786.

Crile G. The fallacy of the conventional radical neck dissection for papillary carcinoma of the thyroid. Ann Surg 1957; 145:317–320.

Martin HE, DelValle B, Ehrlich H, Cahan WG. Neck dissection. Cancer 1951; 4:441–499.

Skolnik EM, King FY, Friedman M, Golden TA. The posterior triangle and radical neck dissection. Arch Otolaryngol 1976; 102:1–8.

LOCAL FLAPS ON THE FACE

FREDERICK R. HECKLER, M.D., F.A.C.S.

Local flap repair of a relatively small excisional skin defect on the face is likely to be one of the first reconstructive procedures performed by the beginning plastic surgeon, and the effort will probably be rewarded with success, at least in terms of flap survival and wound healing. The implication, therefore, is that these procedures require little sophistication or insight and that modest finesse in planning and execution suffice. Certainly, the remarkable vascularity and wound healing potential of facial skin can compensate for multiply compounded errors in both local flap design and technical execution. Despite this apparent ease of success, it has always been my contention that obtaining optimum esthetic results from local facial flaps may require more skill in many cases than that needed for transfer of major flaps for larger defects.

Planning local facial flaps requires a careful analysis of the structural, functional, and cosmetic requirements of the defect; a survey of available local donor sites; and an equally careful selection from the catalogue of flap designs so as to minimize donor site visibility while maximizing the reconstructive benefit. Execution of local facial flap elevation, transfer, and inset necessitates all of the classic attributes of good plastic surgical technique: precision, gentle handling of tissues, and respect for tissue integrity—the same attributes required for success in larger reconstructive areas. In this situation, however, modest errors in either design or execution are more readily apparent, since normal facial skin and features are immediately adjacent as a comparison. Therefore, the "success" enjoyed by the neophyte plastic surgeon may be defined in terms of smooth wound healing and flap viability, but more appropriately should also be defined in terms of ideal structural and cosmetic results. This latter goal is obviously more difficult to achieve and is the subject I wish to address.

To this end, the following discussion will dwell primarily upon general principles of local facial flap surgery, with emphasis upon concepts that have helped me in trying to approach the stated optimal goals more consistently. Specific flaps, ideally suited for reconstructive problems in some specific areas, will be covered in more detail, but only as examples of the application of more broadly based, generally applicable principles. More extensive catalogues of the multiplicity of facial flaps are already available; interested readers wishing to expand their knowledge of these specific techniques are referred to them.

DEFINITION

A local facial flap is defined herein as a skin segment that is transferred to a facial defect from a closely adjacent facial area. Flaps from more distant areas (such as forehead flaps for nasal reconstruction) will not be considered.

ROLE OF LOCAL FACIAL FLAPS

Local flaps are only one item in the list of alternatives available for reconstruction of modest-sized defects in facial skin. Distant flaps from extraregional donor sites and free microvascular transfers may be considered in unusual circumstances, but the alternative choice most often facing the reconstructive surgeon is a skin graft, either split thickness or full thickness. The advantages and disadvantages of local flaps with particular attention to the potential alternative of skin grafting are considered in the following sections.

Advantages of Local Flaps

The use of immediately adjacent or nearby skin to reconstruct a skin defect ensures the closest possible match in color, texture, and thickness. Skin grafts, even full thickness grafts, cannot hope to equal local flaps in any of these aspects in the overwhelming majority of situations. Local flaps are also more desirable in situations where soft tissue resection has been carried down to bone or where the recipient area is otherwise less than ideal for graft take. Free skin grafts to the face do enjoy an enviably high success rate in terms of graft survival. In my experience, however, the properly executed local facial flap has been even more reliable.

Disadvantages of Local Flaps

Jackson has very aptly stated that "the greatest drawback to the use of skin flaps is that they require planning and experience." Mistakes in planning or surgical execution of local flaps can add unnecessary, inappropriate, or excessive facial scarring, thereby defeating the purpose for which the flap reconstruction was initially undertaken. A major drawback to the use of local facial flaps as opposed to skin grafts is the additional scarring incurred on the face at the donor site. However, if carefully planned as to locale and orientation, the donor site deformity always has a favorable outcome compared to the deformity of mismatch of color, thickness, and texture to be seen in the great majority of skin grafts. For this reason, I have, over the years, gradually shifted away from the use of skin grafts for small defects on the face, with local flaps assuming a far more predominant role than skin grafts in my own facial reconstructive armamentarium.

The most frequent indication for skin grafts now is in situations where I am not confident of the adequacy of resection of skin neoplasms. In these cases, skin grafts are applied and a less than ideal esthetic reconstruction is accepted temporarily, with the expectation of replacing the graft at a later date with a local flap once lack of tumor recurrence is assured.

The intellectual exercise required to analyze the small facial defect and to sort through the various local flap options, in order to select the flap most likely to yield the best result with the least donor defect, can be one of the most enjoyable experiences in plastic and reconstructive surgery.

GENERAL PRINCIPLES

Anesthesia

I distinctly prefer local anesthesia for both excision of facial lesions and for local flap repair. Patients under local anesthesia are comfortable, the absence of endotracheal tubes and supporting apparatus facilitates access to the operative field, and the hematoma-engendering coughing and retching sometimes seen with emergence from inhalation anesthesia are avoided. If the procedure is prolonged, as in situations where multiple frozen sections are required, or if the patient is apprehensive, intravenous sedation is helpful.

If only a small area of anesthesia is required, then direct local infiltration is used. In all other situations, I prefer the use of regional nerve blocks combined with supplemental local infiltration for vasoconstriction and hemostasis. I like to give the required combination of supraorbital, infraorbital, and mental nerve blocks prior to scrubbing, prepping, and draping. These blocks do not distort the immediate operative field and take effect by the time surgery commences. Skin markings for excisional measurement and flap planning are then outlined, and local infiltration in the now pain-free field is accomplished.

If a longer procedure is anticipated, or postoperative prolongation of analgesia is desired, a longer-acting agent such as bupivacaine is used for the nerve blocks.

Planning of Excision and Reconstruction

Excision

Most local facial flaps are employed in the repair of excisional defects for skin neoplasia, with less frequent application to traumatic or congenital defects. It is essential that considerations of flap design be considered secondary to complete tumor excision, even if the preferred flap may be compromised in order to assure adequate resection margins. To this end, I prefer to first draw out on the skin the planned excision, usually using 3.5× loupe magnification. Consideration of local flap options and of final flap design are then done; followed by infiltration of the operative area with local anesthetic, tumor excision, frozen section histologic evaluation of margins if necessary; and lastly, flap reconstruction. Some recommend that lesion excision precede flap design. I find that the dynamic and elastic qualities of skin distort and change the original dimensions of the excisional design and, therefore, prefer the order of procedure stated.

RECONSTRUCTION

The *ideal* local flap would exactly match the recipient area in color, thickness, and texture. It would be hairbearing or not as required. Its orientation on the face would allow all resulting scars to run in, or at least parallel to, adjacent skin creases and lines. The site from which the flap is derived would have enough excess skin to allow primary donor site closure without distortion of local structures or features and would be without tension. Flap transfer should be accomplished in one stage without need for delays or secondary pedicle divisions. Potential for complications, including flap necrosis and "pincushioning" with required secondary revisions, would be minimal to absent. This is a tall order! However, the challenge of local flap reconstruction is in trying to sift through all options so as to approach these goals as nearly as possible.

Procedure

1. After outlining the planned excision, determine whether or not primary undermining and closure are possible. *This is almost always preferable to any local flap.* Facial scarring is minimized, and the geometric scar patterns that result from local flap transfer are avoided. Pinching the skin adjacent to the defect together with the fingers usually indicates whether enough laxity is present to permit direct suture. If it is not clear whether primary closure is possible, draw the excisional lenticular design that would be required for primary closure and dog ear elimination, and then in addition, draw the preferred local flap. Skin undermining *at the same level as for flap construction* can then be done, skin advanced, and a few temporary construction sutures placed. If excess tension or distortion of facial features are evident, the sutures are removed and the additional incisions for flap construction are made. Flap *elevation* has usually already been accomplished by the previous undermining, thereby leaving it a simple matter to rotate the flap and close all incision lines.
2. If primary closure is not possible, the first thing to assess is which anatomically adjacent areas possess enough skin laxity or excess to be considered as donor sites. The most important characteristic of potential donor sites, after that of quantitative availability, is skin character in terms of thickness, color, texture, and presence or absence of hair (beard). The ability to reconstitute these characteristics supercedes, in my opinion, the importance of scar placement either at donor or recipient sites. More specifically, it is best to replace cheek skin with cheek skin, nasal skin with skin from the nose, chin skin with chin skin, and so forth. Replacement with skin from other esthetic units, such as cheek skin with cervical flaps or nasal skin with cheek-derived nasolabial flaps, is still usually better than using a skin graft, but is not ideal.
3. Assess normal skin lines and creases in both donor and recipient sites (Fig. 1), and then try to design a flap that allows as many surgical scars as possible to mimic these natural lines by being situated parallel to or within them. A frustrating realization is that the great majority of small facial defects allow such ideal positioning in only a portion of the scar lines created by excision and flap reconstruction.

Transposition Flaps

Transposition flaps are probably the most commonly used local facial flap. Other local flaps such as bilobed (Zimany) (Fig. 2) and trilobed flaps, Limberg rhomboid flaps, and Dufourmental flaps are basically geometric variations in transposition flap design; the planning and construction of all of these can therefore be discussed collectively.

Most local transposition flaps are roughly rectangular in shape, having two longer sides and two shorter sides, one of which constitutes the flap base, and this is not incised. The relationship between these long and short sides constitutes the traditional "length-width ratio" that basically expresses how long a flap can be created with the expectation of reliable flap tip viability. On the face, this ratio is usually three to one and occasionally can exceed this, a reflection of the excellent vascularity in the facial region.

Surgical scars result along each incised margin of this rectangular configuration and, except at rare areas where normal facial lines intersect at right angles, it is virtually impossible to design a flap that has *all* scars sited ideally. However, with most transpositional flaps it should be possible to make a design that, at the very least, permits the two longer, more obvious scars bordering the flap to lie ideally. Planning efforts should also extend to placing the

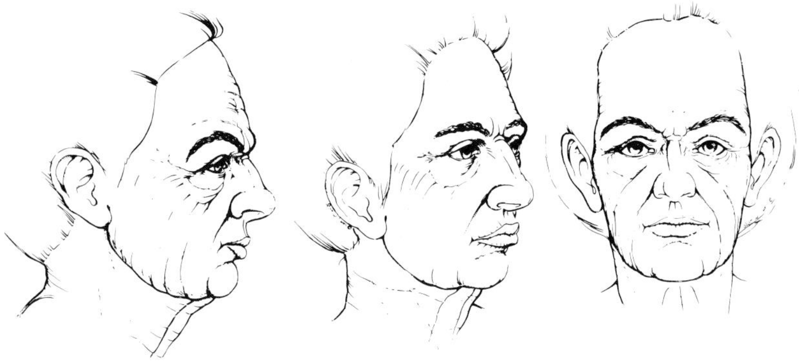

Figure 1 Normal facial skin lines and creases. Facial skin lines and creases assume a fairly typical and reasonably consistent pattern. They tend to run perpendicular to the line of pull of the underlying facial mimetic muscles. Lines and creases are more obvious in the elderly, but can be visualized in younger patients by requesting the patient to assume extreme postures of facial expression, such as forced smiling or squinting. Elective incisions and scars should be placed, if at all possible, either within these lines and creases or at least parallel to them.

donor site scar in normal skin lines, creases, or other anatomically concealed sites (Fig. 3).

Other Options

A number of flap options are available in addition to the classic transposition flap and its several variations. These include rotation flaps, several forms of advancement flaps, and subcutaneous and vascular island pedicle flaps. The basic considerations discussed for transposition flaps in terms of donor site selection and siting of resultant scars also apply, in essence, to all of these. I will, therefore, only discuss several personal favorites among these other options, to illustrate their utility and their place in the overall spectrum of local flap reconstruction possibilities.

Personal Favorites for Problem Defects

Advancement Flaps

These flaps are constructed by undermining skin adjacent to the defect and then stretching the undermined skin forward to close the defect. Rotation or transposition are not used; rather stress relaxation and creep, the visco-

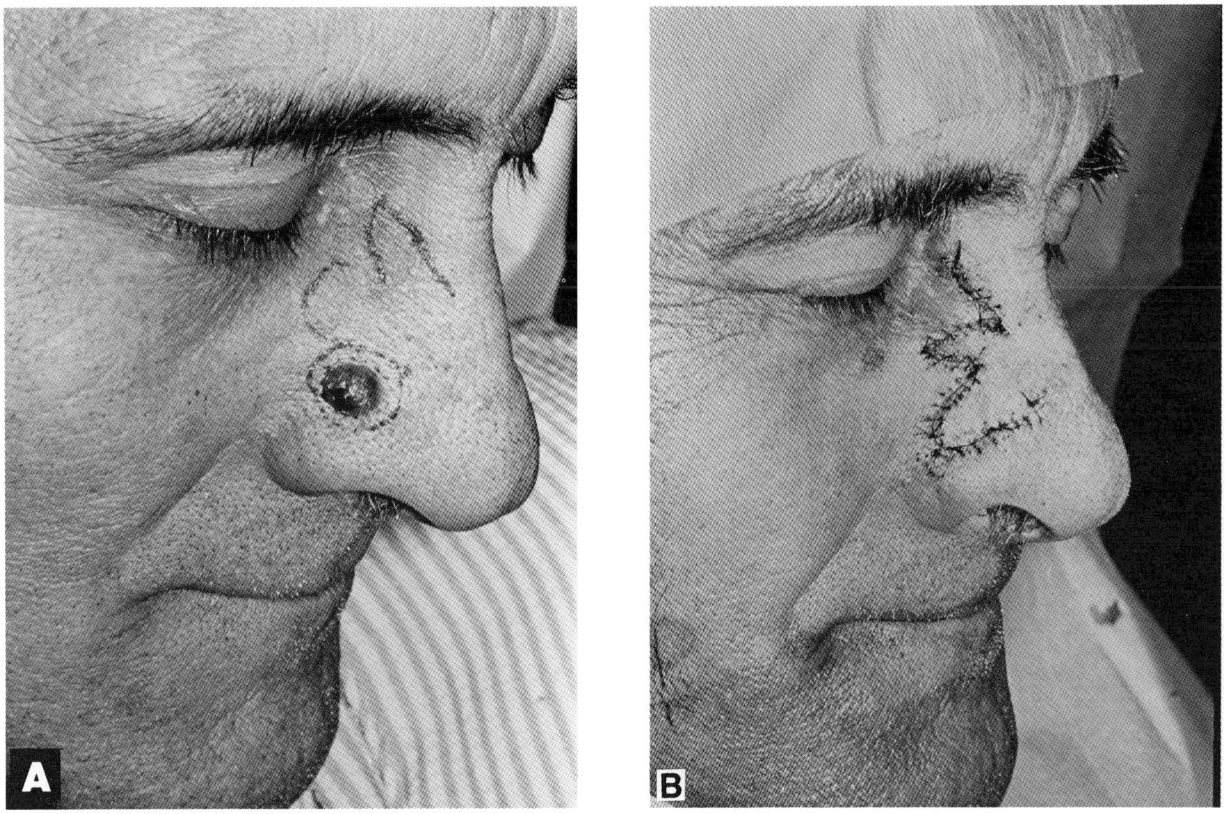

Figure 2 Bilobed flap (Zimany). *A*, Basal cell carcinoma of the nose. Planned resection is indicated as well as bilobed Zimany flap reconstruction outline. *B*, Bilobed flap has been rotated in to reconstruct the nasal defect. The primary, larger flap fills the resection defect and the secondary, smaller flap fills the primary flap donor defect. This variation of a transposition flap in effect transposes the donor defect higher onto the nose towards the glabellar area, where there is more loose skin to allow primary closure of the donor defect.

Figure continues on following page

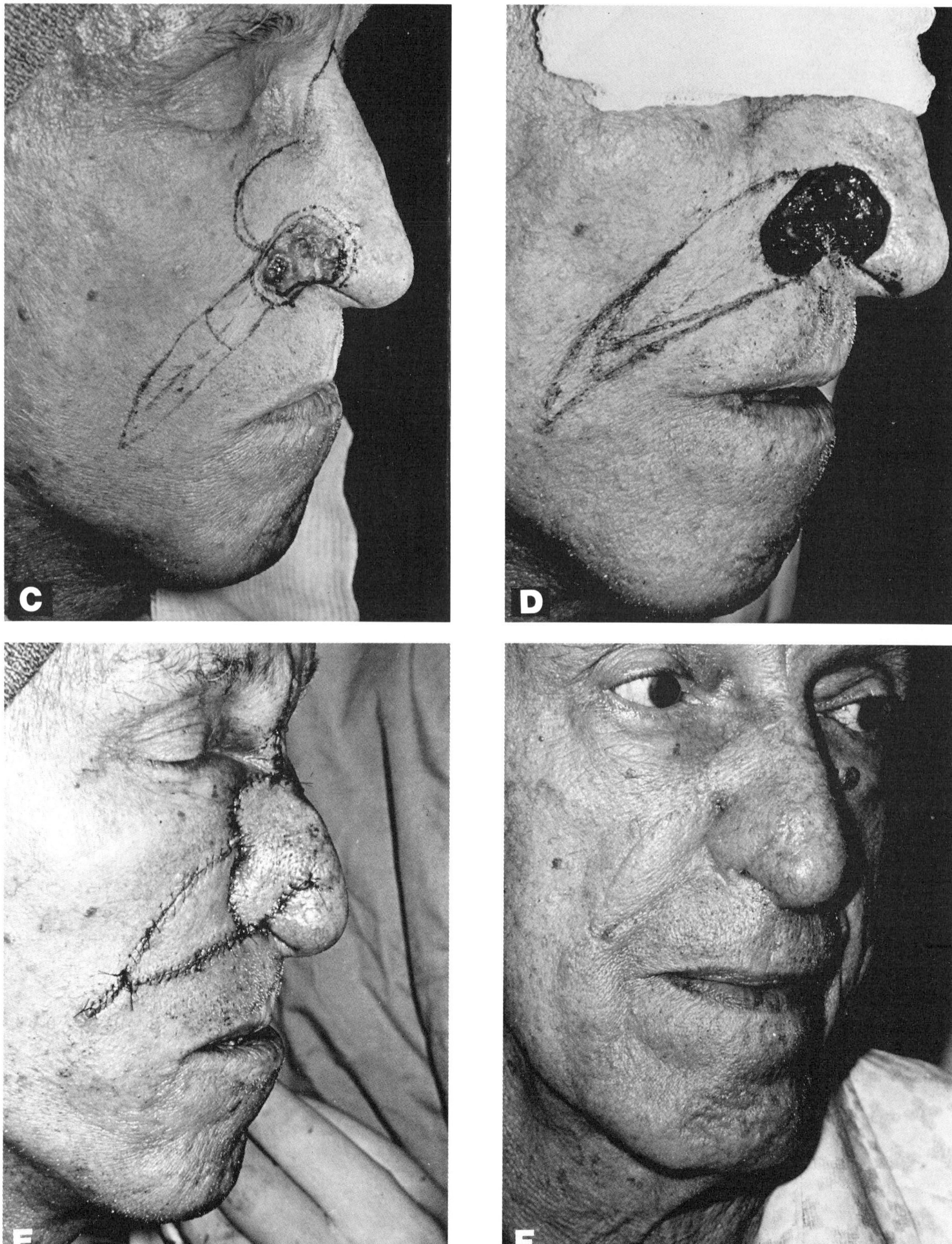

Figure 2 (continued) *C*, A larger basal cell carcinoma in the same general area. This tumor involves both the lateral side of the alar base and the subjacent perialar lip and cheek skin. A combination of flaps will, therefore, be utilized. A Zimany bilobed flap from the nasal dorsum will be transposed to reconstruct the alar defect, and a subcutaneous island pedicle flap from the nasolabial area will be utilized to reconstruct the cheek and lip defect. *D*, The excisional defect involves both the lateral ala and the adjacent perialar cheek and lip skin. Reconstruction of this area with a single flap will not permit retention of the distinctive alar-facial groove. Two flaps are therefore required. *E*, The bilobed flap has been rotated into position with the smaller segment of the bilobed flap reconstructing the donor defect of the larger segment and the glabellar area being closed primarily. The subcutaneous island flap has been advanced in V—Y fashion. *F*, Postoperative result at one year.

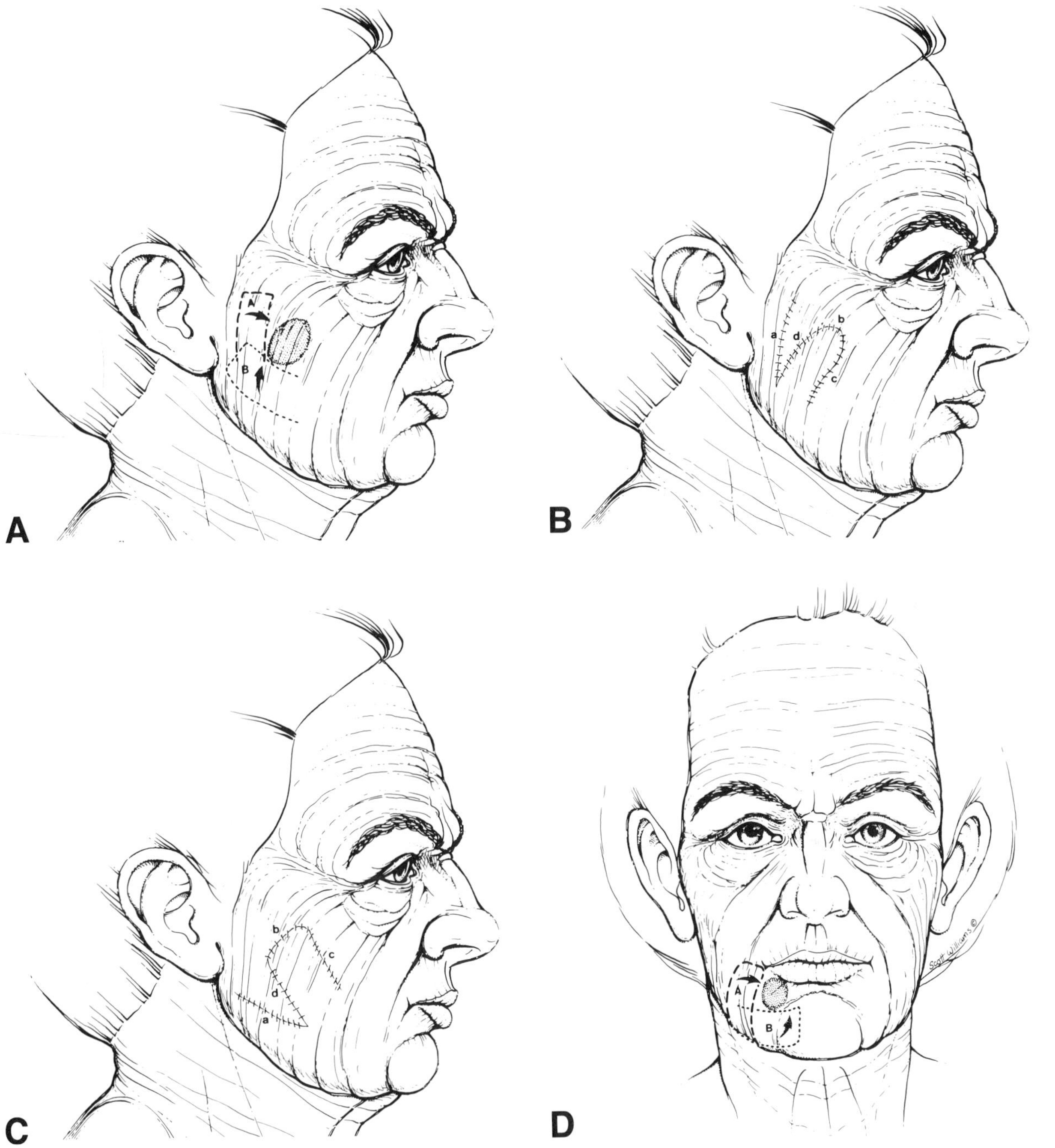

Figure 3 Planning local transpositional flaps on the face. *A*, Two possible flap reconstructive options for an excisional defect on the cheek (stippled area) are indicated. One should choose the flap that permits placement of the majority of resulting scar lines within or parallel to normal facial skin lines and creases. *B*, The resulting scar pattern to be expected from utilizing flap option A. Anticipated scar lines a, d, and c all lie within or parallel to facial lines and creases. Only scar line b is in an inappropriate direction. The majority of these scar lines should thus heal favorably. *C*, Anticipated scar pattern resulting from utilization of flap option B. In this situation, scar lines a, d, and c all run against the direction of normal facial lines and creases and only scar line b is in an appropriate direction. The preferred choice between these two flaps would, therefore, be option A. *D*, Two possible flap options for reconstruction of a defect just below the vermilion border of the lateral third of the lower lip (stippled area).

Figure continues on following page

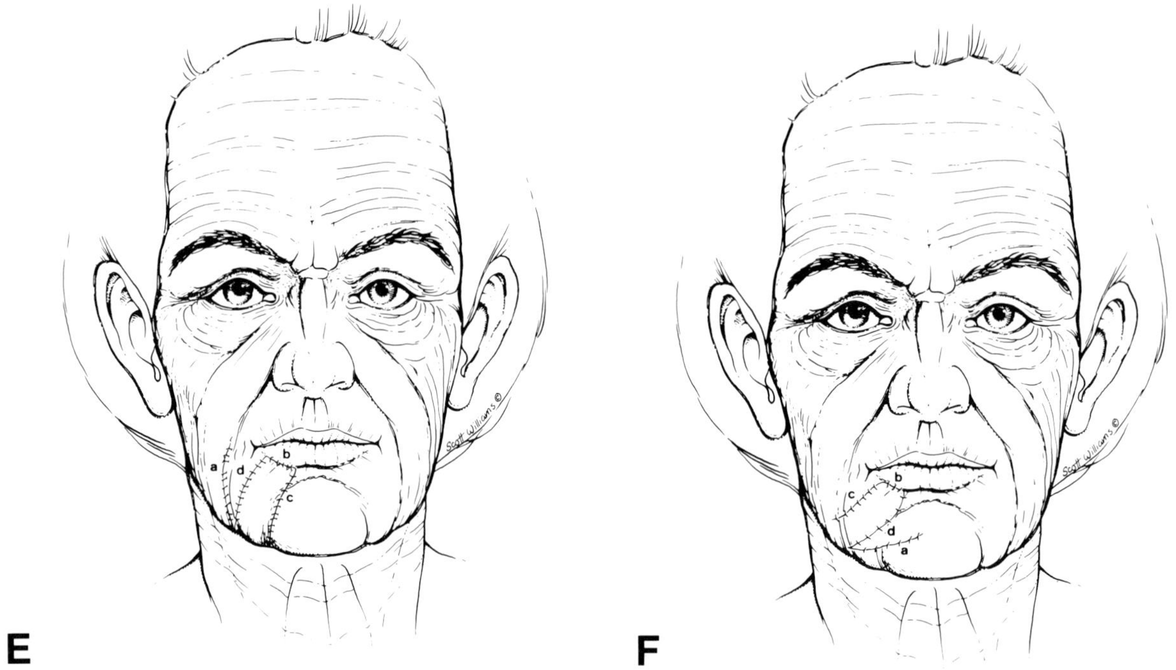

Figure 3 (continued) *E*, Expected scar pattern resulting from use of flap option A. Lines a, d, c, and b all lie predominantly within or parallel to normal facial skin lines and creases. *F*, Expected scar pattern from utilization of flap option B. Lines a, c, and d all lie at least partially counter to normal creases. Only line b is completely in a favorable direction. Therefore, the better of these two particular options would be flap A.

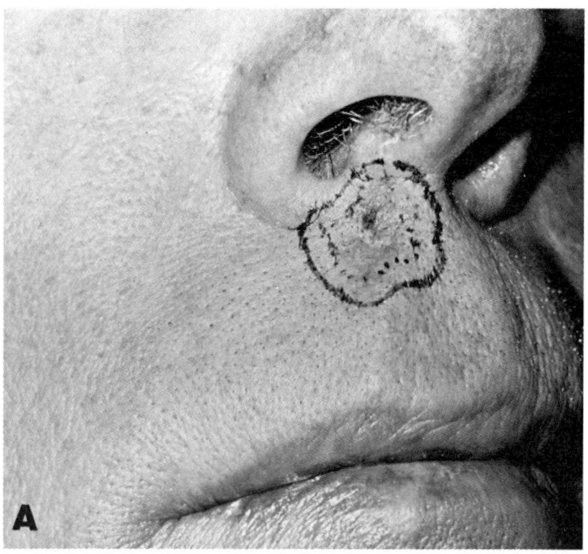

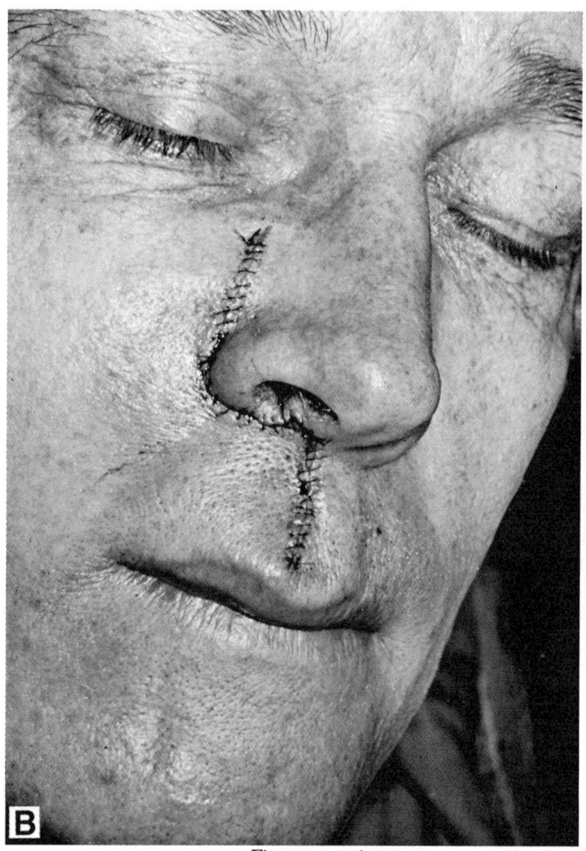

Figure 4 Perialar crescentric advancement flap. *A*, Basal cell carcinoma located on the upper portion of the lateral third of the upper lip also involving the nostril sill. *B*, The excisional defect has been closed by undermining and advancing cheek and lip skin. A crescent of normal skin has been excised from the cheek skin as it advances around the alar base to allow it to fit appropriately. The scar lines are, therefore, placed along the alar-facial groove and the inferior nostril sill. The dog ear from the advancement of the skin is excised and closed along the right philtral column. All lines will therefore be in favorable locations.

Figure continues on opposite page

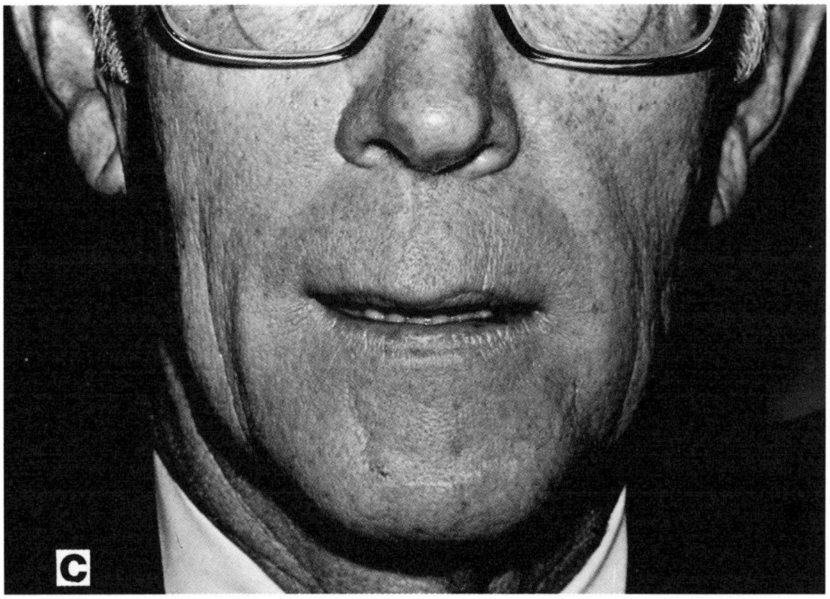

Figure 4 (continued) *C*, Postoperative result at 10 months.

elastic properties of skin, are invoked. Adjunctive incisions in various forms may be used to gain additional release and more extensive advancement. A balance must be struck between the closure tension inherent in all advancement flaps and the resulting compromise in flap circulation caused by this tension. The limitations of permissible tension unfortunately can only be subjectively evaluated, and clinical experience and judgment must be the prime determinants. Suture breaking strength can serve as a rough guide to permissible tension: if a 6–0 nylon breaks during attempted closure, tension is probably excessive. The perialar crescentic advancement flap, described by Webster and elaborated upon by Jackson is a particularly elegant version and should be a prime consideration for defects of the lateral third of the lip (Fig. 4).

Subcutaneous Island Pedicle Flaps

These flaps may be constructed either as transposition flaps, in which case subcutaneous tissue forms the

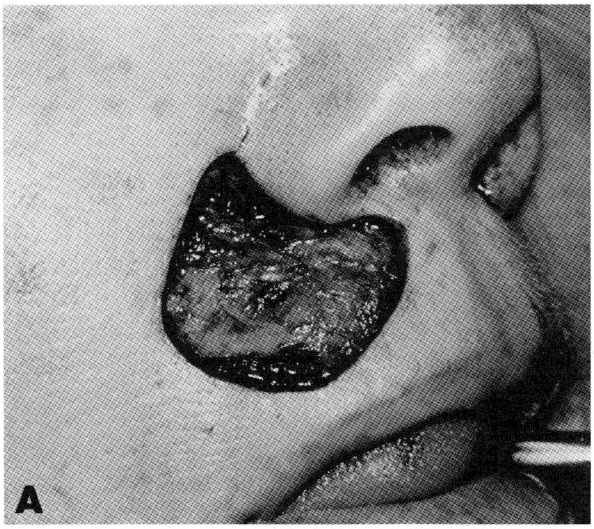

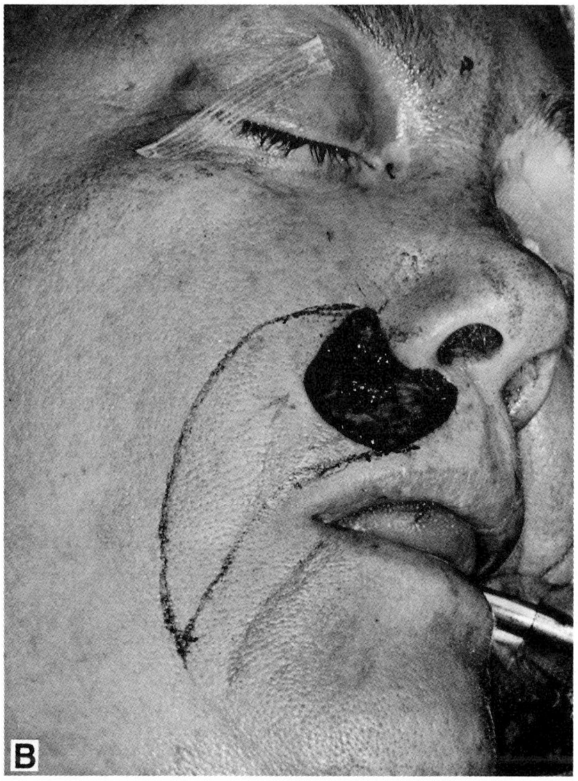

Figure 5 Subcutaneous island pedicle flap. *A*, Excisional defect from resection of a basal cell carcinoma. *B*, Nasolabial subcutaneous island pedicle flap outlined. The flap will be incised peripherally, thereby leaving it based upon subcutaneous blood supply only. The flap is then advanced in V—Y fashion into the defect.

Figure continues on following page

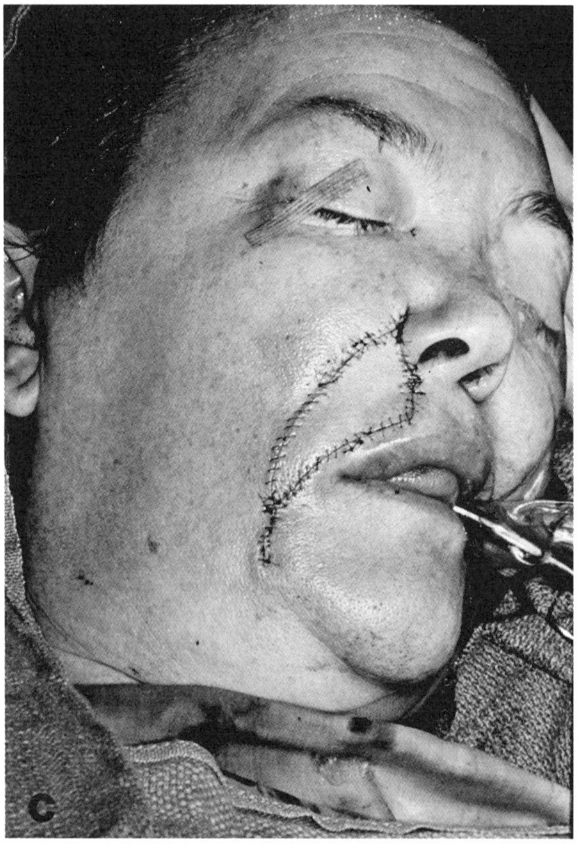

Figure 5 (continued) *C,* The flap has been advanced and the donor site closed in V—Y fashion. The majority of scar lines will be within or parallel to the nasolabial crease and the alar-facial groove or will parallel the vertical lines adjacent to the right philtral column. These flaps are particularly useful in the perialar and nasolabial regions.

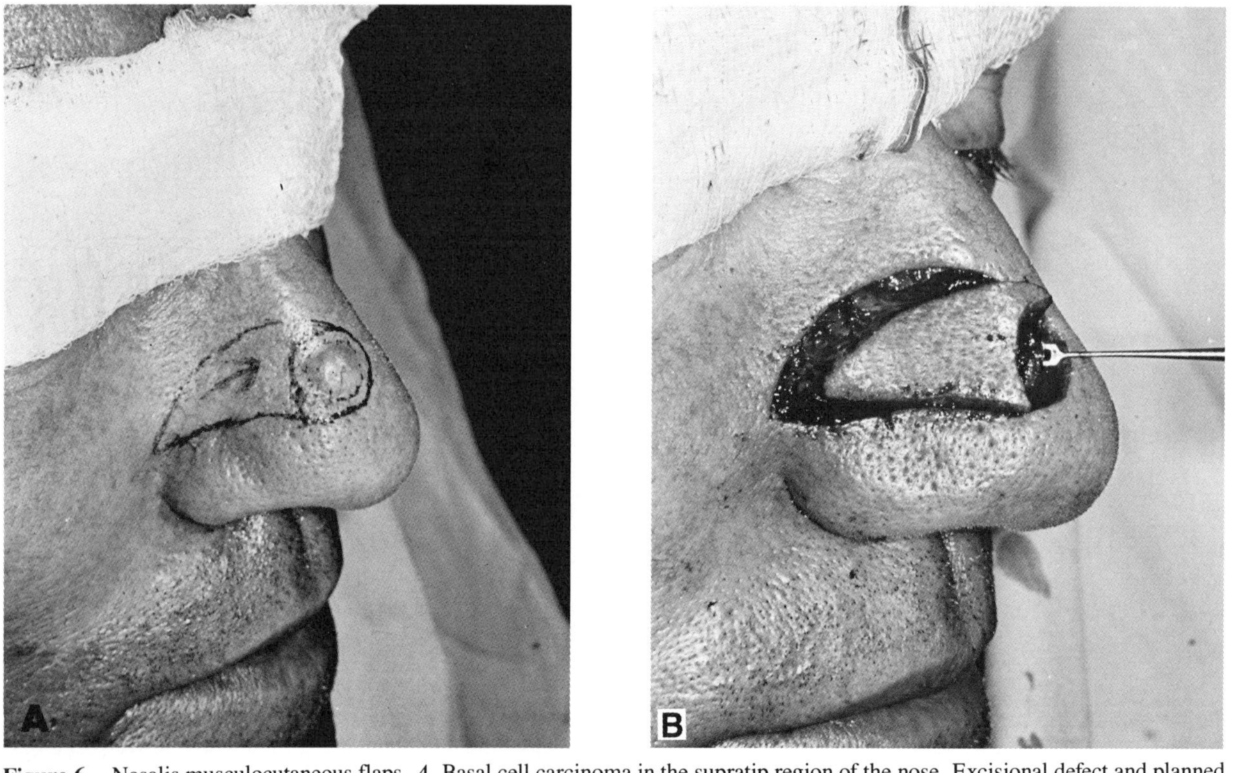

Figure 6 Nasalis musculocutaneous flaps. *A*, Basal cell carcinoma in the supratip region of the nose. Excisional defect and planned island musculocutaneous flap are outlined on the skin. *B*, The skin island has been mobilized as has the underlying nasalis muscle. Blood supply to the skin is, therefore, musculocutaneous in character. This is a particularly hearty flap that is excellent for repairs in this region.

Figure continues on opposite page

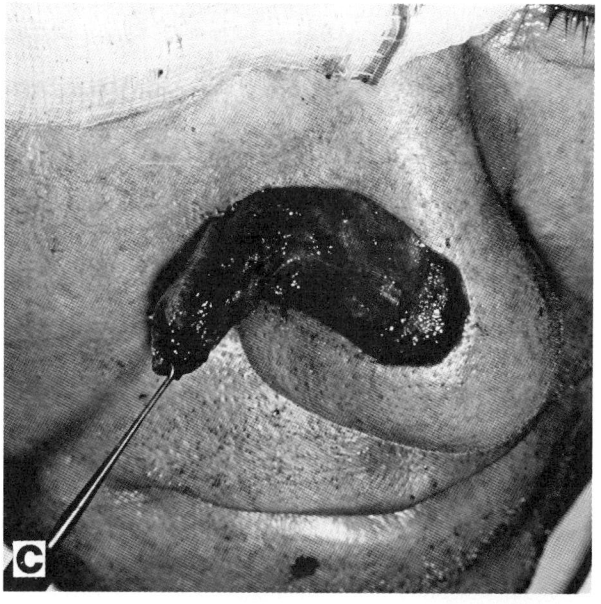

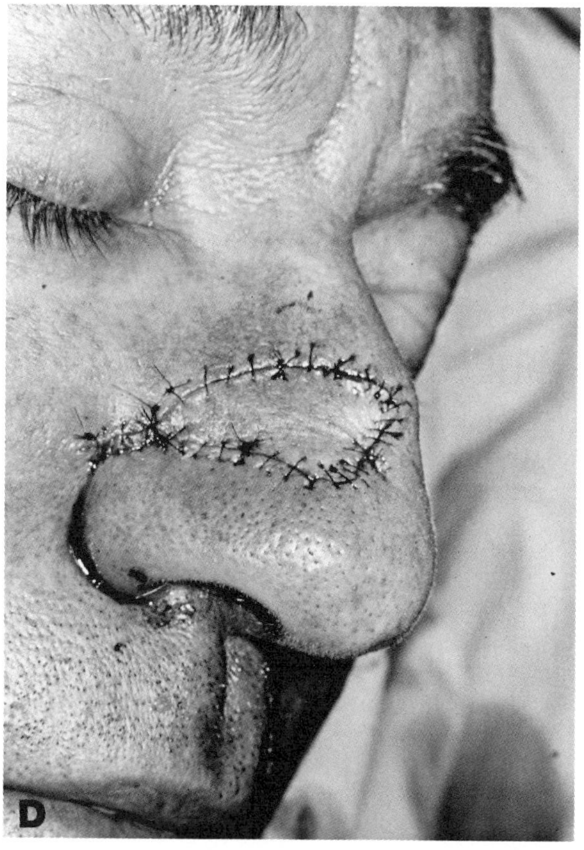

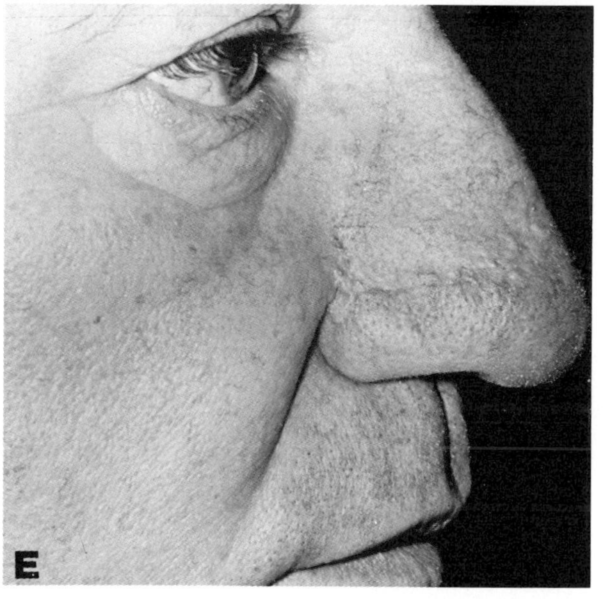

Figure 6 (continued) *C*, The underlying nasalis muscle is mobilized, but left attached laterally, thereby leaving intact its blood supply from the blood vessels near the alar-facial groove. *D*, The flap is advanced in V—Y fashion. Scar lines again run within the alar groove or parallel to it. The majority of scar lines also lie within normal facial creases, which might be seen upon wrinkling the nose. The exception is the most medial scar near the dorsum of the nose. *E*, Postoperative result at fourteen months.

pedicle, or as a form of advancement flap. The former is limited in its arc of rotation by the necessity of keeping the pedicle fairly short, since no definite vessels are included within the pedicle. I have not found frequent situations where these flaps seem to be the best therapeutic option. Conversely, the advancement type of subcutaneous island pedicle has proven to be extremely useful, particularly in the nasolabial area (Fig. 5). In repair of defects in the perialar region and near the nasofacial angle, these flaps approach the ideal, with near perfect color and texture match and with *all* scars lying in favorable lines. Flap reliability has been excellent.

Nasalis Musculocutaneous Flaps

This ingenious flap is excellent for the nasal supratip and tip (Fig. 6). It is also an island flap, based on the nasalis muscle. It may be used for moderate-sized defects in these areas and approaches the criteria noted previously in our "ideal flap" description. Color and texture match are excellent, and scar lines are almost all in natural skin lines.

SUGGESTED READING

Herbert DC, De Geus J. Nasolabial subcutaneous pedicle flaps. II. Clinical experience. Br J Plast Surg 1975; 28:90–96.

Jackson IT. Local flaps in head and neck reconstruction. St. Louis: CV Mosby, 1985.

Lister GD, Gibson T. Closure of rhomboid skin defects: the flaps of Limberg and Dufourmental. Br J Plast Surg 1972; 25:300–314.

McGregor JA. Fundamental techniques of plastic surgery and their surgical applications. New York: Churchill Livingstone, 1980.

McGregor JC, Soutar DS. A critical assessment of the bilobed flap. Br J Plast Surg 1981; 34:197–205.

Rybka TJ. Reconstruction of the nasal tip using nasalis myocutaneous sliding flaps. Plast Reconstr Surg 1983; 71:40–44.
Sprira M, Gerow TJ, Hardy SB. Subcutaneous pedicle flaps on the face. Br J Plast Surg 1974; 27:258–263.
Webster JP. Crescentic perialar cheek excision for upper lip advancement with a short history of upper lip repair. Plast Reconstr Surg 1955; 16:434–464.

ROLE OF THE PLASTIC SURGEON IN MOHS' MICROGRAPHIC SURGERY

ROBERT J. DEMUTH, M.D.
STEPHEN H. MILLER, M.D.
PETER E. GOODKIN, M.D.

In 1932, Frederick Mohs, while a medical student at the University of Wisconsin, described a treatment for difficult epithelial neoplasms that utilized zinc chloride paste for in vivo fixation, followed by histographic excision (Fig. 1). Microscopic control of margins permitted selective removal of neoplasms that extended for unexpectedly long distances beyond the clinically visible borders of skin involvement. Systematic examination of the entire undersurface, as well as the lateral margins of each specimen, was thought better than standard cross-sectional histologic techniques, which might miss finger-like projections of tumor. This technique was recommended for large lesions, those in difficult anatomic areas, and recurrent lesions. The drawback of this technique was the prolonged time needed for in situ fixation, namely 4 to 24 hours. Although in vivo fixation allowed excision without pain or bleeding, the time for excision and tumor clearance was excessive. Mohs now recommends the fixed tissue technique only for large lesions, those on vascular areas, and for melanoma in selected areas where tissue preservation is crucial.

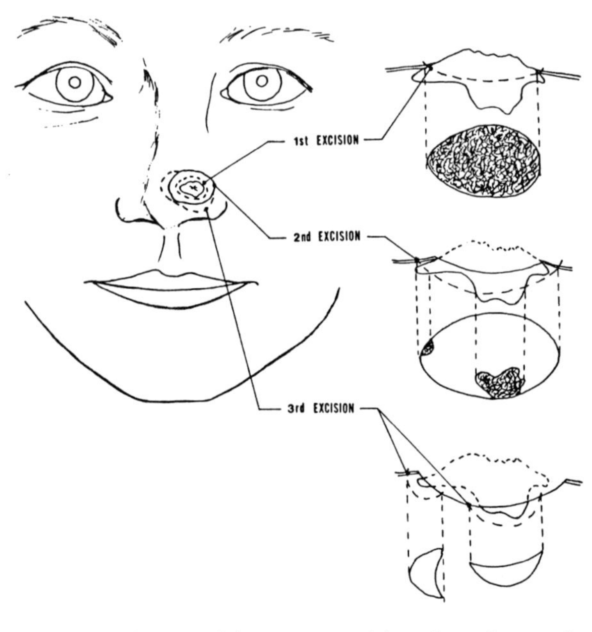

Figure 1 Diagram of three-stage excision of nasal tumor by Mohs' technique.

In 1974, Tromovitch described the fresh tissue technique using the same system of excision, with local anesthesia and microscopic examination of frozen section, thereby avoiding paste fixation. Bleeding was controlled by cautery, ligature, and pressure dressings. After a cancer-free wound was achieved, healing was by secondary intention, or through immediate reconstruction. These modifications saved time and eliminated some of the problems inherent in the paste technique, i.e., wounds that required the development of granulation tissue or dehiscence of the eschar prior to reconstruction.

The goals of treatment are to minimize recurrence and to achieve quality primary wound healing for the best esthetic result. The fresh and fixed tissue techniques are attempts to decrease recurrence rates following the treatment of skin neoplasms. These are as high as 12 to 25 percent in critical esthetic anatomic areas such as the nose, lip, ear, or eyelid. The cause of this high recurrence rate may be the reluctance of treating physicians to create the deformity that is necessary for adequate tumor ablation in these critical areas. Upon recurrence, regardless of the primary treatment modality, decisions regarding secondary treatment are not easy because of the difficulty and inaccuracy involved in visual assessment of the tumor margins.

The second goal of treatment is to achieve quality primary wound healing and the best possible esthetic result. Many defects in the soft parts of the face are easily excised and closed primarily, and do not require a team approach. Unacceptable esthetic results are often produced if one allows wounds to heal by contraction after simple linear closure in critical facial areas such as ear helix, eyebrow, hairline, vermilion white junction line of the lip, nasal nares, canthal margin, or hair-bearing areas. Tissue defects that require flaps, grafts, or sculpturing techniques have led to a team approach to achieve the best esthetic results. Figure 2 shows a distortion of vital structures caused by contraction and epithelialization, with poor end result. This could have been prevented with immediate plastic surgical closure.

Over the past 7 years, 1980–1987, we have treated approximately 250 patients. Recurrent disease was the primary indication for Mohs' excision in a majority of these patients. The dermatologist, trained in Mohs' concept of resection, has treated over 1,000 cases during this

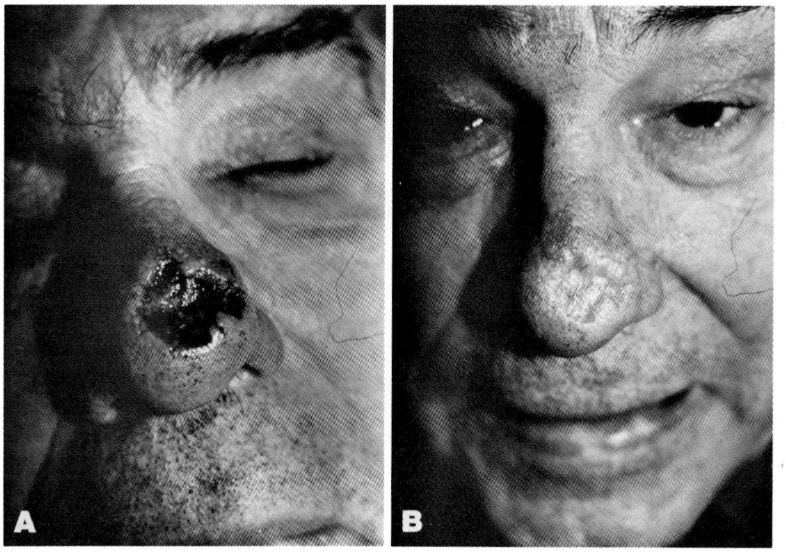

Figure 2 *A*, nose defect from basal cell carcinoma removal. *B*, result after 6 months with contraction and epithelialization.

period, which indicates that not all of these patients required a team approach. After the dermatologist completes the resection and clear margins are verified, a decision is made regarding closure. If closure cannot be achieved simply, the plastic surgery team is called to review treatment procedures, alternatives, and risks according to the needs and desires of the patient and family. A range of alternatives, from the simplest to the more complex, are presented to the patient.

The simplest treatment is still to allow the defect to heal by contraction and epithelialization. This option exists if the defect is small enough and in an appropriate area.

A slightly more complex technique is to close the wound by direct suture after undermining the edges. When simple closure without distortion is possible, our dermatologist closes the defect. If he feels a more elaborate repair is necessary, the patient is referred to the plastic surgeon. The wound is then removed by standard techniques so that the residual scar conforms or is parallel to the lines of facial expression. Occasionally, the central portion of this closure is too tight, and the resected dog ear is trimmed and placed in the tight central area as a full-thickness color matched skin graft. This is demonstrated in Figure 3. The technique was used to prevent eyebrow and hairline distortion. If a more substantial full-thickness graft is needed, donor sites utilized include postauricular, preauricular, upper eyelid, or supraclavicular skin. Split-thickness skin grafts from distant areas can be harvested with local anesthesia, and are sometimes used for closure of inconspicuous areas, such as the nasal lining, ear concha, or postauricular defects. Split-thickness skin grafts are also used as temporary repairs after treatment of more aggressive tumors. If the tumor has not recurred after a minimum of one year, a more definitive repair is then performed. If direct closure or grafting is inappropriate, then direct pedicle transfer combined with W-plasty, Z-plasty, or V-Y advancement and grafting are used. These techniques use similar tissue to achieve primary wound healing, and thereby minimize distortion and scar formation. Donor flaps and suture lines are designed to leave residual scarring in areas of natural creases. Careful attention to lack of tension prevents scar spread. Typical flap design in the central portion of the face is demonstrated in Figure 4. Particular attention is paid to the specific type of tissue transferred. The thickness of the nasal skin varies greatly from one anatomic part of the nose to another, and defects in different locations, therefore, have different requirements for reconstruction. The oily, glandular skin on the tip of the nose cannot be adequately replaced with grafts, nasolabial flaps, or other adjacent thinner skin, because of the poor quality of the color match and thickness. Nasolabial flaps swung across the nasal alar—cheek groove, obliterate the groove, are bulky, and often require secondary thinning. The diagram with Figure 4 demonstrates the use of adjacent, thick, oily nasal tip skin technique transferred by the "tip flip" technique in an effort to maintain the bulk of the nostril flare. Symmetry is maintained, and the donor site, on or near the midline of the dorsum of the nose, is often inconspicuous.

Staged reconstructions were rarely used in our series but are necessary for large defects. In these more complex cases, the reconstructive techniques must include replacement with identical tissue to rebuild lining, support structures, and skin cover. Figure 5 demonstrates a large nasal defect resulting from excision of a recurrent squamous cell carcinoma. A composite ear graft was used for lining and cartilaginous support, and the forehead was selected for external skin cover to achieve proper color match and thickness. Figure 6 shows a more complex case that required general anesthesia for reconstruction. This was a rare instance in which split-thickness skin graft was applied to the middle of the face because of the patient's age and overall medical condition. Split-thickness skin is generally not preferred because its color and texture differs from that of facial skin. This elderly patient also required reconstruction of the nasal lacrimal system which involved intubation of the residual lacrimal system after removal of the punctum and medial canthus. Figure 7 demonstrates

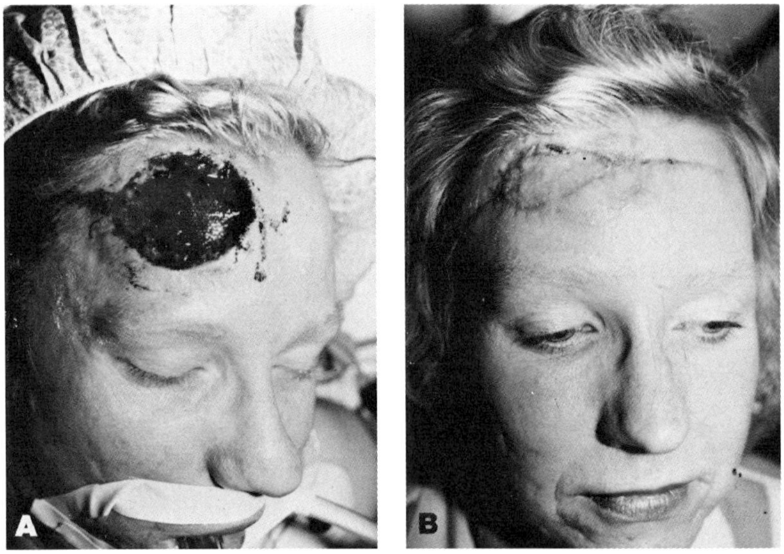

Figure 3 *A*, intraoperative final tissue defect. *B*, early result showing advancement closure utilizing dog ear tissue as a full-thickness skin graft in the central portion of the closure.

the use of a Mustardé flap for lower eyelid and cheek reconstruction, thus preventing ectropion in a large recurrent lesion.

The Mohs' chemosurgery technique is not necessary in the treatment of most skin cancers. Simple, nodular basal cell carcinoma, or well-circumscribed squamous cell carcinomas, have excellent cure rates and esthetic results with other treatment modalities. We feel that the technique is useful, however, where preservation of tissue is essential to prevent unnecessary destruction of vital facial features in the morphea- (sclerosing) type basal cell carcinoma, in recurrent lesions, and in areas known to have a high rate of recurrence around the nose, ears, and eyelids with standard techniques. Team treatment is a successful approach in facial regions prone to high recurrence rates.

In over 1,000 cases treated by our team dermatologist, there have been fewer than 30 recurrences. In our

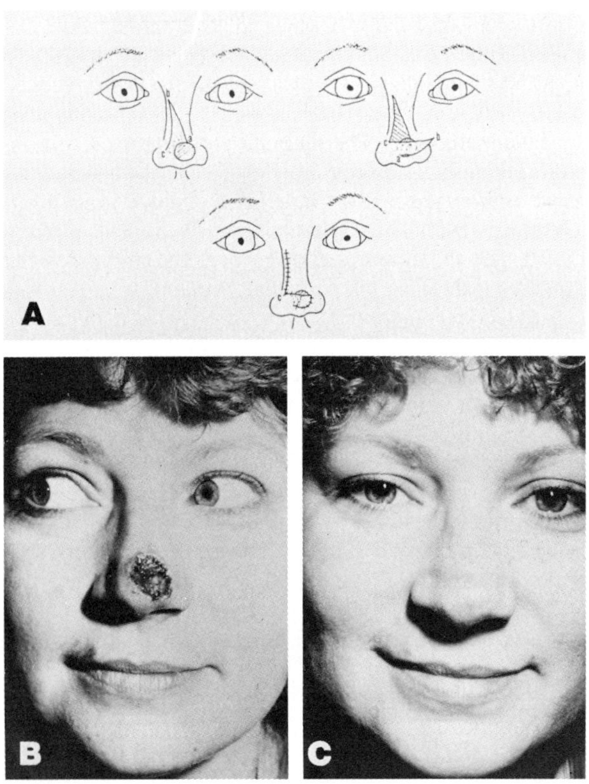

Figure 4 *A*, diagrammatic representation of "tip flip" reconstruction of nasal tip deformity. *B*, intraoperative defect. *C*, final result 1 year after surgery.

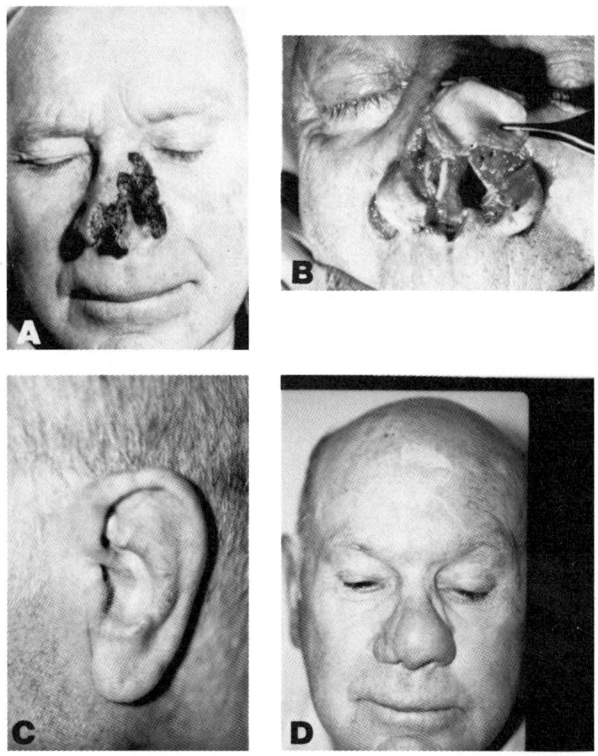

Figure 5 *A*, tissue defect following excision of carcinoma of nose and septum. *B*, beginning of reconstruction using left ear concha composite graft. *C*, left ear donor site 1 year after reconstruction. *D*, overall front view appearance 1 year after surgery.

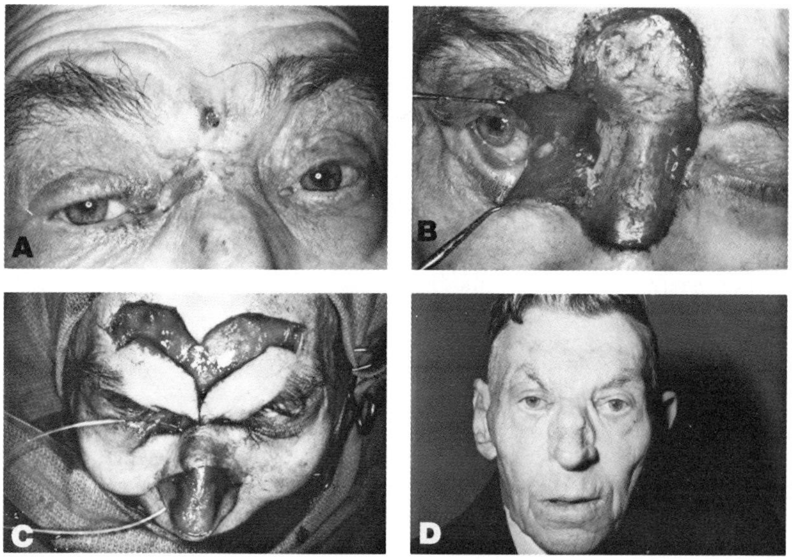

Figure 6 *A*, preoperative recurrent basal cell carcinoma. *B*, tissue defect following Mohs' resection. *C*, intraoperative view showing forehead pedicle flaps rotated to close glabella in association with bipedicle nasal flap. *D*, final result 2 years after one-stage reconstruction.

joint series of 250, there have been four recurrences. Occasional complications of flap necrosis, or partial take of skin grafts, have occurred, leading to some distortion of the planned reconstruction in spite of careful attention to design, hemostasis, and surgical technique. Outpatient care has been the primary goal, and hospitalization has rarely been required. Antibiotics are given only in those cases in which contaminated skin is encountered; in particular with transfer of nasal skin, which contains large crypts filled with secretions and bacteria in abundance. Open wound care is recommended as much as possible, postoperatively, for simplicity and management on an outpatient basis. Patients are followed by the plastic surgery team until primary wound healing is achieved and then follow-up is carried out by both teams for several months until a satisfactory esthetic result has been verified. The dermatologist on the team then follows the patient for a minimum of 5 years at regular intervals to verify cure.

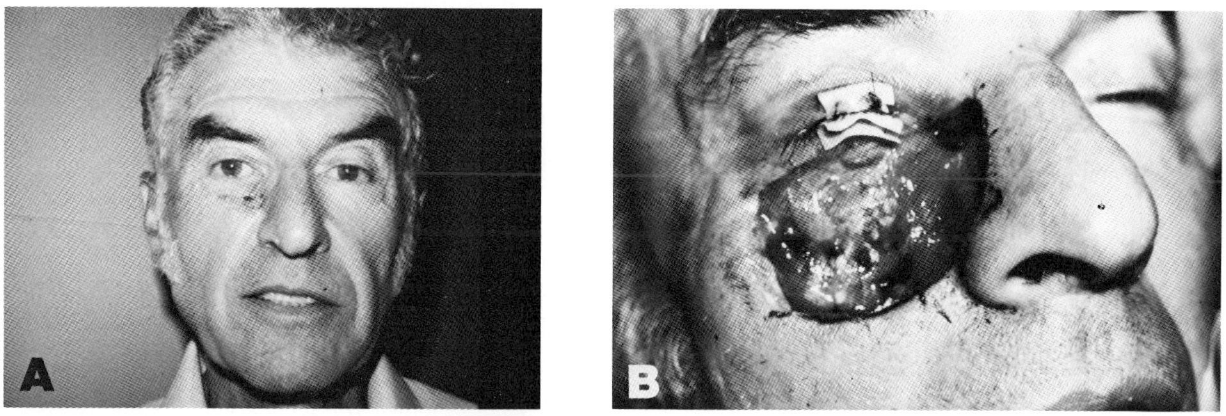

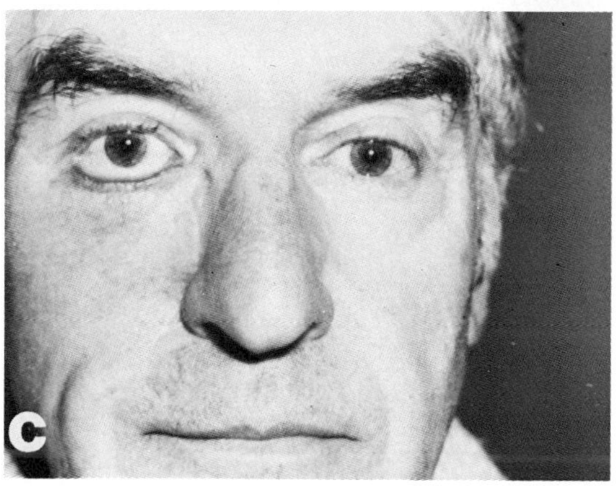

Figure 7 *A*, preoperative appearance of recurrent basal cell carcinoma of the right infraorbital cheek area. *B*, defect at time of Mohs' resection. *C*, primary wound heal following Mustardé flap reconstruction in primary healing at 6 months.

Referring dermatologists from geographic areas adjacent to our treatment center often assume the primary responsibility for follow-up care. Details of the treatment are always transmitted to facilitate accurate inspection of the treated area.

The majority of our patients must travel more than 1 hour by car to visit our treatment center. If our treatment team feels that there is any doubt regarding the family's ability to transport the postoperative patient to a home environment, arrangements are made at a nearby low-cost overnight facility within easy reach of our hospital, to ensure that problems encountered can be managed adequately. Preoperative instructions include directions for abstinence from complicating medications such as steroids, aspirin, or other anticoagulants prior to the excision. It is requested that a member of the family always be available for immediate postoperative care. Supportive families have been most cooperative due to the cost-cutting advantages of outpatient care.

There are several disadvantages to this team approach. The degree of difficulty and resection time with the Mohs' technique cannot be accurately predicted, and this requires the plastic surgical team to be available on-call. Our team works on a 1 day per week basis with 1 to 3 patients treated weekly. Occasionally, primary reconstruction is not carried out on the same day and this requires hospital admission and operating room scheduling on short notice. Conflicts in scheduling occur when emergency or elective case load is high, thus forcing considerable adjustment of daily schedules. A second disadvantage is that the patients are often first seen by the plastic surgeon after the resection is completed and the tissue defect present. Ideally, the surgeon would have the patient's history and physical examination performed by his own team, but in these cases we must depend on medical clearance by another physician. This sometimes requires the rapid establishment of a physician-patient relationship and quick evaluation of the patient's medical status and ability to care for himself or have such care provided by family members. Despite these difficulties, considerable information can be obtained and good rapport developed. The ability to complete the care of these patients under local anesthesia enables the surgical team to get to know the patient's medical status by observing response to the surgical procedure. During the verbal discussion of the operative procedure and follow-up care with the patient, we are able to analyze the ability of the patient and family to follow directions for the strict requirements in early postoperative care. If there is any doubt about these capabilities in our treatment team's assessment, then hospitalization is arranged on a semi-emergency basis.

The advantages of the system include a high cure rate, limited deformity, and a quality esthetic result in treatment of areas of esthetic importance that have a high recurrence rate. A combination of the skills of the Mohs' surgeon and the reconstructive skills of the plastic surgery team has achieved good results in our treatment series.

SUGGESTED READING

Burg G, Hirsh RD, Konz B, et al. Histographic surgery: accuracy of visual assessment of the margins of basal-cell epithelioma. J Dermatol Surg Oncol 1975; 1:21–24.

Koplin L, Zarem HA. Recurrent basal cell carcinoma: a review concerning the behavior and management of recurrent basal cell carcinoma with emphasis on the incompletely excised lesion. Plast Reconstr Surg 1980; 65:656–664.

Mohs FE. Chemosurgery: a microscopically controlled method of cancer excision. Arch Surg 1941; 42:279–295.

Mohs FE. Chemosurgery. Clin Plast Surg 1980; 7(3):349–360.

Shanoff LB, Spira M. Hardy SB. Basal cell epithelioma: a statistical approach to natural management. Plast Reconstr Surg 1967; 39: 619–624.

Tromovitch TA. Stegman SJ. Microscopically controlled excision of skin tumors: chemosurgery (Mohs) fresh tissue technique. Arch Dermatol 1974; 110:231–232.

NONMICROSURGICAL RECONSTRUCTION OF POSTABLATIVE HEAD AND NECK DEFECTS

MARK E. KRUGMAN, M.D.

Head and neck reconstruction represents the ultimate challenge to the plastic reconstructive surgeon. Nowhere else in the body does the integration of form and function play such an important role. Nowhere else is the lack of form and function more difficult to conceal.

Although microvascular reconstruction has been the most dramatic advance in head and neck reconstruction, most defects can be suitably managed with nonmicrovascular methods.

The surgeon should have available to him the full range of reconstructive methods. The nonmicrovascular surgeon should work with a microvascular surgeon. Tumor resection should never be compromised at the expense of the reconstructive result. One must always plan and be prepared for a "worst case" scenario. This chapter deals principally with post-tumor-ablation defects of the upper aerodigestive tract. In general, I attempt definitive reconstruction at the time of tumor ablation. Staged reconstruction allows tissues to shrink and scar down, thereby making secondary reconstruction much more difficult.

LIP DEFECTS

Small defects, less than 25 percent, may be treated by direct closure. A shield-shaped defect is preferred. The tattooing of the vermilion border and use of local anesthesia facilitate the reconstruction. Abbe-type flaps have been well described and are used for intermediate defects. Larger defects are reconstructed with modified Bernard-Burow's repair, as described by Madden. While the Karapandzic flap preserves function, it does create a microstoma. For this reason, it is not preferred for large defects.

ORAL DEFECTS

Small defects of the oral cavity may be closed directly. Larger floor-of-mouth defects may be reconstructed with inferiorly-based nasolabial flaps. Split-thickness skin or mucosal grafts may also be used. I prefer to quilt the graft, as described by MacGregor, rather than to bolster. An excellent source of mucous membrane for a variety of purposes may be harvested from the maxillary sinus.

Partial thickness buccal lesions have been traditionally grafted (Fig. 1). Given the severe degree of trismus that occurs when the pterygoids are resected, I have recently begun to use the parascapular free flap (Fig. 2). Palatal island flaps, based on the greater palatine vessels, and random palate flaps may be used to cover palatal defects and oroantral fistulas. Partial thickness defects in the hard palate are usually allowed to heal secondarily. Tongue flaps may be used for anterior palatal defects. Although I rarely employ them, they are a valuable method in selected patients.

I prefer to reconstruct hemiglossectomy defects by sewing the contralateral anterior tongue to the posterior defect. This results in a shorter but wider tongue. The functional and esthetic results are superior to simple closure.

Large oral defects are best reconstructed with myocutaneous flaps. The workhorse has been the pectoralis major (PMC) flap (Fig. 3). The PMC flap has made obsolete the donor-deforming forehead flap. The deltopectoral flap, formerly the reconstructive keystone in the head and neck, is now used infrequently.

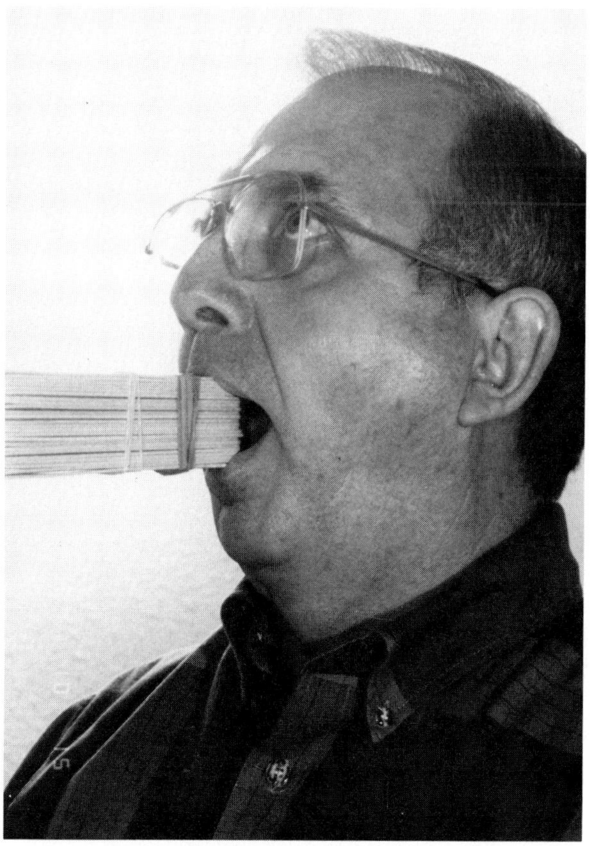

Figure 1 Patient is performing tongue blade incentive exercises to prevent trismus after skin grafting.

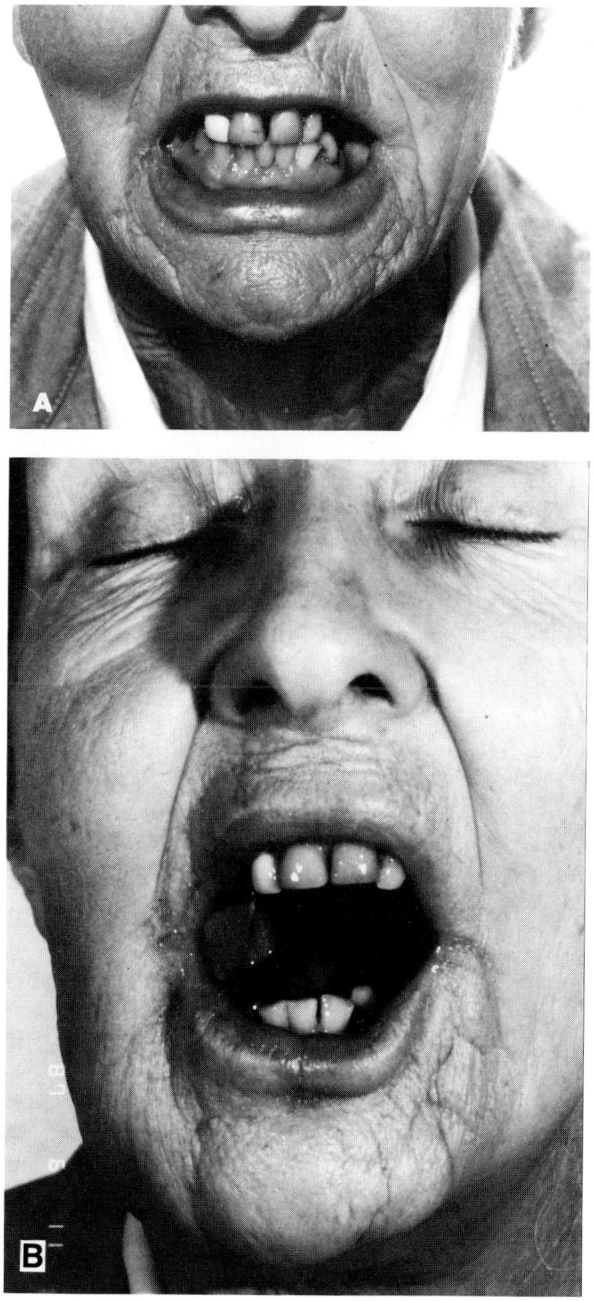

Figure 2 *A,* Severe trismus followed resection of posterior oral tumor and skin grafting, which has been corrected, *B,* With partial mandibulectomy and parascapular free flap.

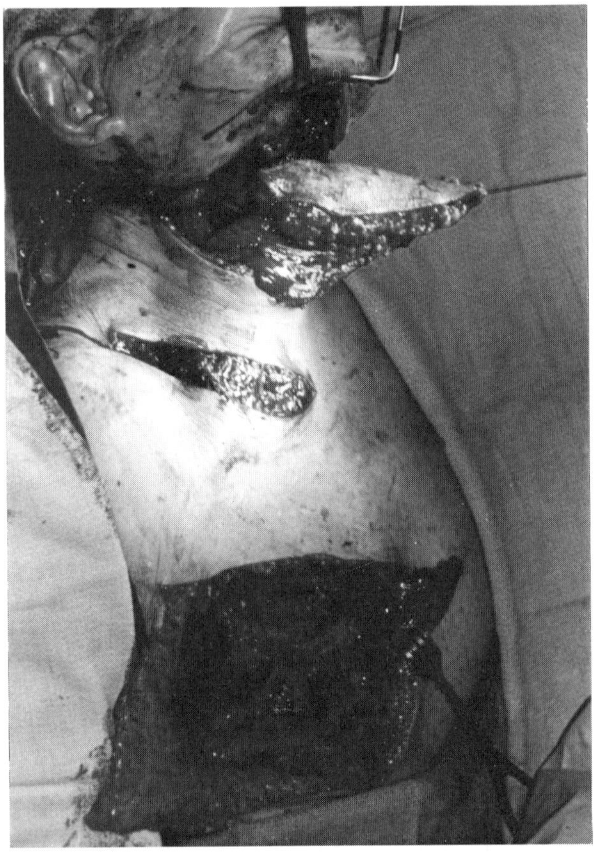

Figure 3 Pectoralis myocutaneous flap is elevated after resection of oral cancer.

When a small, bony, mandibular defect exists in a nonradiated field, I prefer a titanium wire basket filled with cancellous bone.

The key to success in alloplastic reconstruction is adequate soft tissue coverage. When the field has been irradiated, or where there is a soft tissue deficiency, I prefer a microvascular composite flap. My early experience of the PMC flap over an alloplastic implant or nonvascularized autografts was very poor. Similar results were reported by others. When the titanium basket is used, I attempt to cut the basket in a shallow fashion and set back the distal segment a small amount to maximize the soft tissue cover.

Several other myocutaneous flaps have been used in the oral cavity. The sternocleidomastoid flap, as described by Ariyan, has had limited usefulness in the hands of myself and colleagues. The skin paddle survival has been inconsistent and flap viability cannot be depended upon if a radical neck dissection (or most modified radical neck dissections) is done. Similar circumstances limit the use of the platysma myocutaneous flap for oncologically-oriented reconstructions.

PHARYNGEAL DEFECTS

Smaller pharyngeal defects may be closed with primary closure or tongue flaps. Traditionally, commando or composite resection types of procedures were closed primarily. Removal of the posterior bony framework, with ability to collapse soft tissue cover, permitted direct closure. The PMC flap offers a number of advantages over primary closure composite resections. Its bulk preserves a more normal external contour and allows a more secure closure and carotid artery protection. Its skin paddle maintains a better physiologic relationship in the oropharynx. The bulk of the pectoralis is a distinct disadvantage in the hypopharynx, and the trapezius flap is a less bulky alternative. This latter flap, however, has the disadvantage of a compromised blood supply when a radical neck dissection is performed. More recently, my colleagues and I have been exploring thinner, free microvascular flaps for hypopharyngeal resurfacing. Lesions localized to the posterior pharyngeal wall may be skin-grafted postablation.

PARANASAL SINUS AND ORBITAL DEFECTS

Prosthetics has been and continues to be the mainstay of maxillary sinus reconstruction. Close association with a skilled maxillofacial prosthodontist is essential for the head and neck surgeon. Raw areas such as the pterygoids may be skin-grafted. Orbital defects may be reconstructed with temporalis muscle. I prefer cured, preshaped Silastic placed through a coronal approach for nonradiated front sinus defects with healthy skin. Reconstruction of the implant with the aid of three-dimensional

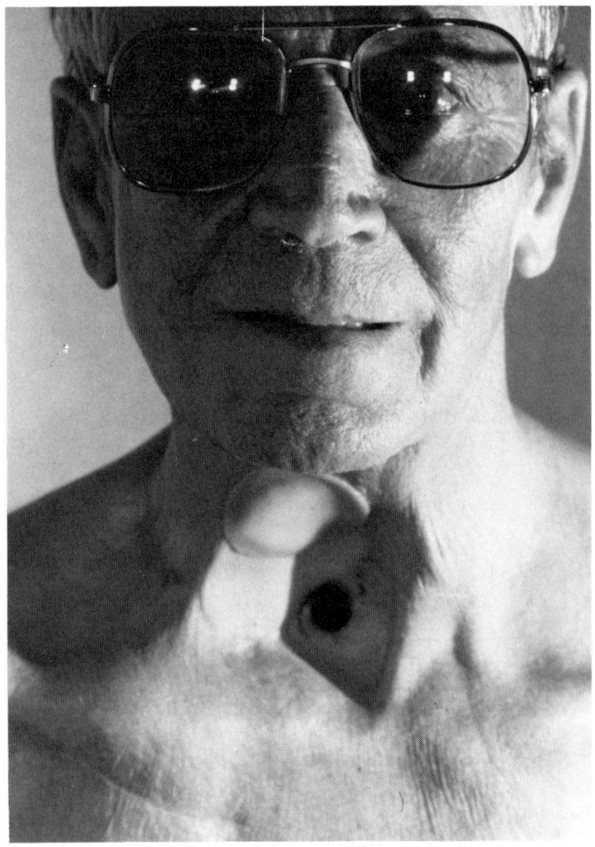

Figure 4 Stomal adhesive covers pharyngocutaneous fistula.

computerized tomography (CT) reconstruction has been helpful.

NECK DEFECTS AND FISTULAS

Small oro- or pharyngocutaneous fistulas may be managed temporarily with enterostomal hydrocelluloid materials, such as Duoderm or Restore (Fig. 4). These materials are also useful to close off irregularly-shaped permanent tracheostomy stomas during the day in obstructive sleep apnea patients. Small fistulas are often successfully managed with local tissue. Turnover flaps are used for the oral or pharyngeal layer, and advancement flaps resurface the skin. Larger defects with exposed vessels or fistulas are closed with myocutaneous flaps. Again, the PMC flap remains the standard. Partial defects of the neck without great vessel exposure may be skin-grafted. I have found hyperbaric oxygen therapy a valuable adjunct to conventional wound care in the preparation of the recipient bed.

It is generally true in plastic surgery that there is no substitute for experience and planning. No individual can encompass all ablative and reconstructive skills. A skilled microvascular surgeon, maxillofacial prosthodontist, oral surgeon, and speech pathologist are important skilled members of the head and neck reconstructive team. Resection of the tumor is only the first step. Reconstruction demands an ecumenical team approach for normalization of form and function.

SUGGESTED READING

Ariyan S. One stage reconstruction for defects of the mouth using a sternomastoid myocutaneous flap. Plast Reconstr Surg 1979; 63:618–625.

Madden JJ, et al. Reconstruction of the upper and lower lip using a modified Bernard-Burow technique. Ann Plast Surg 1980; 8:100–107.

McGregor IA, McGregor FM. Cancer of the face and mouth. New York: Churchill Livingstone, 1986:410.

MAJOR CRANIOFACIAL DEFECTS: ROLE OF FREE TISSUE TRANSFER

ROBERT A. HARDESTY, M.D.
VERNON L. YOUNG, M.D.

Patient with extensive loss of skin and soft tissue that involves the face, scalp, and neck are among the most difficult problems encountered by the reconstructive craniofacial plastic surgeon. We recently presented a two-institution series of 27 patients who had ablative resections or traumatic loss that resulted in major soft-tissue or composite defects of the head and neck; all of these were reconstructed with microvascular free tissue transfer. Any cutaneous defect larger than 100 cm^2 was considered "gigantic." From this experience, the principles that evolved in the management of such complex and massive defects are presented and discussed.

ETIOLOGY OF THE DEFECT

The vast majority of gigantic defects in our series were secondary to ablative resections for tumor. A combination of patient delay, inadequate initial treatment, and primary tumor aggressiveness was responsible for tumor size of such magnitude. Typically, recurrent or deeply invasive tumors tend to invade adjacent structures prior to distant metastatic spread. The outlook is usually considered poor when these neoplasms have invaded bone, brain, or other vital structures. Many deeply-penetrating or locally-invasive tumors were once considered inoperable because resection would produce a large ablative cutaneous defect with exposure of multiple vital structures. Recent reports that suggest improved palliation, together with the experience gained from skull base surgery, craniofacial surgery, and microsurgery have allowed ablation of tumors that were once thought unresectable. By combining these different techniques and surgical approaches, truly radical and, it is hoped, curative resections can now be successfully performed. These combined techniques in a select subset of patients can also afford planned palliation and relief of intractable pain and the morbidity of progressive local cutaneous disfigurement.

In addition to the advanced cancer, large composite defects of face and scalp may be traumatically induced, thereby resulting not only in major cutaneous deficits but also in acute exposure of vital structures, especially the brain or dura. Trauma cases and burns accounted for 11 percent of the presenting etiology.

RECONSTRUCTION OPTIONS

Reconstruction choices for such major defects have traditionally included skin grafting, local rotation flaps, and delayed tubed pedicle flaps. The discovery of the deltopectoral flap and the subsequent commencement of the pedicled, regional, musculocutaneous flap era revolutionized reconstruction of head and neck defects. Specifically, myocutaneous flaps provide a reliable, expeditious reconstructive choice for gigantic defects of the lower one-third of the craniofacial skeleton. The reach of regional flaps can be extended to cover large defects of the middle third of the facial skeleton, however, with fixed pedicles and limited arc of rotation, they become increasingly limited as the defect size increases and the location progresses to the vertex of the skull.

Microvascular free tissue transfer is the latest addition to the armamentarium of the reconstructive craniofacial surgeon. It uniquely allows immediate and complete coverage of virtually any defect of almost unlimited size with greater flexibility than prior reconstructive methods. Microvascular free tissue transplantation has a number of distinct advantages: (1) avoidance of size and reach limitations imposed by regional flaps, (2) one-stage reconstruction is possible without resorting to multistage procedures, (3) essentially unrestricted donor possibilities as compared to the local or regional flaps, and (4) greater flexibility to design and transfer composite tissue. However, microsurgery is not without its attendant problems, risks, and complications. These include: (1) the need for special training and equipment, (2) extended operating time, and (3) the fact that completion of a successful tissue transfer is based entirely on a patent microvascular anastomosis. In our series, and in centers where routine use of microvascular tissue transfer are used in age- and disease-equivalent populations, the success rate of 90 percent or greater is quoted. This compares favorably with the morbidity of regional flap transfer.

We do not advocate free flap closure for all large defects of the head and neck. The simplicity of skin grafting and local pedicle myocutaneous flaps make them appropriate for the majority of patients who undergo reconstruction. However, in select subsets of patients with massive defects and exposed vital structures, such alternatives may not suffice. Limitations of skin grafts, local flaps, distant pedicled myocutaneous flaps, and donor site restrictions may not allow for immediate or complete closure of these difficult wounds. Skin grafting may not reliably provide stable wound coverage when radiotherapy or chemotherapy is anticipated. The use of certain local flaps is precluded by the size and location of the defect. Inherent inadequacies of all regional pedicle flaps for head and neck reconstruction include limitations of reach based on arc of rotation, flap size, limited flap choice, bulkiness, lack of reliability in transferring blocks of composite tissue (skin, muscle, and bone) to the cranial vertex, and the necessity to extend flap reach by delay procedures. When local or regional pedicle flaps are unsuccessful or inadequate, free tissue transfer can consistently be used as the "bail out" reconstructive option. Our experience shows that microvascular free tissue transfer provides the greatest flexibility in the reconstruction of large complex head and neck defects. Careful planning and measurement of the defect size in relationship to donor-recipient vessels can allow accurate design and execution of free flap harvest and inset while optimally maximizing the usable surface area of the transferred tissue (Fig. 1).

In our series, the majority of patients underwent immediate reconstruction, which was necessitated by exposed dura, dural grafts, brain, or incontinuity defects between the cranial cavity and oropharynx. The approach to all ablative resections that undergo immediate reconstruction is frozen-section control of the margins and additional resection from the margins for permanent histology. In those selected cases where no vital structures are exposed, microvascular reconstruction is delayed until the final pathology report is obtained to assure completeness of resection. The rationale that reconstruction should be delayed so that recurrences are not buried under a flap may appear at first logical and sound. However, in this particular subset of patients with advanced or recurrent cancer, radical surgical ablation may represent a final salvage attempt to free the patient of disease; and further surgical resection may not be compatible with life. The goal should be to complete both ablative and reconstructive surgery expeditiously in one stage. We feel the patient can better tolerate adjuvant radiotherapy or chemotherapy with less morbidity if vital structures and massive defects are closed with vascularized flap coverage rather than a mere skin graft. Lastly, the patient's perspective should not be overlooked. The value of a single-stage ablation and reconstruction that requires one hospitalization cannot be discounted. Despite size, location, or type of defect created, the ablative surgeon need not be limited in his resection by reconstructive constraints, because of the availability of a wide array of free flap donor sites.

PATIENT EVALUATION

All patients should be evaluated clinically to determine the extent of local tumor invasion and to ascertain if they can tolerate general anesthesia. The length of anesthesia for combined ablation and microvascular reconstruction varied between 8 and 18 hours in our series. However, the major risks of general anesthesia occur during the induction and extubation periods. Thus, after our evaluation, if there are any additional concerns regarding the patient's cardiovascular system, we routinely consult preoperatively with our colleagues, the internists, cardiologists, and anesthesiologists.

Sophisticated diagnostic aids are essential to detect the presence and define the extent of intra- or extracranial extension of tumor. The minimal diagnostic workup should include high-resolution narrowly-columnated computed tomography (CT) scan. Delineation or obliteration of normal soft-tissue plans can be enhanced further by the use of magnetic resonance imaging (MRI). Occasionally, when lesions are suspected of invading intracranial venous or arterial structures, an angiogram of the carotid system with both arterial and venous phases can be obtained. Evaluation for unsuspected distant metastasis includes a thorough clinical evaluation, routine radiologic examination of the chest, and biochemical serum analysis. These different diagnostic modalities, when needed, allow a fairly accurate assessment of location, extent, invasion, and resectability of the tumor.

Optimally, these advanced lesions are best treated by a multidisciplinary surgical team that includes a neurosurgeon, head and neck surgeon, and reconstructive microsurgeon. These procedures by the nature of the size,

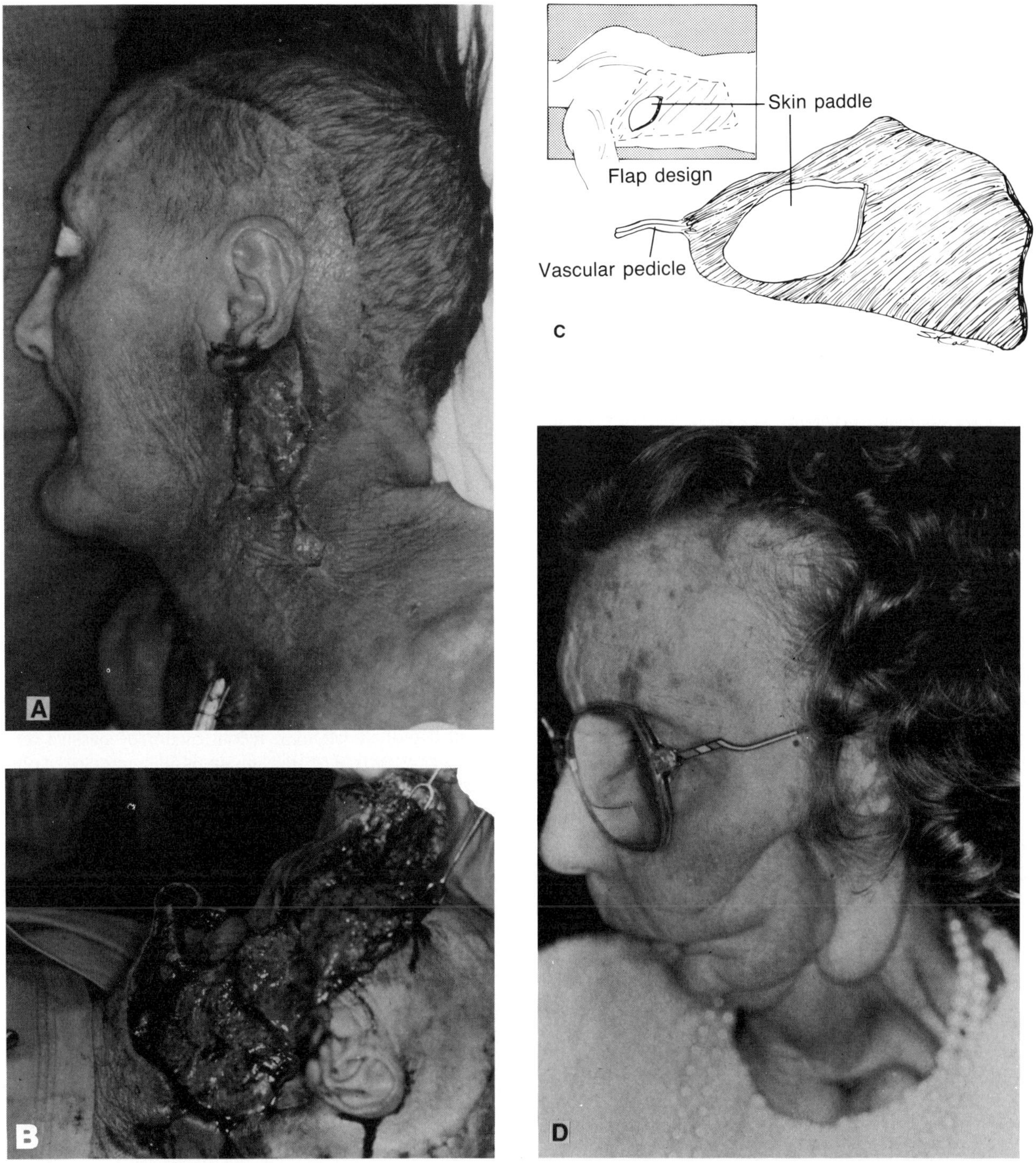

Figure 1 *A,* A 76-year-old female presented with a recurrent malignant mixed parotid tumor that required infratemporal fossa resection, partial maxillectomy, partial mandibulectomy, and left neck dissection. She received postoperative adjuvant radiation therapy. A pectoralis major myocutaneous muscle flap had been used for reconstruction and subsequently partially necrosed. *B,* She presented to the plastic surgery service in a cachectic state 3 months postsurgery with a widely-patent orocutaneous fistula that resulted in continuous salivary soiling. Elevation of the flaps prior to débridement resulted in a gigantic cutaneous defect as well as exposure of a long segment of carotid artery. *C,* A latissimus dorsi myocutaneous free flap was designed to provide well-vascularized muscle cover for the exposed carotid artery, as well as cutaneous reconstruction of the skin deficit. *D,* A postoperative view following reconstruction with a latissimus dorsi myocutaneous free flap.

location, operative time, and technical requirements lend themselves to a team approach. Preoperatively, each member independently examines the patient and evaluates the diagnostic tests. The interdisciplinary team then meets to discuss approaches, alternatives, and sequencing of surgical procedures. Thus, a well-planned premeditated definitive plan for ablation and reconstruction can be formulated. We have found that this preoperative planning session not only expedites patient care and coordinates the involved surgeons but, in addition, provides an educational and "cross-fertilization" experience for all members of the team.

Postoperatively, all patients should be followed up with routine regular physical examination to evaluate any local or regional spread of disease. Physical examination alone is not sufficient for evaluation of recurrence in these deep and insidious tumors due to their nature, location, and size. Regular monitoring with serial MRI or CT scans is recommended. Free flap coverage, in our experience, does not decrease the sensitivity of these diagnostic modalities.

FREE FLAP SELECTION

The literature is replete with descriptions and anatomic dissections of the most common free flap donor sites. Additional free flap donor sites are continually being described in various locations, and their applicability is diverse. It is beyond the scope of this chapter to describe each individual free flap available, but our approach to these massive defects is presented and discussed next.

The choice as to which free flap to use is dependent upon: (1) the reconstructive goals, (2) donor site availability, (3) type of tissue to be replaced (skin, muscle, bone, or composite), and (4) familiarity of the operative surgeon with donor flaps. In our series, six different types of microvascular free tissue transfer were utilized (latissimus dorsi flap, scapular flap, rectus abdominis flap, radial forearm flap, groin flap, and the omental flap). In general, we have found that when the resultant defect is large and cavernous, the latissimus dorsi and rectus abdominis muscles, with or without their cutaneous paddles, allow coverage of the cutaneous defects as well as provide a three-dimensional vascularized muscle "bulk" to fill the ablative dead space. When composite tissue (skin and bone) or pliable skin are needed to restore contour, our flaps of choice are the microvascular scapular or the radial forearm flaps. They provide both reliable donor vessel anatomy and composite tissue transfer capability. Skin paddles and bony components can be designed and harvested in various positions within their defined vascular territory, and thus, allow a greater degree of freedom in composite transfer design. Furthermore, the scapular flap, with its osseous component, can be elevated to include the latissimus dorsi muscle on one vascular pedicle (subscapular artery). In our experience, the groin flap and omental flap, though clinically useful when needed, are used only under unusual situations.

Analysis of our data identified, in addition to the gigantic cutaneous defect, two distinct clinical groups of patients based on their reconstructive needs: (1) patients with exposed vital structures and (2) those with contour deformity. Sixty percent of patients had some type of vital structure exposed that required immediate coverage. This included exposed brain, dura, or dural grafts. Large composite tissue resections often create contour irregularities and large cavities with potential dead space in need of obliteration. Three patients had direct intraoperative continuity between the oronasal cavity and the cranial contents. Separation of the oronasopharynx and intracranial structure was of utmost concern. The presence of a direct communication between aerodigestive tract and intracranial contents not only added to the three-dimensional complexity of the reconstruction but, more important, conventional regional or local flaps did not adequately provide a dependable reconstructive barrier between the brain and the aerodigestive tract due to limitations of size or arc of rotation. The potential for catastrophic sequelae is high, especially when the dura has been resected or grafted. This separation is facilitated by moving the microvascular pedicle closer to the defect so that the surgeon is able to take advantage of a much greater area of the usable flap. This allows latitude in flap orientation, positioning, and inset that is not possible with local or pedicle flaps.

While six different types of microvascular tissue transfer were utilized, the latissimus dorsi continues to be the "workhorse" flap when major size defects are encountered. Its expansiveness, constant vascular anatomy, ease of harvest, and minimal donor site problems make it our flap of choice in the reconstruction of massive head and neck defects. The free latissimus dorsi muscle not only meets the reconstructive requirements of size and rich vascular supply to cover vital exposed structures, but also provides malleable tissue that can be manipulated in multiple planes to fill potential dead spaces. The tissue can be sculptured, contoured, and folded to achieve specific reconstructive goals.

The following case presentation underscores the advantages of microvascular reconstruction. A 70-year-old, hypertensive, insulin-diabetic patient presented with a recurrent Marjolin's ulcer secondary to thermal injury in childhood. She had undergone seven previous procedures, including a full course of therapeutic radiation. She exhibited radiation field effect on local skin and soft tissue, which precluded the use of local flaps as a means of reconstruction. The resection resulted in loss of bony architecture as well as skin and soft tissue. In addition, immediate coverage of surgically-exposed right frontal dura was needed. A latissimus dorsi free flap achieved all of these goals and allowed completion of the reconstruction in a one-stage procedure, thus demonstrating the flexibility of microvascular free tissue transfer. In situ sculpturing of the flap and application of split-thickness skin graft provided definitive cover as well as an esthetically acceptable result (Fig. 2).

Extensive neoplasms with origin in the skin of the face or the maxillary sinus may invade the bony planes of the cranio-orbital skeleton to involve the cranial base. Resection of such tumors is now possible. However,

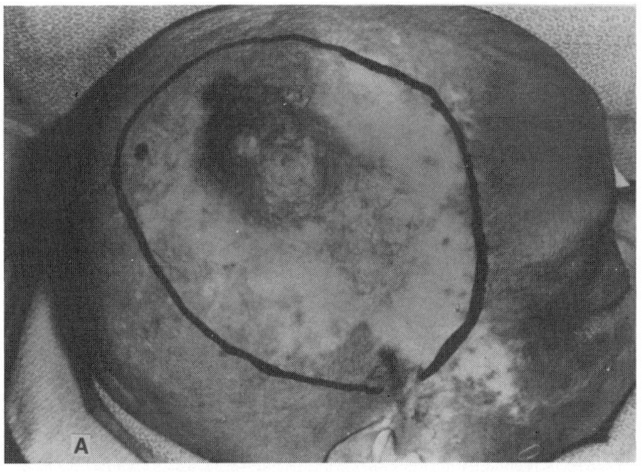

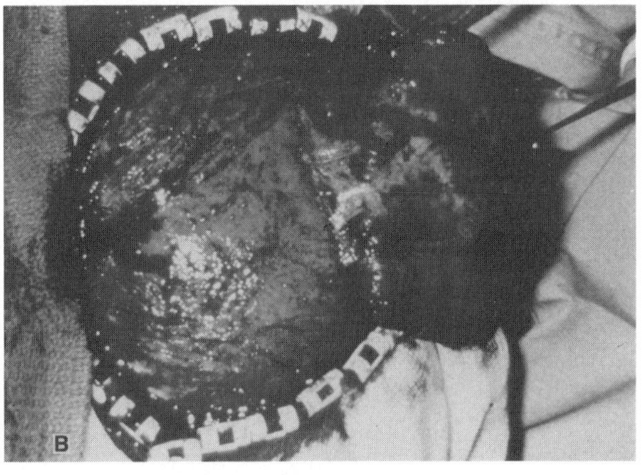

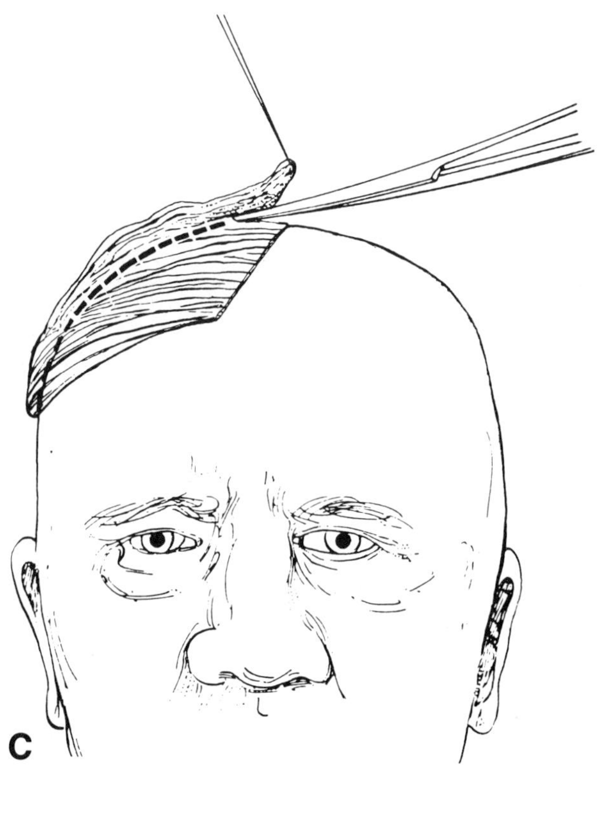

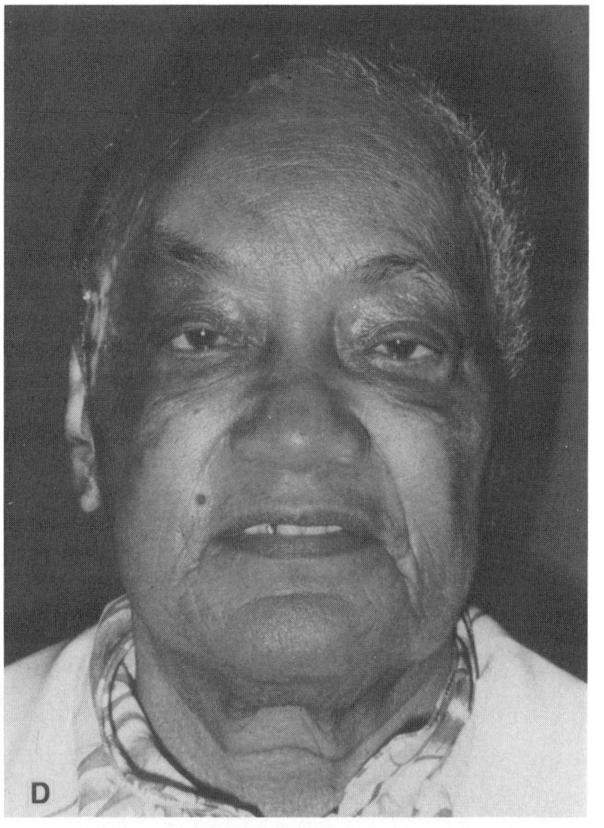

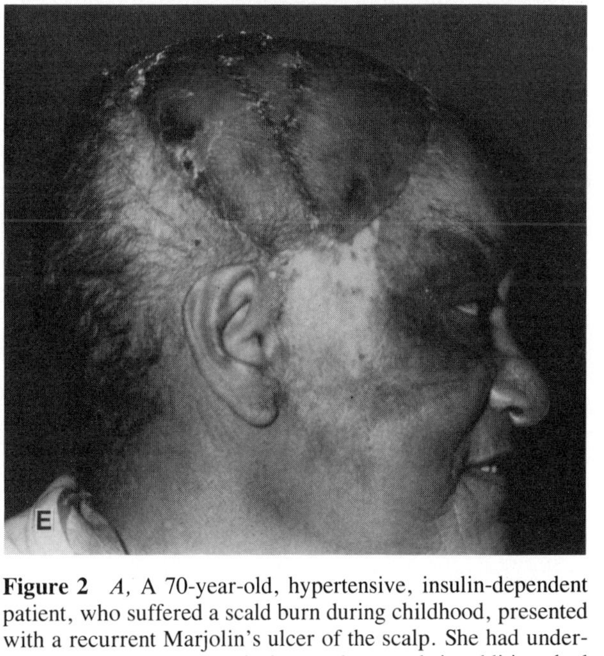

Figure 2 *A,* A 70-year-old, hypertensive, insulin-dependent patient, who suffered a scald burn during childhood, presented with a recurrent Marjolin's ulcer of the scalp. She had undergone seven previous surgical procedures and, in addition, had received 6,000 rad of therapeutic radiation. She exhibited radiation "field effect" on local skin and soft tissue, thus limiting the usefulness of local flaps. *B,* A composite resection was completed and resulted in not only a large cutaneous defect but also exposed dura. *C,* A latissimus dorsi muscle onlay free flap was inset. Sculpturing of the flap and partial-thickness, nonmeshed skin graft allowed a one-stage esthetic reconstruction. *D* and *E,* The patient is shown 5 months postoperatively.

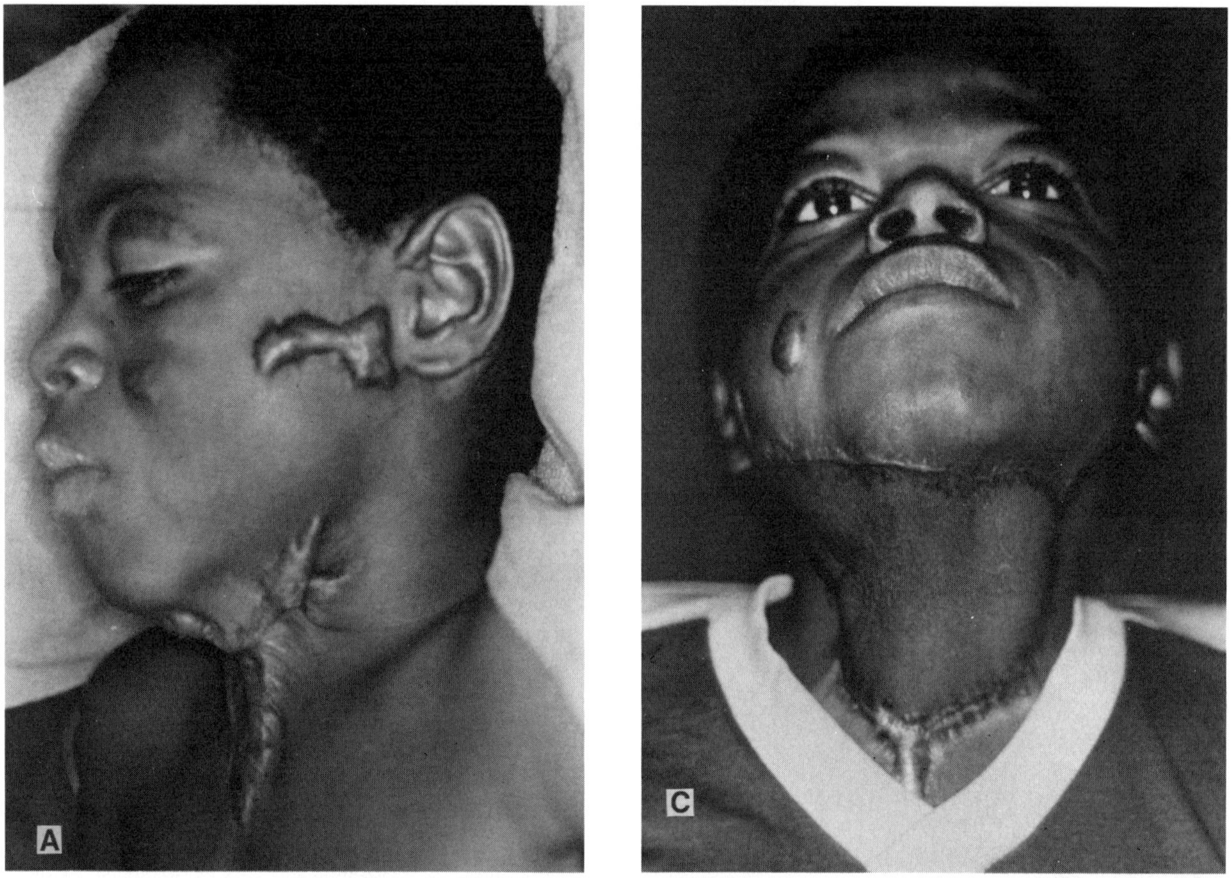

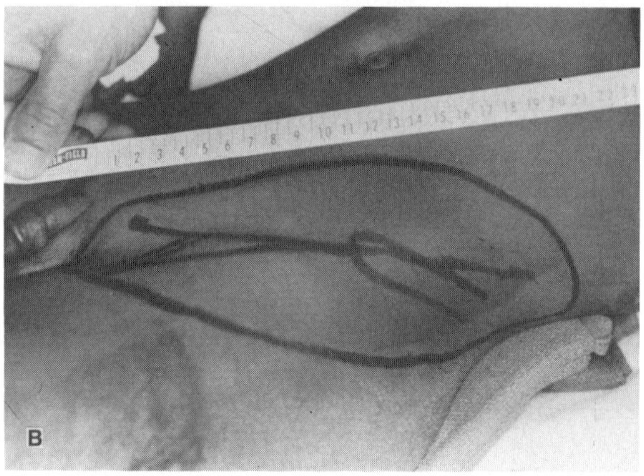

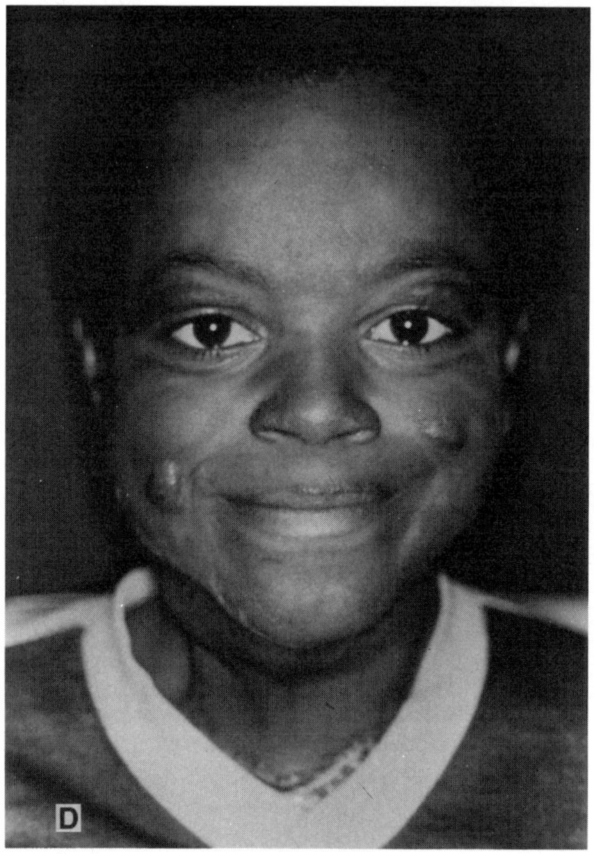

Figure 3 *A*, a 10-year-old black male suffered a thermal injury to face and neck resulting in a cicatricial scarring and keloid formation. *B*, In addition to the unsightly keloid formation, the contractile forces of wound healing resulted in a functional impairment. With his propensity to form keloid, a hidden free flap donor site was chosen. *C* and *D*, The patient 1 year following free tissue transfer with near total extension.

following resection the dura or dural grafts covering the brain are in direct communication with the nasopharynx and oral cavity. Cerebrospinal fluid leakage, with ascending infection, could result in a catastrophic outcome. In addition, those patients who have undergone a combination of ablative surgery and aggressive radiation therapy are at a high risk for nonhealing orocutaneous and cutaneous fistulas. In our series, the lack of infection is noteworthy. There were no postoperative donor or recipient site infections, cerebrospinal fluid leaks, or signs of meningitis. There has been no fistula formation or draining sinus tracts. This is significant because of the nature of the surgery, the size of the defect created, duration of surgery, exposed vital structures, patient population, oronaso-pharyngeal-cranial contamination, and prior radiation or surgery.

Figure 1 exemplifies a typical scenario of fistula formation and its untoward effects. A 76-year-old female had undergone resection of a recurrent malignant mixed parotid tumor that required infratemporal fossa resection, partial maxillectomy, partial mandibulectomy, and left neck dissection. She received postoperative adjuvant radiation therapy. A pectoralis major myocutaneous flap used for primary reconstruction subsequently partially necrosed. The patient presented to the plastic surgery service 3 months postoperatively in a cachectic state. In addition to the skin defect, there was a widely-patent, high, orocutaneous fistula that resulted in continuous salivary soiling. She required tube feedings for nutritional support. The patient underwent wide débridement that produced a gigantic cutaneous defect as well as exposure of a large segment of carotid artery. For reconstruction, a latissimus dorsi myocutaneous free flap was designed and tailored to reconstruct and obliterate the various constituent parts of the defect. The skin paddle was used to replace the cutaneous defect, while the muscle provided a well-vascularized cover for the exposed carotid artery.

In patients with massive defects and significant contour deformity, restoration of function and form are paramount after attainment of wound coverage. Microvascular tissue transfer offers a wider choice of alternatives when specific defect deficits are to be reconstructed. Composite tissue (skin, subcutaneous tissue, muscle, or vascularized bone) can be transferred independently, or in any combination needed. Free tissue transfer allows the reconstructive surgeon various options in the selection of specific tissue composition, of appropriate design and dimensions, from different donor areas. This specificity allows for a better tissue match and, thus, a better esthetic reconstruction. Free tissue transfer uniquely allows donor site choice based not only on reconstructive tissue needs but also on esthetic and functional considerations. A graphic example is presented in Figure 3. This 10-year-old flame burn victim suffered secondary cicatricial scarring that resulted in keloid formation and functional deformity. Release of the scar contracture produced a gigantic cutaneous defect. Because of the boy's propensity to form keloid, a less conspicuous donor site was chosen. A free groin flap fulfilled all reconstructive needs as well as providing a hidden donor site.

SUGGESTED READING

Hardesty RA, Ramasastry SS, Young VL, et al. Refinements in microvascular tissue transfer for major craniofacial resection. American Association of Plastic Surgeons Annual Meeting, Nashville: May 6, 1987.

Jones NF, Schramm VL, Sekhar LN. Reconstruction of the cranial base following tumor resection. Br J Plast Surg 1987; 40:155-162.

Quillen CG. Latissimus dorsi myocutaneous flaps in head and neck reconstruction. Plast Reconstr Surg 1979; 63:664-670.

Swartz W, Banis JC, Newton ED, et al. The osteocutaneous scapular flap for mandibular and maxillary reconstruction. Plast Reconstr Surg 1986; 77:530-545.

Webster MHC, Soutar DS. Practical guide to free tissue transfer. London: Butterworth, 1986.

PAROTID TUMORS: DIAGNOSTIC PROCEDURES AND RADIOTHERAPY

MARK S. GRANICK, M.D., F.A.C.S.
DWIGHT C. HANNA, M.D.

DIAGNOSTIC TECHNIQUES

Our diagnostic evaluation of parotid tumors is based on the experience of having evaluated and treated some 1200 salivary gland neoplasms. There are numerous tests and studies available, but few of them are clinically useful. This review will discuss the relevant diagnostic maneuvers and suggest a practical approach to parotid neoplasms.

The most critical tool in evaluating a parotid mass is the patient's history and physical examination. No clinician is capable of making a histologic diagnosis on the basis of a clinical examination, but there are many clues that give important hints to the patient's condition.

Most parotid tumors present as a painless mass. A history of pain or facial weakness is highly suggestive of malignancy. A history of intermittent enlargement of the mass suggests a possible branchial cyst or inflammatory disease (Fig. 1). Some patients report a history of a prior or concurrent tumor, such as breast, prostate, renal carcinoma, or melanoma, which may be a source for metastases to the parotid. A history of radiation treatment in childhood for acne or thymus enlargement predisposes the patient to salivary and thyroid tumors.

The physical examination must be systematic. Even if the presenting problem seems obvious, a thorough ex-

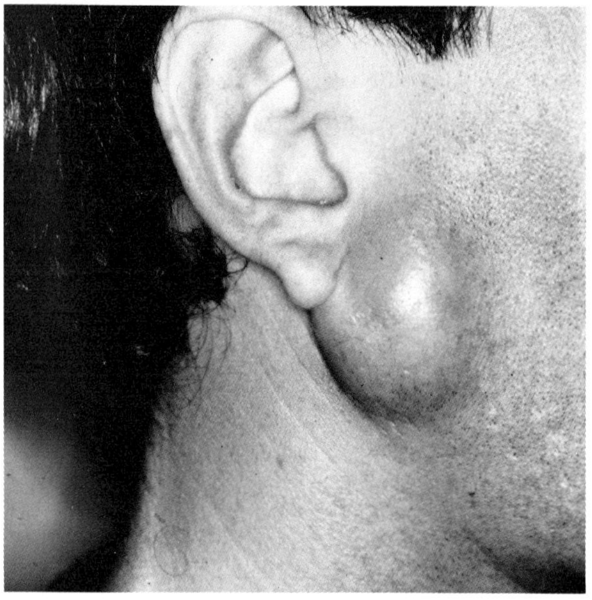

Figure 1 This 27-year-old man complained of intermittent swelling, redness, and tenderness of his right cheek. His history revealed a prior incision and drainage performed by his family doctor. Lesion was removed and, as expected, was a first branchial cleft cyst.

amination of the facial and scalp skin, intraoral and pharyngeal areas (Fig. 2), and neck must be performed on every patient. A primary melanoma, squamous cell carcinoma, or eccrine carcinoma with metastases to the parotid may be detected. The presence of skin fixation to the tumor suggests extraglandular extension of a malignancy (Fig. 3). A fixed hard tumor is likely to be a squamous carcinoma, whereas a spongy cystic-feeling mass in a middle-aged man will probably be a Warthin's tumor. Facial nerve dysfunction is another hint that the tumor is likely to be malignant (Fig. 4).

All of the tests that are potentially helpful deal with imaging. On occasion, plain x-ray films may delineate a sialolith. The best use for sialograms (injection of contrast media via a cannulated Stensen's duct) is to evaluate inflammatory disorders of the parotid. Sialograms have no clinical value in assessing the status of a tumor. Ultrasound studies and radionuclide scanning rarely add any clinically useful information. Computed tomography (CT) and magnetic resonance imaging (MRI) are worthwhile when used selectively. The indication for CT or MRI is to determine the extent of spread of a large extraglandular or recurrent tumor.

There are many biopsy techniques available. Core-needle biopsy and incisional biopsy are rarely indicated, because of the potential for inadvertent facial nerve injury and the possibility of tumor seeding. Fine-needle aspiration biopsy has been reported to be a reliable technique. We, however, have found several major shortcomings to this technique. Due to the diverse range of histopathology in salivary gland tumors, the structure of the tumor, rather than the individual cell types, is often critical to the diagnosis. Needle aspiration destroys the tumor organization and allows only a cytologic examination. Another objection is that the technique is only reliable in an institution where the pathologists encounter a large number of salivary gland specimens, and there are few such programs. An additional caution is that regardless of the result of these biopsies, the tumor still needs to be removed in almost all cases.

Our recommended biopsy technique is parotidectomy. In most instances, removal of the tumor along with the superficial parotid is both the definitive diagnostic maneuver and adequate treatment for the tumor. We rely on frozen section analysis of the operative specimens for immediate feedback as to the tumor type. Frozen sections

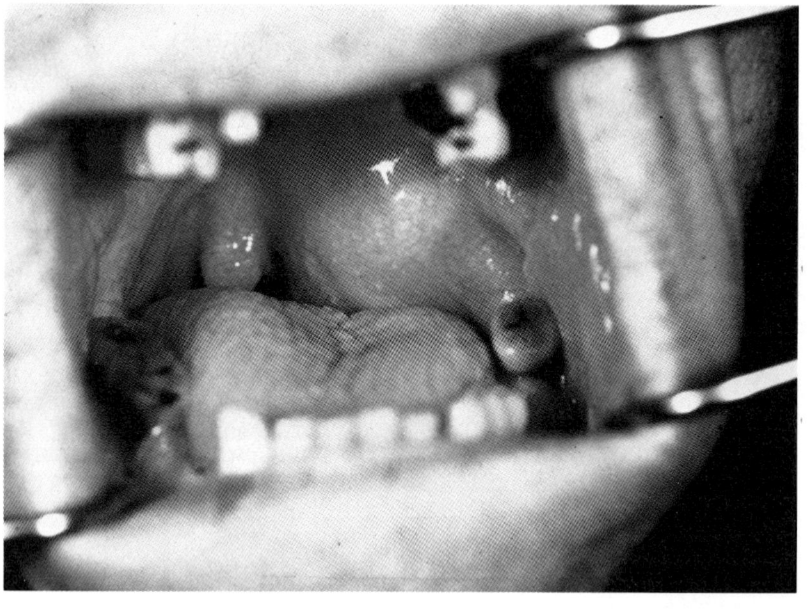

Figure 2 Intraoral examination shows swelling in left oropharynx, and demonstrates deep lobe involvement in this patient's left parotid tumor.

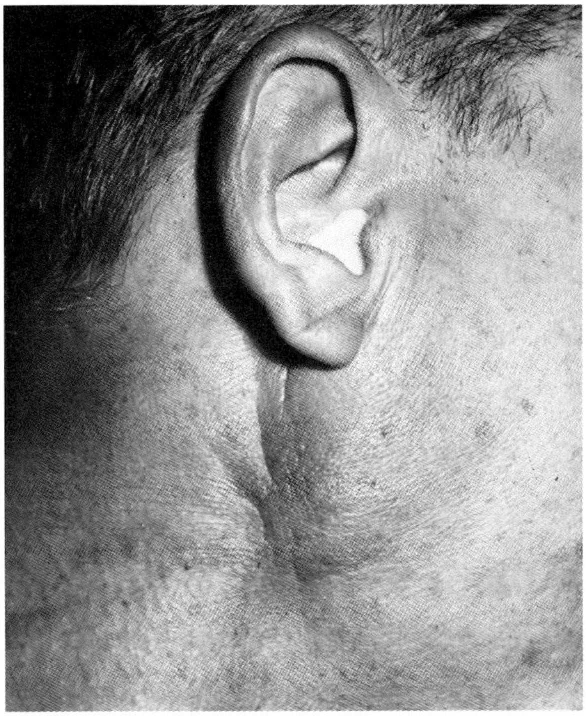

Figure 3 Examination of patient's facial skin revealed fixation of the skin to an underlying parotid tumor, suggesting extraglandular extension of a malignancy. The patient underwent parotidectomy and wide resection of the involved skin for primary adenocarcinoma of the parotid.

have been very reliable in our experience. This information can be helpful in determining the necessary extent of surgery in terms of managing the deep parotid lobe, the neck, and the facial nerve (Fig. 5).

Consequently, a practical approach to the patient presenting with a parotid mass is first to establish that the patient indeed has a parotid neoplasm. The history and physical examination is the most important part of the patient's diagnostic evaluation. If the tumor appears to have significant extraglandular extension, then CT or MRI studies are indicated. The next step is parotidectomy. The surgeon should be prepared to handle a total parotidectomy, facial nerve resection and nerve graft reconstruction, neck dissection, mandibulectomy, or wide skin resection and reconstruction, as the situation dictates. The patient, of course, should be informed preoperatively of all possibilities in his particular case.

RADIOTHERAPY

Radiation therapy plays a critical role in the total care of the parotid tumor patient. While surgery remains the primary treatment modality, radiotherapy is an important adjunct in many situations (Table 1). The following is a surgeon's perspective of radiation treatment for parotid disease.

Radiation exposure is a powerful treatment modality for microscopic salivary gland disease. It is generally not effective in treating large salivary tumor loads. Consequently, with the exception of parotid lymphoma, radiation is reserved for postoperative adjunctive therapy. The treatment also alters normal tissue within the exposure portals, and leaves local potential for malignant transformation with an induction time of 15 to 20 years. Consequently, radiation treatment should only be used when there are appropriate indications.

Radiation therapy should be considered in two clinical settings. Patients with gross disease, who either cannot or refuse to undergo surgery, should be treated with radiotherapy. Secondly, patients with presumed subclinical tumor should be considered for radiation treatment. These patients include those who have had surgery for malignant tumors and have histologically positive margins, or those whose tumor is presumed to be close to the surgical margin. In this category we include all high grade

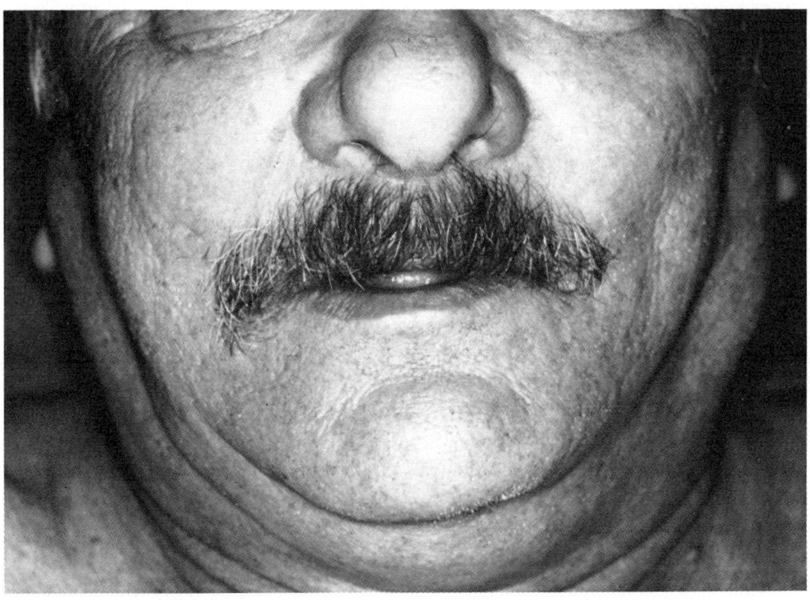

Figure 4 This 54-year-old man presented with longstanding asymptomatic left parotid mass. Preoperative examination revealed a subtle loss of left lower lip depressor muscle function, suggesting a malignant parotid neoplasm. Note the slight lower lip asymmetry with left-sided lower lip elevation and decrease in visible vermilion. Tumor was an acinic cell carcinoma involving the marginal branch of the facial nerve.

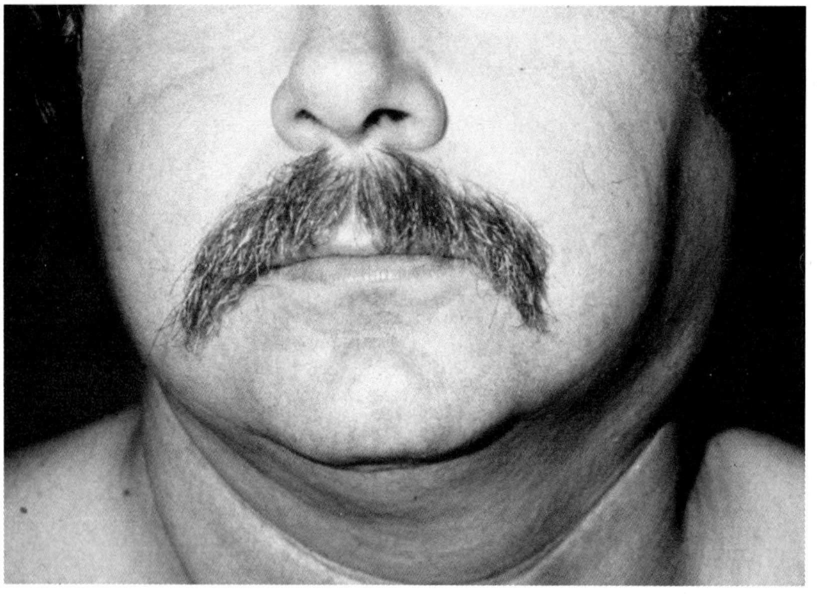

Figure 5 This 24-year-old man had a 4-year history of a gradually enlarging left parotid mass. At surgery, the tumor was pale gray, friable, and completely enveloped the facial nerve. Frozen section analysis of a tumor sample revealed it to be a lymphoid malignancy, at which point the parotidectomy was aborted. The tumor turned out to be a Stage I nodular sclerosing Hodgkin's lymphoma, and he was treated with radiotherapy.

malignancies, all adenoid cystic carcinomas, all patients with tumor involving the facial nerve, all cases of extraglandular tumor extension, most recurrent tumors (including pleomorphic adenoma), and all patients with metastatic tumor in the neck.

The area to be treated should include the entire surgical site and scar. The neck is included in the field in high grade tumors, and following neck dissection for metastatic cervical disease. Patients should optimally receive 6,000 to 6,500 rad in 6 to 7 weeks.

Megavoltage equipment is required for treatment. Cobalt and low-power linear accelerators (4 to 8 mev) produce photon beams that are effective against tumors and have a skin-sparing effect. Photon therapy is limited, however, due to risk of spinal cord injury with a direct beam. Consequently, when cobalt alone is used, tangential wedge fields are required to treat the parotid bed. Unfortunately, this necessitates the inclusion of a greater area of normal tissue. High power linear accelerators (>12 mev) produce electron beams that spare the spinal cord when a direct parotid field is used. Electrons, however, produce a much higher skin dosage than cobalt. Therefore, the ideal treatment plan at this time is to combine cobalt and electron therapy to maximize parotid bed dosage, and minimize damage to skin, spinal cord, and adjacent normal tissue.

TABLE 1 Indications for Radiotherapy

Indications
Gross Disease
Patient not medically able to tolerate surgery
Patient refuses surgery
Parotid lymphoma
Microscopic Disease
Highly malignant tumors and all adenoid cystic carcinoma
Extraglandular tumor extension
Stage N_1 disease
Parotid deep lobe involvement
Positive margin of resection
Tumor adjacent to facial nerve
Following resection of recurrent tumor

There are a number of significant complications that can occur as a result of radiation treatment of the parotid area. These can be grouped into acute and chronic problems that are the direct result of radiation therapy. A sore throat seems to be the most irritating of the acute side effects. It can occur during treatment and may last several weeks following therapy. Acutely, the skin becomes red and sore, tinnitus frequently occurs, there is a transient taste distortion, and a moderately dry mouth.

The late complications happen infrequently when the proper dosage and fields are used. Clearly, the worst outcome is tumor induction, usually a sarcoma, as mentioned previously. Other complications can be devastating as well, such as osteoradionecrosis of the mandible or temporal bone. Radionecrosis can usually be avoided by adhering to the following precautions: combining cobalt (photon) and electron therapy, limiting the field size, and providing prophylactic dental care before commencing the irradiation. Trismus due to fibrosis of the muscles or temporomandibular joint capsule is dose-dependent and can occur when more than 6,000 rad are administered. Chronic auricular chondritis is seen only in patients treated entirely by cobalt. This is due to the necessity of irradiating greater areas of normal tissue, including the auricle, when photon beam therapy alone is used. Other potential problems are less dangerous but, nonetheless, very annoying to patients and include: decreased hearing due to thickening of the tympanic membrane and/or serous otitis, chronic dry mouth, loss of skin appendages, and dry tight skin in the treatment field. Facial nerve function and regeneration, even through a nerve graft, is generally unaffected by radiation. Compromised facial nerve function due to compression by tumor can be improved, but not if tumor invades the nerve.

A number of factors come into play when referring a parotid tumor patient for adjunctive therapy. Treatment planning is quite complex. Just as in surgery, different radiotherapists have different viewpoints, do things somewhat differently, and get different results. When treating a parotid tumor, a radiation oncologist experienced with head and neck tumors will most likely obtain the best outcome. The radiation facility can also limit the quality of treatment. Current state-of-the-art treatment requires that the facility have electron beam capability.

The social aspects of a therapy program must also be considered. Treatment sessions take place daily over a two-month period. In spite of the inconvenience that a distant facility may impose upon a patient and his family, appropriate treatment is so crucial that it is well-worth the effort to obtain treatment at the best installation and by an experienced radiotherapist. This important facet of patient care is best handled by a head and neck cancer center that provides a team approach to patient management, including physicians of various specialties and experienced paramedical personnel. A head and neck team can best coordinate multidisciplinary therapies into a program that is socially acceptable to the patient and family.

The authors would like to thank Dr. Raymond Leen and Dr. Judith Figura who have provided excellent radiation therapy for our patients and have taught us the basics of radiotherapy.

SUGGESTED READING

Cohen MB, Ljung B-ME, Boles R. Salivary gland tumors: fine-needle aspiration vs. frozen-section diagnosis. Arch Otolaryngol Head Neck Surg 1986; 112:867–869.

Fitzpatrick PJ, Theriault C. Malignant salivary gland tumors. Int J Radiat Oncol Biol Phys 1986; 12:1743–1747.

Granick MS, Hanna DC, Erickson ER. Accuracy of frozen section diagnosis in salivary gland lesions. Head Neck Surg 1985; 7:465–467.

Granick MS, Hanna DC, Newton ED. Management of benign and malignant primary salivary gland tumors. In: Georgiade N et al, eds. Essentials of plastic, maxillofacial, and reconstructive surgery. Baltimore: Williams & Wilkins, 1986:162.

Guillamondequi O, Byers RM, Lapley NduV. Malignant tumors of salivary glands. In: Fletcher GH, ed. Textbook of radiotherapy. Philadelphia: Lea & Febiger, 1980:433.

SQUAMOUS CARCINOMA OF THE EXTERNAL AUDITORY CANAL

CLAUDE C. COLEMAN Jr., M.D., F.A.C.S.

Although primary cancers of the external ear canal are relatively uncommon, neglected tumors of the external ear, surrounding scalp, parotid gland, and metastatic cancers to the parotid lymph nodes involve it secondarily. It is often impossible to say with certainty where the primary cancer arose. Such cancers extend clinically to involve the dura and brain and widespread involvement of the petrosa, and middle and posterior fossae of the skull is seen ultimately in neglected cases. In 1959, an operation was developed in the surgical laboratory at the University of Virginia that was designed to remove the ear and temporal bone through a combined intra- and extracranial approach. That operation, herein described, was monobloc in principle and followed all of Halsted's criteria. Subsequent studies performed on fresh material in the laboratory of the State Medical Examiners' office at the Medical College of Virginia further amplified and perfected the procedure.

PATHOLOGY

Most cancers of the external ear canal and temporal bone are epidermoid in nature. Patients with such cancers have been followed for many years. Repeated attempts at surgical excision, with multiple courses of radiotherapy, have been utilized in most of the patients who underwent definitive resection (Fig. 1). Pain on the affected side with tinnitus and facial nerve paralysis often were presenting symptoms. Invasion of the mastoid and surrounding scalp produced marked lateral displacement of the ear (Fig. 2). Involvement of bone, as shown on x-ray films, was present in over one-third of the cases treated.

Neglected basal cell carcinoma of the external ear occasionally involved the bony ear canal and mastoid. Such tumors very often had been treated initially by inadequate surgical excision. The erroneous opinion that basal cell carcinoma is an innocuous skin cancer gave such patients a false sense of security until pain mandated a wide three-dimensional resection.

SURGICAL TREATMENT

Prior to positioning the patient on the operating table, a large-caliber polyethylene catheter is introduced into the subarachnoid space via a spinal needle. A free flow of cerebrospinal fluid (CSF) must be obtained before further preparation for surgery is begun. Any question regarding the anesthesiologist's control of the CSF necessitates cancellation of surgery. The tumor is surgically outlined in a circular fashion with the involved ear at the center of the circle. A vertical extension on the upper lateral neck affords access to the upper jugular lymph nodes and also gains wide access to the infratemporal fossa (Fig. 3). Access to the upper portion of the internal jugular vein allows the graceful inclusion of the contents of a homolateral radical neck dissection. The circular skin

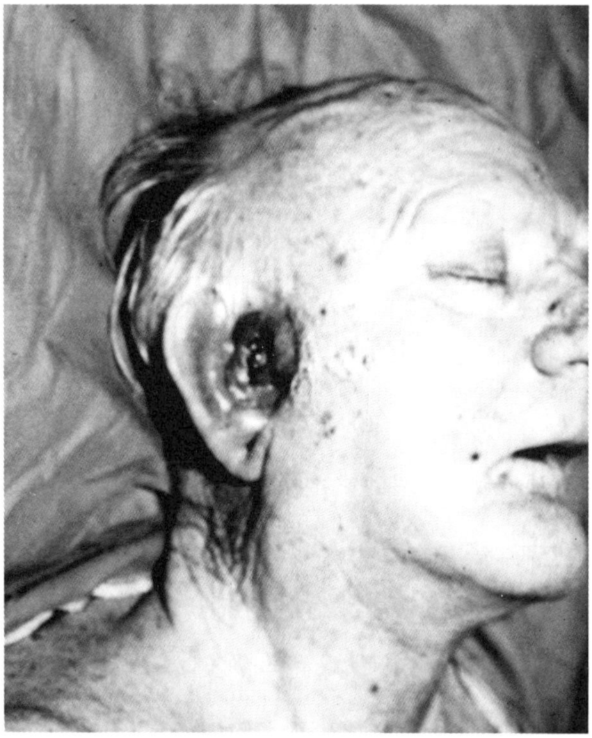

Figure 1 Extensive squamous cell carcinoma of external ear canal with deep invasion of mastoid and temporal squama. Patient underwent incision and graft and received 6,000 rad of radiation.

incision is carried down to the temporal squama anteriorly and superiorly. Posteriorly, the deep soft-tissue cut extends to the occipital bone. Inferiorly, the cut that joins the anterior and posterior incisions is of the greatest importance. Through this approach the upper sternocleidomastoid is swept from the mastoid, thereby exposing the posterior belly of the digastric muscle, which is also taken out of its groove in the inferior surface of the mastoid. Thorough muscle elimination is mandatory in order to develop a clean, unobstructed view of the skull base and the jugular foramen.

Subperiosteal dissection of the temporalis muscle, anteriorly and superiorly, gains wide access to the temporal squama. The occipitalis and posterior scalp muscles are reflected widely to expose the mastoid and occipital bones. Anteriorly, the zygomatic arch is divided and, if the temporomandibular joint is to be removed, the neck of the condyle is divided.

BONE EXCAVATION

Two or more trephine holes are made to the dura (Fig. 4). With an olive-tipped burr, bone cuts are made to join the burr holes and, gradually, the trenches are widened with rongeurs until the temporal lobe above and the cerebellum posteriorly can be seen. At this stage of the operation, cerebrospinal fluid is withdrawn from the

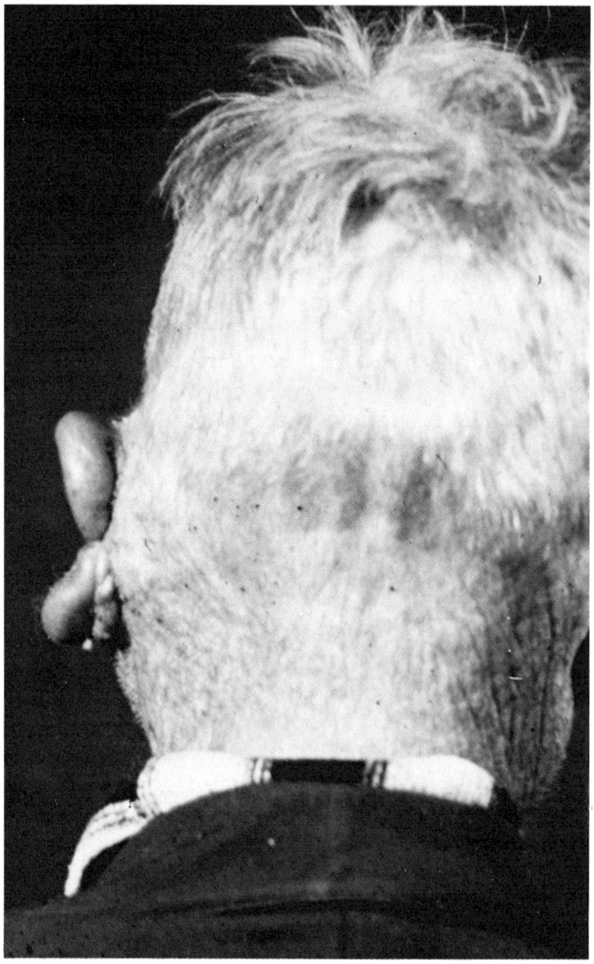

Figure 2 Extensive recurrent squamous cell carcinoma of the external ear with invasion of mastoid and parotid gland. Total facial nerve paralysis with tinnitus and deafness implicated the middle ear and petrosa.

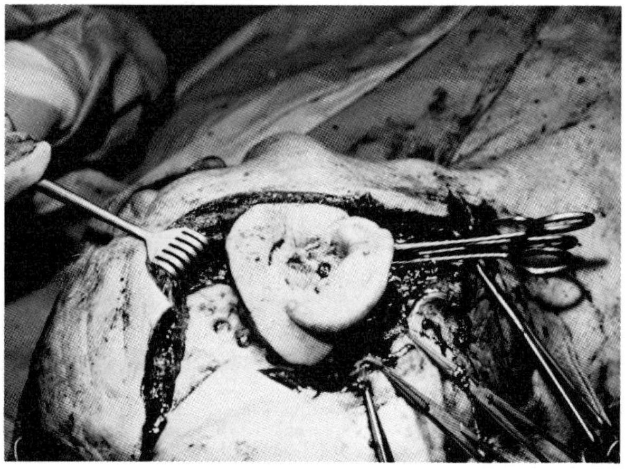

Figure 3 Wide exposure of the temporal squama and occipital bone is foremost in the combined approach. Burr holes can be seen superior to the soft tissue.

subarachnoid indwelling catheter. Fluid is allowed to run into a sterile container throughout the intracranial portion. After the temporal and occipital lobes have become sufficiently softened, the brain can be displaced medially, and exposure of the sigmoid sinus is obtained by thoroughly unroofing it with rongeurs in the posterior fossa (Fig. 5). At this stage of the procedure, the emissary vein of the mastoid is encountered and has to be ligated. The transverse and sigmoid sinuses must be totally liberated from the deep sulcus in the occipital bone. Bone division of the temporal squama is developed anteriorly and the trench is widened down to the zygomatic arch, which is divided (see Fig. 4). With the temporal lobe retracted, the dura is stripped from the floor of the middle fossa and the petrous pyramid is exposed medial to the tympanic antrum. The vertical cut in the posterior fossa is carried down to the floor just posterior to the sigmoid groove. The base of the skull is exposed and the occipital bone is cut through the digastric groove with the high-speed drill (see Fig. 4). The cut is extended anteriorly between the tympanic plate of the mastoid and the styloid process to join the cut in the middle fossa. It is essential that these cuts through the middle and posterior fossae be *complete* before division of the petrous pyramid.

The superior petrosal sinus runs in a shallow groove along the summit of the pyramid and must be electrocoagulated before division of the petrosa is begun. The pyramid is cut through at 45 degrees to the skull base with a high-speed drill. As the base of the pyramid is approached, careful observation of the sigmoid sinus orients the operator with regard to the jugular bulb. The petrous ridge is divided at the cut demonstrated in Figure 6.

After removal of the specimen, many small veins entering the jugular or inferior petrosal sinus must be secured by cautery or ligature. Tears in the dura are closed with nonabsorbable sutures that incorporate small fragments of muscle to control cerebrospinal fluid leaks.

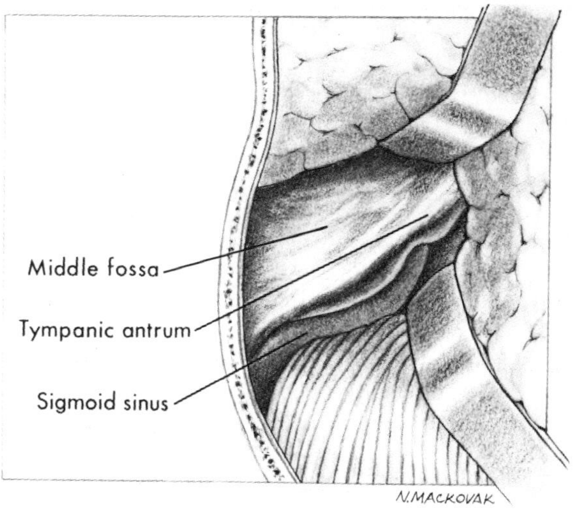

Figure 5 Intracranial exposure of the petrous ridge afforded by continuous decompression of the ventricles. Retraction of the cerebellum gives exposure to the transverse sinus and its sigmoid extension.

WOUND RECONSTRUCTION

After removal of the specimen, a portion of the temporal lobe, cerebellum, and dural sinuses is exposed in an irregular defect in the lateral skull. The use of the pectoralis major island myocutaneous flap has served admirably in the reconstitution of such wounds (Fig. 7). Despite extensive liberation of the acromiothoracic artery, the distance from the clavicle to the upper edge of the scalp and skull defect strains the pectoralis major pedicle and the

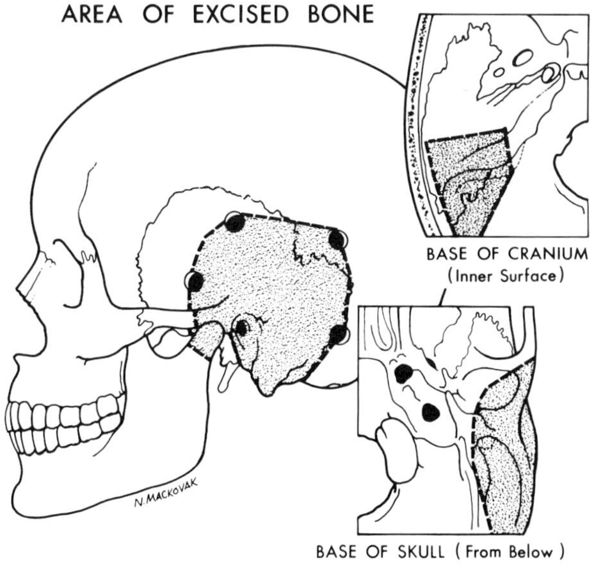

Figure 4 Artist's schematic drawings outline bone removal in three dimensions.

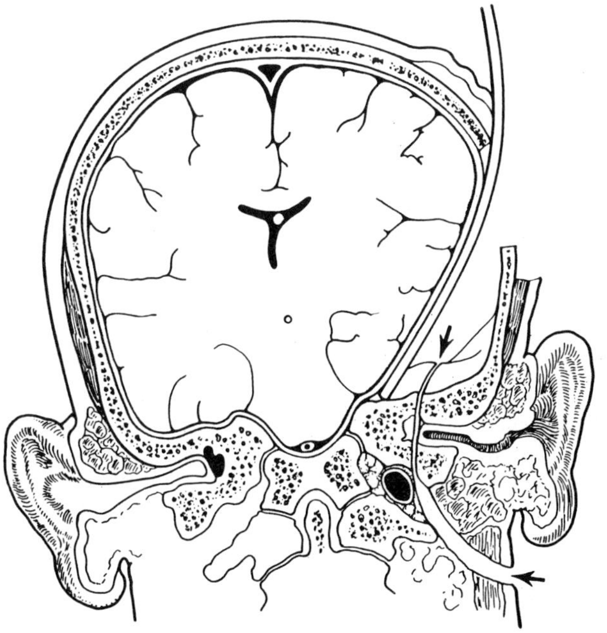

Figure 6 Bone cut through the petrous pyramid, just lateral to the jugular bulb, permits removal of the specimen in one piece.

head should be turned to the operated side. Suction drainage must be accurate and unimpeded during the early postoperative period. A first compression dressing to the operated side is mandatory in order to enhance the effect of wound drainage.

DISCUSSION

Although primary cancers of the external auditory canal are relatively uncommon, the structure is often involved in neglected cancers of the external ear and surrounding structures. Previous reports of the surgical procedures have varied considerably. Such cancers were at one time treated by piecemeal removal, with or without the use of intracavitary radium. The wounds were left open, and patients often were subjected to long periods of painful drainage from osteonecrosis. A radical monobloc removal of the temporal bone was advocated, but such a procedure was not reported. More recently, Gaisford and Mladick reported their results with piecemeal removal. Although Gaisford had a negligible incidence of wound complications, his local recurrence rate was not clearly defined.

The operation herein described was first reported in 1959 and it was designed to remove the involved temporal bone in one piece. Such procedures are technically difficult and the graceful development of the intact specimen is impeded by the enormous blood vessels that surround the temporal bone.

Primary cancers of the temporal bone are rare and are not likely candidates for temporal bone resection. Such tumors arise in a bony vault deep in the substance of the brain. They are not diagnosed early and, when they are discovered, the tumor generally has broken through its bony walls and extends into dura and brain. We have encountered cylindroma of the middle ear that presented through a perforation in the tympanic membrane. This was the only patient who developed a local recurrence and a distal metastasis. In management of such patients, a preliminary examination of the middle and posterior fossae through a subtemporal decompression should be performed before an extensive monobloc removal of the temporal bone is embarked upon. Extension of tumors in such patients can, thus, be ascertained and definitive resection obviated. Wound closure in these patients has been greatly improved by use of the myocutaneous flap. The pectoralis major island flap covers the temporal defect and is far more acceptable from an esthetic standpoint than the large hair-bearing scalp flaps first described.

An essential part of the temporal bone resection is the decompression of the cisternae and ventricles of the brain via a subarachnoid catheter. After the induction of anesthesia, a large indwelling catheter is introduced through a malleable spinal needle and fluid flow is controlled by the inclusion of a stopcock, readily accessible to the anesthesiologist. Flow of CSF should be determined before the procedure is begun and any adjustments in catheter position should be made at that time. The operation demands adequate and graceful exposure of the petrous pyramid and the adjacent fossae of the skull bone.

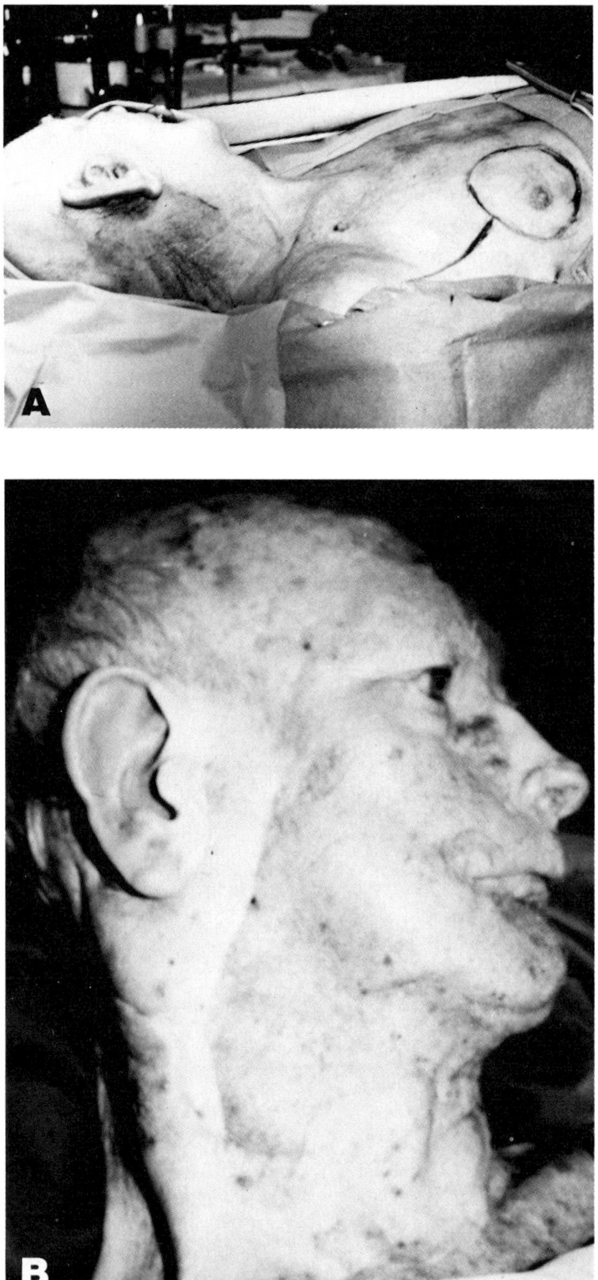

Figure 7 *A*, Incisional markings for circumauricular ablative excision, neck dissection extension, and pectoralis major island myocutaneous flap in patient with ear canal carcinoma. *B*, The patient is shown 2 years following temporal bone resection resurfaced with pectoralis major island myocutaneous flap and latex ear prosthesis.

Such immediate exposure is only possible by mechanical reduction of the brain tension by the steady release of CSF. The intravenous injection of sucrose or other high molecular substances is time-consuming and unreliable. It has been my policy to terminate the operation in any patient in whom free egress of spinal fluid cannot be unequivocally established prior to the soft tissue cuts.

The application of Halstedian principles in the treatment of advanced cancers of the ear and mastoid was first advocated by me in 1956. Since that time, the operative mortality has remained about 11 percent. On the other hand, intraoperative hemorrhage has remained at 24 percent. That finding compares favorably with Conley and others. Despite the improvement in technique and the development of highly sophisticated power tools, one still has to cope with the removal of a bony vault that is secured on all sides by large veins. Conley has stated that one must expect a high incidence of hemorrhage during the operation. The terminal part of the operation is concerned solely with avoidance of injury to the jugular bulb while still performing an honest tumor resection.

Other investigators have advocated a discontinuous removal of the specimen. They have also advocated piecemeal removal of the temporal bone in the same manner reported by Eldridge Campbell in 1951. In that case, the patient's wound was never closed, and she died from local recurrence.

Despite the hazards of terrifying hemorrhage, monobloc removal offers the best chance of cure. In primary cancer of the middle ear, it is unlikely that any method of treatment will be successful since the tumor generally is out of control when pain and facial weakness occur.

The disfigurement from such procedures is considerable. Fascial sling stabilization of the face and improvement of the wound closure have reduced the stigmata of the procedure.

Attempts to salvage the facial nerve have been recommended by Ariyan and others. We strongly oppose such a maneuver in any patient with clinical evidence of extension into the petrosa. The margin of safety is too narrow in an operation designed to remove the major portion of the petrous pyramid. Partial to subtotal removal of the temporal bone has been reported, depending on the findings from x-ray films and computed tomography. Even with a formal craniotomy prior to temporal bone resection, extension of tumor into the mastoid is impossible to determine. I have routinely divided the petrosa through the tympanic antrum in all patients with extension into the bony auditory canal. That otological philosophy is comparable to House's approach for the removal of cerebellopontine angle tumors via the mastoid approach.

From the Department of Surgery, Medical College of Virginia, and Henrico Doctors Hospital, Department of Plastic Surgery, Richmond, Virginia.

SUGGESTED READING

Coleman CC Jr, Khuri A. A rational approach to the treatment of advanced cancers of the external ear and temporal bone. VA Med 1959; 82:21.

Coleman CC Jr. Removal of the temporal bone for cancer. Am J Surg 1966; 112(4):583–590.

Coleman CC Jr. Tumors involving the cranio-facial skeleton. In: Converse JM, ed. Reconstructive plastic surgery: principles and procedures in correction, reconstruction, and transplantation. 2nd ed. Philadelphia: WB Saunders, 1977:2757.

Conley JJ. Cancer of the middle ear. Ann Otol Rhinol Laryngol 1965; 74:555.

Ariyan S, Sasaki CT, Spencer D. Radical en block resection of the temporal bone. Am J Surg 1981; 142:443–447.

House WF. Trans-cochlear approach to the petrous apex. Trans Amer Acad Opth Laryngol 1977; 84:927–931.

Gaisford JC, Hanna DC, Susen AF. Major resection of the scalp and skull for cancer with immediate complete reconstruction. Plast Reconstr Surg 1958; 114:235.

Mladick RA. The core resection of the auricular areas and subjacent bone. Plast Reconstr Surg 1974; 53:281.

LIP RECONSTRUCTION

GORDON R. TOBIN, M.D.

Partial or total lip loss and congenital deformities that produce oral incompetence or facial disfigurement require lip reconstruction. The most common cause of lip loss is resection for cancer, which is usually squamous cell carcinoma of the vermilion in the lower lip and basal cell carcinoma of the skin in the upper lip. Trauma is the second leading cause of lip loss. The most common congenital lip defect, cleft lip, is discussed elsewhere in this book.

The role of the lips in appearance and in the functions of speech, eating, and salivary continence places severe demands on reconstructive methods to achieve both pleasing form and satisfactory function. A lip reconstructive technique must restore missing skin cover, oral lining, a semblance of vermilion, a labial sulcus, commissure definition, adequate stomal diameter, sensation, and a competent oral sphincter. Of the many described techniques for lip reconstruction, few provide all of these requirements, particularly the functionally essential elements of sensation and sphincter function.

RECONSTRUCTIVE OPTIONS

Surface Reconstruction

Defects of only skin, vermilion, or mucosal surfaces that do not involve the orbicularis oris muscle are replaced with grafts or local flaps with surfaces similar to the missing tissue. Nasolabial skin flaps are especially useful for large surface defects. Inferiorly-based nasolabial skin flaps are useful to replace missing upper lip lateral element skin, and either superiorly- or inferiorly-based nasolabial skin flaps are useful to replace missing lower lip skin. Vermilion is replaced either by advancement of adjacent labial mucosa or by flaps from the tongue undersurface leading edge.

Direct Closure

Wedge excision with direct defect closure was first described by Celsus in 25 B.C. This technique remains the preferred procedure for defects of either lip up to approximately one-fourth of lip length.

Innervated Myocutaneous Flaps

Innervated myocutaneous flaps are composite flaps based on perioral muscles with overlying skin, underlying mucosa, and preserved motor and sensory innervation. The functional advantages of preserving motor and sensory innervation are substantial and make these flaps the preferred choice for many lip defects.

Innervated Orbicularis Oris Myocutaneous Flaps

Karapandzic described the first flap of this type, which is comprised of the orbicularis oris muscle with overlying skin, vermilion, and mucosa. This flap is mobilized on neurovascular pedicles that contain the fifth and seventh cranial nerves and is advanced from either or both sides into the lip defect. This technique is applicable to defects of either lip in all locations, and the preserved innervation produces an excellent functional reconstruction. The principal limitation of this technique is the increasingly severe microstomia that results with progressively larger lip defects.

Innervated Depressor Anguli Oris Myocutaneous Flaps

These flaps reconstruct the lower lip and oral sphincter with a composite flap of the depressor anguli oris (triangularis) muscle with overlying skin, underlying mucosa (for both oral lining and vermilion), the motor nerve (seventh-mandibular marginal) and the sensory nerve (fifth-mental). Cover, lining, vermilion, sulcus, commissure, circumference, sphincter function, and sensation are restored to the lower lip. I prefer this procedure for reconstruction of lateral lower lip defects more than one-fourth lip length, or for total lower lip loss. One flap restores loss of one-half of a lower lip (Figs. 1 and 2), and bilateral flaps restore loss of an entire lower lip (Fig. 3). The length of the mental nerve sensory innervation does not permit transfer of this flap to the upper lip, thus limiting its use to lower lip defects.

Innervated Levator Anguli Oris Myocutaneous Flaps

This flap is used for reconstruction of large upper lip defects. It contains the levator anguli oris muscle with overlying skin and underlying mucosa (for lining and vermilion). Branches of the sensory (fifth-infraorbital) and motor (seventh-buccal) cranial nerves that enter the flap along its lateral border are preserved. The flap is based distally at the oral commissure. The muscle is detached from its origin on the maxilla and transferred with encompassing skin and mucosa into the lip defect. This flap restores cover, lining, vermilion, sulcus, commissure, circumference, sphincter function, and sensation to the upper lip. For total upper lip reconstruction, I prefer bilateral levator anguli oris flaps in conjunction with a midline Abbe philtral reconstruction (Fig. 4). The motor and sensory nerves that enter the lateral flap border tether the flap to an extent that it cannot be used for lower lip defects.

Oral Circumference Advancement Flaps

Oral circumference advancement flaps reconstruct upper or lower lip full-thickness defects by circumferential advancement of adjacent lip tissue as composite flaps. The simplest example of this technique is direct closure of a wedge-shaped defect. More complete examples of

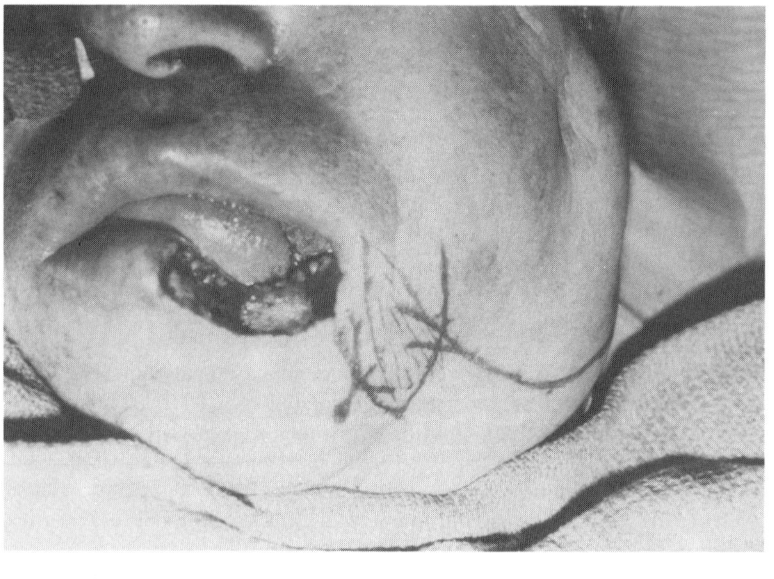

Figure 1 An innervated depressor anguli oris myocutaneous flap. The relationships of the skin incision (''V''), muscle (parallel line), motor nerve (seventh-lateral), and sensory nerve (fifth-medial) are shown.

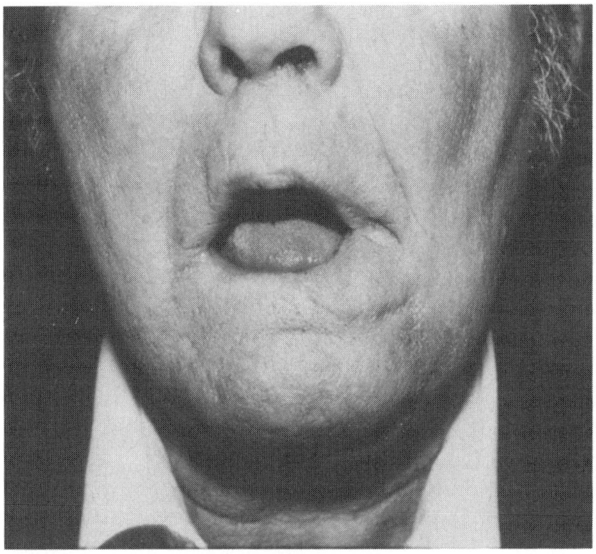

Figure 2 An innervated depressor anguli oris flap reconstruction restores normal oral circumference, sensation, and a functional sphincter. Postoperative result is shown.

such flaps are Karapandzic's innervated orbicularis oris myocutaneous flaps and Gillies' fan flap. Gillies' fan flap was the first described oral circumference advancement flap. It has historic significance but little current application, unless modified to preserve innervation. Oral circumference advancement flaps do not restore oral circumference, and thus produce microstomia when used for large defects.

Cross-Lip Flaps

Cross-lip, or "lip-switch" flaps (Sabattini, Abbe, Estlander, Stein, and Kazanjian) transpose full-thickness lip wedge flaps to opposite lip defects on vermilion pedicles that contain the coronary vessels. These flaps produce denervated reconstructions and denervate the orbicularis oris medial to the donor sites, although partial reinnervation subsequently occurs from axonal ingrowth. They also fail to restore oral circumference. In spite of these shortcomings, the Estlander flap is still widely used in lip reconstruction. I find little merit in these techniques, except for the Abbe flap, which is the procedure of choice for philtral reconstruction in both congenital and acquired defects. Also, Burget and Menick have described an excellent method for upper lip lateral element reconstruction that uses a midline Abbe flap designed with precise lateral element dimensions (Fig. 5).

Nasolabial Flaps

Nasolabial flaps based distally (Dieffenbach, Von-Bruns, DeNonvilliers, Nelaton and Ombredanne, and "island nasolabial flaps") and proximally (Malgaigne and Sedillot), restore lip loss with full-thickness flaps from the ipsilateral nasolabial fold. These flaps, however, are denervated, and they denervate the lips and face medial to the donor site. Based on design of the skin paddle, the levator anguli oris myocutaneous flap can also be classified as a distally-based nasolabial flap, but it differs substantially from other nasolabial flaps because of careful attention to inclusion and inset of the levator anguli oris muscle and careful preservation of motor and sensory innervation.

Cheek Flaps

Reconstruction of lip losses has been done with bilateral cheek flaps by advancement of laterally-based pedicles (Lisfranc, Bernard, "modified Bernard flaps," Burow, and "modified Burow flaps") and by transposition of inferiorly-based pedicles (Dieffenbach). Cheek flap reconstructions transect the orbicularis oris muscle at the commissure, fail to reconstruct the sphincter, and denervate the opposite lip, except for neuromuscular-sparing modifications, such as described by Freman and Webster.

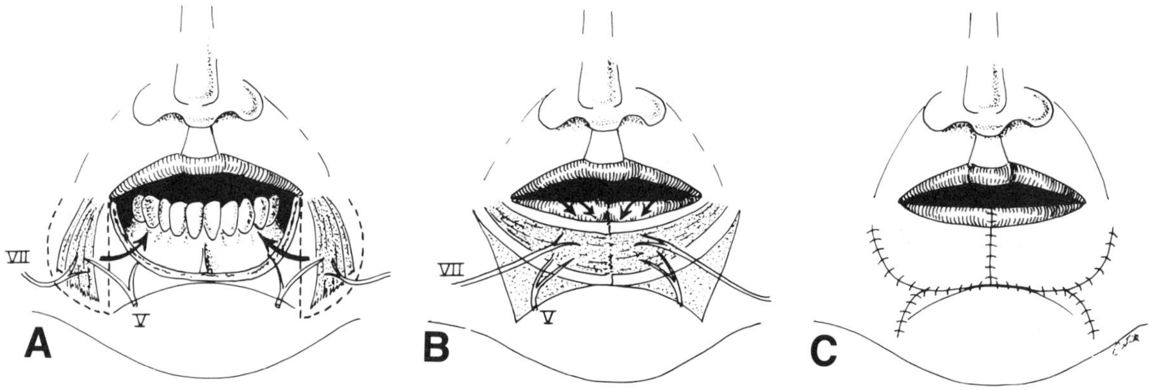

Figure 3 A bilateral depressor anguli oris total lower lip reconstruction. *A,* The flap design shows the relationships of the incisions, muscle, motor nerve (seventh), and sensory nerve (fifth). *B,* Flap transposition reorients the depressor anguli oris to become the lower lip oral sphincter. Vermilion is restored by mucosal advancement. *C,* Flap inset and direct donor defect closure completes the reconstruction.

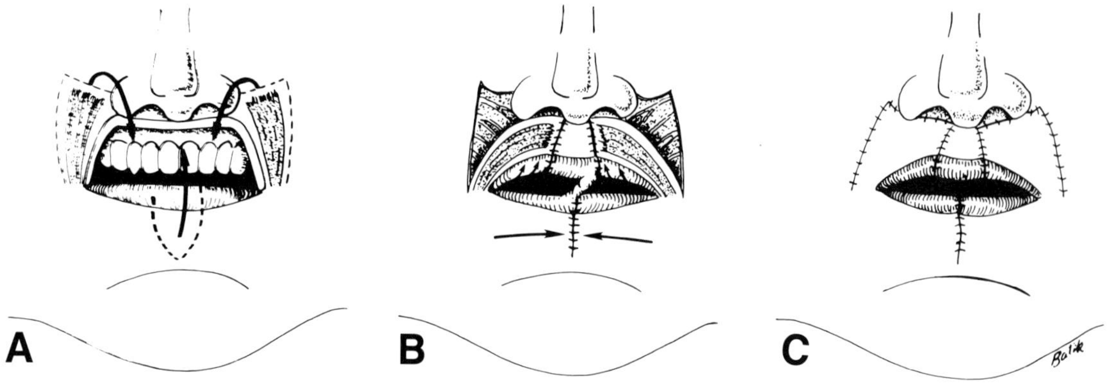

Figure 4 A levator anguli oris myocutaneous flap upper lip reconstruction. *A,* The flap design shows the relationship of the incision and the levator anguli oris muscle. *B,* Flap transposition reorients the muscle to become the upper lip oral sphincter. Motor and sensory innervation as it enters the lateral flap border is carefully preserved. Vermilion is restored by mucosal advancement, and the philtrum is reconstructed with an Abbe flap. *C,* After flap inset and direct donor defect closure, division of the Abbe flap vermilion pedicle completes the reconstruction.

Distant Flaps

Distant flap reconstructions (Taliacotius, Cole, New) fail to provide sensation and motor function and are inferior to regional flaps in texture and color match. Accordingly, they are used only when extensive tissue loss makes local flaps unavailable.

PREFERRED APPROACHES

For reconstruction of defects larger than those that can be closed directly, the vast majority of described procedures fail to provide sensation or reconstruct a functional oral sphincter. In the absence of either sensory or motor function, speech and eating are difficult, and a high incidence of salivary spillage occurs. Accordingly, I prefer fully innervated reconstructions, such as those provided by innervated myocutaneous flaps. Except for the Abbe flap from the lower lip midline, I avoid cross-lip flaps, as they denervate the lip medial to their donor site and fail to increase lip circumference. Although I use nasolabial skin flaps for reconstruction of both external and internal surface defects, I avoid the use of full-thickness nasolabial flaps because they transect the motor and sensory nerves to the muscles of facial expression and the central face skin medially. Cheek flap reconstructions have been replaced by innervated myocutaneous flaps, except in cases of massive defects in which the perioral myocutaneous units are lost. The Freman modification of the Bernard design, however, remains a useful option for midline lower lip defects. Distant flaps are reserved for massive defects where there are no other options.

Patient Selection

Patients are selected for specific reconstructive techniques according to the size and location of the lip loss. My preferred approaches for specific defects are described in the following paragraphs.

Small Defects of Either Lip

Defects less than approximately one-eighth of oral circumference (one-fourth of either lip) can be closed directly, as the resultant asymmetry and loss of oral

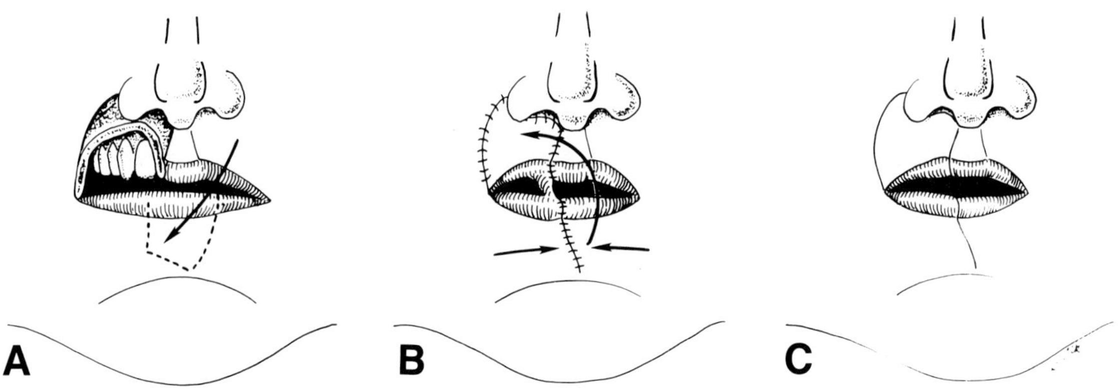

Figure 5 Upper lip lateral element reconstruction by the technique of Burget and Menick. *A,* The Abbe flap pattern is taken from the contralateral lateral element. *B,* The entire lateral element medial to the oral commissure and lateral to the philtral column is replaced, and the donor defect is closed directly. *C,* Division and inset of vermilion pedicle completes the reconstruction.

circumference is functionally and esthetically acceptable. A small defect that ablates the philtrum, however, destroys a significant esthetic anatomic feature, and this is best reconstructed with an Abbe flap from the lower lip midline.

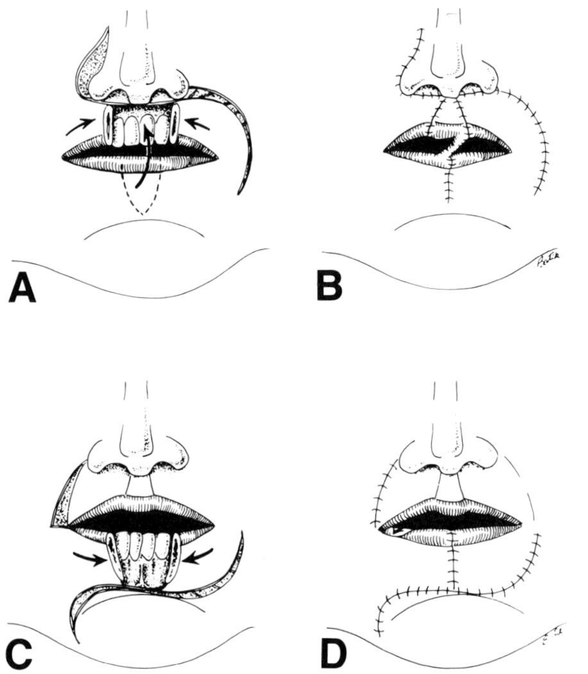

Figure 6 Composite illustration of midline subtotal lip defect reconstruction shows alternative techniques. On the right, the residual lateral lip is advanced medially by innervated orbicularis oris myocutaneous flaps. On the left, the lip is advanced as a laterally-based advancement flap with "Burow's triangles" skin excisions placed in esthetic unit borders. *A* and *B* show midline subtotal upper lip reconstruction. The philtrum is made from a lower lip midline Abbe flap. On the left, the lateral element is made by an advancement flap with perialar skin excision, as described by Webster. On the right an innervated orbicularis oris myocutaneous flap is used. *C* and *D* depict midline subtotal lower lip reconstruction. On the left, the residual lateral lip is advanced by the method described by Freman. On the right, an innervated orbicularis oris myocutaneous flap is used.

Lower Lip Reconstruction

Innervated depressor anguli oris myocutaneous-mucosal flaps provide the preferred reconstruction of large lateral defects of the lower lip (see Fig. 1). In addition to restoration of sensation and sphincter activity, this reconstruction prevents microstomia by completely restoring oral circumference (see Fig. 2). For total lower lip reconstruction, bilateral innervated depressor anguli oris myocutaneous-mucosal flaps provide a superior functional reconstruction compared to other described methods (see Fig. 3). In subtotal lower lip losses in the midline, either bilateral innervated orbicularis oris myocutaneous flaps or the Freman modification of Bernard cheek advancement flaps is chosen (Fig. 6), provided the defect size is small enough that the resultant microstomia is not too severe.

Upper Lip Reconstruction

For total upper lip reconstruction, I prefer bilateral innervated levator anguli oris myocutaneous flaps for the lateral elements and a midline Abbe flap for the philtrum (see Fig. 4). For a subtotal defect that involves only one lateral element, I prefer either a midline Abbe flap with the exact dimensions of the preserved lateral element, as described by Burget and Menick (see Fig. 5), or a unilateral innervated levator anguli oris myocutaneous flap with dimensions designed according to the same principles. Midline subtotal defects are best reconstructed with a midline Abbe flap philtral reconstruction and medial advancement of the remaining portion of the lateral elements, either as innervated orbicularis oris myocutaneous flaps or as laterally-based advancement flaps facilitated by excising "Burow's triangles" of crescentic perialar skin (see Fig. 6), as described by Webster. Abbe flap philtral reconstruction is done simultaneously with lateral element advancement for symmetrical defects, but it usually needs to be delayed for asymmetrical defects in order to place it in the precise midline, the previous closure lines being ignored.

Timing of Therapy

Reconstruction of lip defects is best done at the time of cancer excision, if tumor excision is confirmed as complete. If there is uncertainty about complete tumor excision at the time of resection, reconstruction is temporarily delayed until complete excision is histologically confirmed.

Principles and Technique

The methods of lip reconstruction described above are based on the following principles: (1) Motor and sensory innervation to a flap should be preserved, and the use of denervated flaps avoided whenever possible. One exception to this principle is the midline Abbe flap, when used for either philtral or lateral element reconstruction. In these instances, partial reinnervation follows, and the advantages of this flap for these specific defects outweigh the residual denervation. (2) The oral sphincter is always reconstructed, if possible. For large defects, this is done by transposition of innervated perioral muscles into the sphincteric ring, as in depressor anguli oris and levator anguli oris flaps. (3) Reconstruction is done by esthetic units, as advocated by Burget and Menick, thus allowing inset and donor defect scars to lie along esthetic unit borders. The techniques for developing and transferring innervated myocutaneous flaps are as follows:

1. *Innervated depressor anguli oris myocutaneous-mucosal flap lower lip reconstruction* (see Figs. 1 to 3). The cutaneous component of the flap overlies the depressor anguli oris muscle and is based superiorly at

the level of the oral commissure. After skin and subcutaneous tissue incision, the facial nerve marginal mandibular (motor) branch is dissected free from surrounding tissues back to the mandibular angle. This dissection is approached by a horizontal incision within skin creases in the shadow area beneath the mandibular body. The incision also provides access for a submental and upper cervical (supraomahyoid) lymphadenectomy, if indicated. Distally, the motor nerve is carefully dissected into the lower lateral border of the depressor anguli oris muscle. Next, the mental (sensory) nerve is approached by incising the medial edge of the flap to allow entry into the loose areolar plane deep to the muscle. The mental nerve is identified as it exits from the mental foramen, and its branches to the flap are dissected free from surrounding tissues to permit transfer. Once the nerves are identified and dissected, the muscle is dissected along its lateral border and detached distally. The mucosal lining of the flap is then incised along lines of the skin component, but it is made 1 cm wider than the skin flap medially to provide mucosal tissue for vermilion replacement. Transposition of the composite flap reorients the depressor anguli oris muscle to provide the missing oral sphincter, and the motor and sensory nerves are carried with the flap during transposition. Vermilion reconstruction is provided by advancement of flap mucosa over the medial flap border, in a fashion similar to reconstruction of vermilionectomy defects. Mucosal, muscle, and skin layers are closed individually, and the donor defect is closed directly.

2. *Innervated levator anguli oris myocutaneous flap upper lip reconstruction* (see Fig. 4). Innervated levator anguli oris myocutaneous flaps are designed directly over the muscle to ensure its inclusion. The muscle runs from the oral commissure to the maxilla above the canine fossa, and it lies directly under the nasolabial crease. The flaps are designed in the shape of an upper lip lateral element and are based distally at the oral commissure. Following incision of the skin and subcutaneous tissue, the levator anguli oris is detached from the maxilla and bluntly dissected from surrounding muscles in order to preserve the motor and sensory nerves that enter the flap at multiple points along its lateral border. The mucosal lining is incised along the lines of skin incisions, but is made 1 cm wider medially to provide vermilion reconstruction. The nerve filaments that enter the flap lateral border are carefully dissected and preserved during transfer into the upper lip defect. The philtrum is reconstructed by an Abbe flap.

Tricks and Traps

For the upper lip, an Abbe flap philtral reconstruction is done at the same time as the lip reconstruction if the defect allows the Abbe flap to lie precisely in the midline. If the upper lip defect is asymmetrical, and the orbicularis oris flaps are closed out of the midline, philtral reconstruction is done at a later time and the flap is placed in the upper lip midline, with the previous closure line being disregarded.

In cases where oral commissure definition is lost, such as produced by orbicularis oris myocutaneous flaps, reconstruction of the commissure can be done by any of several methods, such as the one described by Freman.

Outcome

The reconstructions described earlier incur minimal risk. These techniques result in restoration of lip anatomy, sensation, and oral sphincter function and make them substantially better than historical precedents. Careful attention to sphincter reconstruction and to preservation of both motor and sensory nerves is crucial to the best possible outcome.

SUGGESTED READING

Bakamjian V. Use of tongue flaps in lower lip reconstruction. Br J Plast Surg 1964; 17:76–87.

Burget GC, Menick FJ. Aesthetic restoration of one-half of the upper lip. Plast Reconstr Surg 1986; 78:583–593.

Freman BS. Myoplastic modification of the Bernard cheiloplasty. Plast Reconstr Surg 1958; 21:453–460.

Karapandzic M. Reconstruction of lip defects by local arterial flaps. Br J Plast Surg 1974; 27:93–97.

Smith JW. The anatomical and physiologic acclimatization of tissue transplanted by the lip switch technique. Plast Reconstr Surg 1960; 26:40–56.

Spira M, Hardy B. Vermilionectomy. Plast Reconstr Surg 1964; 33:39–46.

Tobin GR. Lower lip and oral sphincter reconstruction with innervated depressor anguli oris flaps. Proceedings, American Association of Plastic Surgeons, 62nd Annual Meeting, April 1983; 17.

Tobin GR. Functional lower lip and oral sphincter reconstruction with uninnervated depressor anguli oris flaps. In: Grabb W, Vasconez LO, Strauch B, eds. Grabb's encyclopedia of flaps. Boston: Little, Brown, in press.

Webster JP. Crescentic peri-ala-cheek excision for upper lip flap advancement with a short history of upper lip repair. Plast Reconstr Surg 1955; 15:434–464.

Webster RC, Coffey RJ, Kelleher RE. Total and partial reconstruction of the lower lip with innervated muscle-bearing flaps. Plast Reconstr Surg 1960; 25:360–371.

SURGICAL APPROACH TO THE MOUTH

IAN A. McGREGOR, D.Sc., Ch.M., F.R.C.S., F.R.A.C.S., F.A.C.S.

One of the keys to precise, accurate surgery is generally considered to be adequate exposure of the operative site and this applies in surgery of the mouth just as in other surgical fields. While surgery of the anterior part of the oral cavity can be carried out using the open mouth as the sole access, the adequacy of that access rapidly diminishes with passage towards the back of the oral cavity, the lower lip and the mandible constituting the bar to access. Until recently the problem was not a major one since hemimandibulectomy was frequently carried out as part of intraoral resections for tumor, although in many of the clinical situations the bone was, in fact, free of tumor. Today there is increasing recognition that the maintenance of an intact mandibular arch contributes substantially to the excellence of the result achieved after an intraoral resection, viewed in terms both of function and cosmesis. Unless the mandible is involved by tumor its resection is no longer acceptable. With the consequent current trend towards mandibular conservation, the problem of access has become one of greater significance.

If adequate access to the oral cavity and good exposure of its contents are to be obtained without resecting bone, the solution would appear to lie in dividing the lip and carrying out an osteotomy of the mandible. Osteotomy of the mandible and division of the soft tissues which attach the body to the floor of the mouth on the side of the tumor allow the entire hemimandible to be rotated laterally, exposing the structures lying within the concavity of the mandibular body—the "mandibular swing" approach.

DIVISION OF THE LIP

The standard way in which the lip has generally been divided has been by using a vertical incision through the midline, often continued down into the submandibular element of a neck dissection incision. Such a lip-splitting incision is used, either without associated mandibular osteotomy, as an approach to the anterior floor of mouth, or as a preliminary to mandibular osteotomy.

Used without an associated mandibular osteotomy, lip-splitting is usually carried out in order to facilitate exposure of the anterior floor of mouth. A straight incision used for such an approach requires considerable retraction of the tissues on each side of the divided lip below the lower labial sulcus with stripping of the soft tissues off the outer aspect of the mandible on each side of the symphysis. Stripping of the soft tissues in this way can be avoided if the lip incision is modified, dividing it in the mid-line only as far as the base of the chin prominence. If the incision is then continued laterally on each side along the line encircling the chin prominence for approximately 3 cm, its line runs almost along the same level on the skin as the lower labial sulcus intraorally. Deepening the skin incision to this sulcus creates a full-thickness lower lip flap on each side. Retraction of the two flaps laterally exposes the anterior floor of mouth effectively without the need to strip any soft tissue off the symphyseal mandible (Fig. 1).

Used as a preliminary to osteotomy, the straight lip-splitting incision can be deepened without further soft tissue dissection to reach the symphyseal site, if this has been the site chosen for the osteotomy. Choosing the osteotomy site will be discussed below, but even assuming that the symphyseal site has been selected, the straight vertical incision gives a less than optimal cosmetic appearance, continuing as it does over the prominence of the chin. A better cosmetic result is achieved if the incision is modified so that, instead of continuing downwards over the chin prominence, it stops at the hollow between the lower lip and the chin prominence, turns at a right angle and follows the curve round the base of the chin prominence, reaching the symphysis below the lower border of the mandible. As with the straight incision, it can then continue on as the submandibular component of the neck dissection incision. If such modification is to be combined with a symphyseal osteotomy, the soft tissue hemiprominence of the chin has to be elevated as far as the midline, but this has not created problems of skin survival.

THE OSTEOTOMY SITE

The osteotomy site most frequently used today is symphyseal, and when the intraoral lesion is in the vicinity of the midline, it is the logical site to select (Fig. 2). In the past, even when the pathology was on one or other side of the mouth, it was considered to have advantages. Until recently, the most frequently used method of reconstituting the continuity of the mandible was by wiring the bone ends together. The results were often less than perfect, only fibrous union being regularly achieved, but

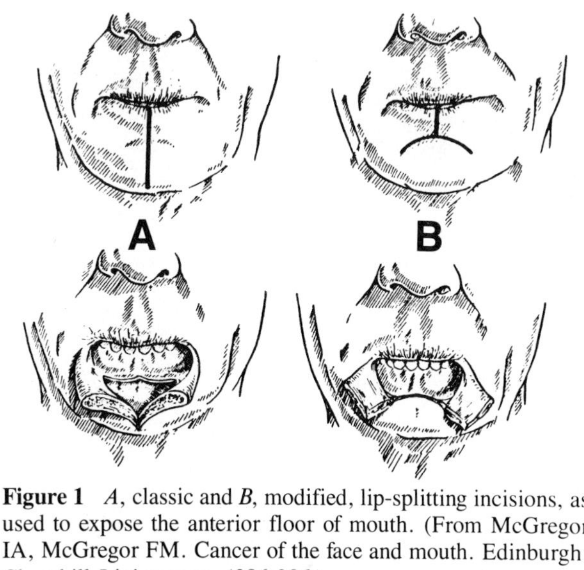

Figure 1 *A*, classic and *B*, modified, lip-splitting incisions, as used to expose the anterior floor of mouth. (From McGregor IA, McGregor FM. Cancer of the face and mouth. Edinburgh: Churchill Livingstone, 1986:386.)

despite this the functional result remained satisfactory because the forces acting on the two sides of the symphyseal site remained largely equal and stresses which might tend to cause disruption at the site of the osteotomy were minimal. Methods have been recently developed which allow the mandible to be fixed much more effectively and this has made it possible to take a fresh look at the osteotomy site with a view to determining its optimal position on the bone (Fig. 3).

When an osteotomy is carried out, the object is to allow one side of the mandible to swing laterally, and, in order to achieve this, certain of the structures which hold the bone in its normal position have to be divided. When the symphyseal site is used the structures which are divided on the side of the osteotomy are the geniohyoid and genioglossus muscles, the anterior belly of digastric, mylohyoid, and the mucosa along the floor of the mouth. If the site of the osteotomy is moved laterally beyond the tongue muscles, it becomes possible to avoid dividing genioglossus and geniohyoid, and if the line selected is immediately in front of the mental foramen, the anterior belly of digastric can also be left undivided. The only structures which are divided to allow the swing to take place become mylohyoid and the mucous membrane along the floor of the mouth (Fig. 4). On the grounds of reducing the amount of soft tissue dissection and damage, therefore, the lateral site would appear to have significant advantages, particularly since the exposure which both provide is similar. There will naturally be occasions, largely influenced by the site of the lesion within the mouth and its pathology, which will determine which osteotomy site is appropriate, the symphyseal or the lateral, but in practice the symphyseal site has overriding virtues only on rare occasions.

FORM OF THE OSTEOTOMY

The bony cut can be straight vertical or stepped. When the method of fixing the osteotomy was limited to direct wiring the use of a stepped cut was a modification designed to improve subsequent stability of the osteotomy, but it does have certain undesirable aspects compared with a straight cut. The stepped cut is technically more difficult and involves a greater amount of periosteal stripping. Periosteal stripping has a devitalizing effect on the bone which is bared, though admittedly the effect is not a major

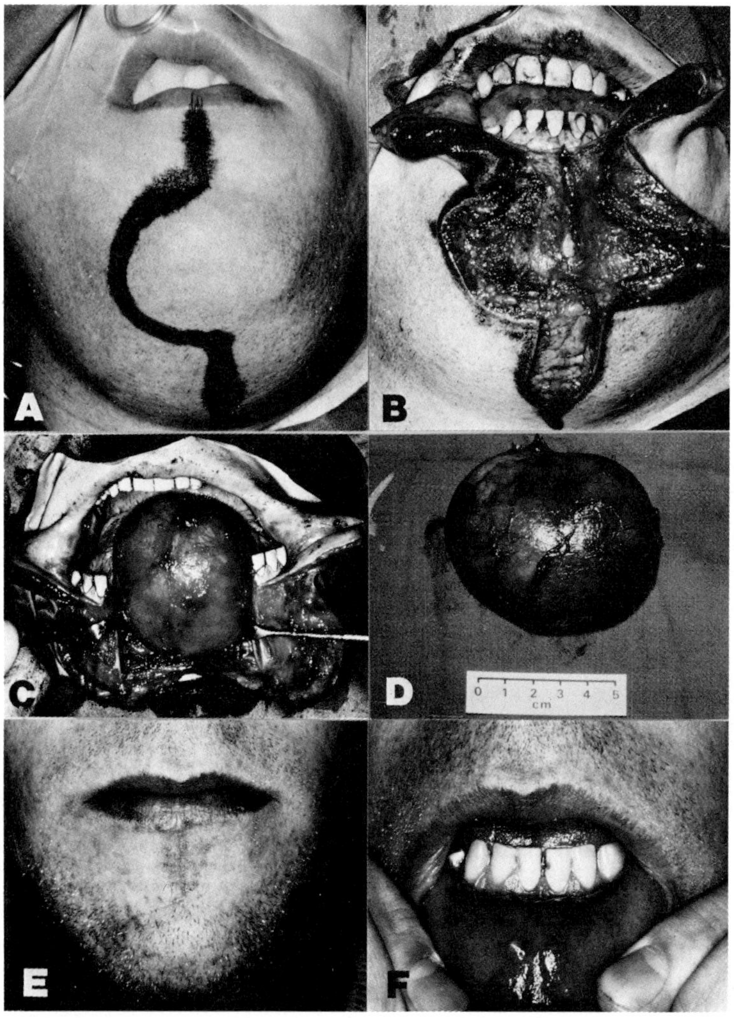

Figure 2 The symphyseal osteotomy approach to the anterior floor of mouth and tongue, used to expose a large sublingual dermoid cyst. *A*, The lip-splitting incision outlined on the skin. The submental swelling created by the dermoid cyst can be seen. *B*, The lip split and the symphyseal mandible exposed, ready for the osteotomy cut. *C*, The symphyseal osteotomy completed, and each side of the mandible retracted, exposing the cyst prior to its enucleation. *D*, The dermoid cyst, 7.8 cm broad, after enucleation. *E*, The external appearance 3 weeks postoperatively. *F*, The mandibular continuity restored without the sacrifice of a tooth.

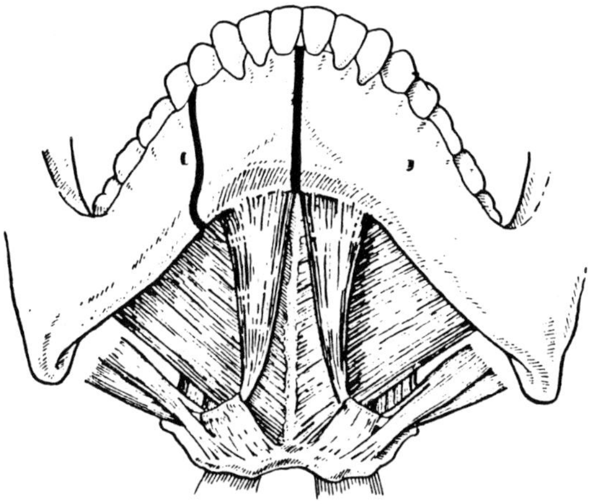

Figure 3 The alternative sites for mandibular osteotomy—symphyseal and lateral—placed between the mental foramen and the insertion of the anterior belly of digastric. (From McGregor IA, McGregor FM. Cancer of the face and mouth. Edinburgh: Churchill Livingstone, 1986:390.)

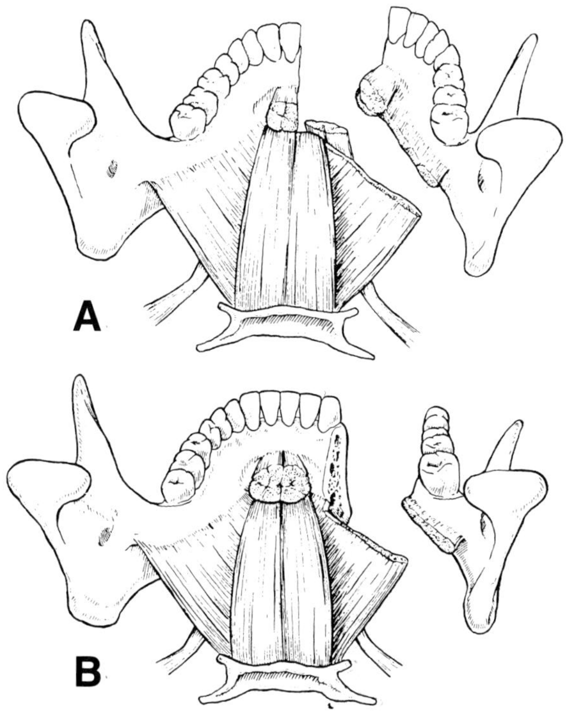

Figure 4 The structures which are divided in carrying out an osteotomy to allow the body of the mandible to "swing" laterally. *A*, At the symphyseal site, the main attachment of the tongue to the mandible, genioglossus, is divided together with geniohyoid, the anterior belly of digastric, mylohyoid and the mucous membrane of the floor of the mouth. *B*, At the site between the mental foramen and the insertion of the anterior belly of digastric, the only structures divided are mylohyoid and the floor of mouth mucosa. (From McGregor IA, McGregor FM. Cancer of the face and mouth. Edinburgh: Churchill Livingstone, 1986: 391.)

one. Stepping of the osteotomy is also not readily applicable to the dentate mandible since it puts the roots of the teeth at risk. In the dentate mandible this is an important factor, since it is when teeth are present that osteotomy is so valuable because the floor is deep and relatively inaccessible unless exposed by osteotomy. In many ways, the main virtue of the straight bony cut is that it can be applied to all mandibles, dentate or edentulous, and does not call for a change in technique depending on whether or not teeth are present. The obvious potentially unsatisfactory aspect of the straight cut concerns subsequent fixation and stability of the osteotomy.

When the fixation methods available were restricted to wiring, the stabilization of a straight bone cut was certainly inadequate, but alternative fixation methods are available today which are capable of providing complete stability even after a straight bone cut.

These methods consist of *compression plating* and *combined direct wiring and transfixing K-wire*. Compression plating is being used increasingly in craniofacial surgery and maxillofacial trauma, and for those familiar with the technique it is extremely effective. Equally effective, and suitable for the surgeon who is inexperienced in the use of plates, is the combination of direct wiring and the transfixing K-wire.

PRACTICE OF THE OSTEOTOMY

In most instances of squamous carcinoma where the osteotomy is being used for access, the lateral site, in front of the mental foramen and behind the insertion of the anterior belly of digastric, is the preferred site (Fig. 5). The skin incision, curving round the chin prominence, has the incidental virtue that the vertical part of the curve directly overlies the osteotomy site and it requires only to be deepened to expose the bone. With the bone exposed, the periosteum is stripped back on each side for 1 to 2 mm, sufficient to allow room for the saw blade. Holes are bored on each side of the projected line of the bone cut, just above the lower border, in preparation for the subsequent insertion of the wire loop. In the case of the edentulous bone, the incision of the mucoperiosteum is extended up and over the occlusal ridge. In the dentate mandible (Fig. 6), a site between two suitable teeth is selected, a preoperative occlusal film having been taken to ensure that the roots are reasonably straight and unlikely to be damaged by the saw. The interdental papilla is incised vertically with a scalpel, dividing it equally between the two teeth. The incision should be deepened down to the bone and extended down along the lingual side as well as on the buccolabial side. The mucoperiosteal incision on the buccolabial surface is then continued down beyond the buccal sulcus to meet the periosteal incision. The splitting of the interdental papilla by the scalpel in this way is necessary to avoid tearing the papilla off the teeth on either side as the bone ends separate when the cut is complete. The fine saw blades which are available today make it possible to cut the bone between the two teeth without any need for extraction. I have not found it necessary to extract a tooth in any instance.

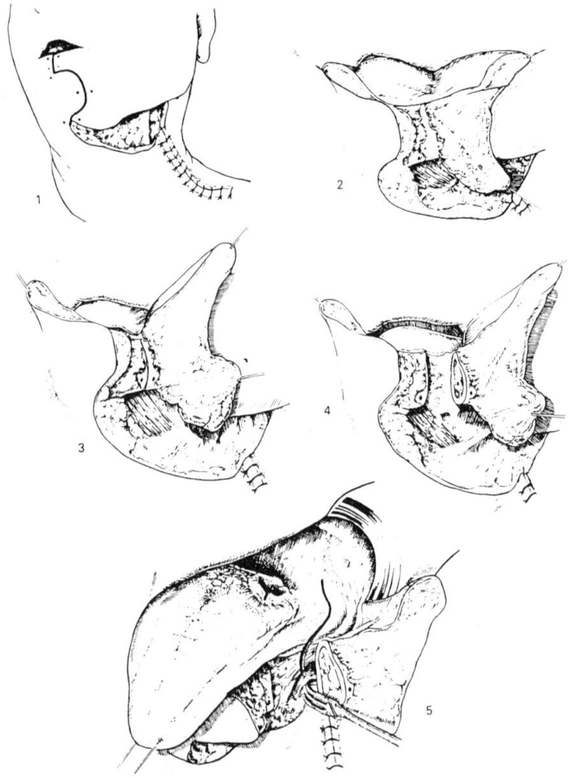

Figure 5 Mandibular osteotomy, used in exposing the posterior third of the tongue. The lip-splitting incision (*1*), curving round the chin prominence, overlies the mandible at the site of the osteotomy (*2*), and allows the bone to be exposed and divided with a minimum of soft tissue stripping (*3*). Division of the periosteum on the lingual surface allows the two bone fragments to separate (*4*), and division of mylohyoid allows the bone to "swing" laterally exposing the tumor of the posterior third of the tongue (*5*). (From McGregor IA, McGregor FM. Cancer of the face and mouth. Edinburgh: Churchill Livingstone, 1986:392.)

When the bone has been completely divided, the two ends separate to expose the lingual mucoperiosteum, and this also is divided. The bone of the mandible behind the osteotomy is retracted laterally, defining the mylohyoid muscle. As it is divided, together with the overlying mucous membrane, the swing increasingly takes place, exposing the posterior oral cavity.

The technique which has been described is equally applicable to the symphyseal site, except for the added structures, genioglossus, geniohyoid, and digastric, which require to be divided in order to allow the hemimandible to swing laterally.

RESTORATION OF BONY CONTINUITY

When the combination of direct wiring and transfixing K-wire is used to restore continuity of the body of the mandible, the first step is insertion of the K-wire into the symphyseal side of the osteotomized surface. The type of K-wire which is used is short and sharpened at both ends, primarily designed for use in hand surgery. The osteotomy site, being already exposed and visible, allows both the point of insertion and the direction of insertion to be decided very precisely. In theory, the greater the distance between the site of the wire loop and the point of insertion of the K-wire, the greater the control of torque, but with the curve of mandibular body and the fixity of the condyles in the temporomandibular joint, torque has not created a problem in practice (Fig. 7).

The K-wire is driven through the bone and emerges through the skin of the chin. It is then drawn further through until it is just visible at the osteotomy site. The wire loop is then inserted, the "fracture" is reduced and the loop is tightened to hold the bone in its reduced position. Steadying the bone with the fingers, the K-wire is

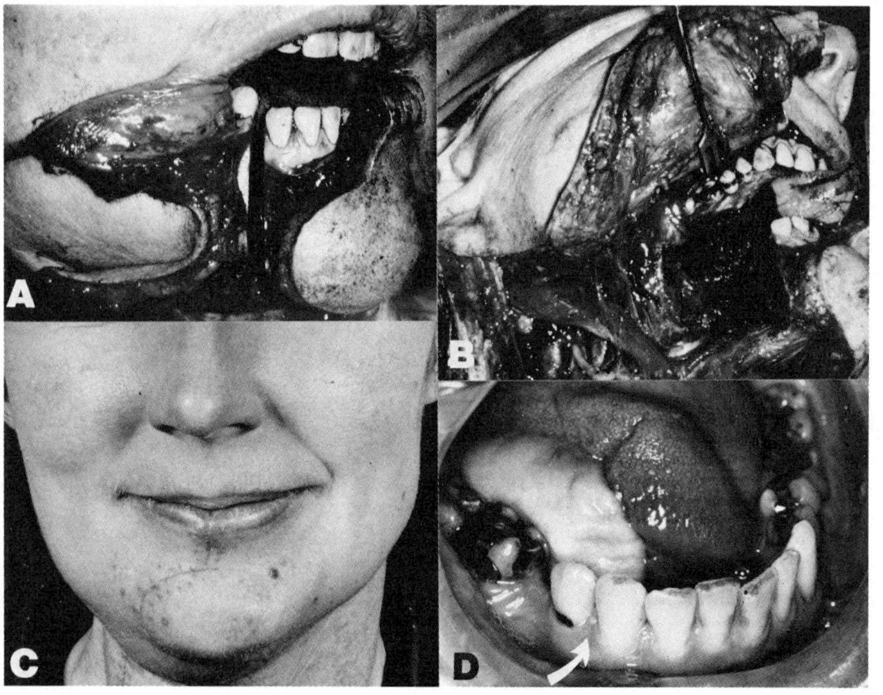

Figure 6 Mandibular osteotomy, as shown in Figure 5, used in the dentate mandible. *A*, Shows the lip-splitting incision and the division of the bone, the interdental papilla divided with the scalpel, the bone with the fine oscillating saw. *B*, Shows the exposure provided by the upward retraction of the osteotomized ramus. *C*, Shows the appearance of the patient 3 weeks postoperatively. *D*, Shows the reconstitution of the interdental papilla, the osteotomy site indicated by the arrow.

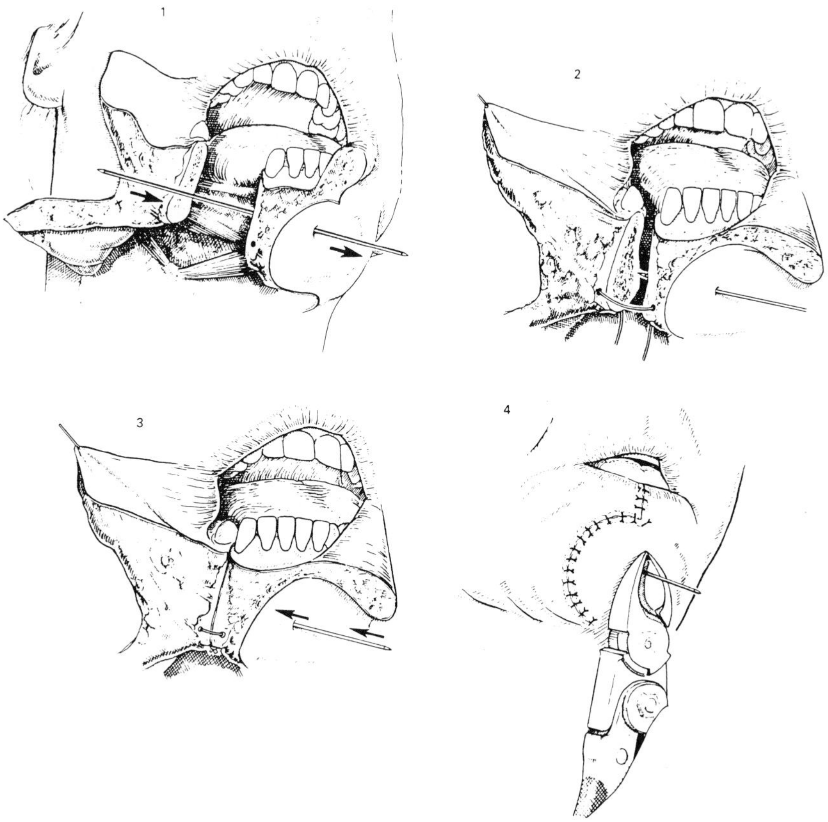

Figure 7 Reconstitution of mandibular continuity following osteotomy. Prior to carrying out the osteotomy, drill holes are bored on each side of the site selected, as shown in Fig. 5, in preparation for interosseous wiring. The short K-wire, sharp at both ends, is driven into the symphyseal side of the osteotomy and emerges through the skin (*1*). It is then pulled through until its tip is just visible at the cut end of the bone (*2*). The bone ends are wired together (*3*), held steady in correct alignment, and the K-wire is driven across the osteotomy site, engaging the bone opposite and stabilizing it. The K-wire is cut short (*4*), leaving the end palpable under the skin for easy subsequent removal. (From McGregor IA, McGregor FM. Cancer of the face and mouth. Edinburgh: Churchill Livingstone, 1986:393.

driven across the osteotomy site until it engages solidly with the bone behind the osteotomy. The stability which results is total, and no other fixation is required. The K-wire is cut short so that, while it is deep to the skin, its tip can be felt emerging from the bone. This allows it to be removed under local anesthesia once the union of the osteotomy has taken place.

When compression plating is used, the bone on each side of the selected osteotomy site has to be cleared of its periosteum over the area to which the plate is going to be applied. The plate is placed in position and appropriate eccentrically directed drill holes are made before carrying out the osteotomy in preparation for the subsequent compression fixation, making sure that the screws are sufficiently long to engage the lingual cortex of the bone. After completion of the excisional and reconstructive surgery the bone ends are approximated, the plate is placed in position and the screws are inserted and tightened, compressing the bone ends together. Once bony union has occurred the screws can be removed with the screwdriver, working through a stab incision in the skin directly over the plate. The plate itself can then be removed by incising the lower buccal sulcus. The plating technique is an excellent one in the hands of those expert in its use, but it is the more technically demanding of the two methods.

In the edentulous mandible the mucoperiosteal margins can be sutured together when bony continuity has been restored, even over the occlusal ridge. In the dentate bone the attachment of the mucoperiosteum to the bone increases as it approaches the interdental papilla and no suturing is possible in that area. Despite this the mucosal margins lie close together and the interdental papilla is restored to a surprising extent (see Fig. 6). Its complete restoration is remarkably rapid, so much so that it quickly becomes impossible on clinical examination to say where the mucosal incisions were made.

SUGGESTED READING

Carraway JH, McGregor IA. Restoration of mandibular continuity after symphyseal osteotomy. Br J Plast Surg 1981; 34:392–394.

Domarus HV. Stabilization of the mandible by AO compression plating after mandibulotomy. Br J Plast Surg 1981; 34:389–391.

McGregor IA, MacDonald DG. Mandibular osteotomy in the surgical approach to the oral cavity. Head Neck Surg 1983; 5:457–462.

McGregor IA, McGregor FM. Cancer of the face and mouth. Edinburgh: Churchill Livingstone, 1986.

Spiro RH, Gerold FP, Strong EW. Mandibular "swing" approach for oral and oropharyngeal tumors. Head Neck Surg 1981; 3:371–378.

HYPOPHARYNX AND CERVICAL ESOPHAGUS RECONSTRUCTION

JACK FISHER, M.D.

Circumferential resection of the pharynx or cervical esophagus may be necessary for the treatment of neoplasms and caustic or traumatic strictures. Numerous techniques have been described for reconstruction of these defects. Early techniques for pharyngoesophageal reconstruction used cervical skin to line a reconstructed pharynx. This procedure, described by Wookey, had many disadvantages that included poor healing, multiple stages, and a high stricture rate at the mucocutaneous suture lines. The deltopectoral flap improved overall results, but still had major disadvantages. The development of pedicled, visceral reconstructions, such as gastric transposition, significantly improved reconstructive results primarily in patients after laryngopharyngectomy. Although numerous techniques are available for reconstruction of the hypopharyngeal and cervical esophageal area, my preference is free intestinal reconstruction using jejunum.

Free jejunal transfer by microvascular technique has a relatively long history, but its acceptance was delayed until standard microsurgical methods made this a highly reliable and safe procedure. Free vascularized transfer of the bowel into the cervical region of experimental animals was reported as early as 1903.

In 1959, Seidenberg and associates reported the first-clinical case in which a patient had reconstruction of the cervical esophagus with a free jejunal transfer. Other reports of the use of this technique appeared in the 1960s and early 1970s. Presently several large series of reconstructions of the cervical esophagus with free jejunal transfer have confirmed the efficacy and reliability of this reconstructive technique.

Reconstruction is required when a circumferential segment of the pharynx and cervical esophagus must be replaced. The requirements for successful reconstruction are a posterior wall, an anterior wall, and adequate skin coverage. Also needed for successful reconstruction is a widely patent connection between the reconstructed segment and the remaining pharynx and esophagus. A wide-open stricture-free connection is essential since most reconstructions are either nondynamic r uncoordinated so that tongue thrust and gravity must initiate propulsion of food. Normal swallowing is impeded with a narrow connection or stricture.

In discussing reconstruction of the pharynx and cervical esophagus, several criteria can be established for the ideal reconstruction. In patients with a limited life expectancy, a one-stage procedure is preferable. The method should be predictable, safe, and compatible with either pre- or postoperative radiation therapy. The ideal method should be able to fill a gap of essentially any size. As will be discussed, free jejunal transfer comes as close as any technique in approaching the ideal reconstructive procedure in cervical esophageal reconstruction. Experience has shown that transfer of jejunum using standard microsurgical technique is resistant to stricture formation at the anastomotic site, provides adequate rehabilitation of swallowing, allows freedom to repair defects at any level of the cervical esophagus and pharynx, and has a relatively low complication rate. Since this method provides a reconstruction with a rich blood supply, radiation therapy appears to be well tolerated. In benign strictures, a major advantage to free jejunal transfer is the ability to work around an intact larynx.

THERAPEUTIC ALTERNATIVES

The cervical skin procedures are rapidly becoming of only historic interest because of three major disadvantages: they are multistage procedures, they are not compatible with radiation therapy, and they can fill only limited defects in the neck. The prototype of the chest wall skin flap procedure for pharyngeal and cervical esophageal reconstruction is the deltopectoral flap using Bakamjiams method. The skin flap is tubed upon itself with the skin side in. This flap is predictable and does not involve a delay, but it does require a two-step procedure. However, difficulties with the lower anastomosis of the tube flap can result in more stages, delayed swallowing, and a prolonged hospitalization.

The tube pectoralis major myocutaneous flap is a one-stage procedure and has less incidence of necrosis than the deltopectoral flap. However, this flap can be extremely bulky in some patients. When tubed and placed under the neck skin, the pectoralis flap may have a limited lumen, thus resulting in delayed swallowing. The visceral interposition procedures include the gastric pull-up and the colon interposition. In the gastric pull-up procedure, the stomach and the duodenum are both mobilized. After the esophagus is mobilized in the chest, the stomach is brought up through the posterior mediastinum into the neck. an opening is made in the gastric fundus and the gastric fundus is anastomosed to the pharynx. Thus, with this technique, the chest is violated to accomplish a reconstruction limited to the neck area. If stomach is not available or appropriate, the colon can be used in similar fashion. However, there is a significant incidence of necrosis and stricture formation associated with colon interposition.

These surgical alternatives have an appropriate place in reconstruction of the pharynx and the cervical esophagus and individualization of treatment is important. These alternatives have been briefly discussed since they are important in the reconstructive armamentarium. However, in the majority of patients with a defect after esophagolaryngectomy or with a benign stricture that is limited to the cervical esophageal region, my preferred approach is reconstruction with free jejunal transfer using microsurgical technique.

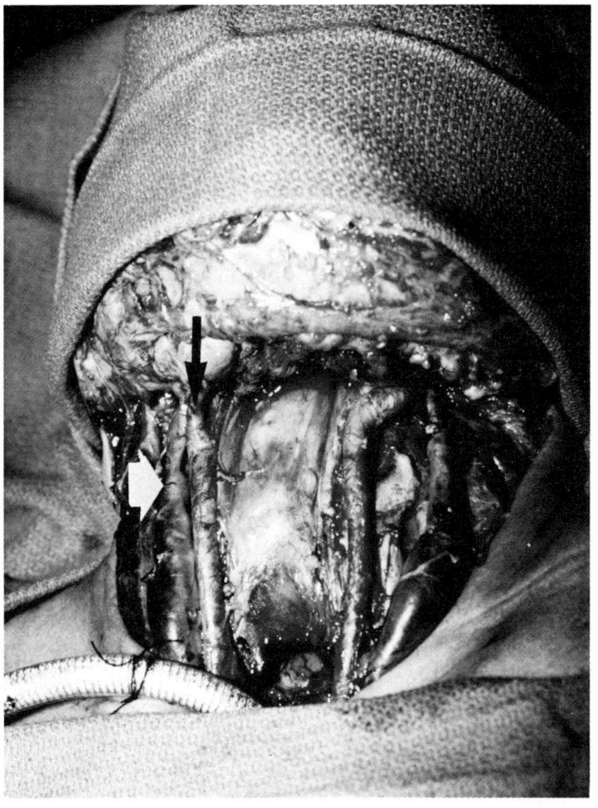

Figure 1 Patient after completion of esophagolaryngectomy with bilateral neck dissection and sparing of internal jugular veins. White arrow indicates right internal jugular vein; black arrow indicates base of right external carotid artery.

PROCEDURE

A two-team method is used in reconstruction of the pharynx and cervical esophagus with free jejunum (Fig. 1). In patients with cancer, one team performs the resection, while another performs a laparotomy for harvesting of the free jejunal segment. A midline laparotomy incision from xyphoid to umbilicus usually provides adequate exposure for harvesting the donor bowel. A self-retaining retractor is inserted to free the surgeon and his or her assistant for dissection of the small bowel. Typically a segment of the jejunum 40 cm distal to the ligament of Treitz is selected. At this level, the jejunum has a diameter approaching that of the cervical esophagus and the mesenteric vessels are of adequate size and length.

The jejunum is brought out of the abdomen and inspected. In thin individuals, the vascular pedicle can be easily seen coursing through the mesentery, whereas it may only be palpable in obese patients. Shining an operating room light behind the mesentery frequently will highlight the vessels. The mesentery is marked on either side of the selected vascular pedicle. Using clamps with silk ties, the mesentery is serially divided to either side of the vascular pedicle (Fig. 2). It is important to maintain the isoperistaltic orientation of the bowel, so the distal end of the jejunal segment is marked with an appropriate suture at the beginning of the dissection. It is also important to divide the mesentery carefully to avoid a hematoma in the mesentery wall. Even a small hematoma can later present a problem in dissection of the vascular pedicle during the microvascular anastomosis.

Once the mesentery is divided to the base of the vascular pedicle, the jejunal artery and vein are dissected and

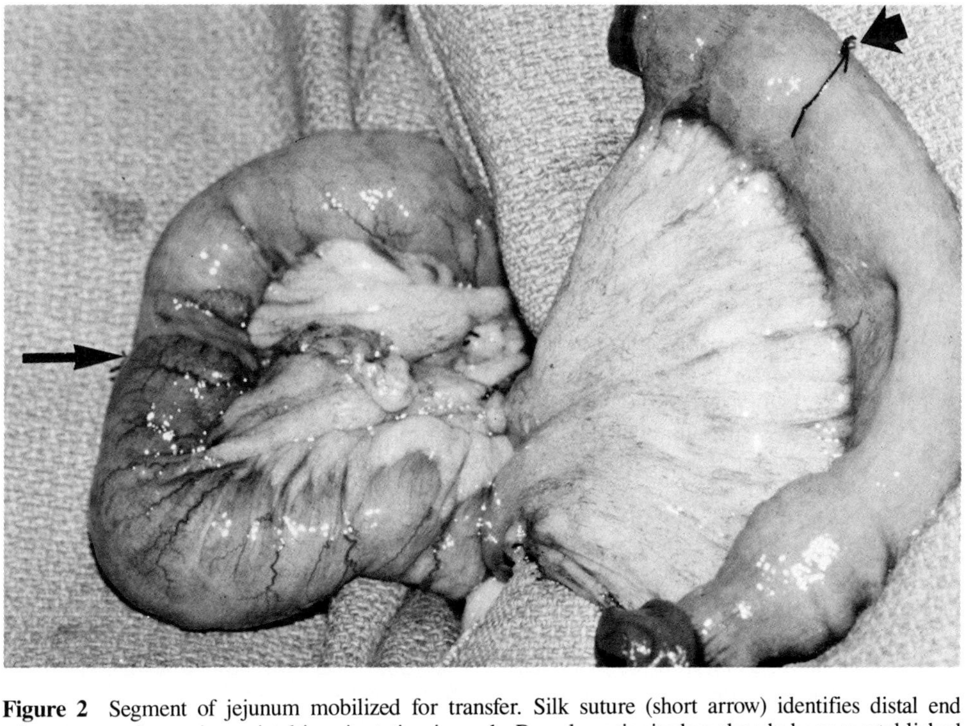

Figure 2 Segment of jejunum mobilized for transfer. Silk suture (short arrow) identifies distal end of segment to insure isoperistaltic orientation in neck. Bowel continuity has already been reestablished in abdomen (long arrow), while resection is being performed in head and neck.

tagged with silk sutures. This dissection of the vascular pedicle at its base is usually performed under 2.5 to 3.5 loupe magnification. Next the intestine is divided after bowel clamps have been placed proximally and distally on the jejunum. No bowel clamps are directly applied to the isolated segment that is to be transferred.

A common error is to isolate a segment of jejunum that is far longer than the defect in the neck. After measuring the esophageal defect in the neck, the intestine in the abdomen should be placed under stretch and a segment of slightly greater length harvested. With the isolated segment of jejunum attached only by its vascular pedicle, intestinal continuity in the abdomen is restored. Once the resection in the head and neck area is complete, the appropriate recipient artery and vein in the head and neck area are isolated.

Selection and Preparation of Recipient Vessels

One of the most critical steps in successful transfer of free jejunum is appropriate selection and preparation of the recipient vessels in the head and neck area. Failure to choose the correct recipient vessel and poor location are probably the most common errors. Although the surgeon performing the resection usually exposes most of the recipient vasculature, it is important for the reconstructive microsurgeon, using appropriate technique, to perform the definitive dissection of these recipient vessels.

Of the various stages in the entire reconstructive procedure, I spend the greatest amount of time in choosing and preparing the recipient vessels The most common recipient artery is the external carotid or one of its branches. Whenever possible, it is preferable to perform an end-to-side mocrovascular anastomosis between the jejunal artery and external carotid artery or its branches. The chances of arterial occlusion because of either vessel spasm or thrombosis are less in an end-to-side anastomosis, especially when working with atherosclerotic or radiated vessels. Using loupe magnification, the surrounding soft tissue is cleared off the external carotid and its proximal branches. Enough length must be obtained so that occluding clamps are not placed too close to the site of the end-to-side microvascular anastomosis. If only a short segment of the recipient vessel is isolated, then the surgeon will find clamps interfering with the microanastomosis under the microscope.

One important pitfall when performing an end-to-side anastomosis to either a recipient artery or vein is the occurrence of torsion of that recipient vessel once the occluding clamps have been applied. A simple maneuver is to place a small dot with a marking pen on the anterior wall of the recipient vessels prior to applying the vascular clamps. Small cerebellar vascular clamps are useful for occluding the external corotid or its branches. If the jejunal artery is large and of similar caliber to the recipient artery, then an end-to-side microvascular anastomosis may be used. Often the superior thyroid artery is smaller than a jejunal artery, and I tend not to use it as a recipient vessel. If the external carotid and its branches are not available, another choice of recipient vessel is the transverse cervical artery.

Finally, the common carotid artery can be used in selected patients. It is necessary to completely cross clamp the common carotid when anastomosing the jejunal artery to it in an end-to-side fashion. In most patients, there is some atherosclerotic plaque in the common carotid, and it is better to fracture the plaque transversely well below and above the site of the microvascular anastomosis. Although a side-biting clamp that would allow flow through the carotid system seems logical, this maneuver makes a microvascular anastomosis extremely difficult. It is imperative to be able to look into the lumen of the recipient vessel when performing a microvascular anastomosis between a small donor artery and a large recipient vessel. It is particularly critical to be able to see clearly into the common carotid artery's lumen, which is frequently thick-walled and atherosclerotic. Many techniques are available for monitoring cerebral blood flow during carotid artery occlusion. One of these methods should be used if it is necessary to cross clamp the carotid.

When surturing the jejunal artery end-to-side to the common carotid, the microsuture should first be passed through the jejunal vessel outside inward and then passed inside outward on the carotid. this maneuver reduces the chance of dissecting a plaque off the artery wall. Although it is infrequent that the common carotid artery is required as a recipient vessel in head and neck microsurgery, there are situations where it may be the only appropriate vessel. This procedure can be safely performed with careful selection of patients and intraoperative monitoring.

Selection of the recipient vein is the next important step. In most cases, the internal jugular is used in an end-side fashion. Torsion of the internal jugular vein occurs easily once it is mobilized, it is helpful to mark the anterior wall prior to applying the occluding clamps. A set of pediatric cardiovascular clamps are useful in head and neck microsurgery, particularly for occlusion of the jugular vein. The deep facial branch of the internal jugular vein is often present after extirpative surgery and matches the size of must jejunal veins for an end-to-end microvascular anastomosis.

A small, self-retaining rectractor in the neck and a small suction drain deep to the recipient vessels are useful devices. Once everything is prepared correctly in the recipient area, attention is returned to the abdomen when the jejunal segment has been perfusing on its vascular pedicle. The warm ischemic time of the bowel can be significantly reduced by insuring that everything is ready in the recipient area. Heavy silk ligatures are placed at the base of the jejunal artery and vein. The vessels are now ligated and divided. The free jejunal segment is brought to the head and neck area while another team closes the abdomen.

Proximal Bowel Anastomosis

The next step is to perform the proximal bowel anastomosis between jejunum and the pharynx or upper cervical esophagus. An important maneuver is fixation of the bowel in the appropriate position prior to the microvascular anastomosis. This insures both stability of the bowel during the microvascular anastomosis and proper positioning of the recipient vessels. The worst scenario is to perform a microvascular anastomosis first and then to discover that the bowel does not reach or fill the defect. With bowel laid into the defect, proper positioning of the jejunal vessels in relation to the already prepared donor vessels can be confirmed.

The jejunum is anastomosed with 3–0 interrupted Vicryl sutures initially beginning on the posterior wall. In my experience, the single most common complication has been fistulas at the proximal anastomosis between the jejunum and pharynx. This is particularly frequent when an anastomosis is performed between the base of the tongue and the jejunum. Although these fistulas will close spontaneously, it is preferable to avoid them. The situation can be remedied by adding a second layer of silk sutures between the base of the tongue and the jejunum. Most of these fistulas are probably related to traction of the mobile tongue on the jejunum, and an extra reinforcement in this area is helpful. The posterior interrupted Vicryl sutures are tagged and tied after the posterior wall is completed, thereby providing better visualization of the bowel anastomosis. However, the anterior sutures can be tied as they are placed.

Vessel Anastomosis

With the proximal bowel anastomosis completed, the microscope is brought into the operative field. There is no particular rule as to whether the artery or the vein should be anastomosed first. Usually it is easier to do the deeper anastomosis followed by the more superficial. When using the external carotid artery and the internal jugular vein as the recipient vessels, the artery usually lies deep to the vein. The jejunal artery is anastomosed to the recipient artery by standard microvascular technique, usually with 9–0 microvascular suture. In patients with particularly large vessels, 8–0 microvascular suture may be appropriate. After completion of the arterial anastomosis, usually the jejunal vein is anastomosed to the internal jugular in an end-to-side fashion. In many patients, the jejunal vein is extremely large, and a running 8–0 nylon suture can give an excellent and meticulous microvascular venous anastomosis. It is easier to do the posterior wall of the vein intitially, followed by the anterior wall anastomosis. With the microvascular anastomosis completed, the vascular clamps are removed from the vein and then from the artery. Immediate peristalsis with abundant mucous production is usually seen with revascularization. Finally, the distal bowel anastomosis is performed between the jejunum and the lower cervical esophagus with 3–0 Vicryl interrupted sutures (Fig.3).

In most patients after pharyngolaryngectomy, the skin flaps close easily without tension over the free jejunal segment. However, in noncancer resections where the larynx is present, closure of the neck may compromise the free jejunal transfer. A simple skin graft on a portion of the jejunum is a safe and simple solution.

Postoperative Procedure

The free jejunal transfer can be monitored by leaving a piece of bowel exposed or by freeing up a small segment of bowel on its mesentery and leaving it exteriorized as a monitoring patch. Acland described this later technique and I have found it useful.

As experience with microsurgery increases, fewer drugs are being used by most microsurgeons to prevent thrombosis. Our patients receive aspirin pre- and postoperatively. Although dextran was used previously with these patients, this practice has essentially stopped. The most important factor in improving patency rates of small

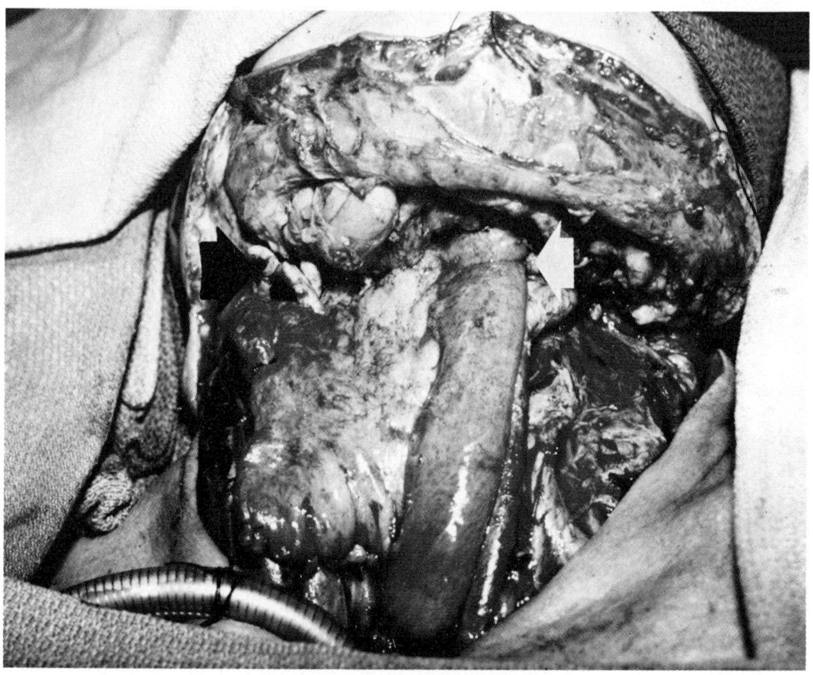

Figure 3 Completion of free jejunal transfer. Proximal jejunum has been anastomosed to pharynx (white arrow) and distal portion of jejunum to lower cervical esophagus. The jejunal artery has been anastomosed to the right external carotid artery and the jejunal vein to the right deep facial branch of the internal jugular vein (black arrow).

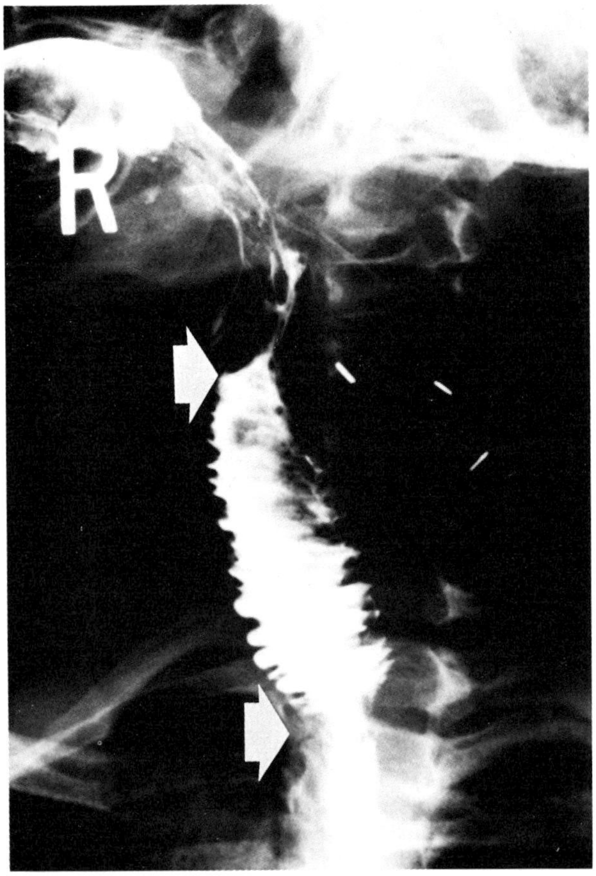

Figure 4 Gastrografin swallow 10 days postoperatively showing flow through jejunal segment. Upper arrow shows proximal anastomoses; lower arrow shows distal bowel anastomoses between jejunum and lower cervical esophagus.

vessel anastomosis is good microsurgical technique, not drugs.

The advantages of free jejunal transfer forreconstruction of pharyngeal and esophageal defects are resistance to stricture formation at the anastomotic site, excellent swallowing rehabilitation, freedom to repair defects at any cervical level of the esophagus and pharynx, and excellent survival of the transferred segments. In benign strictures, reconstruction can be accomplished without resection of the larynx using the free jejunal transfer technique. This technique allows for a single-stage reconstruction and is particularly useful in patients who had previous failed reconstructions. It can be used in patients who have had radiation and in those who are about to receive radiation after the procedure. A vascularized segment of bowel provides an excellent blood supply that promotes healing of the surgical wound. Also, after laryngoesophagectomy, many patients have a limited life span; therefore, a predictable one-stage method that allows alimentation to be resumed seems preferable (Fig. 4).

SUGGESTED READING

Bakamjian VY. A two-stage method for pharyngoesophageal reconstruction with a primary pectoral skin flap. Plast Reconstr Surg 1965; 36:173–184.

Hester TR Jr, McConnel FMS, Nahai F, Jurkiewicz MJ, Brown RG. Reconstruction of cervical esophagus, hypopharynx and oral cavity using free jejunal transfer. Am J Surg 1980; 140:487–491.

Hiebert CA, Cummings GO Jr. Successful replacement of the cervical esophagus by transplantation and revascularization of a free graft of gastric antrum. Ann Surg 1961; 154:103–106.

Jurkiewicz MJ. Vascularized intestinal graft for reconstruction of the cervical esophagus and pharynx. Plast Reconstr Surg 1965; 36:509–517.

Seidenberg B, Rosenak SS, Hurwitt ES, Som ML. Immediate reconstruction of the cervical esophagus by a revascularized isolated jejunal segment. Ann Surg 1959; 149:162–171.

Ong GB, Lee TC. Pharyngogastric anastomosis after oesophago-pharyngectomy for carcinoma fo the hypopharynx and cervical oesophagus. Br J Surg 1960; 48:193–200.

Peters CR, McKee DM, Berry BE. Pharyngoesophageal reconstruction with revascularized jejunal transplants. Am J Surg 1971; 121:675–678.

Wookey H. The surgical treatment of carcinoma of the pharynx and upper esophagus. Surg Gynecol Obstet 1942; 75:499–506.

LARYNGEAL CARCINOMA

EDWARD A. LUCE, M.D.

Approximately 9,000 new cases of carcinoma of the larynx are diagnosed annually in the U.S.A. The disease is responsible for an estimated 3,500 deaths per year: the sex ratio is five to one, male to female. Considerable global variation exists in the incidence of laryngeal cancer. The highest rates have been reported in India, where the incidence in older males may be 10 times that reported in the United States. Within the United States, the rates are highest in New Orleans and lowest in New Mexico and Utah. Studies of the incidence of laryngeal cancer over the past 40 to 50 years reveal an overall increase, presumably attributable to an increase in smoking (particularly in women) and to improved reporting.

The principal risk factor in the development of cancer of the larynx is smoking. Both tobacco and alcohol are strongly associated with elevated risk and interact to a greater degree than either additive alone. Other environmental factors, such as occupation, are of much less importance than tobacco and alcohol. Overall, epidemiologic studies indicate that a few occupations, such as the metal and asbestos industries, may be at increased risk from occupational exposure.

Squamous cell carcinoma is the histologic type in 98 percent of carcinomas of the larynx. Atypical squamous cell abnormalities, not unlike that found in the bronchial tree in heavy smokers, are present in the larynx of smokers. Keratosis with atypia, carcinoma-in-situ, and microinvasive cancer are precursors of clinically evident cancer. Verrucous carcinoma of the larynx is a distinct clinicopathologic entity, similar to that of the buccal cavity, and represents less than 1 percent of all laryngeal cancers.

The larynx-hypopharynx is subdivided into three broad anatomic areas: glottis, supraglottis, and subglottis. These areas have distinct types of cancer with different anatomy, clinical behavior, and therapeutic implications. The supraglottic larynx consists of the epiglottis, the aryepiglottic folds, the arytenoids, false vocal cords, and the ventricles. The glottis includes the true vocal cords and anterior commissure. The subglottis begins 5 mm below the margin of the vocal cords and ends in the inferior border of the cricoid cartilage. The pyriform sinuses and postcricoid areas compose the hypopharynx and are often included in the supraglottis. Lesions that arise primarily in the subglottis are uncommon and compose only 5 percent of all laryngeal cancers.

Intrinsic, or glottic, cancers tend to be symptomatic early in the course of the tumor. Voice dysfunction and hoarseness produced by small, early lesions may motivate the patient to seek medical care. In contrast, supraglottic lesions arise in clinically more silent areas and may reach substantial size before producing symptoms of dysphagia or hoarseness. In addition, the vocal cords are characterized by a sparse lymphatic supply, and nodal metastases are uncommon until the lesion extends out of the glottis. The supraglottic larynx has a rich vascular and lymphatic supply, and the initial presentation may be a metastatic node in the neck.

Classification and staging are performed with TNM classification (Table 1). The particulars of TNM staging are used to compose a broad clinical classification (Table 2).

TABLE 1 TNM Classification and Staging

Supraglottis	
Tis	Carcinoma-in-situ
T1	Tumor confined to region of origin with normal mobility
T2	Tumor involving adjacent supraglottic site(s) or glottis without fixation
T3	Tumor limited to the larynx with fixation or extension to involve the postcricoid area, medial wall of pyriform sinus, or preepiglottic space
T4	Massive tumor extending beyond the larynx to involve oropharynx, soft tissues of neck, or destruction of thyroid cartilage
Glottis	
Tis	Carcinoma-in-situ
T1	Tumor confined to vocal cord(s) with normal mobility (includes involvement of anterior or posterior commissures)
T2	Supraglottic or subglottic extension of tumor, with normal or impaired cord mobility, or both
T3	Tumor confined to the larynx with cord fixation
T4	Massive tumor with thyroid cartilage destruction, or extension beyond the confines of the larynx, or both

TABLE 2 TNM Stage Grouping

Stage I	T1 N0 M0
Stage II	T2 N0 M0
Stage III	T3 N0 M0
	T1 or T2 or T3, N1, M0
Stage IV	T4, N0 or N1, M0
	Any T, N2 or N3, M0
	Any T, Any N, M1

DIAGNOSIS

As mentioned, early symptoms in glottic cancer are those related to voice changes. Unfortunately, a delay in diagnosis often occurs because of inadequate examination. In the past, the average patient who was hoarse because of laryngeal carcinoma saw three physicians and waited an average of 8 months before the larynx was examined and a diagnosis established. The hoarseness of carcinoma is unrelenting and not usually intermittent. Hoarseness that persists for longer than 3 weeks should be investigated vigorously. Ear pain, dysphagia, and airway compromise, as well as a neck mass, are all late findings in glottic carcinoma.

Carcinoma of the supraglottic area tends to remain asymptomatic until the lesions have reached considerable size. Voice changes do occur, but hoarseness is late in onset. Pain on swallowing may be initially mild and often can be lateralized by the patient to a specific side or site. Ear pain may be referred by the vagus nerve, but unilateral ear pain, associated with a sense of fullness, may be due to the involvement of the eustachian tube orifice in the lateral wall of the nasopharynx.

The key element of the physical examination is inspection of the larynx by indirect laryngoscopy, mirror examination, or flexible endoscopic examination. The vast majority of patients can be adequately examined by indirect mirror laryngoscopy as a screening procedure. Patients with positive findings or the occasional difficult mirror examination, can be examined more thoroughly with a flexible endoscope. At our institution we have utilized the 3.2 mm nasopharyngoscope for ease of passage and excellent patient tolerance.

In the past, laryngeal imaging was accomplished by xeroradiography, tomography, and contrast laryngography. All these imaging techniques have been replaced and surpassed by the computed tomography (CT) scan. CT scans are not indicated for small, well-localized lesions of the true vocal cords, particularly of the mid-cord region. The principal value of the CT scan is to define the extent of larger lesions, particularly cartilage invasion or extensive soft tissue spread.

Definitive examination and biopsy is obtained in the operating room under general anesthesia, accomplished with a small (5.5 mm) endotracheal tube. Direct laryngoscopy with any of the operating laryngoscopes provides inspection of inaccessible areas: the recesses of the pyriform sinuses, postcricoid areas, and cervical esophagus. Careful inspection of the anterior commissure and region should be done in cases of smaller glottic carcinomas.

TREATMENT

The selection of a treatment modality—radiation therapy or surgery—is based on the optimal combination of the best functional result and the highest cure rate. In general, radiotherapy is utilized for small, well-defined exophytic lesions, and surgery directed toward more advanced disease.

In glottic carcinoma, management of carcinoma-in-situ and microinvasive carcinoma has been controversial. Our management has been by microlaryngoscopy and cord stripping, with thorough pathologic examination. Careful follow-up is mandatory, and every effort should be directed toward cessation of smoking.

Glottic Cancer

Radiotherapy is recommended for T1 lesions of the mobile, true vocal cord. Extension of the gross tumor into the anterior commissure or arytenoid is viewed with concern, since such findings have been associated with a higher recurrence at our institution. T2 lesions with normal cord mobility are usually managed with conservative laryngeal surgery: vertical hemilaryngectomy. Detailed discussions with the patient are essential in these instances to balance the pros and cons of the decision to elect for radiotherapy or surgery.

More advanced lesions, T3 or T4, require a total laryngectomy and neck dissection. Selective T3 lesions may be approached with an extended hemilaryngectomy and neck dissection. The decision to perform less than a total laryngectomy for a T3 carcinoma is a sophisticated one, and should be reached only by those surgeons with considerable experience in this area.

Supraglottic Cancer

As described, the opportunity to treat an early (T1) lesion of the supraglottis is infrequent. When the lesion is ulcerative in type, the suspicion of occult extension of the tumor should be high. An exophytic T1 lesion can be managed by radiotherapy.

Larger lesions, T2 and T3, can be encompassed with partial laryngeal surgery; a supraglottic laryngectomy. In my experience, the oncologic and medical indications for horizontal or supraglottic laryngectomy must be scrupulously inspected. Often tumor extends beyond the apparent margins and the opportunity for cure may be compromised. The difficulties with recurrent aspiration and secondary pulmonary infection are considerably greater with supraglottic conservative surgery than with partial laryngectomy for glottic cancer. The association between cancer of the upper aerodigestive tract and chronic obstructive lung disease is high, and such an association may preclude supraglottic laryngectomy.

Large, bulky, or infiltrating lesions (T4) are managed by total laryngectomy and bilateral, modified neck dissection.

In selected patients with a pyriform sinus primary and extension to the medial laryngeal wall and epiglottis, we have combined a vertical laryngectomy with a supraglottic resection, thereby preserving cord and arytenoid. The resultant defect has been reconstructed with a flap of pectoralis or sternocleidomastoid muscle. In a small group of patients, the results, both in terms of voice preservation and tumor control, have been encouraging.

Combined Therapy

Combined therapy has been advocated to reduce the significant local, regional, and distant failure in large, advanced lesions of the larynx and hypopharynx. Little evidence exists to support the contention that preoperative radiotherapy, followed by surgery, will accomplish that goal. We have reviewed our experience in patients with advanced cancer of the larynx and hypopharynx to determine the efficacy of preoperative radiation. We cannot demonstrate an improved survival rate with preoperative radiation (5,000 to 6,000 rad) over that of radical surgery alone. Currently, we employ postoperative radiation, initiated 10 to 14 days after surgery. Postoperative radiation should also not be applied indiscriminately, since a distinct complication rate is associated with full-dose radiation therapy. The indications include extracapsular nodal extension, multiple node involvement, positive margins on permanent section at the primary site, and massive primary disease that extended into the extra laryngeal soft tissue.

Chemotherapy, either single-agent or multiple-agent, as a combined primary therapeutic modality with either radiotherapy or surgery, remains in the experimental protocol stage.

COMPLICATIONS

The acute complications of extirpative surgery of the head and neck are secondary to the inevitable contamination, the wide planes of dissection, and the tenuous nature of oropharyngeal and pharyngeal suture lines. Yet, because of the rich vascularity of the area, extirpative and reconstructive surgery is accomplished with a surprisingly low complication rate. Prior radiation alters this balance substantially. The review of our experience with advanced cancer of the larynx and hypopharynx also included a comparison of complications and morbidity between preoperative radiotherapy plus surgery versus surgery alone.

Postoperative complications, including the incidence of pharyngocutaneous fistula, flap slough, and carotid artery rupture were all significantly higher in those patients who had been previously irradiated. All postoperative deaths occurred in the same group (Table 3).

Other complications associated with conservative laryngeal surgery include inadequate airway and recurrent aspiration.

A persistent complication that has plagued surgeons since the performance of the first total laryngectomy has been the inadequate or stenosed tracheal stoma. Operative techniques probably play a major contributory role in determination of the likelihood of stenosis. Mechanical handling of the tracheal mucosa, poor approximation

TABLE 3 Postoperative Complications

Operative Complications	*Patients with Preoperative Radiation Therapy (N=53)*	*Surgical Patients with No Radiation (N=28)*
Pharyngocutaneous (PC) fistula	15 (28%)	5 (18%)
Flap slough	8 (15%)	1 (4%)
Carotid rupture*	7 (13%)	0
Mortality*	4 (8%)	0

* All carotid artery ruptures occurred in the presence of PC fistula; all deaths occurred in carotid artery ruptures.

or excessive tension at the mucocutaneous suture line, devascularization of the trachea, and inadequate removal of the strap muscles have all been implicated in the process. Beveled tracheostomies, Z-plasties, and split stomas with large lateral flaps have been proposed to avoid the complication of tracheal stenosis.

We reviewed our experience to clarify the etiologic factors in postoperative stomal stenosis. From a technical standpoint, a single vertical transection of the trachea at the time of laryngectomy and suture to the skin resulted in the highest incidence of stenosis. A beveled stoma reduced the incidence to one-half, but the lowest incidence was associated with a primary effort to interrupt the straight line contracture, as with a Z-plasty or posterior V-flap. The use of postoperative radiotherapy also increased the incidence substantially, but, curiously, preoperative radiotherapy had little effect.

RESULTS AND FOLLOW-UP

Cure in cancer of the larynx varies tremendously from a 90 percent 5-year survival in T1 glottic cancer to a 10 percent figure in T4 of the hypopharynx with nodal metastases. The significant variables are those of site, primary size, and the absence or presence of nodal metastases. General survival figures for glottic cancer are plus 90 percent for T1, 80 percent for T2 lesions, with a decline to 55 percent for T3, and 25 percent for T4 lesions. Table 4 shows our institutional experience with 3- and 5-year survival of laryngeal cancer, both crude and adjusted for death due to other causes.

TABLE 4 Survival Rates (Crude and Adjusted for Other Causes of Death)

	Stages			
	I	*II*	*III*	*IV*
3 year crude	80%	58%	60%	27%
3 year adjusted	—	66%	56%	39%
5 year crude	63%	52%	26%	09%
5 year adjusted	76%	66%	50%	29%

Rehabilitation of the laryngectomee is unsuccessful unless the patient can communicate by some method other than writing. Development of esophageal speech is considerably facilitated by preoperative education and early postoperative enrollment in speech therapy. Nevertheless, more than half the patients do not develop effective esophageal speech. Various mechanical hand-held devices are available, either of the transcervical or transoral types. Transcervical appliances are not satisfactory if the soft tissues of the neck are rigid from postoperative or radiation changes. The transoral type is conspicuous in use and often becomes clogged with saliva.

Voice rehabilitation in the aphonic laryngectomee is accomplished most satisfactorily, in our experience, with a Blom-Singer trachoesophageal fistula and appliance. This procedure is performed on a delayed or secondary basis.

SUGGESTED READING

Cann CI, Fried MP. Determinants and prognosis of laryngeal cancer. Otolaryngol Clin North Am 1984; 17:139–150.

Griffith GL, Meeker WR, McMahan A, Luce EA. Management of carcinoma of the larynx. J Ky Med Assoc 1979; 77:169–172.

Griffith GR, Luce EA. Tracheal stomal stenosis after laryngectomy. Plast Reconstr Surg 1982; 70:694–698.

Luce EA. The irradiated wound. Surg Clin North Am 1984; 64:821–829.

Luce EA, Meeker WR. Comparison of pre-operative irradiation vs primary surgery in treatment of advanced cancer of the larynx-hypopharynx. Presented to the Society of Head and Neck Surgeons, Pittsburgh, April 1979.

Million RR, Cassisi NJ. The larynx. In: Million RR, Cassisi NJ, eds. Management of head and neck cancer. Philadelphia: JB Lippincott, 1984:315.

Pearson BW. Sub-total laryngectomy. Laryngoscope 1981; 91:1904–1912.

Romm S. Cancer of the larynx: current concepts of diagnosis and treatment. Surg Clin North Am 1986; 66:109–118.

Wells HE, Luce EA. Recurrence rate in T. laryngeal cancer managed with radiotherapy. Unpublished data.

SCAPULAR OSTEOCUTANEOUS FREE-FLAP MANDIBULAR RECONSTRUCTION

JOSEPH C. BANIS Jr., M.D.
WILLIAM M. SWARTZ, M.D.

Composite reconstruction of mandibular and maxillary defects with associated soft tissue deficits as a result of tumor extirpation or trauma remains a major challenge to the reconstructive surgeon. If one excludes the many well-recognized problems of obtaining adequate amounts of well-vascularized soft tissue with which to reconstruct a defect, one can identify certain basic requirements in donor flap tissue for optimum restoration of function and form.

Soft tissue requirements for external coverage include variable amounts of bulk, as well as color and hair absence to match the face. Soft tissue requirements for internal lining reconstruction usually include thin, pliable, non-hairbearing skin. Donor sites for soft tissue reconstruction have frequently been problematic due to the esthetic results.

Mandibular reconstruction has been plagued by problems with: (1) the obtaining of adequate bone stock and bulk, (2) the long time needed for "creeping substitution" to solidify nonvascularized bone grafts, (3) nonunion and fibrous union, (4) internal and external fixation devices and techniques, (5) the presence of implanted hardware and its effect on subsequent radiation therapy, (6) the ability to proceed with early postoperative therapeutic radiation of defects reconstructed with nonvascularized bone grafts, (7) use of nonvascularized bone graft or cancellous bone graft methods of reconstruction in previously irradiated defects, or defects with poor soft tissue coverage or availability, (8) potential for osteomyelitis or osteoradionecrosis, and (9) poor function and esthetic result in spite of technical success of the reconstruction.

Microsurgical techniques of free tissue transfer have vastly increased the reconstructive surgeon's choice of donor tissue for well-vascularized soft tissue as well as bone. The osteocutaneous groin flap based on the deep circumflex iliac artery and vein, the dorsalis pedis—second metatarsal bone osteocutaneous territory, and the radial forearm osteocutaneous flap have all found a place in composite mandibular reconstruction; but all have certain limitations.

Teot and Bossé et al demonstrated the potential for composite microsurgical vascularized bone reconstruction of the mandible with the use of bilateral scapulae for mandibular reconstruction. Their initial experience with this flap and cadaver studies that demonstrated a rich vascularity of the scapular cutaneous territory and the lateral border of the scapula itself, have led to the clinical use of this osteocutaneous donor territory as one of our preferred flap donor sites for major head and neck reconstruction.

ADVANTAGES

The scapular osteocutaneous free flap donor territory has many advantages to recommend it in mandibular reconstruction and soft tissue reconstruction in the head and neck. The territory is large, generally hairless, and results in a medium-thickness flap. It can be divided into multiple flaps (up to three independent cutaneous flaps in the authors' clinical experience) (Fig. 1). The color match for use in the head and neck region is generally very acceptable. Anatomic characteristics of this flap include a reliable and very rich vascularity, with extremely high blood flow compared to various other territories.

ANATOMIC CHARACTERISTICS

An almost straight, bony segment of the lateral border of the scapula can be harvested, generally 2- to 2.5-cm wide, shaped similarly to the normal adult mandible. This bony structure has sturdy cortical component, combined with a well-vascularized and structurally stable cancellous cavity centrally, in the cross-sectional configuration of a steep isosceles triangle. The gentle typically convex curvature of the scapula makes the contralateral scapular border an ideal donor site for a body of mandible reconstruction with an intended posterior (near the anatomic angle of mandible) vascular connection to upper neck ves-

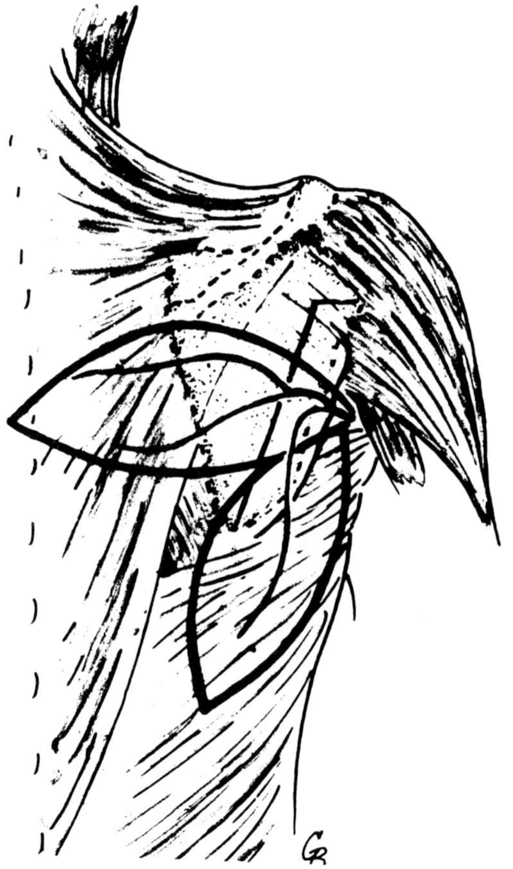

Figure 1 Schematic of multiple cutaneous flaps and lateral scapular osseous flap.

sels. Segments of bone up to 10 to 15 cm in length from the glenoid fossa to the scapular tip can be harvested (in petite females up to large adult males respectively).

The pedicle is long and constant and provides up to 10 cm of vascular pedicle length for the cutaneous flap only, and up to 5 cm of pedicle length when the vascularized lateral border of scapula is used, with another 5 cm of independent mobility on a vascular pedicle for independent placement of skin flaps about the bone. The anastomosable vessels are of large (up to 3.0 mm) diameter. The donor site has proved to be relatively free from functional deficits or consequences even when the bony harvesting is carried out.

Of major importance in selection of this flap for osteocutaneous mandibular reconstruction is the ability to develop multiple flaps on a single pedicle and to place the cutaneous flaps in an independent fashion relative to the bony reconstruction. This is possible due to the long vascular leash that connects the bone to the skin flap, or flaps.

Compared to these attributes relative to soft tissue coverage, the groin-iliac crest soft tissue territory is often excessively bulky, restricted in mobility and placement with respect to the underlying bone, sometimes of uncertain hardiness of vascularity (depending on how one elevates and contorts the cutaneous territory to fulfill the needs of the defect), and does not allow for development of multiple cutaneous flaps upon a single vascular pedicle. The color match of this territory for use in facial reconstruction is fair, but generally not as good as the scapular territory. Attributes of the groin-iliac crest cutaneous territory are significant and include: (1) nonhairbearing skin, (2) no significant long-term functional deficit and a minimal esthetic defect, especially important when reconstructing defects in young females, (3) a medium-large cutaneous territory, (4) a reliable vascular anatomy and pedicle, and (5) the ability to position the patient for expedient two-team simultaneous procedures.

The dorsalis pedis cutaneous territory (compared to the scapular territory) is of medium size, is only moderately mobile relative to its underlying bone, thus allowing for minimal independence of soft tissue flap placement, does not allow development of multiple independent skin flaps, and has a major color mismatch for external facial use in the Caucasian. This flap also may be difficult to dissect due to some anatomic variability of its vasculature. Attributes of the dorsalis pedis flap are: (1) it is an extremely thin flap, excellent for anterior oral and floor-of-mouth reconstruction, (2) it is generally hairless or minimally hairbearing, (3) it is supplied by an indefinitely long and large vascular pedicle with reliable and easily assessed preoperatively vasculature, and (4) its donor site defect is minimal in regard to functional and esthetic outcome when properly managed, and is usually hidden by footwear.

The radial forearm flap cutaneous territory, as compared to the scapular territory, results in a more significant and less easily hidden donor defect that usually requires skin grafting and does not allow for development of multiple independent flaps on a single vascular pedicle. Advantages, however, include: (1) a large available territory (not as large as the scapular flap but probably able to cover almost all facial defects), (2) excellent color match for facial use, (3) reliable flap vasculature with a long and large vascular pedicle, and (4) minimal hairiness as a rule.

TECHNIQUE OF OSTEOCUTANEOUS MANDIBULAR RECONSTRUCTION

The scapular osteocutaneous flap usually requires two position changes when it is used for immediate reconstruction of extirpative tumor defects—one following extirpation of the tumor (creation of the defect) in the supine position, and another from the lateral or prone position after flap dissection. On occasion, in the case of a delayed reconstruction of a tumor or traumatic defect, the surgeon may have a predetermined knowledge of the flap requirements (by prior measurements or computed tomography [CT] scan computer-generated acrylic model) that allow for flap dissection as the initial operative maneuver in the lateral or prone position, with only one position change back to the supine position for inset and osteosynthesis. It has not been possible in the authors' experience to do extirpation, flap harvest, and reconstruction in one position, or as a simulataneous two-team procedure.

After tumor resection, the specimen is carefully measured in order to reproduce on sterile, clear x-ray film the exact dimensions of the soft tissue and bony territory resected, including the angle of osteotomies on the mandible. This greatly facilitates reconstruction, since the orientation, dimensions, and spatial relationships of the mandible and soft tissue segments are distorted once the tumor is removed. Alternatively, if possible, a CT scan computer-generated milled acrylic model of the bony segment can help accomplish this with less difficulty.

Once extirpation has created the defect, the patient must be placed in the lateral or prone position. The cutaneous vessels have usually been identified preoperatively by Doppler examination to ascertain the dominant cutaneous vessel locations prior to outline of the cutaneous flap, or flaps. Cutaneous flaps are incised and elevated in the usual fashion for elevation of a cutaneous scapular flap. The cutaneous flaps can be elevated at the level of the subcutaneous fat-muscular-fascia junction from the medial approach, with a search for the cutaneous vessels at the lateral border of the scapula. Alternatively, one may identify the circumflex scapular vascular pedicle initially at the lateral border of the scapula as it emerges from the triangular space, and then elevate the cutaneous flaps after these vessels have been identified and protected.

The usual technique of dissection of a cutaneous scapular flap is altered, however, when one approaches the circumflex scapular artery and vein at the lateral border of the scapula. In the dissection of the scapular osteocutaneous flap, the vascular connections to the lateral border of the scapula are preserved with preservation of the superficial and deep periosteal vessels. The entire pedicle is carefully dissected as far proximally as desired, i.e., generally to the branching of the subscapular artery into the thoracodorsal artery and the circumflex scapular artery, or the subscapular artery origination from the axillary artery. This dissection preferably is carried out as much as possible prior to bony dissection since the bloody nature of the bony dissection after the osteotomies are completed would hinder subsequent vascular pedicle dissection.

Once the vascular pedicle has been dissected, the teres major and teres minor muscles are dissected free from the lateral border of the scapula, taking care to preserve periosteal vascular integrity of the vessels that supply the bone. The infraspinatus muscle is divided approximately 2.5 cm medial to the lateral border of the scapula (at the junction of the sturdy lateral scapular bone with the thin bone of the central plate of the scapula), and bluntly dissected down to the thin plate-like medial extension of scapular bone, medial to the lateral border being harvested. All muscles may be dissected under well-visualized conditions immediately down to the periosteum, provided the periosteal vessels are kept intact, i.e., an actual muscle cuff is not required as long as the periosteal vessels are protected. The muscle dissection to identify the periosteum on the lateral border of the bone segment desired may be made to just below the glenoid fossa, with care taken not to violate the joint. The dissection can be carried through the scapular tip to give up to 15 cm of bone in a large adult male. When the periosteum has been visualized, an oscillating saw is used to make the longitudinal cut and the transverse cut just below the glenoid fossa. Osteotomes may be required for the final fracture and bony separation. The subscapular and serratus anterior muscles usually are sturdy structures that minimize the tendency of the bone to separate until these muscles are completely dissected free on the anterior surface of the scapula. Once the dissection of these muscles has been completed, the bone is freely mobile and can then be removed in continuity with the previously dissected skin flaps.

Donor site reconstruction can be carried out with absorbable or permanent suture, using a continuous suture technique to reattach the teres major and teres minor muscles to the remaining lateral segment of infraspinatus musculature. This part is usually completed quickly. The cutaneous closure usually is carried out as a primary closure with skin grafting avoided if possible. This is a difficult area in which to obtain primary take of skin grafts; a much improved appearance results with primary donor site closure.

The patient is then repositioned and the mandibular defect is created or more often, the previously created defect is reopened. After removal of the flap, the next step is to fashion as exact a neomandible analogue of the resected mandible as possible. As discussed previously, this is greatly facilitated by exact drawings on x-ray film of the dissected specimen before it leaves the room, or by having obtained preoperatively a computer-generated milled acrylic model from CT scan examination and data. With the information at hand regarding the dimensions and angles needed within the bone, one can quietly set to modifying this vascularized bone flap into a mandibular analogue. The work is done on a back bench with several good assistants and adequate lighting. A Freer or Joseph elevator is used to elevate the periosteum gently and delicately over the intended sites of osteotomies. A high speed side-cutting burr is used to create wedge osteotomies, carefully and accurately fashioned to create the angles necessary for the symphyseal and mandibular angle reconstructions. Care is taken to keep the bone well irrigated to prevent thermal devitalization in the areas of osteotomy. Very sturdy (0.045 or 0.062 inch) Kirschner pins and 0.022 inch stainless steel wire are employed for osteosynthesis for torsional rigidity and compression respectively. The sturdy bony stock of the scapular cortex and compact cancellous cavity allows considerable tightening of the compression wires and secure placement of the pins, so that clinically rigid stability is provided by these conventional techniques. Several cases have been completed that employed plate and screw fixation techniques. These newer fixation methods show promise and have several advantages. When using these techniques, however, one must be sure to avoid devitalization of distal segments of bone by compression of the soft tissue that carries the vascularity to them. It is also necessary to avoid periosteal stripping to place these plates. During this portion of bony modeling, every attention and effort is directed toward preservation of the periosteal-soft tissue vascular bridge that maintains blood supply to those distal segments no longer in bony continuity because of the osteotomies. External fixation devices are rarely necessary.

When intra-flap contouring and osteosynthesis have been completed, the osteocutaneous flap is moved to the patient. A decision must be made as to whether osteosynthesis to the remaining segments of the patient's mandible should be carried out before or after the vascular anastomoses have been completed. This depends on logistical considerations with respect to the position of the vascular anastomosis relative to the mandible, the accessibility of the vessels after osteosynthesis has been completed, and consideration of the length of ischemic time. The flap may be cooled by topical methods with bags of ice chips or sterile slush in order to prolong a safe ischemic time. Osteosynthesis to the remaining mandible may be carried out in similar fashion to the intra-flap osteosynthesis with K-pins and intraosseous wires, or plates and screws as appropriate. The vascular anastomoses are carried out in standard fashion. The preferred vascular arrangement in our unit is end-to-side arterial anastomosis to the external carotid artery, and end-to-side venous anastomosis to the jugular vein. In any given situation, a number of other vascular arrangements and recipient vessels may be considered and used.

A particular note should be made regarding the use of cutaneous paddle flaps for both internal lining and external coverage. The logistics of insetting an internal paddle are frequently quite involved; the internal cutaneous paddle generally requires insetting prior to osteosynthesis of the neomandibular segment to the residual mandible. The surgeon should do a step-by-step mental "dry run'' to ensure that the order of flap insetting, with its multiple parts, is such as to make the rest of the procedure as technically easy as possible. Difficulties with this procedure have often been related to an inadequate mental review of how each step will impact the rest of the steps. There is a definite learning curve involved in this aspect of the operation and the first few may well take longer than subsequent cases.

CASE STUDIES

The scapular osteocutaneous flap has proved to be a versatile and reliable method for composite reconstruction of tumor and traumatic defects of the head and neck. Its rich vascularity has proved useful in infected and irradiated wounds. These cases illustrate the exceptional versatility of mandibular reconstruction with this tissue.

Case 1 (Fig. 2) is a 62-year-old male who had recurrence of a previously irradiated squamous cell carcinoma of the right retromolar trigone region which involved the buccal mucosa. His extirpative surgery involved full-thickness resection of buccal mucosa, right hemimandible from the right midascending ramus in the right parasymphyseal region, and a large territory of external cheek skin overlying the mandible. The reconstruction with the scapular osteocutaneous flap used two separate fasciocutaneous flap territories for internal lining and external cover, overlying the bone.

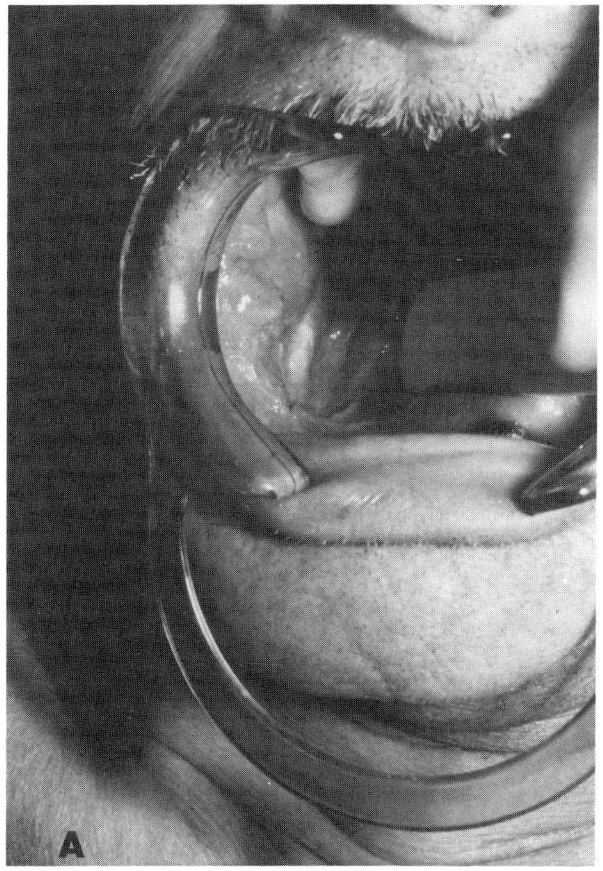

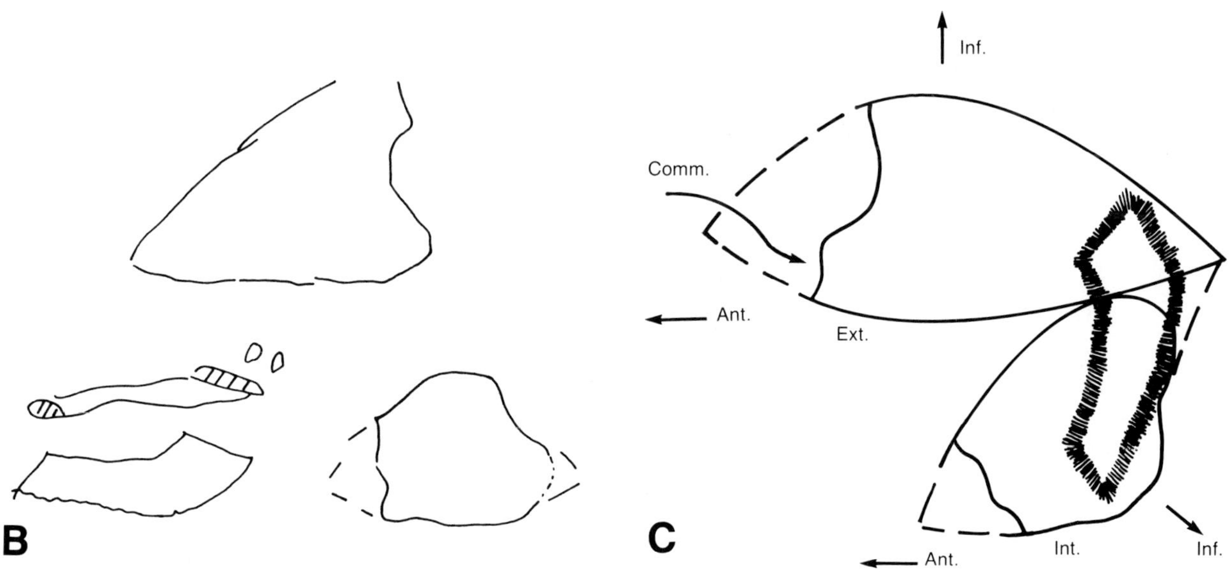

Figure 2 Case 1, A 62-year-old male with recurrent, previously irradiated tumor in right retromolar trigone region. *A*, Shows the rather unimpressive appearance of the invasive tumor in the buccamucosal region. *B*, Template representation of the skin, mucosa, and bone dimensions is drawn from the resection to fashion the neomandible and flaps. *C*, These flap representations are then further transferred into a single composite, which helps the surgeon identify the exact lines of incision and orientation of the flap.
Figure continues on following page

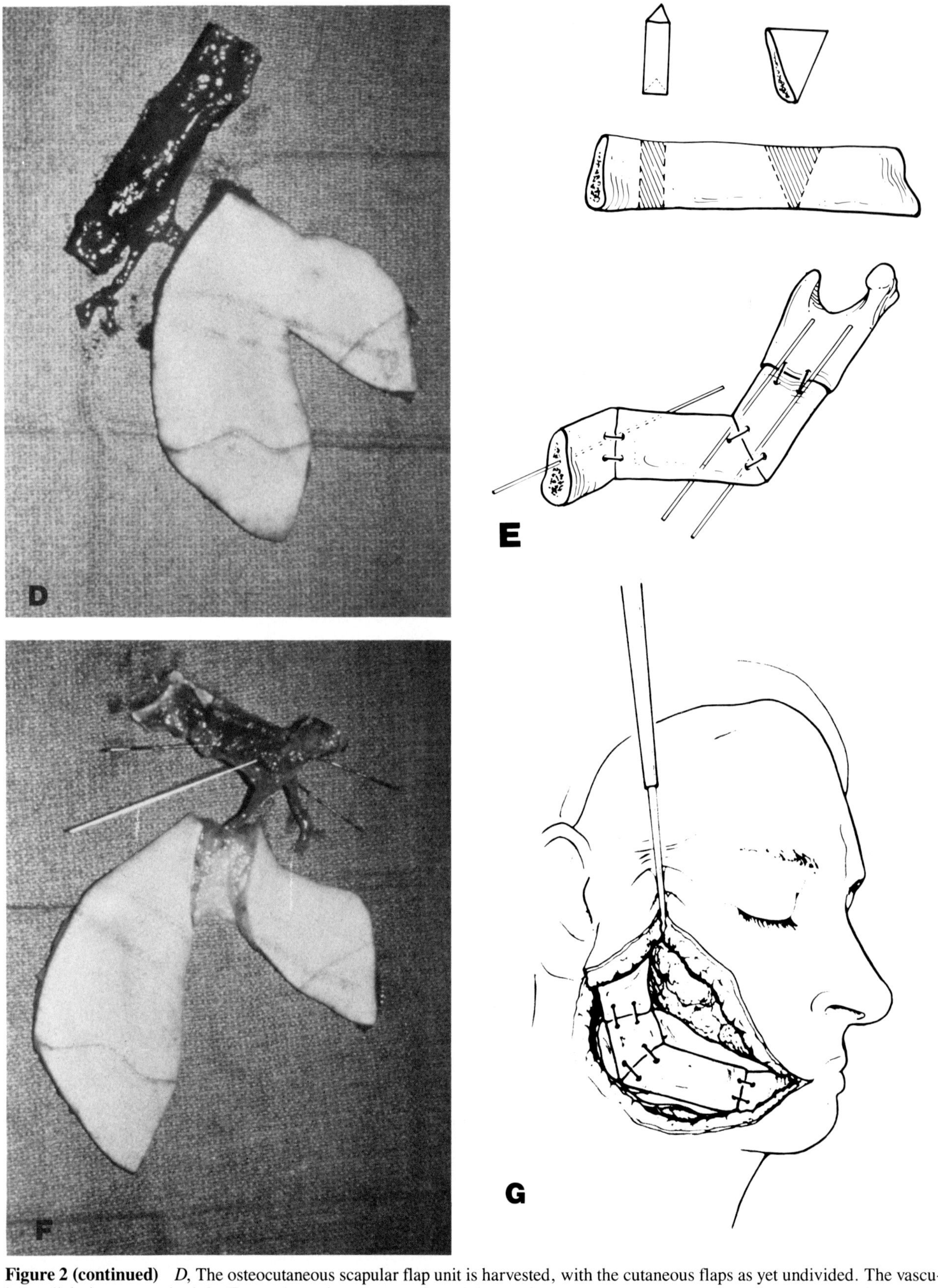

Figure 2 (continued) *D,* The osteocutaneous scapular flap unit is harvested, with the cutaneous flaps as yet undivided. The vascular pedicle is seen to the left. *E,* A schematic representation of the closing wedge osteotomies for recreation of symphyseal and mandibular angles is depicted along with the K-pin and interosseous wire reconstruction, and *F,* the actual flap with osteosynthesis pins and the split cutaneous flap is seen in the lateral projection. *G,* The schematic depiction of the inset of this osteocutaneous unit is demonstrated.

Figure continues on opposite page

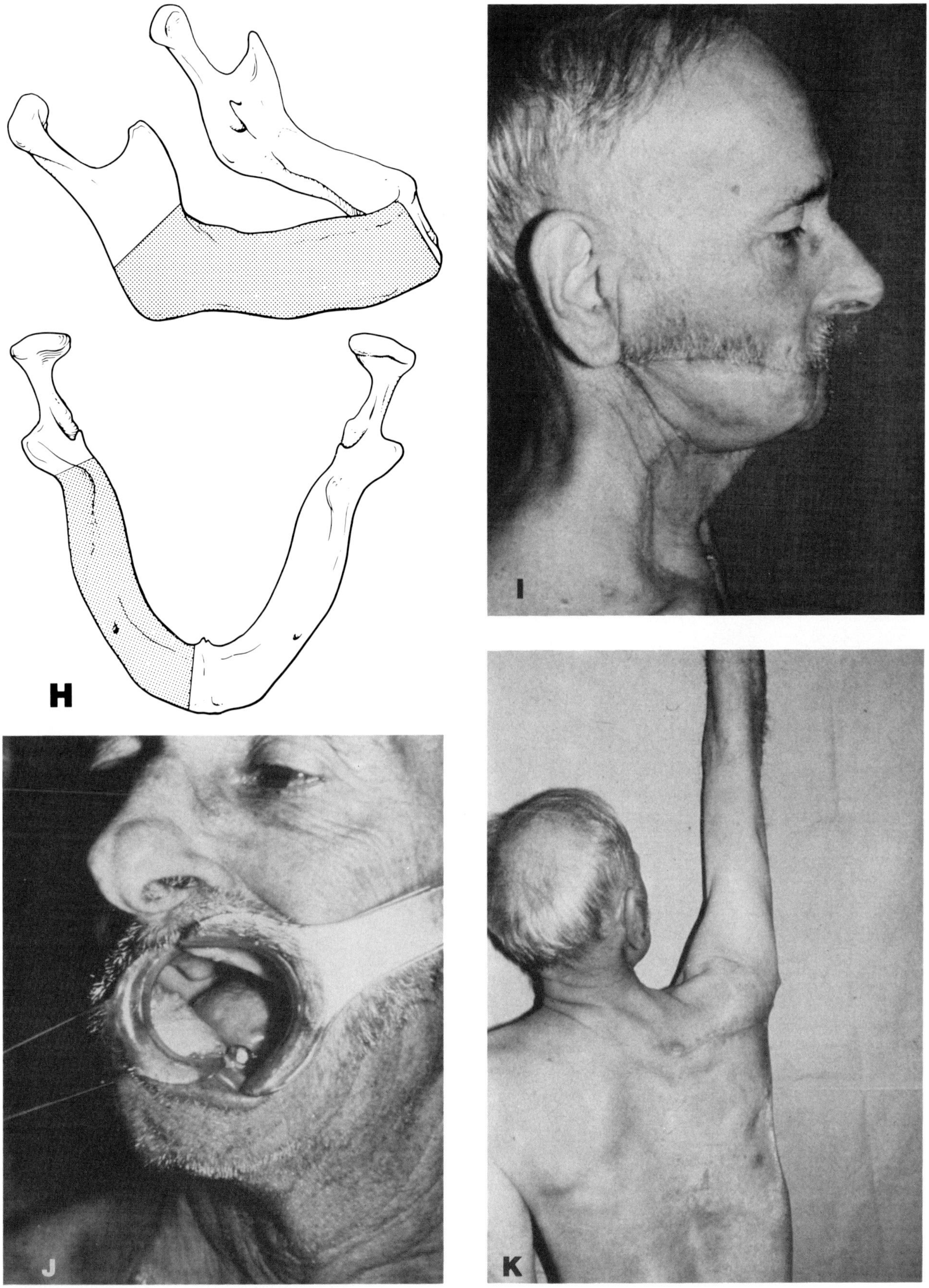

Figure 2 (continued) *H*, A schematic representation of the extent of the mandible resected and reconstructed *I*, Postoperative skin coverage. *J*, Shows the quality of the intraoral lining flap. *K*, The range of motion of the right shoulder region is normal, and without pain or loss of strength.

The patient experienced a smooth and unremarkable postoperative course with primary healing of the intraoral and external skin flaps as well as primary bony union. Furthermore, he began postoperative radiation therapy 3 weeks postoperatively as it was thought that all previously maximally irradiated tissue has been resected and replaced with the nonirradiated free flap tissue. The radiation therapy did not clinically affect healing.

Case 2 (Fig. 3) is a 52-year-old male who had previously undergone resection of a stage 4 squamous carcinoma of the tongue, floor of mouth, and mandible from right midbody to left midbody. Bilateral pectoralis major flaps had been used for attempted reconstruction, with sequential failure of both. He presented with two draining pharyngocutaneous fistula wounds, both growing greater than 10^5 organisms of a polymicrobial flora on quantitative biopsy cultures.

His requirements included internal lining for undersurface of tongue, floor of mouth, and coverage of a neomandibular segment if possible. The scapular osteocutaneous territory was chosen due to its healthy vascularity and the ability to obtain both a thin intraoral flap and sturdy bone.

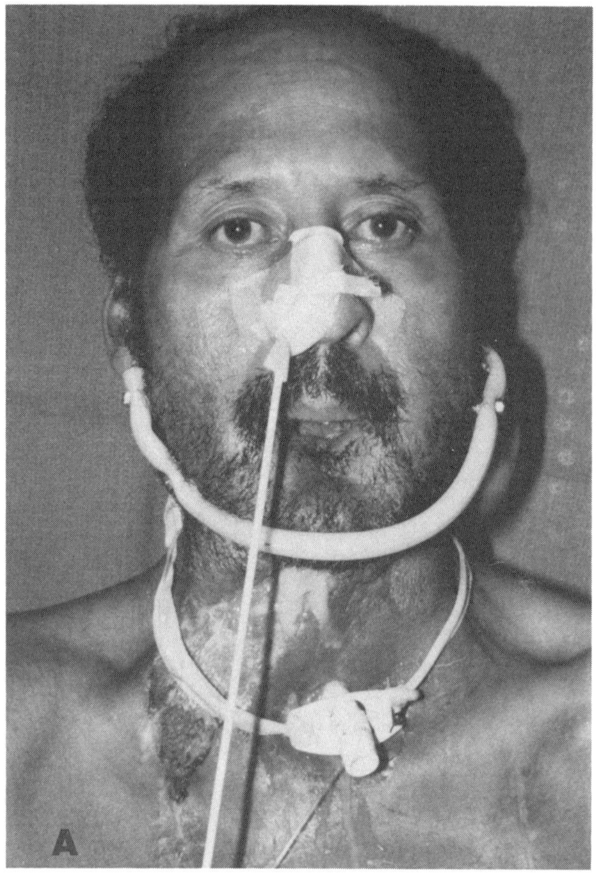

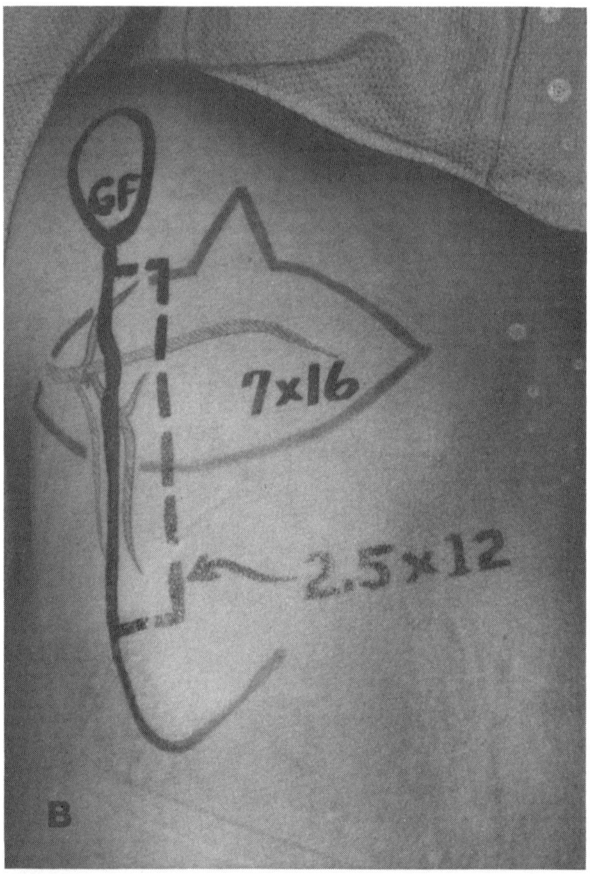

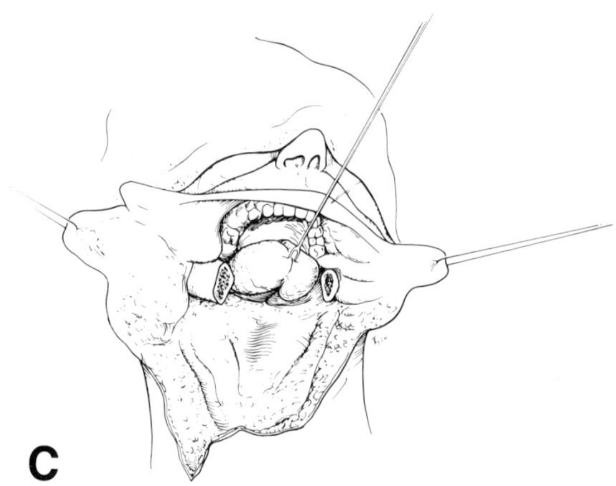

Figure 3 Case 2, *A*, A 52-year-old male presents with biphasic mandibular stablization device following tongue, floor of mouth, and anterior mandibular resection, and failed pectoralis major myocutaneous flaps bilaterally with infected pharyngocutaneous fistulae. *B*, The schematic representation of the intended harvest of the lateral border of the scapula is shown as well as the fasciocutaneous flap from the left shoulder region. *C*, The intraoperative extent of resection, including complete surgical excision of all infected areas of the wound, is demonstrated schematically.

Figure continues on opposite page

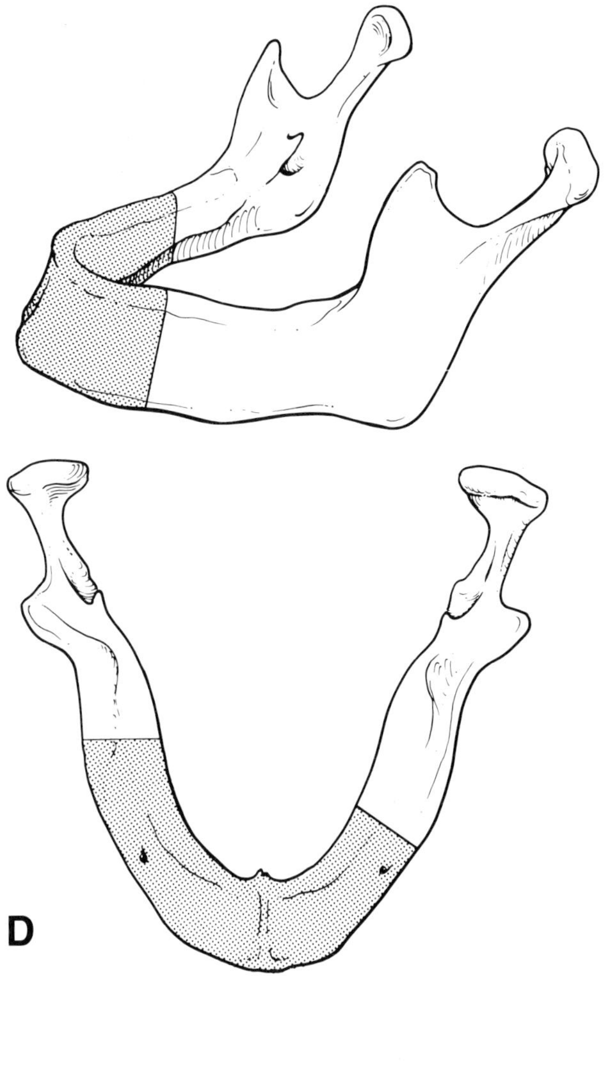

D

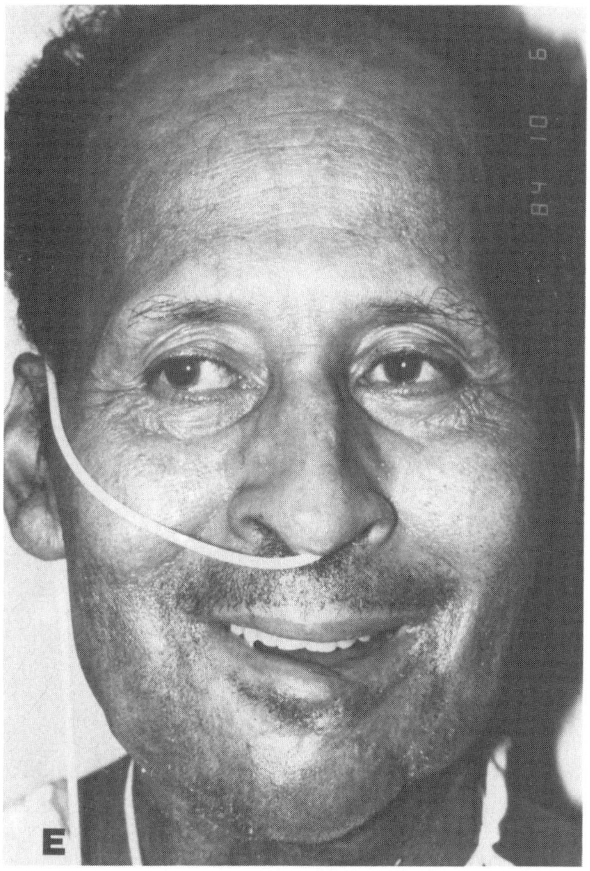

Figure 3 (continued) *D,* A schematic of the amount of bony resection and reconstruction. *E,* The patient's postoperative appearance.

This patient experienced good wound healing except for a minor wound infection in the anterior neck flaps (not part of the flap reconstruction itself) where they had been closed under some tension. This required local revision and repair. A bleeding episode deep in the neck required exploration and suture ligation of an eroded small arterial vessel, presumably due to the infection. Bony healing and union was unaffected by the infection. The mandible remained viable and stable at all times postoperatively. The patient had primary healing of his reconstruction and was able to have full course postoperative radiation therapy begun within 6 weeks of reconstruction.

In case 3 (Fig. 4), a 60-year-old male with a history of identification of an intra-socket squamous cell carcinoma of the mandible underwent a hemimandibulectomy, including condyle, and immediate reconstruction with a scapula osteocutaneous free flap. His postoperative course had uneventful wound healing. He subsequently underwent split-thickness skin graft vestibuloplasty, followed by dental prosthetic restoration with the use of osseointegrated vitanium implants. He has experienced an excellent return to dental function, notices essentially no difference in functional use of his mandible and teeth compared to preoperatively, and can eat sticky, hard, and crunchy foods equally well.

In all of these patients, early bone scans documented viability of the vascularized bone. In no case did postoperative radiation therapy affect the apparent clinical healing. Solid primary bony union was demonstrated clinically and radiologically.

DISCUSSION

The scapular osteocutaneous flap has found a significant place in the armamentarium for mandibular reconstruction. The anatomic characteristics that lend themselves well to this application include the large vessels and long vascular pedicle. The fasciocutaneous nature of the cutaneous flaps makes for an extremely well-vascularized, robust flap. The rich blood supply of the lateral border of the scapula similarly makes this very healthy vascularized bone territory. The mechanical properties of the lateral border of the scapula provide for a sturdy segment of bone, with similar appearance and properties to the normal mandible. The cortical cancellous nature of the bone has allowed placement of osseo-

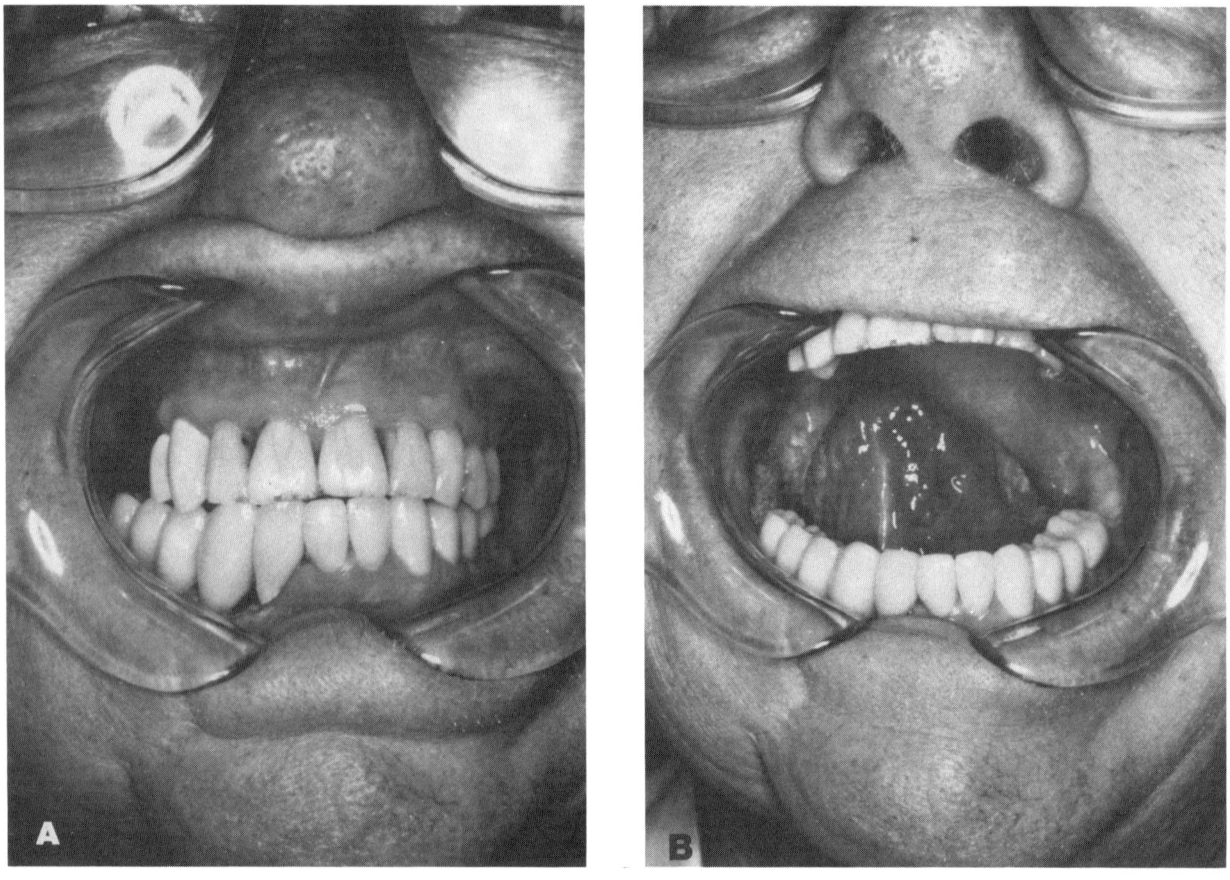

Figure 4 *A*, A 60-year-old male, following right hemimandibulectomy and scapular osteocutaneous free flap reconstruction that included an intraoral lining flap, demonstrates near-centric occlusion. *B*, Excellent oral apperture and mandibular motion following osseo-integrated vitanium dental implants for prosthetic dental restoration.

integrated dental implants directly into the bone, with resultant stable denture fitting and function.

The absolute indication, in our units, for a scapular osteocutaneous reconstruction of the mandible is when an internal lining flap, as well as an external cover flap, is needed in addition to the bony reconstruction of the mandible. No other territory currently available so readily provides multiple skin flaps that can be placed independently about the central bone flap.

The disadvantages of this territory include logistical considerations of patient positioning and the extra time needed for completion in a sequential rather than two-team simultaneous fashion intraoperatively. Females may find the donor site scarring objectionable, and the benefits of the procedure for young women must be weighed against this concern. The functional outcome with regard to shoulder mobility and use, however, has been outstanding.

It has been possible to obtain nearly absolute centric occlusion in patients with remaining dentition. In cases that involve condylar head resection, the neomandibular condyle has been constructed without use of interpositional Silastic temporomandibular joint arthroplasty or prosthesis, with no measurable restriction of mandibular motion or oral aperture.

SUGGESTED READING

Banis JC, Abul-Hassan HS. Cutaneous free flaps. In: Georgiade N, Garwick W. Riefkohl R, eds. Essentials of plastic maxillofacial, and reconstructive surgery. Baltimore: Williams & Wilkins, 1987; 835.

Banis JC, Acland RD. Clinical applications of the scapular skin and osteocutaneous flap. Transactions, Eighth International Congress of Plastic Surgery, Montreal: 1983; 137–139.

Silverberg B, Banis JC, Acland RD. Mandibular reconstruction with microvascular bone transfer. Am J Surg 1985; 150(4):440–446.

Swartz WM, Banis JC, Newton ED, et al. The osteocutaneous scapular flap for mandibular and maxillary reconstruction. Plast Reconstr Surg 1986; 77(4):530–544.

Taylor GI, Miller GD, Ham FJ. The free vascularized bone graft. A clinical extension of microvascular techniques. Plast Reconstr Surg 1975; 55:533–544.

Teot L. Bossé JP, Moufarrege R, Papillon J, Beauregard G. The scapular crest pedicled bone graft. Int J Microsurg 1981; 3:257–262.

RADIAL FOREARM FLAP IN HEAD AND NECK RECONSTRUCTION

DAVID S. SOUTAR, Ch.M., F.R.C.S.(Edin), F.R.C.S.(Glasg)

Defects in the head and neck, as a result of tumor excision, remain a problem for the plastic and reconstructive surgeon. Difficulties arise from the lack of available tissue in this region of the body and from the specialized nature of the structures involved.

There is now a wide variety of reconstructive techniques available to import tissue into the head and neck. Two-stage methods of reconstruction, such as the deltopectoral flap or forehead flap, remain popular in many countries, but have largely been superseded by single-stage techniques that use myocutaneous flaps such as the pectoralis major, trapezius, latissimus dorsi, and sternocleidomastoid. These pedicled flaps require a donor site in close proximity to the head and neck, which may not always be desirable.

The advent of microvascular surgery has opened up a wide variety of donor tissues that can be transferred to the head and neck in a single stage. The forearm is such a donor site and the free radial forearm flap has proved to be a useful and reliable method of reconstruction. The technique first gained widespread acceptance in reconstruction of postburn contractures of the neck and, subsequently, its role in head and neck surgery was extended—particularly to reconstruction of the oral cavity.

Advances in reconstructive surgery have allowed the excisional surgeon greater freedom with regard to tumor extirpation, and have moved the emphasis away from delayed or staged reconstruction toward primary reconstruction at the time of tumor excision.

THERAPEUTIC ALTERNATIVES

I am in the privileged position of carrying out both the excisional surgery and the reconstruction, two aspects of head and neck surgery that go hand in hand. The pathology and natural history of the disease, together with the prognosis and likelihood of cure, must be considered along with the projected cosmetic and functional results of surgery. Despite advances in reconstructive techniques, our enthusiasm to prolong life must be tempered by consideration of the quality of life and of alternative treatments.

Benign conditions that are non–life-threatening allow a greater time scale for reconstruction and, therefore, singe-stage techniques and immediate reconstruction assume less importance. Therefore, I confine the use of the radial forearm flap in head and neck reconstruction almost exclusively to the treatment of malignancy. In such cases, alternative treatments, such as chemotherapy and radiotherapy, should be considered as should combined modalities of treatment that incorporate chemotherapy, radiotherapy, and surgery.

PREFERRED APPROACH

I favor excision and primary reconstruction in the treatment of malignancy, using a single-stage technique followed by early, radical radiotherapy when appropriate. The aim of surgery is to achieve primary wound healing with a rapid return of function and an acceptable cosmetic appearance. This is particularly important in cases when the prognosis is limited and where it is difficult to justify a prolonged stay in hospital. This approach also permits combined modality treatment (particularly radiotherapy and/or chemotherapy) to be given in the early postoperative period. If such combined modality treatment is to be effective, then the method of surgical reconstruction must offer rapid and effective wound healing with the import of well-vascularized tissue and subsequent minimal scarring.

PATIENT SELECTION AND REJECTION

Age per se is not a contraindication to the use of microvascular surgery, and this particularly applies to the radial forearm flap. The radial artery appears to be remarkably free from arterial disease, even in the very elderly patient. It is essential to perform an Allen's test preoperatively to ensure that the hand will maintain its viability once devoid of radial arterial input. In the rare cases of a positive Allen's test, an alternative method of reconstruction should be used.

PRINCIPLES OF TREATMENT

The radial forearm flap is a fasciocutaneous flap that offers thin, pliable skin suitable for reconstructing defects of large or small surface area. It is not an effective method of dealing with volume defects where bulk is required. The technique has, therefore, proved most useful in reconstruction of the skin surface of the neck and face, and also the mucosal surface—particularly the oral cavity and pharynx. Furthermore, because of its pliable nature it is possible to fashion a tube for reconstruction of circumferential defects in the pharynx and upper esophagus.

The forearm donor site also allows composite tissue transfer by the inclusion of a segment of vascularized tendon (Fig. 1), vascularized nerve, or, more commonly, a segment of radius as a vascularized bone graft. The latter has proved useful in reconstruction of the horizontal ramus of the mandible at the time of tumor excision.

The radial forearm flap can be raised at the same time as the excisional surgery is performed in the head and neck, without the need to alter the position of the patient on the operating table. The use of two surgical teams working simultaneously can often shorten the operating time.

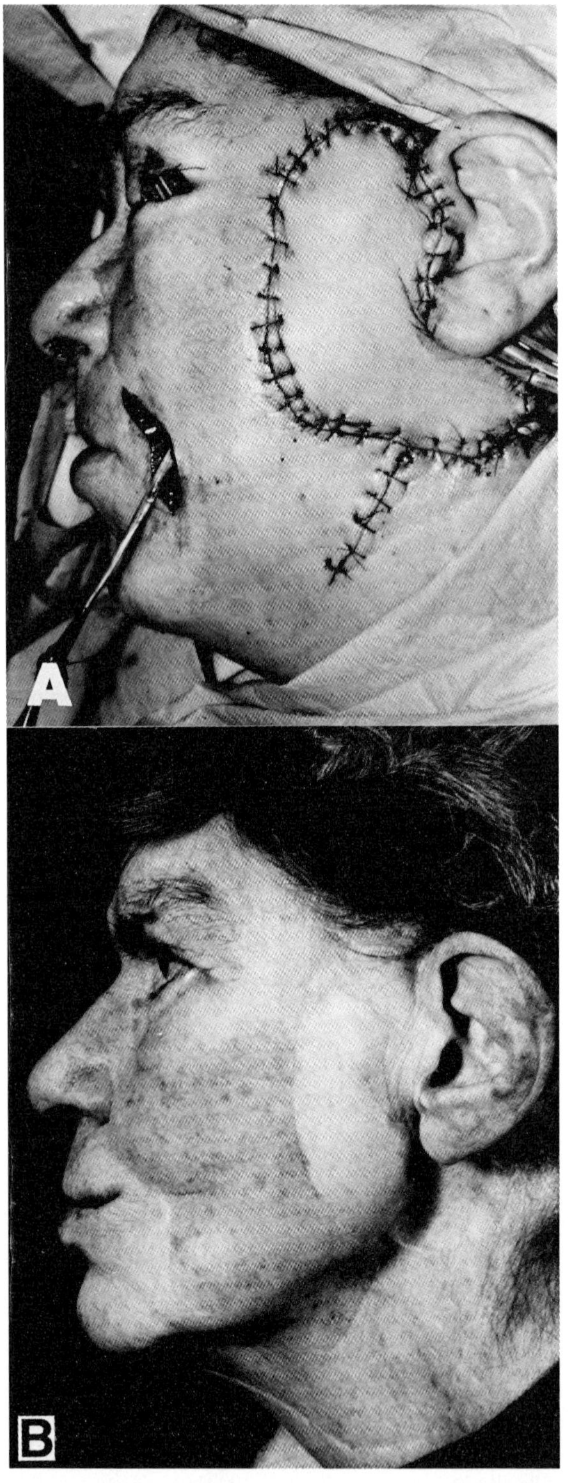

Figure 1 *A*, This radical parotidectomy for anaplastic carcinoma included the overlying skin, facial nerve, and muscle so that nerve grafting was not possible. A radial forearm flap was used to reconstruct the skin and included a segment of vascularized palmaris longus tendon, which was anastomosed to the temporalis muscle proximally and to the commissure of the mouth distally. A lateral tarsorrhaphy was also performed as part of the primary reconstruction for facial paralysis. *B*, The patient underwent radical postoperative radiotherapy. Three years following treatment the skin contour is satisfactory and the angle of the mouth is maintained in a good position.

Excision

It is important that excisional surgery is not compromised by the proposed method of reconstruction. Since the radial forearm flap is mainly used for surface defects that are affecting either skin or mucosa, it is relatively simple to design the appropriate shape and size of skin paddle to reconstruct the excisional defect.

DESIGN OF THE RADIAL FOREARM FLAP

The radial artery is palpated and its course in the forearm is marked. Variation in design of the flap is possible depending on the amount of tissue required for reconstruction. The more distally-sited flaps have the thinnest skin and are, therefore, the most pliable. Proximal flaps contain more subcutaneous fat and offer slightly more bulk.

The flap is raised in a subfascial plane to reveal tendons distally and muscle bellies proximally. It can be designed to incorporate a segment of vascularized palmaris longus, or vascularized radial nerve if a vascularized nerve graft is required. A segment of radius can be included; sited distal to the insertion of pronator teres. A preoperative x-ray film of the arm is mandatory to exclude any pathologic conditions of the radius and to assess the thickness of the cortex and the suitability of the radius as a donor site for bone. A boat-shaped segment of radius should be removed, with right-angled cuts avoided since these have proved to be sites of weakness and possible fracture. Only a relatively thin strip of cortex is required for reconstruction of the mandible or facial bones and, certainly, no more than 40 percent of the circumference of the radius should be removed. The bone is straight and is most suitable for reconstruction of the horizontal ramus. It is, however, possible to perform an osteotomy to change the direction of the segment of radius and this can be used successfully in symphyseal reconstruction.

Donor Defect

Muscle is readily graftable and for this reason some authors advocate design of the flap in the proximal region of the forearm. There is no doubt that grafting over tendon is difficult because of shearing strains and because damage to the paratenon can often result in tendon exposure with delayed wound healing. To minimize problems of exposed tendons, the donor defect is most often closed directly by mobilization of the forearm skin in a subfascial plane and transposition of a flap based on perforators from the ulnar artery (Fig. 2). In this way, the cosmetic deformity of the donor defect is minimized and rapid, primary wound healing achieved. Problems of tethering and adherence of tendons to skin graft are also avoided.

The donor defect can be closed simultaneously with the insetting of the flap into the head and neck region. Postoperatively, the donor arm is immobilized in plaster and can virtually be ignored in the early postoperative period while attention is focused on problems in the head and neck. Where bone is removed, it is essential to immobilize the arm in an above-elbow plaster cast. Subsequent mobilization is dependent on the postoperative

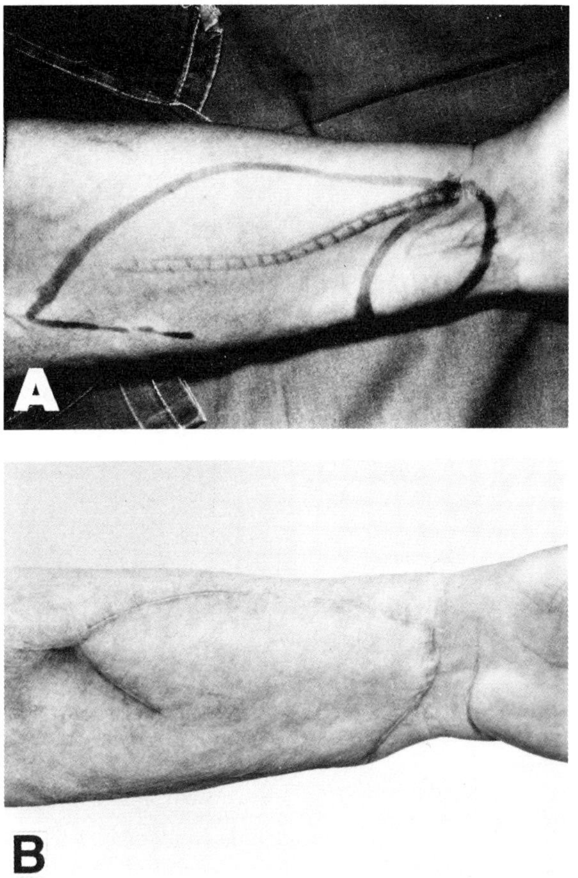

Figure 2 *A*, A distally-sited radial forearm flap is designed and the incision and back cut of the ulnar transposition flap is outlined. *B*, Effective primary wound closure is achieved and the wound is soundly healed by 3 weeks.

appearance in radiographic examination. Should a fracture of the radius occur, it is essential to prevent angulation so that function is maintained. I have found external fixation to be a useful procedure in such cases.

ADVANTAGES OF THERAPEUTIC APPROACH

Despite the problem of healing in the donor defect and cosmetic considerations, I favor the distal region of the arm since it provides the thinnest, most pliable skin and permits a long vascular pedicle.

It is the reliability of the vascular pedicle and its ability to sustain both large and small flaps that single out the forearm as one of the most useful free flap donor sites. In addition to the size of the vessels, the length of vascular pedicle also simplifies the microvascular aspects of the surgery, so that excision can be performed without the need to preserve adjacent vessels for anastomosis. It is often advisable to site the anastomosis at a distance from the zone of trauma, e.g., if there has been preoperative radiotherapy or in cases where the tumor is associated with gross infection.

The microvascular anastomosis can be sited in the opposite side of the head and neck so that excision, which may include a radical neck dissection, is never compromised.

The forearm donor site allows simultaneous operation at two different sites in the body with relative ease. In addition, immobilization of the arm in the early postoperative period results in a relatively pain-free donor site, even when bone is removed. This greatly facilitates the early postoperative recovery of patients who have undergone major head and neck surgery.

RESULTS

I have used the radial forearm flap extensively in head and neck reconstruction. The technique probably undergoes its most severe test when used for immediate reconstruction following excision of intraoral tumors. Local problems of oral contamination, salivary leak, and previous treatment in the form of surgery or radiotherapy conspire against reconstructive surgery. In addition patients tend to be elderly, with medical problems often associated with alcohol and tobacco abuse.

A recent analysis of 100 consecutive cases of intraoral reconstruction in which the free radial forearm flap was used, comprised patients from 34 to 85 years old, with a mean of 58.9 years. Despite this, the operative mortality was only 2 percent with a total hospital mortality for the group of 4 percent. There were nine cases in which the free flap was unsuccessful, but only five of these required a further method of reconstruction. There was no correlation between the patient's age and the incidence of microvascular problems.

In the 91 successful flaps, only one case has ever developed a fistula (1.1 percent). Additional evidence of rapid primary wound healing was provided by the return to oral diet, which varied from 6 to 30 days with a mean of 12.3 days. Furthermore, the postoperative hospital stay, when this technique was used, varied from 8 to 51 days with a mean of 19.5 days. Both the establishment of oral feeding and the length of postoperative stay appeared to parallel the extent to which intraoral excision was prolonged in composite tissue reconstruction that involved the mandible.

Sixty intraoral radial forearm flaps in this series underwent elective postoperative radical radiotherapy. Patients received either 6,000 rad in 30 fractions over 6 to 8 weeks, or 5,400 rad in 18 fractions over the same period of time. Radiotherapy commenced within 6 weeks of surgery, and all flaps tolerated this radical dose with no evidence of intraoral wound breakdown or fistula. Similarly, composite osteocutaneous flaps where a segment of radius was used to reconstruct the mandible, tolerated this radical radiotherapy with no extrusion or sequestration of the radius (Fig. 3).

The radial forearm flap can be assessed preoperatively and has proved to be one of the simplest and most reliable free flaps currently available. Its use has to be balanced with the cosmetic deformity that results in the arm, but this can be minimized by careful design, by aiming at primary wound closure, and by avoidance of the use of skin grafts. There is no additional scarring in the head and neck region except that required for excisional

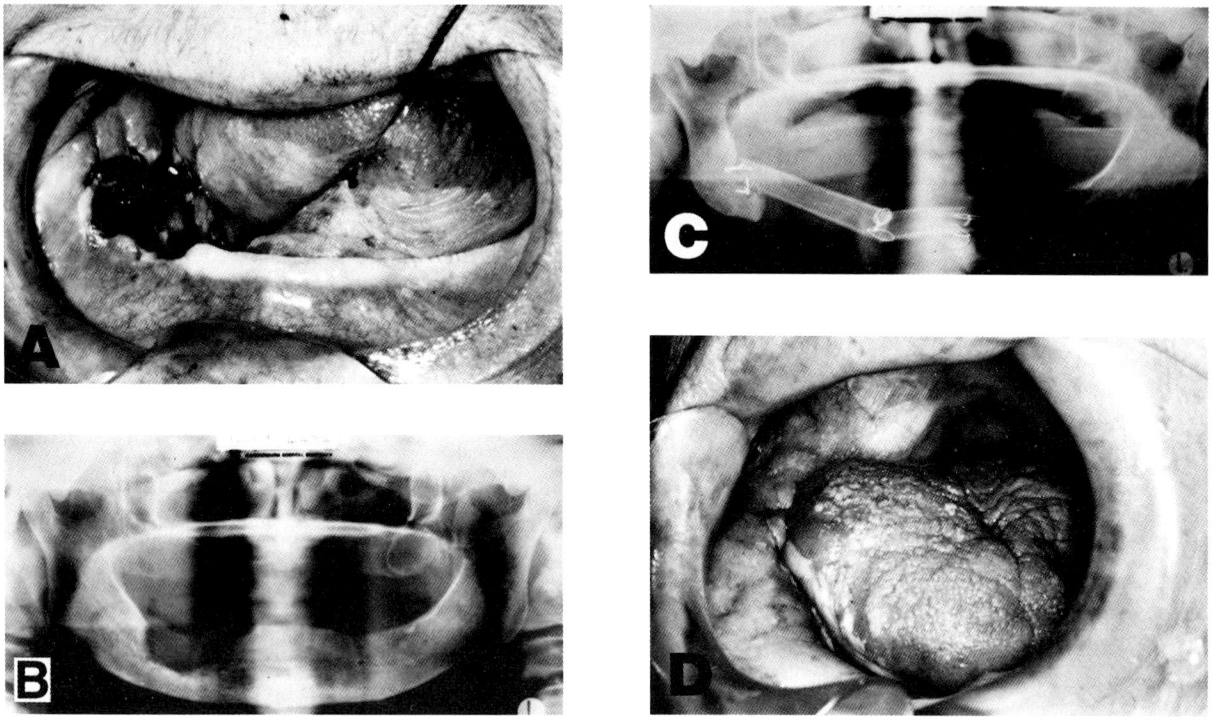

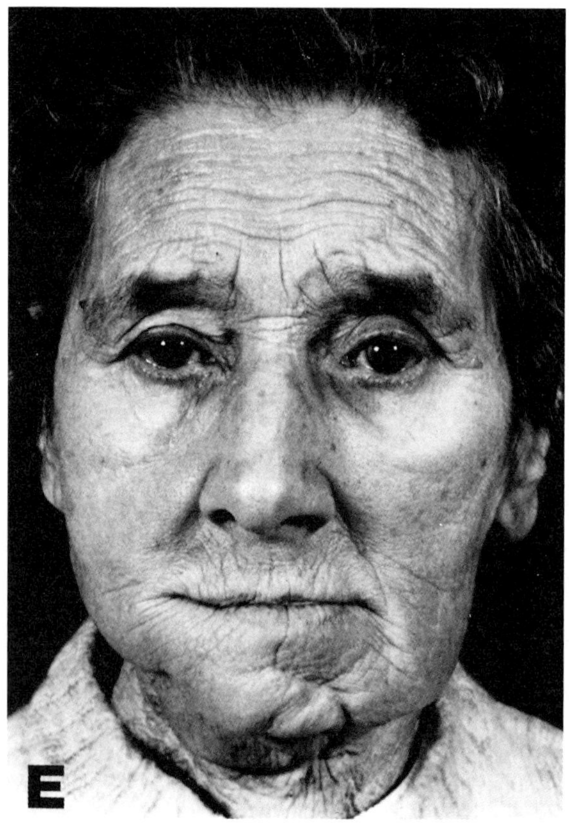

Figure 3 *A*, This 75-year-old female patient presented with a T4N0 squamous carcinoma of the right, lower alveolus. *B*, The extent of bone invasion is seen in the preoperative orthopantograph. *C*, The defect was reconstructed with composite radial forearm flap that incorporated a segment of radius to reconstruct the mandible. *D*, The patient underwent radical postoperative radiotherapy 6 weeks after surgery. The flap conforms well to the contours of the oral cavity and maintains the tongue in a good position. *E*, The patient remains well 2 years following treatment.

surgery. The length of operating time, which averages 8 hours, should not serve as a contraindication and the technique is not associated with any increased risk to the patient.

The radial forearm flap does appear to offer a method of immediate reconstruction in head and neck cancer. It provides well-vascularized tissue that enables primary wound healing with minimal scarring, and can be used in combined modality treatment with early, postoperative, radical radiotherapy. It is probably most useful in intraoral reconstruction where the thin, pliable nature of the skin conforms well to the contours of the oral cavity and acts as a suitable replacement for the mucosa.

SUGGESTED READING

Boorman JG, Brown JA, Sykes PJ. Morbidity in the forearm flap donor arm. Br J Plast Surg 1987; 40:207–212.

Harii K, Ebihara S, Ono I, et al. Pharyngoesophageal reconstruction using fabricated free forearm flap. Plast Reconstr Surg 1985; 75:463–470.

Song R, Gao Y, Song Y, Yu Y, Song Y. The forearm flap. Clin Plast Surg 1982; 9:21–26.

Soutar DS. The radial forearm flap in intra-oral reconstruction. Ch.M. Thesis, University of Aberdeen, 1986.

Soutar DS, McGregor IA. The radial forearm flap in intraoral reconstruction. The experience of 60 consecutive cases. Plast Reconstr Surg 1986; 78:1–246.

Soutar DS, Scheker LR, Tanner NSB, McGregor IA. The radial forearm flap. A versatile method for intraoral reconstruction. Br J Plast Surg 1983; 36:1–8.

Soutar DS, Widdowson WP. Immediate reconstruction of the mandible using vascularized segment of radius. Head Neck Surg 1986; 8:232–246.

Yang G, Chen B, Gao Y, et al. Forearm free skin flap transplantation. Natl Med J China 1981; 61:139–141.

CRANIAL BASE TUMORS

IAN T. JACKSON, M.D., F.R.C.S., F.A.C.S.

The newer developments inherited from craniofacial surgery for congenital deformity have enabled cranial base surgery for tumors to be more effective, safer, and systematic. In the past, some excellent surgery was carried out for cranial base tumors, but unfortunately, it was hazardous and often insufficiently radical. As a result, survival figures were depressing. The advances that have taken place in this area have been a classification of the skull base in relation to surgical approaches, improvement of exposure, the introduction of exposure osteotomies, the galeal frontalis flap, microvascular free tissue transfer, and the team approach. The latter has been an extremely important and significant development. The team consists of the cranial base surgeon, the neurosurgeon, the oncologist, the radiotherapist, and the maxillofacial prosthetist. In addition, inherited from the congenital deformity craniofacial team, there is a social worker used to handling patients who have had major head and neck procedures; a psychiatrist who can be helpful in preoperative preparation and postoperative support; and nurses, both on the floor and in the operating room, who have experience in dealing with these patients. An additional important facility is the intensive care department, since many of these patients may have significant airway problems and immediately postoperatively may have tracheostomies or indwelling nasal or orotracheal airways.

CRANIAL BASE CLASSIFICATION

In devising surgical approaches, it is helpful to divide the cranial base into distinct areas. These are the *anterior cranial base area*, which is the anterior cranial fossa; the *middle area*, which is the middle cranial fossa; and the *posterior area*, which is the posterior cranial fossa. The middle cranial fossa is complex in its anatomy, thus, it is useful to further subdivide this area into a segment that lies anterior to the petrous temporal bone and another segment consisting of the petrous temporal bone itself.

In the anterior area lie the frontal lobes, the orbits, the nasopharynx, the frontal sinuses, the ethmoid sinuses, and the sphenoid sinus. In the anterior segment of the middle cranial fossa lie the temporal lobes, the cavernous sinus, the pituitary, the foramen ovale for the trigeminal nerve, and the foramen rotundum and spinosum; the optic foramina are in the anteromedial area. The posterior segment of the middle cranial fossa contains the entry of the carotid canal, the canal itself within the petrous bone, and the exit at the apex of the petrous bone; the cochlear nerves; and the facial nerve within the petrous bone. The posterior cranial fossa has posterior lobes; the cerebellum and brain stem; the jugular foramen for transmission of the jugular vein; the transverse sinus; and the glossopharyngeal, vagus, accessory, and hypoglossal nerves. The anterior cranial fossa is the portion of the cranial base most commonly affected with tumor pathology, either malignant or nonmalignant; next is the middle cranial fossa. The incidence of tumor involvement of the posterior cranial fossa base is extremely low.

TUMOR TYPES

Almost every conceivable variety of malignant and nonmalignant tumors has been encountered, and these are listed in Table 1. Many of the malignant lesions are recurrent, after treatment by either conventional resection, Mohs surgery (with adjuvant radiotherapy alone or after surgical resection), or chemotherapy. Many of the tumors are extremely aggressive, and a large proportion of patients have

TABLE 1 Pathology of Operated Skull Base Tumors

Nonmalignant		*Malignant*	
Fibrous dysplasia	18	Squamous carcinoma	16
Osteoma	2	Basal cell carcinoma	12
Meningioma	12	Anaplastic carcinoma	2
Lipoblastoma	1	Malignant melanoma	1
Neurofibroma	13	Adenocarcinoma	5
Pleomorphic salivary adenoma *	3	Adenoid cystic carcinoma	12
Adamantinoma*	2	Mucoepidermoid carcinoma	2
Keratocyst*	1	Osteosarcoma	2
Inverting papilloma*	1	Chondrosarcoma	3
		Neurofibrosarcoma	2
		Liposarcoma	1
		Neurosarcoma	2
		Rhabdomyosarcoma	3
		Retinoblastoma	1
		Aesthesioneuroblastoma	2
		Malignant teratoma	1
		Schwannoma	2
TOTAL	53		69

* Locally aggressive

never been tumor free since the original diagnosis. The vast majority of tumors are extracranial, invasive, and penetrate the cranial base region.

INVESTIGATIONS

Standard roentgenograms are of little help. Polytomography is not used. The main investigations are CT scanning and MRI scanning; both of these have useful features. The CT scan illustrates both soft tissue and bony tissue abnormalities, whereas the MRI scan is helpful in showing soft tissue tumors. Three-dimensional CT scanning is being investigated and may have a considerable amount of potential in the future as new programs are developed to specifically deal with tumor related diagnostic and planning problems. Carotid angiography is essential in many of the malignant tumors in order to assess the tumor's proximity to the carotid vessels. Where there is any indication of necessity to sacrifice the carotid, crossflow studies with compression of the involved carotid artery are performed during angiography. A careful assessment of cranial nerve function is carried out, since involvement of a cranial nerve is an adverse prognostic indicator. Numbness and pain in the relevant distribution can be significant. Endoscopy is a routine part of head and neck assessment. The nasal cavity, palate, pharynx, and larynx are systematically examined. General assessment for metastasis, both lymph node and otherwise, is undertaken, and a tissue biopsy is obtained if possible.

SURGICAL APPROACHES

Anterior Cranial Fossa

Any tumor arising in and around the nose, nasopharynx, orbits, maxilla, and frontal sinuses is potentially an anterior cranial fossa tumor and, certainly in the case of malignant tumors, must be considered as such until proved otherwise. It is only by using this philosophy that one can ever hope to perform adequate oncologic surgery in these areas. Unless there is to be a lower soft tissue and bony resection, e.g., orbital exenteration or midface resection, the most common approach is by a coronal flap. This is performed in the standard way as for correction of a congenital craniofacial anomaly, thereby allowing adequate exposure of the nasal and orbital area. An exposure of the anterior cranial base can be obtained with the addition of a frontal craniotomy. If possible, the craniotomy is limited. On many occasions, it is possible to resect midline lesions through a central trephine craniotomy. The reason for reducing the amount of cranial bone removed is that only the minimal amount of bone will be lost rather than a whole frontal bone flap if there is a postoperative infection.

Nonmalignant Tumors

In midline, nonmalignant lesions such as fibrous dysplasia, the unaffected bone is removed for access and the involved bone is resected (Fig. 1). This will frequently leave a communication between the nasopharynx and the anterior cranial fossa. If this communication is not closed securely, there frequently will be ascending infection or an extradural abscess. If there has been a dural repair, either by suture or with fascia, meningitis can develop and even death can ensue. Therefore, the nasal cavity and floor of the anterior cranial fossa are closed by raising a galeal frontalis flap based on the supraorbital or supratrochlear vessels. This flap is sutured down along the floor of the anterior cranial fossa using drill holes through the free bone edges. If further bone graft reconstruction has to be performed on the orbits, then it is essential that these areas are also covered with vascularized tissue, and a further galeal frontalis flap from the contralateral side may be used. Orbital wall bone grafting is performed with split skull grafts and, if necessary, the floor of the anterior cranial fossa is reconstructed. The removed glabellar bone and the frontal trephine are replaced and wired in position.

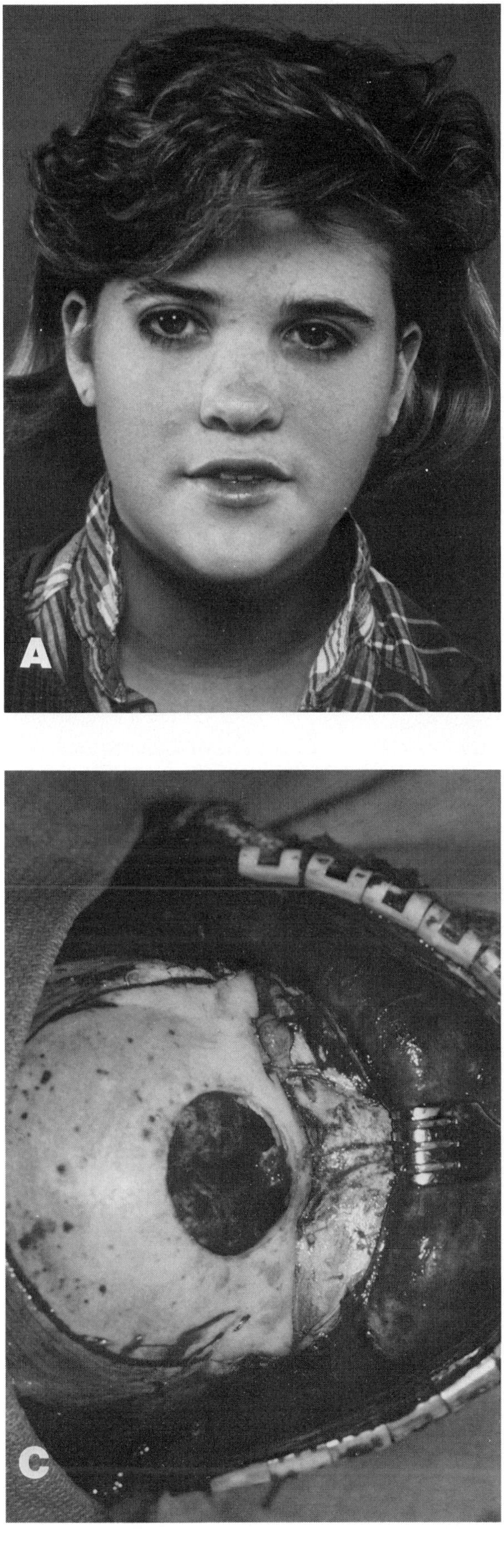

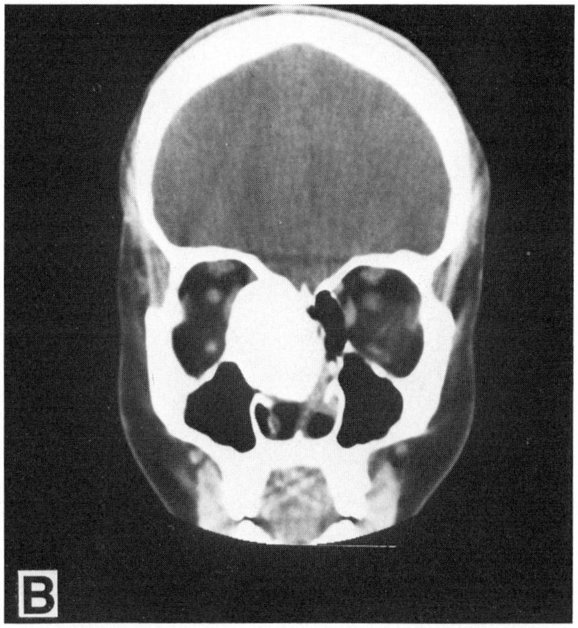

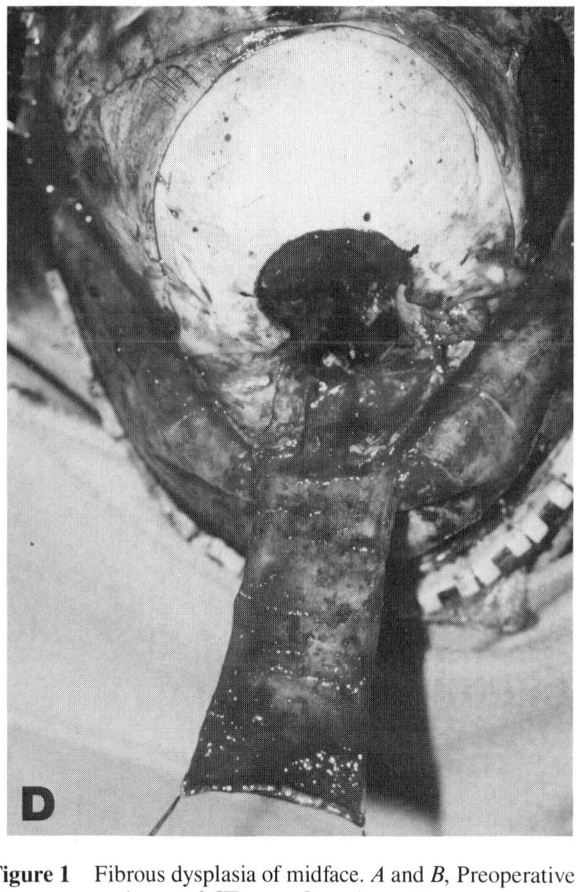

Figure 1 Fibrous dysplasia of midface. *A* and *B*, Preoperative appearance and coronal CT scan of a patient with a nasoethmoid orbital fibrous dysplasia causing headaches and diplopia. *C*, Coronal flap elevated. Trephine craniotomy to allow exposure of the anterior cranial fossa. *D*, The floor of the anterior cranial fossa, ethmoid sinuses, medial wall of right orbit are resected. Galeal frontalis flap elevated to separate the anterior cranial fossa from the nasopharynx.

Figure continues on following page

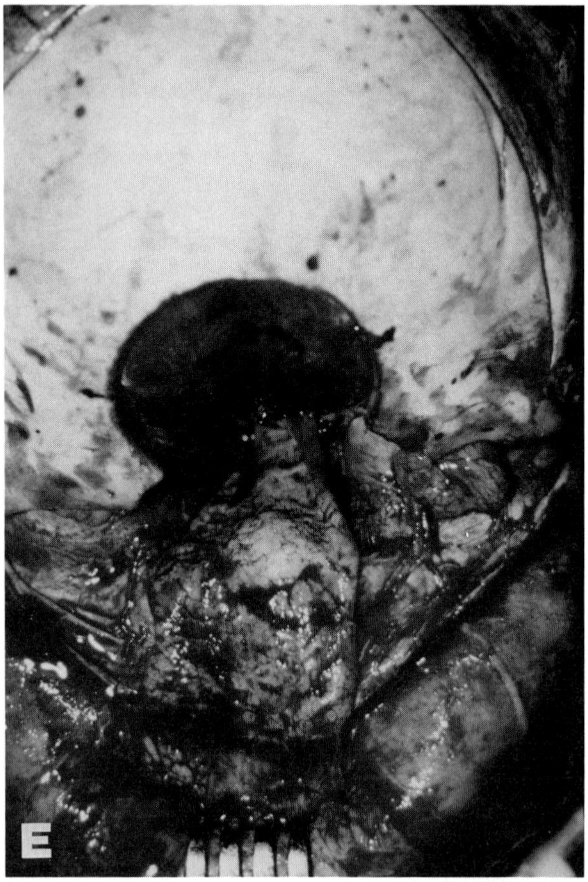

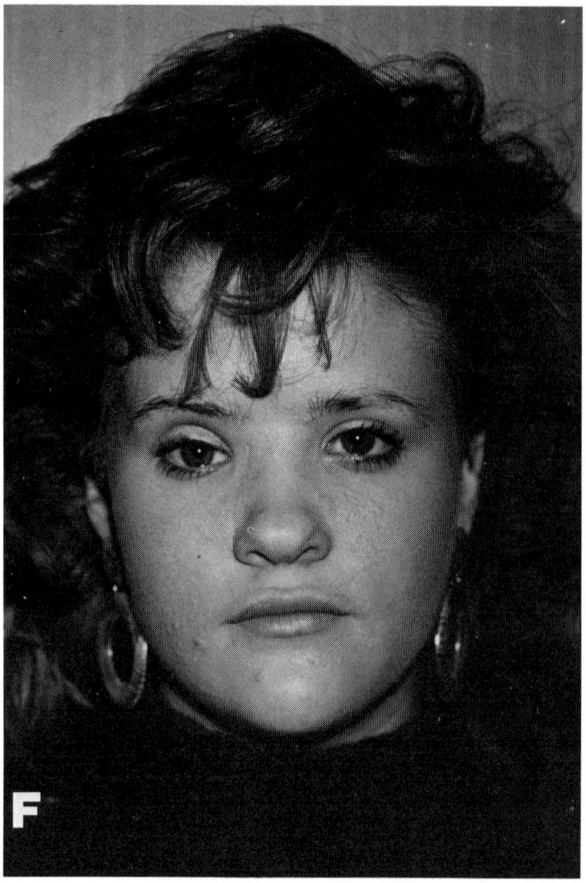

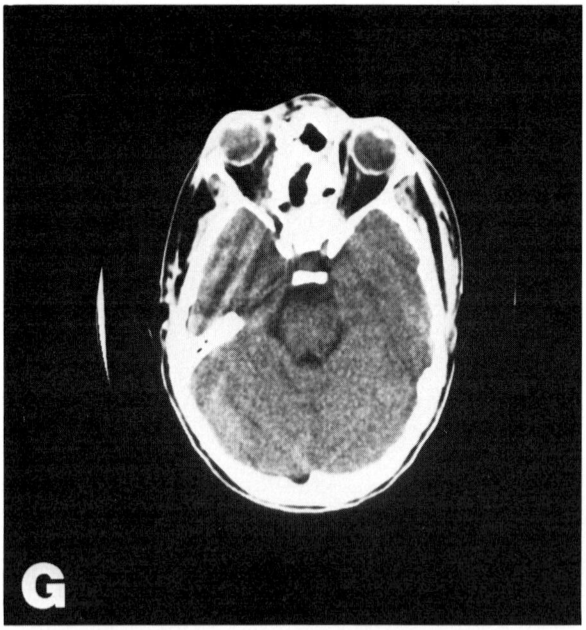

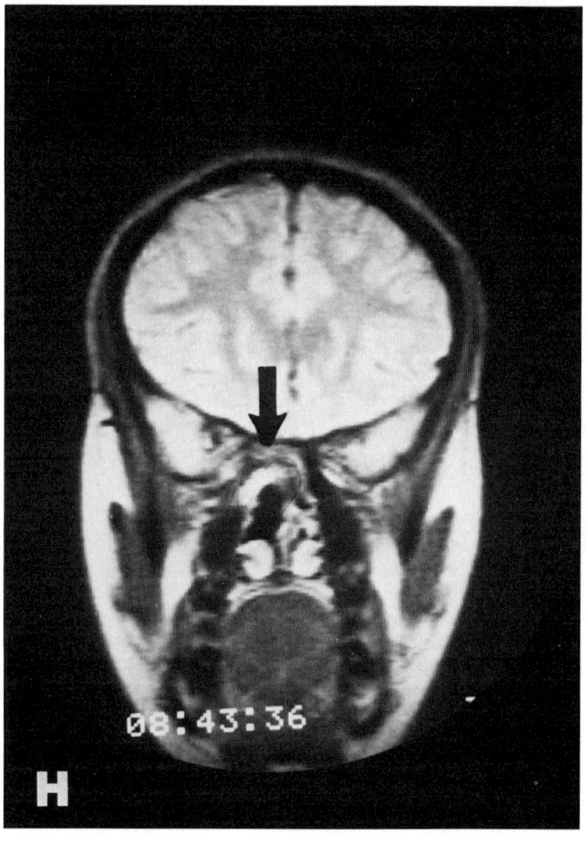

Figure 1 (continued) *E*, Galeal frontalis flap in position. Cranial bone grafts to floor of anterior cranial fossa and medial wall of the orbit. These bone grafts are protected by the galeal frontalis flap. *F* and *G*, Patient and axial CT head scan 1 year after surgery. There has been a total alleviation of symptoms. *H*, Coronal MRI scan showing the position of the galeal frontalis flap (arrow).

Malignant Tumors

In malignant cases, a similar approach may be employed, particularly if so much orbital and maxillary bone has been removed that there may be displacement of a retained eye with the development of troublesome double vision (Fig. 2). Again using galeal frontalis flaps and split skull grafts, a satisfactory reconstruction may be effected.

It is our custom to leave recurrent, aggressive carcinomas unreconstructed, particularly when these recur following radiotherapy and where bone is extensively involved. It is considered eminently safer to excise the lesion radically. This may involve removal of the whole of the midface with one or both maxillae, together with the medial walls of the orbit, floor of the anterior cranial fossa, ethmoid sinuses, and sphenoid sinuses. Closure in these cases was initially achieved using an extended glabellar flap, but now is obtained using the galeal frontalis flap or, on one occasion where this was not available, a temporalis muscle flap was used. In several other cases, the pectoralis muscle flap was employed. This somewhat conservative approach has been used in 18 cases of recurrent midface tumors. Of these, followed up for a maximum of 8 years, four patients have died of recurrent tumor, one died of unrelated causes, and the others are still alive and well. None of these patients have wished extensive reconstruction. The osseointegration techniques of Branemark have proved to be extremely satisfactory in the patients who have been willing to undergo this type of reconstruction.

Some midface tumors are located in a more posterior position; in order to get at these, it may be necessary to split the face and to remove bony segments of the face, i.e., "exposure osteotomies" to gain access to the lesion. Once the tumor has been resected, the nasopharynx is closed off using the galeal frontalis flap, either unilateral

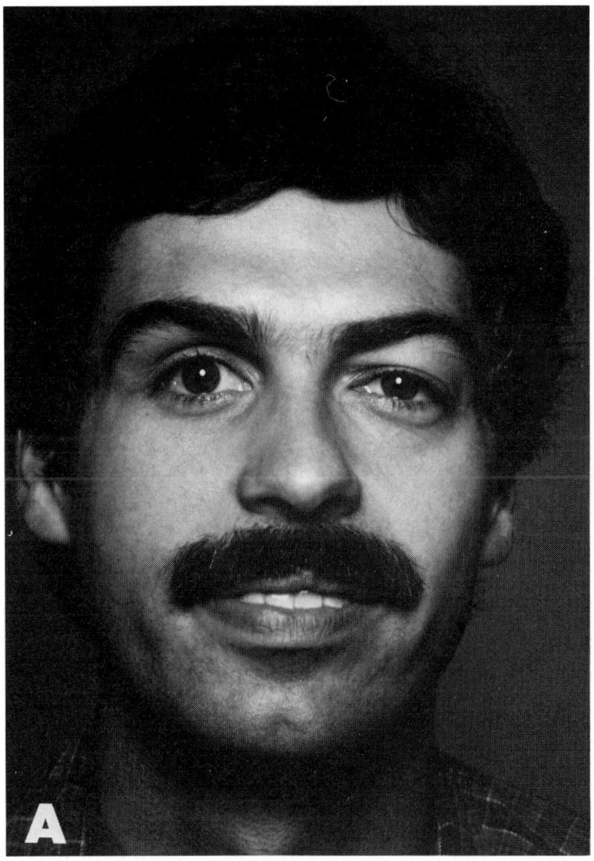

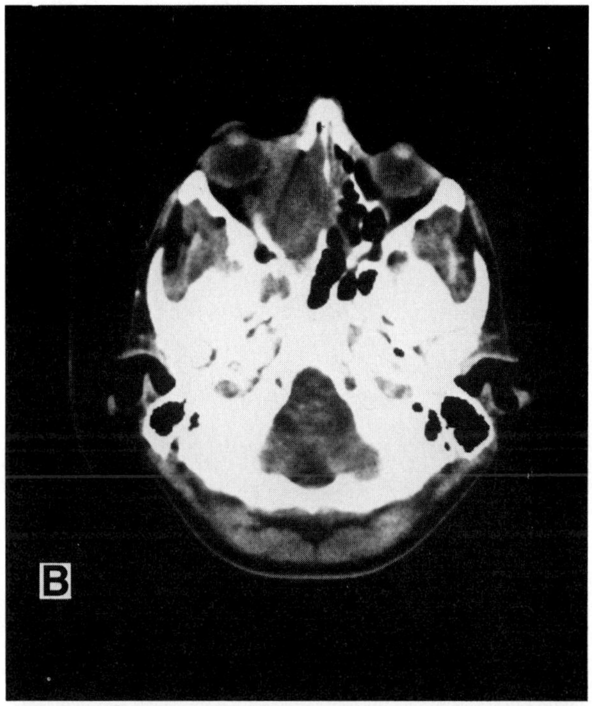

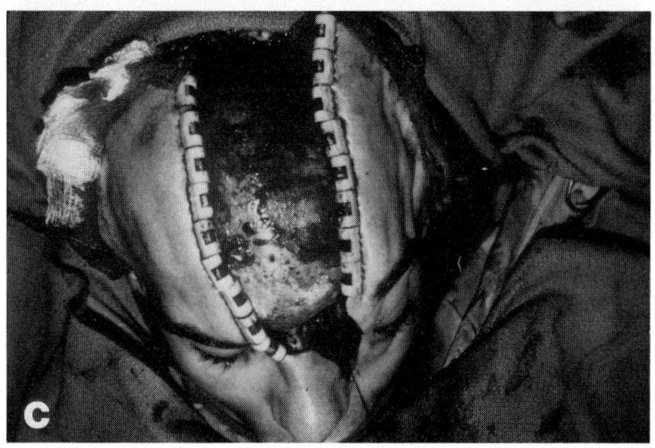

Figure 2 Rhabdomyosarcoma of midface. *A* and *B*, Preoperative appearance and axial CT scan of a patient with a left frontonasal orbitomaxillary rhabdomyosarcoma. Note proptosis of left eye. *C*, Surgical approach using a coronal flap and a partial face-splitting incision. The orbital contents were dissected away from the tumor, which was well encapsulated in the orbital area. There was total resection of orbital floor, medial wall of the orbit, nasal septum, and maxilla from orbital floor to just above tooth roots. The approach to the anterior cranial base was through a frontal trephine craniotomy.

Figure continues on following page

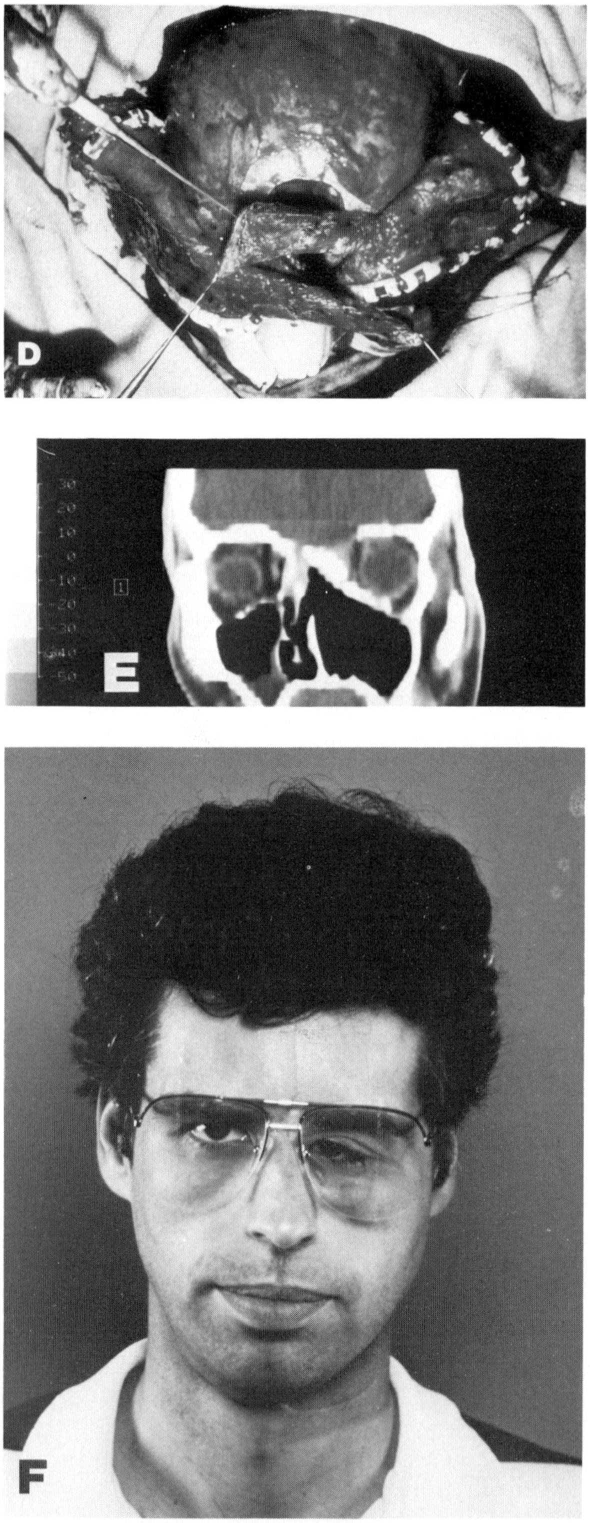

Figure 2 (continued) *D*, Bilateral galeal frontalis flaps were used to close the floor of the anterior cranial fossa from the nasopharynx and to close the orbit and maxilla from the nasal cavity. Bone grafting of floor of anterior cranial fossa, medial wall of orbit, and floor of orbit was done to maintain the eye in reasonable position. *E*, A coronal CT scan shows the bone graft from the floor of the anterior cranial fossa to the medial wall of the orbit and to the floor of the orbit. The black area below the grafts is the area of resection. *F*, Appearance 3 years post surgery, radiotherapy, and chemotherapy.

or bilateral, and the exposure osteotomy is then replaced and wired or plated into position. The face splitting incision heals satisfactorily.

As one moves laterally, it may be necessary to sacrifice the orbital roof or orbital walls. Again in the condition of fibrous dysplasia, these are immediately reconstructed. In cases of superior orbital tumors or meningiomas that are invading the orbit, an orbitozygomatic osteotomy exposure osteotomy may be performed (Fig. 3). The tumor is then resected and the bony defect is reconstructed with split-skull bone graft. The exposure osteotomy is wired or plated back in position. In this way, it is possible to remove even malignant tumors without causing undue deformity to the patient's face.

This technique is particularly effective in patients who have tumors involving the region where the anterior cranial fossa, orbit, and middle cranial fossa abut on one another. The removal of the orbital roof, lateral orbital wall, and a portion of the zygomatic arch allows access to these three cavities, so that it is possible to completely excise both malignant and nonmalignant tumors with as much immediate reconstruction as is judged wise. If the frontal sinus is opened, a galeal frontalis flap is used as a vascular filling material to prevent any intracranial infection.

ANTERIOR SEGMENT OF MIDDLE CRANIAL FOSSA

Nonmalignant Tumors

Although one can encounter benign lesions in this area, the vast majority are malignant. Occasionally, meningioma or neurofibroma may escape through one of the foramina in the floor of the middle cranial fossa. These are approached by doing a temporal craniotomy; through this the foramen from which the neurofibroma is escaping can be identified. It is frequently necessary for exposure purposes to osteotomize the zygomatic arch and to remove the anterior aspect of the ascending ramus of the mandible. In this way, the base of the skull can be dissected at a subperiosteal level and removed until the tumor is encountered. Removal can usually be accomplished by blunt dissection.

Malignant Tumors

With malignant tumors, the approach is much more complex (Fig. 4). These tumors are most commonly infratemporal fossa tumors such as recurrent adenoid cystic carcinomas, squamous carcinomas, or sarcomas. The tumor may involve the ascending ramus of the mandible, the posterior portion of the maxilla, the orbit, and the skull base. Access to these lesions is particularly difficult. A hemicoronal or full coronal flap is elevated and the incision is continued down through the preauricular area and into the neck. Enough of a neck dissection is performed to locate the carotid artery and the internal jugular vein. A total parotidectomy is performed with preservation of facial nerve. The ascending ramus of the mandible is removed, as is the zygomatic arch. The whole infratemporal fossa is now exposed, and it is possible to dissect cranial-

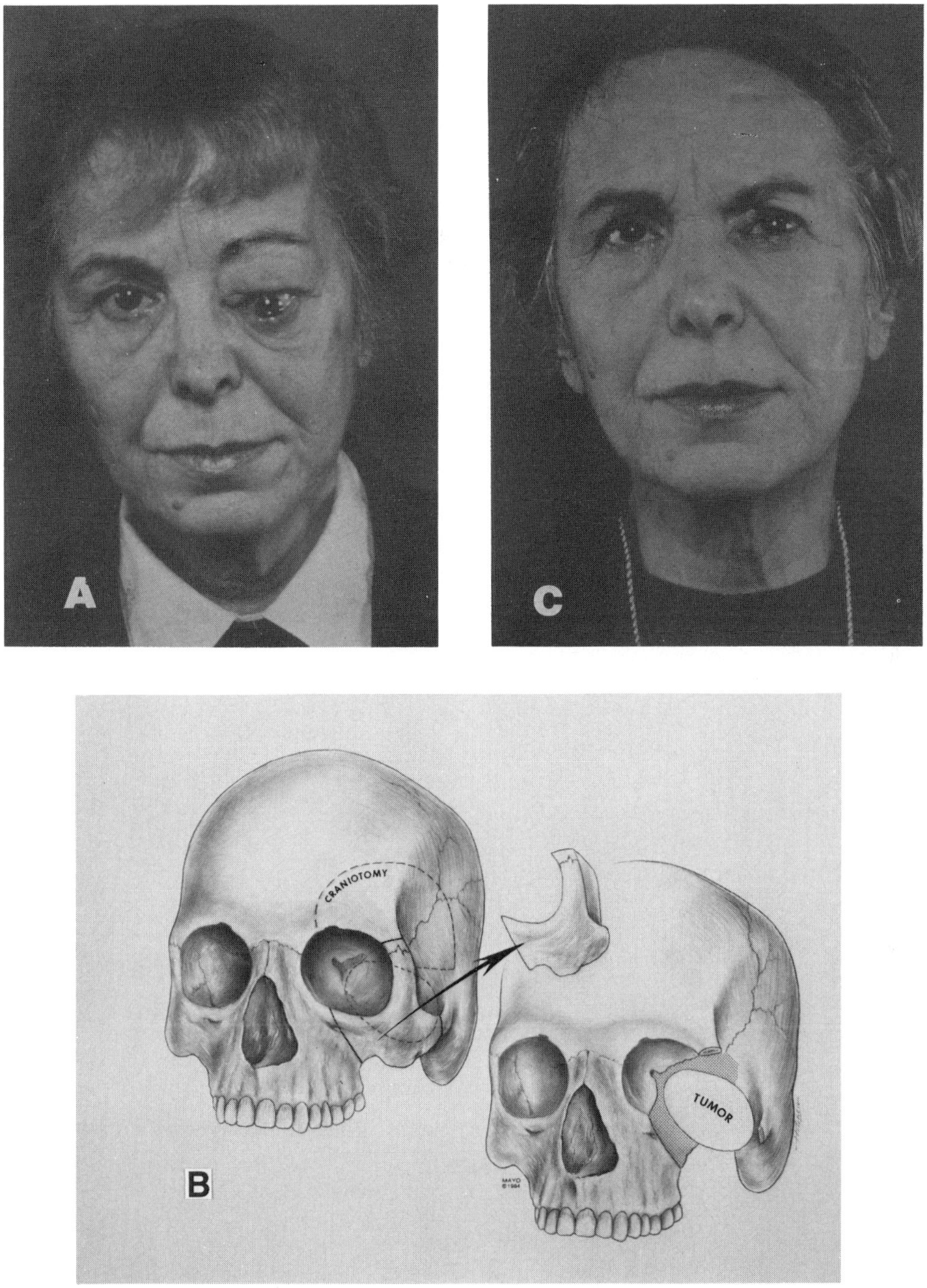

Figure 3 Recurrent meningioma, anterior and middle cranial fossa and orbit. *A*, Patient with meningioma involving anterior cranial fossa, middle cranial fossa, and orbit with proptosis and downward displacement of left eye causing severe diplopia. *B*, Exposure osteotomy: removal of orbitozygomatico-maxillary complex with temporal craniotomy. *C*, Postoperative appearance 18 months after surgery. Diplopia is much improved.

ly along the carotid artery and jugular vein and so remove the tumor. The mass usually lies external to the styloid process, and therefore there is little danger of injury to the internal carotid artery. On occasion, the artery may be involved; in such cases, the results of cross-flow studies are necessary in order to decide whether the carotid artery may be resected or not. The cranial base is resected as extensively as is necessary to remove the tumor. It is then possible to remove the resected specimen from behind and below the facial nerve.

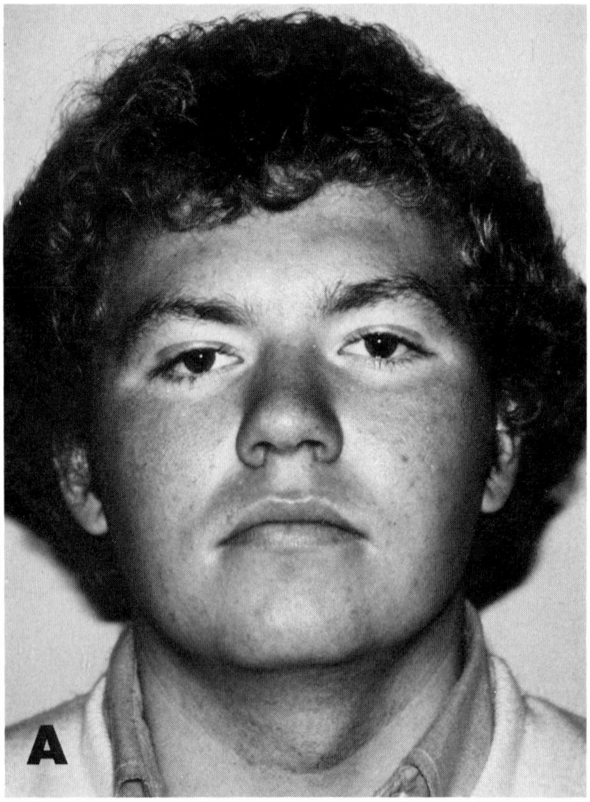

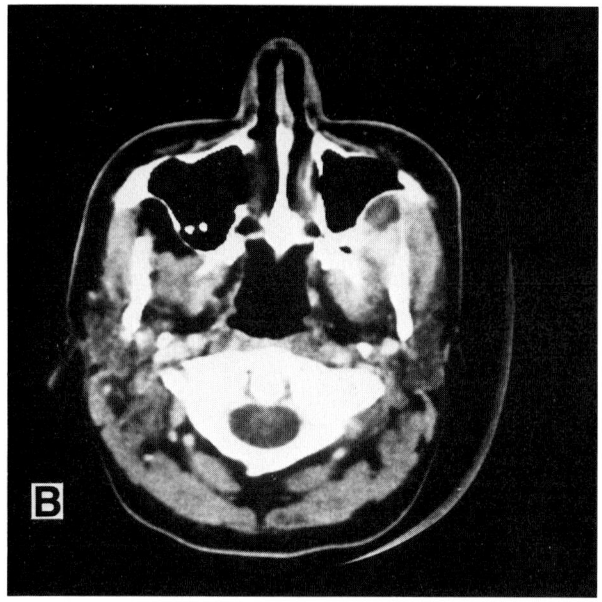

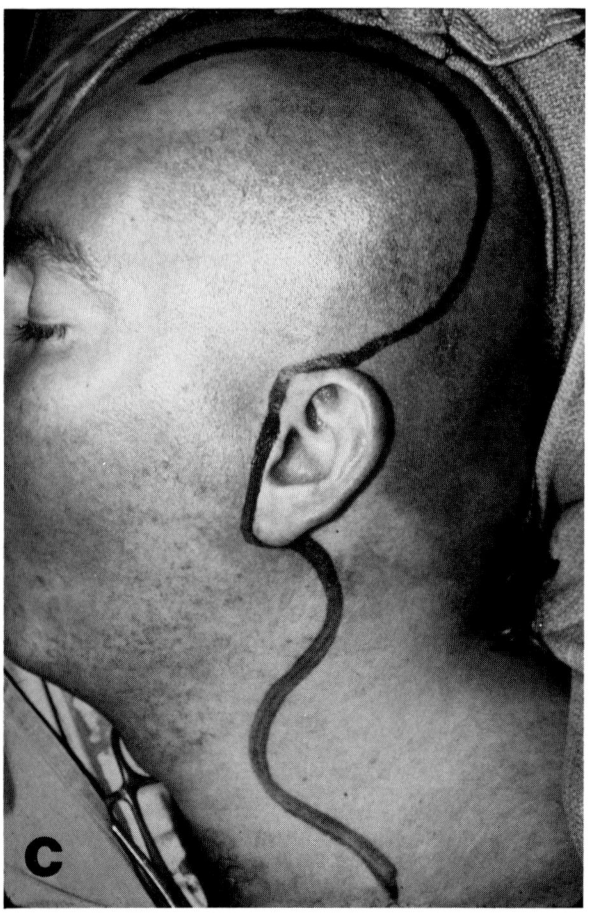

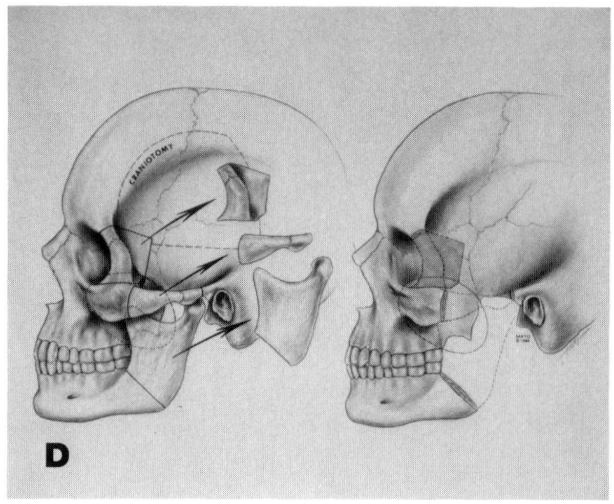

Figure 4 Liposarcoma middle cranial fossa and infratemporal fossa. *A*, Preoperative appearance. *B*, Axial CT scan of a patient with a left-sided liposarcoma involving the posterior maxillary area, infratemporal fossa, and base of middle cranial fossa. *C*, Standard approach to infratemporal fossa and anterior middle cranial fossa tumors. *D*, Exposure osteotomy for resection of infratemporal fossa tumors, consisting of the orbit, zygomatic arch, and ascending ramus of the mandible.

Figure continues on opposite page

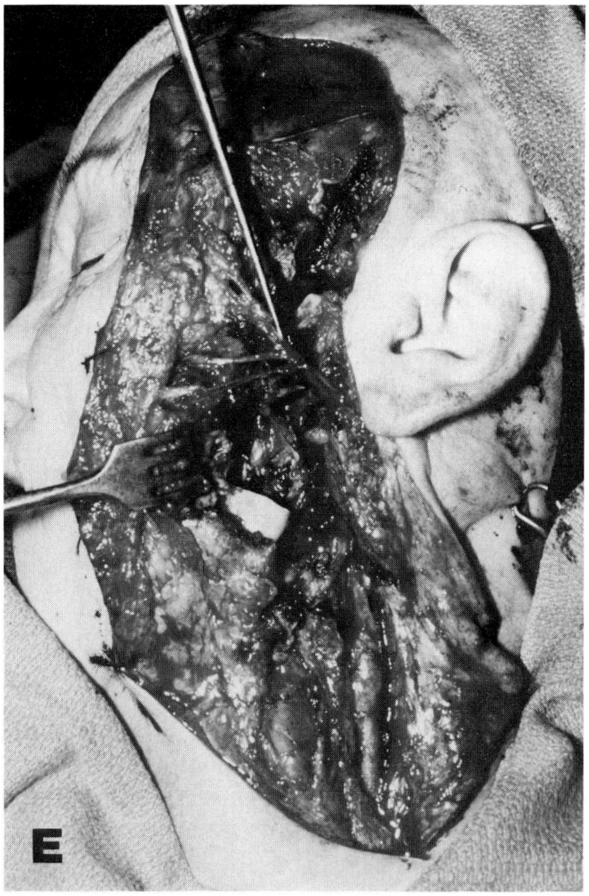

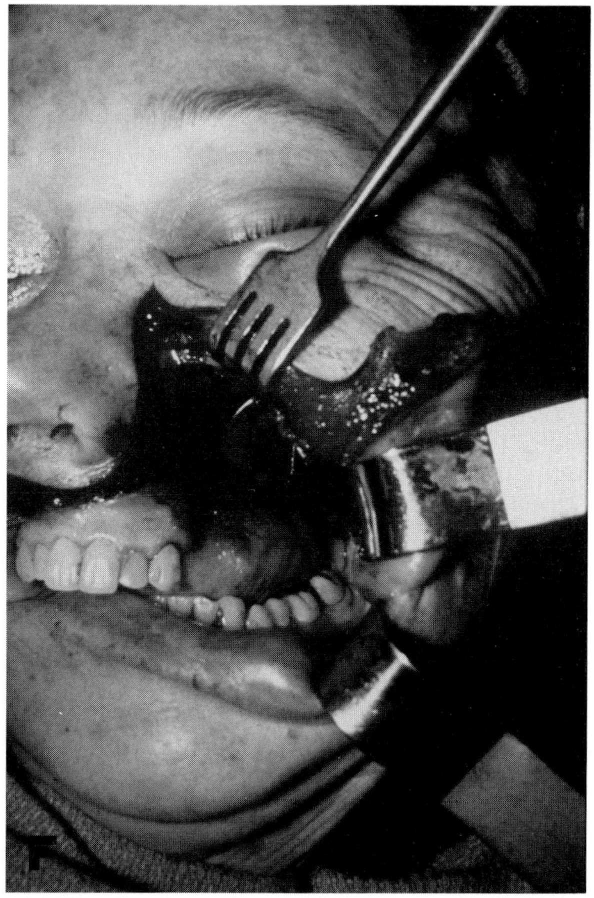

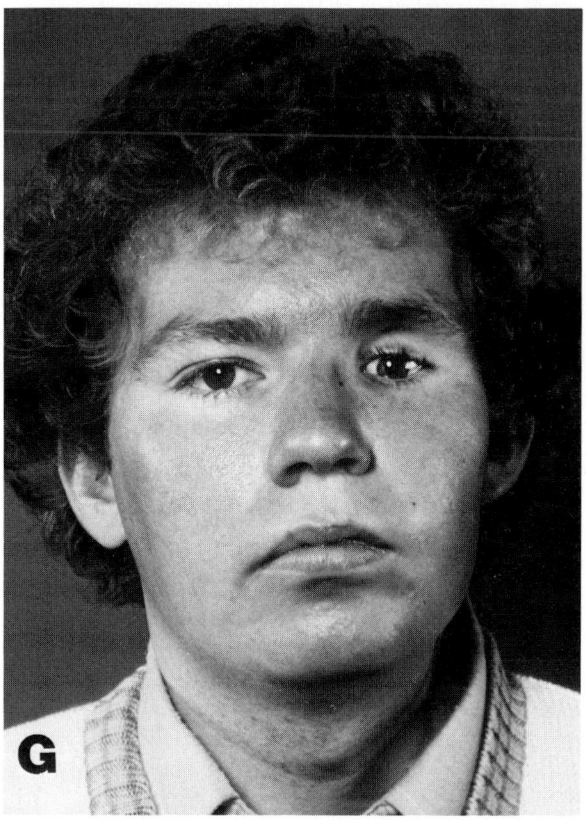

Figure 4 (continued) *E*, The entire facial nerve is retracted. The ascending ramus of the mandible has been removed, and the tumor is now visible. *F*, Following dissection of the tumor in the middle cranial fossa and in the infratemporal fossa, the maxilla is approached through a partial Weber-Ferguson incision, a maxillary osteotomy is performed to resect the tumor invading the maxilla. An en bloc tumor removal can now be accomplished from the lateral approach bringing the tumor out between the transected angle of the mandible and the facial nerve. *G*, Appearance 2 years after surgery. The patient died 6 months later with spinal metastasis of the liposarcoma.

Resection is extremely difficult when the posterior part of the maxilla or the orbit is involved. In this situation, it is best to elevate the temporalis muscle with the infratemporal fossa contents; by dissecting deep to the muscle, the lateral orbital wall and the posterior portion of the maxilla in continuity with the remainder of the infratemporal fossa contents may be removed. If necessary, the orbital contents may be included in the block. With some difficulty, an en bloc removal can be performed. If there is extension of the tumor into the orbit, the maxillary antrum, and toward the ethmoid sinuses, a midline Weber-Ferguson incision is advocated, either in the classic fashion or by extending the incision up over the midline of the forehead. In this way, the orbital and maxillary block as required can be added to the resection of the contents of the infratemporal fossa. In these cases, it is necessary to have vascularized muscles, particularly to close off entry into the oral cavity. To this end, we have used the sternomastoid muscle based on its superior vascular pedicle. In other cases, the sternomastoid muscle has been used in this way to fill out the cosmetic contour defect left by resection of the ascending ramus of the mandible. It is unwise to replace the latter since the dead space and the connection into the oral cavity will often result in sequestration. A galeal frontalis flap is used if there is any connection with the nasopharynx.

Unfortunately, almost all of the tumors presenting in this area are recurrent. They are biologically extremely aggressive and extensive, and so the prognosis is not particularly good. In patients with involvement of the floor of the middle cranial fossa, it is our custom to first do a temporal craniotomy and biopsy the trigeminal nerve ganglion as it lies in Meckel's cave. If the biopsy is positive, we would not proceed with any resection, unless the patient is opposed. This is because, not only would there be no cure of the lesion, but the resection would cause both severe esthetic and functional deformities.

POSTERIOR SEGMENT OF MIDDLE CRANIAL FOSSA

Tumors of the posterior segment of the middle cranial fossa include those in relation to the petrous temporal bone. In our practice, these are always malignant and are frequently recurrent, except in the case of middle ear carcinoma. The tumors are usually basal cell or squamous cell carcinomas of the external ear that invade inward, together with a few malignant melanomas. Parotid tumors, such as adenocystic, anaplastic, and mucoepidermoid carcinomas, may invade along the ear canal and so involve the middle ear. The remaining tumors are primary squamous carcinomas of the middle ear. All of these tumors require petrosectomies of various types, with resection of variable amounts of skin and ear. In external ear tumors, the ear is resected to obtain adequate clearance, and a *partial petrosectomy* is performed. If necessary, a temporal craniotomy is performed and the temporal lobe is elevated; this allows the floor of the middle cranial fossa to be resected as necessary for removal of the tumor. A similar approach is used in *subtotal petrosectomy*. This is best done with a neck dissection to locate the internal jugular vein and the internal carotid artery. If there is extension anteriorly along the petrous bone, the ascending ramus of the mandible and the zygomatic arch may have to be removed for exposure. In a subtotal petrosectomy, this is not taken deep to the styloid process and so there is little danger of injuring the internal carotid. In a *total petrosectomy*, which is carried out for deeply-penetrating tumors and for middle ear carcinomas, a neck dissection is again performed to locate the great vessels. The internal carotid artery is followed up to its entry into the petrous bone, its entry into the middle cranial fossa is located intracranially, and a resection of the petrous bone is carried out through the carotid canal. Any potentially-involved bone in relation to the canal itself is resected separately. If necessary, and if cross-flow studies are satisfactory, the carotid artery can be resected. The results of resection of external ear and parotid tumors have been satisfactory, but those for middle ear carcinomas have been dismal.

Posterior Cranial Fossa Tumors

Tumors of the posterior cranial fossa are unusual. Neurofibromas may occur and may escape through the jugular foramen to present as parotid tumors. They usually involve the cranial nerves at the cerebellar-pontine angle and at the glossopharyngeal, vagus, accessory, and hypoglossal nerves. There may be hoarseness and wasting of the sternomastoid and trapezius muscles. Occasional involvement of the base of the posterior cranial fossa is seen together with sarcomas in relation to the muscles attached to that structure. A standard neurosurgical posterior cranial fossa approach is undertaken with wide resection to the jugular foramen; in the case of neurofibroma, it is usually easy to remove a tumor by a mixture of blunt and sharp dissection.

LIMITS OF RESECTABILITY

This is an important consideration in skull base tumors, but is often difficult to determine. If angiography shows that the cavernous sinus is involved, then these malignant tumors are felt to be unresectable. Extensive involvement of the optic nerves with bilateral blindness is unlikely to result in curative resection. Involvement of the trigeminal nerve ganglion in the middle cranial fossa indicates brain extension, and curative resection is therefore unlikely. Involvement of the skull base in relation to the cavernous sinus obviates total resection. In these cases, radiotherapy selectively directed to where residual tumor has been left can be employed, but the prognosis remains poor. Unfortunately, many of these tumors are aggressive: they have recurred after failure of other therapeutic modalities and may always be likely to recur. However, in our own experience, we have been pleasantly surprised at the survival statistics. Unless there is an obvious contraindication, we will always give the patient the benefit of the doubt and at least proceed with an intracranial exploration as the first step to assess resectability.

RECONSTRUCTION

As has been mentioned already, reconstruction is often as simple as possible to allow for regular follow-up with unrestricted examination of the area of tumor excision. Galeal frontalis flaps, temporalis fascia flaps, skin grafts, and local flaps are preferred when possible. Deltopectoral, pectoralis myocutaneous cutaneous, and scalp flaps are used when indicated.

Microvascular free tissue transfer is preferred in nonmalignant tumors, palliative resections, and secondary reconstructions. The flaps used are latissimus dorsi, scapular, radial forearm, rectus abdominis, and occasionally omentum. In complex three-dimensional problems, external prostheses using osseointegration techniques have been used.

COMPLICATIONS

With the experience gained in the whole field of craniofacial surgery, the incidence of complications has been low. The potential problems are death, CSF leak, extradural abscess, meningitis, blindness, trismus, and facial palsy when a total parotidectomy is performed for exposure. Death is rare and, if it occurs, it is usually related to some condition other than the cancer or the resection. The incidence of significant infection has dropped considerably over the years; this is because of two factors. The first is a great reduction in operating time as a result of increasing experience. The second is an increased understanding of the mechanism of intracranial infection and its causes. Coupled with this is the use of vascularized material in the form of galeal frontalis, temporalis muscle or fascia, and free tissue transfer to close off connections between the nasopharynx and the extradural space. This latter maneuver is especially necessary when a dural repair has been carried out. Infection has also been reduced because the smallest possible craniotomy consistent with good exposure is being used to remove the tumor, autogenous fascia are used for dural repair, and the wound is irrigated with dilute Betadine.

Postoperative atelectasis and chest infection have been greatly reduced by the use of cranial bone for reconstruction rather than rib or iliac crest. This allows earlier mobilization and better toleration of chest physical therapy.

If a CFS leak continues over 7 to 10 days in spite of spinal taps, reexploration is indicated. This, in our experience, rarely ever happens if the following conditions are met. The exposure to dural repairs should be adequate, the repair must be watertight, and it should be augmented by a galeal frontalis, temporalis muscle, or fascia flap. In some cases (middle cranial fossa) the sternomastoid muscle is used.

Blindness does not occur unless by design, e.g., by exenteration. When there is any danger of corneal exposure postoperatively, the recommended measures should be instituted—Frost suture or temporary tarsorrhaphy, ophthalmic ointment, or, if necessary, cover with a plastic dome.

In some cases, diplopia will occur because of changes in eye position after removal of segments of the orbit. There is little to do for this. The patient may eventually accommodate or may be improved with orbital reconstructive measures. In some cases, diplopia occurs because of muscle imbalance resulting from muscle entrapment, damage or resection, trochlear disruption, or nerve damage. These cases should be referred to the ophthalmologist.

Lacrimal drainage problems require careful assessment; treatment should be by dacryocystorhinostomy, by insertion of Lester Jones tubes, or by other varieties of lacrimal drainage system reconstruction. Upper eyelid ptosis may occur; this is dealt with by freeing the levator muscle and shortening the aponeurosis as indicated. Prior to this, the Bell's reflex and corneal sensation should be checked. If these are defective, the question of ptosis correction must be carefully considered. If there is no eye, full-thickness lid resection is indicated in some cases. If the lower eyelid is lax transversely, it may be tightened with a Kuhnt-Szymanowski procedure or by the insertion of conchal cartilage for support.

Unless the facial nerve is transected, any facial weakness should recover. However, it should be remembered, that a large block of resected tissue is mobilized and manipulated out from under the nerve. This involves considerable stretching of the nerve; thus, neuropraxia is common. In the elderly patient, recovery takes longer and may not be absolutely complete. This is probably vascular in nature.

If the nerve is divided and it is possible to insert a nerve graft, this should be done at the initial procedure. The necessity for postoperative radiotherapy is no contraindication to this. If nerve grafting is not possible, serious consideration should be given to immediate temporalis and masseter transfer. If these muscles are not available, an alternative is a static fascial sling. Lagophthalmos can be corrected with a gold weight (1.5 to 1.8 g). It is probably best to wait and do this later on an outpatient basis with local anesthesia, when the required weight of implant can be accurately assessed.

Carotid damage or ligation can cause hemiplegia. This should not occur inadvertently. Any carotid surgery should be anticipated, cross-cerebral flow studies should be available, and the vascular team should be alerted if carotid replacement seems likely. Carotid invasion by tumor does not necessarily negate tumor resection.

POSTOPERATIVE MANAGEMENT AND FOLLOW-UP

The majority of these patients are managed immediately postoperatively in the neurosurgical intensive care area. They are carefully watched for airway problems, CSF leaks, bleeding, and signs of infection.

If progress is satisfactory, the majority will leave hospital within a week to 10 days. Patients with malignant tumors are followed up at regular intervals, initially 3 months and then 6 months, later extending to a year. At each return, complete examination of the head and neck is undertaken with nasendoscopy and laryngoscopy. Any suspicious area is biopsied. At 6-month intervals, chest roentgenography and CT or MRI scans are performed. Care should be taken in the interpretation of these investigations; not infrequently, recurrence is reported, which at biopsy is found to be granulation or scar tissue. If indicated, adjuvant treatment can be commenced when healing is complete; it should not be delayed longer than a month to 6 weeks. Treatment may be radiation therapy or chemotherapy. If a patient has had a postradiotherapy recurrence and the whole area is resected and replaced with well-vascularized tissue, further radiation can be given if indicated.

SUGGESTED READING

Albrektsson T, Branemark PI, Jacobsson M, Tjellström A. Present clinical applications of osseointegrated percutaneous implants. Plast Reconstr Surg 1987; 79:721–730.

Curioni C, Toscano P, Clauser L, Padula E. Facial and craniofacial resections and reconstruction techniques for tumors involving the orbital walls. Chir Testa e Collo 1984; 1:15–36.

Derome P. Les tumeurs sphéno-ethmoidales: possibilités d'exérèse et de réparation chirurgcales. Neurochirurgie 1972; 18(Suppl 1):1–164.

Jackson IT, Adham MN, Marsh WR. Use of the galeal frontalis myofascial flap in craniofacial surgery. Plast Reconstr Surg 1986; 77:905–910.

Jackson IT, Hide TAH. Systematic approach to tumors of the base of the skull. J Maxillofac Surg 1982; 10:92–98.

Jackson IT, Laws ER Jr, Martin RD. A craniofacial approach to advanced recurrent cancer of the central face. Head Neck Surg 1983; 5:474–488.

Jackson IT, Marsh WR, Bite U, Hide TAH. Craniofacial osteotomies to facilitate to skull base tumour resection. Br J Plast Surg 1986; 39:153–160.

Jones NF, Sekhar LN, Schramm V. Free rectus abdominis muscle flap reconstruction of the middle and posterior cranial base. Plast Reconstr Surg 1986; 78:471–477.

SURGICAL RESTORATION OF THE NOSE

GARY C. BURGET, M.D.

A tacit promise exists in the lay literature and media that plastic surgeons can replace a missing nose. This promise has not been kept, for though we can assemble upon the face a conglomerate mass of tissues held together with collagen glue, such a lump can only *appear* to be a nose, and then *only if its surface contour is precisely correct*. Nasal reconstruction has passed through the stages of cover, lining, and support. Its newest stage, the stage of contour, has already begun. The present era of nasal reconstruction may see us abandon, once and for all, the creation of formless tissue masses. Lining, support, and cover do not make a nose. Rather, it is the manner of shaping and assembling these materials that gives contour to the lump and *the visual impression of a nose*.

CASE REPORT

The surgical restoration in our case report exemplifies principles and techniques necessary to restore normal contour to most large nasal defects. It may be used as a prototype. The patient presented (Fig. 1) with a large recurrent basal cell carcinoma excised in stages with microscopic control of the wound margins. The extirpative surgeon, June Robinson, M.D., was asked to decide the timing of reconstruction, since she possessed the greatest understanding of the tumor's potential for recurrence. Immediate restoration was recommended.

The patient was given a choice of management. Alternatives to surgical restoration of the nose—healing by contraction, skin graft, prosthesis—which are simple and inexpensive, were rejected by the patient. This fastidious and valiant schoolteacher, who faced her classes nearly every day during the course of the surgical reconstruction, wished the dignity of a normal-appearing nose and would accept nothing less. However, she was made to understand that the restoration would require one operation under general anesthesia and two further operations over a period of at least 6 weeks. Another 4 to 6 months would be required for scars to soften and fade.

Early restoration of the nose may be undertaken the day after excision of the tumor, before tissue reaction is severe, or 5 days later, when edema has subsided and a fibrin barrier lines the wound. It should not be done in the period when bacterial contamination and wound edema are maximal. This patient chose to begin her reconstruction 2 weeks after tumor excision.

THE FIRST OPERATION: ASSEMBLY

A Platform

The nasal defect often extends onto the adjacent lip and cheek. It is a tempting shortcut to fill the single concavity with a single flap and later worry about contour. Free flaps employed in this way have at times turned the horrible concave deformity into a ridiculous convex one. In such cases, the patient is told that numerous operative stages will follow, during which the shapeless pendant will be changed into a nose. These operations seldom come to pass, for hardly anyone knows how to do them; in addition, the patient, who has by now had a generous taste of plastic surgery, has lost his or her appetite for it. The patient fades out, often to the great relief of the surgeon.

The ala of the nose sits upon the platform of the lip and cheek at a precise position and angle. If both the platform and the alar base are constructed at one operation, then postoperatively, the platform will drag the alar base laterally or inferiorly across the face as it shifts and settles. Additional stages of surgery will be necessary to

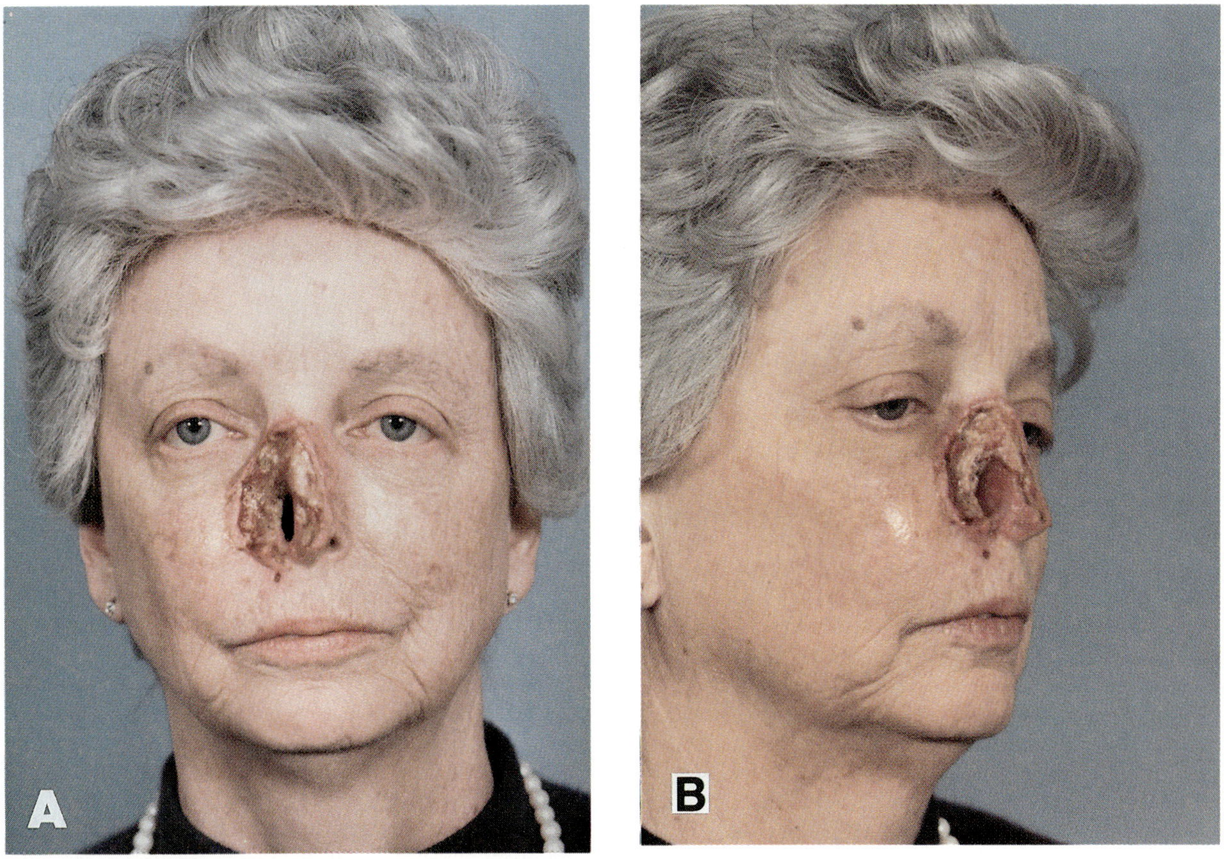

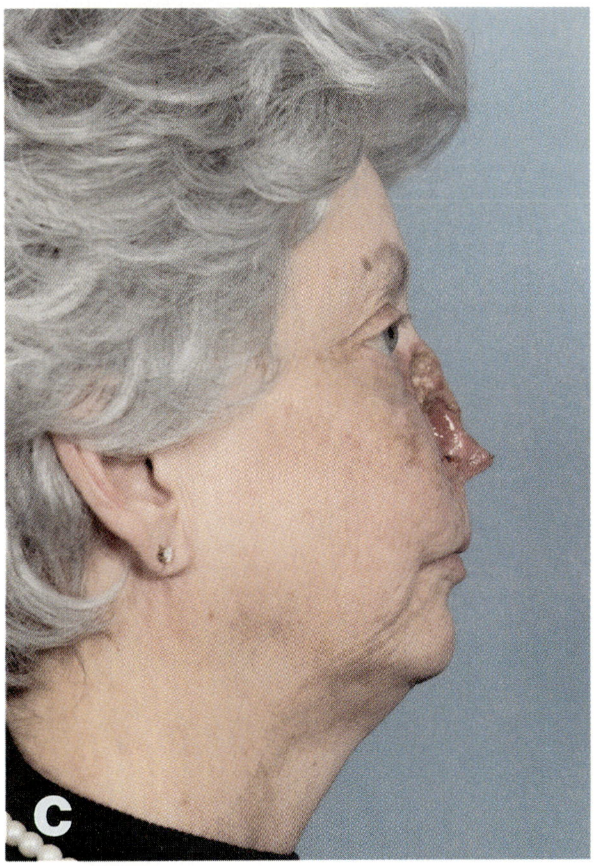

Figure 1 April 2, 1987. The defect shown in different views (*A*, *B*, and *C*) following tumor excision.

replace the ala in its normal position. But if the lip-cheek platform is established first and the nose unit is added later when the platform has become stable, the course of reconstruction is shortened and a normal contour can be achieved at the outset.

The surface of the lip-cheek platform can be made from a rotation flap of cheek skin based superiorly for small defects or inferiorly for large ones. Where the defect is deep and extends down to the anterior wall of the maxilla, a local flap of fat can act as filler. Though the patient did not require it, the swinging or flip-fat flap of Gillies, Aymard, and Millard will fill the depression and create a sweeping transition from cheek to nose.

In this case, because the margins of tumor excision were favorable, the extirpative surgeon urged early reconstruction. This was undertaken on an inpatient basis under general anesthesia with the invaluable assistance of plastic surgeon Diane Gerber, M.D. The wound was first débrided of fibrin and ligatures, infiltrated with epinephrine solution, and totally excised (including its base) with a 1-mm margin of normal tissue. The remaining skin of the involved topographic subunits of the nose was then excised as we described in 1985 (Fig. 2). The excision included a small piece of the right alar base, the remaining portion of the left nasal tip, the dorsal subunit, and the entire left alar subunit. The left ala was sacrificed because it had been resurfaced some years before with a full-thickness skin graft. An inelastic contracted skin graft abutting a nasal defect is best excised, since unpredictable tensions in these old scars can distort the final nose. The lines of subunit excision followed normal shadowed valleys on the nasal surface so that, if the final nasal scars healed poorly and cast linear shadows, these shadows would seem a part of the normal nasal surface.

The lip-cheek platform was, for the most part, intact in our patient. There was soft tissue overlying the anterior maxilla so that a local fat flap was not needed. Furthermore, the junction of the right alar base and the lip was normal so that the cheek and the ala could be repaired in one stage without fear of postoperative distortion. A superiorly-based rotation flap was designed in the fine wrinkle line of the nasolabial crease with a 1.0-cm back-cut at the level of the oral commissure. The flap, 8-mm thick, was elevated off the underlying fat for 5-cm laterally, rotated counterclockwise into the defect, and anchored to the edge of the pyriform aperture. The margin of the rotation flap was then trimmed so that the donor scar would lie exactly in the nasolabial wrinkle line, and the donor site was closed in layers. A No. 19 suction drain hooked to a vacuum tube was brought through the incision and a fine mattress suture was positioned to close the hole after the drain was removed.

The Lining Sleeve

Thin, flexible, vascular nasal lining flaps are in short supply—but nothing else will do. Thick lining flaps bulge inward and outward, thus making a potato shape inevitable even before support and cover are added. Lining flaps with poor vascularity may themselves survive, but will not nourish the primary cartilage grafts needed to impart normal contour to the nose. In such cases, the cartilage grafts liquify and drain out. Rigid lining flaps, such as composite grafts, placed under a forehead flap weeks before it is formed into a nose maintain the shape they are given on the forehead. When the new nose is assembled, the preplaced lining does not conform to the contour of the nose, but rather dictates that contour itself. Only lining flaps from intranasal donor sites (the vestibule, the middle vault, and the septum) are thin enough to preserve shape and the airway, vascular enough to nourish primary cartilage grafts, and soft enough to conform to the contour of the new nose.

The lining sleeve for our patient was made from ipsilateral and contralateral septal mucoperichondrial flaps (Fig. 3). Both sides of the septum were infiltrated with 1:50,000 epinephrine. The mucoperichondrium of the entire right anterior septum was elevated. A flap 2.0 cm high

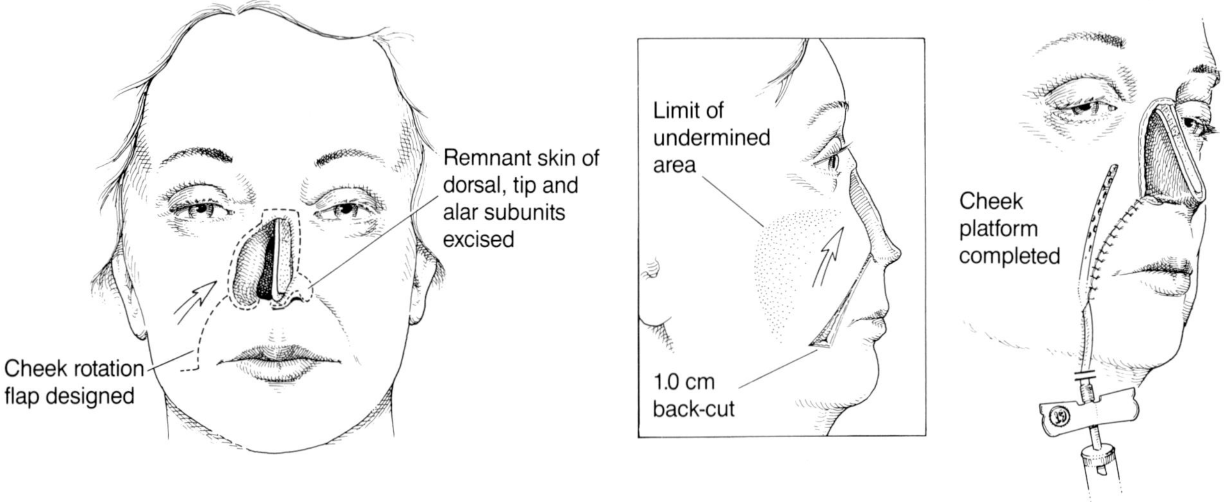

Figure 2 The remaining skin of the involved topographic subunits of the nose was then excised.

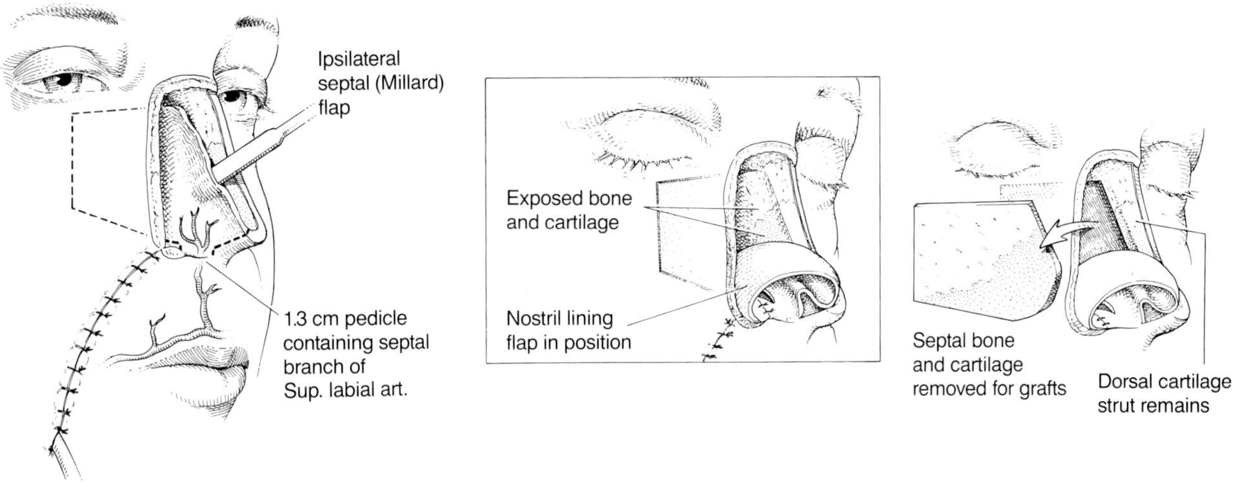

Figure 3 The lining sleeve for the patient was made from ipsilateral and contralateral septal mucoperichondrial flaps.

and 2.5 cm deep was cut loose from the right side of the septum, but left attached by a 1.3-cm pedicle based in a zone between the lower edge of the pyriform aperture and the anterior plane of the upper lip—the region of the nasal spine. It is in this zone that the septum receives its major anteroinferior blood supply through the septal branch of the superior labial artery. When left attached in this strategic zone, the septal mucoperichondrium may be twisted, manipulated, and transposed without fear of necrosis. This ipsilateral septal flap was bent laterally and sutured with 5-0 gut into the lining defect of the vestibule. The pedicle of the flap temporarily obstructed the nasal airway until 3 weeks later, when it was sectioned with a scalpel. The flap was then allowed to lie limp in the nasal cavity until the next important surgical step.

This ipsilateral septal flap is identical to the flap described by Millard in 1967, except that (1) it includes the entire anterior septal mucosa, (2) it is based on a narrow pedicle centered strategically on a named artery, and (3) it becomes a composite flap when a scaffolding of carefully-shaped bone and cartilage grafts is fused to its submucosal surface. All available bone and cartilage were removed from the anterior septum except for an 8-mm dorsal strut left for support.

A contralateral mucoperichondrial flap (Fig. 4) was designed with its base dorsally (anterosuperiorly) in a zone containing uninjured branches of the left anterior ethmoidal artery. This flap, also 2.0 cm wide and 2.5 cm deep, was hinged across the midline like a swinging door, pulled caudally, and sutured to the mucosal edge of the right pyriform aperture with 5-0 gut sutures. This is the time-honored flap of DeQuervain (1902) employed over the years by Gillies, Kazanjian, and Millard. The two septal flaps (right and left) were then sutured together and allowed to collapse onto the nasal floor to await the addition of a bone and cartilage chassis to their submucosal surfaces.

A Fabricated Composite Flap

If it is to contribute support and contour to the new nose, the lining sleeve must first be converted to a composite flap (Fig. 5). Pieces of septal and conchal cartilage and bone are shaped to resemble nasal surface subunits. With the precision required to build a model airplane, the pieces are fastened to the submucosal-perichondrial surface of the nasal lining. The sleeve depends upon the grafts for its rigidity and shape; the grafts will not survive unless they are in contact with the vascular lining sleeve. When complete, the fabricated composite flap is a microform of the external nose, having the same contour, but reduced in all dimensions by 2.5 mm. The normality or

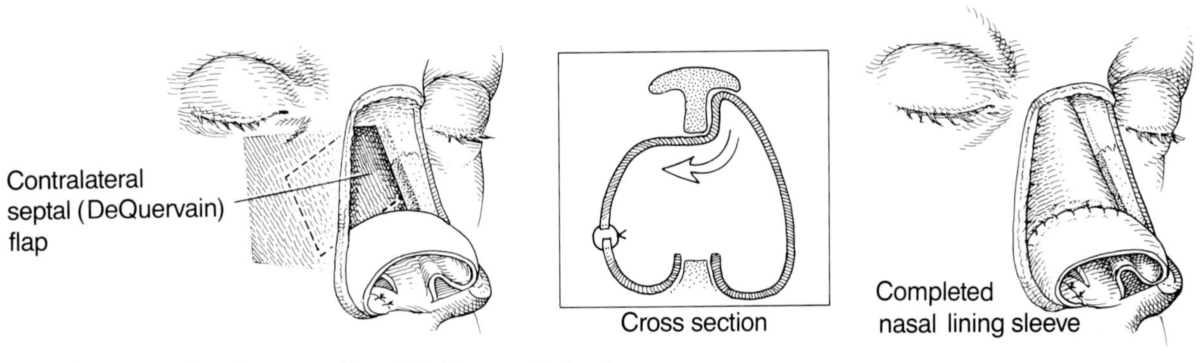

Figure 4 A contralateral mucoperichondrial flap was designed.

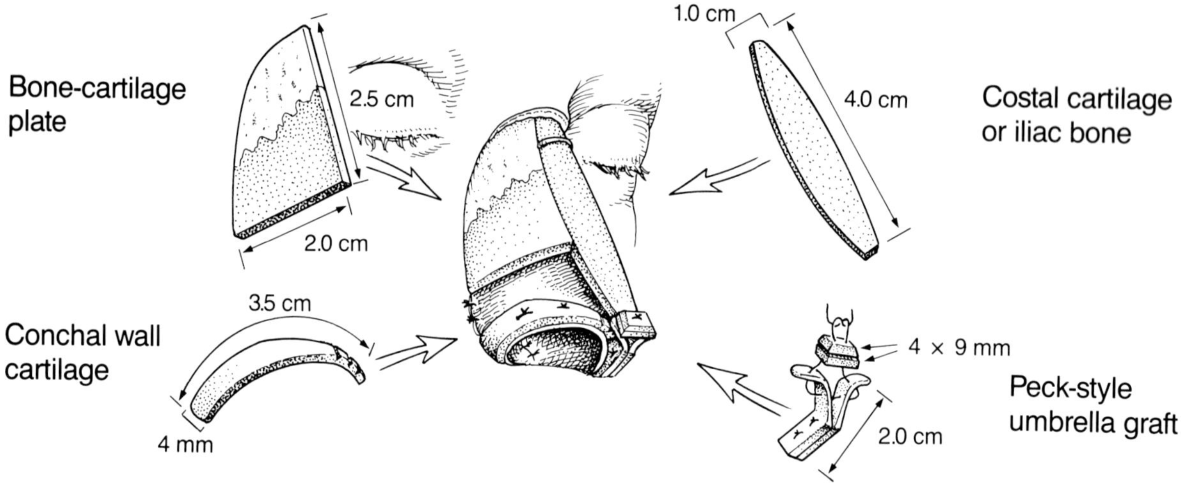

Figure 5 The lining sleeve is converted to a composite flap to contribute support and contour to the new nose.

beauty of the final visual impression depends upon the contour of this modeled scaffold.

Four different hard tissue grafts are required for a major nasal restoration: a buttress, a strut, a brace, and a batten. Each piece serves to fix the underlying mucosal lining in position and imparts shape to a specific subunit of the nose.

Here is how the internal chassis was constructed in our patient:

The Columellar Strut

Cartilage from the walls and floors of both auricular conchae was removed through anterior incisions. Two new alar cartilages were cut from this material, each measuring 4.0 mm wide and 3.5 cm long, with the normal 50 degree columellar-lobular angle of rotation described by Sheen. The two strips were fastened to each other and to the stumps of the original medial crura with 6-0 clear sutures. Their projecting ends were scored and bent laterally and sutured to the lining of the vestibular domes. In this position, the strips supported the vestibules and the nasal tip and lent a normal angular contour to the columella. Tip contour was provided by a double-layered conchal cartilage graft measuring 4 by 9 mm fastened atop the new alar cartilages with a 6-0 clear mattress suture. It is not surprising that this complex of columellar and tip grafts is identical to the umbrella graft used in esthetic rhinoplasty by George Peck. Both grafts restore normal contour to the nasal tip and columella.

A Flying Buttress for the Bridge

The entire right eighth costal cartilage was removed and carved with a No. 15 carbon steel scalpel blade until it was shaped precisely like a normal osseocartilaginous dorsal hump 1.0 cm wide, 4.0 cm long, and 8 mm thick. It was wired to the nasal bones with a single 3-0 wire suture. Iliac bone would have been the chosen graft material if this patient had been less than 40 years old, since costal cartilage slowly warps in young patients, even when it is carved in a balanced manner. Likened by Millard to the "bony gnomon" of a sundial, this dorsal graft is an architectural flying buttress. It prevents the biologic force of wound contraction acting on the tip from shortening the nose. At the same time, the dorsal graft gives a shape to the nasal bridge.

A Brace for the Middle Vault

A large piece of ethmoid perpendicular plate and attached septal cartilage was trimmed to a trapezoidal shape and placed over the lining of the middle vault. This formed a replacement for the right nasal bone and upper lateral cartilage. Such a graft braces the nasal sidewall against upward contraction and the middle vault against collapse. Patients who wear eyeglasses are especially appreciative of this bony platform.

Alar Battens

The remaining conchal cartilage was shaved thin and formed into two delicate strips. Each strip was carved to resemble a bulging alar lobule and fastened along the lower edge of the lining sleeve from the alar base to the apex of the new nostril with 6-0 clear sutures. As a thin strip of wood stretches a sail, so these alar battens stiffen the edge of the nostril. They also render shape to the alar subunit.

When complete, the bone and cartilage chassis enveloping the mucosal lining sleeve stood erect by itself, felt rigid to the touch, and embodied the desired curves and bulges of an ideal external nose.

A Skin-Tight Skin Flap

Construction of the structural nasal framework requires the talents of a model airplane builder, while the design of the forehead skin drape demands the skill of a tailor. In the design of a forehead flap, there is a thin line between too scant and too full. A tight flap can collapse the scaffold. An overly generous one allows centripetal contraction to obscure all contour.

The pattern for a made-to-measure skin flap is fashioned from heavy aluminum foil such as that used to package sutures or petrolatum gauze (Fig. 6). There is a tendency to make the flap fit the nasal defect. However, the defect has been enlarged and distorted by edema, wound contraction, and local anesthetic injections. Its shape on the operating table does not reflect that of the skin missing from the nose. The defect should be made to fit a flap of ideal shape. Such a flap can be designed from the remaining normal subunits of the opposite side of the nose or (when these have been lost) from a model of an ideal nose. The pattern for the flap is cut to fit entire topographic subunits—an entire ala, dorsum, or tip—so that the small amount of trap-door contraction, inevitable in any flap, will mimic the normal bulge of an ala, dorsum, or tip.

To preserve its axial quality so that it may be thinned without fear, the forehead flap is designed vertically. An angle as slight as 15 degrees off the vertical will cut across branches of the supratrochlear and angular arteries and make thinning of the flap risky. Even if extra length is needed to reconstruct the columella, a vertical axial flap is preferable to an oblique random flap. When elevated, the hairbearing columellar extension of a vertical flap may be thinned of fat and frontalis muscle and each hair follicle may be clipped from behind. A vertical flap will easily bear such rough treatment; an oblique random flap may be neither thinned nor depilated.

The surface defect of the nose in our patient was enlarged to cover entire topographic subunits: the dorsum, right sidewall, both alae, and the tip. Since contralateral normal subunits were not present to serve as a mirror-image template, the nasal pattern was made to reflect an ideal nasal shape. The heavy aluminum foil of a petrolatum gauze package was cut, bent, and crimped until it fit over the nose like a custom-tailored garment. The three-dimensional pattern was then flattened to two dimensions and placed vertically on the forehead in line with the frown crease just medial to the eyebrow on the right side, the side on which the nasal defect was largest. A Doppler pulse amplifier confirmed the location of two arteries in the pedicle. In order to gain flap length, the columellar portion of the flap extended into the hairbearing skin of the frontal scalp. With the forehead skin on a slight stretch, the pattern was traced in methylene blue dye. The base of the flap was tapered so that it measured only 1.5 cm wide at the orbital rim. As the pattern was incised on the forehead, the cut was made on the inside of the blue line to avoid taking even 0.5 mm of marginal excess. The distal 1.5 cm of the flap were then elevated off the frontalis mus-

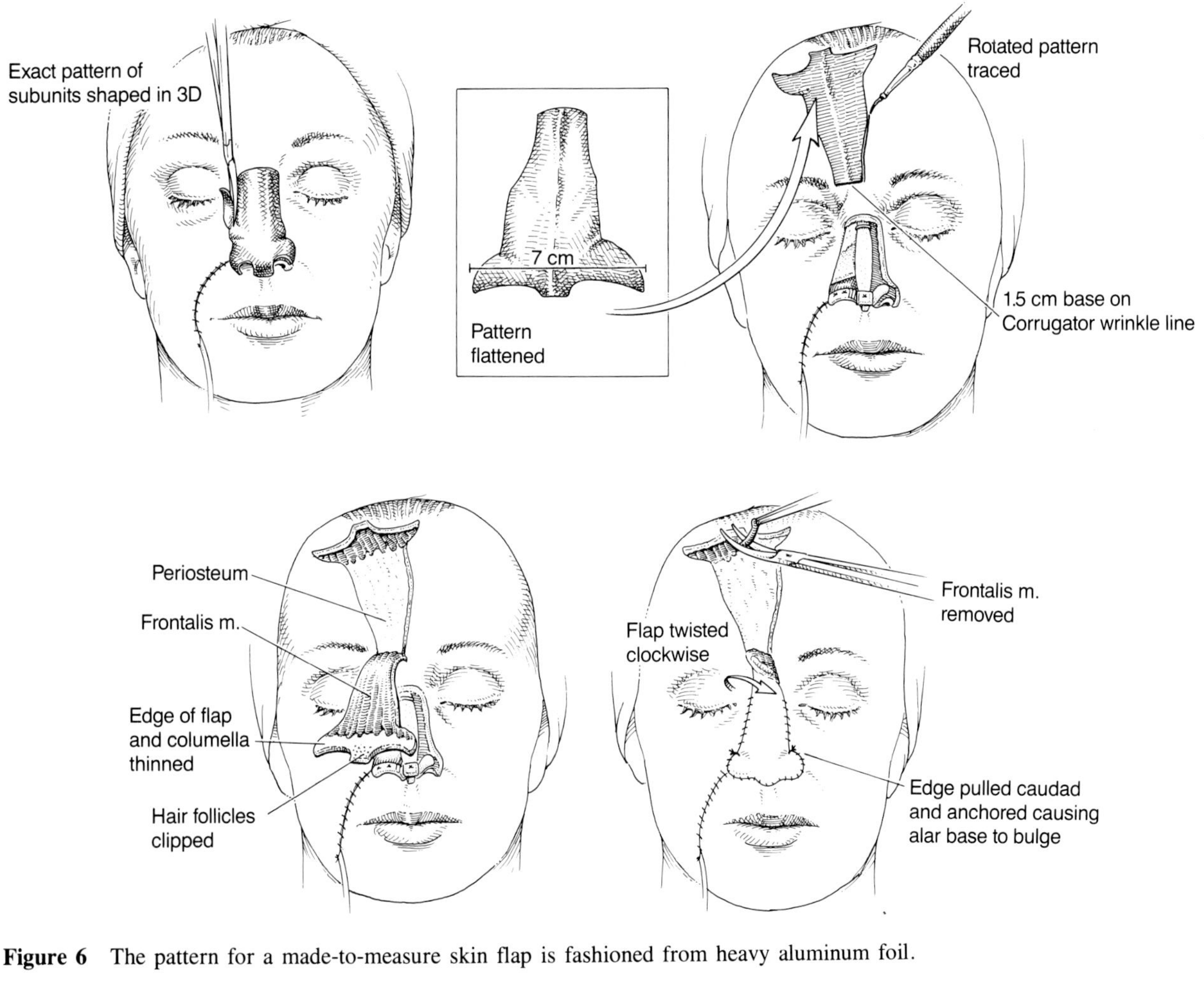

Figure 6 The pattern for a made-to-measure skin flap is fashioned from heavy aluminum foil.

cle, and at that point the scalpel sank deeply to the periosteum and the frontalis muscle was lifted up with the proximal pedicle. The margins and distal portions of the flap were thinned with a curved Joseph scissors. During thinning, the several axial vessels visualized in the subcutaneous fat were preserved. Using magnification, each hair follicle in the hairbearing columellar extension of the flap was exposed in the subcutaneous layer and clipped off with a fine scissors.

If, in spite of all precautions, this flap had been too short, its base could have been lengthened. This is accomplished by extending the pedicle over the supraorbital rim and sectioning fibers of the corrugator muscle tethering its base, while preserving branches of the vessels.

The thinned vertical paramedian forehead flap was then twisted clockwise (a left-sided flap would have been twisted counterclockwise) and transposed onto the osseocartilaginous chassis. The edges of the flap were adjusted to enhance the shape of the nose during positioning with 6-0 sutures.

Autoexpansion Closes the Forehead

The forehead is forgiving. Although the donor site frequently cannot be closed with sutures, skin grafts, rotation flaps, or tissue expanders are not needed. In fact, they compound the deformity. Wound contraction can be relied upon to close defects as wide as 3 cm by tissue autoexpansion.

In our patient's operation, the frontalis muscle remaining in the donor defect on the central forehead was removed. The forehead and scalp surrounding the donor site were elevated from the periosteum of the frontal bone for 7 cm bilaterally and superiorly (Fig. 7). Four heavy simple sutures tied under moderate tension brought together the four limbs of the cross-shaped defect. These four key sutures, placed close to the wound edge to minimize their stitch marks, were removed 10 days later. Distal dogears were excised from the lateral and superior extensions of the donor site and closure was completed in layers. As is usual, a central donor defect remained. The exposed periosteum in this defect was protected from desiccation with petrolatum gauze. No contraction occurred in the forehead wound for a lag period of 3 weeks; the wound then rapidly and totally closed during the fourth and fifth postoperative weeks. The biologic force of wound contraction autoexpands the adjacent forehead skin during this period, thus making surgical manipulations or mechanical tissue expansion unnecessary (Fig. 8).

In this case, the raw surface of the forehead pedicle was covered with a split-thickness skin graft 0.012 in thick. Though this is not strictly necessary, it simplifies wound care and minimizes the number of postoperative office visits.

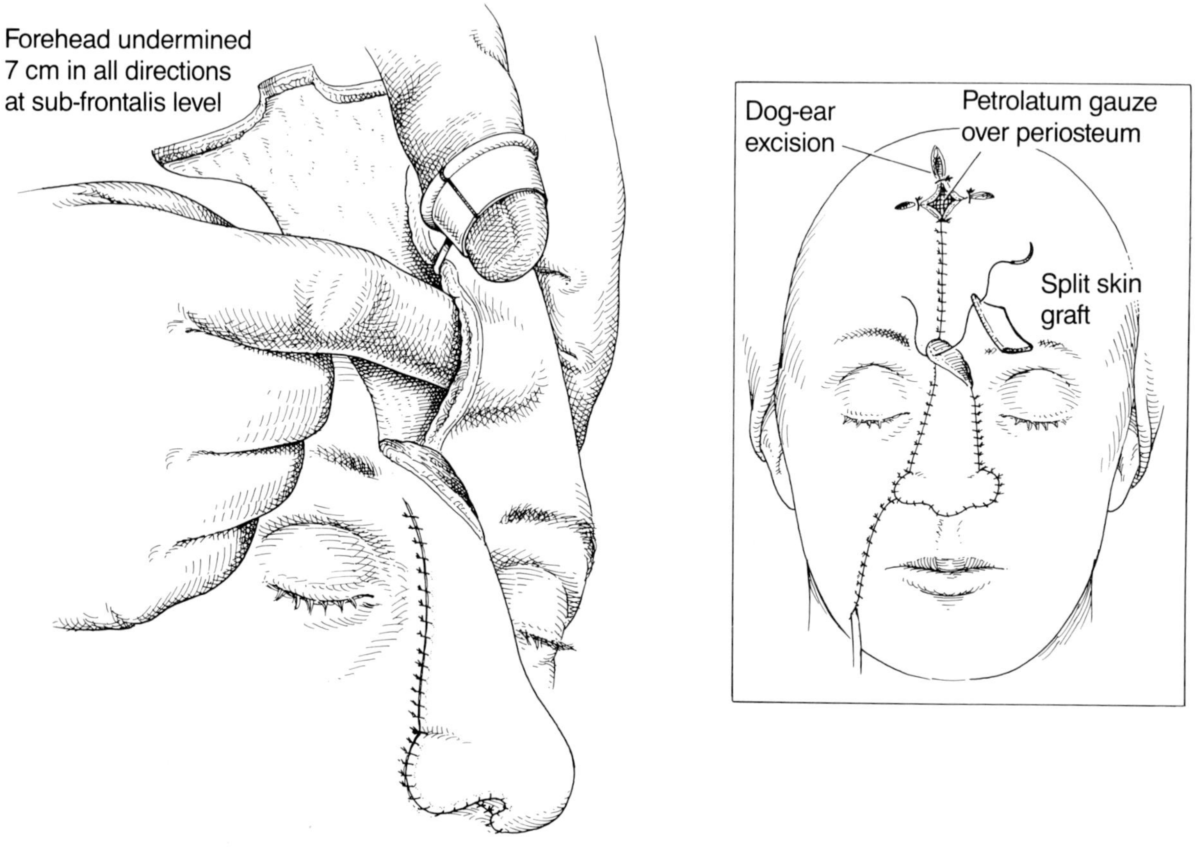

Figure 7 The forehead and scalp surrounding the donor site were elevated from the periosteum of the frontal bone.

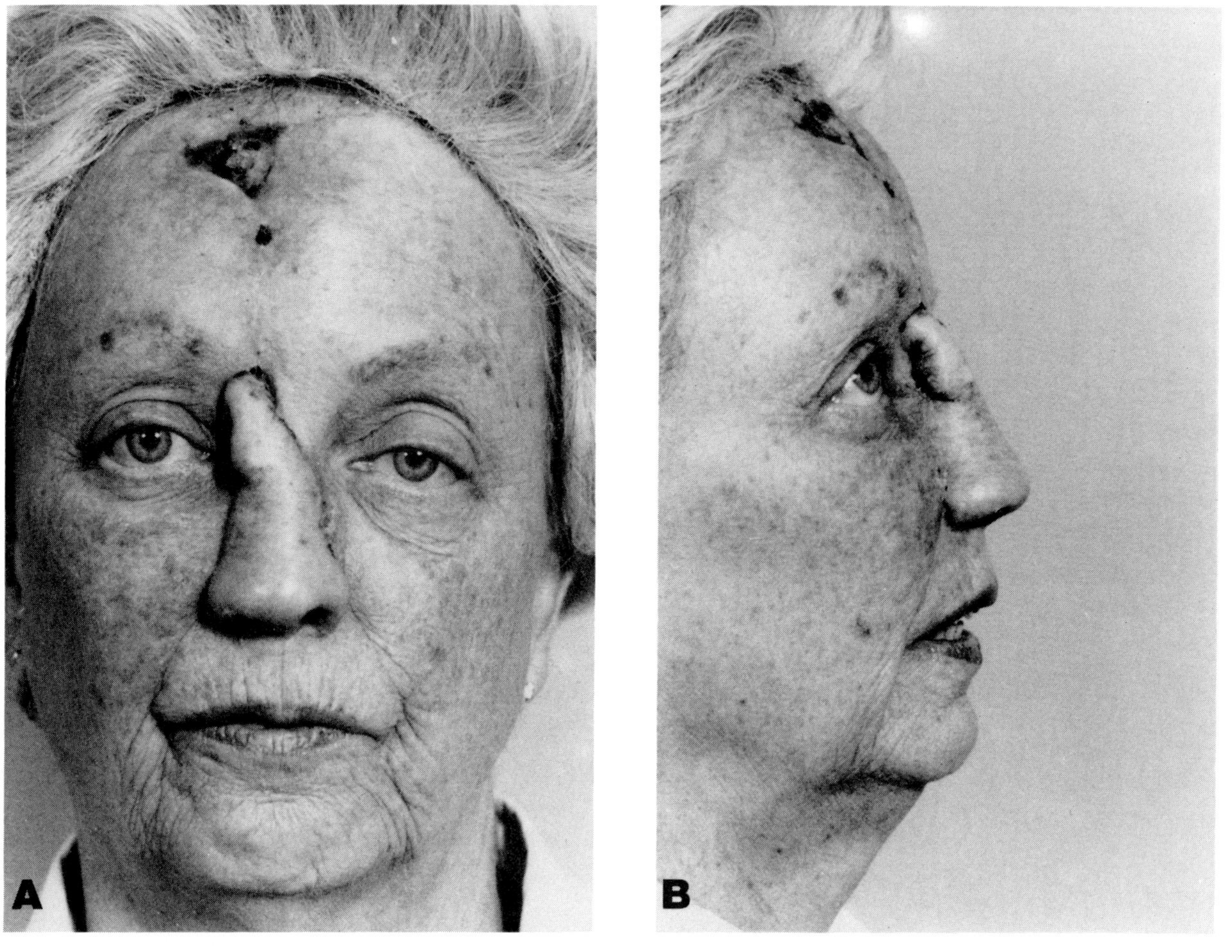

Figure 8 *A* and *B*, May 9, 1987. The nose before the intermediate operation to refine its contour.

Postoperative Details

Most skin sutures were removed between the second and fifth postoperative days. Only the four key forehead sutures remained until the tenth day. A 1-inch square band-aid was kept over the forehead wound. Eyeglasses were suspended from the forehead for 1 week to avoid strangulating the pedicle.

The postoperative complication of flap necrosis is rare except in patients with longstanding radiation damage to the face and in those who smoke. Hematoma is uncommon unless one has scored the galea-frontalis in attempting complete forehead closure. Infection occurs most often in patients with acne rosacea or rhinophyma.

THE SECOND OPERATION: REFINEMENT

In any plan for major nasal restoration, it is useful to include an intermediate operation between assembly and pedicle division. The numerous intersecting planes of scar in a major nasal restoration contract and bring about unpredictable changes in contour that do not occur in small segmental reconstructions. Rather than return to the nose in piecemeal fashion over a period of months and years, it seems wiser to follow Millard's expedient example of 1974 and adjust the nasal contour while the skin pedicle is yet intact. The skin flap may be boldly lifted off the nose, the entire subcutaneous surface sculpted, and additional cartilage grafts added where required. This intermediate stage eliminates the need for the many secondary operations that have generally followed reconstructive rhinoplasty.

In our patient, the intermediate operation was done 8 weeks after the first, though it has been done as early as 3 weeks.

At this stage, the lateral border scars and those along the nostril rims were excised and the entire flap was elevated off the nose at a superficial plane, thus leaving it attached at only the columella and its pedicle. The central axis of the flap, left bulky at the initial operation, was thinned with a curved Joseph scissors; the axial branches of the supratrochlear and angular vessels, which were seen running in the subcutaneous layer just above the frontalis muscle, were carefully preserved. The underlying scar and fat of the nose were then shaped to bring out the normal concave slope of the nasal sidewall, the gentle valley of the alar groove, the specific slope and bulge of the alar lobule, the linear depressions lying along the nasal dorsum, and the gentle indentation between the alar lobule and the nasal tip (Fig. 9). The rubbery subcutaneous tis-

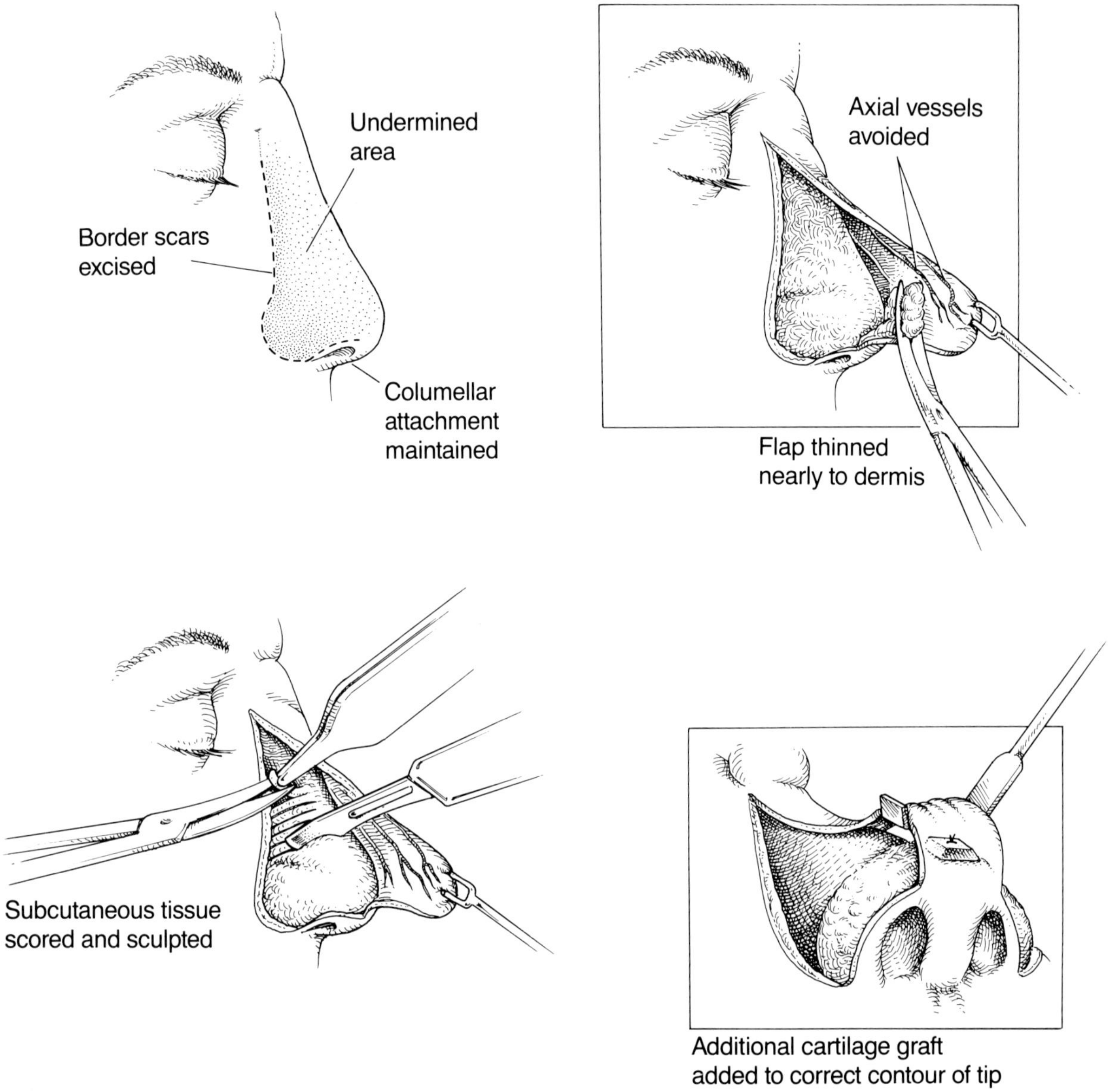

Figure 9 The intermediate operation to refine contour.

sue was scored in parallel strips 1-mm wide and each strip was dissected off with a fine forceps and scissors. This maneuver, which requires patience and a visual aptitude, was repeated again and again until the desired nasal shape was achieved. Because the nasal tip did not project sufficiently, an additional tip graft, styled to Peck's specifications, was implanted atop the nasal scaffold, now solidly imbedded in subcutaneous fat and scar. The newly-thinned forehead flap was then replaced over the nose, employing 6-0 clear subcuticular sutures to anchor it into the alar groove and to strengthen the marginal closure. As a final step, a scalpel was inserted into the right nostril and the Millard ipsilateral septal pedicle was divided, thus opening the airway (Fig. 10).

THE THIRD OPERATION: PEDICLE EXCISION

If the skin pedicle is sectioned and replaced on the forehead, it will remain there permanently as a trap-doored nubbin. It is far more artistic to thin the proximal stump and to trim it to a small inverted V-shape, which is inset just medial to the eyebrow (Fig. 11). The distal part of the forehead pedicle (the part attached to the nose) may be raised up and thinned without trepidation. Even when it is elevated off the nose for 1.5 cm, the cephalic edge of the divided flap bleeds freely.

It may seem prudent to carry the dorsal unit of the nasal flap all the way to the root of the nose. In reality,

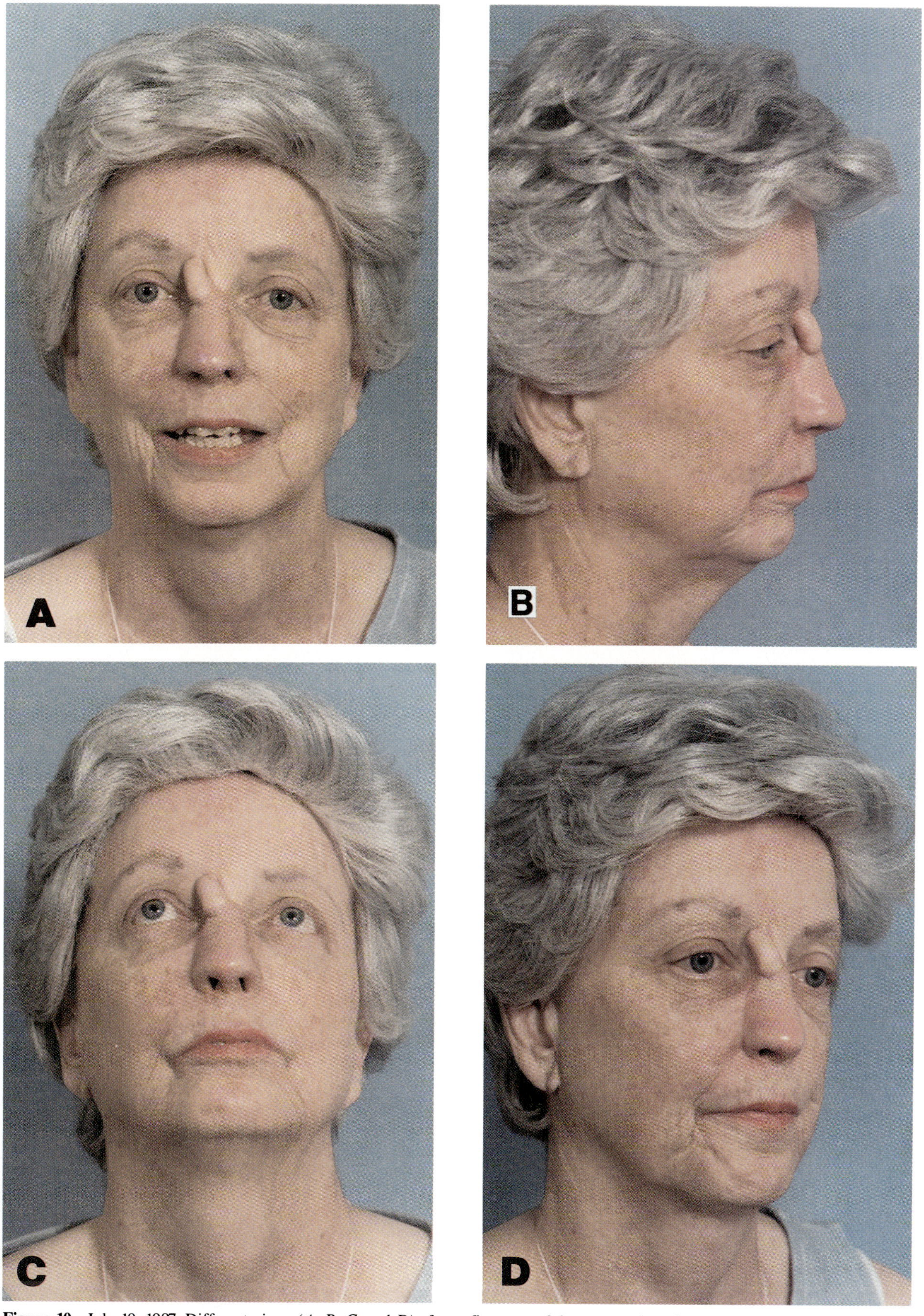

Figure 10 July 10, 1987. Different views (*A, B, C,* and *D)* after refinement of the contour by subcutaneous sculpting and an additional cartilage graft.

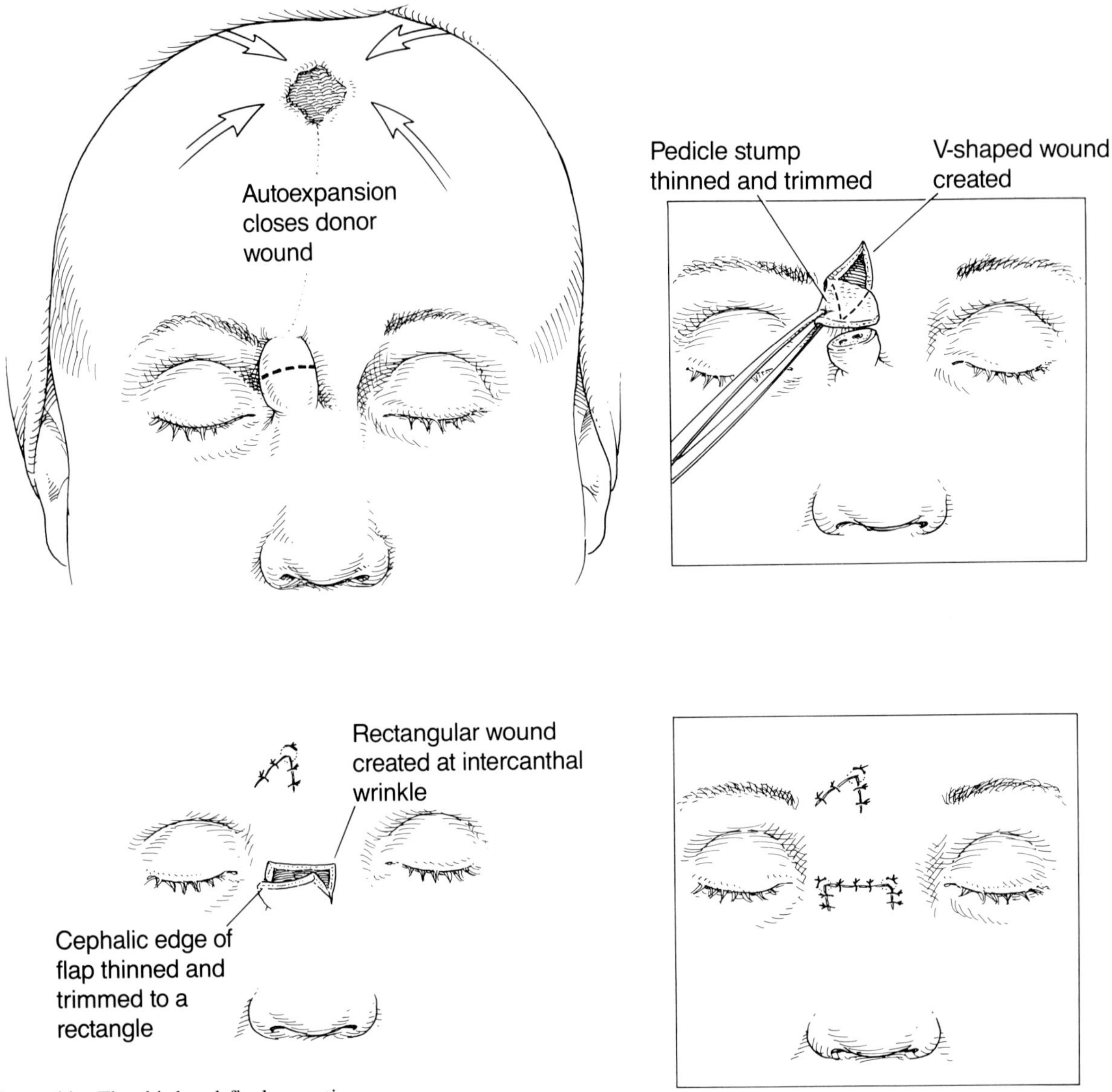

Figure 11 The third and final operation.

it is better to place the superior border of the flap in the inverted U-shaped wrinkle line that runs across the nasal dorsum from canthus to canthus. Then also, the skin flap should remain rather wide and patulous near the root of the nose, and some procerus or frontalis muscle should be preserved over the bone as in a normal nasal root. If this loose, mobile tissue is not preserved, the nasal flap will have the odd appearance of being stuck to the bridge of the nose.

In our patient, an additional 7-week interval passed before the skin pedicle was excised, although 3 weeks is sufficient. The proximal stump and distal end were thinned and trimmed, the bed of scar and fat near the nasal root was shaped, each corner of the squared skin flap was drawn into its angle with a three-point, half-buried mattress suture, and the incisions were closed with simple 6-0 sutures. Several lightly-tied basting or quilting sutures held the flap to its bed.

The Postoperative Period

This patient had understood that a period of collagen hypertrophy and maturation would ensue, during which time the flap would bulge and the border scars would indent, and that the nose would not approach its final shape for at least 4 months (Fig. 12). During this maturation period, she wore a soft, oval silicone tube in each nostril while she slept to brace against scar contraction. Crusting of excess mucous in the large, single nasal cavity required daily cleaning. However, repeated examinations revealed a pink, well-healed cavity and septal edge after 3 months. This restored nose, like all previous ones, had become self-cleansing.

The Era of Contour

Nothing more than lines and patches of light and lines and patches of shadow create the visual impression of a

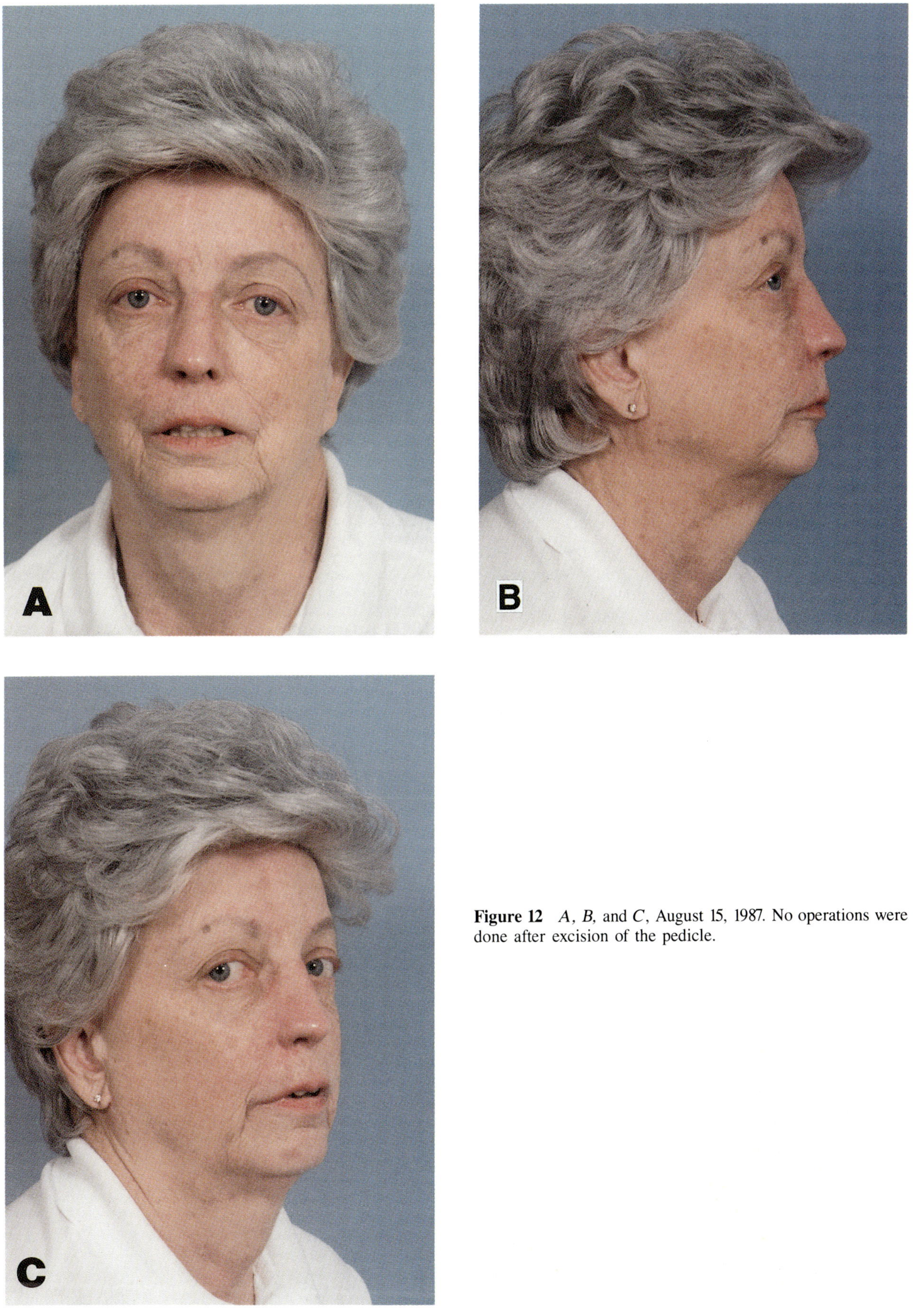

Figure 12 *A*, *B*, and *C*, August 15, 1987. No operations were done after excision of the pedicle.

nose from a lump of transplanted tissues. These alone communicate to our eye that here is a specific shape—palpable and measurable. The creation of meaningful contour requires a visual and artistic aptitude that is not to be confused with intellectual or academic ability or with manual dexterity—it is the capacity to visualize forms in space. Many intelligent and manually adept people do not develop this aptitude, while some dull and manually inept ones do.

Here are four dicta for the era of nasal contour:

1. Choose good materials, i.e., those that are nearly identical to the missing tissues: internal nasal lining flaps, a cartilage graft to replace each missing cartilage, forehead skin cover designed vertically so that it may be thinned and depilated.
2. Demand ideal contour from the outset. It can be achieved at the first operation by careful measurement and a good eye. Carve cartilage grafts to resemble surface units of the nose and assemble from them a frame with a nasal shape. Using an ideal nose or the patient's opposite side as the model, cut a tailored three-dimensional pattern. Then flatten it to two dimensions and use it to achieve a sartorially exact fit. Take no excess with the flap.
3. Anticipate the unrelenting effect of the myofibroblasts. Brace, batten, and buttress all the flimsy lining tissues against their inexorable contraction with cartilage and bone grafts. Design the forehead flap to cover whole units so that the slight inevitable bulge of trapdoor contraction mimics the normal convexity of a dorsum, tip, hemitip, or ala.
4. Do not take lightly the effect of a half millimeter. Our eye makes sophisticated contour judgments of a half millimeter at 30 ft across a crowded room. Judging deformity or beauty is easy and automatic. Knowing what contour has created the visual impression is difficult. As you carve, cut, and stitch each half millimeter, remind yourself that it is shadows cast by these small distances that tell the eye in a half second "Here is a nose, it is normal, it is ideal, it is beautiful."

Armed with these directives, diligence, and a glimmer of visual aptitude, you can evoke from a lump of transplanted tissues the visual impression of a nose. You will know you have been successful when your patient returns months later asking questions about "my nose." He will have to be reminded that it is *not* a nose, nor ever will be. It is gratifying to have fooled the public; but to have fooled the patient, upon whose face the "nose" plainly sits, is the plastic surgeon's finest hour.

SUGGESTED READING

Burget GC, Menick FJ. The subunit principle in nasal reconstruction. Plast Reconstr Surg 1985; 76:239–247.

Gillies HD. Plastic surgery of the face. H. Frowde, London: Hodder & Stoughton, 1920:30.

Menick FJ. Artistry and aesthetic surgery: aesthetic perception and the subunit principle. Clin Plast Surg 1987; 14(4):723–735.

Millard DR. Hemirhinoplasty. Plast Reconstr Surg 1967; 40:440–445.

Millard DR. Reconstructive rhinoplasty for the lower half of the nose. Plast Reconstr Surg 1974; 53:133–139.

Sheen JH, Sheen AP. Aesthetic rhinoplasty. St. Louis, MO: CV Mosby, 1987:38.

AESTHETIC SURGERY: FACE

INTERVIEWING THE PATIENT

JAMES H. WELLS, M.D., F.A.C.S.

Most plastic surgeons spend their training years learning the technical aspects of their craft. Yet one of the most critical areas in dealing with patients is frequently overlooked—the patient interview. Without some interviewing ability, all the marvelous skills that doctors have spent years developing may go for naught. The interview begins, however, long before the physician ever sees the patient. It starts with the receptionist who answers that first phone call, responds to a patient's questions, and schedules the appointment. These activities set the tone for the forthcoming interview.

Each doctor should decide what is his goal for the interview. Some surgeons see this as a time for the hard-sell approach to surgery. Others give a great deal of time to providing information and allowing the patient to get to know them. The interview also allows the physician to know the patient. Patient selection, after all, is one of the most important criteria for a successful surgical outcome. Some physicians utilize a patient counselor or coordinator who conducts the initial interview, while the physician follows up near the end. I am opposed to this. This style gives a very impersonal aspect to the interview, which should, on the contrary, be a very personal activity. Patients should be treated in the manner one would wish to be treated oneself.

The front office is the starting point for the interview. Subsequent to a patient's phone call and appointment scheduling, he or she should be mailed either patient brochures about a particular procedure or general information about the office. General costs regarding the consultation and a confirmed date and time of appointment also should be provided. Many physicians have this information in a standard format. This initial part of the interview is carried out on behalf of the physician. The office should avoid making the patient wait more than 2 weeks for a consultation. Once personal contact with the patient has been established, it may be alright to wait longer between the initial interview and the surgery. This allows adequate time to evaluate the problem and agree upon the proposed surgery and its goals.

Other than contact with the office by telephone, the patient's next impression of the office begins with the waiting room. It should be personalized, comfortable, and nonintimidating. Indirect lighting often allows a more relaxed, homelike environment, thus allowing patients to relax rather than become apprehensive. A second waiting area for postoperative patients, separate from that for new patients, is desirable. New patients do not need to see the immediate postoperative bruising of recent surgery. This may add to their apprehensions and fears. One should give consideration to scheduling new patient visits and postoperative follow-ups at different times to avoid this contact. A second entrance into the office for postsurgical patient visits is helpful.

The patient should not be kept waiting. The doctor must try to remain within 15 minutes of the scheduled appointment time and must allow enough time for the consultation. This varies from 15 to 45 minutes depending on the patient, the problem, and the technique and style of the individual physician. One should apologize, if late, upon entering the consultation room. The patient's anger about waiting could be diffused either by waiving the consultation fee or by paying for his or her parking to show that one cares about one's patients and their time commitment. In the event the appointment has to be cancelled, the patient should be given as much advance notice as possible. The return visit should be rescheduled to accommodate the patient. Again, one should consider waiving the consultation fee for such cancelled appointments.

The examining room is the most usual site for consultations. This is adequate for patients with noncosmetic problems. Cosmetic patients prefer a more casual environment; either the physician's office or a separate consultation room decorated much like a home environment. This area allows soft lighting and facilitates intimate discussions regarding the personal nature of cosmetic surgery. It may be an area where photographs can be taken or other techniques presented to show the patient the nature of the problem and what the proposed correction might entail. This area should convey a suggestion of the physician's own personal tastes and sense of esthetics. There should be adequate space for the patient and at least one family member. I encourage a family member to attend, particularly in noncosmetic surgical cases. Occasionally, one may get a family and many small children. Families should be urged to leave small children at home. If one has a practice of a reconstructive nature where a large number of children are seen, then an area might be provided where children could spend their time with minimal distractions to the interview process. I suggest seeing families with children either early or late in the day in order to minimize office disruptions.

How to address patients is of concern, particularly to older patients. They should be addressed as "Mister" or "Mrs.," along with their last name. Respect should be given for their seniority. Neither front office personnel nor physicians should use a patient's first name unless so directed. Additional terms of endearment such as "dear," "honey," or "sweetheart," are inappropriate forms of address. Each patient has a name and an identity and should be accorded appropriate respect by using that name. It should not be assumed that new patients always know who one is, particularly in an office with multiple physicians. Always introduce oneself upon entering the consultation area and, as mentioned before, if late for the consultation, an apology must be made. Most patients will accept a simple explanation regarding the delay and their anger will be dissipated.

The interview should be conducted while seated. When the physician remains standing, the patient senses that he is in a hurry to get on to the next patient. He should sit down, be relaxed, and indicate that the patient has his undivided attention and no interruptions will be tolerated. Office personnel should be instructed on the policy for phone calls and interruptions. The interview can continue uninterrupted if one takes emergency-only or physician-only phone calls. When the interview begins to take longer than anticipated, it may be necessary to interrupt it to see other patients who require limited time. This may be done by moving the patient to another examining room, to change clothes, to obtain photographs, or to consult with other office personnel regarding fees, scheduling of surgery, cosmetic care, or makeup activities. The physician may then return as appropriate and complete the consultation.

Physical appearance is important. Patients prefer to see a physician dressed in a white lab coat and normal clothing. A recent survey indicated that patients do not care to see physicians in operating scrubs during a consultation. One should be conservative in dress and style. Multiple gold chains around the neck, a flashy appearance, and too slick a look tend to detract from one's image as a physician and from the respect patients would like to give their doctor. Most patients still view the physician conservatively in the old "family doctor" way.

Many physicians have their receptionist inquire of the patient as to the reason for the consultation. Some topics, however, are very private and patients may give a totally different reason for the consultation to the front office. One should not assume that what the receptionist was told is the true reason for the visit, so one should ask the patient again why he or she has come. The interview may start with a statement such as "How can I help you?" My inclination is to listen first. We were all taught in medical school that the patient will tell his or her story and indicate what the problem is and we must allow time for this. After listening to the patient, I am impressed that surgeons do not need to "sell surgery." A patient would not be in the office unless he or she were considering surgery. The patient's purpose is to tell his or her story, obtain information, learn about the physician as a surgeon and compare him with other surgeons who may have been consulted, and see how attentive the office is to patient needs. If their agenda is fulfilled, most patients will schedule with that physician.

A little small talk before the formal interview begins does several things. It helps relax the apprehensive patient and allows him or her to know the physician a little better, while at the same time the latter obtains a sense of the patient's values. For example, knowing what the patient does and whether he or she is employed or unemployed, gives an idea where he or she perceives him or herself to be on the socioeconomic scale. A better idea may emerge of how important it is for this particular patient to have a facelift and be accepted in her social circles, or whether it is being done for job retention. This should come out in the interview with the patient in any event. When a child is the patient, one should talk to the youngster in a playful manner to ease any fears. Parents want to know how a physician relates to their child. When they sense compassion and caring, a great deal has been done toward establishing a patient–physician relationship that will endure.

Brochures can be helpful. As part of the interview process, they should be mailed by the front office at the time of scheduling. The patient thereby gains insight about the procedure before meeting the physician. Brochures are available through national specialty societies, prepared commercially, or written individually to reflect personal preferences. If some type of printed material is given to all patients, it has been known to support a physician's informed consent concept in litigated cases. The use of photographs for difficult problems that the patient may have trouble conceptualizing may be alright. However, one must be careful about implied guaranteed results. The few times that I have shown patients pre- and postoperative photographs of other patients, they have focused on the results illustrated, and totally disregarded the possible outcome of their own surgery. When they did not get exactly the same results, they were extremely unhappy. If one were to be totally honest with regard to photographs, I feel one would have to show pictures of all patients treated and let the new patients decide the outcome and results for themselves. This is clearly an unrealistic choice. A little bit left to the patient's imagination regarding the final outcome has, in my experience, provided a more satisfied patient. The use of image computers, currently very popular, is a two-edged sword. Some patients realize this is merely an idea-tool that suggests a possible surgical result. Others focus on the image created by the computer and interpret it as their own expected surgical result—only to be left disappointed postoperatively. Disclaimers must be made! Patients must understand that this is merely a tool to help them visualize the possible results of surgery. It must not be an implied result of the proposed surgery.

Semantics during the consultation are important. I try to avoid words that suggest pain, disfigurement, or prolonged illness. Alternative wording that still conveys the seriousness of surgery, or possible untoward results, is better accepted. If asked about complications, one must not be afraid to admit that they do occur. However, this should be followed with an explanation of how that complication may be dealt with to obtain the desired result. The patient must understand that one is prepared to take care of him or her in any event.

Preparation of the patient for examination may be done by oneself or the staff. When the patient needs to disrobe, one should indicate what clothing needs to be removed. Alternative cover-up clothing should be provided. When the examination is to be in another room, the patient should be transferred there before disrobing. The physician should leave the room while the patient changes and should not merely tell the patient to remove her blouse or lift her skirt to show the area of concern. New patients should never disrobe before meeting the physician. It is advisable to have a female attendant present for examination of all female patients. Photographs of breasts or full body shots where total nudity is required may best be done by someone of the same sex, or with an attendant present. Immediately after the photography, the patient should be allowed to cover up or get dressed. If the patient's problem can be discussed after he or she has dressed, the doctor should step out of the examining room and return for the discussion a few minutes later. During the examination, any asymmetries and variations of body parts from the normal should be pointed out. This is often a surprise for patients, who frequently do not appreciate the amount of asymmetry each of us exhibits. Photographic documentation of "before and after" surgery is an important part of this interview process. Nelson and Krause's recently published book is an excellent and complete discussion of this topic.

A second consultation is often held several weeks after the first. This allows the patient time to consider the proposed surgery; its risks and benefits. It allows time for additional thoughts, both by the patient and surgeon. For rhinoplasty consultations, I frequently ask patients to return with photographs of noses esthetically pleasing to them. Not infrequently, their initial expectations are unrealistic as seen from the photographs they have selected. This allows me adequate time to help them lower these unrealistic expectations to an acceptable level. It also allows me to exclude the potential problem patient, whom I may have missed on my first interview, from my list of surgical candidates. I encourage the patient to bring a spouse or family member to the second consultation. This gives me the opportunity to meet the family before the immediate postoperative period. If any problems should occur during surgery, which I need to discuss with the family, a previously developed rapport proves most helpful. If one does not take time to develop this rapport before surgery, there will never be time to develop it afterwards. There is no rush to schedule elective surgery. The preoperative period is the time for careful thought and preparation for what one hopes will be an uncomplicated and successful surgical outcome. I do not charge for this second visit as I consider it a continuation of my initial consultation.

Discussion of fees is a difficult problem for most physicians. Most of us prefer to leave the business end of the practice to our front office and deal personally only with the surgical aspect. That is my preference. My front office has indicated to me that I tend to give surgery away when I get involved in the discussion of surgical fees. For that reason, when patients ask me the cost of surgery, I refer them to my office manager who gives them a written quotation. Once the fees are written down and the financial relationship with the office is established, we have very few problems regarding fees. It is also important to be a patient advocate in the event of an underpaid insurance claim. The writing of letters on behalf of patients to an insurance company or to insurance review committees is beneficial with regard to establishing rapport.

Within that initial consultation, some provision for secondary surgery needs to be made. The patient needs to understand what the possibility is for a secondary procedure and what his or her financial obligation might be. One must be very clear as to what one expects of the patient as well. If one wishes to waive all surgical fees, that is fine, but it must be made clear. If one wishes to charge for supplies only, again it must be made very clear so the patient understands his or her financial obligation.

Follow-up to surgery is another part of the interview. Clearly, when the patient is pleased with the results and with the surgeon, many referrals follow. "Before and after" photographs, given to the patient after surgery, allow him or her to show and convey feelings about you and the experience. I believe this is an extension of the interview process. If, on the other hand, the patient is unhappy with the surgical results, one should listen carefully and not write the patient off as just another complainer. This situation requires a willingness to listen to criticism of one's work and the outcome. If a simple secondary procedure can solve the problem, it should be done and the costs absorbed. When the problem is something anticipated within the possible outcomes of surgery during the first interview, then provision should have been made to handle it during discussions about possible secondary procedures.

It helps during the interview to establish a time period in which the physician will return phone calls or answer additional questions. I encourage patients to call back following their initial consultation to clarify points or ask additional questions. I do not expect any of them to remember everything that is discussed and I tell them this. One of the most difficult things is to refuse to do surgery. But there are occasions when surgeons must not operate and, in fact, must bluntly and firmly indicate to patients that surgery is not indicated and that they are poor candidates for it. Financial considerations must not cloud surgical judgment. This may be the most difficult thing to do for a surgeon just beginning his practice.

My previous comments make it plain that I try to run a very open office and make both my staff and myself very accessible. This takes a great deal of time. However, I feel good that my patients and I are able to establish an excellent rapport before the surgery as a result of this style of practice. I believe it has generated many referrals and, in the event of surgical complications, we have been able to work through the problem with patient and family.

A final comment as regards fees and the cost of

delivering health care. Although we are all experiencing an increase in the cost of delivering health care, fees should be established at a reasonable level that avoids "nickel and diming" patients. They should preferably not be billed for every activity performed on their behalf. Fees should be written off if one feels it appropriate. Fee discussion may be delegated to the office manager but the physician must maintain control and awareness of what is happening in the office. There are numerous stories of embezzlement and fraud perpetrated within offices in the name of physicians.

One should put oneself in the position of the patient and decide how one would like to be treated. The idea of undergoing elective surgery for whatever reason should be made as pleasant and as comfortable as possible. The patient interview and the initial contact with the physician and office staff establish the tenor of all current and future relationships with patients.

SUGGESTED READING

Nelson GD, Krause JL Jr. Clinical photography in plastic surgery. Boston: Little, Brown, 1988.

OFFICE SURGERY

GUSTAVO A. COLON, M.D., F.A.C.S.

Ambulatory surgery in the past 10 years has risen rapidly because of consumers' needs for less expensive health care of excellent quality and convenience. The major stimulus for its conception and maturation has been a savings in health care cost, which is passed on to the patient. Three ambulatory surgical concepts have developed. The first one is a hospital outpatient facility, attached to the hospital's operating rooms, which may have separate beds or recovery units for ambulatory or outpatient surgery. The second is a freestanding surgical facility, not associated or attached to any hospital, which treats ambulatory surgery patients but has no facilities for overnight or long-term recovery. The third concept is the office surgical facility, which is usually a specialty facility attached to a physician's office.

Obviously, the reason for ambulatory surgical facilities is to decrease the cost to patients. There is no question that outpatient surgery decreases the ultimate cost to both the patient and third party payers. Patients, in particular, like the global, or total, charges because they know exactly what the surgical procedure, anesthesia, and recovery room costs will be. These costs are less because office and ambulatory surgical facilities require fewer staff than hospitals.

GENERAL PATIENT SELECTION AND CRITERIA

Elective procedures for cosmetic surgery lend themselves extremely well to outpatient office surgery. The only limiting factors are medical contraindications that may require hospitalization. However, all office facilities must be equipped to handle any necessary medical or surgical emergency. Age should only be a consideration if the patient's general health warrants careful postoperative monitoring in a hospital setting. Otherwise, if the patient's general health is good, I do not hesitate to treat patients in ambulatory surgical settings, unless they need to have other procedures performed, either at the time of the initial operation or secondarily, that would require hospitalization.

It is imperative that all outpatients have someone drive them home. Also, the patient should arrange to have someone spend the day and evening of surgery with them, as well as the following day. All patients are called by the office staff during the evening after surgery and the following day to check on their condition. Specific postoperative orders are given to the patient. These orders are given, both written and verbally, to the individual who will take care of the patient when he or she is discharged from the surgical ambulatory facility. Patients who come from out of town are sent either to convalescent care centers or to their hotel. Occasionally, a patient will request transfer to a hospital after the ambulatory surgery. This is arranged with the hospital, so that the patient can be admitted for a one or two-day hospitalization after the surgery.

Coexisting medical problems must be evaluated preoperatively. While they may not contraindicate outpatient surgery, each case has to be evaluated individually. Heart disease, pulmonary disease, diabetes, or any chronic illness that may require hospitalization or intensive postoperative care, certainly negate ambulatory surgery. Also, patients who seem to be high anesthetic risks should not be treated in an ambulatory surgical facility. Office surgical suites should be a safe surgical environment where elective surgery assures predictable results.

SURGICAL PROCEDURES

Category of Operations

1. Many reconstructive plastic surgical procedures that do not invade body cavities and do not require long-term care or multiple procedures can be done on an outpatient basis.
2. Most esthetic surgery can be done safely and economically for the patient in an office surgical suite.

3. Hand surgery is very amenable to outpatient surgery since many procedures can be done under local or regional block anesthesia. Most elective hand surgery today is done on an outpatient basis in either a hospital ambulatory surgical setting or a freestanding surgical facility.
4. Pediatric plastic surgery can be done on an outpatient basis. Pediatric operations are one of the most common types of outpatient surgery e.g., tonsillectomy, herniorrhaphy. These procedures generally are done in a freestanding surgical facility or the hospital outpatient facility. I have found that in an office surgery facility the recovery facilities for children are not as adequate as in the hospital. Office facilities have physical restraints in equipment size, i.e., they are designed for adults. Therefore surgeons with office operating facilities generally do not do a great volume of pediatric surgery.

SUPPORTING FACILITIES

Radiologic diagnostic facilities and pathology (either frozen of permanent sections) are contracted to outside consultants. These consultants service, supply, and support these outpatient facilities. Blood and blood substitutes are included.

INSPECTION AND ACCREDITATION

Inspection and accreditation of hospital facilities has been primarily done by the Joint Commission for Accreditation of Hospitals (JCAH). Freestanding ambulatory surgical facilities also are inspected by the JCAH as well as by the Accreditation Association for Ambulatory Health Care Facilities (AAAHC). This is an association that can accredit both freestanding surgical facilities and office facilities. Specialty facilities such as plastic surgery are now being accredited by the American Association for Ambulatory Plastic Surgical Facilities (AAAPSF). This association classifies office facilities into:

Class A A facility in which minor plastic surgical procedures are performed under local, regional, or topical anesthesia.

Class B A facility in which both minor and major plastic surgery procedures are performed under intravenous or parenteral sedation: analgesia or disassociative drugs.

Class C A facility in which major plastic surgical procedures are performed under general anesthesia that requires external support of vital body functions.

No facilities are accredited for elective surgery of major body cavities. Certain states, such as the state of Louisiana, have specific accreditation criteria and licensing for ambulatory surgical facilities. Accreditation of freestanding surgical facilities and hospital facilities generally requires acquisition of a certificate of need from a state licensing board. However, at the present time, office facilities do not require this type of certification, nor do they require state licensing.

Applicable State and City Laws Regarding Such Facilities

At present, there are no federal guidelines for ambulatory surgical facilities. In 1983, the Federal Government outlined guidelines for reimbursement from Medicare to ambulatory surgical facilities. Individual states have rules and regulations for Medicaid reimbursements to ambulatory surgical facilities. These may vary from state to state. It is imperative, at the present time, that all physicians who do outpatient surgery make both State and Federal Governments aware of the cost savings that can be incurred through encouragement and promotion of outpatient surgery.

REIMBURSEMENT

At the present time, all ambulatory surgical facilities are well regarded by the insurance companies, which feel that ambulatory surgery is cost-saving for the third-party payers. It minimizes hospitalization and, obviously, the cost to the patient and the insurance company. One of the factors that has made reimbursement to free ambulatory surgical facilities and office surgical facilities very desirable to insurance companies is that these facilities can offer global, or total, procedure charges, i.e., charges per operative procedure rather than charges per time, unit or operation, or per item used in the outpatient facility. Reimbursement for outpatient surgery in hospital facilities and freestanding facilities is now routinely done by third-party payers. Office surgical facilities, as they become more numerous and accredited, are being treated by insurance companies in the same fashion as freestanding and hospital facilities.

ADVANTAGES AND DISADVANTAGES

Hospital outpatient surgical facilities are patient effective in that they increase the volume of patients processed through the hospital operating room, but they are not really cost effective. Because hospital outpatient facilities are usually very successful, they begin to help carry the financial losses in other parts of the hospital. This causes the charges for ambulatory surgery to rise. Ultimately, the cost of outpatient surgery equals the cost of inpatient surgery, without the costs of hospital room.

Freestanding surgical facilities have paved the way for ambulatory surgery and they have succeeded because:

1. They reduce health care cost.
2. More than 40 percent of all elective surgical procedures, can be performed on an outpatient basis.
3. The charges of freestanding surgical facilities can be at least half the comparable hospital outpatient costs.
4. They are financially viable. Ambulatory surgical facilities can lower community costs because: (a) they eliminate overnight hospital stay, thereby decreasing personnel cost; (b) some unnecessary diagnostic tests and non essential drugs can be eliminated; (c) they uti-

lize their facilities and staff much more efficiently; and (d) there is an easier recovery period at home for the patients.

Office and specialty facilities have other specific advantages in that they not only reduce the cost of surgical care but they also make more effective use of physician's time because:

1. Time consuming hospital formalities are reduced.
2. There is more efficient time use because the physician is in his office; between operations he can do some office work and even see other patients.
3. Freestanding ambulatory surgical and office facilities provide a comfortable setting for patient and family.
4. These facilities streamline the delivery of surgical services because the operations can be patient specific and procedure specific, with less waste and more privacy. This has a great patient appeal, as well as convenience for both the patient and surgeon.
5. There are economic advantages to the patient because secondary procedures can be done in an office facility at, perhaps, no charge to the patient.

Ambulatory surgical facilities stress that they have a lower infection rate than hospitals because they are dealing with a more healthy patient population.

Office surgical facilities have the same experience. Not only do they have a healthier population, but, since fewer doctors use the facilities and the procedures are usually unispecialty, the infection rate is even lower. In our surgical facility, surgi-unit, in over 2,000 procedures done over 9 years we have had no infections.

The disadvantages of outpatient office surgery are:

1. Patients' resistance because they are used to going to the hospital.
2. Physicians' resistance because they are used to operating in more familiar surroundings, and are creatures of habit.
3. Reduced hospital income.
4. Loss of contact with colleagues in the hospital.

ESTHETIC PROCEDURES THAT CAN BE DONE IN OFFICE SURGICAL SUITES

While many minor surgical procedures can be done on an outpatient basis, experience shows that many more procedures of esthetic surgery can be done in our office surgical facility. The program that we have in our surgi-unit involves informing the patient completely about preoperative arrangments. The patient is seen in the first office visit by our patient coordinator, who instructs and advises him or her about the operative procedures and shows them videotapes—not only of the facility, but also of the procedure that is to be performed. The patient is then scheduled for surgery and, during a preoperative visit, he or she is given the *postoperative* medication. There is no *preoperative* medication given except at the time of initial evaluation on the morning of surgery. The patient has the following laboratory work done: urinalysis, complete blood count, partial thromboplastin time test, electrolytes, electrocardiogram, and chest x-ray study, as necessary and required by the physician. Preoperative instructions are given at that time. On the morning of surgery, the patient comes in and has taken no medication. He or she is given Ativan, per body weight, intravenously 20 minutes before surgery; then, if local standby anesthesia is to be used, he or she is given a combination of Ativan and Sublimaze (Tables I and II). The patient then undergoes the surgical procedure. Since our surgi-unit is a class C facility, procedures can be done either with local standby anesthesia, or general anesthesia, with or without intubation.

Facial esthetic procedures that can be done in the office facility are facelifts with coronal lifts, blepharoplasties, rhinoplasties, otoplasties, liposuction of the head and neck, mentoplasties or chin implants, scar revisions, dermabrasions, excision of multiple facial lesions, and reconstruction. Body contouring procedures can also be done—usually under general anesthesia. These procedures are liposuction of the trunk, abdomen, and extremities. Even a small, lower abdominoplasty can be done. As regards breast surgery, breast augmentation is certainly done on an outpatient basis in our facility, as well as mastopexies, small reduction mammoplasties, breast reconstructions with expanders or with implants, and removal of gynecomastia.

We find that many more operative procedures that fall within the armamentarium of the plastic surgeon can now be done within an office surgical facility because of the increase in third party payers who require outpatient surgery for cost containment.

The office surgical facility receives the third party reimbursement.

The future of office surgery is limitless. We, as the leaders in office surgery, must inspect, accredit, and strive for excellence, safety, and security for our patients in all

TABLE 1 Sedation Dosages

Ativan (Lorazepam) 0.04 mg/kg	Intravenously push slowly 20 min preoperatively.
Sublimaze (Fentanyl) 0.05 mg/cc	½ cc intravenously push initially before surgery and ½ cc every half hr as needed Total Range: 2–6 cc

TABLE 2 Procedures Done in Surgi-Unit Using Ativan-Sublimaze

1981–1983 (36 Months)

Augmentation mammoplasty	207	Mentoplasty	14
Mastopexy	27	Coronal lift	15
Breast reconstruction	10	Otoplasty	5
Rhytidectomy	62	Gynecomastia	7
Blepharoplasty	71	Suction lipectomy	28
Rhinoplasty	135	Other local/standby surgical procedures	286

Total Procedures 867

office surgical facilities, and zealously guard against the lure of entrepreneurism and unqualified office surgical facilities.

SUGGESTED READING

Bredlove B. Successful management of ambulatory surgery programs. American Health Consultants, 1985.

Courtiss E. Office surgery. Clin Plast Surg 1983; 10(2):221–359.

Coleman WP III, Colon GA, Davis S. Out-patient surgery of the skin. New York: Medical Examination Publishing Co., 1983.

Goldsmith SB. Ambulatory surgery. Rockville, MD: Aspen Publishers, 1977.

O'Donovan TR. Ambulatory surgical centers: development & management. Rockville, MD: Aspen Publishers, 1976.

Schultz RC. Out-patient surgery. Philadelphia: Lea & Febiger, 1979.

ANESTHESIA FOR COSMETIC SURGERY

NECITA ROA, M.D.

Anesthesia for cosmetic surgical procedures should provide a smooth and complication free anesthetic, optimal perioperative conditions without invasive monitoring, minimal perioperative patient discomfort, and short anesthesia recovery period without side effects. These can be achieved by: (1) considerable attention to detail, (2) optimal preoperative preparation, (3) optimal sedation for surgical procedures under local anesthesia, (4) use of techniques to avoid bucking, coughing, and vomiting during anesthetic emergence and tracheal extubation, (5) maintenance of low-normal blood pressure and slow heart rate intraoperatively to provide a relatively dry surgical field, (6) judicious use of local anesthetic and vasoconstrictor drugs, and (7) use of techniques, drugs, and drug dosages that permit a rapid and nearly complete anesthesia recovery with minimal side effects.

PREMEDICATION

Premedicant drugs are usually not given preoperatively, since patients are not seen by the anesthesiologist until shortly before surgery. For maximal effectiveness, these drugs should be given at least an hour before the procedure.

Sedative and anxiolytic drugs are not given preoperatively to ensure rapid recovery from anesthesia, to enable the anesthesiologist to do a thorough preanesthetic evaluation and discuss with the patient the planned anesthetic management, and to obtain informed consent. If indicated, these drugs are administered as soon as the intravenous is started. If the patient is extremely apprehensive, diazepam (0.1 to 0.2 mg per kilogram) or midazolam (0.08 to 0.1 mg per kilogram) is given orally 1 to 2 hours preoperatively with a sip of water.

Despite the usual overnight fasting, cosmetic patients usually have large acidic gastric fluid volumes because of preoperative apprehension and anxiety. Since these patients are at risk for aspiration, those who require deeper sedation and general anesthesia are given histamine H_2-receptor antagonists (cimetidine or ranitidine) and metoclopramide preoperatively, orally or intravenously. This drug combination is effective in reducing gastric volume, raising gastric pH, and reducing the incidence of postoperative nausea and vomiting.

Cimetidine is the most commonly used histamine H_2-receptor antagonist. The recommended dose regimen is 300 mg, orally or intramuscularly, 1 to 1.5 hours prior to anesthesia and surgery. Peak effects following oral or intramuscular administration are usually achieved in 60 to 90 minutes and last for approximately 4 hours. Despite its slightly more rapid onset intravenously (45 to 60 minutes), intravenous administration of the drug is usually avoided because of the possibility of bradycardia and hypotension with rapid administration.

We prefer to use *ranitidine*, rather than cimetidine, with metoclopramide preoperatively because of its longer action, lower incidence of adverse reactions, and less interference with the metabolism of other drugs. It is usually given orally with a sip of water 1 to 2 hours preoperatively at a dosage of 150 mg. If this is not possible, 1 mg per kilogram of ranitidine is given as soon as the intravenous is started. Maximal effect occurs in 60 to 90 minutes and lasts for approximately 6 to 8 hours.

Metoclopramide increases lower esophageal sphincter pressure, speeds gastric emptying time, and has antiemetic properties. It is usually given orally 1 to 2 hours preoperatively, if feasible, or as soon as the intravenous is started. Effects are evident 30 to 60 minutes after oral administration and 1 to 3 minutes after intravenous injection. For maximal efficacy, the drug is given in combination with H_2-receptor antagonists at least an hour preoperatively and prior to the administration of narcotic analgesics.

Metoclopramide has been proven to be relatively safe in the dose range commonly employed (10 to 20 mg). Agitation, irritability, and extrapyramidal symptoms may occur with rapid intravenous injection, especially in children and at higher dosages. These adverse effects are infrequent with the oral dosage and with slow infusion of the drug. Because of its dopaminergic receptor-blocking property, the drug is not used in elderly patients and is contraindicated in patients with Parkinson's disease.

To avoid exaggerated perioperative elevations in blood pressure, *antihypertensive medications* are given orally with sips of water on the morning of surgery and continued up to the time of surgery. To avoid rebound hypertension postoperatively, clonidine is given until immediately prior to surgery.

LOCAL ANESTHESIA WITH SEDATION

Most cosmetic surgical procedures are done under local anesthesia for cost containment, for its simplicity and inherent safety, and because of the surgeon's fear of bucking, straining, and vomiting during emergence from general anesthesia and in the immediate postoperative period. Simple procedures such as scar revision, excision of cysts and nevi, and revision of pierced ears are done under local anesthesia without sedation. Intravenous sedation is indicated for procedures such as rhytidectomy, blepharoplasty, rhinoplasty, coronal lift, and chin augmentation to minimize the patient's discomfort and awareness during the infiltration of the local anesthetic and to enable the patient to lie still comfortably on the operating table for the duration of the procedure.

Optimal sedation can be achieved by a combination of drugs, carefully titrated to the point where the patient appears to be asleep, yet is fully oriented and cooperative when spoken to. A properly sedated patient is drowsy but cooperative, amnesic, analgesic, and with no circulatory or respiratory depression. Our practice is to give carefully titrated doses of the following drugs:

1. For procedures 2 hours or less: intravenous fentanyl (1 to 2 μg per kilogram) followed 3 to 5 minutes later by titrated doses of diazepam (in 2.5-mg increments every 2 to 5 minutes up to total dosage to 0.15 to 0.2 mg per kilogram) or midazolam (in 1-mg increments every 1 to 2 minutes up to a total dosage of 0.1 mg per kilogram). Supplemental doses of diazepam (2.5 to 5.0 mg) or midazolam (1.0 to 2.0 mg, in 1-mg increments) are administered as necessary to maintain the desired level of sedation throughout the procedure.
2. For procedures 4 hours or more: intravenous lorazepam (0.03 to 0.04 mg per kilogram; maximum dosage of 2 mg), followed 20 to 25 minutes later by morphine sulfate (in 2-mg increments up to total dosage of 0.1 to 0.15 mg per kilogram) and 1.25 mg of droperidol to prevent nausea and vomiting.
3. Intravenous thiopental (1 to 2 mg per kilogram) or methohexital (0.25 to 0.5 mg per kilogram) is usually given in addition to the above sedation to produce a brief period of sleep during the injection of the local anesthetic.
4. Subanesthetic or analgesic dose of ketamine (0.5 to 0.7 mg per kilogram) intravenously during extensive local anesthetic infiltration or painful block, to minimize the dose of narcotic analgesics.

Diazepam is the most frequently used benzodiazepine in anesthesia and is a valuable adjunct to local anesthesia. Intravenously, it provides short-term light sleep and anterograde amnesia, reduces perioperative anxiety, and increases convulsive threshold for local anesthetics. It has a wide margin of safety; clinically significant respiratory and cardiovascular depression are usually not seen with a carefully titrated intravenous dose of 0.2 mg per kilogram. Its main drawbacks are pain on injection, increased incidence of thrombophlebitis, and prolonged drowsiness with repeated injections because of the cumulative effects of its pharmacologically active metabolites.

In combination with narcotic analgesics, the dosage of diazepam is significantly reduced. To avoid significant respiratory depression, it is titrated in 2.5-mg increments (1.25-mg increments in the elderly) until slurring of speech occurs. Anterograde amnesia and soporific effects are usually achieved within 3 to 5 minutes and last for at least 30 minutes. To maintain optimal level of sedation, additional doses of 2.5 to 5 mg are usually required every 30 to 60 minutes.

Midazolam is a water-soluble short-acting benzodiazepine, 1.5 to 2 times more potent than diazepam. Like diazepam, it increases convulsive threshold for local anesthetics and produces a short period of light sleep, mild sedation, and anterograde amnesia. The duration of amnesia produced is dose-dependent—20 to 30 minutes with 5 mg, 40 minutes with 0.15 mg per kilogram, and 60 to 90 minutes with 0.2 to 0.25 mg per kilogram. Its advantages over diazepam include: (1) rapid onset, (2) it can be given intramuscularly and intravenously without producing pain on injection, (3) lower incidence of venous irritation and thrombophlebitis, and (4) less cumulative effect and more rapid recovery after multiple doses (shorter elimination half-life and lack of active metabolites).

The use of midazolam intramuscularly preoperatively is not recommended, especially in the elderly, because of the unpredictable response of the patient to a given dose of the drug. Loss of consciousness and significant respiratory depression have occurred. At a dose of 0.07 to 0.08 mg per kilogram, sedative effects are evident in 15 minutes, with peak sedation occurring 30 to 60 minutes after injection.

For conscious sedation, midazolam can be used alone or in combination with a narcotic immediately before the procedure. In combination with narcotic analgesics, the drug is carefully titrated to avoid significant respiratory depression, or apnea, and hypotension. It is given intravenously in 1-mg increments, every 1 to 2 minutes, until the desired effect is reached. Sedation is usually achieved within 3 to 5 minutes. Additional doses are usually required every 20 to 30 minutes, one-quarter of the initial dose, to maintain the desired level of sedation.

Lorazepam provides the sedation required for long surgical procedures such as rhinoplasty and rhytidectomy. It produces a unique type of sedation wherein the patient appears to be asleep, yet is fully oriented when spoken to. Sedation after intravenous injection is usually achieved in 15 to 30 minutes (in 2 hours after oral or intramuscular administration) and lasts for 6 to 8 hours. The duration of amnesia with lorazepam alone is 30 minutes with 2 mg and 4 hours with 4 mg. Because of its prolonged clinical half-life, repeated doses are unnecessary.

To avoid oversedation and prolonged recovery, we

limit the dosage to a maximum of 2 mg intravenously. Additional sedation is provided by morphine sulfate (0.1 to 0.15 mg per kilogram), droperidol 1.25 mg, and subanesthetic doses of thiopental or methohexital, if indicated. This regimen provides consistent anterograde amnesia for at least 1.5 to 2 hours.

Ketamine produces a dissociative state characterized by catalepsy, light sedation, amnesia, and marked analgesia. Onset of anesthesia is rapid following intravenous injection (within 60 seconds) but is not clear-cut, as patients appear to gaze into space and may not close their eyes for several minutes. Sleep is usually accompanied by nystagmus, lacrimation, and involuntary movements of the extremities. The analgesic effect of ketamine outlasts the duration of sleep. Consciousness usually returns in about 10 to 15 minutes after an intravenous dose of 2 mg per kilogram, but the analgesic effect persists for about 40 minutes. Because of the possibility of intraoperative excitatory phenomena and the high incidence of postanesthetic emergence reactions, that range from less than 5 to greater than 30 percent, the use of this drug in cosmetic surgical patients is usually avoided unless absolutely necessary.

Satisfactory operating conditions, minimal postanesthetic side effects, and rapid recovery from anesthesia can be achieved if subanesthetic doses of ketamine are used in combination with lorazepam or diazepam and low-dose narcotics, and administered only to produce brief amnesia and profound analgesia during infiltration of local anesthetics. The onset of analgesia with low-dose ketamine (0.5 to 0.7 mg per kilogram intravenously) occurs within 1 minute and lasts for about 5 to 8 minutes. Excitatory phenomena, unpleasant dreams, and hallucinations occur infrequently with this technique. Intraoperative excitatory phenomena may be terminated by lowdose thiopental (1 to 2 mg per kilogram intravenously).

To achieve optimal sedation, *narcotics* are used in combination with either benzodiazepines or barbiturates. These drugs enhance the effects of sedative drugs and minimize discomfort during infiltration of the local anesthetic.

In combination with lorazepam, *morphine* proves optimal sedation for rhinoplasty and rhytidectomy. It should be given intravenously, in carefully titrated doses, 20 to 30 minutes after the intravenous administration of lorazepam. Its analgesic effect starts immediately and peaks in 20 minutes. Respiratory depression occurs approximately 7 to 10 minutes after intravenous administration, peaks in 15 to 30 minutes, and may last for as long as 4 to 5 hours.

Fentanyl, a synthetic opioid, is 50 to 100 times more potent than morphine. It is given intravenously in dosages of 1 to 2 μg per kilogram. Its peak analgesic effect occurs within 2 minutes and lasts for 30 to 60 minutes. Respiratory depression is maximal in 5 to 10 minutes and returns to normal in 1 hour. With these dosages, the incidence of nausea and vomiting is very low.

GENERAL ANESTHESIA

Abdominoplasty, augmentation mammoplasty, mastopexy, reduction mammoplasty, and suction lipectomy are done under general anesthesia. In our unit, rhinoplasties and an increasing number of procedures combining rhytidectomy, blepharoplasty, and brow-lift are now done under general endotracheal anesthesia instead of local anesthesia with intravenous sedation. General anesthesia ensures adequate oxygenation and ventilation, minimizes the risk of aspiration, shortens surgical time, and permits a more rapid discharge from the recovery room to the self-care unit.

The choice of general anesthetic techniques depends on the skill and experience of the anesthesiologist and the medical condition of the patient. Anesthetic techniques should provide optimal operative conditions, ensure a prompt and nearly complete recovery with minimal side effects, and minimize the possibility of postoperative bleeding and hematoma formation. These goals can be accomplished by: (1) administration of a smooth general anesthetic, (2) maintenance of low-normal blood pressure and slow heart rate intraoperatively to provide a relatively dry surgical field, (3) smooth anesthetic emergence and endotracheal extubation, (4) use of minimal dosage of anesthetic drugs to ensure rapid anesthetic recovery, and (5) use of minimal dosage of narcotics to avoid postoperative nausea and vomiting.

Premedication

Sedative-anxiolytic drugs and narcotic-analgesics are not given preoperatively. The only medications given preoperatively are: (1) cimetidine or ranitidine, (2) metoclopramide, and (3) antihypertensive medications.

Induction

Anesthesia is induced with minimal doses of an ultrashort-acting barbiturate (sodium thiopental or methohexital) 3 to 5 minutes after the intravenous administration of fentanyl (1 to 2 μg per kilogram) and glycopyrrolate (0.2 mg). As soon as the patient is unconscious and ventilation by mask is possible, a nondepolarizing muscle-relaxant drug is administered to facilitate endotracheal intubation. The patient is then ventilated by mask with nitrous oxide (N_2O) and O_2 (50:50) and 2 to 4 percent enflurane or isoflurane until sufficient depth of anesthesia for endotracheal intubation is attained. A smooth and expeditious intubation is then performed under deep anesthesia to attenuate the hemodynamic responses to laryngoscopy and endotracheal intubation (hypertension and tachycardia).

Maintenance of Anesthesia

Anesthesia is maintained with enflurane or isoflurane, nitrous oxide, incremental doses of nondepolarizing muscle relaxant, and controlled ventilation. Minute ventilation is adjusted to maintain normocardia, which helps prevent tachyarrhythmias caused by the topical use of cocaine and local infiltration of epinephrine. To ensure a smooth and prompt awakening, the technique is converted to a balanced anesthetic toward the end of the surgical procedure. Patients are then maintained on $N_2O:O_2$ (70:30) and controlled ventilation until the procedure is completely finished and the dressings have been applied.

Emergence from Anesthesia and Endotracheal Extubation

Patients are awakened at the end of the surgical procedure with minimal stimulation to avoid a stormy anesthetic emergence and are extubated awake and responsive, with minimal coughing or bucking. This can be accomplished by: (1) maintaining the patient on controlled ventilation with $N_2O:O_2$ until there is adequate reversal of the neuromuscular junction blockade and resumption of spontaneous ventilation, (2) no unnecessary manipulation of the head and neck after the reversal of the neuromuscular blocking agent, and (3) no oropharyngeal suctioning until immediately prior to endotracheal extubation. This practice helps minimize postsurgical bleeding and hematoma formation.

PERIOPERATIVE ANESTHETIC COMPLICATIONS

Problems include oversedation, overdose of local anesthetic, overdose of vasoconstrictor agents (cocaine and epinephrine), perioperative hypertension, and postoperative nausea and vomiting.

Oversedation During Local Anesthesia

To avoid patient discomfort and to provide amnesia for the entire surgical procedure, the surgeon administers a heavy premedication to produce a state of general anesthesia. This practice is unwise and unsafe without an anesthesiologist in attendance and without the use of a pulse oximeter. It is associated with snoring, significant respiratory depression, depression of airway reflexes, and the possibility of aspiration. Snoring is a sign of respiratory obstruction and usually associated with hypoxia and hypercarbia.

Inadequate Sedation

It is much safer to undermedicate than to overmedicate patients. Additional sedation can be given intravenously in the operating room, carefully titrated to the desired effect. Increasing restlessness is not always an indication of inadequate sedation. It could be due to: (1) hypoxia and hypercarbia, (2) full bladder, (3) inadequate local anesthesia, (4) local anesthetic toxicity, or (5) overdosage of epinephrine. These problems should be ruled out or corrected before administering more sedation.

Overdosage of Local Anesthetic

It is not uncommon to exceed the maximum suggested dosage of local anesthetics, especially during rhytidectomy and rhinoplasty. Toxic reactions following an overdose of local anesthetics usually occur within 5 to 20 minutes. They are manifested clinically as circumoral and tongue numbness, tinnitus, lightheadedness, visual and auditory disturbances, restlessness, garrulousness, slurred speech, nystagmus, shivering, and muscular tremors or twitching. Systemic toxicity can be avoided by staggering the dosage and by using the weakest effective solution if extensive local infiltration is required.

Management of the early signs of systemic toxicity is mainly supportive. It includes: (1) discontinuance of local infiltration to prevent progression to convulsions, (2) administration of oxygen, (3) cardiovascular monitoring, and (4) maintenance of adequate ventilation.

Overdosage of Vasoconstrictor Drugs (Cocaine and Epinephrine)

This problem can be minimized by strict adherence to the suggested dosage, use of 4 percent instead of 10 percent cocaine solution or cocaine flakes, and use of less concentrated solution of epinephrine. The maximum safe clinical dose for cocaine is 3 mg per kilogram and for epinephrine, 200 μg per kilogram. Under general anesthesia, the maximum suggested dose for epinephrine depends on the anesthetic agents used: (1) halothane—1.5 μg per kilogram, (2) enflurane—4 μg per kilogram, and (3) isoflurane—4 μg per kilogram.

The clinical manifestations of cocaine and epinephrine toxicities are restlessness, excitement, talkativeness, tachycardia, hypertension, and ventricular arrhythmias. These can be controlled by: (1) labetalol, 10 to 20 mg intravenously, given in 5-mg increments over 10 minutes, (2) propanolol, 2 to 5 mg intravenously, given in 1-mg increments, and (3) adequate ventilation.

Intraoperative Hypertension

Persistent elevation in blood pressure intraoperatively is undesirable because of increased surgical bleeding. This is uncommon in a well-managed general anesthetic. It is more likely to occur in patients with history of hypertension, especially during surgical procedures under local anesthesia. It can be avoided by the administration of antihypertensive medication up to the morning of surgery, judicious use of cocaine and epinephrine, adequate sedation with local anesthesia, maintenance of sufficient depth of general anesthesia, adequate ventilation, and use of Foley catheter to avoid bladder distention in long surgical procedures.

Postoperative Hypertension

Hypertension in the immediate postoperative period is common after a general anesthetic. It is a major concern among plastic surgeons and, more often than not, is blamed for postoperative surgical bleeding and hematoma formation. Common causes include pain, bladder distention, hypercarbia, hypoxia, hypothermia, fluid overload, and emergence delirium.

Therapy should be directed at the cause, rather than

the symptom. Management includes narcotics for pain, bladder catheterization to relieve bladder distention, airway support, oxygen therapy, aggressive warming, and physostigmine for emergence delirium. If these conservative measures are ineffective, sublingual nifedipine (10 mg) or intravenous labetalol (10 to 20 mg) may be given.

Postoperative Nausea and Vomiting

These are distressing problems in cosmetic surgical procedures. Etiologies include narcotic-analgesics, air in the gastrointestinal tract from assisted or controlled ventilation, sudden movement or position changes, anesthetic drugs, history of motion sickness, and obesity. These can be minimized by: (1) preoperative use of cimetidine or ranitidine and metoclopramide, (2) prophylactic use of droperidol (1.25 mg intravenously), (3) minimal use of narcotic-analgesics, (4) gastric decompression prior to endotracheal extubation, and (5) use of Transderm V-scopolamine in patients with history of motion sickness.

SUGGESTED READING

Ameer B, Greenblatt DJ. Lorazepam: a review of its clinical pharmacologic properties and therapeutic uses. Drugs 1981; 21:161–200.

Gibbs CP, Modell JH. Aspiration pneumonitis. In: Miller RD, ed. Anesthesia. New York: Churchill Livingstone, 1986:2033.

Jaffe JH, Martin WR. Opioid analgesics and antagonists. In: Gilman AG, Goodman LS, Gilman A, eds. The pharmacological basis of therapeutics. New York: Macmillan, 1980:494.

Reves JG, Fragen RJ, Vinik HR. Midazolam: pharmacology and uses. Anesthesiology 1985; 62:310–324.

Stoelting RK. Pharmacology and physiology in anesthesia practice. Philadelphia: Lippincott, 1987:117.

White PF, Way WL, Trevor AJ. Ketamine: its pharmacology and therapeutic uses. Anesthesiology 1982; 56:119–136.

White PF. Ketamine—its use as an intravenous anesthetic. Clin Anaesthesiol 1984; 2:1:43–64.

INJECTABLE COLLAGEN

HARVEY A. ZAREM, M.D.

Augmentation of the soft tissue continues to be a frustrating challenge to the plastic surgeon. The most prominent clinical problem through the decades has been the request for breast augmentation. Efforts to correct the deformed breast (usually from congenital asymmetry or from removal of a large benign tumor) prompted surgeons to transplant fat as early as the 1900s. Ironically, our specialty is now back to the same point. Efforts to augment soft tissue with autogenous tissues have presented two major problems—scarring at the donor site and failure of the transplanted tissue to survive. Exogenous tissue and synthetic materials are ready solutions to the problem of scarring, but persistence of a foreign tissue or tolerance of a foreign body remain constant biologic challenges.

If one excludes tissues or organs transplanted to sustain life (such as kidney, heart, and liver), in which immune suppression is appropriate, the perseverance of nonautogenous soft tissue in the nonimmunosuppressed human has been unsuccessful. Although documentation is sparse (and understandably so when one considers the difficulty of such documentation in humans), inert tissue, such as cartilage, and "denatured" tissue, such as bone, have the most successful clinical record of persistence as exogenous tissue transplants. Soft-tissue transplantation is thought to have been conspicuously unsuccessful by many clinicians.

Another goal in soft-tissue augmentation is the desire for a transcutaneous (nonincisional) malleable material for small, subtle defects. Prior to the availability of injectable collagen, alloplastic materials were used for skin contour defects. A popular substance, especially in the Orient, was paraffin. Subsequently, liquid silicone became available. As part of a legitimate study in the United States, 10 investigators were designated to use Dow Corning's medical grade silicone (Silastic) in a clinical trial. The results of this trial remain controversial. However, the majority of the investigators have continued to report the success of injections of medical grade Silastic into humans. Although many clinicians have experienced significant problems with patients who have been injected with what has been reported as "silicone," the legitimate investigators have insisted that these problem patients are victims of injections of nonmedical grade silicone. Judging from articles in some of the "scientific" journals that represent nonqualified pseudoplastic surgeons, there seem to be many clinicians in the United States who are currently injecting nonmedical grade silicone into patients. A biologic material such as injectable collagen has its definite appeal and a potential role in the armamentarium of the plastic surgeon and the dermatologist because of concern on the part of the medical profession as to the safety of the injection of alloplastic materials, such as silicone.

Knapp et al reported the first clinical trial of injectable collagen in 1977. In the ensuing 12 years, two additional generations of injectable collagen, Zyderm II and Zyplast, have evolved. The issues that were raised in the beginning—perseverance and body tolerance of the material—have continued to be the focus in assessment of the role of injectable collagen in human use.

The first generation of injectable collagen was bovine dermis, subjected to pepsin hydrolysis. This soluble form of collagen forms fibrils on warming to 37° C. The liquid collagen is thus transformed into a white, cohesive mass. In the concentration of 35 mg per milliliter (Zyderm I), immediate resorption of the water results in a significant loss of bulk. The second generation of injectable collagen, Zyderm II, was made available in a concentration of 65 mg per milliliter. It is the most popular collagen preparation for intradermal injection. The technique of placing the Zyderm in the superficial dermis has resulted in the transient correction of superficial skin wrinkles and the supplementation of attenuated dermis in skin scars. A third generation of injectable collagen, Zyplast, represents a product that has resulted from crosslinking the fibrillar collagen with glutaraldehyde.

Since they recognize the advantage of a readily available exogenous material that can be injected into the skin and subdermal tissues to correct wrinkles of the skin or small contour defects, clinicians have been quick to utilize this material. An extensive experience has evolved. According to figures from the Collagen Corporation, more than 350,000 patients have received injectable collagen. In addition, collagen material crosslinked with glutaraldehyde has been used in a variety of clinical situations that include resorbable sutures, fabrication of heart valves, vascular prostheses, and a number of hemostatic agents.

Ten years of experience with Zyderm has placed it into some perspective. The technique of placing the soluble collagen in the superficial dermis has resulted in transient correction of wrinkles of the skin and this allows supplementation of the attenuated dermis and skin scars. The temporal persistence of Zyderm remains an unknown. There is a distinct clinical impression amongst some users that the injected collagen fibrils form the framework for the laying down of autologous collagen to a limited degree, thereby resulting in a cumulative gain of dermal collagen after repeated injections. This clinical speculation has not been documented histologically. Tolerance is essentially the issue of antigenicity of injectable collagen.

The recent introduction of Zyplast (a crosslinked collagen with glutaraldehyde) has not provided us with sufficient experience to comment with any degree of certainty on the intended enhanced persistence. However, the Zyplast is intended to be injected subdermally, or at best in the very deep portions of the dermis, rather than intradermally as the Zyderm. When the Zyplast has been injected intradermally, beading and nodularity have been observed to persist for a few months.

HYPERSENSITIVITY

Using symptoms of hypersensitivity at the treatment site as a criterion, DeLustro has reported an incidence of hypersensitivity of approximately 1 percent in a group of 200,000 patients. All patients subjected to injectable collagen were pretested with an intradermal skin test. Approximately 3 percent of those tested exhibited a localized hypersensitivity reaction to collagen and did not receive further injections.

DeLustro et al further report that 56 percent of the reactions occur following the first treatment, 28 percent following the second, 10 percent following the third, and 6 percent following subsequent exposures. ELISA is considered to be an extremely sensitive test for the existence of antibodies. Using ELISA, sera from human subjects who had been injected with bovine collagen showed an 88 percent incidence of antibodies against bovine collagen, but no reaction was detected against human collagen in this group. The data reported by DeLustro et al further suggests that the relative risk of a hypersensitivity reaction to Zyderm implant does not increase with multiple exposures.

In contrast to the reports by DeLustro et al, Frank, Ozkan, and Fisher reported in the plastic surgical forum in October, 1986, that the highly sensitive ELISA assay can detect antibodies to modified bovine dermal collagen, and that multiple injections can produce rising antibody titers to animal collagen. The authors found that in humans the titers to anti-Zyderm antibodies rise in some patients as repeated administrations are received. Evidence suggests that the immune response against the bovine origin is specific for bovine collagen. Hypersensitivity reactions appear to be localized to the site of injection, and there is no evidence to date that the antibodies to the bovine collagen appear to be associated with any immunity to human collagen.

Sensitivity to the collagen antigen and the potential problems from such humoral sensitivity are concerns for the physician who is considering injectable collagen for a patient. Another issue of concern is the persistence of the injected material.

PERSISTENCE

Several recent papers have investigated the histologic reaction of injectable noncrosslinked collagen (Zyderm) and glutaraldehyde crosslinked collagen (Zyplast). The persistence of the implanted collagen has been shown by McPherson et al to demonstrate, in guinea pigs, a fourfold increase in wet weight of Zyplast over Zyderm at 39 days, when injected subcutaneously. Kligman and Armstrong have investigated the histologic reaction to injected collagen in humans. Zyderm collagen was dispersed among host collagen fibers and gradually lost the appearance of a cohesive implant by 90 days. Evidence of host colonization by host fibroblasts was absent. In contrast, the glutaraldehyde crosslinked collagen, Zyplast, remained as a distinct focus for 6 months. The crosslinked collagen became invaded by host fibroblasts and collagen was laid down. Both types of implants induced an inflammatory reaction that lasted 6 months and included edema and fibroplasia in the superficial papillary dermis. The inflammatory reaction may, in part, explain the loss of skin wrinkles. Persistence of injected collagen remains an issue in dispute. However, if the crosslinked collagen, Zyplast, induces a fibroplasia by the host, a net gain of collagen may result without the actual persistence of the exogenous collagen.

At this writing, one would have to conclude from the reports in the literature that the ultimate fate of Zyderm and Zyplast in the human is undetermined from both experimental and clinical evidence.

CLINICAL EXPERIENCE

Klein et al have described the details of an extensive clinical experience in the techniques of using collagen. If one assumes the safety of injectable bovine collagen in humans, the clinician's concern focuses on the persistence of the material injected, whether intradermally or subdermally. A thorough review of the literature fails to reveal any data to substantiate the persistence of injectable collagen to any significant degree. Experience with the Zyderm I and the Zyderm II for the past 10 years, and with Zyplast over the past 2 years, is subjective. With the patient's own assessment used as a guide, the clinician must conclude that the effect of the injectable collagen persists for no more than 8 to 10 months. A recent survey of my own patients indicates that the majority of patients return for further collagen injection to correct deep nasolabial folds at approximately 6 to 8 month intervals. Most of these patients have sought the collagen injection on their own initiative. When confronted with the apparent status of the effects of collagen that persist for approximately 6 to 8 months, many patients feel that the time and cost involved is worth it. From the patient's standpoint, correction of specific wrinkles and of the nasolabial fold cannot be accomplished in any other fashion than by the injection of collagen. Therefore, the time and cost involved in repeated injections have already been considered by the patient and the decision made.

The failure of clear evidence that the injectable collagen persists has led clinicians to pursue again the possibility of injectable fat. Injection of autogenous fat, aspirated from other areas of the body (such as the lower abdomen), has become a popular technique designed to approach some of the problems that are currently being addressed with injectable collagen. However, intradermal injection of fat to correct the specific wrinkles within the skin has not replaced the continued interest in collagen injection. Although the injection of synthetic exogenous material such as silicone has not been condoned by legitimate plastic surgeons, its use continues around the country by some physicians. One of the most common uses of silicone injections has been to cover up contour defects of the nose after rhinoplasty. The fate of injectable silicone remains another issue. The majority of clinicians have seen enough long-term problems with the inflammatory reaction and edema associated with silicone injections that this mode of therapy remains unattractive. In view of the lack of significant complications, and the apparent relative safety of injectable collagen, the clinician understandably chooses this material for correction of small contour defects and facial wrinkles over other existing modalities.

As long as the patient is fully aware of the temporary nature of the collagen implant and that the associated problems with injectable collagen continue to be limited to the local injection sites, the use of collagen would appear to be reasonable in the informed patient.

SUGGESTED READING

DeLustro F, Smith ST, Sundsmo J, et al. Reaction to injectable collagen: results in animal models and clinical use. Plast Reconstr Surg 1987; 79:581–594.

Frank DH, Ozkam AN, Fisher JC. Plastic Surgical Forum, Vol. IX, ASPRS Annual; Scientific Meeting, Oct, 1986. Discussion (Medical Letter) Plast Reconstr Surg 1987; 79:593–594.

Klein AW, Rish C. Injectable Collagen Update, J Dermatol Surg Oncol 1984; 10:519–522.

Kligman AM, Armstrong RC. Histologic response to intradermal Zyderm and Zyplast (glutaraldehyde crosslinked) collagen in humans. J Dermatol Surg Oncol 1986; 12:351–357.

Knapp TR, Kaplan EN, Daniels JR. Injectable collagen for soft tissue augmentation. Plast Reconstr Surg 1977; 60:39–45.

McPherson JM, Sawamura S, Armstrong R. An examination of the biologic response to injectable, glutaraldehyde crosss-linked collagen implants. J Biomed Mater Res 1986; 20:93–107.

MALE PATTERN BALDNESS

JOHN DEVINE Jr., M.D., F.A.C.S.
PAUL S. HOWARD, M.D.
ERNEST K. MANDERS, M.D.
LEO McCAFFERTY, M.D.

EVALUATION OF THE PATIENT

There is no substitute for clinical judgment and an in-depth personal interview of all patients seeking esthetic surgery. During the interview, as Millard has said, the plastic surgeon should "seek insight into the patient's desires." At the end of the interview for male pattern baldness, the surgeon should know the period of time over which balding has occurred, the motivations for surgery, whether the expectations are realistic, and how the patient's family and friends support his decision for surgery. It is well documented that men seeking cosmetic surgery can be psychologically unstable; therefore, we must investigate these patients carefully, searching for the telltale signs of instability that will lead to the unfavorable result and the dissatisfied patient. We explain that many men, including politicians, actors, and athletes, are bald and, in many instances, use their baldness as an advantage. Multiple operations are the rule as the balding process proceeds, so motivation and courage by both patient and surgeon are necessary to achieve the desired result. Hair styling and dye-colored sprays are useful adjuncts to camouflage the sequelae of surgery, but all patients must be warned that, even with the best results, diving into a swimming pool will unmask the scars and remaining baldness.

Patient selection should include a detailed clinical examination of the scalp and remaining hair to rule out dermatologic scalp disease and to determine the adequacy of the occipital and parietal hair for flap or round graft use. The donor hair should be of a density to allow transplantation (14 to 20 hairs per 4 square millimeters) without compromise of the secondary donor site. Round grafts should be harvested only from the occipital scalp so as not to interrupt a future temporoparieto-occipital flap, if one is necessary. Examination should include Doppler analysis of the superficial temporal artery and particularly of its posterior branches.

The patient desiring esthetic improvement for male pattern baldness should be offered the currently available techniques. We are emphasizing long temporoparieto-occipital flaps as the surgical treatment of choice. These flaps have recently been described by Ellenbogen with no delay and with no flap loss or distal alopecia, although we still prefer to delay these flaps. Round grafts are used more as an adjunctive procedure than for primary creation of a hairline. We have not yet utilized free scalp flaps or Nataf's vertical flap. When careful attention is given to grooming, a reasonable hairline is possible regardless of the direction of the hair follicles in the flap.

Once the decision is made to proceed with the operation, the proposed frontal hairline is carefully studied along with the patient, wife, mother, and girl friend, and a final determination is made prior to surgery. This determination should be considered permanent as the hairline is extremely difficult to correct at a later date.

ROUND GRAFTS

Round grafts, first described by the Japanese and subsequently popularized by Orentreich, were the first procedures used for the operative treatment of male pattern baldness. The technique and its variations have been described by Stough et al, Norwood, Unger, and others, including a detailed description of the technique by Devine and colleagues.

If hair density is less than 10 to 14 hairs per 4 square millimeters, the potential for visible scarring and for poor hair growth after transplantation is increased.

The salient operative details include local anesthesia with epinephrine and proper harvesting of the grafts with sharp circular punch instruments oriented so as to minimize follicle damage. The grafts (Fig. 1) must be trimmed fastidiously under magnification and sorted so the plugs with the greatest number of follicles can be used at the hairline. Less dense plugs are placed behind this row. Careful attention must be given to hemostasis at both the donor and recipient sites. Finally, the grafts must be inset in the proper direction.

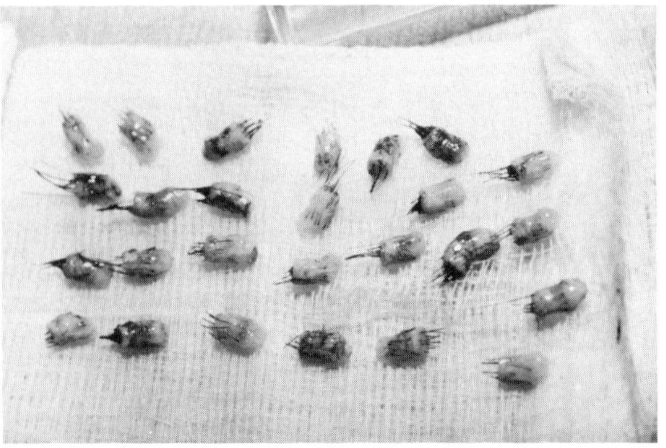

Figure 1 Round grafts.

The patient is seen at 24 hours to determine if hemostasis is adequate and whether the grafts are still in the proper direction. It is during the first 24 to 48 hour period that a good graft take will be insured. The hair will initially shed, to be followed by returned growth at 12 weeks.

SQUARE AND STRIP GRAFTS

We find little use for these techniques and do not presently recommend them. Strip grafts are useful in the reconstruction of the eyebrow. These are usually harvested from the parietal scalp and may preclude the use of scalp flaps.

Satisfactory results can be accomplished using this technique (Fig. 2).

SCALP REDUCTION

Blanchard first described scalp reduction in 1976. Since then, reductions have been devised in many patterns depending on the area of alopecia to be reduced (Fig. 3). The principle of reduction is the same as for serial scar excisions. The area of alopecia to be excised is subdivided into excisable areas with care taken not to be overly ambitious in each scalp excision as wide unsightly scars may result. These wounds are closed under moderate tension so as to use the intrinsic elasticity of the adjacent scalp to make up for the excised skin. Extensive subgaleal undermining is performed so that skin tension is minimized. Good surgical judgment is necessary to avoid excessive tension that creates wide scars and further alopecia. A patient managed with scalp reduction and round grafts is illustrated in Figure 4.

TEMPOROPARIETO-OCCIPITAL SCALP FLAP

Scalp flaps are the primary procedure for reconstruction of the frontal hairline. These are long, arterialized flaps that can be transferred without delay when the posterior branch of the superficial temporal artery can be located within the flap for most of its distance. We prefer to delay these flaps so as not to risk any distal alopecia. Careful operative technique is necessary to minimize scarring and to insure follicle survival. Therefore, those who are not familiar with flap procedures and plastic surgical techniques should probably be wary of these flaps. A template is used to help in the design of the flap for the delay procedures. The flap is based on the parietal branch of the temporal artery as determined by Doppler flow. We have found the Shaw hemostatic scalpel (Oximetrix Co.) a useful aid in hemostasis. The flap is inset 14 days after the first delay and the donor site is closed, primarily with wide undermining. The carefully inset flap may have a minimal dogear, which will require revision 3 weeks postoperatively. The direction of hair growth seems to be less important when appropriate styling is utilized. Therefore, we have not attempted flap design to change the direction of follicle growth. Figure 3 shows a 28-year-old physician who returned to work the day after surgery with "instant-hair."

MICROGRAFTS

The micrograft technique has been credited to Nordstrom. Using the operating microscope, the micrografts are dissected from the round graft to include three hair follicles per graft. The grafts are transplanted into stab wounds created with an 11 scalpel blade. Nordstrom shows impressive results after seven sessions with the micrograft technique.

SCALP EXPANSION

Scalp expansion of the available hairbearing tissue increases the area of this tissue, but necessarily decreases the density of the hair follicles. Austad has shown that the hair follicles and other epidermal appendages are not damaged by careful expansion.

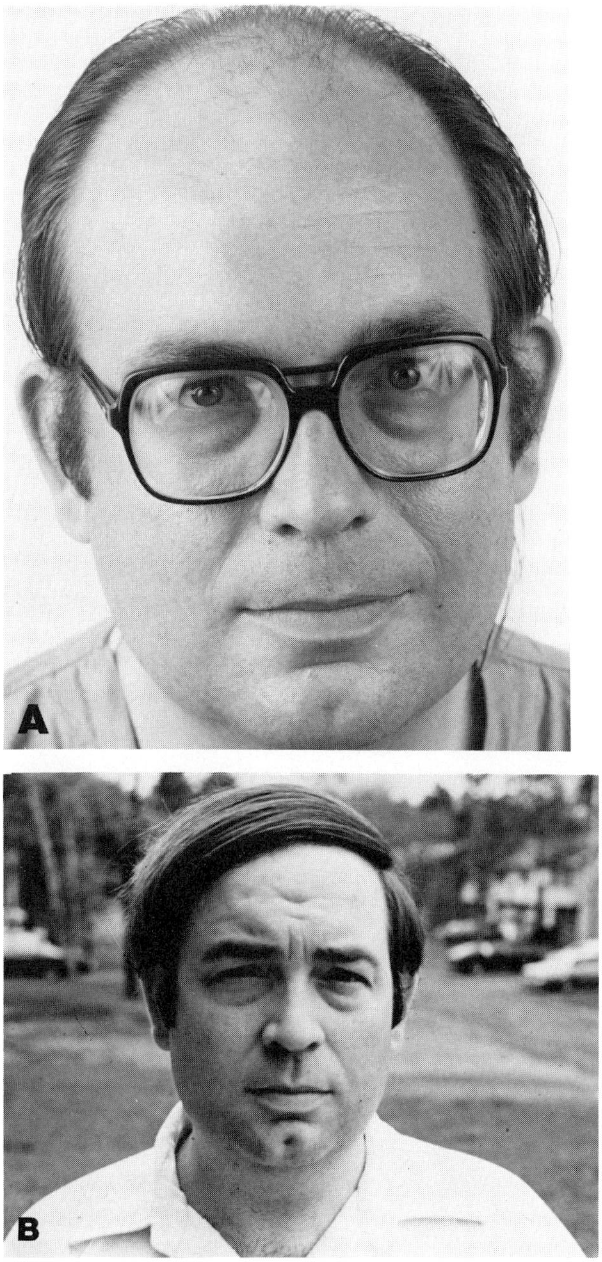

Figure 2 *A*, Preoperative view, before strip and square grafts. *B*, One year post operation.

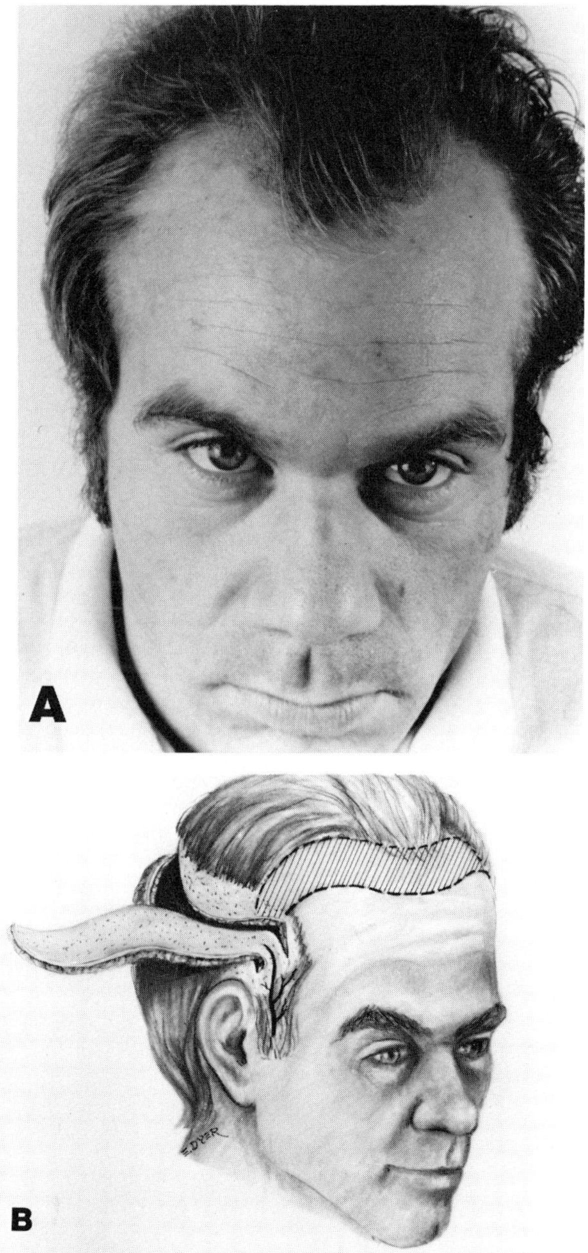

Figure 3 *A*, Preoperative view. *B*, Flap elevation.

Figure continues on following page

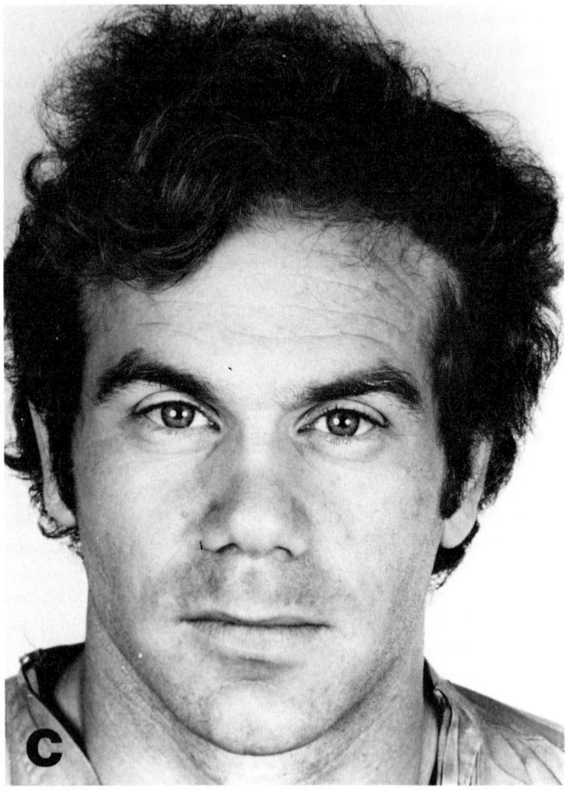

Figure 3 (continued) *C*, Postoperative view.

The tissue expanders are placed in the subgaleal plane without scoring the galea. Expansion proceeds weekly over 2 to 4 months with two expanders placed under the temporoparieto-occipital scalp. Should the expansion prove to be insufficient after the trial closure, the expander can be deflated and the scalp reexpanded to a greater area. Measurement will allow some confidence in timing the advancement. Most men require expansion to a distance of 48 to 52 cm from ear to ear.

Inflation is usually well tolerated physically, but some men are extremely self-conscious during the period of temporary deformity in the late expansion stage. Though temporary deflation during working hours is an alternative, none of our patients have opted for this. Success depends in part on the emotional support the surgeon gives his patient.

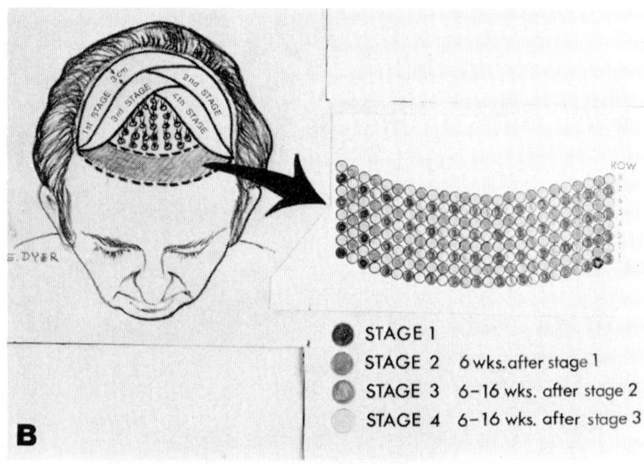

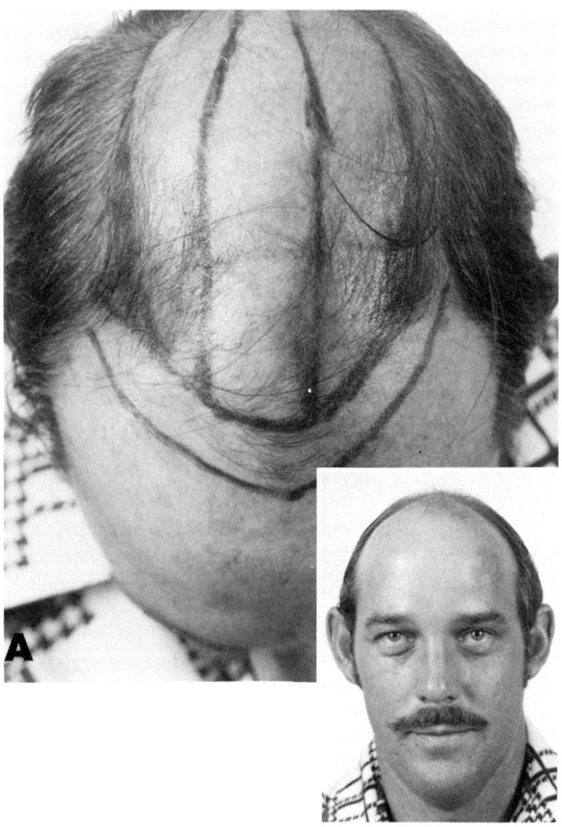

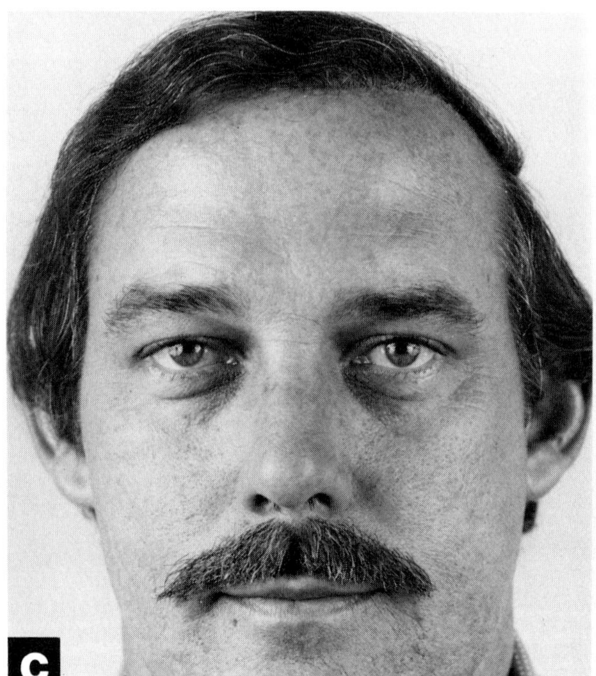

Figure 4 *A*, Preoperative scalp reduction plan. Inset: full-face preoperative photograph. *B*, Schematic illustration of reduction plus round grafting. Note the intervals necessary for the desired result with round grafting. *C*, Postoperative view.

Dow Corning-Wright (Arlington, TN) has recently manufactured a differential tissue expander utilizing an end-to-end differential in envelope thickness designed to allow greater expansion and larger scalp flaps in the temporal region. This is also a concept credited to Manders.*

Complications attendant to expansion include deflation, skin erosions, hematomas, seromas, and infections. The most common problem is exposure from overzealous inflation in an attempt to shorten the period of expansion. Patients and surgeons must proceed slowly. If conducted with care, soft tissue expansion can be of great benefit to patients seeking reconstruction for male pattern baldness.

---

* U.S. Patent No. 4,574,780. Tissue Expander and Method. The authors wish to state that one of us (EKM) will receive benefits from the use of the differential expander described herein.

SUGGESTED READING

Austad ED, Pasyk K, McClatchey KD, et al. Histomorphic evaluation of guinea pig skin and soft tissue after controlled tissue expansion. Plast Reconstr Surg 1982; 70:704.

Blanchard G. Reduction of bald spots (detonsuration): new concept in the surgical treatment of baldness. Union Med Can 1976; 105(4):618.

Devine JW, Howard PS, Nordstrom REA. Treatment of male pattern baldness: update. Adv Plast Reconstr Surg 1986; 3:273.

Manders EK, Friedman M. Scalp expansion for the elimination of male pattern baldness. Plast Reconstr Surg, in press.

Norwood OT. Hair transplant surgery. Springfield, IL: Thomas CC, 1984.

Okuda S. Clinical and experimental studies on transplanting of living hair. Jpn J Dermatol Urol 1939; 46:135-138.

Orentreich N. Autografs in alopecias and other selected dermatological conditions. Ann NY Acad Sci 1959; 83:463.

Rimmetto, Stubel A, Ellenbogen R. Male baldness: intermediate single—stage rotation of very long arterralimed temporoparieto-occipital flaps. Plast Reconstr Surg 1986; 77:215.

RHINOPLASTY: THE BONY VAULT

ROLLIN K. DANIEL, M.D., F.A.C.S.

Traditionally, modification of the nasal bony vault was designed to establish a new dorsal profile line and close the secondary open roof deformity. However, numerous variations are now required as the rhinoplasty operation has progressed from very large hump removals to an operation of more finesse. Three factors must be considered when one looks at the bony vault and its attendant cartilaginous component: (1) establishment of a new profile line, (2) alternation in the base width of the lateral walls, and (3) closure of the open roof. Each of these entities will be considered separately.

DORSAL PROFILE LINE

One can elevate, modify, or lower the profile line.

Elevation

In 100 consecutive primary esthetic rhinoplasties done by the author, the raising of the entire profile line was extremely rare, and occurred in less than 1 to 2 percent of patients. As described by Gunter, elevation can be done most easily by utilizing a septal graft and making it into a "V" or a "U" shape. Longitudinal partial-thickness cuts are made in the cartilage, then the graft is fractured at the desired point. The principle is that the perichondrium on the opposite side remains intact and provides support. Recently, Sheen has discussed the low radix concept, which implies a depressed radix area that can arbitrarily be defined as the area ± 3 mm from the intercanthal line. If one fills the radix with a crushed cartilage graft, then the hump reduction is reduced. This latter concept of raising the radix is extremely important as it lessens the apparent hump deformity, and allows a finesse rhinoplasty.

Modification

Modification of the dorsal line is a more unusual concept, and usually occurs where the lateral profile is near ideal proportions, but where irregularities exist at the keystone area or the dorsum is exceedingly broad. In narrowing the broad dorsum, one can make parallel cuts to convert the "Y" septum to a straight "I," and then mobilize the lateral walls inward (Fig. 1). Sheen has taken a different approach whereby one defines the ideal dorsum and then takes out lateral segments. This assumes that one will have a union between the lateral bony wall and the dorsum, which introduces another variable into the healing equation.

Lowering

By far the majority of profile lines need to be lowered, and fall into two broad categories, hump removal versus modification of the nasofrontal angle area (Fig. 2). Traditionally, hump removal consisted of two steps; first, the cartilaginous vault was incised and then the bony hump was disarticulated with an osteotome, thereby permitting en bloc hump removal. This method is certainly a quick and elegant technique when done by an experienced surgeon. However, for the majority of surgeons and noses, the incremental technique is a much more controlled and graded method. The bony hump is rasped down, then the cartilaginous vault is excised with a Number 11 blade. The author has tried both sequences; the classical excision of the cartilaginous vault first, before rasping of the bone, as well as the recommended method of rasping the bone first followed by excision of the cartilage. With the exception of the large "beak," or the severely deviated nose, there is a more controlled result from rasping the bone

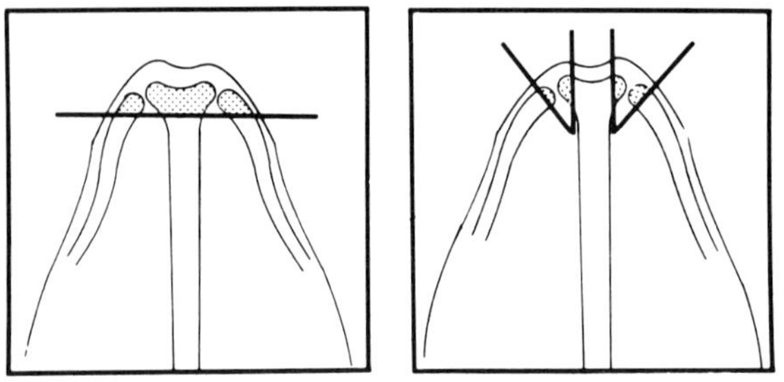

Figure 1 Modification of nasal hump width can be accomplished by either transverse excision, which lowers the overall profile line, or vertical wedge excision which preserves profile height.

down first followed by a gradual reduction of the cartilaginous vault with a Number 11 blade. Deepening of the nasofrontal groove area has classically been done by one of three methods: (1) avulsion of muscle, (2) burring out of bone, or (3) en bloc removal. The en bloc removal with disarticulation can produce the definitive dorsal line—or it can be excessive and requires reinsertion as a modified Skoog graft. This technique is diagrammatically easy, but technically difficult. It is better to separate hump removal and deepening of the nasofrontal angle into two distinct procedures. Deepening of the nasofrontal groove is done either with a gouge or burring down of bone. Avulsion of muscle should not be done as this eliminates concealing cover for the disrupted bony vault.

OPEN ROOF

It has long been accepted that lateral osteotomies and mobilization of the lateral walls result in closure of the open roof. However, computed tomography (CT scan) analysis indicates that the open roof is rarely closed and that the normal, natural curvature with its tripartite configuration is lost forever—either rasped to dust or placed in a specimen bottle. For most esthetic purposes, dorsal reduction is limited to 2 to 5 mm, and the open roof can be minimized by mobilization of the lateral nasal walls. In the very large nose, hump removal can, in the best of hands produce a sawed-off dorsum, or, in the worst of hands, result in an inverted "V" deformity with visual separation of the bony and cartilaginous vaults. Therefore, some form of dorsal graft reinsertion should be considered in the case of very narrow, high-arched noses, or those with secondary deformities. Dorsal augmentation may be accomplished by utilizing an osseocartilaginous graft, a modified Skoog rhinoplasty, or a retractable roof rhinoplasty.

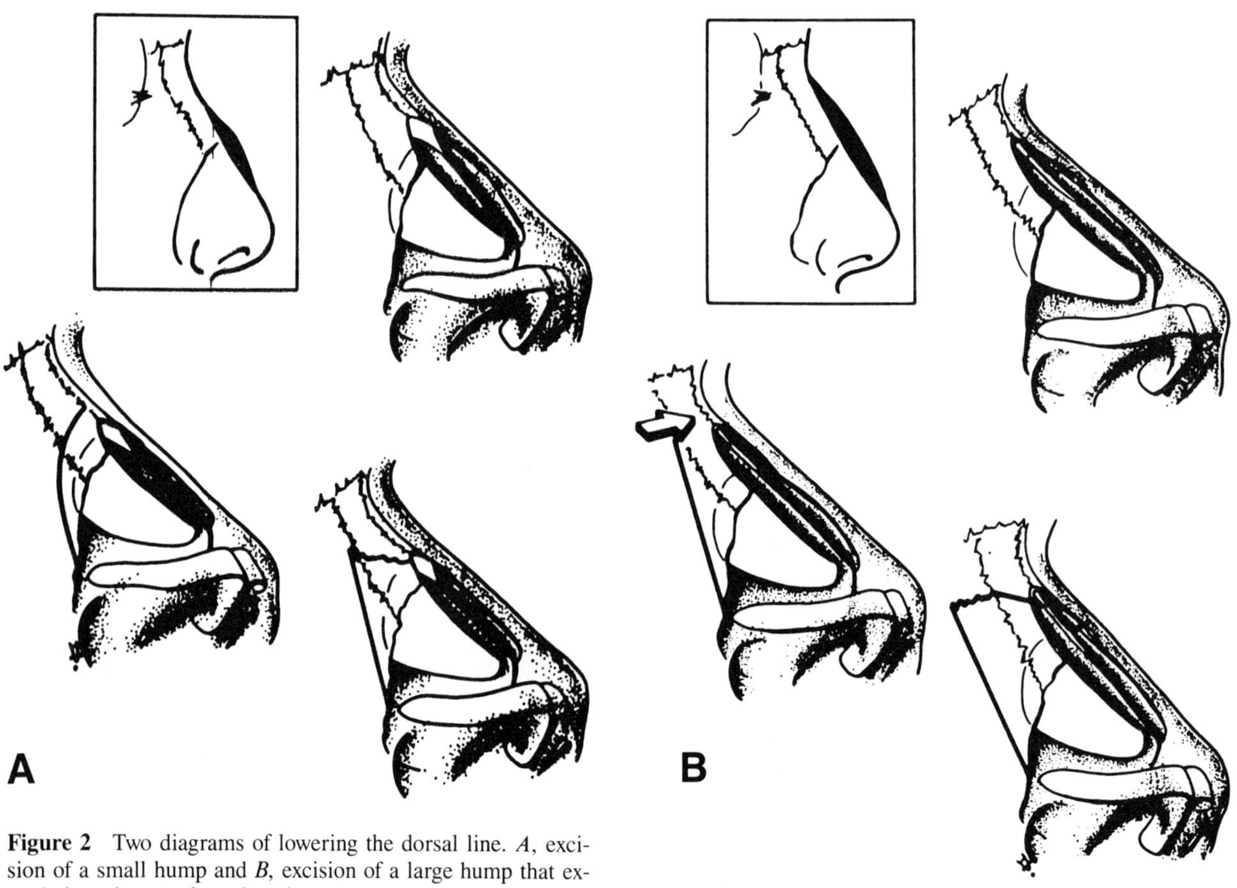

Figure 2 Two diagrams of lowering the dorsal line. *A*, excision of a small hump and *B*, excision of a large hump that extends into the nasofrontal region.

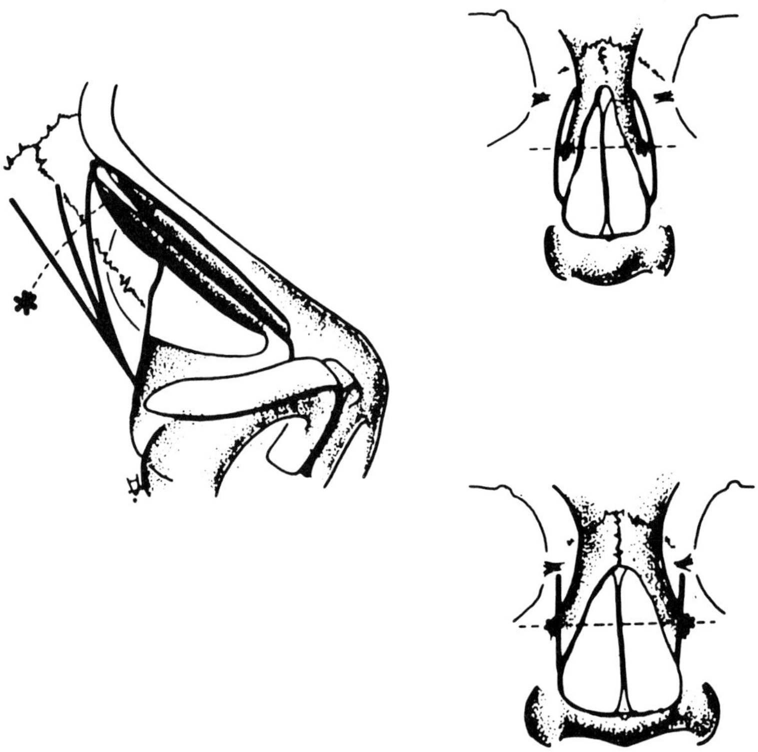

Figure 3 Lateral osteotomies can be low-to-low, low-to-high, or angulated.

BONY VAULT WIDTH

The wide bony vault is a frequent patient complaint. Traditionally, a combination of osteotomies was done, which began with lateral osteotomies to accomplish infracture, followed by medial osteotomies to allow an outfracture. These maneuvers mobilized the nose, but often resulted in a collapsed bony vault with dropping of the nasal bones into the airway. Based on the work of Peck and others, retention of the periosteal and overlying skin connections prevents the bones from dropping into the bony vault, thereby leading to more conservative osteotomies. Preoperatively, one must decide on the number, type, and sequence of osteotomies. The base width of the bony vault is usually marked on the seated patient and location of the point of maximum width determines how low the osteotomy must be. If this point is in the lower or mid-

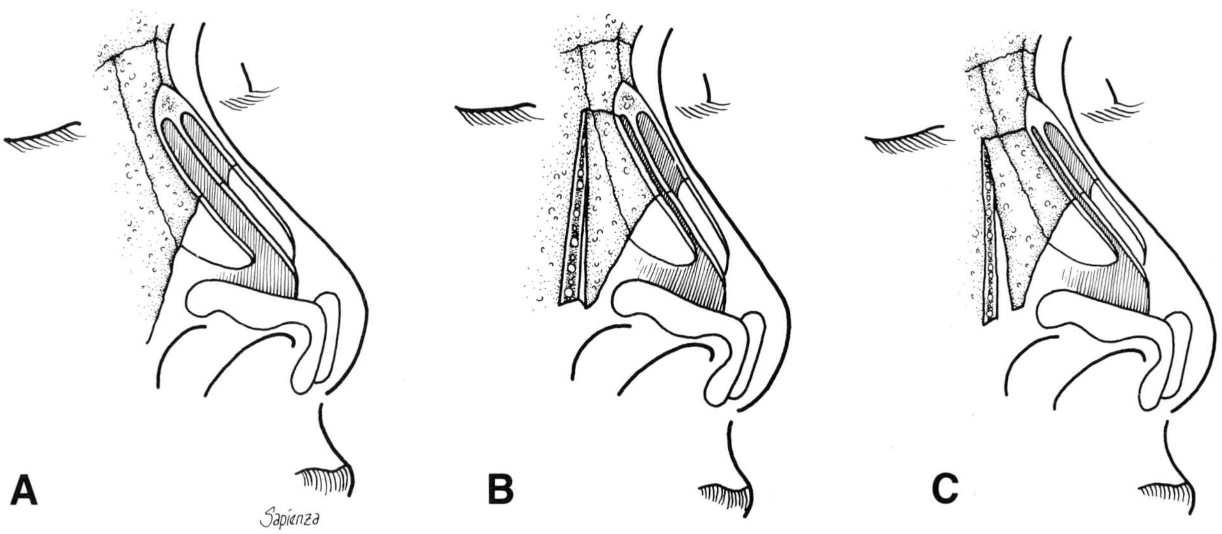

Figure 4 Closure of the open roof. *A*, the open roof. *B*, low-to-high osteotomy with tilt of the lateral wall, and *C*, low-to-low osteotomy with significant movement of the lateral wall.

portion of the distance from intercanthal line to pyriform aperture, a low-to-high osteotomy will suffice, but the closer the widest point of the bony vault extends above the infraorbital rim, the more likely one is to utilize a low-to-low osteotomy (Figs. 3 and 4). If a lateral osteotomy has been done and mobilization is not complete, a small transverse 2 mm osteotomy is done, followed by digital pressure. Medial osteotomies are generally reserved for those cases where the bone is either exceedingly wide or thick and rigid, as it is in males. Preoperatively, if it appears that mobilization will be difficult, a medial oblique osteotomy is done first in order to break the thick bony triangle, and this is followed by a lateral osteotomy.

SUGGESTED READING

Daniel RK, Ethier R. Rhinoplasty: a CT scan analysis. Plast Reconstr Surg 1987; 80:175.

Daniel RK, Lessard ML. Rhinoplasty: a graded aesthetic-anatomical approach. Ann Plast Surg 1984; 13:436.

Daniel RK, Letourneau A. Rhinoplasty: nasal anatomy. Ann Plast Surg (In press).

Gunter JP, Rohrich RJ. External approach for secondary rhinoplasty. Plast Reconstr Surg (In press).

Peck GC. Techniques in aesthetic rhinoplasty. New York: Thieme-Stratton, 1984.

Regnault P, Daniel RK. Aesthetic plastic surgery. Boston: Little, Brown, 1984.

Sheen JH, Sheen AP. Aesthetic rhinoplasty. 2nd ed. St. Louis: CV Mosby, 1987.

DEVIATED NOSE

JACK P. GUNTER, M.D.
RODNEY J. ROHRICH, M.D.

PHILOSOPHY

In most externally deviated noses, there is an associated deviation of the nasal septum. If the deviation is not severe, it may be possible to effect the correction with osteotomies alone, or with camouflage procedures such as onlay grafts. However, if the septal deviation is significant, surgical modification of the septum is required to produce the best functional and esthetic results.

Our philosophy on the correction of the deviated nose is to be conservative in the surgery on the external framework, but be prepared to be radical on the septum.

GENERAL PRINCIPLES

Mobilize All Deviated Structures

Any structure that is out of place should be freely mobilized so that it can be placed back in its correct position without a tendency to return to its preoperative position. If the nasal bones are deviated, osteotomies must be performed; if the upper lateral cartilages are displaced, they should be freed from the septum and the lower lateral cartilages; and all deviated portions of the septum must be mobilized so they can be placed in the midline.

Keep Maximal Attachment of Mucoperichondrium

Preservation of mucoperichondrial attachment helps in two ways. It maintains a blood supply to the cartilage so that it is less vulnerable to resorption, and helps support the mobilized cartilage segments so they are not completely detached and fall to the back of the nose.

Maintain Septal Support

While radical septal surgery may be necessary, it is essential to maintain support of the septum for the lower one-half of the nose. If septal support is lost during the operation, it must be reestablished.

Plan Osteotomies Precisely

Accurately planned lateral and/or medial osteotomies along previous fracture sites, or at the periphery of developmental asymmetries, aid in restoration of symmetry to the nasal pyramid. Hump removal and septal straightening should be completed before the osteotomies, while the nasal dorsum is still stable. Minimal bony rasping and incremental cartilage incisions can be performed after the osteotomies.

SURGICAL TECHNIQUE

Surgery on the External Framework

The nose is exposed through a complete transfixion incision that is connected to intercartilaginous incisions. If lower lateral cartilage alteration is necessary, it is usually performed by making a marginal incision along the caudal border of the medial and lateral crura and delivering the cartilages. An external approach (transcolumellar incision to connect the medial ends of the marginal incision) is used occasionally, but only when there are unusual or complicated tip deformities.

The skin of the dorsum is undermined and submucosal tunnels are made between the upper lateral cartilages (ULC) and the nasal septum, so that the septum can be freed from the ULC. If hump removal is indicated, it is easier to resect a small cartilaginous hump with a knife blade before dissection is started on the tunnels. This separates the junction of the septum with the ULC, but leaves the mucosa intact. The mucosa is then easily elevated from the incised edges of the septum and ULC, and this allows for further reduction, if necessary, with angled scissors. At this point, the mucosa still serves as an interconnection between the septal cartilage and the ULC and should remain attached to one side of the septum during the surgery to aid in stabilization.

After the dorsal septum and the ULC are trimmed to the desired height, the bony hump is removed, if indicated. Adjustments are then made to achieve the desired dorsal profile. The next step is the septal surgery, with the osteotomies performed last.

Septal Surgery

In all cases, except those requiring an external approach, a complete transfixion incision is made, and the mucoperichondrium is elevated on one side or the other, but not both. We usually elevate on the side of the major deviation, because it is easier to work from that side. When the septum is shifted off the bony crest, the mucosa on that side must be freed to allow the septum to be placed back on the nasal spine and/or maxillary crest. The only elevation of mucoperichondrium on the opposite side of the septum is performed in areas where the septum is to be resected, or in areas where the adherence to the septum prevents desired movement of the cartilage—usually at the anterior cartilaginous septum-maxillary crest junction.

At the junction of the anterior maxillary crest with the septum, it is difficult to avoid perforation of the mucoperichondrium during the elevation. The reason for this is that the mucoperichondrium of the septum and the mucoperiosteum of the crest fuse with each other and travel between the cartilage and the crest to connect with their counterparts on the opposite side. For intact elevation, it is recommended that the mucoperichondrium (superior tunnel) and mucoperiosteum (inferior tunnel) be raised separately to the junction. A knife blade, or sharp scissors, is then placed submucosally to incise the fused tissue where it starts between the maxillary crest and cartilaginous septum.

If the mucoperichondrium is elevated intact, it is usually desirable to perforate it posteroinferiorly on one side. This allows drainage of any bleeding that may occur between the flaps, behind the area of splinting and/or packing.

After the mucoperichondrium is elevated, it must then be decided what to do to correct the septal deformity. Several options are available: resection, morselization, segmental through-and-through cross-hatching, and swinging-door flaps.

Resection

This can be performed safely for most deviations along the maxillary crest. The resection may include both septal cartilage and maxillary crest. As much cartilage as possible is preserved, but if there are problems with the correction, a large amount of cartilage, perpendicular plate of the ethmoid, vomer, and maxillary crest may be resected, provided an "L" strut of cartilage from the dorsum and caudal septum is left in place (Fig. 1). The "L" strut should be at least 1 cm in width and the ends should remain attached to the perpendicular plate and the nasal spine.

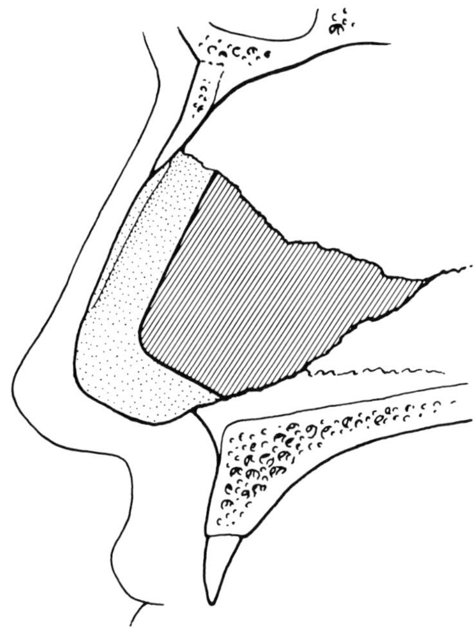

Figure 1 "L" strut. (Figures 1 to 5 are reproduced, by permission, from Gunter JP, Rohrich RJ. Management of the deviated nose: the importance of septal reconstruction. Clin Plast Surg 1988; 15:43–55.)

Morselization

This is a way to crush a segment of cartilage to erase its cartilage "memory" and prevent its return to the original position. The main disadvantage of morselization of the cartilage is that it weakens the morselized area. If any part of the "L" strut is morselized, it should be splinted in the desired position for 1 week. Morselization also tends to increase the surface area of the cartilage, which may or may not be a disadvantage.

Segmental Through-and-Through Cross-Hatching

This accomplishes the same thing as morselization, when done through cartilage but not mucosa, and has the same disadvantage of weakening support. It differs from morselization in that elevation of the mucoperichondrium is necessary only on one side of the cartilage, and the incised segment of cartilage is completely separated from the adjacent cartilage. The attachment of the mucoperichondrium on one side helps to keep the cartilage segments in position after the cross-hatching.

Swinging-Door Flaps

These are used to reposition large pieces of flat, but angulated, cartilage that are displaced. A cartilage flap is outlined with through-and-through incisions along the edges of the displaced portion, and the section that is not displaced or deviated (base of the flap) is left intact. To reposition this flap of cartilage, the intact base must be weakened so that it can act as a hinge on which the displaced portion can swing back to the midline. The weakening is usually accomplished by morselization, or incisions partially through the base. As much of the base as possible should remain intact, but if the flap has a tendency to return to its original position, it may have to be completely incised. When this is the case, the mucoperichondrium should be intact on one side to help maintain control of the freed cartilage segment, and splinting will be necessary if the segment is needed for support of the nose.

DIFFICULT ANATOMIC PROBLEMS

Correction of a Deviated Caudal Septum

When the caudal septum is off the nasal spine, it must be repositioned on the spine. This is usually managed with a swinging-door flap, so that the septum can be placed on the spine and stabilized with a figure-of-eight suture (see description below). This suture (4–0 or 5–0 catgut) starts through the space between the cartilage and the spine and passes through the mucosa of the opposite side. It is passed back through the mucosa at the level of the inferior edge of the spine and passes under the spine, thereby catching a bite of periosteum. It then goes back through the space between the cartilage and the spine, through mucosa, back more cephalad through mucosa and cartilage, and is then tied to the free end.

If the caudal septum has a curved deviation, a swinging-door flap does not work. Such a case requires morselization, segmental cross-hatching, or multiple through-and-through incisions with splinting.

Correction of a Dorsally Deviated "L" Strut

If the deviation of the "L" strut is angular, a swinging-door flap is used. An incision is made at the area of the deviation. It starts ventrally and extends dorsally to within 2 to 3 mm of the dorsal border (Fig. 2). If the deviated portion can then be positioned in the midline without reversion toward the deviated side, it is splinted and nothing further is needed. However, if it tends to move toward its original position, splints are placed on both sides and secured with at least two through-and-through 3–0 nylon sutures. The incision is then continued through the dorsal edge of the strut. The splints stabilize the interrupted strut and prevent both segments from displacing backward into the nose.

If the "L" strut has a curved deviation, it is preferably managed by morselization or multiple through-and-through incisions. Again, the strut must be partially incised and splinted before the incisions are completed. When a displaced caudal septum prevents the dorsal strut from remaining in the midline, it also requires correction.

SPLINTING TECHNIQUE

Nasal Septal Splints

These splints are used routinely for splinting the septum following septal surgery. This eliminates the need for packing (unless turbinate resection has been performed), which the patient appreciates; but more important, the splints position the septum in the midline during the initial stages of cartilage wound healing.

The splints are made of soft Silastic and have an airway along the side. The airway is important, not because it allows the patient to breathe, but because it is wedged between the flat surface of the splint and the inferior and middle turbinates. This pushes the flat part of the splint toward the midline and stabilizes it in that position. If the turbinates on one side are enlarged and pushing the splint past the midline, they may be reduced by partial resection, or a portion of the splint airway can be removed. The splints are left in place for 1 week.

SCRAMBLING

Figure-of-Eight Suture

When used correctly, a figure-of-eight suture (Fig. 3) helps to stabilize, reposition, or correct overriding of car-

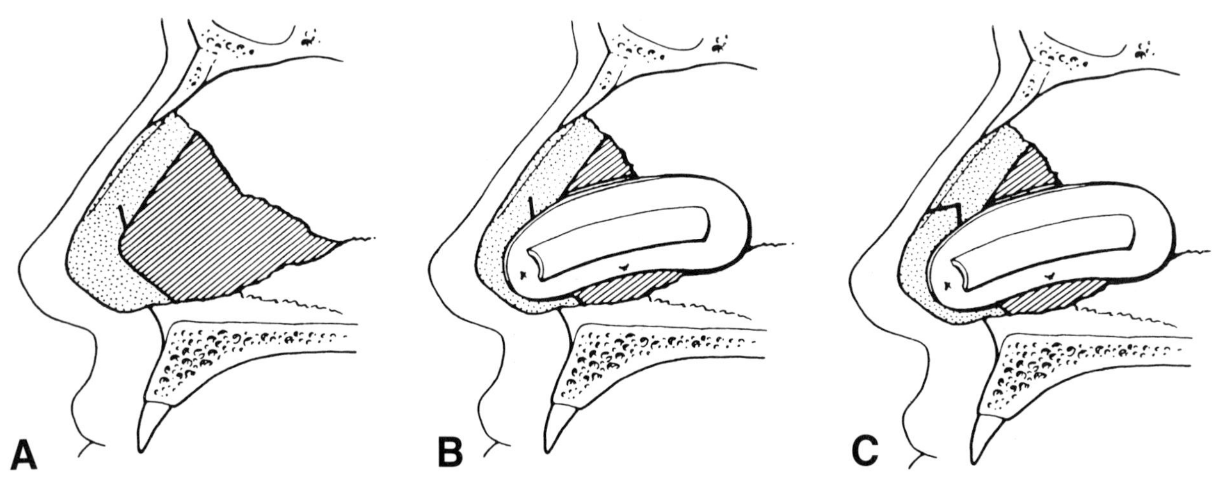

Figure 2 *A*, Incision partially through "L" strut. *B*, Splints applied for support. *C*, Transection completed after splinting.

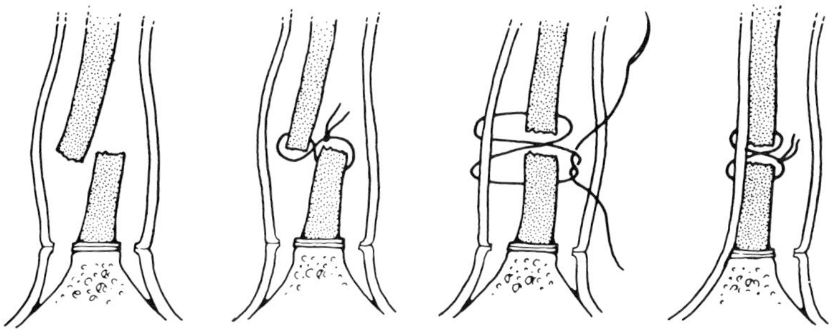

Figure 3 Figure-of-eight suture. The inclusion of mucoperichondrium in suture, *center, right,* prevents overriding of cartilage edges, *right.*

tilage edges. The type of suture we use for this is a 4–0 or 5–0 plain catgut on a short, straight needle. It is passed submucosally on one side, between the edges of the cartilages, and through the mucosa of the opposite side. It is then passed back through the mucosa and one of the pieces of the cartilage. It then travels back between the cartilage edges and through the mucosa, near the first area penetrated, then back through the mucosa and other piece of cartilage, and is tied to the loose end. As it is tightened, it snugs up the mucosa and brings the edges together without any overlap. It is important that the mucosa on one side be included in the suturing, otherwise there will be a tendency for the edges to overlap.

Loss of Support of the "L" Strut

About the worst thing that can happen in septal surgery is for the "L" strut to break before the splints are applied. When this happens the cephalic edge of the caudal segment has a tendency to fall back into the nose (Fig. 4).

This problem is managed by placing a 4–0 nylon suture, with a needle on each end, submucosally through the cephalic end of the caudal segment. Each end is then passed through the dorsal skin and pulled away from the nose to place the displaced segment back into position. As an assistant holds the suture, a 4–0 plain catgut figure-of-eight suture is placed at the fracture site to stabilize the fracture. The 4–0 nylon suture is then passed through a plaster of Paris splint as it is placed on the nose. When the splint dries, the suture ends are pulled snugly and tied over the splint.

If the cephalic segment also tends to fall back into the nose after fracture of the "L" strut, another 4–0 nylon suture, that passes through the dorsal skin and catches the cephalic cartilage segment, is used to lift the segment while the figure-of-eight is placed. It is then tied over the plaster splint in the same way as the caudal suture.

Mucoperichondrial Perforations

The mucoperichondrium may be perforated accidentally during elevation. If there is no perforation at the same position on the opposite side, closure of the perforation is not necessary; if there is an opposing perforation, one of them should be closed. Closure is best accomplished by passing a 5–0 plain catgut suture through the mucoperichondrium at the anterior portion of the nose, so that it can be tied with the free end left long (Fig. 5).

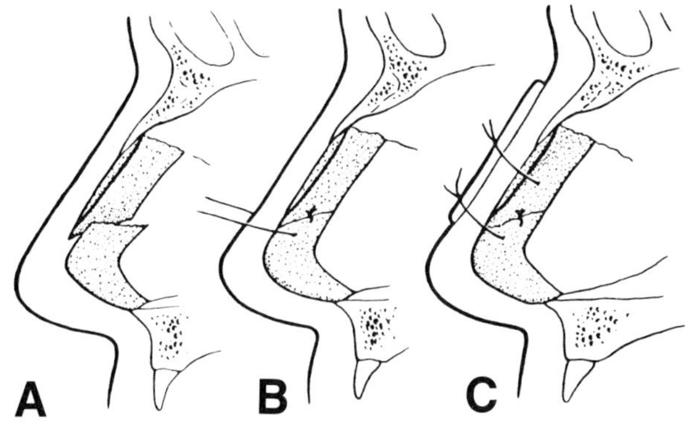

Figure 4 *A,* Fractured "L" strut. *B,* Traction suture through skin and caudal segment and figure-of-eight suture to stabilize fracture line. *C,* Traction sutures through, and tied snugly over, a plaster splint.

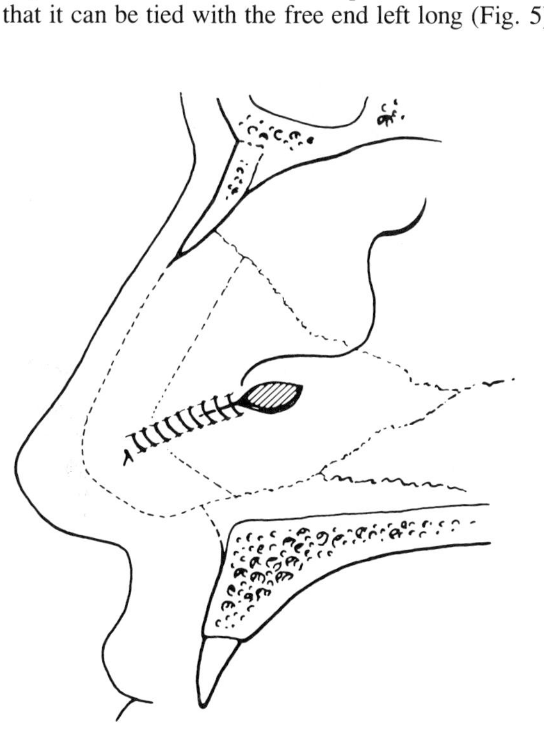

Figure 5 Closure of perforation of mucoperichondrium. Suturing starts anteriorly, proceeds past perforation, and then returns anteriorly to be tied to remaining long end of suture.

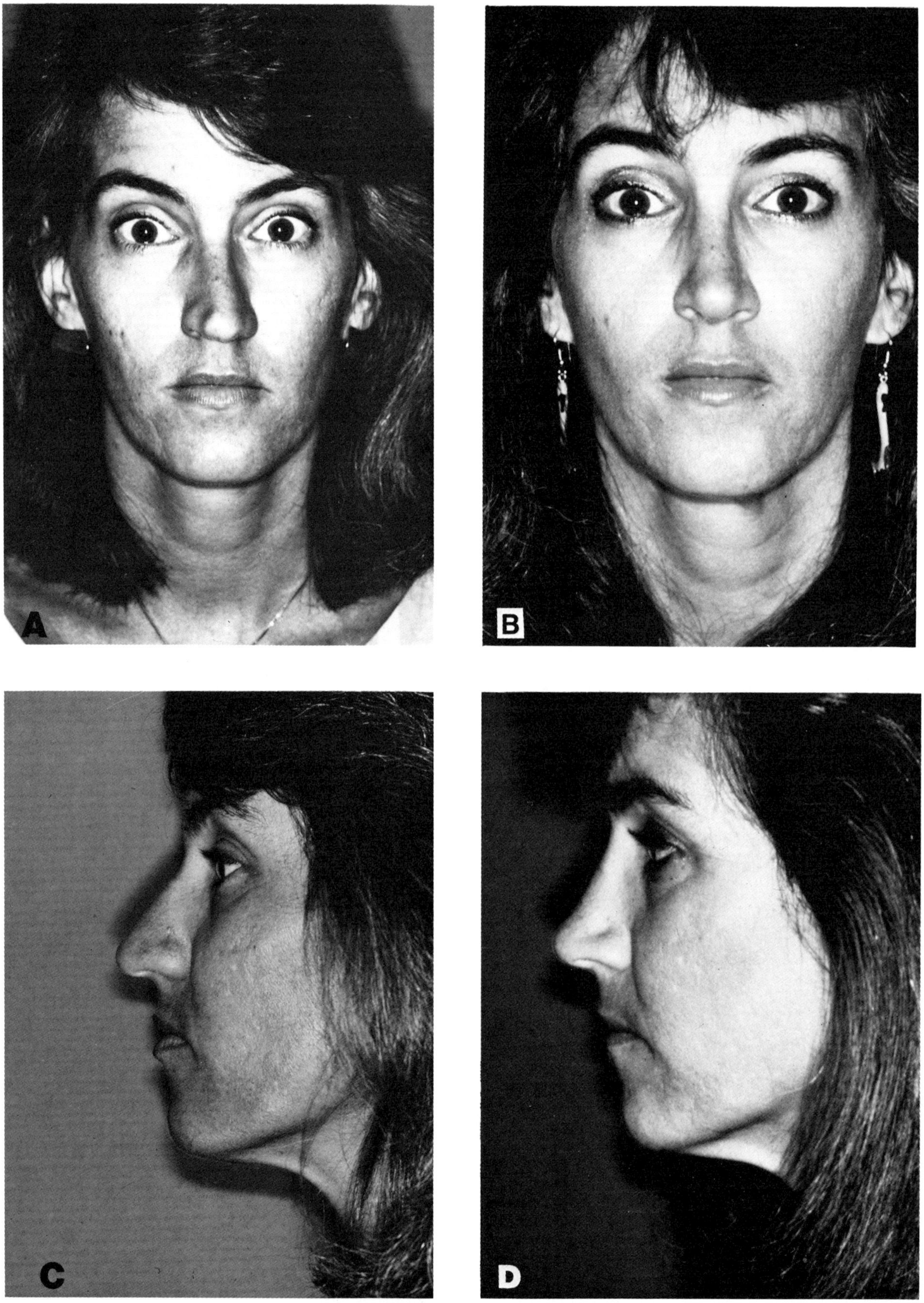

Figure 6 *A* and *C*, Preoperative and *B* and *D*, Postoperative views (9 months).

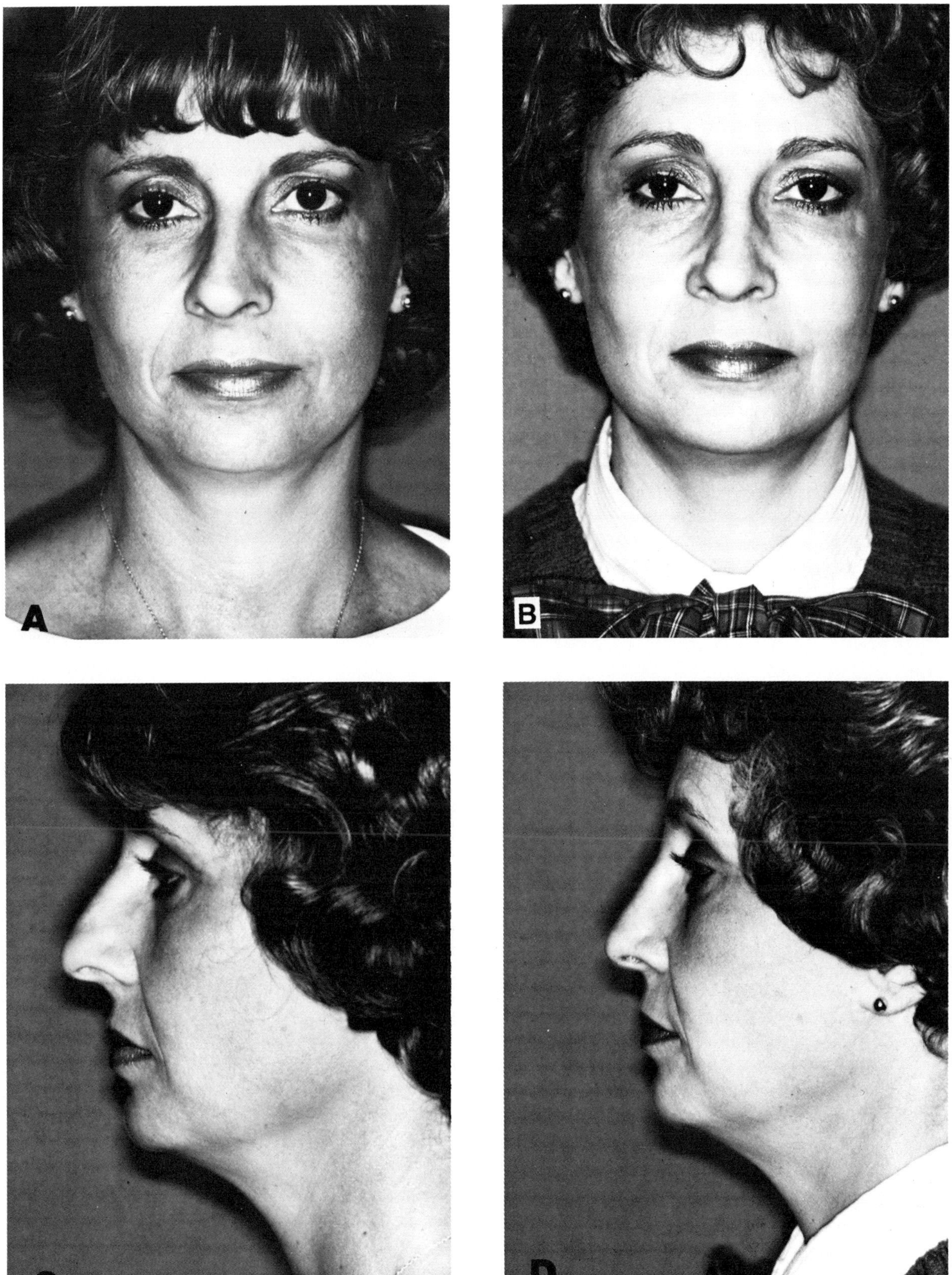

Figure 7 *A* and *C*, Preoperative and *B* and *D*, Postoperative views (14 months).

The suture is then run in a baseball-stitch fashion to the perforation and continued to close the perforation. It is then run back to the point of origin and tied to the remaining long end.

Enlarged Turbinates

Chronically hypertrophied turbinates that cross the midline make it impossible to place the septum in the center of the nasal cavity. The turbinates have to be corrected by outfracturing and/or resection. We prefer to *partially* resect the anterior end of the turbinates and outfracture the posterior segment. The reasoning for this is that there is less space anteriorly, where resection will give a larger airway, and posteriorly, where the nasal vault is larger, resection, in our hands, has resulted in increased postoperative hemorrhage. Overzealous resection of the turbinates can result in atrophic rhinitis with chronic crusting and bleeding, and we recommend resecting only what is necessary. After resection of the anterior end of the turbinates (usually only the inferior turbinate has to be resected), cauterization and packing with a hemostatic agent controls any postoperative oozing.

ILLUSTRATIVE CASES

Two representative cases are presented to illustrate results obtained from using the previously described techniques. The first case (Fig. 6) represents the correction of a deviated caudal septum with use of partial resection and a swinging-door flap. The second case (Fig. 7) was corrected with sectioning of the "L" strut.

SUGGESTED READING

Brain DJ. The management of the deviated nose. J Laryngol Otol 1981; 95:471–486.

Conrad K. Correction of crooked noses by external rhinoplasty. J Otolaryngol 1978; 7:32–42.

Gorney M. Septum in rhinoplasty. In: Millard DR, ed. Symposium on corrective rhinoplasty. St. Louis: CV Mosby, 1976; 13:180.

Gunter JP, Rohrich RJ. Management of the deviated nose. Clin Plast Surg 1988; 15:43–55.

Johnson CM, Anderson JR. The deviated nose—its correction. Laryngoscope 1977; 87:1680–1684.

Planos J. The twisted nose. Clin Plast Surg 1977; 4:55–67.

THE SEPTUM IN RHINOPLASTY: FORM AND FUNCTION

MARK GORNEY, M.D., F.A.C.S.

Contrary to the classic architectural dictum, function is almost wholly dependent on form. In septorhinoplasty no-one's septum is really straight. Heredity, birth, and repetitive trauma all combine to give most of us some degree of septal irregularity. As long as the nasal vault is adequate, it does not bother us. However, it is self-evident that any narrowing or lowering of that vault, without simultaneous correction of the deviated septum, will lead to some limitation of air flow. The externally deviated nose cries out for both esthetic as well as functional correction. What I am concerned with here is the essentially straight, or slightly deviated, nose inside which there is a potential for both functional and esthetic disaster. You cannot straighten a crooked nose without correcting the septum; you can create a crooked nose if you do not.

It is almost superfluous to state that a structurally sound and straight septum is the foundation of a satisfactory rhinoplasty result. There is still, however, substantial disagreement among plastic surgeons on appropriate corrective techniques. There is also some misunderstanding of nasal physiology, particularly around the valve area, and sometimes a cavalier disregard for the integrity of the nasal airway. I suspect a much higher degree of obstructive complications than those officially reported in the literature. In other words: it is nice to make them beautiful; but can they breathe?

The ear, nose, and throat literature is replete with references on the septum that go back to the turn of the century. There are volumes written on the functional aspects of nasal surgery. Neither this material nor the internal anatomy or physiology of the nose will be belabored here, and attention will be limited to one facet of a broad field, namely, a simplified overview of the functional and structural aspects of septoplasty as related to cosmetic rhinoplasty.

NASAL PHYSIOLOGY

I will focus on several limited, but critically important, facets of internal nasal physiology of significance to the plastic surgeon.

The way in which air currents traverse the nasal conduits—their direction, their shape, and speed of the stream—is determined as much by nasal configuration as by the natural anatomic constriction found approximately 2 cm inside the nostrils. This area, commonly referred to as the "valve," is the confluence of the caudal edge of the upper lateral cartilages and the septum (overlapped by the upper border of the alar cartilages). This constriction acts like the nozzle of a hose. The length and capacity of a hose mean nothing; the stream that it throws, and direction of same, is modified by the shape of the nozzle.

On normal inspiration in the intact nose, the air is directed upwards and backwards, arches up between the septum, and turbinates to the face of the sphenoid, down through the choana and into the pharynx. Relatively little passes along the floor. The choana has essentially no effect on the stream.

Over the turbinates, air becomes humidified to approximately 90 percent relative humidity before it reaches the larynx.

On expiration, air passes through the lower choana and is thrown into eddies by the baffle effect of the posterior aspect of the turbinates and the nozzle effect of the nostrils.

As the air currents are moved over the ciliated surfaces, particulate matter is deposited, probably by electrostatic principles. The mucosal glands deposit a lubricating blanket that is moved by the cilia and carries off debris. Tear flow assists.

Cilia line the inner surface of the nose, except for the olfactory areas. One must visualize a house, through the center of which run two corridors covered with thick, velvet-pile wallpaper. The dust that enters the house is passed along the wall, ceiling, and floor, down the corridor, through the back door, and into the ashcan—a complete trip in 20 minutes. This self-cleaning wallpaper works 24 hours a day unless something happens. Cilia are tough and have only one natural enemy: dryness. This incapacitates their ability to function and move mucus.

The principal iatrogenic enemy of cilia is scars; hurdles over which cilia cannot move the mucosal blanket. Annular scars not only bar the flow but further narrow the nozzle, thus creating a mechanical as well as a physiologic barrier.

The valves must be of sufficient size to allow free flow of respiration, and both should be nearly alike. If very disproportionate amounts of air are allowed to enter one side only, it will tend to dry and undergo metaplasia. This may be reported by the patient as a feeling of nasal obstruction. Underventilation will lead to constant mucus accumulation.

The important relationships between the superior edge of the alar cartilage and the caudal edge of the upper laterals is illustrated in Figure 1. The legend explains the anatomic-physiologic correlation, as well as the valve or nozzle concept. Any uncorrected or iatrogenic septal deviation at this point automatically aggravates obstruction on inspiration and virtually assures dissatisfaction.

ARCHITECTURAL SIGNIFICANCE OF THE SEPTUM

If one drops an imaginary line from the nasion to the nasal spine, anything posterior to that line can be resected from floor to ceiling without fear of collapse. Anything anterior to it must be resected with discretion and forethought, lest insufficient support and subsequent functional (and esthetic) distortion occur. Even if there seems to be an adequate dorsal cartilaginous support remaining, beware of the effect of contracture of the mucosal leaves and the plane of scar between them. If there have been perforations, this is even more significant.

If one considers the upper laterals as the wings sprouting from the upper edge of the septum (an embryologically correct concept), then if the upper edge of the septum is deviated, it must be freed from the wings that tether it. If one fails to do this, their guywire effect eventually redeviates the dorsum. This separation should be done at the submucoperichondrial level. If one keeps the mucoperichondrial flap attached to the underside of the upper laterals, except where they join the septum, then the mucoperichondrial flaps will not sag. In this way, one can avoid cutting away the upper laterals, mucosa and all. In my opinion, this maneuver always creates scar and synechiae, which later may restrict inspiratory air flow (Fig. 2).

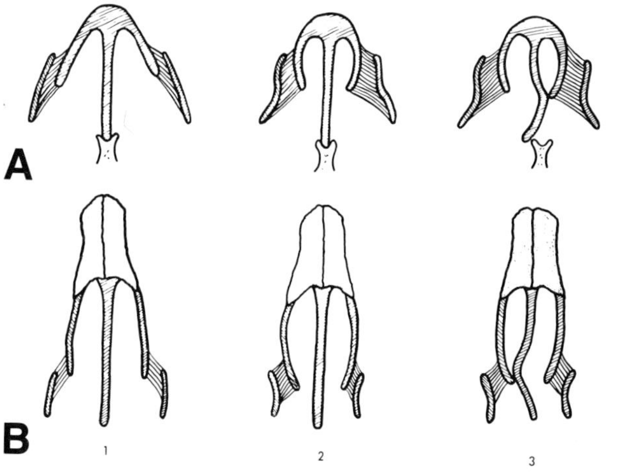

Figure 1 Anatomic and physiologic relationships in valve area. Upper edge of the alar cartilage slightly overlaps lower edge of upper laterals. There is tenuous fibrous attachment between them. *A*, Cross section and *B*, sagittal sections—column 1, quiet inspiration, midsagittal septum, column 2, forceful inspiration, midsagittal septum; column 3, forceful inspiration, deviated septum. There need be no external deviation visible. When nose is narrowed, problem becomes more disturbing.

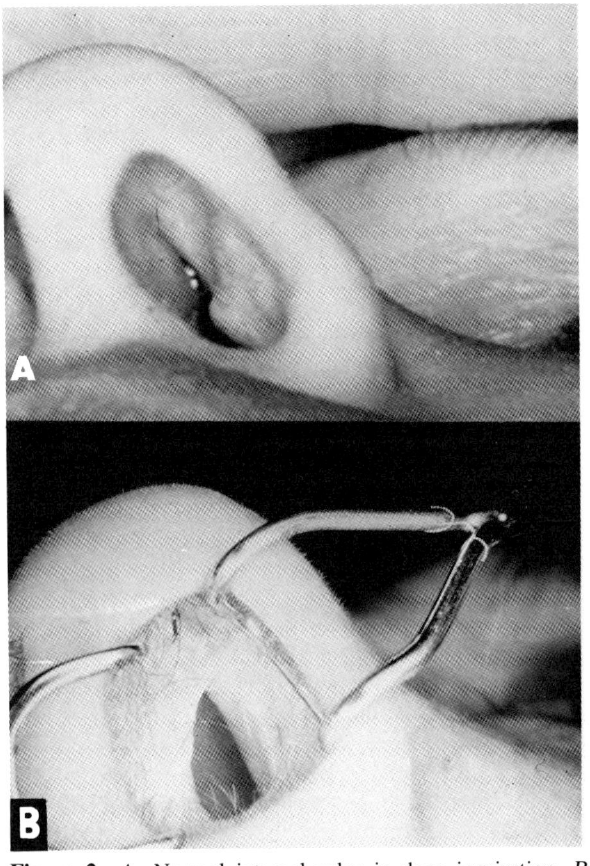

Figure 2 *A*, Normal internal valve in deep inspiration. *B*, Postoperative annular cicatricial constriction.

High septal deflection, often undetected, can frustrate a perfect rhinoplasty. The hump, which is in the normal midsagittal plane, may be covering a septum just under it that is quite crooked. (It is easy to miss these in cursory preoperative examinations.) Operative edema may deceive the surgeon. When the infracture has been completed, one has brought together the nasal bones and upper laterals against an undiscovered deviation of the upper border of the septum. Two weeks later, when the edema recedes, the beautiful result at the end of the operation may look distinctly off-center. (Fig. 3).

The sequence of the septal correction at surgery is important. Figure 4 shows a typical subluxation and override of the septovomerine junction at the anteroinferior corner of the quadrilateral cartilage. What happens here can have a profound effect on the new profile line. If one frees up the dislocated lower edge of the vomer bone and replaces the inferior edge of the septal cartilage within it, this tends to lift the lower end of the nose. If, on the other hand, one has to cut off the extremely deviated lower edge of the septum and/or chisel the vomer groove out to replace the septum in the center, one may end up by lowering the tip of the nose, whose support depends on the remaining cartilaginous strut (see Fig. 4). Thus, the surgeon must know what he or she is going to do ahead of time. It is poor planning to make a beautiful profile and then fix the septum, only to find it lowered in the tip area. I try to do the correction first, and leave more than adequate dorsal buttress so that corrections along the profile line, or shortening of the nose, can still be done at the end of the rhinoplasty without weakening the remaining support. If in doubt, obviously, the hump resection and dorsal correction must be done first and then septoplasty, so that enough cartilage is left behind to guarantee integrity of the profile line. I also find that it is much easier from the standpoint of visibility, neatness, and safety to do the septum first, particularly if it is badly bent.

The hump may be relative or absolute. A large Arabic or Romanesque hump can be characterized as an absolute one. If the profile line suddenly dips below the end of the nasal bones, this is a relative hump and is almost invariably caused by septal abnormality. If the septum has been distorted severely enough to require almost total removal, this will affect the profile line significantly. This is the nose in which it is wise to consider use of the

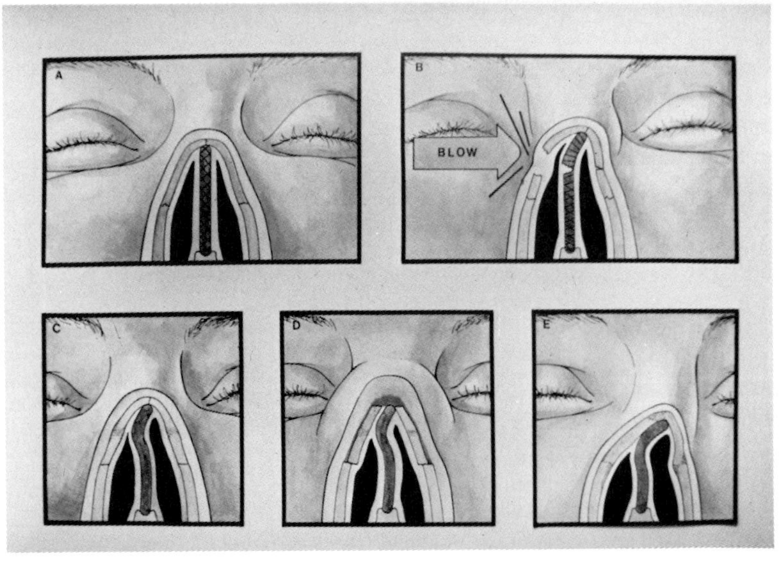

Figure 3 *A*, Normal nasal configuration; *B*, Trauma deviates dorsal portion of cartilage; *C*, After reduction, cartilage remains deviated and may not be seen; *D*, Lateral walls are moved in during rhinoplasty and joined to undetected deviation; and *E*, entire alignment appears deviated after edema subsides.

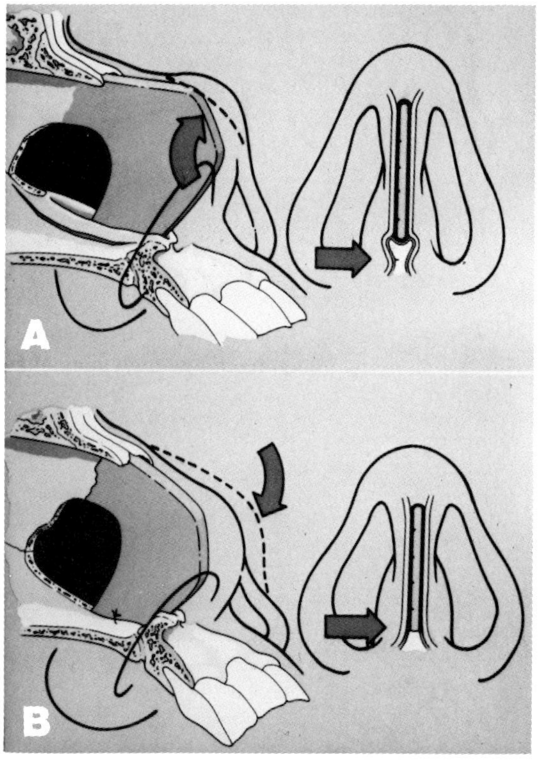

Figure 4 Effect on the nasal tip height from *A*, restoration of the vomer groove to the midline and mounting of the septal cartilage on it, versus *B*, resection of the vomer and drooping lower of the septal cartilage, which causes tip of the nose to drop also.

resected septum to bridge the sag between the self-supporting tip and the end of the nasal bones.

In severe internal deviations, the remaining L-shaped strut may remain deviated. If the surgeon fails to straighten it, a redeviated nose is almost guaranteed. Until recently, most authors advised various maneuvers to score, cut, crosshatch, or remove strips vertically from the convex side of the deformity, with the idea of allowing the remaining septum to swing back into the midline. There are also a number of maneuvers described to keep it there. In my experience this has been, at the very best, chancy. As many, or more, have redeviated as have stayed improved. The existence of interlocking stresses within cartilage is well-known, as is the tendency of cartilage to curl to the opposite side to that in which scored. For the past few years, I have always scored on the concave side. If the deviation is a complex one, both sides are scored but always on the concave portion. The obvious improvement in long-term follow-ups has been gratifying (Fig. 5).

Recently, in particularly badly deviated septums, I have taken to reinforcing the scoring by suturing a small batten of curved, surplus septal cartilage on the unscored side to act as a reinforcement. This curved cartilage batten on the opposite side acts as a counterspring to the residual curvature in the remaining strut. This maneuver is illustrated in Figure 6. The results so far have been gratifying.

TECHNICAL SUGGESTIONS

No one operation can correct a deformity so infinite in its variables. Several authors have pointed out that the classic submucous resection is, per se, hardly ever the complete answer. What must be done is an operation that will: (1) restore function, (2) correct deviation, and (3) prevent saddling, columellar retraction and tip droop.

The principle of the operation is to divide every attachment of the cartilaginous septum, except for a mucosal flap on the one side (to maintain the blood supply), and to release the interlocking stresses in the twisted cartilage. The goal should be maximum mobility with the least possible removal of tissue. My approach to the problem is an amalgam of many standard techniques with a few personal modifications. There are a few caveats as follow:

1. If an *inter*cartilaginous incision is to be made, it is far better to do so 1 mm below the actual valve. Strong upward traction on a double hook on the nostril margin, while the upper lateral cartilage is stabilized with the middle finger, will reveal the actual inferior edge of the upper lateral. One should not cut there, but slightly below in order to minimize the annular contracture directly at the valve.
2. The secret to avoiding perforations is to undermine at the right level—subperichondrially. In the distal 1 to 2 cm of cartilaginous septum, the mucosa is intimately attached to the cartilage. After incision along the protrusive leading edge, a very sharp elevator is useful to find the correct plane. It is easy to start down

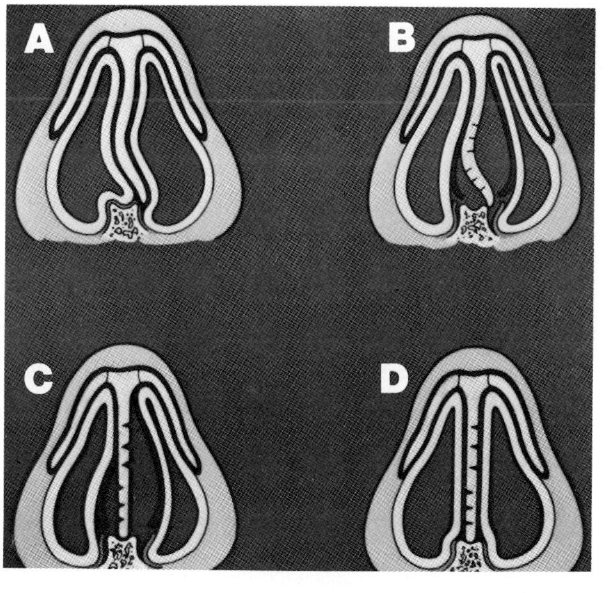

Figure 5 *A*, Typical biconvex deviation with subluxation. *B*, Mucoperichondrial flap is elevated on left side. Right side is left partially attached for blood supply. *C*, Shows release of interlocking stresses by scoring on each concave surface and restoration on vomer groove. Trimming may be necessary to allow septal cartilage to swing back. *D*, Replacement of mucosal cover. Mattress sutures may be indicated.

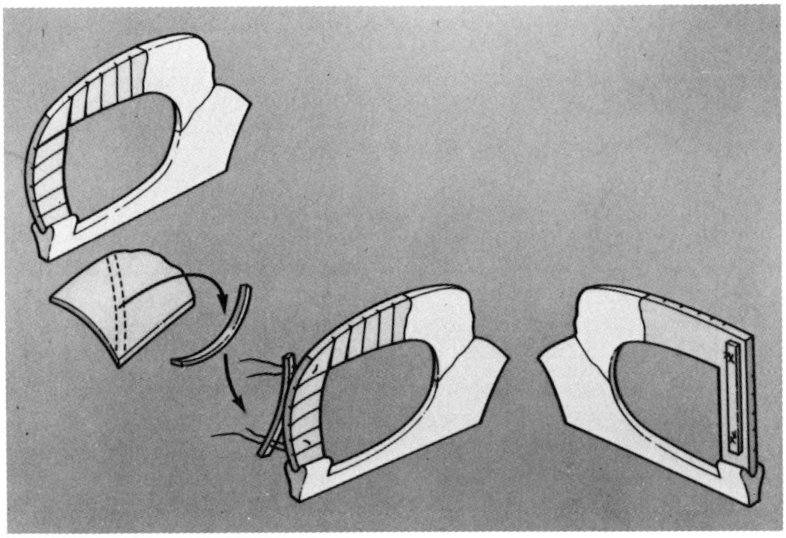

Figure 6 If the remaining strut shows persistent deviation, it should be scored on the concave side and deviation counteracted by fabrication of countercurved "batten" from resected, deviated cartilage. Batten should be fastened in place.

the wrong one, and this virtually guarantees perforations and tears, particularly along the spurs, crests, and ridges where the mucosa is as thin as wet tissue paper. There is a very characteristic gray-bluish reflex visible when one enters the right plane. There is also a clean, smooth feel on the instrument, which will glide along quite easily. When the instrument passes from the cartilage to the vertical plate of the ethmoid, there is a characteristic change in the feel of the scraping. It is best to proceed in semicircular upward motions rather than push straight and back. One should not try to go past the angle of deviation or around ridges. This also produces perforations. (Small perforations are of no consequence unless they are back-to-back on both mucosal leaves, which produces a permanent perforation).

3. Along the inferior anterior aspect of the cartilaginous septum, where it fits in the vomerine ridge, it is very difficult to pass down from the subperichondrial space of the cartilage to the subperiosteal space of the vomer. The quadrilateral septal cartilage is invested completely by perichondrium, even along its lower edge, which sits in the vomer groove. The vomer ridge, in turn, has periosteum tightly adherent over it. Therefore, after undermining from the roof of the nose to the septovomerine ridge, one should not try to continue inferiorly but should back off and begin a new tunnel under the periosteum of the vomer. It is much easier to join these two spaces without tearing once they have been independently developed.
4. If cartilage is excised, it should be done with the certain knowledge that enough dorsum is left behind to prevent a saddle nose. One must remember that the plane of contracting scar between the leaves of mucosa will exert a powerful pull inferiorly and may create a saddle by distortion of a weak or detached dorsal strut. The plane of cut is set by the inclination of the hand that holds the scissors. The cartilage should not be cut with the scissors parallel to the wrist. The scissors should be inclined inferiorly and cut on a plane parallel to the nasal dorsum.
5. This operation is like making a watch in a drainpipe. The most useful instruments to ease this sometimes difficult procedure are a combination suction-elevator and Blakely alligator forceps, (model No. N3000 made by Stortz). The former eliminates the need to keep changing instruments at critical moments. The latter is much easier to use because its fulcrum is at the tip of the instrument and only the business end opens, thus making it easier to work in restricted posterior spaces. Both save a lot of time.
6. A deflected vomer can often be "greensticked" into the midline by placing a 1 mm chisel on the nasal floor and scoring along one side of the base of the deviated vomer ridge. A little pressure by opening a long thin speculum along the floor of the nose often does the trick.
7. If the vertical element of the remaining L-shaped cartilage support is still crooked, one should not depend on columellar pockets or transfixation devices to straighten it. Not only will it not work, but it will carry the tip of the nose with it when it redeviates. It should be scored on its concave side and, if need be, stiffened on the intact (convex) side with a thin cartilage batten (see Fig. 6). Figure 7 shows a typical case of severe internal distortion where the remaining cartilage was prevented from recurving by a batten on the right side.
8. At the end of the procedure I use Xomed's internal Teflon splints, held in place by two mattress sutures. This, alone, may do the job. If in doubt, one should pack the nose lightly. What was the convex side should be packed first. (If the nose deviates to the right, pack the left side first). The "cram-jam" technique should not be used. One should pack carefully from the floor up and use just enough material to put the mucosal leaves back to back. One nasal length should be put in at a time and tamped down by opening the specu-

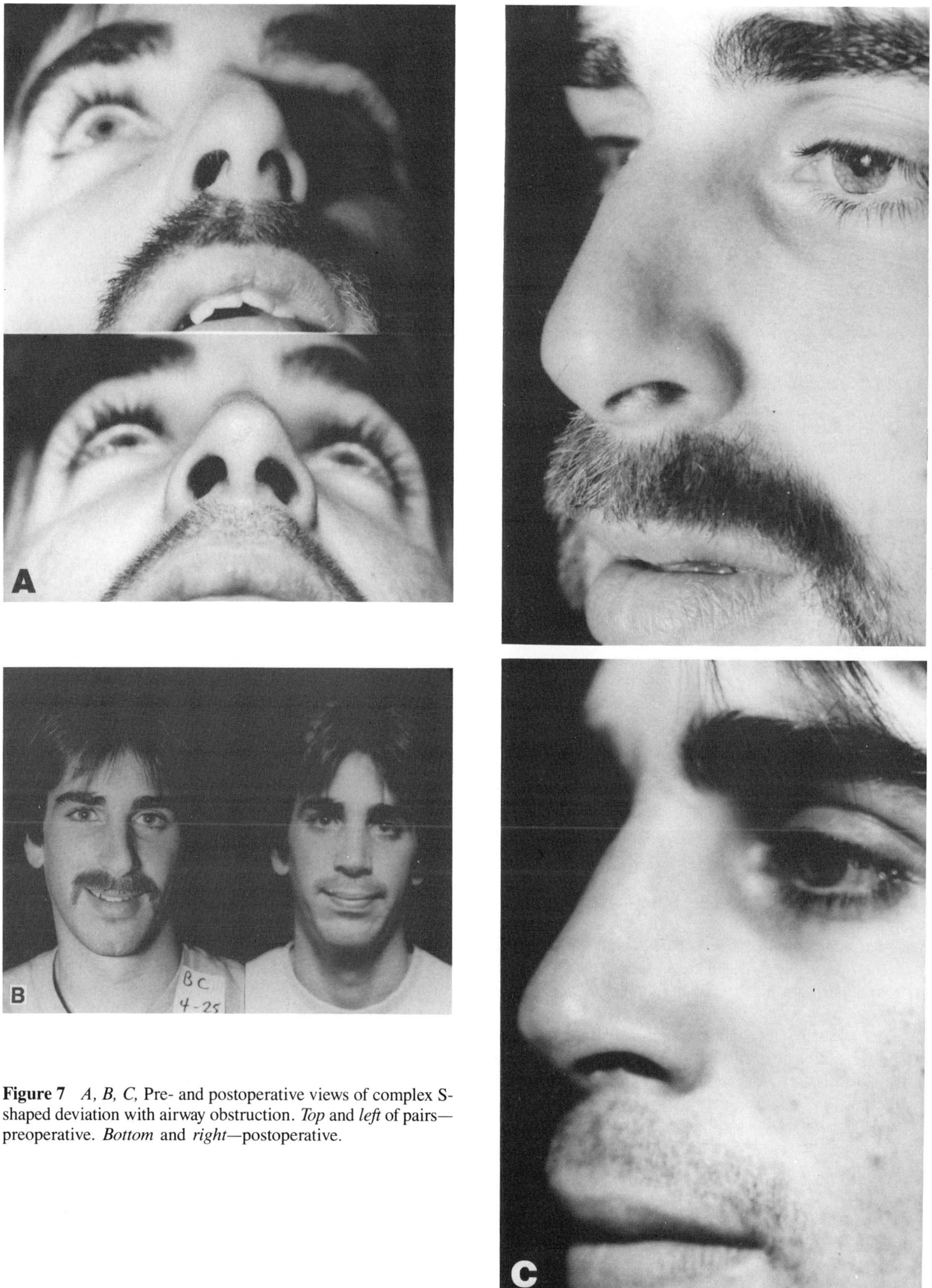

Figure 7 *A, B, C,* Pre- and postoperative views of complex S-shaped deviation with airway obstruction. *Top* and *left* of pairs—preoperative. *Bottom* and *right*—postoperative.

lum. It should be borne in mind that an overall splint will bring things further together, and too much packing may tend to separate the nasal bones. The pack stays in for 2 days. If there is bad deviation and obstruction, the pack may be pulled from the old obstructed side 1 day later than the other. The splints can stay in for a whole week.

9. Totally intact, accurately-closed mucoperichondrial leaves, if inadequately packed, may be dangerous. Septal hematomas are not uncommon and, if not evacuated properly, can give a very thick, obstructive septum. If in doubt, there is no harm in making a couple of stab wounds with a No. 5 blade at separate sites on either side at the base of the mucoperichondrial flaps for drainage. Stab wounds should not overlap.
10. The turbinates are often part of the problem. Time and space do not permit a detailed account of this aspect. However, it may be appropriate to deal with troublesome turbinates at the time of surgery by several simple maneuvers. They can be outfractured by forceful pressure with a long speculum, cauterized along their edge, or trimmed away. Overenthusiastic treatment should be avoided. Turbinates respond nicely to intranasal corticoids, injected directly into the submucosa at the end of the operation.

SUGGESTED READING

Brent B. Case No. 7. In: Brent B, Brent B, eds. The artistry of reconstructive surgery: selected classic case studies. St. Louis: CV Mosby, 1987.

Freeman BS. Facial palsy. In: Converse JM, eds. Reconstructive plastic surgery: principles and procedures in correction reconstruction and transplantation. Vol 2. Philadelphia: WB Saunders, 1977:1124.

Fry HJH. The importance of the septal cartilage in nasal trauma. Br J Plast Surg 1967; 20:392–402.

Goldman IB. Rhinoplastic sequelae causing nasal obstruction. Arch Otolaryngol 1966; 83:151–155.

Gorney M. Correction of the deviated nose. Clin Plast Surg 1981; 8:201–210.

Horton CE. Combined septoplasty and rhinoplasty. In: Masters FW, Lewis JR Jr, eds. Symposium on aesthetic surgery of the nose, ears, and chin. St. Louis: CV Mosby, 1973.

BLEPHAROPLASTY

ARTHUR G. SHIP, M.D., D.M.D.

Blepharoplasty is generally thought of as a simple, easily executed operation that almost invariably produces good results. While all surgery demands skill, this procedure requires thorough patient evaluation and treatment planning, precise anatomic knowledge, and meticulous execution.

A successful blepharoplasty removes redundant skin and muscle, eliminates bulging fat tissue, and establishes a well-defined orbital-palpebral sulcus with a smooth expanse of pretarsal skin. Scars are symmetrical and inconspicuous. The correction of ageing or "tired" eyes contributes to a youthful and fresher appearance.

Prior to surgery, the surgeon should review with the patient the anticipated results and benefits of blepharoplasty, and should avoid facile promises. The risks involved, and alternative methods of treatment, should be discussed. The possibility of secondary surgery deserves mention. The patient should be aware that a full recovery may require 6 to 12 months.

PATIENT EVALUATION

Careful preoperative evaluation is essential to surgical planning. A systematic examination that includes vision testing is performed upon the seated patient. If this is done while the patient observes him or herself in a mirror, findings can be shared. The initial evaluation notes eye shape, lid attitude, fat protrusion, scleral show, skin and muscle excess, degree of brow ptosis and whether it influences perceived upper lid ptosis. The resting position of the upper lids is observed for unilateral or bilateral ptosis or lid lag. The surgeon documents the varying amounts of excess skin, muscle, and fat in the upper lids, as well as a poorly- or well-defined orbital-palpebral sulcus. The texture and dimensions of the pretarsal and upper lid skin are appreciated. Laxity of the lower lid and scleral show may reflect atonicity of the tarsus and lateral canthal tendon. This is demonstrated by the "snap-back" test described by Rees. Any excess of skin, muscle, and fat of the lower lids is noted. Gentle pressure on the globe demonstrates the location of fat pockets. When the patient rolls the eyes upward and outward, fat protrudes in the lower lateral compartments opposite to the direction of gaze. Other findings such as festoons, deep furrows, smile lines, and malar fat pads may be present. Their correction may not be possible during primary surgery.

All findings are charted and a diagram based upon Flowers' design is valuable (Fig. 1). Finally, photographic documentation is obtained.

SURGERY PLANNING

In formulating a plan for surgery, each component of the procedure is designed to accommodate the degree of deformity and the causal mechanisms. Descent of the brows below the bony prominence increases the extent of hooding and compromises the result of upper lid skin resection. Correction of brow ptosis may be indicated,

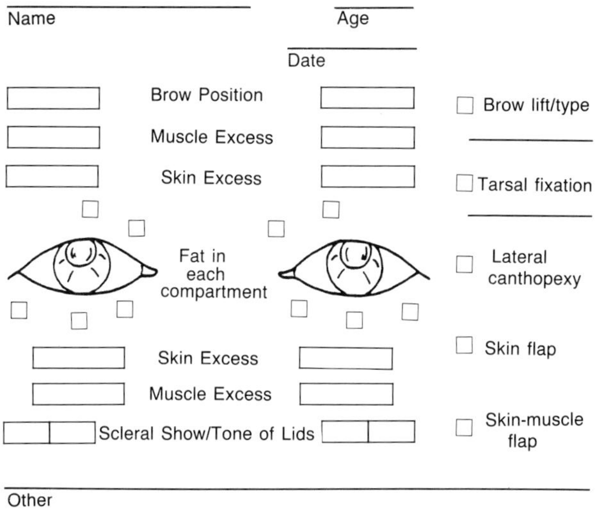

Figure 1 Schematic employed for charting clinical findings and treatment planning.

coincident with blepharoplasty, or as a preliminary procedure via a coronal, hairline, forehead skinfold, or direct supra-brow resection. Lid lag may reflect the residue of thyrotoxicosis, or excessive skin removal during prior surgery. Blepharoplasty will not correct this deformity.

Upper lid ptosis may be congenital, or the result of cataract surgery and the disruption of the levator aponeurosis. Tarsal or levator advancement can be incorporated into the blepharoplasty.

Deep-set orbital-palpebral sulci may be aggravated by resection of fat from the upper lids, or may require pedicled fat grafting from the medial fat compartments.

The resting level and tone of the lower lid and extent of scleral show may be related. A cicatricial ectropion requires appropriate correction prior to cosmetic blepharoplasty. Loss of tone or senile ectropion require a lateral canthopexy with fixation of the lower tarsus and/or lateral canthal tendon to the lateral orbital rim. The Kuhnt-Szymonowski procedure (tarsoconjunctival resection) is obsolete. Scars that indicate previous blepharoplasty suggest caution, because repeat surgery may result in a postoperative ectropion, even when no skin is removed.

Heavy lids may indicate excess muscle. This can be determined by having the patient squint. This especially well demonstrates discrete muscle excess in the lower lid. When selective muscle resection or limited thinning is indicated, a skin flap is essential.

The choice of a skin flap also may be dictated by the presence of festoons or crepiness of the lower lid skin. When muscle redundancy contributes to the formation of festoons, separate skin and muscle flaps are preferred. Under certain circumstances, a skin flap may be elevated for approximately 5 mm after which the muscle is penetrated and the dissection continued to the infraorbital margin as a skin–muscle flap. When only a skin flap is utilized, the excess must be trimmed conservatively, because skin will contract upon healing and produce an ectropion—at least initially.

TECHNIQUE

Immediately prior to surgery, the patient is reexamined in a seated position, looking straight ahead to locate the medial and lateral limits of skin excess. The lateral cutaneous redundancy forms an identifiable fold; the upper and lower borders of which are marked. Similarly, the medial redundancy is marked at the junction of orbital and nasal skin (Fig. 2). The patient is then placed in the supine position and prepared for surgery. Skin marking is continued. It is customary to address the upper lid first. The line for the lower incision should correspond to the cephalic border of the tarsal plate, usually situated 8 to 10 mm above the ciliary border and easily identified by everting the lid. The medial and lateral limits of the incision have been previously determined and marked. Skin excess may be measured by pinching the skin with a forceps. Preferentially, the skin is lightly grasped with a fine-tooth forceps 4 to 5 mm above the line of the caudal incision and pulled upward until the seal between the lids is broken. This displaces the newly marked line of incision. Without releasing the forceps, the skin is now pulled downwards and marked at a point that corresponds to the point of cephalic displacement of the lower incision. This maneuver accommodates the differing modulus of elasticity of the pretarsal skin and of the crepey excess of the upper lid. The ink mark at the upper border is then extended in a gentle arc to join the previously placed markings.

The lower lid incision is then marked. Only the lateral 5.0 mm of subciliary incision need be inscribed with a 5.0 mm lateral extension that extends out at an obtuse angle into, or immediately adjacent to, a normal skin crease.

Local anesthesia of the upper and lower lids is obtained through a single injection site approximately 1.0 cm beyond the lateral canthus. Eight to 10.0 cc of 1 percent lidocaine with 1:100,000 Adrenalin (or 1:200,000) is infiltrated, *subcutaneously only*, utilizing a flexible 27 gauge 1½″ needle. Surgery is delayed for 6 to 7 minutes to permit full vasoconstriction. The upper lid incisions are made using a 15C blade.* The skin between the incisions is sharply dissected; the underlying muscle is left *in situ*. Hemostasis is secured with thermocoagulation (the Concept^R battery-operated disposable high temperature cautery† is preferred). A 3- to 6-mm wide strip of subjacent orbicularis oculi muscle is removed in the lower third of the wound (see Fig. 2B). This facilitates the formation of a well-defined orbital-palpebral sulcus by the adhesion of the denuded tarsal dermis to the levator expansion. Formal tarsal suture fixation is thereby unnecessary in most patients.

* Martin Steril 15C (Gebruder Martin D-72, Tuttlingen, W. Germany.)
† Concept^R Accu-Temp^R Cat. No. 4200

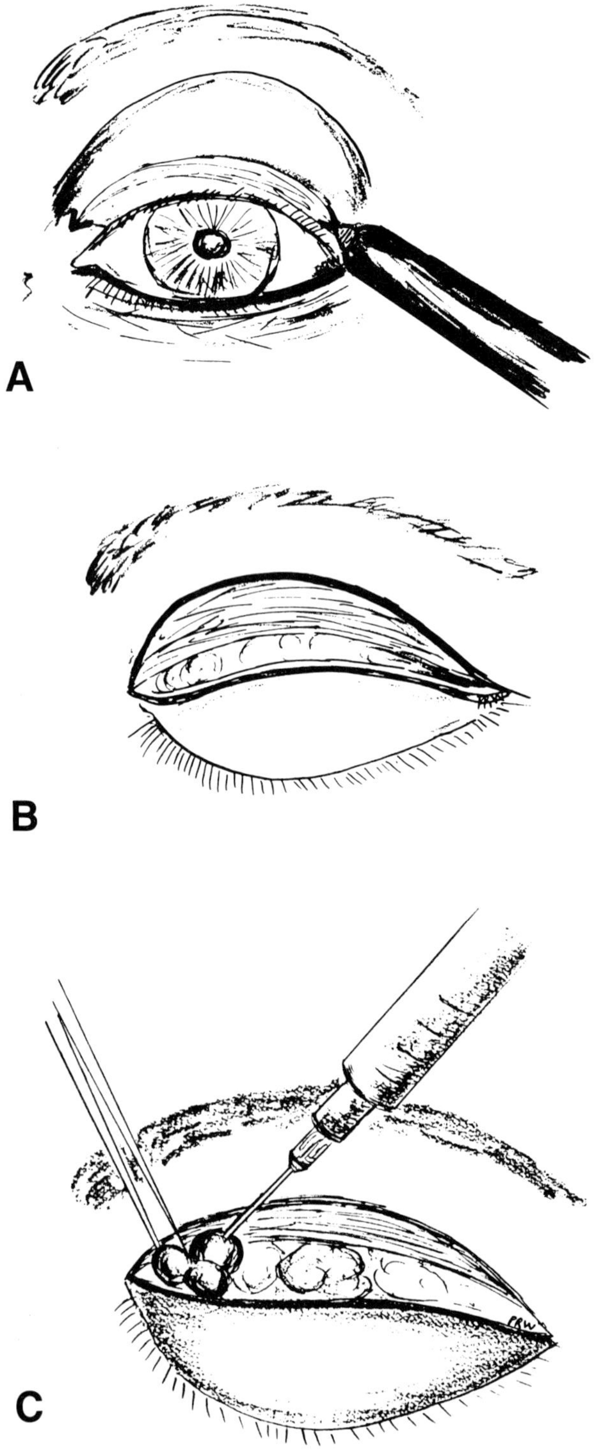

Figure 2 *A,* Shows the medial and lateral extent of upper lid skin redundancy being marked in the seated patient just prior to surgery. *B,* The orbicularis oculi muscle has been resected from the lower third of the skin defect. *C,* Injection of the medial fat pad is illustrated, prior to mobilization, to avoid pain, bradycardia, nausea, and vomiting.

At the cephalic level of the muscle resection, the septum orbitale presents. It is gently elevated with a fine forceps and incised at the lateral border of the central fat compartment. The entire septum orbitale is opened with Stevens tenotomy scissors (one blade is placed below the septum; the scissors extend the incision through the central compartment directly into the medial compartment). Two distinct fat masses will be present; one centrally, tan–white, that is loose and pliable, and one medially, more dense and golden–yellow with a firm globular consistency. The fat may be confined by a tense membrane that requires a separate incision. Light pressure is placed on the globe, and the fat is gently teased. Protruding fat is cross-clamped, amputated sharply, and thermally coagulated. Prior to performing this maneuver on the medial fat pad, it is important to inject 0.25 cc of lidocaine to block the nerves that supply this compartment (see Fig. 2C) to avoid pain associated with bradycardia, nausea, and even vomiting. The base of the amputated compartment should be grasped with a fine forceps upon release of the clamp, to prevent retraction of a vessel that may otherwise be difficult to retrieve and control.

Attention is then directed to the lower lid. The two 5.0 mm limbs of the incision, described above, are made with the 15C blade. To create a skin-muscle flap, scissors are inserted directly on the lateral orbital rim; the tips are guided to slide down below the orbicularis oculi muscle. The entire lower lid is then mobilized by blind dissection, caudally to the level of the infraorbital rim. This is generally an avascular plane, and the dissection proceeds without appreciable bleeding. A fine single hook is then placed at the junction of the two incision limbs and sharp curved serrated scissors or a knife are utilized to complete the infraorbital incision, approximately 0.5 to 1.0 mm below the ciliary border. The hook provides countertraction while the assistant pulls down on the cheek and the patient looks upward. The assistant sweeps the cilia upward. The cut surface of the skin is then grasped with a small four-finger rake, or double hook. If a skin-muscle flap at the level of the skin incision is desired, tenotomy scissors are used to incise the muscle. Eversion of the mobilized skin-muscle flap then permits hemostasis to be secured. A 6–0 black silk suture is placed through the soft tissue at the ciliary border, left long, clamped, and used to retract the lower lid upward and protect the globe. When a skin flap is desired, sharp dissection is carried out to the level of the infraorbital rim. Fine capillary and arteriolar bleeding will occur. The high temperature battery-operated cautery is effective.

The lateral fat compartment is entered first. It is readily located, since the septum orbitale has not been violated and the infraorbital fat contents have not been decompressed. It presents at a higher level than the central and medial fat compartments and is situated 5 to 8 mm below the lateral border of the lower lid. Gentle pressure on the globe demarcates the position of this fat pad. The septum orbitale is incised, as is the small sac immediately surrounding the fat, thus permitting it to herniate. It is infiltrated with 0.25 cc of lidocaine to avoid pain and its sequelae. The presenting fat is then removed as described above. Only after the lateral fat compartment has been reduced should the central and medial fat compartments be addressed. They are entered in a manner identical to that described for the central and medial compartments of the upper lid. Once the septum orbitale has been widely opened, redundant fat presents and is removed. The surgeon is cautioned to anesthetize the medial compartment prior to mobilization, crossclamping, and amputation. Again, the base should be grasped with a fine forceps to prevent retraction of a vessel.

When adequate hemostasis is assured, a cold compress is placed in the lower wound. The suture that retracts the lower lid cephalically is now repositioned to retract it caudally. The upper lid wound is inspected to assess the adequacy of skin excision. Heavy-lidded patients may require more extensive resection of muscle. Indeed, in the upper lid, orbicularis muscle can be resected to the same extent as overlying skin. When orbicularis oculi is excised, care must be taken that the subjacent levator expansion is not inadvertently incised, or ptosis may result. The fat compartments are reevaluated; the globe is gently pressed to determine if additional fat presents. At this point, tarsal fixation or ptosis correction, if appropriate, should be completed. Minimal to moderate degrees of upper lid ptosis can be corrected by some form of tarsal fixation. Suture of the pretarsal dermis to the levator expansion is preferred to suture of pretarsal muscle. Three or more sutures of 5–0 or 6–0 white Mersiline are used. The patient is then placed in a sitting position, and the degree of correction is assessed by observing the level of the upper lids. When further correction is indicated, the sutures are removed and replaced at a higher or lower level. Congenital ptosis, secondary to weakness of the levator, may require aggressive correction before reasonable symmetry is produced. The upper lid is closed with a running suture of 6–0 black silk, buttressed with two or three interrupted sutures.

The redundant skin and muscle of the lower lid is then assessed by employing a maneuver that the patient has rehearsed preoperatively. The patient is asked to look backward and open the eyes and mouth widely. The stretched lower lid tissues are then gently mobilized over the now concave surface of the wound, avoiding medial or lateral displacement. The redundant skin (and/or muscle) is accurately excised in a single continuous motion with the curved serrated scissors, so that it lies exactly at the level of the incised ciliary border. (Some surgeons prefer to incise the redundant tissue at right angles to its leading edge and remove it segmentally.) There should be no gap. Prior to suturing, the cut edge should be inspected for bleeding. The wound is then closed with a minimum of interrupted 6–0 black silk sutures. The wide-open eye and mouth maneuver is performed again to assess the tissue in the area of the lateral triangle. This is tailored and approximated with a suture 2 to 3 mm from the lateral border of the incision to avoid the need to "chase a dogear." A final suture is placed at the apex of the triangle.

Nonantibiotic ophthalmic ointment is placed in the fornix and on the suture lines, and cold, moist eye pads are applied to the corrected eye while the second eye is addressed. If, after completion of the blepharoplasty, other surgical procedures are performed, compresses are renewed periodically. Compression dressings are avoided. Postoperatively, ice-cold, moist eye pads are applied and renewed frequently. The patient is instructed to cleanse the suture lines gently, to protect them with nonantibiotic ophthalmic ointment, and to sleep on extra pillows. All sutures are removed in 48 to 72 hours. No tape splinting is employed. Application of frequent cold compresses is recommended for several weeks, especially upon rising, to counteract morning periorbital edema. Patients are advised to wear tinted glasses for 7 to 12 days and are permitted to use cosmetics beginning 5 days after surgery. They are reminded that swelling, scar induration, minimal asymmetry, etc., are part of the healing process and may require as long as a year to resolve.

After surgery, persistent edema, early thickening of scars, and minimal contour irregularity can be expected to improve or disappear with the passage of time. Lid lag may be manifest for up to a year, or permanently if excessive upper lid skin and muscle has been resected. Pigmentation of lower lids is rarely a consequence of surgery alone, and is usually evident to some degree preoperatively. Four to 5 percent hydroquinone cream, applied twice daily for 6 weeks or more may reduce cutaneous pigmentation. Crepey skin that persists after blepharoplasty can be corrected by application of a phenol chemical peel, without taping. Postoperative hematoma should be treated aggressively. Failure to do so may result in appreciable asymmetry.

LATERAL CANTHOPEXY

Lower lid laxity (Fig. 3A) has traditionally been treated by some variant of the Kuhnt-Szymonowski procedure. This requires development of a skin flap, resection of a full-thickness wedge of muscle, tarsus, and conjunctiva, followed by direct repair of the marginal defect and redraping of the skin. Direct lateral canthopexy is simpler and is the preferred technique for such correction. It is readily executed during cosmetic blepharoplasty and requires little additional instrumentation or time. The lateral limb of the upper lid incision permits direct access to the lateral orbital rim (Fig. 3B). The periosteum is incised longitudinally and gently stripped, medially and laterally, for 4 to 5 mm. Two or more holes are drilled close to the leading edge of the bone, at approximately the level of the medial canthi. (The Concept^R battery-operated dermabrader[††] fitted with a Jacobs chuck and wire passing bit is adequate for this purpose.) A No. 5–0 white Mersiline or clear nylon suture is backed through

---

[††] Concept^R Mini-dermabrader No. 5000

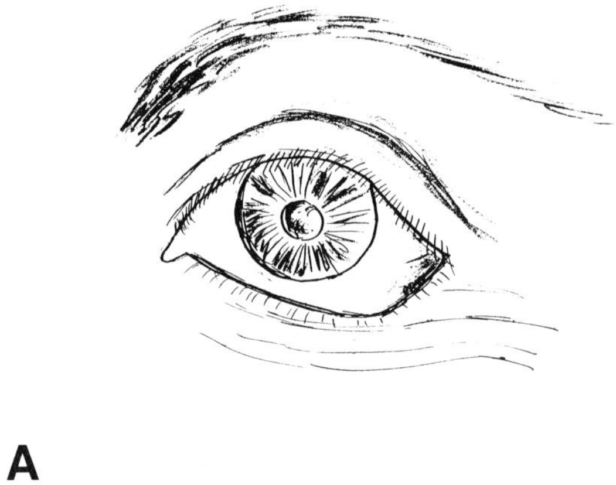

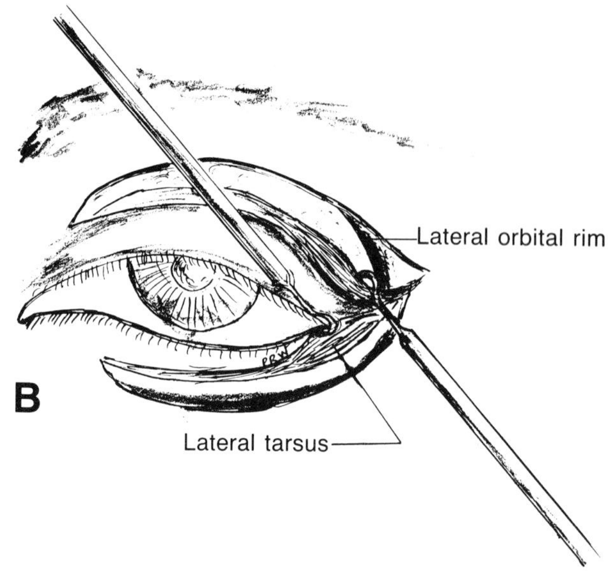

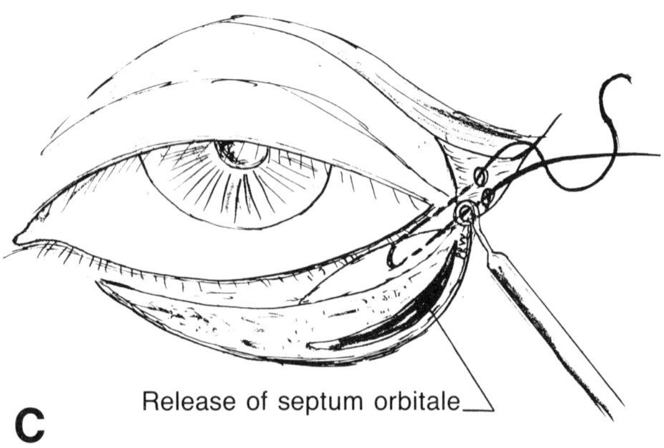

Figure 3 *A,* Excessive scleral show between the inferior limbus and lower eyelid ciliary margin at rest. *B,* Technique of correction of lax lower eyelid is depicted: exposure of the lateral orbital bony rim through the upper eyelid incision and exposure of the lateral tarsus of the lower eyelid through the lower eyelid incision. *C,* The lateral tarsus is sutured to the bony orbit through fixation holes in the lateral orbital wall. Note the release of the septum orbitale.

one hole and is sutured to the tendinous portion of the lower tarsus. The needle is then passed through the second pre-drilled hole (Fig. 3C). The septum orbitale must be incised through the lateral half of its attachment to the infraorbital rim. The lateral canthal ligament, a tenuous structure at best, can be left intact or transected. The degree of correction is assessed by snugging up the suture. Adjustment of the height of advancement may require that a third hole be drilled, to elevate or depress the level of attachment. In a primary blepharoplasty, lateral canthopexy produces substantial correction of lower lid laxity. It elevates the lateral canthal insertion for cosmetic improvement. As a secondary corrective procedure, its success depends upon adequacy of skin and/or muscle. When these are deficient, correction will be compromised.

SUGGESTED READING

Castanares S. Blepharoplasty for herniated intra-orbital fat. Anatomical basis for a new approach. Plast Reconstr Surg 1951; 8:46–58.

Flowers R. Blepharoplasty. In: Courtiss E, ed. Male aesthetic surgery, St. Louis: CV Mosby, 1982:207.

Rees TD. Surgical procedures. In: Rees TD, ed. Aesthetic plastic surgery. Philadelphia: WB Saunders, 1981:470.

FOREHEAD LIFT: COMPOSITE MUSCULOAPONEUROTIC GRAFTS

BRUNO RISTOW, M.D., F.A.C.S.

HISTORY AND EVOLUTION

The contrast between a surgically rejuvenated face and ptotic eyebrows or wrinkled foreheads led several surgeons, whose work I admire, to address the problem.

The early division of involved muscles, the selective removal of muscles, and electrocoagulation of small islands of muscle were among notable improvements to the sole redraping of skin. In the quest to rejuvenate aged foreheads, I have used all the above operations. It was the desire to improve results further that led to the technique outlined below.

The original seeds for an autograft technique began to germinate as I perceived the broadening horizons created by grafts in modern rhinoplasty. A brief sketch of my evolving thoughts on grafting was first presented at the instructional course on Facial Rejuvenation at the American Society for Aesthetic Plastic Surgery in Boston in 1985. Observation of late postoperative results convinced me that it was impossible to exert control over the relentless and disorganized attempts of the healing procerus and, in particular, corrugator muscles to reconnect. The most meticulous division of these muscles still led, in a small but still significant number of patients, to late asymmetrical results upon muscle contraction.

The second evolutionary stage came with the conviction that the bulk of the corrugators and procerus should be *removed*, which, per se, led to a depression contour deformity. One attempt was made with this technique, and the contour deformity proved permanent. Just above the procerus and corrugators, however, were the fanning frontalis muscle and a central portion of the galea aponeurotica. With progressive boldness, the removed bellies of corrugators and procerus were replaced by fragments of galea and frontalis. Not a single complication followed, and the long-term results confirmed my antevision that these fragments would scar and, thus, effectively insulate the tenacious procerus and corrugators from their attempts to recreate the objectionable lines. These long-term pleasing results encouraged me to advance from observing the benefits in private practice to reporting it to colleagues.

Up to now, more than 380 patients have benefited from this approach. At least 65 percent of our patients who undergo facelifts are also improved by concomitant forehead lifts.

INDICATIONS

The indications are: ptosis of the eyebrows; ptosis of the entire complex of forehead and eyebrows (the Beethoven look); notable discrepancy between the apparent age of the forehead and a previously-done face-lift; scowling appearance; worried appearance caused by semipermanent contraction of the frontalis in order to elevate the eyebrows; or any combination of the above conditions.

TECHNIQUE

I use a closed-system neuroleptic anesthesia with tracheal intubation, subsequently supplemented by local infiltration of the incisional lines, the frontalis between the left and right neurovascular bundles (NVB), and the region of the procerus and corrugators. The solution injected is Ringer's lactate with concentrations of 0.36 percent of cardiac lidocaine and 1:350 of epinephrine.

A traditional gullwing coronal incision is made and placed 5 to 6 cm behind the hairline. The forehead is elevated by sharp dissection. It is important that the knife blade is angled approximately 30 degrees in its sweep between the periosteum and the overlying galea-frontalis complex, thus affording protection against laceration or avulsion of the periosteum. This small precaution is essential in order to provide tissue in which to secure the graft later. Small emissary veins can also be controlled if sufficient tissue is left surrounding them. For larger emissary veins, which have to be divided, a small fragment of muscle inserted at their emergence from the frontal bone has proved useful.

Upon approach of the NVB and the orbital rim, a sponge dissector (peanut) is used to complete the elevation. A glance at the preoperative medical photographs of the patient determines if the dissection should go *over* the orbital rim (if notable elevation of the eyebrows is indicated) or remain just at the rim (when slight elevation is desired). A careless approach by the surgeon to this area may result in the patient's most feared deformity: too high a position of the eyebrows.

A Joseph nasal scissors is then gently inserted behind the right supraorbital NVB and progressively spread (Fig. 1). The nerves and vessels become visible, and the intertwining corrugator fibers are divided. This leads to anterior stumps of muscle that are attached to the dermis and to a posterior group of stumps, attached to the pericranium. An important observation is that the NVB structures are *within* the muscle and, therefore, the graft, when placed later, should mimic this anatomic condition. Precisely the same approach is used on the supratrochlear NVB. Since there are no nerves at the procerus level, the muscle is simply divided and the respective stumps trimmed (Fig. 2). A similar approach is used on the left NVB group.

The muscle stumps are meticulously retracted from between nerves and vessels, and their excess trimmed (Fig. 3). At the conclusion of this maneuver, one should have intact nerves and vessels and only a very thin layer of remaining muscle if any, at the flap side. A saline-soaked gauze is placed over these delicate structures and attention is directed to the harvesting of the composite graft.

Over the years, one design proved superior. My personal impression is that this is for two main reasons. The

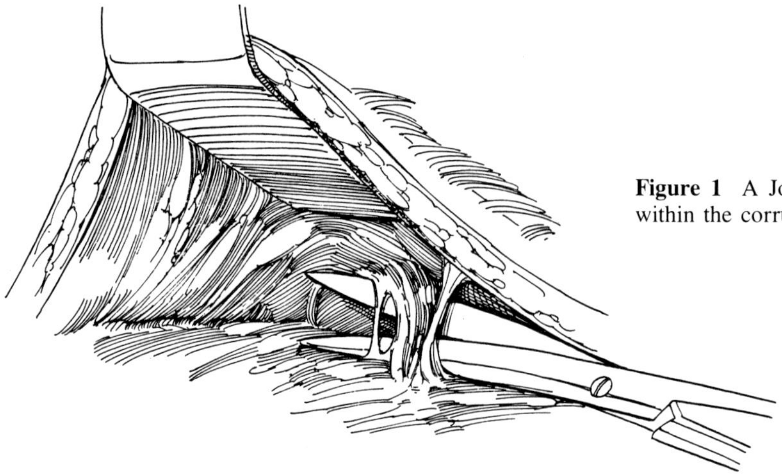

Figure 1 A Joseph scissors exposes the nerves and vessels within the corrugator muscle.

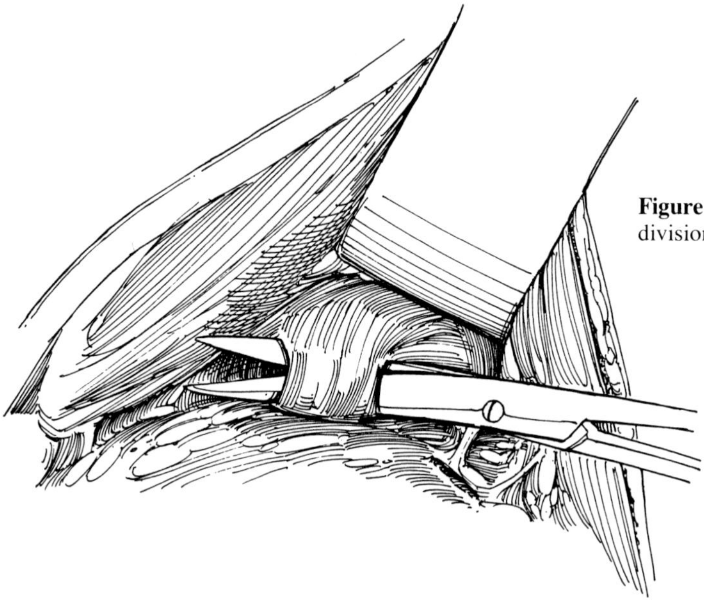

Figure 2 A Joseph scissors isolates the procerus prior to its division.

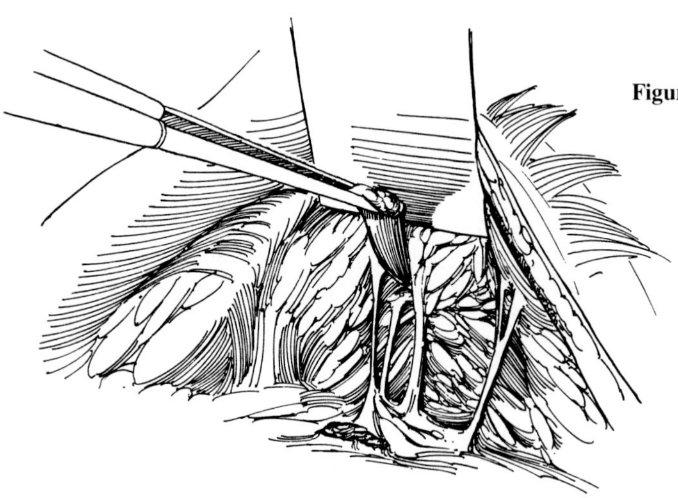

Figure 3 Muscle stump is retracted just prior to its trimming.

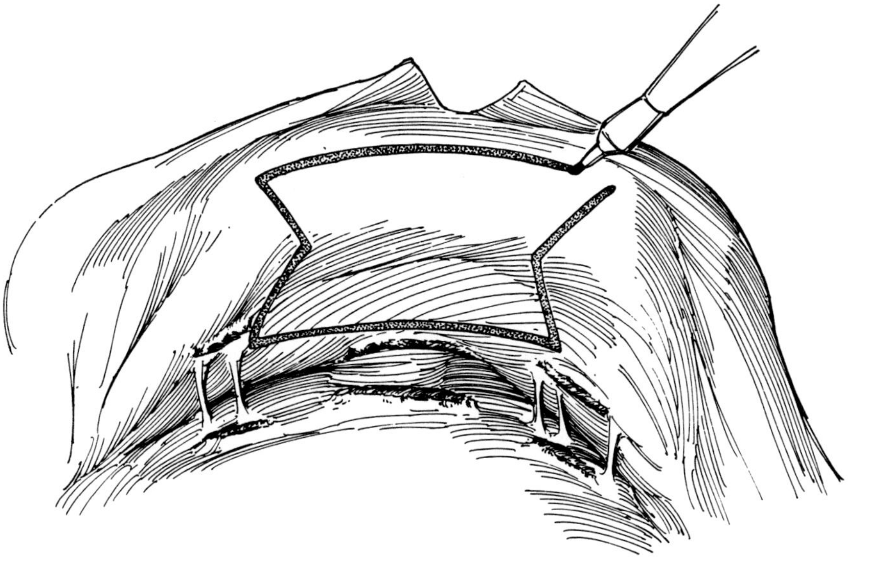

Figure 4 Outline of the composite galea-frontalis graft.

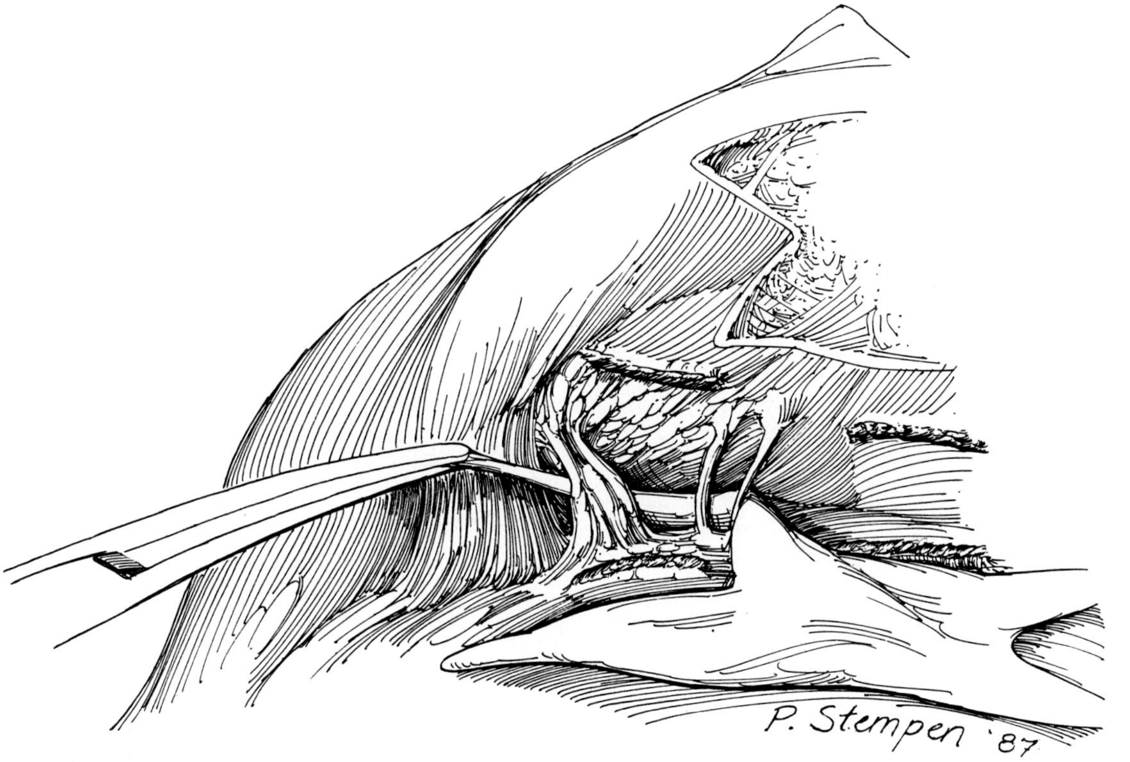

Figure 5 Caudad graft limb being positioned behind NVB.

first is that it is better to remove the frontalis partially rather than to cut it selectively; the second is that the lateral border of the graft, where it parallels the NVB, should not be straight but in the form of a "Z" (Fig. 4). This precludes a perceptible demarcation line on the forehead and, upon animation, transmits some movement to the midline.

The sole purpose of the local anesthetic infiltration of the frontalis now becomes apparent. It facilitates removal of the graft because it increases the graft's volume and decreases bleeding at the time of removal. The composite graft is then further incised at each end. One of the graft limbs is then gently passed behind the supratrochlear and supraorbital NVBs and the other limb is laid cephalad to these structures (Fig. 5).

Sutures of 5–0 plain catgut secure the graft in place. It is important to further anchor it to the caudad stumps of the procerus and superiorly to the pericranium (Fig. 6). A Jackson-Pratt thin silicone drain is placed horizontally, immediately superior to the graft, and exits through the lateral scalp. It is removed the following morning.

Closure is with very moderate tension, determined with the help of Pitanguy's clamp. Plain catgut, 3–0 and 4–0, is used exclusively.

RESULTS

The explanation for the pleasing long-term results can be summarized as follows:

1. Inability of the stumps of corrugators and procerus to reconnect effectively and, therefore, recreate lines.
2. No late contour deformities due to the bulk of the graft substituting for muscle excised.
3. Healing of the entire forehead at a slightly higher level, especially at the excised frontalis-periosteal interface.
4. The degree of expression left on the patient's forehead is at the control of the surgeon. He may choose, during the dissection, to leave some muscle, or remove most of it.

COMPLICATIONS

Infections have been entirely absent. One patient experienced an immediate postoperative graft displacement that necessitated repositioning. Subsequent adoption of sutures to anchor grafts limited this complication to one case. Paresthesias, if present, are temporary and subside with the passage of time. Remnant paresthesia can, however,

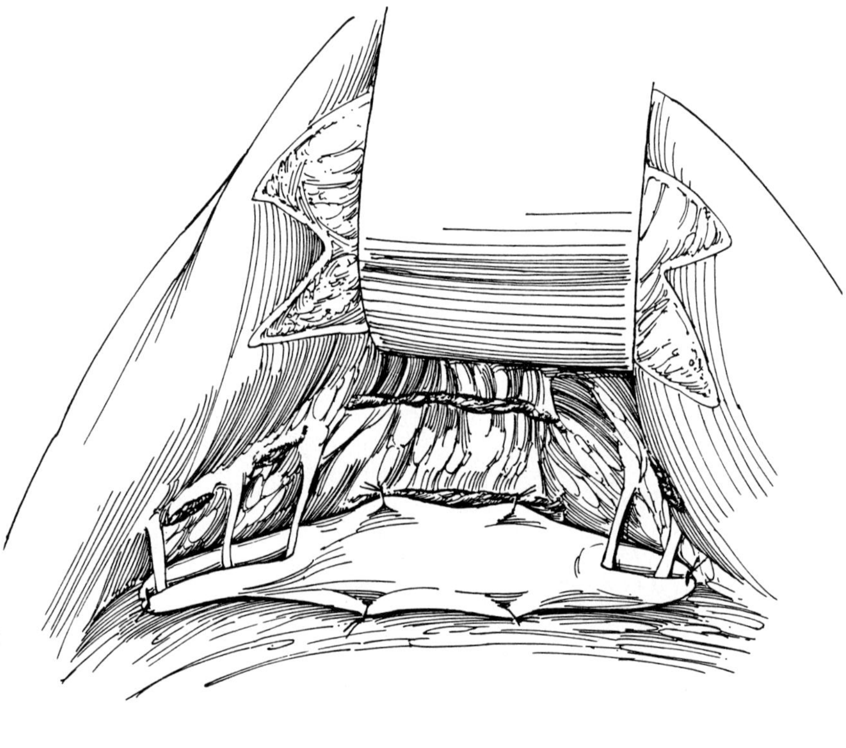

Figure 6 Composite autograft sutured in place.

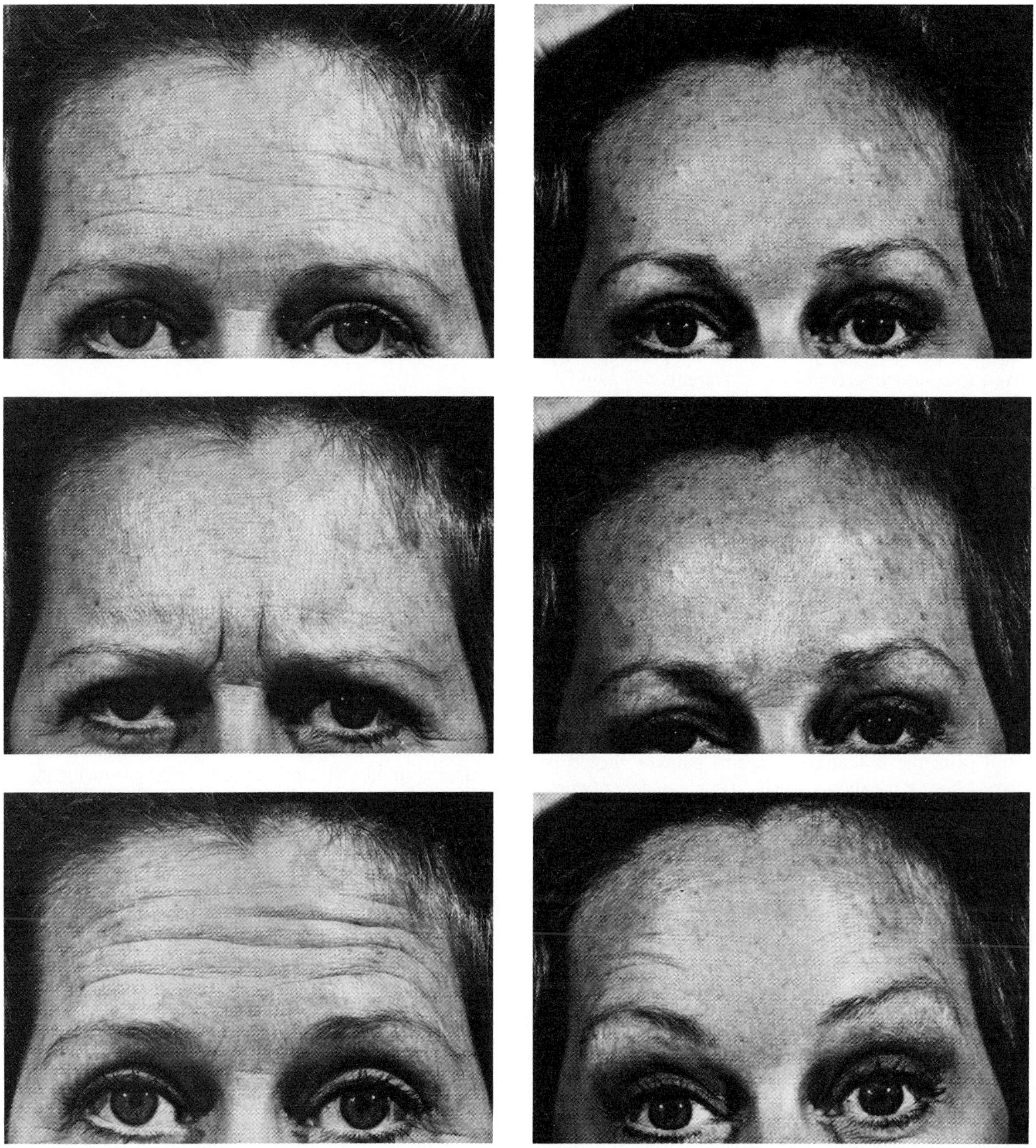

Figure 7 The left column depicts the preoperative condition. From top to bottom: at rest, with animation of the corrugators and procerus, with animation of the frontalis. Photos in the right column are corresponding postoperative results.

be a consequence of an abnormally high emergence of one or more nerves, which necessitated their division. Only two such abnormal emergences were encountered. A caveat to such patients of the inevitability of such a division poses no problem between a genuinely attentive surgeon and a well-selected patient.

SUGGESTED READING

Conley J. Frontal rhytidectomy, plastic and reconstructive surgery of the face and neck. Vol I. New York: Grune & Stratton, 1972:31.

Kaye BL. Forehead and brow. In: Rees TD, ed. Aesthetic plastic surgery. Vol. 2. Philadelphia: WB Saunders, 1980:731.

Pitanguy I. Forehead lifting, aesthetic plastic surgery of head and body. New York: Springer-Verlag, 1981:202.

Ristow B. Facial rejuvenation surgery. Instructional Courses, ASPRS Meeting. Atlanta:1987.

Ristow B. The surgery of facial rejuvenation. Instructional Courses ASAPS Annual Meetings. Boston: 1985, New Orleans: 1986, Los Angeles: 1987.

Ristow B. The value of musculoaponeurotic grafts in forehead lifts. Presentation & Film, ASPRS Meeting, Los Angeles: 1986.

NATURAL FACELIFT

RICHARD ELLENBOGEN, M.D.

Facelift is the one operation from which every living human may one day benefit. The surgeon must realize that the patients who request facelift are requesting both an emotional and physical improvement. They want to look better, younger, and refreshed—not surgically done, different, pulled, or strange. Therefore, the operation I perform is a direct attempt to minimize the surgical tip-offs that a procedure has been performed. Over many years and after many criticisms, my procedure has evolved into one where almost all patients are satisfied and almost none complain of either looking like another person or "operated upon". It is an evolution of good techniques, and a gradual extinction of those associated with the surgical look. I do all facelifts as an office procedure after the patients are cleared by an internist, who is on call during the procedure. Prior to surgery, I go over photographs with the patient and show what I can do, may be able to do, and cannot do. I do this before premedications as a reinforcement of my consultation.

SELECTION OF PATIENTS

Facelift patients, who range from their mid-thirties to over eighty years, include both men and women. The general principle is that good facelift patients should be realistic about what they will get. They can accept complications and not expect more than is surgically possible. During the consultation, the doctor must determine whether the patient is realistic. The complications must be discussed, both ethically and legally. The hoped for projected result is demonstrated in the mirror, with no guarantees given. If the overall attitude of the patient is "do your best, I don't expect miracles," one can feel safe in operating. Patients in their late thirties and forties almost always have this outlook and are generally the happiest patients postoperatively. Avoid patients who do not listen to you, patients who demand how many years can be taken off, or patients who must be healed by a specific date. Obesity is not a contraindication and, in many cases, gives an excellent result.

I have found that patients who call the office continuously, re-asking questions previously answered, will only be a drain on doctor and staff after surgery and should be avoided. If ever I feel the patient should visit a psychiatrist to see if his or her expectations are realistic, I refuse surgery. One's own gut reaction, bolstered by experience, should suffice and not require outside help. One should listen to one's staff, who can frequently spot a malcontent or a litigious personality.

Certain organ diseases and other problems cause me to refuse surgery: uncontrolled hypertension, alcoholism, drug abuse, heavy smoking, diabetes (adult or juvenile), past heart attack, past stroke, past Bell's palsy, chronic asthma (cough and straining cause hematomas), history of bleeding, on steroid therapy, cervical disk disease (the neck cannot be adjusted during surgery), chronic brain syndrome, multiple sclerosis,history of carotid occlusion, transient ischemic attacks, vascular tumor of the head and neck, rheumatoid arthritis, certain arrhythmias. After all, this is elective surgery. The doctor should remember that this is a tremendously important decision for patients. They will discuss what they do not like, and the doctor should counter with his solution, its reservations and restrictions. If one cannot visualize what they are describing, one should not operate. The doctor must be confident he has the skill level to correct the defect. If not, surgery must be refused.

PREOPERATIVE MARKING

Marking is performed with the patient seated, with good shadow light. I have never, over the past 12 years, extended the incision above the ear in men or women. It can cause an upward tilt of the lateral eyebrow thus (giving an angry look), a bald visible incision, an obliterated sideburn, and a widened forehead. Some patients lost hair and some complained of a masked, pulled look. My pull is more posterior than superior. I feel that an incision in front of the sideburn is also undesirable. My incision (Fig. 1), extends 2 mm in front of the tragus. The incision inside the ear, in my hands, always pulls the tragus forward, or hides it, thereby exposing the auditory canal. I have been unable to create a tragus that equals a normal tragus with the "in ear incision." The posterior incision is in the postauricular crease and extends almost to the top of the pinna and 3 inches straight back. Placement any lower does not allow a woman to wear her hair up.

The anterior platysma bands are marked for reference, as is the lower mandibular border. A half-inch to three-quarter-inch incision is outlined over the hyoid, in the midline rather than further anterior. This incision's position gives excellent visualization of the platysma, neck, and mandibular border. Also, it stretches when operating and shrinks when healed. It heals imperceptibly.

DISSECTION

With the use of various rhytidectomy scissors, the dissection is as pictured in Figure 2. The dissection extends anteriorly to the nasolabial fold and the marionette mouth (the depressed fold from the corner of the mouth to the mandible resembles that of a marionette), inferiorly to the cephalad aspect of the thyroid cartilage, and posteriorly to the pinna for 3 inches. The inferior margin parallels the jawline to meet the postauricular incision. Sixty to 80cc of quarter percent local Xylocaine, with 1 percent: 200,000 Adrenalin with Wydase, are injected 5 minutes before dissection of that side. I perform the postauricular neck dissection first and connect it to the anterior face dissection. The neck dissection connects at the midline. Hemostasis is then achieved.

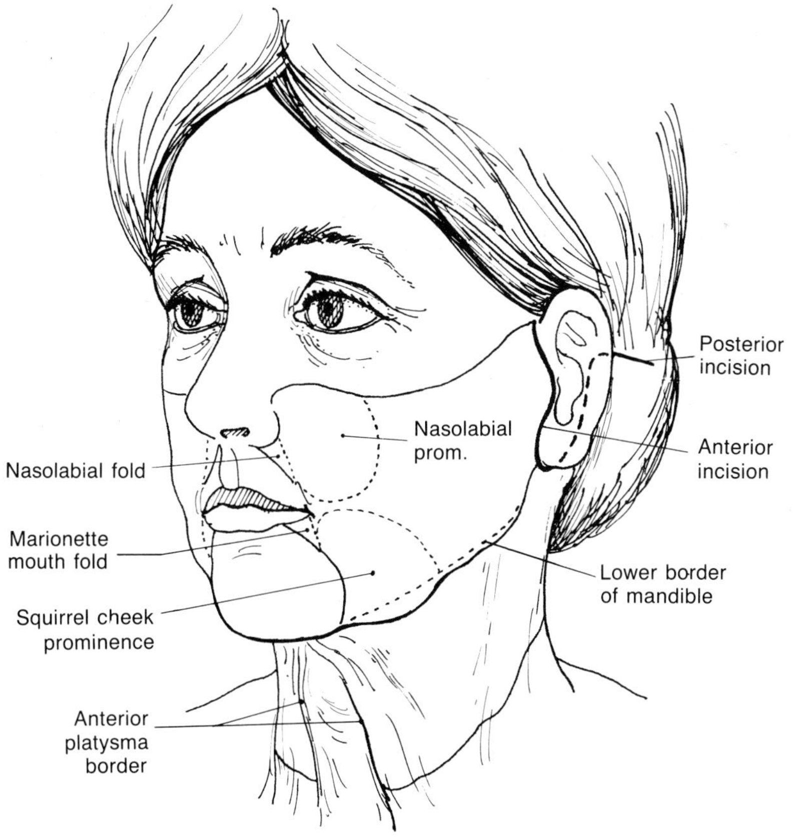

Figure 1 The marking preauricularly extends from top of pinna under the lobe in postauricular sulcus and 3 inches into the hairline slightly curvilinear. Postauricular hairline incision is almost at the cephalad concha. The upper margin of dissection is from cephalad to ala nasi to cephalad to pinna. Anterior dissection is anterior to the nasolabial fold, corner of mouth, and squirrel cheek prominence. The inferior dissection is to thyroid cartilage. For reference, the mandibular border, anterior platysma bands, nasolabial fold and prominence, marionette mouth fold, and squirrel cheek prominence are marked.

FAT CURETTAGE AND REINJECTION

There is a bulging area posterior to the nasolabial folds (the nasolabial prominence) and posterior to the marionette mouth (squirrel cheek prominence). This area has not been corrected successfully by superficial musculo-aponeurotic system (SMAS) plication, skin tightening, or fat suction. I use a 4 mm or 6 mm Fox skin curette and gently curette out the fat in this area, both on the skin flap and face side (see Fig. 2). I check visually under the flap to make sure there is no debris and the surface is flat. This fat, usually 3 to 7 cc is saved and reinjected into the depression of the marionette mouth and the nasolabial fold. A 10 cc syringe with a 14 guage needle is used. After injection, the fat is molded flat by hand. Patients are told they may feel lumpy for up to 3 months. I almost never tighten the SMAS. It has not corrected the nasolabial folds and has given a too tight look in younger patients when in repose, as well as in many patients while talking. Only in very thin, very lax, older patients do I feel a SMAS plication worthwhile as regards overall satisfaction and result.

FAT SCULPTING

I then mark the fat that covers the lower mandibular border under the flap with gentian violet and remove all fat to the upper thyroid cartilage border that overlies the platysma. I have compared open removal to fat suction postoperatively and have even opened necks that had been fat-suctioned to check the comparative efficacy. A significantly cleaner and more efficient removal of fat is done by direct vision. This is manifest in comparable postoperative results. Care is taken over the sternocleidomastoid to avoid the posterior auricular nerve, which, if cut, results in painful neuromas and numb ear lobes. Hemostasis is again checked at this point.

THE PLATYSMA

After trying numerous platysma procedures that include complete transection, removal, lateral displacement, partial excision of anterior bands, etc., I now almost invariably suture the platysma in the midline without removal of anterior bands. In obese individuals the platysma is separated and fat that is deep to the platysma and superficial to the mylohyoid can be safely removed. This area is very vascular and contains numerous lymph glands. The removal of half to three quarters of an inch of anterior bands in many cases made the platysma too tight, thus producing postoperative temporary hoarseness by pressure on the thyroid cartilage, and recurrent platysma bands in the neck rapidly reappeared. I universally use 3–Nylon for the platysma closure. An absorbable material will dissolve and muscles will not heal together. I cut the platysma at the lower hyoid level. I remove three-quarters of an inch of muscle at the cut to prevent platysma from growing back together. I only cut and remove platysma

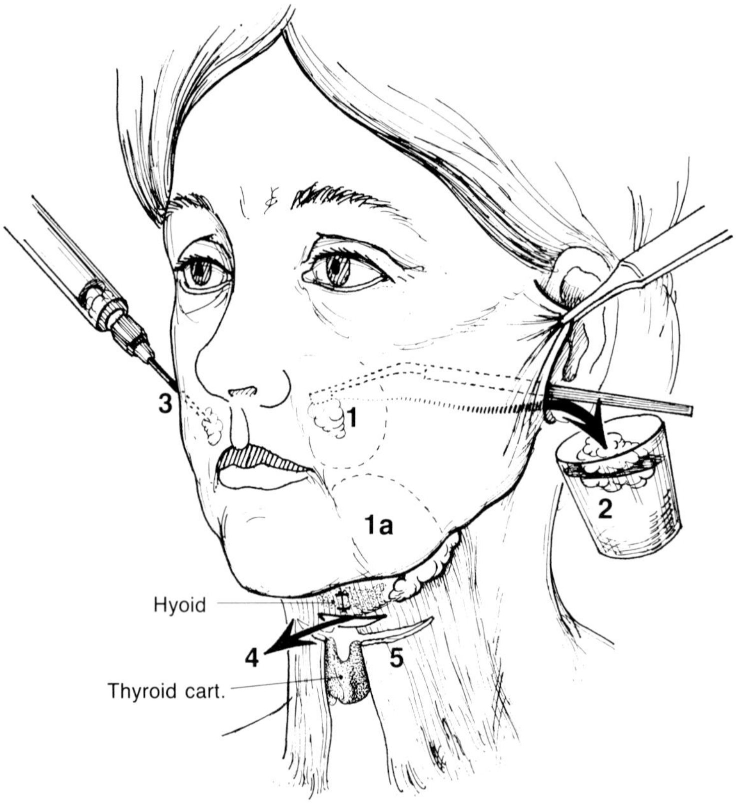

Figure 2 The dissection. After the flap is elevated, fat is curetted out in the nasolabial *(1)* and squirrel cheek prominence (la). *(2)* The fat is collected and *(3)* reinjected into the nasolabial fold and the corner of the marionette mouth fold. *(4)* Fat superficial to the platysma inferior to the mandible is removed while *(5)* the platysma is cut at the level of the cephalad thyroid cartilage with ¾ inch removed. It is sutured at the midline with 3–0 Nylon.

2 inches posteriorly. It is a hemi not a total transection. I no longer suture the platysma posteriorly to the sternocleidomastoid, and rarely do patients complain of stiff neck or difficulty in lateral movement (see Fig. 2).

CLOSURE

After a final hemostasis check, closure is performed. I use small 10 F drains placed in the most posterior part of the postauricular incision. The drain rests in the lowest portion of the dissection and curls up into the face dissection. Drains do not prevent hematomas, but, on removing the drain on day one, I usually discover 10 to 50 cc of tissue fluid, serum, blood, and liquified fat that the postoperative wound does not have to assimilate. The drain, by its suction, does obliterate dead space of the widely undermined face and neck.

The fixed or pulled down earlobe is, I believe, the greatest tip-off of a surgical face (Fig. 3). On the mandibular border marking line, the skin of the face is pulled directly up to meet the cartilaginous auditory canal. A cut is made to this point, and it is connected with a single, buried 3–0 Nylon suture from subcutaneous tissue to cartilage. With the D'Assumpc̆ao skin marker, the anterior hairline of the postauricular flap is pulled directly cephalad, not posteriorly, to exactly meet the hairline above. Posterior pull causes a jog or step off. The skin should blanch with finger pressure. A 3–0 Nylon stitch connects the two edges. The postauricular stitch is then placed to take up the pleating behind the ear. Inferior to the tragus, a stitch of 5–0 Nylon is placed. The pull is directly back and slightly up. The skin overlying the tragus should be defatted to give better tragal definition. Behind the ear, I use plain 4–0 catgut. It dissolves and does not have to be removed, thereby preventing a wound disruption during stitch removal. The ear skin here is sutured both to the postauricular skin and to mastoid fascia deep in the sulcus. This, I believe, creates a bond that prevents the scar being pulled down the neck during postoperative healing. One must check that the pull does not mask the mouth or spread the nose. The flap is also checked for viability. A 5–0 Nylon stitch above the tragus sets the preauricular line.

ANCILLARY PROCEDURES

At this stage I usually do my ancillary procedures such as fat injection, fat grafting, perioral dermabrasion, lesion removal, etc. When performing blepharoplasty and facelift, I always do the facelift first. I can then check again for hemostasis after the blepharoplasty. My respect and fear of the retrobulbar hematoma is genuine. Manipulation of a facelift patient after blepharoplasty is not conducive to good intraorbital hemostasis.

DRESSING

Light compression over the cheek and a tighter compression over the neck are advised. I take off the dress-

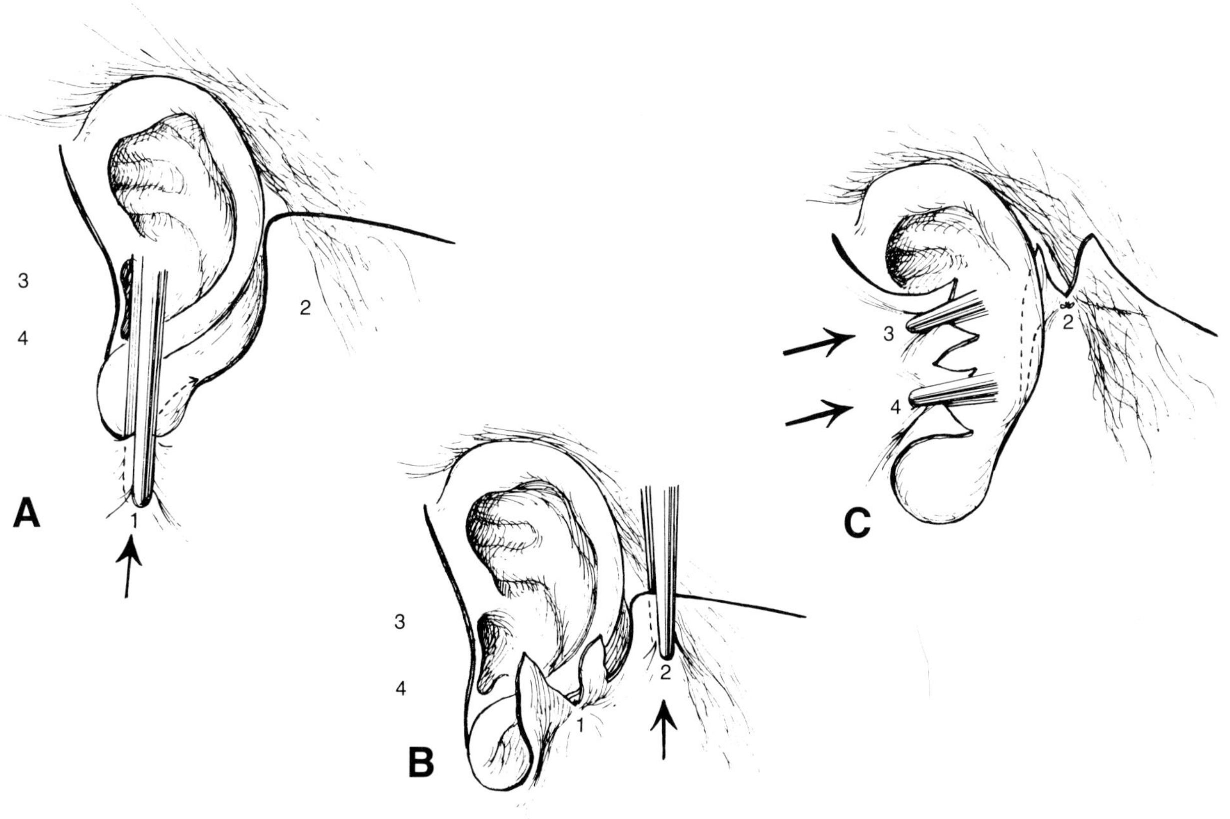

Figure 3 *A*, *B*, and *C*, Skin on the mandibular borderline *(1)* is pulled cephalad to the cartilaginous canal and sutured with a subcutaneous 3–0 Nylon to the cartilage. Hairline to hairline and a cephalad pull is shown at *(2)*. Posterior pull causes a jog in the hairline. The pull of the face is straight back at *(3)* and also at *(4)*.

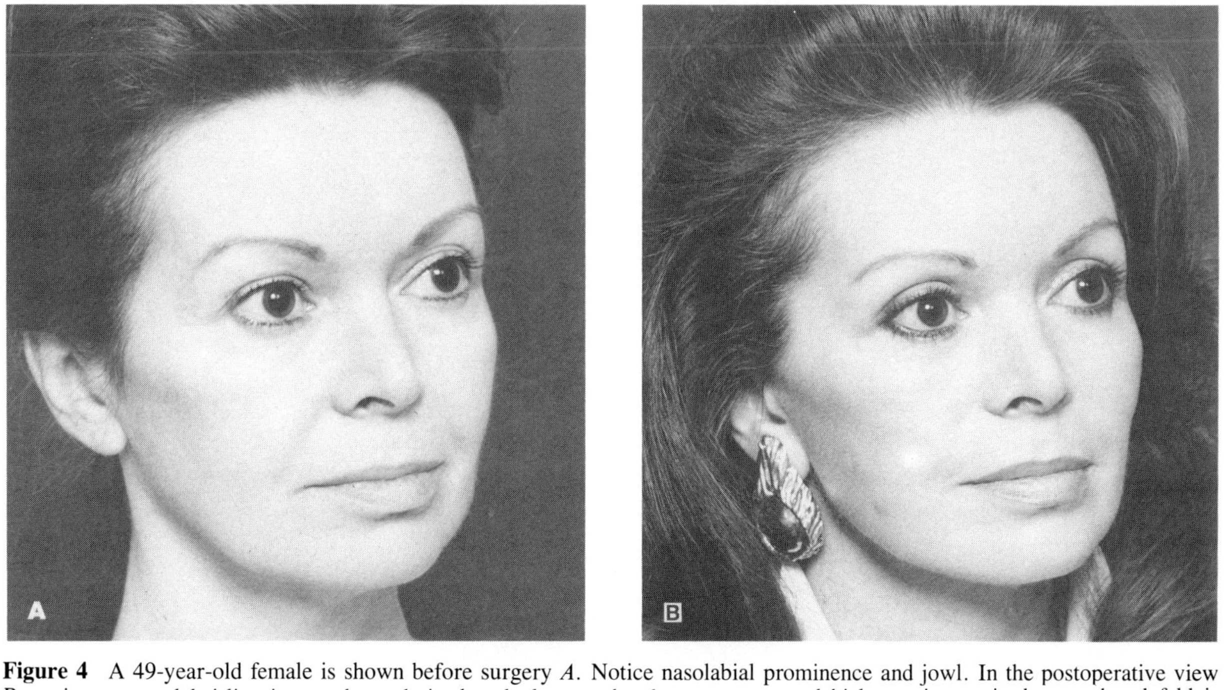

Figure 4 A 49-year-old female is shown before surgery *A*. Notice nasolabial prominence and jowl. In the postoperative view *B*, notice temporal hairline is not changed, jowl and platysma bands are gone, nasolabial prominence is decreased and fold is minimized. Fat injected into corner of mouth reverses preoperative downward point.

ing to remove drains and check for hemostasis on day one and replace it with a neck-only compression for 3 days.

POSTOPERATIVE

Stitches are removed after 1 week. During that time, activity is limited. I give all patients antibiotics. Make-up is permitted after a few days. I limit coffee and forbid cigarettes from 3 days before to 10 days after surgery.

I institute neck exercises from day three. They consist of lifting the neck high and touching left shoulder then right shoulder to prevent some of the stiffness for which platysma procedures are known. A good idea is to have a make-up artist and a hairstylist help the patient reemerge into society at about 2 to 4 weeks. If a patient is afraid of what people will say, a new hairstyle frequently throws the critics off. Camouflage ecchymosis make-up may be begun as soon as day four. See results in Figures 4, 5, and 6.

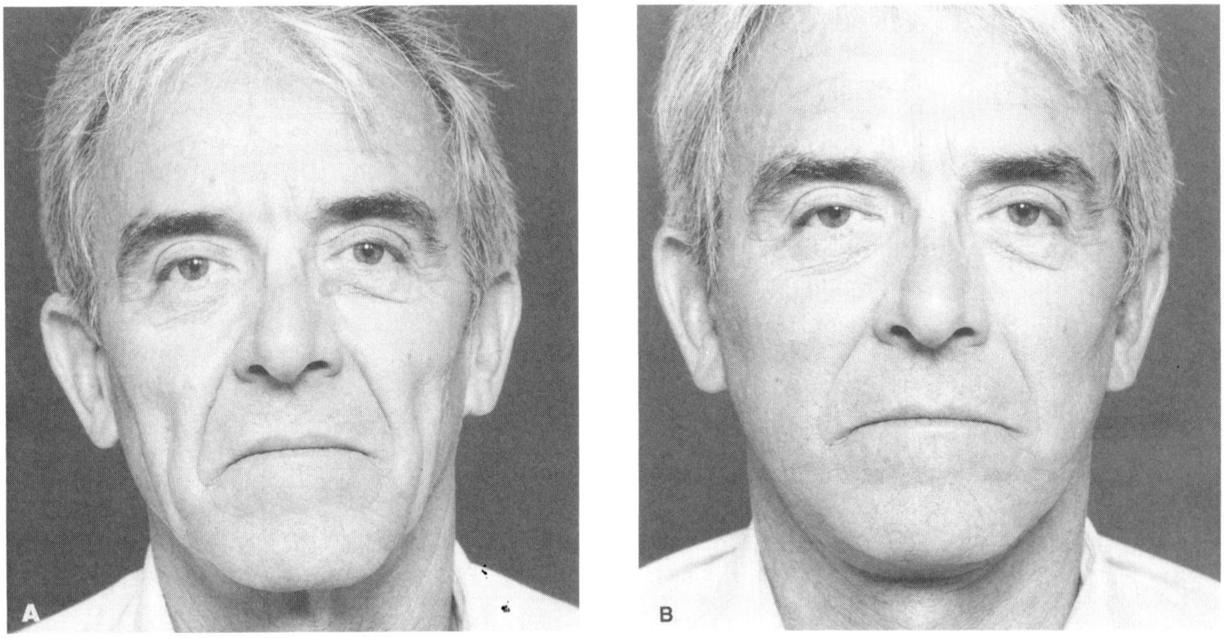

Figure 5 *A*, a 61-year-old man before surgery. Note deep nasolabial folds, hollows of cheeks, left anterior platysma band. *B*, One year post surgery, note sideburns are normal, platysma band is gone, fat curettage and reinjection improved the nasolabial fold. Fat was also injected into the cheek hollows.

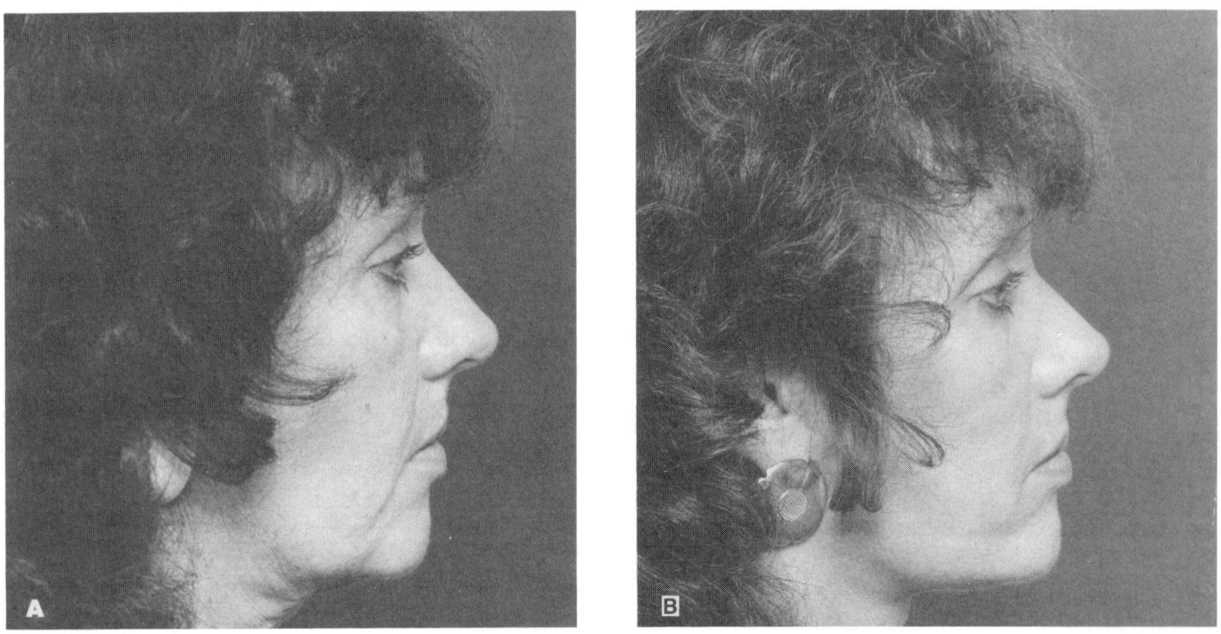

Figure 6 A 47-year-old women is shown *(A)*, with preoperative neck and jawline laxity, squirrel cheek, nasolabial fold and marionette mouth fold. Postoperative view, *(B)*. The idea is to improve each age sign without the patient looking "done" or different.

TABLE 1 Avoidance of Telltale Signs of Surgery

Tipoffs	*Avoidance Techniques*
Wide forehead	Extend incision cephalad only to top of pinna.
Paralyzed eyebrow	Same
Temporal hair loss	Same
Temporal scar visible	Same
Sideburn thin or obliterated	Same
"Masked" look due to extreme temporal pull	Same
Mouth pulled or corner elevated	Same
Lateral eyebrow elevated (angry look)	Same
Nostrils widened	Caused by excessive skin pull on nasolabial fold. Curette out fat in nasolabial prominence and inject into fold. Limit skin pull.
Mouth widened, lips thinned, possible philtrum obliteration	Excessive skin pull or SMAS pull. Depend on fat curettage in nasolabial prominence and corner of mouth
Hidden or unnatural tragus or exposed external auditory canal	Make tragal part of preauricular incision 2 mm in front of tragus point leaving normal shiny skin on apex of tragus. Defat skin over tragus. Preauricular incision will fade.
Pulled down earlobe	Suture subcutaneous tissue of face infra-auricularly to cartilaginous canal with permanent 3–0 Nylon buried suture.
Scars of earlobe	In this area, concentrate on a perfect closure and see that the skin does not invert.
Descending postauricular scar on neck with time	Use dissolving 4–0 catgut behind ear (so stitch removal, which frequently opens the incision, is not necessary). Suture incision to mastoid fascia at postauricular sulcus.
Jog at postauricular hairline	The first pull and tacking suture on closure should be postauricular hairline to hairline. The pull behind the ear should be cephalad not posterior.
Residual jowl	All fat from the inferior margin of the mandible, overlying the platysma, must be excised.
Dents under mandible	The fat excision under the mandibular border must be carefully beveled, not sharp.
Residual turkey gobbler bands in neck	The platysma must be closed in the midline. Transection must be at the hyoid level not lower. Any lower leaves bowstring bands. A piece 3/4″ should be removed to prevent regrowth.
Submental scar	This cannot be avoided if platysma is to be addressed. A 3/4″ scar over the hyoid heals less conspicuously
Scar down the neck	Suture postauricular flap to mastoid fascia deep in sulcus with absorbable suture not skin to skin

TIP–OFFS

A patient who has had a face-lift may have tip-off, or telltale, signs that they have had surgery. The successful surgeon in facial ageing is cognizant of these tip-offs and adjusts his technique accordingly (Table 1).

COMPLICATIONS

No one has recently done a study on the most common complications of facelifts performed today. The classic complications are still there, but newer ones have been added (see Table 1). Hematoma is still the number one problem: both large, early postoperative and small, late-forming cheek bumps. The postoperative hematomas must be scrupulously evacuated and bleeding stopped. An entire new local anesthesia should be instituted and blood pressure monitored and controlled. Skin slough is the number two concern, both major and minor. The realization that smoking contributes to this and its restriction preoperatively have helped. Visible scarring is still a possibility. Hair loss depends on the technique and the individual. Facial weakness, paralysis, paresthesia, and neuromas are less common with experienced operators. Neuromas and severance of the greater auricular nerve are particularly troublesome. Cervical nerve severance in an appropriate host mimics a marginal mandibular palsy. Fortunately, most nerve injuries repair themselves with time. Newer techniques have introduced the possibilities of platysma bands, irregular neck fat contours and facial asymmetries, lumps and bumps, and possible slower healing times.

SUGGESTED READING

Ellenbogen R. Regrowth of platysma following platysma cervical lift: etiology and methodology of prevention. Plast Reconstr Surg 1981; 67(5):616–623.

Ellenbogen R. Visual criteria for success in restoring the youthful neck. Plast Reconstr Surg 1980; 66(6):826–837.

Ellenbogen R. Free autogenous pearl fat grafts in the face: a preliminary report of a rediscovered technique. Ann Plast Surg 1986; 16(3):179–194.

Ellenbogen, R. Pseudoparalysis of the mandibular branch of the facial nerve after platysmal face-lift operation. Plast Reconstr Surg 1979; 63(3):364–368.

FACELIFT: INDICATIONS FOR SUCTION LIPECTOMY

EUGENE H. COURTISS, M.D.

Suction lipectomy is a technique for the removal of fat; it is neither more nor less. However, because it is very dissimilar to traditional methods for removal of fat, such as the knife or scissors, it became controversial. The controversy was fueled by the fact that suction lipectomy is often performed blindly—which is also contrary to the traditional surgical principle of "cut only what you can see." Nonetheless, after the value of the technique for changing contours of the extremities and torso became established, its use to contour the fat of the face and neck became logical. Furthermore, it has been demonstrated by many surgeons, and in many patients, that removal of fat by suction is safer than when cutting instruments are used. As a result, the indication for suction lipectomy, in conjunction with a facelift, is simple: it is performed when removal of fat from the face or neck is desired. The fact that the technique of removal is suction, rather than a scissor or knife, does not change the indication.

The term "facelift" is a misnomer. When a facelift is performed, major changes in the neck are pari passu of the procedure. In fact, the operation should be termed a "face- and necklift." However, since that terminology is most cumbersome, and both the public and surgeons are so accustomed to the term "facelift," an attempt to change the name would be almost impossible. Nevertheless, major contour changes in the neck are part of a facelift.

PATIENT COMPLAINT

When a patient complains about the appearance of her or his face, precise details should be sought. The question should be asked: "When you look in the mirror, what do you see that bothers you?" If the patient complains about fullness in the jowls, cheeks, or neck, those areas should be examined to determine whether the undesired contour is due to fat collection or other causes.

EXAMINATION

A precise, anatomic examination and analysis of the patient's pathologic anatomy is essential to the planning of any operation. When examining a patient who complains about facial appearance, examination of the four layers that may need treatment is essential. Thus, specific attention should be directed to: skin, fat, fascia and muscle, and bone.

If the problem is confined to the skin, a chemical face peel, dermabrasion, or skin lift may be indicated. If excess fat is present, fat removal (by suction) may be indicated. Should general laxity of the cheeks, or anterior neck muscle bands, be present, treatment of the superficial musculoaponeurotic system (SMAS) may be appropriate. Finally, if a change in the bony contour is desired, bone augmentation, reduction, or repositioning may be indicated.

SELECTION OF ALTERNATIVES

When the examination indicates that the problem is due to a collection of fat, the decision must be made whether to remove the fat alone, or whether to remove excess skin also. In other words, when should the patient have suction alone, and when should a facelift (with suction) be performed? The decision may be difficult and there is no absolute answer. However, the following guidelines are helpful. Removal of fat by suction alone (without a facelift) should be performed when the patient has fat that is localized to the neck or face. On the other hand, a simultaneous face- and necklift should be performed when more profound changes are sought. In any case, a face- and necklift can be performed later, but I have never had to do so because of a failure of the skin to contract. The patient's chronologic age is irrelevant.

The following is axiomatic—when the problem is one of fat collection, the fat must be treated; excision of skin alone will not treat excess fat. In many patients, treatment of more than one layer is indicated and any layer that needs change should be changed. The more that is done, the greater will be the change.

PREOPERATIVE

The patient should be instructed to stop taking aspirin-containing medications for 10 days. When a history of bleeding is negative, no bleeding studies are done. However, when the history indicates easy bruising, or bleeding problems, evaluation by a hematologist is arranged. No routine laboratory studies are performed.

Smokers are told to stop smoking for 2 weeks prior to operation. If they refuse, a notation is made and, later, the neck flap is handled differently, with very conservative planning of the amount to be excised. It is better to be conservative and not superimpose tension upon skin the vascularity of which has been compromised by nicotine. This would cause a slough.

TECHNIQUE

Marking. Before the patient receives any sedation or anesthesia, the incisions and extent of dissection are drawn on the skin with marking dye. In addition, the fat collections are sketched.

Anesthesia. Sedation is achieved with diazepam (Valium) or midazolam (Versed), the dose being sufficient to cause the patient's speech to slur. If the patient is normotensive, 1 mg per kilogram of ketamine is administered. If the patient is hypertensive, 0.1 mg (1 cc) fentanyl (Sublimaze) is given. Then the local anesthetic is injected. My preference is 2 vials (100 cc) of 0.25 percent bupivacaine (Marcaine), to which I add fresh epinephrine to make a solution of 1:400,000. In addition, 600 units of hyaluronidase are added to the 100 cc. The local anesthetic is injected before the patient is prepped or I scrub.

Submental incision. A 2 cm incision is made in an anterior submental crease. Then a pair of facelift scissors is inserted and spread in the midline as far as the inferior extent of the skin marking.

Cannula. A suction cannula is inserted. I prefer a 5.0 mm (internal diameter) plastic uterine cannula*, because I can observe what is happening and it is kinder to the tissues. However, other cannulas, such as the small 2 mm metal three-hole "Mercedes," are also satisfactory.

When smaller cannulas are used, less fat is removed. However, in the neck, the intent is to remove as much fat as possible so there is no advantage to smaller cannulas.

Suction machine. Despite claims by the manufacturers, all the pumps I have used (Berkeley, Grams, M.D. Engineering, and Wells Johnson) are equally effective and produce sufficient vacuum to perform the procedure. Should the surgeon wish to remove less fat, the vacuum can be reduced, or a smaller cannula used.

Technique of suction of neck fat. When suction lipectomy of the extremities or torso is performed, the cannula opening is kept down. However, when suction of the neck is performed, it is best to turn the cannula up, i.e., under the skin. Why the difference? The marginal branch of the facial nerve and the external jugular vein are located deep to the platysma muscle; therefore it is safer to keep the cannula under the skin and, thus, superficial to the platysma muscle. If the hole is inward, the cannula may penetrate the muscle and damage those structures. In contrast to sharp instruments, suction will not totally remove the fat under the skin. This observation can be proven during a facelift by examination of the underside of the skin that has been in contact with the cannula. Fat remains. The suction has exploded the cells leaving the cellular membranes.

Work on the SMAS should be done *before* the fat on superficial surface of the platysma muscles is removed. This obviates bringing defatted muscle onto the cheek, and removal of fat from a tight muscle is easier than when the muscle is loose.

Also, in contrast to suction lipectomy of the torso and extremities, a single cavity is created. Most surgeons, when performing a facelift, completely undermine the neck flap. There is no reason to leave any bands. They do not carry nerves or vessels and they restrict contouring of the skin and the neck. Futhermore, the creation of tunnels produces contour irregularities. Even champions of the collapsing tunnel theory make crisscross tunnels to remove more fat.

Treatment of anterior borders of the platysma muscles. These anterior borders are cleaned of fat with the suction cannula tip turned down. Then the anterior borders of the muscles are approximated from just under the chin to the level of the thyroid cartilage with 3–0 Vicryl sutures. Inferior to the last suture, the platysma muscles on each side are divided for 2 cm. This prevents the formation of a single band.

Skin incision. Skin incisions of choice are made in the temple, retrotragal, retroauricular, and scalp areas.

Elevation of cheek flaps. The 5.0 cm uterine cannula, or the three-hole "Mercedes" cannula, is inserted into the cheeks to elevate the cheek flaps. This may be done with the suction turned down or off and the intent is to elevate the cheek fat. The cannula dissection should connect the cheek and the neck (where a cavity had been created during suction of the neck).

Superficial musculoaponeurotic system (SMAS). I perform a SMAS on almost all patients. The SMAS is elevated through an "L" shaped incision. The horizontal limb is 3 cm in length and is located just inferior to the zygomatic arch; the vertical limb is located about 1 cm anterior to the tragus and extends 5 to 6 cm below the mandibular border. The SMAS is elevated from the parotid superiorly. Inferiorly, the dissection is deep to the platysma, with which it is in continuity.

Then, the SMAS is pulled in a cephalad direction and a posteriorly-based triangle is resected. The SMAS is then sutured to itself at the zygomatic arch with 3–0 Vicryl sutures. The SMAS and platysma in the cheek and neck are then pulled posteriorly and the excess is trimmed and sutured with 3–0 Vicryl sutures. Note that the anterior borders of the platysma muscles have already been sutured. This maintains a muscular sling or girdle, which would be difficult to create had the anterior borders not been approximated previously.

Fat removal from the superficial surface of the platysma. After the platysma is tight and stable, the fat from the superficial surface of the platysma is removed. This is best accomplished by means of suction, used with a sweeping action. As noted, if fat is removed prior to suturing the platysma, defatted muscle may be advanced onto the face where it may not be desired, and the procedure is more difficult because the muscle is loose. In any case, the platysma muscle can be defatted completely. Scissors may be used; however, bleeding is greater when vessels are cut by scissors than when they are avulsed by suction.

Removal of fat from jowls. The jowls should be inspected to determine whether additional fat is present that should be removed. If it is, suction lipectomy with the same plastic or metal cannula should be performed.

Hemostasis. This is obtained with electrocautery. However, should facial muscles contract when cautery is used, hemostasis is obtained chemically by use of topical epinephrine or microfibrillar collagen hemostat (Avitene).

Closure. After the excess skin is marked and excised, the scalp incisions are closed with staples. The remainder of the incisions are closed with a single layer of buried 4–0 Vicryl in the anterior auricular region and a running 4–0 blue Prolene in the posterior auricular areas. No drains are inserted; instead, a space is left between two sutures in the retroauricular region.

Dressing. A firm dressing is applied. Cotton soaked in mineral oil pads the ears, 4 × 8 gauze pads contour the neck, and a Kerlix dressing is applied. No antibiotics are used.

---

* Uterine cannula. Catalog No. 280 O.D. 8 mm, Busse Hospital Disposables. Hauppauge, NY.

POSTOPERATIVE

The dressing is removed in 2 to 3 days, at which time patients may wash their hair and an elastic chin support is applied. This is worn day and night for 2 weeks, then for nights only until the edema has been absorbed. The sutures are removed 8 to 10 days after the operation.

SUGGESTED READING

Baker TJ, Gordon HL. Surgical rejuvenation of the face. St. Louis: CV Mosby, 1986.

Courtiss EH. Suction lipectomy of the neck. Plast Reconstr Surg 1985; 76:882.

Goldwyn RM. The favorable result in plastic surgery, avoidance and treatment. 2nd ed. Boston: Little, Brown, 1984.

Rees TD. Aesthetic plastic surgery. Philadelphia: WB Saunders, 1980.

Regnault P, Daniel RK, eds. Aesthetic plastic surgery. Boston: Little, Brown, 1984.

Skoog T. Plastic surgery. Stockholm: Almqvist och Wiksell, 1974.

FACELIFT: MALE PATIENTS

SIMON FREDRICKS, M.D., F.A.C.S.

Male facelift is distinctly different from the comparable procedure in women. Men seeking facelift are frequently performance-oriented, Type A, intense personalities who look to the bottom line. They do not easily give up being in control. On the other hand, they may be middle and upper management executive professionals who view their upward mobility as being threatened by the signs of aging; or, worse, they may have lost their positions and are seeking new employment. The latter suffer from reactive depression and may exhibit displaced hostility or complete dependency. Men, in general, unless they are effeminate, by nature are not disposed to preening and consider it threatening or emotionally uncomfortable. Therefore, men seeking this type of surgery need special handling, understanding, and consideration during the initial consultation and informed consent throughout the surgery and postoperative care. It is advisable to do all preoperative laboratory studies on an outpatient basis so that these patients may remain mobile and productive. However, males by nature are more hypertensive and arteriosclerotic than women, and therefore, they do not do as well in the immediate postoperative period if permitted to be outpatients. As a result, I strongly recommend that all male facelift patients be sedated and observed overnight before discharge.

Statistically, males have a higher postoperative hematoma rate than females. This can be significantly reduced if the following precautions are followed. I do not operate on patients whose blood pressure exceeds 140 systolic and 90 diastolic. If the patient's blood pressure is higher, I do not operate until the blood pressure is reduced by an appropriate medical regimen. I never use adrenalin in patients who are known hypertensives, even if they are now well controlled with medication. Otherwise, these patients will frequently undergo a hypertensive episode in the immediate postoperative period. Furthermore, I prefer to operate on males under general anesthesia so that they can undergo a controlled high oxygen saturation tissue environment. An in-dwelling catheter avoids straining in the immediate postoperative period and therefore diminishes the potential for hematoma. Droperidol given prior to extubation prevents postoperative nausea, and Xylocaine given intravenously prior to extubation reduces coughing. These are the two primary causes of increased Valsalva in the critical postoperative period.

We encourage our patients to discontinue smoking prior to operation. I believe that discontinuing smoking at least 48 hours before surgery makes a significant difference in the microcirculation, and I insist that patients do not smoke in the immediate postoperative period. Smokers certainly have a chronic bronchitis, and their laryngeal secretions and coughing are markedly increased. Furthermore, the oxygen deprivation to the microcirculation makes the difference between prompt and delayed wound healing.

Technically, the main operative differences between male and female facelifts are the direction of pull, the sideburn location, and the presence of beard.

Women should be lifted in a true oblique facial direction to encourage the development of a high, prominent cheek bone. If males are lifted similarly, they look strangely effeminate. Instead, males need to be elevated either vertically and/or horizontally in the facial area to smooth the nasolabial depression and to clean the jaw line (Fig. 1). A harder, sharper jaw line is desirable and youthful-appearing in males and requires careful attention to defatting the neck by sharp dissection and/or suction.

I never perform T or Z procedures for the male central neck. These procedures certainly correct the turkey-like, central neck waddle, but to my mind do so at an unacceptable cost. The scars can be a visible embarrassment and are highlighted when the five o'clock shadow of the beard is present. In my opinion, these procedures are an attempt at a quick fix for a patient who is really better served by a lower facelift and simultaneous refinement of the jaw line.

Central neck laxity of any severity can be eliminated by lateral migration of excess tissue with an easily camouflaged scar. I prefer to place the neck scar at the hairline angled to parallel the hair follicles. This placement gives the maximum amplitude of neck rotation and

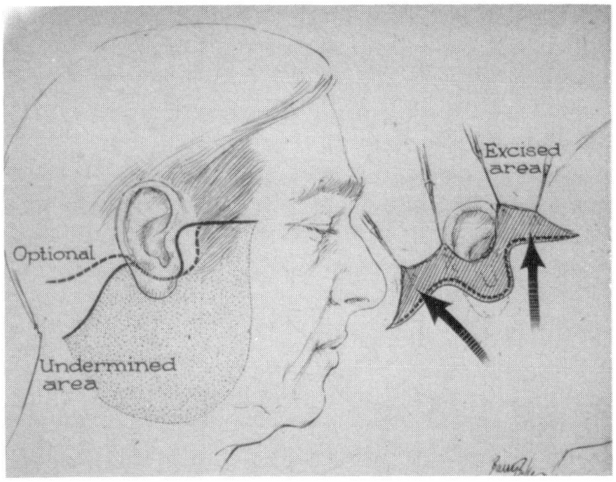

Figure 1 Pattern of incision and undermining for male facelift.

is easily hidden with modern hair styles. If the patient insists on short, severe, crew cut styles, it is necessary to accept a higher placement through the hair of the occiput (Fig. 2).

A conservative subcutaneous musculoaponeurotic system (SMAS) flap tightening is usually performed as well as independent skin rotation. Generally the skin elevation of the neck is taken to the midline. I never completely divide the SMAS, thereby always leaving a good submandibular central SMAS intact. If anterior platysmal cords are prominent, I handle these by a submental incision and suturing of the platysmal sling in the upper neck after incision of the anterior platysma at the level of the hyoid. Occasionally the central subplatysmal fat must be carefully removed. Furthermore, one platysmal anterior fold may be much more prominent than the other. If this occurs, I prefer to resect the thicker fold vertically before incision and central suturing. I leave the resultant V cut open and unsutured effectively to increase the vertical length of the anterior platysmal fold (Fig. 3).

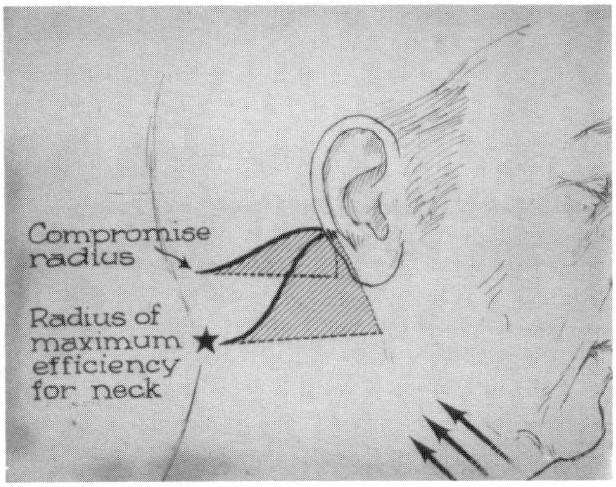

Figure 2 An incision paralleling the submastoid hairline is preferred to one within the hairline to obtain maximum left of the neck.

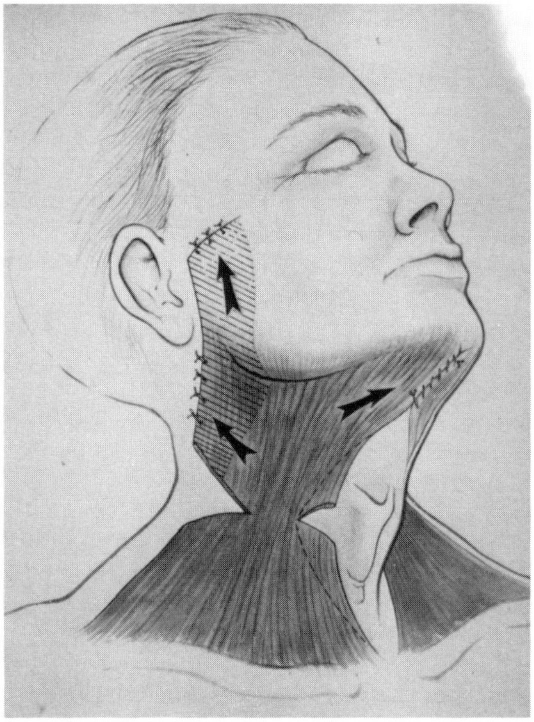

Figure 3 Preferred method of SMAS treatment with superior fixation at the zygomatic arch, posterior fixation of the sternocleidomastoid and submental plication. The platysma is partially divided both anteriorly and posteriorly.

Technically, I find the prominent ptotic brow to be the most difficult part of the aging male face. Direct brow lift results in an unacceptable scar in males. I have been similarly repelled by midforehead horizontal incisions as advocated by others. I find such incisions are usually too permanently prominent.

The coronal approach gives the best result if the patient is not balding. However, men naturally have a more prominent brow, and one should not convert the ptotic male brow into a bizarre-looking, excessively strange, surprised look that is totally unnatural in appearance. It is better to simply accept the lateral brow ptosis.

I never use a tragal edge incision in males as sideburn hair can thereby be migrated too close to the auditory canal. Instead, I prefer the traditional preauricular placement, thus accepting the loss of preauricular skin and the resultant migration of sideburn towards the ear.

In addition, I never use drains, but am scrupulous about hemostasis by pinpoint cautery. Hemostatis is more readily obtained if the procedure is done in the reverse Trendelenburg's position with the head higher than the heart. This avoids the oozing of venous engorgement, which is seen if the head is below the heart level. Furthermore, the procedure is done with the neck in mild anterior flexion, as this is the natural carriage in the erect state. If the head is permitted to fall horizontally or, worse, to be hyperextended, an inadequate lift will result.

I apply a moderate compressive dressing that discourages subflap seroma accumulation for 4 days. I believe that this blood-tinged serum is liberated by drains;

the serum is generally spontaneously absorbed by the fourth postoperative day without drains. Any seroma or hematoma present on the fourth day will be aspirated by a suction machine and 3.7 mm cannula. If this is required, compression dressings are maintained for an additional 48 hours. Normally the dressings are discontinued at 4 days, and the patient is sent for a shampoo and combing. He can then return to sedentary professional and social activity and begin to shave a well-moistened beard carefully and to drive his own vehicle.

I caution males not to have orgasm for 2 weeks and not to engage in sex in a facedown, prone position.

I do not permit pillows in the immediate postoperative period to avoid severe anterior neck flexion that compromises retroauricular circulation. Thereafter, I allow a vertically-placed pillow that falls equally beneath the head and upper back; this maintains the head in an elevated position, but the neck in an extended position.

These patients should sleep on their back for 1 month and stay in cool, air-conditioned environments until their wounds are well healed.

SUGGESTED READING

Baker TJ. Rhytidectomy in the male patient. In: Goulian D, Courtiss EH, eds. Symposium on surgery of the aging face. St. Louis: CV Mosby, 1978:47.

Connell BF. Eyebrow, face, and neck lifts for males. Clin Plast Surg 1978; 5:15–28.

Courtiss EH. Male aesthetic surgery. St. Louis: CV Mosby, 1982.

Fredricks S. Rhytidectomy in men. In: Goulian D, Courtiss EH, eds. Symposium on surgery of the aging face. St. Louis: CV Mosby, 1978:54.

FACELIFT: AVOIDANCE AND TREATMENT OF PROBLEMS

BERNARD L. KAYE, M.D., F.A.C.S.

COMPLICATIONS

Fortunately, complications in facelift surgery are relatively infrequent and usually mild. Many are preventable. Most of them correct themselves or are correctable by reasonable, nonextraordinary measures. Surgeons who do facelift operations find it useful to be familiar with the usual complications of the operation along with their prevention and management.

By-products of Operation

By-products of operation include tightness, edema, decreased sensation or numbness, which is usually temporary, and elevation of hairline. These are best managed by preoperative patient counseling, preferably shortly before the operation.

Ecchymosis

Ecchymosis is not usual, although occasionally bruising may be spectacular (Fig. 1). Bruising subsides in time but may occasionally leave residual pigmentation.

Incision Lines and Scars

Scars are unavoidable biproducts of facelift, as well as all other external surgery. The plastic surgeon tries to minimize them, providing the patient's healing ability will cooperate.

It is important to explain to the patient precisely where the incision lines (I prefer to call them incision lines rather than scars) will be, and that occasionally one might encounter hypertrophic (overgrown) scars in some patients. A history of excessive scarring or keloid is a good indication for a test incision in a nonvisible area many months prior to the facelift operation.

Normally, facelift scars heal with fine incision lines, particularly if one avoids tension, closes exposed incisions

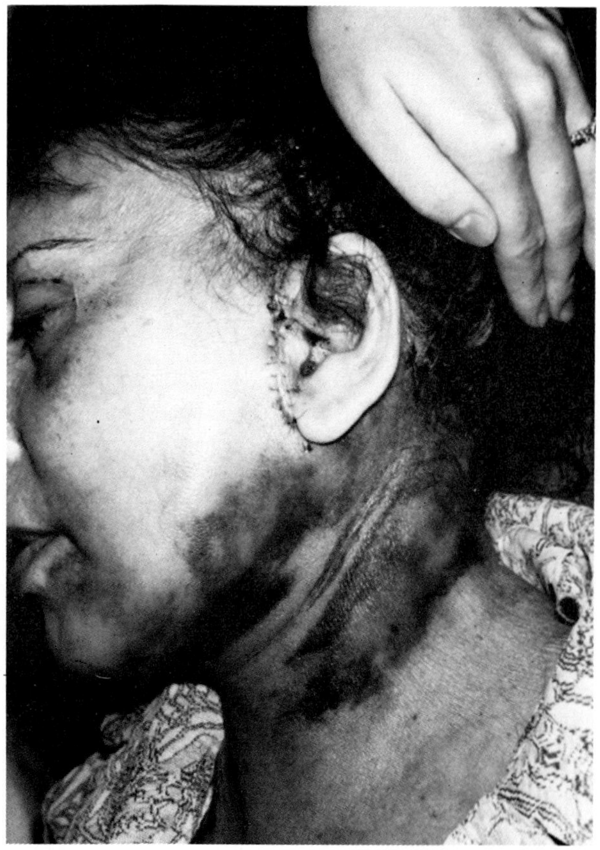

Figure 1 Bruising.

in at least two layers, and leaves sutures in hairbearing areas for at least 10 days to 2 weeks. Hypertrophic scars usually occur in the mastoid postauricular region (Fig. 2) and are more likely to occur in younger patients. Causes of overgrown scars include necrosis that is due to decreased circulation, tension, smoking, or other vascular problem, infection, and keloidal tendencies. Wide, spread scars may be due to subclinical forms of connective tissue disorders, such as Ehlers-Danlos syndrome. Methods to decrease or prevent scarring include placing incisions in favorable locations parallel to normal relaxed lines of skin tension and in hidden areas, avoiding excess tension, closing exposed incision lines in at least two layers, recognizing and pre-evaluating possible keloid formers, and judiciously placing incisions within the hairline. Avoid lateral or central vertical neck incisions that would produce exposed scars (Fig. 3). Treat overgrown scars by frequent, sympathetic postoperative office visits. Counsel the patient about the need to wait for maturation. Judicious use of injectable steroids can help flatten a scar (although it will widen later) that may benefit from excision and/or secondary facelift. Most scars can benefit from later revision when required. Also, the underlying factors that produce the scars should be corrected if they are known (e.g., smoking).

Nerve Injury

The most frequently injured nerve in facelift surgery is the great auricular nerve, probably because of its superficial course over the sternocleidomastoid muscle. It lies 6.5 cm below the external auditory canal on the sternocleidomastoid muscle. Injury to the great auricular nerve is avoided by dissecting over its course under direct vision with adequate light. Dissect in the superficial subcutaneous plane; when you see muscle, you are too deep. The nerve always lies immediately posterior to the external jugular vein.

When you recognize a partial or complete nerve transection, repair it with several epineural interrupted sutures of 6–0 Prolene or finer material. Only slight magnification is required, and, because it is a sensory nerve, successful healing can usually be anticipated.

Motor Nerve Injury

Motor nerve injury is one of the complications most feared by plastic surgeons. Fortunately motor nerve injuries, for the most part, are usually due to factors other than transection. These include edema, pressure, local anesthesia, cautery, sutures, blunt trauma, and hematoma. The vast majority of motor nerve injuries recover spontaneously and are more of an emotional trauma to the surgeon and patient rather than permanent residuals of surgery.

Intraoperatively, motor nerve injury can be prevented by gentle, blunt dissection over the known courses of the nerves. My favorite method of dissection is, with a gauze wrapped finger, dissecting with a peeling motion. Nerves are strong and, in the areas of facelift dissection, are relatively large and unlikely to be injured by gentle, blunt finger dissection, whereas they would not withstand

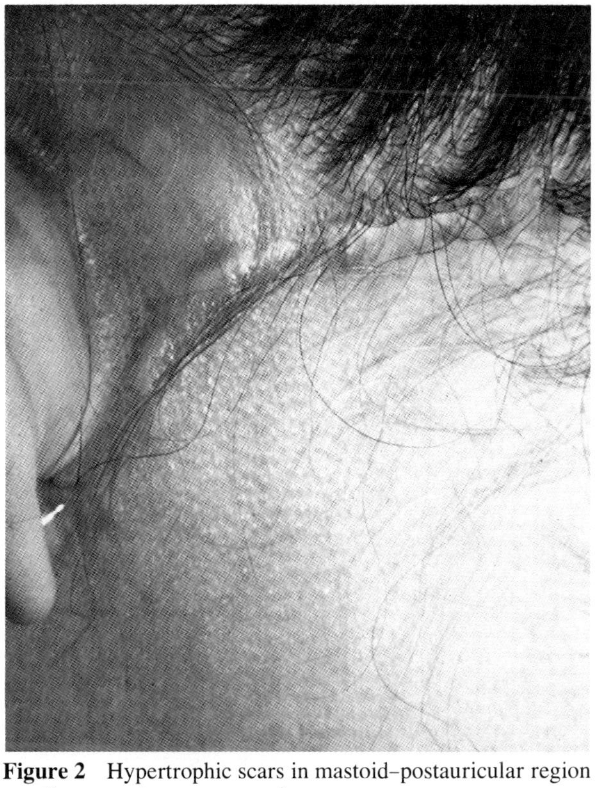

Figure 2 Hypertrophic scars in mastoid–postauricular region usually occur in younger patients.

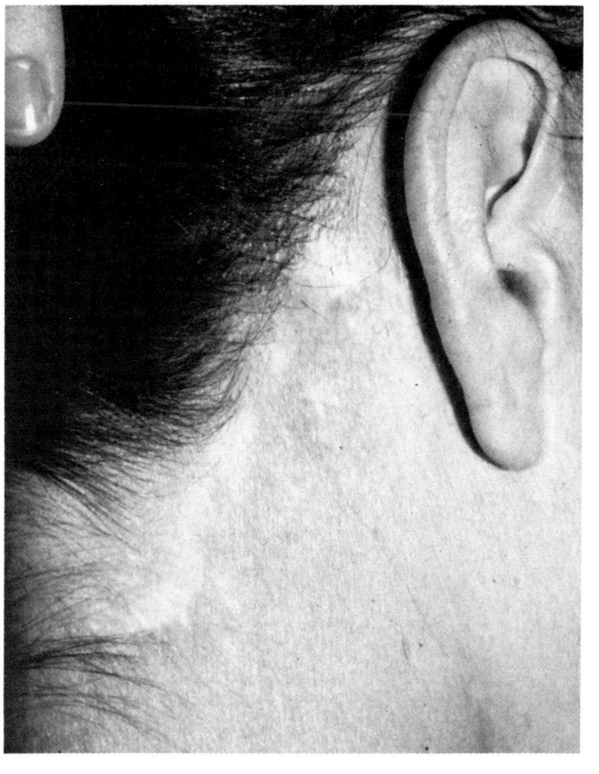

Figure 3 Unfavorable incisions can produce prominent scars.

the onslaught of scissors or knife. Additional preventive measures include use of adequate light and superficial bipolar electrocoagulation. During open defatting procedures, defat *after* underlying tissues (SMAS-platysma) have been transposed into their new positions. This tightens the underlying tissues, which makes tenting of the platysma and cutting of the marginal mandibular branch less likely.

Frontal branch injury (Fig. 4) is best avoided by gentle, blunt finger dissection over the course of the nerve.

Buccal nerve branch injuries result in loss of midface motion and expression and loss of the nasolabial fold on the affected side. These usually recover because of the multiple interconnected branches of the buccal motor nerve.

Marginal mandibular nerve injuries result in lack of depression of the lip on the affected side, and, like other motor nerve injuries, usually recover spontaneously with time.

When you detect an actual motor nerve division intraoperatively, repair it under the best conditions possible. Interestingly, very little has been written about intraoperative detection and repair of motor nerve injury.

Most motor nerve injuries are discovered postoperatively—to the great dismay and anxiety of the surgeon. In such cases, first review all the steps of the operation to see if there was any time or stage where the nerve could have been injured. (It is remarkable how clear our memories of the operative procedure become under these circumstances.) If you have no reason to suspect that the nerve was cut, wait. The vast majority of nerve injuries recover spontaneously and can be managed by frequent follow-up. Neurologic consultation with electrical testing (e.g., electromyography) can be helpful.

Rare, end-stage treatments include re-exploration, attempts at identification and reanastomosis of the nerve, and compensatory surgery such as muscle division or nerve division of the opposite side. Fortunately these extreme end-stage measures are rarely required.

Hematoma

Causes of hematoma include bleeding tendencies, both congenital and acquired. Most congenital bleeding tendencies can be recognized preoperatively because patients usually know about them.

Acquired bleeding tendencies caused by drugs and perhaps foods and vitamins are more difficult to detect. Sometimes even a full standard battery of bleeding tests including prothrombin time, partial thromboplastin time, template bleeding time, and platelet count, are not enough to discover a hidden bleeding tendency.

A great many drugs used today can cause bleeding. In the past aspirin was the chief offender, but we are now familiar with its effects. On the other hand, many other drugs, including anti-inflammatory agents can also cause bleeding.

Preoperative prevention of hematoma includes the medical history. Is there a history of easy bleeding or bruising in the patient or family? What about medications? I believe hypertension is the major cause of hematoma. It is also the most frequent medical finding in patients in the facelift age group. Chronic hypertensives are less of a problem because they know who they are, they are usually on medication for their condition, and, more often than not, their condition is controlled by medical treatment. The dangerous patient is the undetected labile hypertensive.

Consultation in the plastic surgeon's office is an ideal setting for discovering labile hypertensive patients. They are usually apprehensive, and their tendency toward abnormally elevated blood pressures under stress can be detected easily. The plastic surgeon or a member of his staff should check the blood pressure of every new patient who comes to the office.

When I discover such labile hypertensive patients, I contact their physicians to have them treated. Often, you have to educate physicians about the need for medicating such patients, at least during the perioperative period, so

Figure 4 Temporary frontal motor branch injury.

they will not be capable of raising their systolic pressures much above 150, even under stress. After patients have been put on a medication regimen, recheck their blood pressures in *your* office, because your office is where elevated blood pressures and possibly inadequate medication regimens may show themselves.

Hypertension, particularly labile hypertension, is more of a problem in the postoperative period. Monitor blood pressures frequently, especially during the first 6 to 8 hours. Also remember that the two most frequent causes of postoperative hypertension are pain and a full bladder. For long procedures, I have hypertensive patients catheterized so that the full bladder problem is eliminated. Catheterization also allows the anesthesiologist to give intravenous fluids more liberally and to monitor the patient's urine output.

During the immediate postoperative period, I use hydralazine as my primary antihypertensive agent, giving 5 mg intravenously or 10 mg intramuscularly every 30 minutes for systolic blood pressure over 150. My backup agent is usually a beta-blocker such as propranolol (Inderal) in a dose of 1 mg intravenously, repeating it in 5 to 10 minutes if necessary, if the pulse is 70 bpm or more.

In the later postoperative period, make sure the patient has adequate sedation for restlessness and adequate analgesics for pain. Beware if a patient has excessive postoperative pain, which in itself may be a sign of expanding hematoma. Usually, routine antihypertensive medications may be started on the first postoperative day. Some labile hypertensives do not show recurrence of their hypertension and do not need medication after the operation.

Intraoperative causes of hematoma include insufficient hemostasis and unrecognized bleeding vessels. In my opinion, one of the most important methods to prevent hematoma is meticulous hemostasis, not just with one or even with a second look, but with repeat inspection of the operated areas, three, four, or even five or more times. I do not believe that general anesthetic is a cause of excessive bleeding. I have operated on patients under both local and general anesthetic, and, other reports notwithstanding, I have seen no greater incidence of excess bleeding with general anesthesia than with local anesthesia.

Postoperatively, hematomas can be caused by wretching, vomiting, coughing, hyperactivity, and hypertension. Postoperative prevention of hematoma includes the use of antiemetics, antitussives when necessary, careful blood pressure monitoring with use of antihypertensive agents when indicated, sedation for restless patients, and elevation of the head while avoiding flexion of the neck and decreased circulation to the skin. Control pain with analgesics but use them with discretion. As mentioned above, pain can be a sign of expanding hematoma.

Treatment of hematoma varies. Very small hematomas, which are found 10 days to 2 weeks postoperatively, have already organized into scar and will respond to time, massage, and judicious use of steroid injections.

Moderate sized hematomas can be treated by staged aspiration after they have liquified, usually at least 7 days postoperatively, by aspirating every 2 to 3 days for three or four times.

Moderate to larger hematomas can also be treated, as soon as they are discovered, by aspiration with a suction lipectomy cannula (which has the power to suck up the jelly-like clots) accompanied by irrigation.

The most dangerous hematoma is the expanding hematoma. Its manifestations include pain, hardness of the overlying skin, feeling of anxiety by the patient, tightness, trismus and, worse yet, dyspnea due to pressure on the airway. Swelling and discoloration of the lips and buccal mucosa are pathognomonic of an expanding hematoma.

Management of expanding hematoma consists of early recognition and treatment. Take the patient back to the operating room. Preferably under general anesthesia, reopen the incision(s), remove the clots, and control the bleeding vessels. Usually there are multiple fine bleeders, although rarely a single pumping vessel may be the culprit. The incision can then be sutured, sometimes under considerable tension. Usually such management will result in complete, uneventful healing without sequelae.

Failure to discover an expanding hematoma can result in skin necrosis, skin loss, and scarring as well as pigmentation, puckering, and subcutaneous masses, which may persist for months.

Necrosis

The basic cause of necrosis is impaired circulation, which can be due to smoking (both active and "passive"), tension, excessively thin flaps, excessive undermining of tissues beyond the perforating vessels in the cheek, traumatic undermining, and pressure from within (hematoma), or from without (tight dressing).

Prevention of necrosis includes stopping smoking, keeping the patient away from other smokers, avoiding excess tension, dissecting flaps of adequate thickness, sparing important perforators, gentle handling of tissues, avoiding acute angles in flaps (such as an acute postauricular angle) and prompt treatment of expanding hematomas.

Treatment of necrosis generally should be conservative. Do not debride the eschars, which act as a biologic dressing, unless there is obvious liquefaction beneath them. I use Betadine ointment over eschars and allow them to flake off spontaneously. Although the initial scarring can be significant, over months and years this scarring will reduce significantly (Fig. 5A and 5B). A secondary facelift can help remove the scars.

Infection

Fortunately, infection is a rare complication of facelift surgery because of the excellent blood supply to facial tissues. I have seen only two extensive cases of purulent staphylococcal infection with facelift operations. I treated each of these by daily irrigation with a solution of sodium naficillin with a butterfly catheter through a

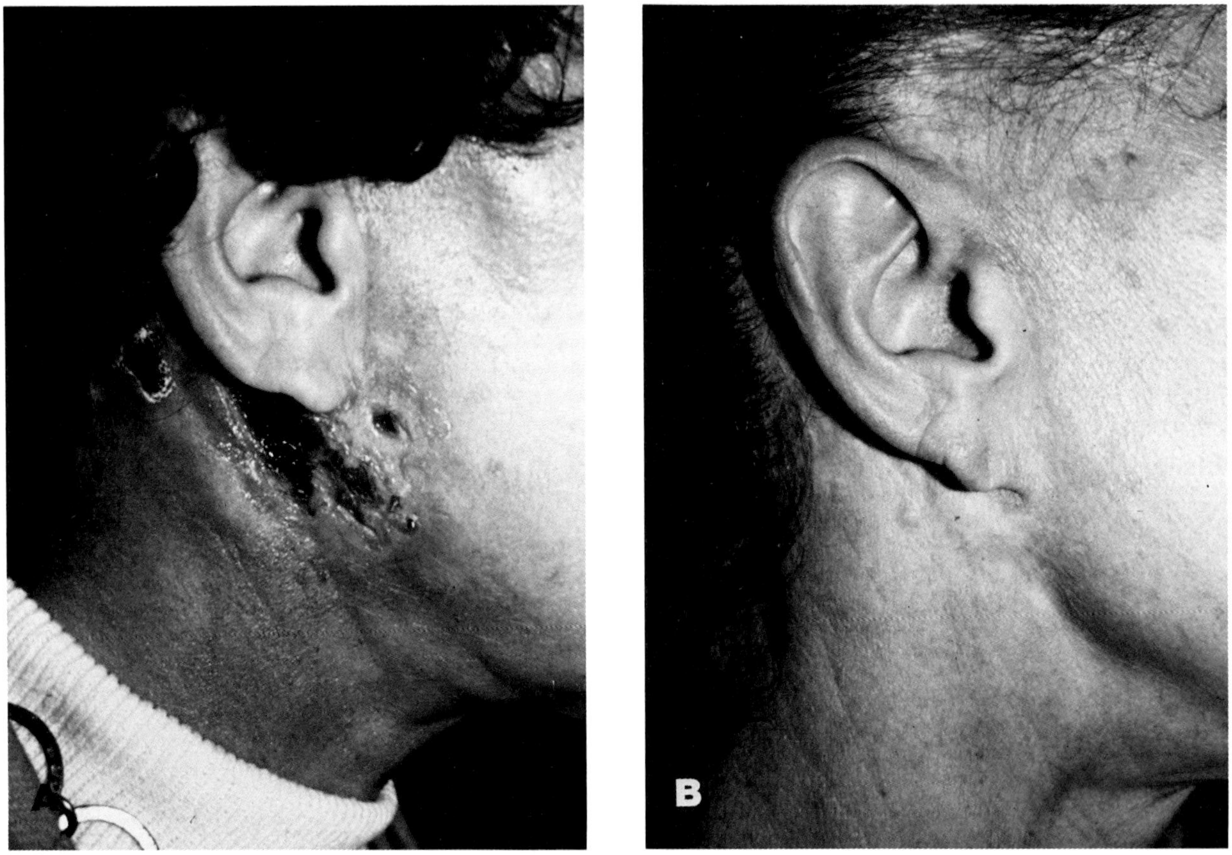

Figure 5 *A*, Necrosis associated with smoking; *B*, Healing 8 years later.

postauricular incision, followed by irrigation with half strength hydrogen peroxide. Infected patients were also given high doses of an antistaphylococcal penicillin along with probenecid (Benamid) to maintain high blood levels of penicillin. Of the two forms of antibiotic treatment, I believe the local treatment was the more important one. Recovery was complete without sequelae (Fig. 6A and 6B).

For prevention, I arbitrarily give an intravenous antibiotic at the start of the operation and continue with oral antibiotics for 1 or 2 days postoperatively.

Hair Loss

Temporary hair loss may occur anterior to an incision line due to nondestructive injury to the hair follicles, which primarily involves decreased circulation. Causes include smoking, tension, mild infection, or an overly thin flap with nondestructive follicle trauma.

Destruction of hair follicles produces permanent hair loss. Causes of such destruction include cutting the bases of the follicles, necrosis of hairbearing skin, and destruction of hair follicles by infection.

Prevent hair loss by having smokers stop smoking, by maintaining good flap circulation with adequate flap thickness, and by avoiding surgical injury of the follicles.

Treatment of hair loss involves waiting at least 3 months for regrowth. When hair loss is in an area of scar, obviously hair growth will not recur and scar excision is required. Reconstructive measures such as hair transplantation plugs or flaps are rarely needed.

Contour Deformities

Contour deformities have become major complications of facial surgery since we have learned to defat faces, either directly or by suction. Contour deformities are best avoided by two measures. First, defat conservatively; even thin faces have a layer of fat between the skin and underlying structures. Second, do most of your defatting *after* the underlying structures (SMAS-platysma) have been transposed and fixed into their new position. By defatting vigorously before these layers have been moved into their new positions, you may find that you have defatted yourself into a hole after you have transposed these underlying structures. Do not remove fat simply because it is there. Remove it only to contour and shape the facial structures. Check carefully in between brief stages of defatting to make sure you are contouring only as much as you want to contour.

If I encounter a contour deficiency intraoperatively, I treat it by grafting fat from elsewhere into the deficiency. If I were asked to treat a late postoperative contour deficiency, my current choice of treatment would be to undermine and loosen the involved area and either graft solid fat or inject particulate fat from aspiration into that area.

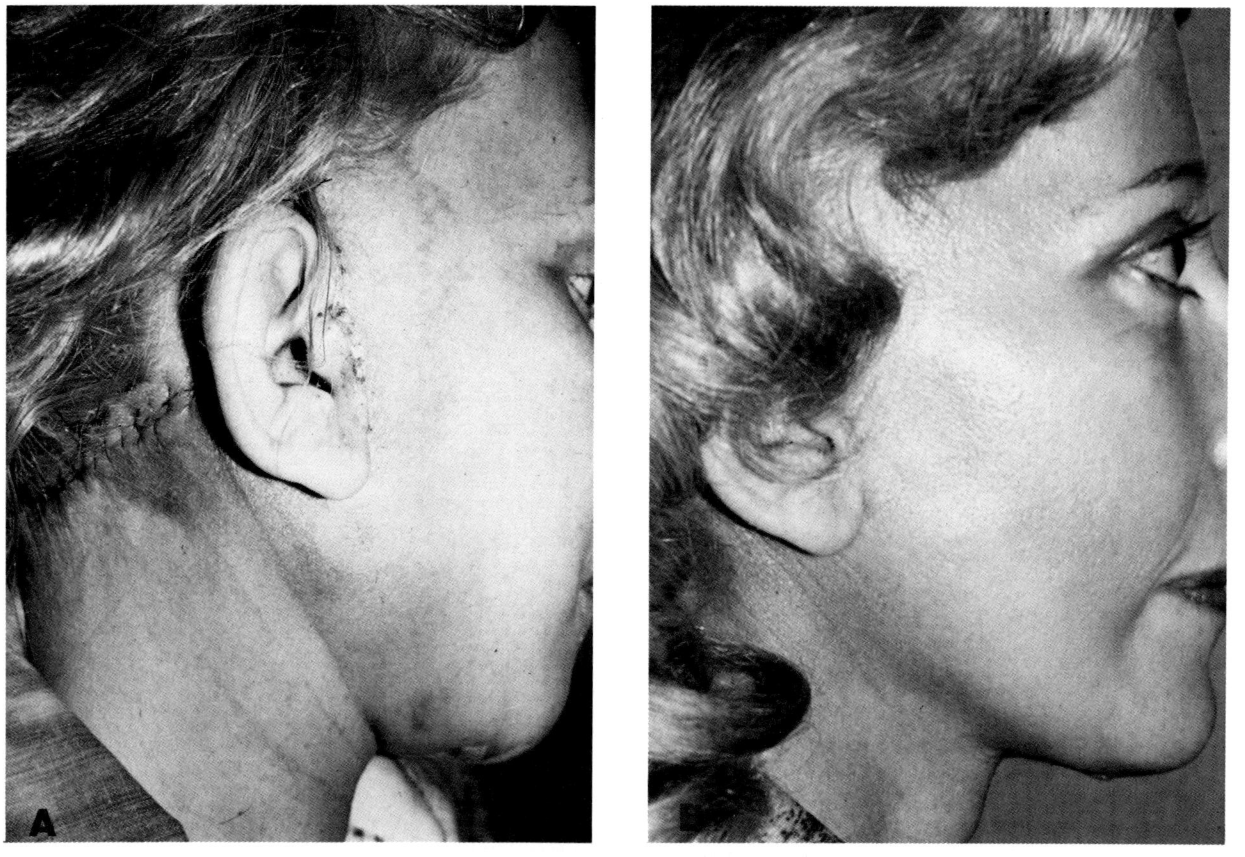

Figure 6 *A*, Purulent staphylococcal infection; *B*, Complete healing after systemic and local treatment.

Early Recurrence of Deformity

Early recurrence of sagging facial tissues can be due to genetic factors, sun exposure, and, in particular, having a facelift at a later age.

It is wise to inform older patients preoperatively, on several occasions, that the results of their operation will not hold as long as those of younger patients and that they will benefit from an early secondary facelift. I have had much less problem with early recurrence, not through better surgical technique, but through preoperative counseling.

Rarely, one may encounter a patient with an undetected connective tissue disorder such as a "forme fruste" of Ehlers-Danlos syndrome. I had one such patient who, 2 months later, looked as if she did not have an operation. She later told me that although she was the youngest of eight siblings, she looked the oldest. She had hyperextensibility of her joints, but I was not able to study her adequately to make the diagnosis.

Postoperative Depression

I believe this complication is mentioned more often in textbooks than it is seen in actual practice and most patients get along quite well emotionally following a facelift. The worst case of postoperative depression I have seen was in a psychiatrist!

Patient Dissatisfaction

Patient dissatisfaction can be due to real or imagined faults of surgery or adverse results. When the adverse results are real it is best to recognize them, form a plan of management, communicate the plan to the patient, and see the patient frequently, spending as much time as is necessary at each visit. Schedule such patients at the end of the day so that you have the time to spend with them.

Patient dissatisfaction due to unrealistic causes must be treated by extensive counseling. Counseling is much more effective preoperatively than postoperatively. What you say preoperatively is considered preoperative education counseling. What you say postoperatively may be interpreted as an excuse for an adverse result.

Let the patients ventilate. Tell them realistically what you can do and what you cannot do. Where indicated, seek consultation from colleagues without hesitation.

SUGGESTED READING

Baker TJ, Gordon HL. Surgical rejuvenation of the face. St. Louis: CV Mosby, 1986.

Fredricks S. Rhytidectomy. In: Courtiss EH, ed. Aesthetic surgery: trouble. How to avoid it and how to treat it. St. Louis: CV Mosby, 1978:118.

Kaye BL, Gradinger GP, eds. Symposium on problems and complications in aesthetic plastic surgery of the face. St. Louis: CV Mosby, 1984.

Kaye BL. Facial rejuvenative surgery: a color photographic atlas. Philadelphia: JB Lippincott, 1987.
McKinney P, Katrana DJ. Prevention of injury to the great auricular nerve during rhytidectomy. Plast Reconstr Surg 1980; 66:675–679.
Owsley JQ. The unfavorable result following face and neck lift. In: Goldwyn RM, ed. The unfavorable result in plastic surgery: avoidance and treatment. Boston: Little, Brown, 1984:591.
Rees TD, Aston SJ. Complications of rhytidectomy. Clin Plast Surg 1987; 5(1):109–119.
Regnault P, Daniel RK. Rhytidectomy. In: Regnault P, Daniel RK, eds. Aesthetic plastic surgery. Boston: Little, Brown, 1984:408.

SPECIAL PROBLEMS IN THE BLACK FACE

W. EARLE MATORY Jr., M.D.

Cosmetic surgery among Black patients has gained increasing popularity over the last 10 years. Two major factors appear to be responsible. First, an increased economic prosperity has brought cosmetic surgery within reach. Second, well-known Black entertainers have made the results of plastic surgery quite visible.

Although the number of Black patients seeking cosmetic surgery has increased, surgeons still have little experience with these patients. Ethnic concerns regarding esthetics are considerable. Individual patient concerns, likes, and dislikes are more variable than in the Caucasian. There are wide-ranging differences in individual anatomy, including marked variations in the relationships of the eyes, nose, and lips to the remainder of the face. While most surgical techniques that I use are identical to those used in the Caucasian, the goal is often quite different. The following five major areas distinguish cosmetic surgery in Blacks from that in Caucasians: (1) criteria of beauty in the Black face, (2) rhinoplasty, (3) lip thinning, (4) managing facial and scalp hair, and (5) the scarring phenomenon.

CRITERIA OF BEAUTY IN THE BLACK FACE

A beautiful female face should have large, widely spaced, soft eyes with long lashes. The nose should be small and slim, the skin clear, pale and smooth and the cheek bones high, the mouth medium sized or small, soft with gentle lips that are not too thick. - Caucasian beauty

Anon

Of significance in black beauty is the facial skeleton, typified by the prominent cheek bones, slightly increased intercanthal distance (separating eyes that pan from amber to dark brown) and immaculate dental arch with ivory-white teeth set in a perfect dental formula. Beauty is the curvilinear contours of that central structure—with its short columella, flaring wings and sentinal tip looking into the "deep" of the filtral dimple—which like a "microwave dish" receives "exhalations" through ovoid, pyriform or round nares. The upper lip is highlighted by the great strength of Cupid's bow and acts in concert with its lower mate forming a calyx of everted melanotic fullness—never true vermilion.

Kenneth McNeill
Tony Jackson

The contrast noted in these interpretations of beauty is striking. In order to improve the looks of a patient who enters the plastic surgeon's office, one must discern a goal, that is, some sense of the definition of beauty. If Caucasian standards of beauty are applied to each Black patient who presents, unrealistic expectations would abound. The plastic surgeon managing the Black patient must, therefore, have a strong sense of what features are esthetic on the Black face.

Black facial features differ from those of Caucasians in several ways. The Black face is fuller, the cheek bones are more prominent, and the broad nose has greater degrees of curvature. The lips are rounded and thick, with a prominent Cupid's bow. In spite of the exaggerated facial curves, the relation of the facial plane to the Frankfort line is always very close to 90 degrees as it is in the "beautiful" Caucasian.

Miscegenation has contributed significantly to wide variations in skin color. Beauty can be displayed by an individual who is reuben black as well as one who is extremely fair. In my experience, a patient with a light complexion is far more likely to develop facial elastosis and require a rhytidectomy. More heavily pigmented patients rarely develop a degree of facial laxity that requires rhytidectomy, unless it is associated with considerable weight loss. Although the latter patient is far more susceptible to abnormal scarring after facial surgery, being fair does not preclude hypertrophic scarring (Fig. 1).

When a patient presents to my office, I try to determine whether the facial features are largely Negroid or largely Caucasoid. This analysis and the patient's desires help determine what alterations of facial features are best for the patient. The nose and lips are primary factors in establishing ethnic facial characteristics, the width of the nose being the most important factor. Features consistent with the Negroid are alar base attachment to the cheek that lies lateral to the inner canthal lines, lip height in excess of 1 cm in the adult. In this category of patient, the most satisfactory surgical approach is simply to soften the exaggerated facial feature. For example, decreasing the alar width by performing the alar cinch procedure and lip thinning will yield pleasant results without compromising ethnicity.

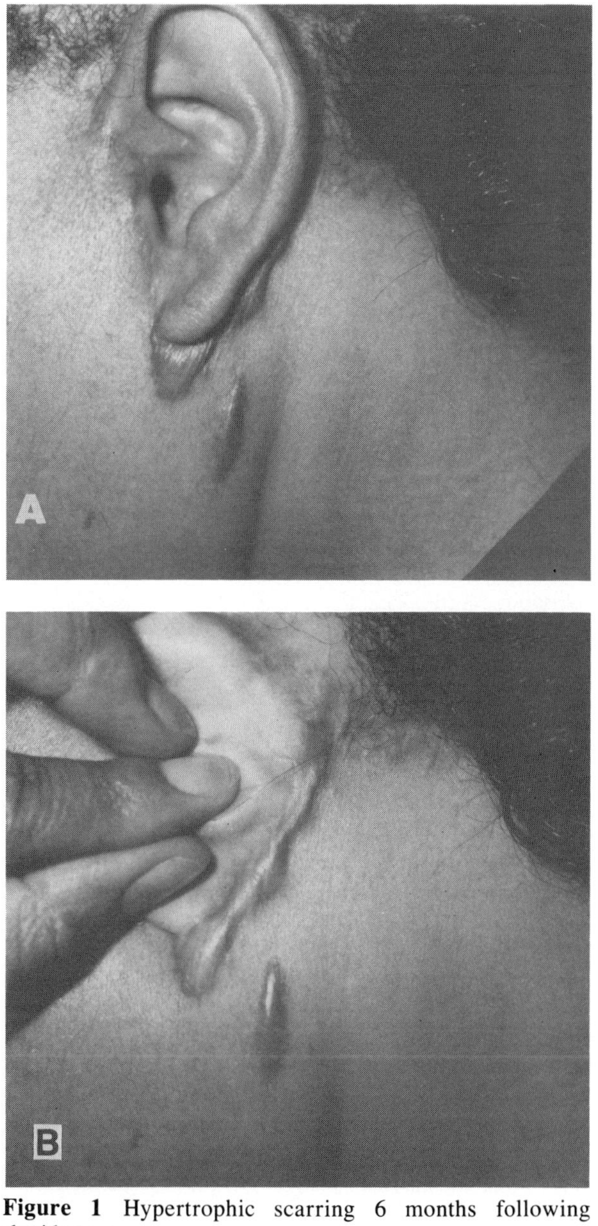

Figure 1 Hypertrophic scarring 6 months following rhytidectomy.

On the other hand, a Black patient who has a fairly narrow nose with alar base attachment well within or close to the inner-canthal lines has nasal and perhaps other facial features that are Caucasoid. These patients often have thin lips with each individual lip height equal to or less than 1 cm. Between these extremes of nasal configurations lie features consistent with Kenneth McNeill's miscegenated ideal composite (MIC). Thus we have identified three Black facial types, the Negroid, Caucasoid, and MIC.

The majority of patients presenting to my office fall within the latter category. According to patient desire, when addressing the MIC and the Caucasoid patient, we can significantly thin and narrow facial features in a fashion similar to what might be done in a Caucasian patient. Alar wedge resection alone to address the alar flare will make a significant difference in altering the nasofacial relationships. If alar base resection alone is performed in a patient with a very wide interalar distance, there is often a resultant distortion of nasofacial relationships.

McNeill points out the contribution of the facial skeleton to Black beauty. His description typifies the esthetic Negroid facial features. Depending upon patient desire, these features represent the goal in the Negroid patient. Most Negroid patients present with an exaggeration of normal ethnic features, columella foreshortening, depressed dorsum, lack of tip support, alar flare, increased interalar distance, and/or thickened lips. The malar eminences are full. The relationships of each respective part of the esthetic Negroid face follow similar criteria of beauty noted in the Caucasian patient.

The female facial symmetry guide (Fig. 2) serves as a guideline for softening exaggerated features in the Negroid patient. A longer preoperative evaluation is indicated in most Negroid patients and especially for the Negroid patient desiring Caucasian features. The additional counseling helps the surgeon understand exactly what changes are requested and allows the patient to understand the physical limitations of surgery.

RHINOPLASTY

Poor bony cartilaginous support of inordinately thick tissues is noted in most Black patients, thus making rhinoplasty far more challenging than in Caucasians. This difficulty is further compounded by wide-ranging differences in individual anatomy, variations in the relationship of the nose to the face, and considerable variations in patient desires.

The following guidelines help to reach a basic goal in all rhinoplasties, that of facial balance and symmetry. As previously described, the nasal index represents the nasal width to length ratio multiplied by 100. The actual numbers are not crucial but they are useful in defining the frontal view of the nose as a triangle. This triangle varies according to racial background and also varies considerably within the three groups: the Negroid, the Caucasoid, and the miscegenated ideal composite. The most common complaint of Black patients who present for rhinoplasty is that the base is excessively wide relative to the whole of the face. The dimensions of the frontal triangle can be altered but care must be taken to maintain ethnicity (for which the concept of nasal alignment is helpful). Ideal nasal alignment according to Broadbent and Matthews is such that the lateral attachment of the ala to the cheek lies within longitudinal lines drawn through the inner canthus. If one brings the elements of the nose to lie within a triangle having a base closer to the inner-canthal lines, nasal features can be improved without ethnic appearance being drastically altered (Fig. 3A). In the Black patient with Caucasian features, having a relatively narrow interalar distance, the nose can be further narrowed to lie well within the inner-canthal lines.

When we look at the inferior view of the nose, a triangle is formed by the tip and the lateral attachments of the ala to the cheek (Fig. 3B). This is most esthetically

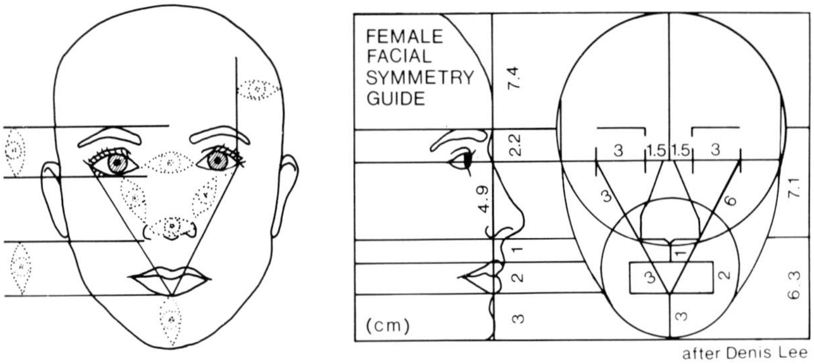

Figure 2 The female facial symmetry guide serves as a guideline for softening features in the Black and in the Caucasian patient.

pleasing when the nose is narrow-based, slightly taller than wide and with minimal alar flare. We define flare as that portion of the ala that extends lateral to the ala attachment to the cheek. By increasing the height of the tip and/or by lessening the flare of the ala, the inferior triangle can be altered.

In the profile, the nose in the Negroid patient and in most MICs, the dorsum is most often depressed, the tip is flat and blunted, and the columella is short. By augmenting the dorsum or raising the tip, the nasal axis may be altered to best suit the patient (Fig. 3C). I prefer to perform most Black rhinoplasties under general anesthesia because of the complicated nature of the procedure.

Table 1 illustrates the numerous operative approaches that I use to alter the frontal, basal, and lateral nasal perspectives. These procedures are discussed in detail elsewhere. The following five major anatomic differences distinguish the Black rhinoplasty from the Caucasian: the depressed dorsum, alar flaring, increased alar width, the fatty tip, and columella foreshortening. Negroid and MIC patients usually need a dorsal augmentation. I prefer to use autogenous bone from the tibia, ulna, iliac crest, or temporal bone. Layered septal cartilage is usually inadequate to augment the dorsum. Infections, displacement and asymmetry are far more common with nonautogenous implants. More recently I have chosen the temporal bone as described by Spear because of its relative straightness, minimal donor deformity, and donor site within the same surgical field. The Black with Caucasian features and occasionally an MIC may have enough dorsal definition to obviate dorsal augmentation. The dorsal pocket is developed through an intracartilaginous incision. The implant is fashioned to contour the depression and extends from the nasion to the distal septum. Extension of the graft to the tip leads to tip irritation or extrusion. Dorsal augmentation followed by nasal infracture significantly improves the frontal triangle.

Alar base resection is indicated in patients with alar flare. The amount of ala to be excised is determined by the amount of flare. Resection of the ala, which results in a straight line between the tip and base, is less than esthetic. Under-resection leaves persistent flare. The optimal resection yields a nice gentle curve. By determining the amount of alar resection that will result in a straight line, and preserving an additional 2 mm of ala, a gentle curve may be achieved (Fig. 4). Prominent alar flare is noted in most Negroid and in some MIC patients. Thus, softening the flare yields a more natural-appearing rhinoplasty.

Reduction of the interalar distance can be performed by two methods. The alar sill advancement as described by deAvelar (as an adaptation of the Cronin ala advancement) can yield a modicum of interalar reduction. This can be highly effective in the Caucasoid or MIC patient in which the alar attachment to the cheek is less than 1 mm lateral to the inner canthal lines. In the Negroid nose that has an alar base attachment more than 2 mm lateral to the inner-canthal lines, an interalar reduction as described by Millard is indicated. Interalar reduction is performed by mobilization, de-epithelialization and suture fixation of the alar base to the distal septum. Alar base resection reduces flaring. Interalar reduction reduces the width of the nose and alters the relationship of the nose to the face. Interalar reduction therefore has significant consequences on the ethnic appearance of the individual. It is important for the surgeon to keep this in mind in establishing patient and surgeon goals.

Tip defatting is a component of almost all Black rhinoplasties. The bulbous fatty tip can be addressed through an intracartilaginous incision. More recently I have noted the ease of the open rhinoplasty technique for defatting, as well as tip sculpturing. Alar base incisions are placed along the alar crease. If an interalar reduction is planned, these incisions are made first. The columella incision is marked along the shadows at the base of the columella. The incisions meet centrally as an inverted "V." Once the lobular skin is elevated, the excess cartilage and fat are excised en bloc preserving a 2- to 3-mm rim of distal lower lateral cartilage. Care must be taken to avoid injury to the subdermal plexus. Serial defatting can result in significant improvement in tip definition. Other methods of enhancing tip definition in these patients include cartilage graft to the tip and to the columella, fixation of the medial crura with simultaneous stabilization of a columella strut, and postoperative splinting. The goals in sculpturing the tip are to alter the basal triangle such that the base is narrow relative to the columella height. By increasing the columella height and by narrowing the interalar distance, resculpturing can be achieved. As is true in the Caucasian, one should avoid allowing the

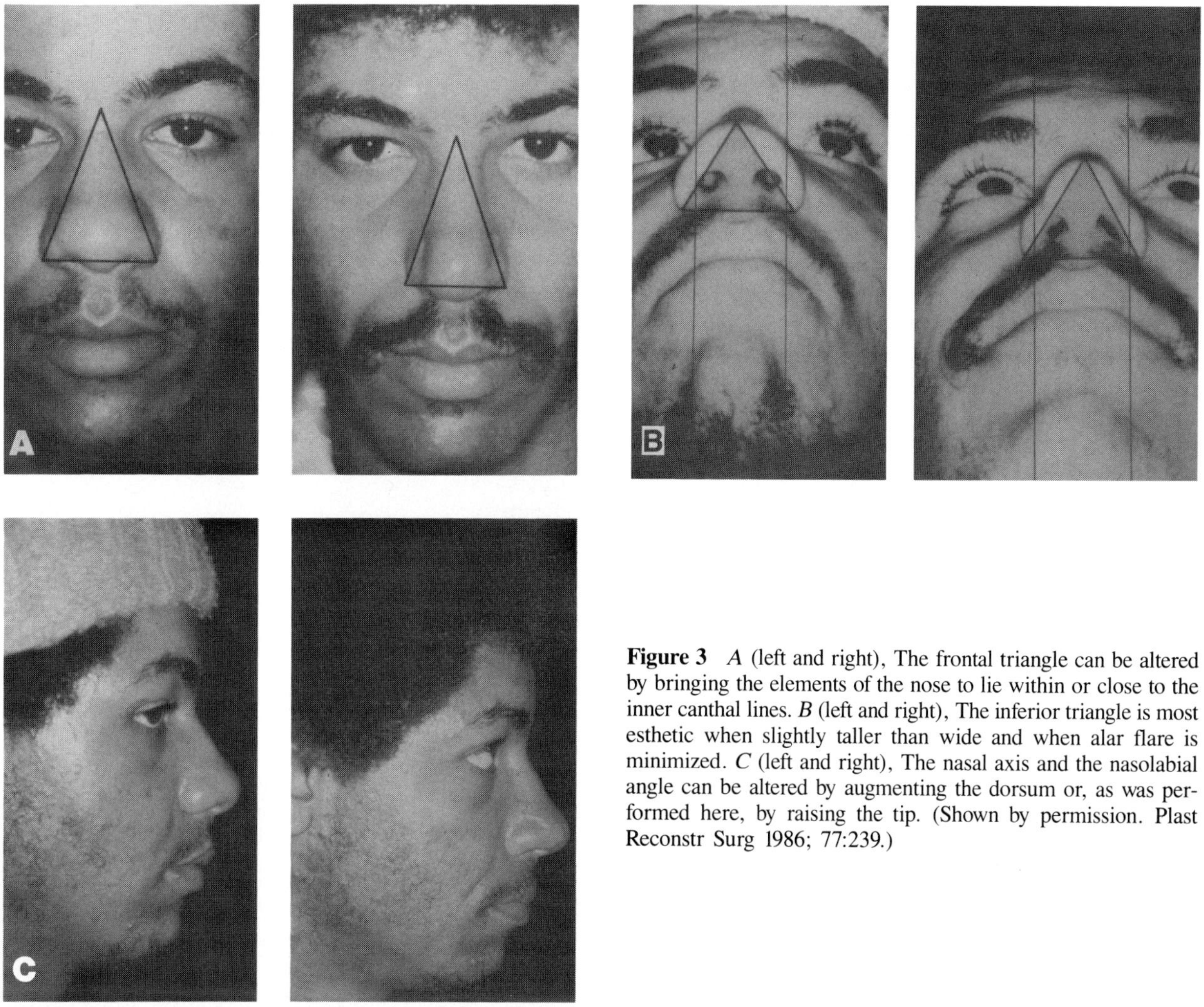

Figure 3 *A* (left and right), The frontal triangle can be altered by bringing the elements of the nose to lie within or close to the inner canthal lines. *B* (left and right), The inferior triangle is most esthetic when slightly taller than wide and when alar flare is minimized. *C* (left and right), The nasal axis and the nasolabial angle can be altered by augmenting the dorsum or, as was performed here, by raising the tip. (Shown by permission. Plast Reconstr Surg 1986; 77:239.)

TABLE 1 List of Operative Techniques

Frontal:	Nasal infracture Dorsal augmentation Alar base resection Interalar reduction
Basal:	Tip sculpturing improving tip projection and definition Defatting Cartilage graft/columellar support Fixation of medical crura Postoperative splinting Alar base resection Interalar reduction
Lateral:	Dorsal augmentation Tip sculpturing Columellar lengthening Alar sill advancement Columellar implants

columella graft to extend to the tip. Graft protuberance at the tip can be softened with a tip implant. The open technique allows precise suture stabilization of the implant and the medial and lateral crura.

In the Negroid and in the occasional MIC patient who has alar flare as well as a wide interalar distance (extending far lateral to the inner-canthal lines), a two-staged procedure yields the best results. The alar base resection along with dorsal augmentation, nasal infracture, tip defatting, and tip sculpturing can be accomplished with the first procedure. A secondary tip defatting and interalar reduction are performed as a secondary procedure (Fig. 5).

For all but the simplest of Black rhinoplasties, a secondary procedure should be planned. The secondary procedure should be deferred, however, until resolution of the nasal edema. In my experience, prolonged edema occurs in approximately 60 to 70 percent of patients and may last for 6 to 18 months postoperatively. Secure but nonrestricting splinting with tape strips and a dorsal splint

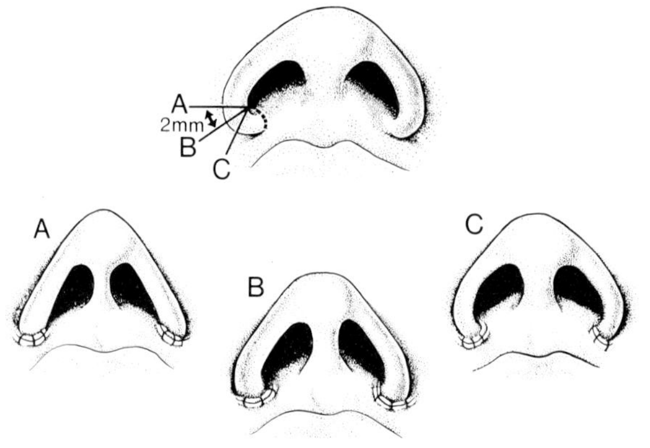

Figure 4 The amount of ala to be resected is determined in the following manner. Alar excision can be performed at point C (center above), yielding persistent flare, or at point A, leading to excessive straightening of the alar rim. Optimal excision is performed at point B, 2 mm inferior to point A, yielding a more natural and gentle curve. (Shown by permission. Plast Reconstr Surg 1986; 77:239.)

are appropriate in the postoperative period. I splint my patients for 3 weeks following surgery. In addition I use Decadron 10 mg IV preoperatively. Serial steri-stripping is helpful in minimizing and in controlling edema.

External scarring in and about the nose has not led to hypertrophic or keloid scarring in any of the patients in my series. An early healing ridge may be noted along skin incisions. This ridge usually resolves with massage. Mild degrees of asymmetry are not uncommonly seen on the alar rim following alar base resection. Asymmetry is minimized by ensuring a detailed preoperative analysis with close study of the preoperative photographs. By doing so, pre-existing asymmetry can be noted and the alar base resection can be adjusted. Alar asymmetry in excess of 1 mm, is noted in over 75 percent of my patients. Excessive resection of the alar base results in too much straightening and exaggerates the smallest degree of asymmetry.

The most peculiar complication to the Black rhinoplasty is what I consider racial incongruity. In the patient with a very wide interalar distance, a nasal infrac-

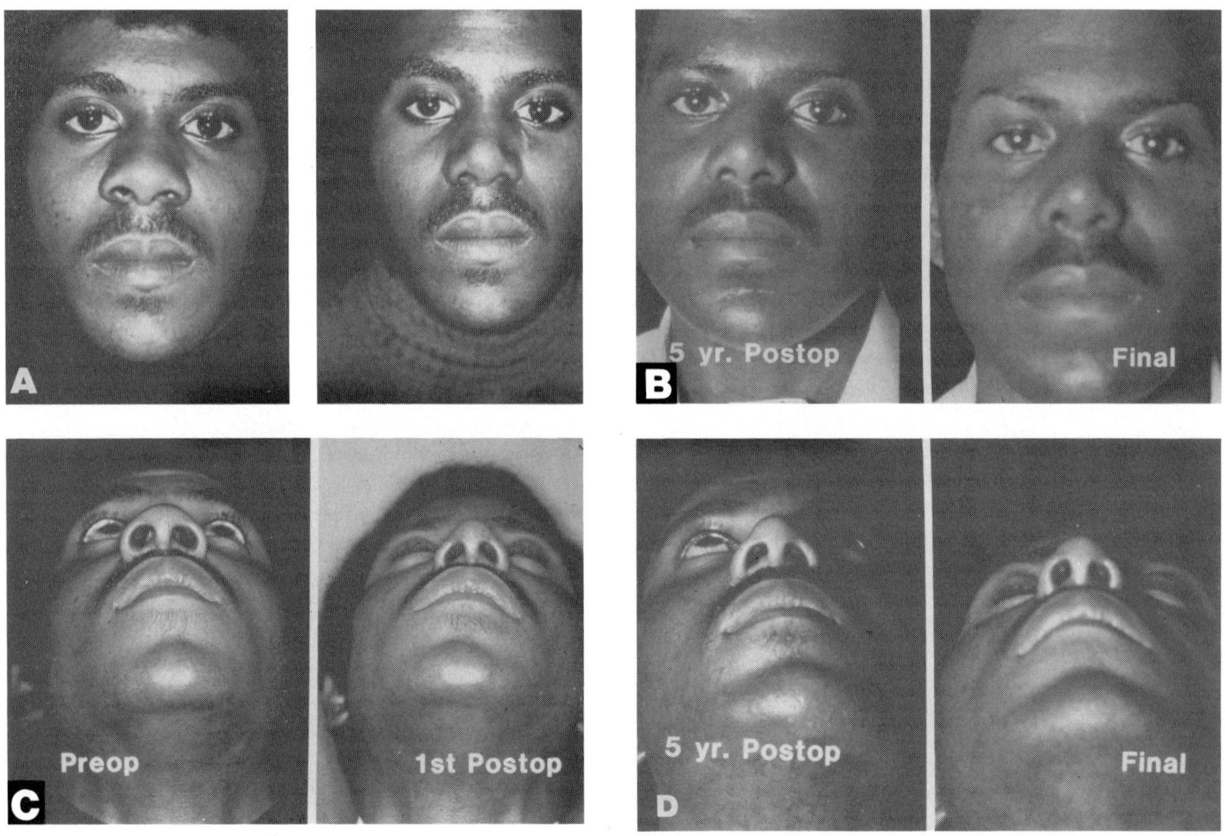

Figure 5 (*A* left, *C* left) A wide nasal pyramid, wide interalar distance, moderate alar flare, and poor tip definition. (*A* right, *C* right) The inferior triangle is better defined and narrowed by tip defatting and alar base resection. Osseous infracture and dorsal augmentation also were performed. (*B* left, *D* left) Five years after nasal surgery there is persistent wide interalar distance, minimal flare, and fair tip projection associated with persistent excess tip fat. (*B* right, *D* right) Two years later, after second rhinoplasty including interalar reduction and additional tip defatting. (Shown by permission. Plast Reconstr Surg 1986; 77:239.)

ture and alar base resection results in a disproportionate narrowing of the dorsum with respect to the lobule width. This results from excessive infracture and from unreduced alar width. One can avoid racial incongruity using the following techniques: (a) limiting the infracture so that it is more proportionate to lobule size at the time of the original surgery—accomplished by elevating the lateral nasal walls and inserting symmetrical nasal packing; (b) simultaneous use of a columella strut and a cartilaginous tip graft—the tip height and the tip definition lessen the accentuation of the alar width; (c) performing a subsequent interalar reduction; or (d) using the alar sill advancement technique to address moderate alar flare and moderate excess alar width.

To summarize my approach to the Black rhinoplasty the following points I feel are crucial. A detailed preoperative, photographic analysis identifying the relationship of the nose to the rest of the face is a must. Determine the physical features and the patient desires with regard to the Negroid and Caucasoid characteristics. Once a set of realistic expectations are determined, primary and secondary procedures can be planned. The Black patient is far more likely to need a second operation. The final results may not be noted for up to 1½ years following surgery.

Beware of the patient with unrealistic expectations. If patient expectations and patient–physician rapport are not optimal, litiginous entanglements can be disastrous.

LIP THINNING

Excessively large lips relative to the remaining portions of the face is a common concern among many Black patients. It is important to note that in most instances the lip enlargement is hereditary. The lip enlargement may also be due to low grade inflammatory reactions, congenital lesions such as hemangiomas or lymphangiomas, or may be due to unknown causes. Protruding lips may also be the result of protruding teeth and malocclusion. A central lip height of greater than 1 cm is commonly noted. In most patients the goal is not directed toward Caucasian features, but simply toward modification of exaggerated lip thickness.

Isolated lip thinning can be performed under local anesthesia, preferably with infraorbital and mental nerve blocks. This approach minimizes lip distortion. The anterior incision is placed posterior to and parallel to the wet line, the area of lip mucosa behind the lip seal region. The incisions should extend lateral to the commissure to avoid unnatural puckering. The incision, however, should not involve the commissures in order to avoid a constricting band. The posterior incision is outlined and a triangular ellipse is excised removing mucosa, underlying glands and a thin ribbon of muscle. Closure is performed in a single layer using horizontal mattress sutures with 5–0 Vicryl to optimize eversion. I have found that a fair number of Black patients react to Dexon, chromic and plain gut. Prolene is less reactive but is irritating when used intraorally. The Vicryl sutures should be removed within 1 week following surgery or sooner if tissue reactivity is noted.

Determining the extent of resection is often difficult. The patient with extremely large lips is usually very pleased following lip thinning procedure. The Caucasoid patient who desires lip thinning is often dissatisfied with the degree of thinning. With these patients a local anesthetic is preferable so that the patient, with the use of a hand mirror, is able to play a role in determining the extent of resection. If the midline lip height is 1.2 cm or less, a 2- to 3-mm wide ellipse is excised. Temporary sutures are placed. Additional resection can be performed if the patient desires.

FACIAL AND SCALP HAIR

The properties of Black skin and hair often require that we alter our surgical technique. In the Caucasian patient, the hair follicles are usually straight above the skin but angled obliquely within the skin. This is true even in the patient with curly hair. In contrast, Black hair forms a tight coil on the surface as well as a curvature of the hair follicle beneath the epidermis (Fig. 6).

Thus the usual practice of angling the surgical incision or the punch biopsy to parallel the follicle may result in shearing neighboring follicles, completely missing some roots, shaft avulsion resulting in hair growing through the side of the graft, frequently not reaching the epidermis. These ingrown hairs may develop an inflammatory foreign body reaction characterized by papules and pustules, known as pseudofollicutitis barbae. One can optimize follicle survival by making skin incision and punch biopsies

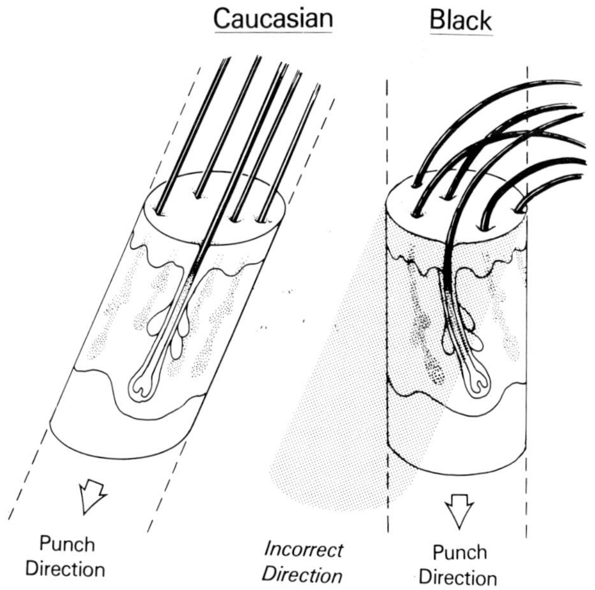

Figure 6 In Caucasian hair, the follicle is usually straight above the skin but angled obliquely beneath the skin. Black hair forms a tight coil on the surface as well as a curvature beneath the epidermis. Thus the angle for punch harvesting must be different for the two races.

nearly perpendicular to the skin. Use of a 4- to 5-mm punch also improves survival.

Hyperpigmentation and hypopigmentation at the recipient site is not uncommon in the Black patient. A leading factor appears to be the gap between the donor graft and the recipient site. This gap is filled with blood and subsequently replaced by abnormal scarring. I prefer to use a recipient site punch that is approximately 1 mm smaller than the donor 4- to 5-mm punch. A 4–0 Nylon suture on a Keith needle can be passed through a row of four or five grafts for stabilization. A second pass in the opposite direction allows ligation. This method of stabilizing the grafts optimizes epidermal to epidermal approximation and prevents the commonly seen cobblestone effect noted frequently in this patient population.

Donor site healing is not infrequently abnormal. Simple closure of a row of donor sites commonly results in a serpiginous thickened scar. I prefer to completely excise the septa separating each respective donor site. I then undermine the skin edges and reapproximate the scalp using dermal suture with 4–0 Vicryl. The skin is precisely aligned and closed with skin staples.

All of the surgical methods used to address alopecia such as hair transplantation, scalp reductions, flap rotations, and tissue expansion can be used in the Black patient. Hypopigmentation, hyperpigmentation, and hypertrophy of the resultant scars can be addressed using hydroquinone, corticosteroid and retinoic acid mixtures as described in the section on the scarring phenomena.

Replacement of hair within the eyebrows and the upper lip is particularly difficult in the Negroid patient for several reasons. No matter how curly the scalp or pubic hair is, the hair in the eyebrows and upper lip areas is usually straight or very slightly curved. The best possible donor site is the contralateral brow or mustache. In the absence of these, strip graft take is poor, often accompanied by poor follicle survival, excessive scarring, hypopigmentation, and hyperpigmentation. I have found temporal transposition scalp flaps very useful for brow reconstruction and partial mustache replacement. Free occipital hairbearing transplant, as described by Walton, is another alternative (Fig. 7). Hair follicle survival is significantly improved and excessive scarring is minimized. The procedure is relatively straightforward. The occipital vessels are localized with the Doppler probe. The scalp flap is outlined based on a template of the recipient site. The orientation should be longitudinal overlying the course of the Dopplered vessel. The hair follicle direction should be oriented so that it is directed away from the nasolabial crease. The flap is then harvested and transferred to the defect. The nasolabial artery and vein, or the facial artery and vein, are used as the recipient vessels. Hair growth is prolific. The hair follicles must be trained and frequently trimmed. Mustache wax or over-the-counter hair relaxers are helpful in softening the curl.

Pseudofollicutitis barbae is a cutaneous infection that occurs following surgical manipulation of the bearded area. This inflammatory foreign body reaction to ingrown hairs occurs in approximately 85 percent of all Black patients who shave. It may occur within the bearded area of the face or at the posterior nape of the neck after shaving. Papules and pustules form at the point of hair penetration and are often accompanied by permanent hypertrophic or keloid scarring. The spiral or helical growth pattern of Black hair results in an ingrowth when the epidermis is incised.

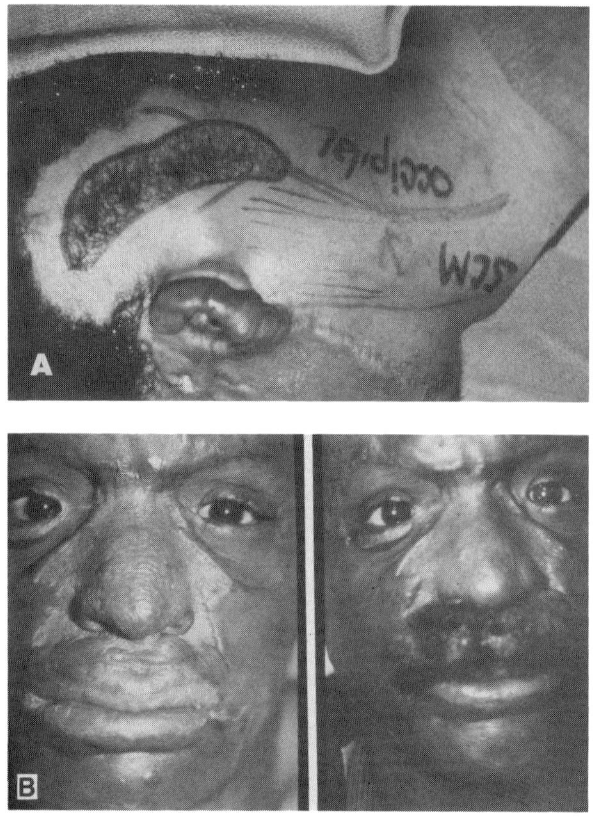

Figure 7 *A*, Identification of the occipital artery course and outline of the flap. *B*, Preoperative and 3 months following free occipital hairbearing flap reconstruction of the upper lip. (Courtesy of Robert L. Walton, M.D.)

Because this is a foreign body reaction to the ingrown hair, initial management consists of pulling out the individual hairs. This can be performed with loupe magnification and fine jeweler's forceps. Prevention of the process is achieved by avoiding incisions of the skin. Use of chemical depilatories, and electric razors designed for black men, and the double-edged foil-guarded blade (American Safety Razor, Verona, Virginia) are very effective. Use of a mild facial soap (Ivory, Dial, Safeguard) or pHisoHex is helpful in diminishing the gram-positive flora, which commonly infects the skin. When the process is extensive with hypertrophic or keloid scarring, a surgical approach is indicated. I excise the skin, dermis and superficial fat to the submuscular aponeurotic layer. Loupe magnification is used to accomplish a meticulous debridement of all residual ingrown hairs.

A split-thickness skin graft, from eighteen to twenty-two one-thousandths of an inch, yields optimal donor and recipient site healing. A thin graft leads to significant contracture at the recipient site. A full-thickness graft is far more likely to develop hypertrophic or keloid scarring at the donor site. The graft is sutured in place, thus minimizing a donor recipient site healing ridge. Postoperatively shaving is usually not necessary but if significant follicular growth ensues, the same preventative techniques should be used.

SCARRING

The greatest fear of patient and surgeon in cosmetic surgery of the black face is resultant excessive scarring. The hypertrophic and keloid scarring that is seen so commonly in the ears, chest, and arms can be quite devastating.

Fortunately certain areas of the face very rarely form such scarring. These include the eyelids, the external and internal nose, and the lips. In a series of several hundred patients, I have noted two patients with excessive scarring in these areas. This was related to infections in both instances. Intraoperative prevention, pressure, steroid injection, topical steroids, hydroquinone, and retinoic acid have been an effective combination in addressing excessive scarring and hyperpigmentation.

Intraoperative Prevention

Rhytidectomy

The Caucasoid Black patient is the most likely to present for rhytidectomy in my practice. Prior to 2 years ago, I felt that the fair-skinned patient was far less likely to develop hypertrophic scars. I have now seen six, in a series of 32 Caucasoid Black patients who have developed some degree of hypertrophic scarring.

My current protocol for evaluating these patients is as follows: I examine these patients to determine scarring tendencies. A test incision can be performed in the postauricular area along the proposed rhytidectomy suture line per patient or physician desires. If abnormal scarring develops within 3 to 6 months, I inject the incision on a monthly basis using Decadron, 4 mg per milliliter for 6 months. (I have found that Decadron is far less likely to result in tissue atrophy or hypopigmentation.) If scarring results are acceptable, I proceed with surgery. While a test incision does not duplicate skin tension and wound healing results, some reassurance can be given the patient and surgeon. The technical details of rhytidectomy and associated suction lipectomy are no different than that in the Caucasian patient. The closure, on the other hand, has been adjusted. I have found that Blacks are far more likely to react to Dexon. Reactivity to Vicryl is less likely but also quite strong. Dexon Plus, Maxon, and Prolene are far less reactive. A reaction to suture material is the most likely precipitant to hypertrophic scarring in my experience. Dermal sutures are placed at the sternocleidomastoid fascia, the mandible, and the malar eminence to minimize skin tension. A running pullout 4–0 Prolene is placed in the dermis along the skin incisions. If necessary, interrupted horizontal mattress suture with 6–0 Prolene ensures epithelial to epithelial approximation. Intradermal injection of Decadron, 4 mg per milliliter, can be performed using the Dermajet as desired. The injections are repeated on a monthly basis for the following 6 months. Skin sutures are removed at 3 days and the dermal suture at 2 weeks.

Following 18 cases of dermabrasion and eight cases of chemical peel in Black patients, I have noted no hyperreactive scarring. I currently use topical Temovate in the postoperative management of these patients. I found that the latter significantly decreases the pigmentary changes that occur following dermabrasion and chemical peel. Hyperpigmentation and hypopigmentation are not infrequent ranging from 8 to 10 percent. These pigmentary changes are usually temporary lasting up to 12 to 18 months. Reconstructive cosmetics have proven extremely helpful during the recovery.

Treatment of Abnormal Scarring

My current regimen for patients who develop keloids is as follows. Patient massaging and use of compression garments are crucial. I advise 5 minutes twice daily for each segment of scar. Intradermal injection with Decadron, 4 mg per milliliter, is given once monthly until resolution of excessive scarring.

Topical 0.05 percent retinoic acid is applied on a twice daily basis. The latter competitively inhibits DNA synthesis within the fiberblast and has proven to be very helpful in decreasing hyperpigmentation and pruritus. Transient redness or scaliness may appear as a result of the ethanol and propylene glycol that are within the agent.

Hydroquinone 4 percent is also a very effective agent in decreasing hyperpigmentation. It is a nonstaining vanishing cream, which when applied twice daily is very effective in decreasing excessive skin pigmentation. I encourage my patients to avoid sun exposure for the first 6 to 12 months following surgery. Exposure to ultraviolet rays is the primary contribution to delayed alterations in pigmentation following chemical peel or dermabrasion.

SUGGESTED READING

Broadbent TR, Mathews VL. Artistic relationships in surface anatomy of the face: application to reconstructive surgery. Plast Reconstr Surg 1957; 20:1–17.

deAvelar JM. Personal contribution to the surgical treatment of Negroid noses. Aesthet Plast Surg 1976; 1:81.

Matory WE Jr, Falces E. Non-Caucasian rhinoplasty: a 16 year experience. Plast Reconstr Surg 1986; 2:239–251.

McNeill K. Personal communications. 1983 and 1984.

Millard DR Jr. Principalization of plastic surgery. Boston: Little, Brown, 1986.

Millard DR. Alar cinch in the flat flaring nose. Plast Reconstr Surg 1980; 65:669–671.

Spear S. Temporal bone as a source of autogenous bone graft. Boston: Northeastern Society of Plastic Surgeons, 1985.

AESTHETIC SURGERY IN THE ORIENTAL: CURRENT TRENDS

ROBERT S. FLOWERS, M.D., F.A.C.S.

Each time I write or speak on the subject of esthetic surgery in the non-Caucasian (or Oriental), I ask myself the question—"Is there truly a significant difference between operating on Caucasians and Orientals?"—and the answer is always an unequivocal affirmative.

There are indeed significant differences, but the first and foremost may be in the approach. In the Oriental, one should always opt for *subtle* changes; placing a premium in all instances on the preservation of ethnic identity.

It is wrong to assume that, because we live in a predominantly Caucasian culture, Caucasian features are the desired goal of all individuals who request change. It is generally a mistake to do procedures that Caucasianize the Oriental face, despite the misconception of some Orientals that Caucasian-type lid folds (those that parallel the lid margin or expose more pretarsal eyelid medially) would enhance their good looks. Such alterations invariably end up looking badly out of place.

Nonetheless it is true today that an international standard of facial esthetics is emerging. A gentle move in that direction can be advantageous—provided the person is not stripped of ethnic identity. Long term "wearability" of facial alterations is far more important than what may be requested at a given moment.

If the above esthetic principles are kept in mind, and if the surgeon has expertise, then it can prove truly satisfactory from an esthetic standpoint to follow these updated trends in esthetic plastic surgery on the Oriental, both from the surgeon's sense of accomplishment and from the patient's satisfaction with the change.

This chapter discusses the current trend in surgery of the Oriental, with occasional comments on geographic variations. However, before dealing with specific anatomic areas, it is germane to address general differences that have a significant impact on surgery.

GENERAL CONSIDERATIONS

Flaps and Fat

The accumulation of vast experience by several surgeons who perform a high volume of plastic procedures on both Orientals and Caucasians has led to significant observations. For years, it has been appreciated that most Orientals have a denser union between skin, subcutaneous tissues, and the deep fascia. The dermis is usually thicker, and the subcutaneous tissue more dense, than in comparable areas of Caucasians. Although the denser vertical connection to the deeper tissues was appreciated by many, the accompanying vascular considerations were not addressed. It has become increasingly evident to those with interracial experience that the blood supply to the skin in Orientals has a more vertical orientation with less collateral circulation than in Caucasians. This means that traditional flaps are more fragile and less prone to survival than flaps of comparable size, shape, and design in other racial groups. Whereas facelift flaps may be dissected widely in Caucasians and extended completely across the midline in the submandibular region and well down onto the neck, with infrequent incidence of skin loss, the same flaps in Orientals suffer a much higher incidence of ischemic problems. Facelifts and abdominoplasties are the two esthetic operations in which this difference has been most commonly, and unfortunately, noticed. The patient in whom the dissection is the most difficult (the one with the most dense connections) is the patient most likely to develop problems. Statistically, these clinical findings are more than coincidental, but they still need microscopic and dye study verification.

This finding has important implications as regards myocutaneous flaps, but the main significance is that clinical experience and injection studies in Caucasians and Caucasian cadavers should not be given "blanket" interracial validity.

Suction-Assisted Lipectomy

Liposuction in the submandibular area has been fairly forgiving in terms of deformity creation. This is true to an even greater degree in Orientals. Their combination of frequent submandibular fat accumulations (in otherwise trim persons), with thicker skin and elastic integrity, makes suction lipectomy a favorable esthetic procedure, especially in view of the vulnerability of traditional flaps. Where the Caucasian often requires a facelift to diminish the slack skin created by submandibular lipoplasty, the Oriental does not.

The greater accuracy for fat removal afforded by direct vision as opposed to aspiration via suction cannula, gives an angularity that is unbecoming to most Oriental faces. On the other hand, suction aspiration preserves some of the vertical blood supply in these collaterally deficient individuals, and lipoplasty's less efficient removal maintains a roundness in the features more commensurate with these patients' other facial characteristics.

The same tendency for fatty accumulation in the neck is also present in the periumbilical areas of the abdomen. Just as the raising of lengthy facelift flaps has an accompanying high incidence of necrosis, the same is true in the abdomen. The preference for suction-assisted lipectomy over abdominoplasty in the Oriental is further boosted by a higher incidence of hypertrophic scars and by the scanty pubic hair that is located much lower than in the Caucasian. The scanty hair means the scars of abdominoplasty are less concealed, but this is compounded by the need for higher placement because of the reduced distensibility of Oriental skin.

Characteristic fatty accumulations are also very common in Orientals in the areas of the iliac crest ("love handles"), but are found with lower frequency in the trochanteric areas ("saddlebags"). Good skin tone and elasticity produce an optimum result after lipoplasty in these two regions.

Fat removal by suction techniques is also more often indicated for the face, e.g., the fatty cheeks and bulging nasolabial folds in the presence of excellent skin turgor, typical of the Oriental race. The clinical observations mentioned earlier concerning collateral circulation give further weight to suction techniques as the preferred treatment over facelift-type techniques.

Although we are less likely to see deforming depressions and irregularities after facial lipoplasty procedures because of the Oriental's thick subcutaneous tissue, we should still expect *some* irregularity, corrugation, depressions, or other deformity to result. Although these problems are characteristically less severe than in the Caucasian, they should always be anticipated in the face, and the worth of the procedure must be assessed against the deformity which may result.

THE EYEBROW AND UPPER LIDS

In the Oriental, there is a new conservatism as regards eyelid surgery. In the years following the Second World War, cosmetic surgery gained popularity in Asia and many patients sought westernization of the eyes. Recently, however, there has been movement in the other direction. It has always been my contention that the Asian desire was simply for more beautiful Oriental lids. Perhaps this was true, but in any case, there is now emerging in the Orient a dislike for procedures that westernize the eyes. The emphasis now is on lid folds that are natural in character and subtle in prominence (which means that the distance between lid fold and lash line stays small).

One way to maintain the natural characteristics of the Oriental eye and avoid any suggestion of surgical alteration is to position the brow upward through a coronal lifting procedure. This freshens and rejuvenates the appearance, and emphasizes the naturally existing lid fold that is usually present. In the Oriental, it is the descent of the thick, juxtabrow tissues in the lateral orbit that gives the eye a tired, weary, and occasionally unhappy appearance. This ptosis of the lateral brow also takes away from the basic Asian design of the orbital region by decreasing the visualized pretarsal portion of the eyelid laterally relative to that in the central or medial portion of the lid. This characteristic is unnatural and rarely occurs in the youthful Oriental. Thus, the person who is interested in only a "refreshening," in other words a very subtle change without a surgically altered appearance to the lids, may be best served by a well-done coronal lift. This is done by resecting primarily from the superior lateral portions of the flap, with very little or nothing removed centrally.

Five or 6 years ago, I presented an essay on the importance of combining coronal lifting procedures with Oriental blepharoplasty in the older person, or one with low positioning of the brow, at an international meeting in Tokyo. This reduction of lateral brow descensus is very important, but coronal lifts should be used very cautiously in patients with *hollowed-out* upper lids. They inevitably increase the visibility and prominence of the hollowed-out, deep-set orbit in the patient with this predilection. When the hollow is deep and prominent, it may be wisest to delete the coronal lift from the list of procedures to be done; even though it may be desirable from the standpoint of lateral brow descensus. During the planning stage the brow should always be checked mechanically and elevated to see if there is an exaggeration of undesirable features. If there is, it should be deleted.

Among Orientals living in Asia and Hawaii, eyebrow tattooing has increased markedly in popularity. Most tattoos are done by non-medical technicians. Often the brows are expertly designed and executed. The popularity of tattooing amongst Orientals no doubt relates to the frequency of scanty brows among their racial types. This allows tattoo artists to position the brow at any point desired, even though the actual brow pad that normally bears the follicles may be resting down on the upper lid. Thus the "brow" may be tattooed on the forehead skin and, although a coronal lift would improve the appearance of the upper lid and the lid fold, it could cause an abnormally high placement of the new eyebrow. In rare instances, the solution to this may be skin excision just beneath the tattoo's caudal margin.

LID FOLD PROCEDURES

Most Orientals have some degree of fold present during youth. Some young Orientals have a prominent fold on one side and none on the other, which raises interesting anatomic questions.

There continues to be much interest in procedures designed to create lid folds. There are those who suggest very simplistic methods of creating them—such as the use of one cutaneously applied nonabsorbable suture running subcuticularly and subconjunctivally, or the simple excision of skin and muscle from the upper lid, or excision of skin and cautery along the muscle. All of the above are invalid methods of obtaining long-term esthetically pleasing lid folds.

There remain two basic techniques: the closed method and the open method. Figure 1 depicts the open method I developed in 1970 and have used since 1972 on virtually all patients. It is increasing in popularity both in the United States and in Asia. Those who have learned the procedure have found it highly effective and it produces consistent and predictably high quality esthetic results. In the anchor technique that I have proposed, the use of an absorbable suture is important. Even the experienced operator occasionally has a suture that transgresses the conjunctiva. It is comforting to know that these "poaching" sutures eventually absorb and that resultant irritation of the cornea or globe is time-limited. It is also reassuring to know that a Nylon, Dacron, or silk suture will not work through the conjunctiva at some late date after surgery.

In my proposed technique the attachment to the tarsus provides an anchor for extra security and checks against lash eversion, which is a common problem after lid fold procedures. Connection to the aponeurosis keeps the pretarsal skin taut. Laterally, where the tarsus dwindles in vertical height, the aponeurosis is attached only

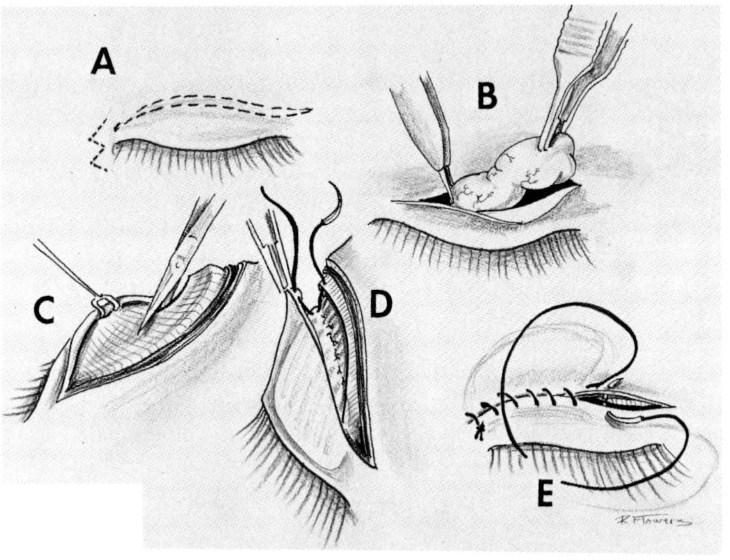

Figure 1 Flowers' technique for lid fold creation in Orientals. *A*, incisions are designed with optional medial epicanthoplasty. *B*, the fat is removed. *C*, the pretarsal extension of the levator aponeurosis is transected. *D*, dermis of pretarsal skin flap is attached to the anterior or superior aspect of the tarsus and to the sectioned aponeurosis. *E*, aponeurosis is also incorporated into skin repair.

to the dermis of the skin flap. Thus, in the far lateral lid, I revert to the basic technique proposed by Dr. Fernandez in 1960.

It is essential that the lid be flipped over and measured preoperatively because the vertical height of the Oriental lid cannot be presumed. The Oriental tarsus is usually 9½ to 10 mm, but may occasionally be as small as 7 mm in vertical height—especially in very petite Asians.

It is always essential to define the desired esthetic characteristics of the eye in both Oriental and Caucasian eyelids. A high quality result is unlikely to occur fortuitously in the absence of a precise plan. For me, the features of such a plan continue to be a fold that begins very close to, but just above, a light, medial epicanthal canopy rises to a maximum divergence from the lid margin near the central eye, and then continues at that level across the remaining portion of the eyelid.

The suture technique has many variations, but the basic technique is depicted in Figure 2. It can produce a nice fold in the thin lid, but generally yields less permanence than the open technique. It allows for no fat removal, which is often a key element of Oriental lid surgery (the medial compartment should not be ignored).

The medial epicanthus continues to require attention, with the best method being my modification of the Uchida split V-W epicanthoplasty, as illustrated in Figure 3. One must ensure that the upper limb epicanthoplasty incision never joins with the upper lid incision but is significantly above it, thereby avoiding combined contracture. The medial extent of the lid fold incision usually approaches within 2 or 3 mm of the lid margin.

The hollowed upper lid produces a dilemma in the Oriental. So far, techniques of injecting autogenous suspensions of fat cells have not been shown to have long-term beneficial effects in the upper orbit. Transposition of the lateral tail of the "lateral" orbital fat to the hollowed-out medial section of the lid, together with the occasional

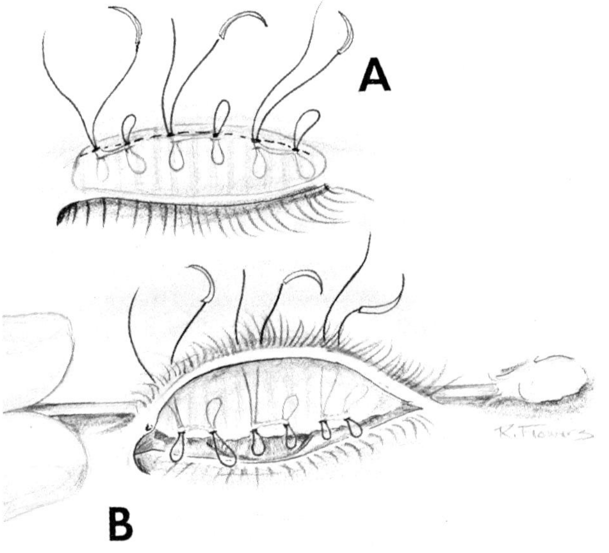

Figure 2 Shows a closed technique for creation of lid folds in Orientals. This is only one of many variations. *A*, external view of suture placement. *B*, view from conjunctival surface, with lid flipped over.

use of prominent medial fat transposed laterally (Fig. 4), will be of benefit. Free grafts of fat have proved less effective than the use of free subgaleal areolar tissue grafts from the scalp, harvested during combined coronal lifting-type procedures.

On the *lower* Oriental lid it continues to be important to avoid raising skin flaps. Avoidance is aided by the fact that in most young Orientals there is little or no skin to be removed. Since skin incisions on the lower lid are much more prominently displayed in Orientals than in Caucasians, the transconjunctival approach to orbital fat continues to be an often preferred technique.

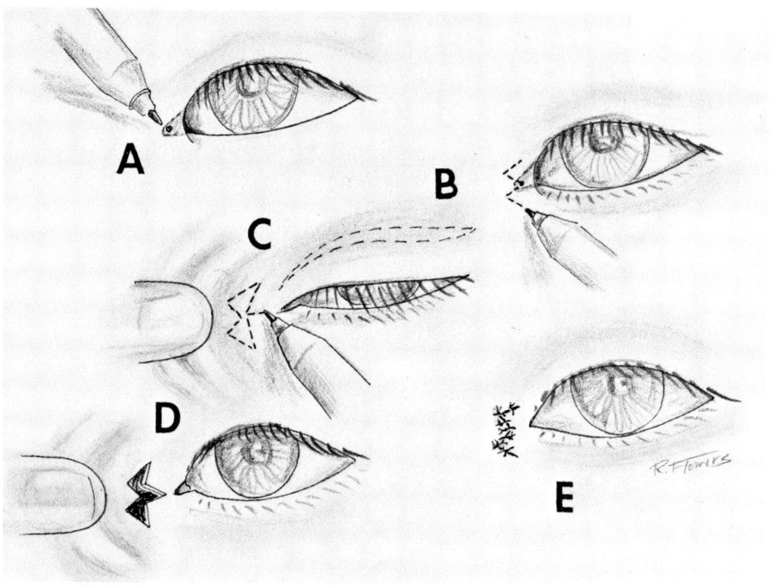

Figure 3 Drawings show recommended technique of medical epicanthoplasty. The upper limb of the W should always be well above the medial lid fold incision, and the W-plasty kept as small as possible. (Flowers' modification of Uchida technique.)

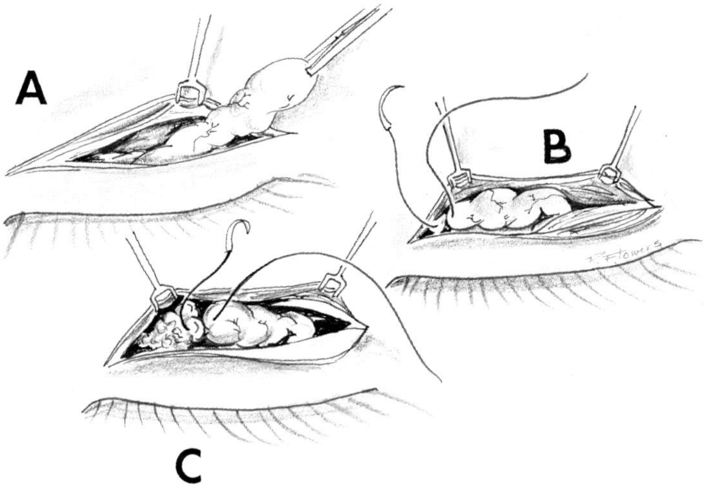

Figure 4 *A* and *B*, transposition of lateral fat to the deficient, hollowed area in the medial lid. *C*, sometimes excessive medial fat can be drawn into the deficient area also.

NOSE

It is important to realize that augmentation by alloplastic implantation is by far the most common method of nasal enhancement worldwide. Bone and cartilage grafts are used occasionally by reconstructive surgeons, but expert alloplastic augmentation of the nasal dorsum (Fig. 5), and occasionally the entire nose, can work extremely well. Complication rates in the thick-skinned Oriental can be less than with autogenous tissues, and operative morbidity is certainly less.

Long-term appraisals of all the new alloplastic materials for the nose are not yet available, but the "old faithful" silicone dorsal implant has proved extremely reliable in my experience, as has the L-shaped prosthesis when it is placed through an intraoral approach, thereby avoiding incisions juxtaposed to the implant. The newly available Implast prostheses are, in my opinion, the best prefabricated products—other than these, my clear preference is for custom fabrication for each individual.

The real improvement in recent years has come through the use of the columellar tip "toboggan graft," which achieves enhancement of the nasal tip (increased projection and refinement) without the need to use foreign materials to achieve additional projection in that region.

Figure 6 shows the preparation of the toboggan graft, which measures approximately 2 cm in length and has a beveled margin that allows rolling of the tip cartilages to avoid visible protrusions and angulations in the tip.

The scant and frequently flimsy septal cartilage in the Oriental often requires reinforcement of the graft with one or more struts to achieve a substantial framework.

The columellar rim incision, which gives access to the recipient pocket, should be long enough to allow insertion without breaking the cartilage. Tip projection should be overcorrected. When there has been resection of supratip, fibro-fatty tissue that has left the pocket for the graft in communication with the dissected space across the dorsum, a Nylon tie-over suture and a bolster maintain the graft in proper position. Where there is an acute

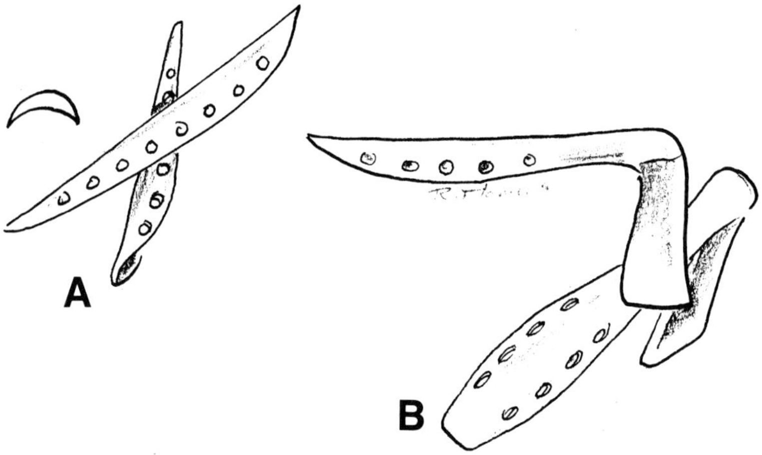

Figure 5 *A*, Implant for the dorsum of the nose only; often combined with "toboggan" cartilage graft to columella-tip. *B*, L-shaped implant, placed through upper muco-labial sulcus incision.

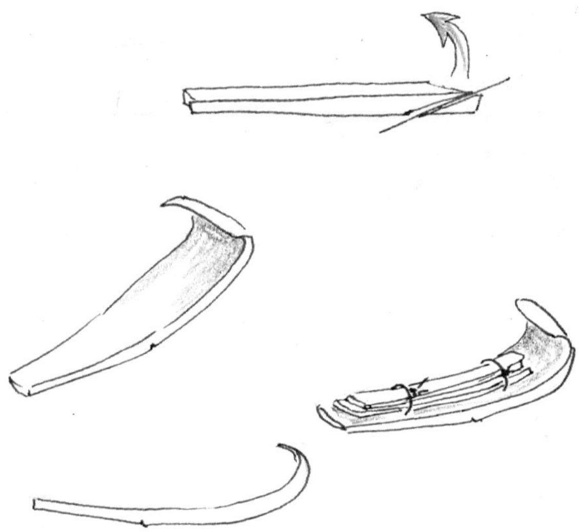

Figure 6 Drawing illustrates the preparation of the "toboggan" graft from septal cartilage. Beveling of the distal end allows rolling and toboggan shape. Often, the scant and flimsy nature of the septal cartilage in Orientals requires reinforcement with multiple layers.

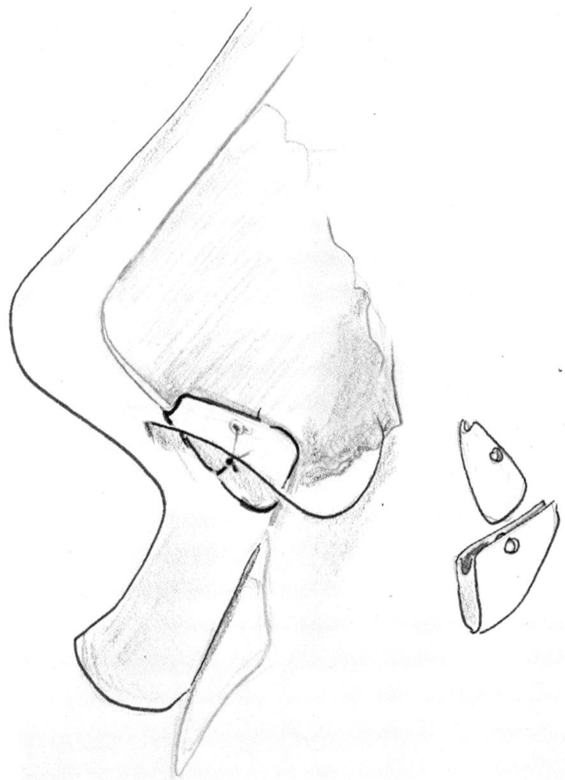

Figure 7 Drawing of maxillary spine graft to open the acute columellar labial angle.

columellar labial angle, the simultaneous placement of an alloplastic graft at the maxillary spine (Fig. 7) helps correct that coexisting problem. When L-shaped implants or grafts are selected, the foot may be left wide to correct the angle, thereby making the maxillary spine graft unnecessary.

The nose that has already turned up nostrils is not suitable for the toboggan graft. Any additional projection of the tip will cause additional upward rotation and result in *more* nostril show and a pig-like appearance. If tip projection is to be increased in such a nose (which usually has a deficiency of skin), there must be a connected dorsal component to check against upward rotation of the graft. This is accomplished most often by an L-shaped implant or graft.

The age old principles applied to nose surgery to prevent complications and morbidity are still valid. They are the avoidance of incisions juxtaposed to alloplastic implants, and only subtle increases in nasal dorsum and projection; usually 1½ to 2 mm suffices. For the dorsal enhancement it is most important to take great care in the construction of a symmetrical pocket and in the preparation and modification of the implant to fit the needs of each patient. One must resist temptation to elongate a nose with alloplastic materials and be fastidious with aseptic technique.

To capsulize the current trends in nasal surgery in the Oriental, the tip usually requires narrowing, sometimes elevation, and, characteristically, an increase in projection. An acute columellar labial angle must be corrected. Most often these changes can be achieved by a columellar tip toboggan graft, plus an occasional implant to the nasal dorsum, possibly combined with a triangular-shaped implant or a graft applied to the maxillary spine (usually inserted through an incision in the upper labial sulcus). In a short turned-up nose with deficient skin, an L-shaped graft or implant must be used to prevent further upward rotation of the tip. Oftentimes, the less done to this latter group of noses, the better.

Lateral osteotomies may be combined with implant augmentation of the nasal dorsum to achieve a narrowed nasal effect.

BIMAXILLARY PROTRUSION AND MIDFACIAL RETRUSION WITH GOOD OCCLUSION

Bimaxillary protrusion is common among many Oriental subgroups. It is usually combined with excellent dentition and good dental occlusion. In such cases, it is difficult to convince patients to undertake extensive orthodontic correction; although in certain cases it is definitely indicated. The condition, however, may be disguised by enhancing projection of the chin with alloplastic augmentation (Fig. 8) or sliding genioplasty, by bringing out the recessed maxilla with an augmentation maxilloplasty, and by nasal enhancement. Chin augmentation is simpler than sliding osteotomy and has less morbidity. Now that longer chin prostheses are available, the esthetic results are improved, but care must be taken to avoid injury to the mental nerves while the longer pocket is being dissected to allow the tails to slide caudal to the nerves.

Thus, augmentation of the recessed maxilla around the pyriform aperture, chin enhancement, nasal augmentation with alloplastic or autogenous materials, and the occasional implant or graft to the maxilla offer an effective correction of typical bimaxillary protrusion deformity without orthodontia or orthognathic surgery.

Sometimes, midfacial retrusion is combined with hypoplastic development of the infraorbital areas of the maxilla, with well developed malar eminences. In such instances, implants designed for the deficient areas may be used to correct the deformity. They are placed either through the lids or upper mucolabial sulcus and are also available from Implast.

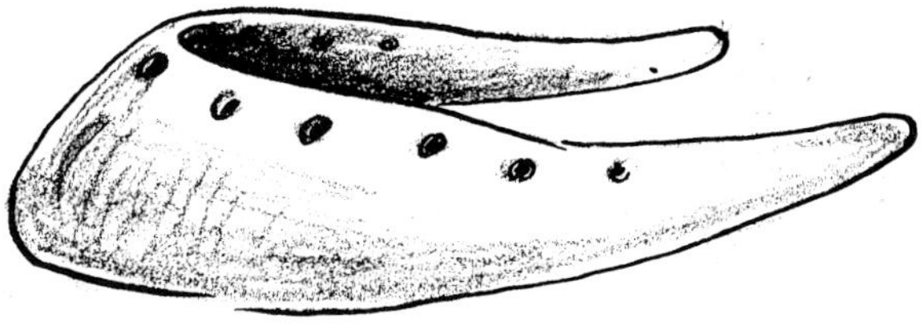

Figure 8 Recommended 8 to 10 cm chin implant, custom fabricated for each patient, or obtained through Implast.

Finally, let us appreciate that aesthetic surgical repair in the Oriental varies in many key ways from aesthetic surgery in Caucasians. Procedures commonly done in Caucasians are inappropriate in Orientals, and some of the procedures that are very appropriate for Orientals may be contraindicated in Caucasians. The differences revolve around the thickness of the skin, the character of the subcutaneous tissue, the blood supply of the skin, and variations in skeletal structure and distribution of subcutaneous tissues.

If these differences are appreciated, anesthetic repair can be most beneficial to patients. The final word of advice that I believe deserves wide dissemination is that repair should be subtle, and by all means conservative. With this as a rule, and surgical expertise as basic equipment, success may be anticipated.

SUGGESTED READING

Fernandez LR. Double eyelid operation in the Oriental in Hawaii. Plast Reconstr Surg 1960; 25:257–264.

Flowers RS. Anchor blepharoplasty in aesthetic surgery of the eyelids. Transactions of the Sixth International Congress of Plastic and Reconstructive Surgery (August 1975). New York: Masson Publishing USA, Inc. 1976; 470–475.

Flowers RS. Nasal augmentation in the intraoral route. Plast Reconstr Surg 1974; 54:570–578.

FEMINIZATION OF THE SKULL

DOUGLAS K. OUSTERHOUT, D.D.S., M.D.

Craniofacial surgery is now a mature subspeciality that, through a natural evolution and increased experience, has been extended from the rare, severe congenital deformity to now include many esthetic conditions. As the ability to correct bony malformations has improved, more subtle deformities now can be approached.

One of the most exciting spin-offs of craniofacial surgery has been recontouring of the craniofacial skeleton to obtain changes for improvement in esthetics. Excessive or diminutive contours are not infrequently a complaint of those wishing esthetic improvement. Nose and chin surgery are common precraniofacial surgery examples. Now the forehead, cheeks, zygomatic arches, and angle of the mandible also can be approached. All of these areas can be augmented as well as reduced.

Esthetic contouring is a large subject: it is the theme of entire symposiums and numerous articles. Rather than being a compendium of various thoughts, this chapter primarily outlines the methods I use to obtain consistent, reliable, long-term results, a low complication rate, and high patient approval. The various Le Fort procedures that are necessary for correction of certain esthetic problems will not be discussed. This chapter is limited to some of the augmentation and reduction procedures utilized for craniofacial contour changing, excluding the nose.

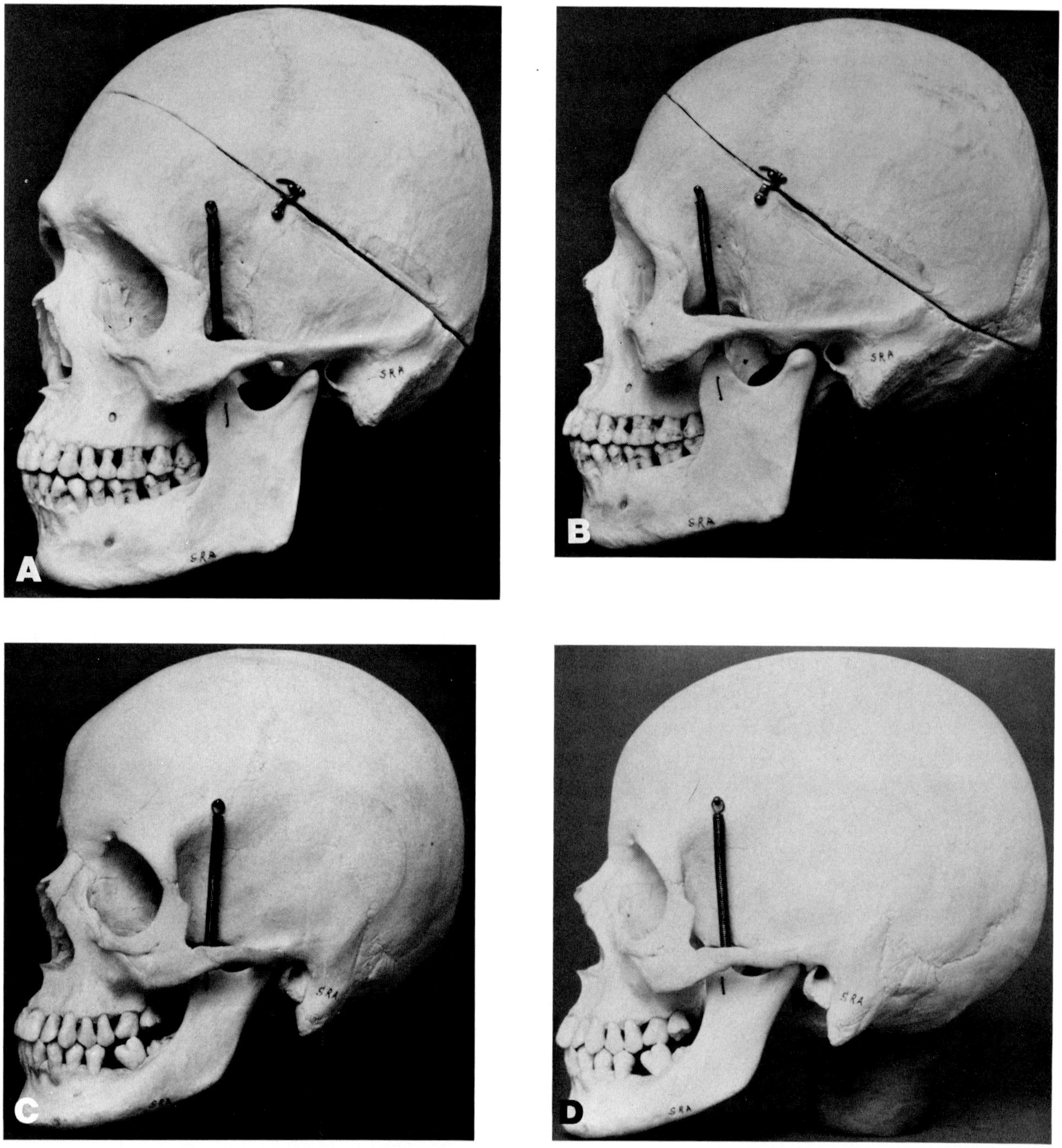

Figure 1 *A* and *B*, Normal male skull: note supraorbital bossing and flat area between bossing in the lower prehead; *C* and *D*, Normal female skull: note minimal supraorbital bossing and continuous curvature to the forehead. (Skulls from Atkinson Skull Collection, University of Pacific Dental School, San Francisco)

FOREHEAD: REDUCTION

Physical anthropologists and forensic pathologists are concerned with the identification and separation of skulls by sex. Prior to the computer and discriminant function analysis, they primarily utilized three skeletal characteristics to identify the male and the female skull: the chin, the nose, and the forehead. Figure 1 shows the skeletal differences of the forehead.

The forehead contour can be reduced (made more feminine) or set back (maintaining masculinity) based on these basic sexual contour differences. Because the degree of the frontal bossing, anterior projection of the orbital rims, and the size of the adjacent frontal sinuses varies, three surgical groups have been classified. In addition, recontouring of the superior lateral orbital angle within the bony orbit has been described as increasing the femininity of the orbital area. This is not something that has been identified as being a more feminine anthropologic characteristic, but it is a procedure that may improve the esthetics of the orbital area in certain cases.

Classification and Methods

Group one includes those patients with normal or slight anterior projection of the supraorbital rims, minimal to moderate contour deformity or bossing, thick skull bone over the frontal sinus, and/or absence of the frontal sinus. These deformities can be corrected by bone reduction alone utilizing a pineapple shaped or methyl methacrylate burr.

Group two includes those individuals with normal or slight anterior placement of the supraorbital rims, but with relatively thin bone over the frontal sinuses, the frontal sinuses generally being of normal size. Correction of the deformity in these patients requires completing as much contouring of the bone as possible without entering the sinus, augmenting the slight remaining concavity above the frontal bossing with self curing methyl methacrylate, and then contouring the plastic until a final desired contour is obtained (Fig. 2).

Group three includes those patients in whom the anterior projection of the supraorbital rims is so excessive that adequate bone reduction contouring is impossible without entering the frontal sinus. In these individuals, the frontal sinus must be opened through an osteotomy, the anterior sinus wall and the contiguous supraorbital rim are removed, and the bone, which is usually divided into several pieces, is then set back to the desired position and stabilized. In addition, bony contouring is completed lateral and superior to the sinus osteotomies as necessary to develop the desired contour (Fig. 3).

Additional contouring with methyl methacrylate must not be completed at the time of the osteotomy to prevent bacterial contamination through the sinus osteotomy. Resultant infection developing around the implant could then lead to osteomyelitis and deformity.

Discussion

Patient satisfaction and final contours have been excellent. The desired contour has been obtained through a single operation. There have been no complications in any of these patients to date.

All of the patients undergoing these procedures have received antibiotics for 8 days postoperatively. The scalp has only been shaved along the line of the incision in order to place gauze with supporting Michele clips along the incision. This has adequately maintained the hair out of the wound, of particular importance when using implant materials. Edema is generally only moderate in amount, as is ecchymosis. The results are seen between 2 and 3 weeks following surgery.

FOREHEAD: AUGMENTATION

Although augmentation of the forehead for cosmetic purposes rarely is requested, both males and females have desired it for improving a deficient contour or asymmetry. To perform a forehead bony advancement for an esthetic purpose would be extremely extensive and expensive surgery. Augmentation of the craniofacial skeleton must be completed in as few procedures as possible, preferably one, have good long-term results, and have as few complications as possible. In general, I do not feel that it is possible to obtain a permanent, significant augmentation with good contour utilizing bone of any origin, e.g., iliac crest, rib, or split skull. When augmentation is to be completed, as described above in the group two reductions or as described in this section, methyl methacrylate is extremely useful. I do not feel that silicone is as easy to contour in the operating room if adjustments are necessary. Long-term results with silicone are not encouraging and apparently all such material must eventually be removed. I also do not feel that the expense of placing a prefabricated CAD-CAM (computer-aided design–computer-aided machined) prosthesis designed from a CT scan is necessary in any but the rare case. The majority of augmentations can be completed by free sculpturing at the time of surgery. New materials, e.g., hydroxyapatite, may become the materials of choice for augmentation in the future.

Methods

Preoperative planning is completed using patient examination and self-review, radiographs, and photographs. The amount of augmentation must be determined preoperatively. The supraorbital rim in the male is generally 8 to 10 mm in front of the cornea; it is approximately 2 to 4 mm less in the female. Augmentation of the forehead can be completed in two manners. Through a bicoronal incision and after exposure of the orbital rims and temporal fossa, methyl methacrylate can be placed directly on the skull and contoured to obtain the desired result. A periodontal probe is used during surgery as a depth gauge to determine the amount of augmentation beyond the supraorbital rim. Once the methyl methacrylate is hard, it is sculpted to develop the desired contour. Male and female differences must be respected. If an individual tends to have a narrow skull, the bitemporal area can be augmented by extending the resin into the temporal fossa and then sculpturing a new superior temporal line and upper temporal fossa. This allows the skull width to be increased so as to avoid giving the skull a pinched look from the augmentation.

If the augmentation is large, e.g., greater than 5 to 7 mm thick, total contouring at the time of the operation may be difficult. In these cases, either a prosthesis designed on a CT scan, a CAD-CAM created model, or a plaster model from an alginate facial moulage may be produced. Both techniques have been used in esthetic and congenital craniofacial problems. The forehead prosthesis can then be gas sterilized and placed directly on the skull with some additional contouring as necessary. Final stabilization of the implant is obtained by using self-curing methyl methacrylate under the implant directly on the skull. Figure 4 shows the result of a forehead augmentation for esthetic purposes.

Results

The results have been pleasing and reliable and can be completed in a minimum of operating time—3 to 5 hours—depending on the extent of the procedure and particularly on the amount of self-curing methyl methacrylate that is utilized. These implants have not shifted or

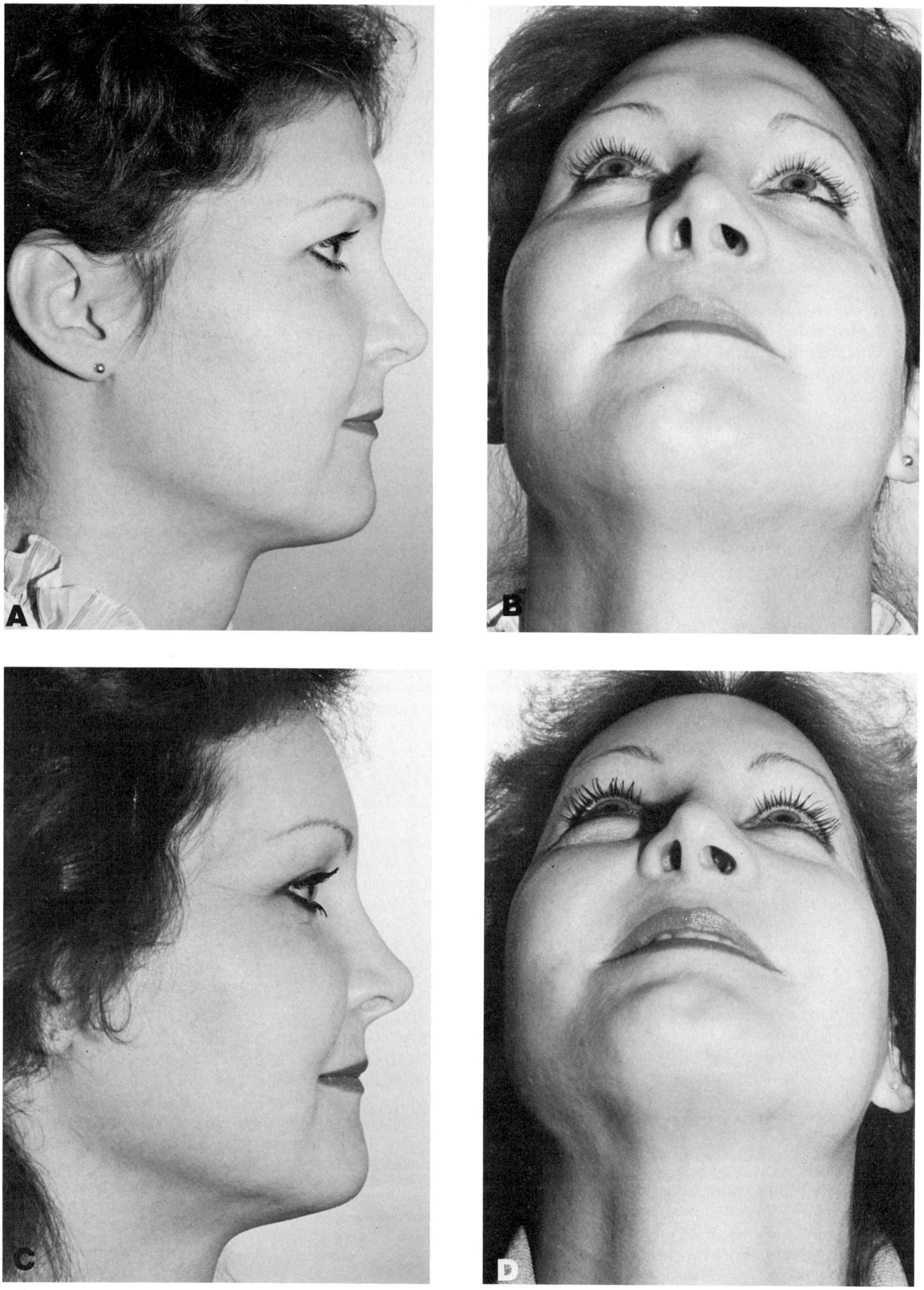

Figure 2 Forehead reduction, group two. *A* and *B*, Preoperative; *C* and *D*, Postoperative.

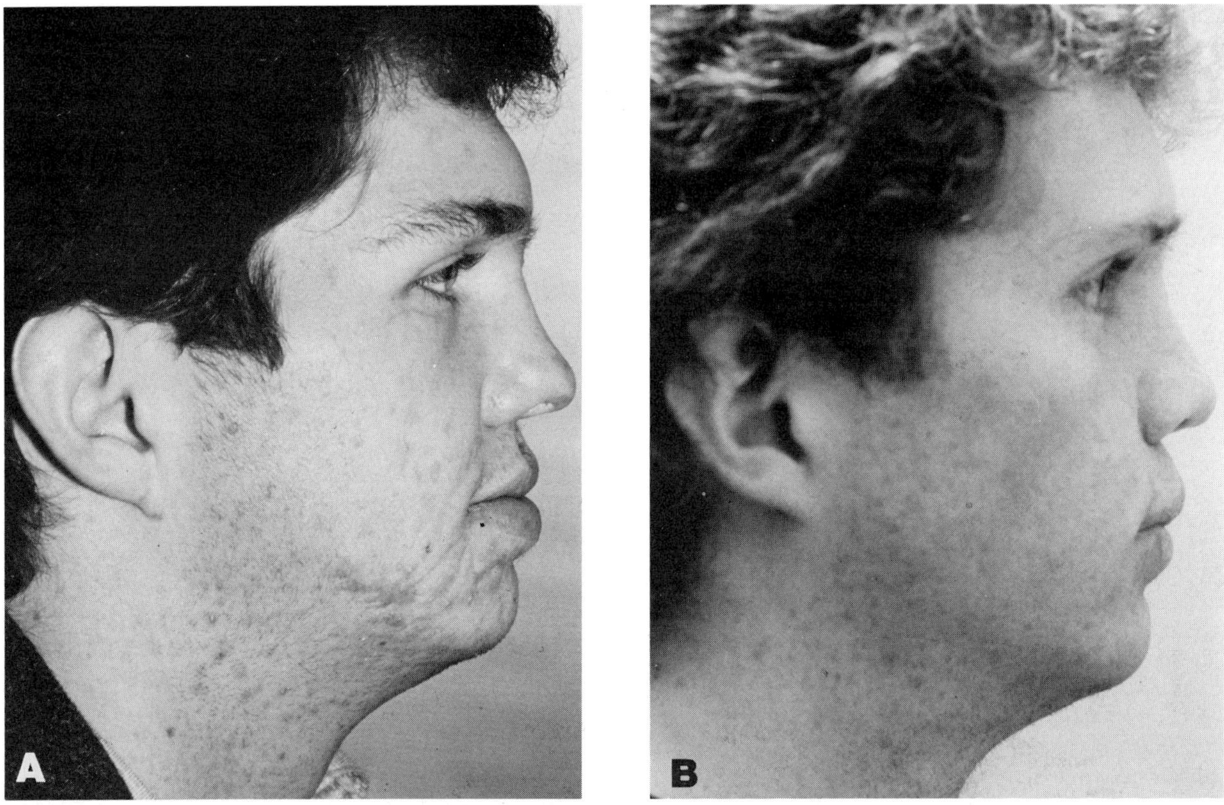

Figure 3 Forehead reduction, group three. *A*, Preoperative; *B*, Postoperative.

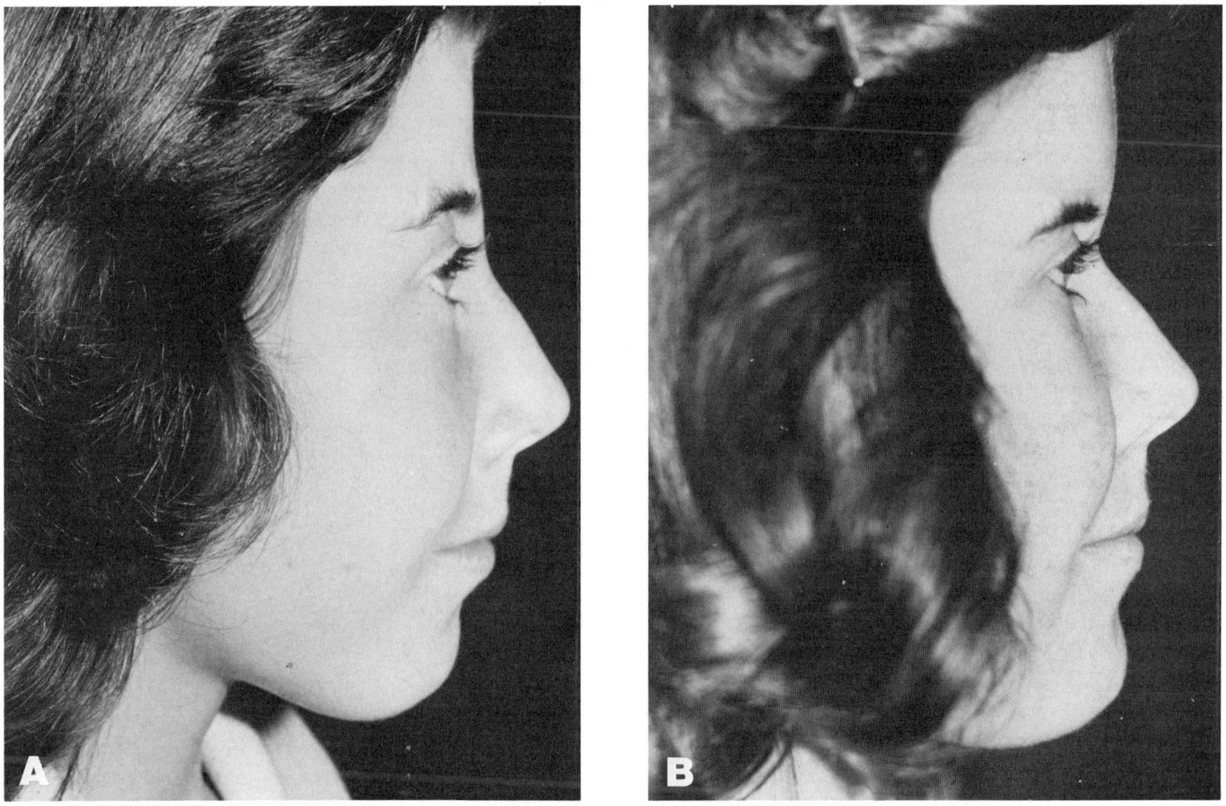

Figure 4 Forehead augmentation, preformed implant. *A*, Preoperative; *B*, Postoperative.

eroded into bone; this is probably because of the exact fit of the implant on the skull by the anchoring layer of methyl methacrylate. The results are as good as one's ability to sculpt.

Complications

Complications have not occurred in this group of patients. There has been an occasional, temporary subgaleal serous fluid accumulation that must be repeatedly aspirated over 4 to 6 days until permanently eliminated. As with the group two patients described above, methyl methacrylate should never be utilized under scars, skin grafts, or within 6 months of a scalp infection.

CHEEKS: AUGMENTATION

Cheek augmentation is a frequently requested procedure. Many patients requesting cheek augmentation refer to magazine photographs in which there is an obvious area of fullness that extends from the lateral alar rim upward and laterally over the zygomatic prominence of the cheeks onto the zygomatic arch toward the anterior attachment of the ear helix. I find the cheek implant designed by Whitaker, made of Proplast, the most successful for obtaining this appearance. Small modifications for individual requirements can be completed on the prosthesis in the operating room prior to saturation with antibiotic. Other implant designs may be indicated; many varieties and shapes are available.

Methods

Implants are preferably placed through a buccal sulcus approach under local anesthesia. The implant is saturated with an antibiotic solution prior to implantation. A blepharoplasty incision may be the preferred route if smaller implants are utilized.

Results

There is a postoperative period of edema generally lasting for 2 to 3 weeks. These implants have not shown any evidence of migration or of penetration into the underlying bone.

Patients' satisfaction with cheek implantation is extremely high. On rare occasions, there is some asymmetry that requires reexposure of the prosthesis and repositioning. Whitaker has described rare cases of late infection, at which time the implant has been easily removed. The wrap-around implants described above have a natural-looking appearance in those patients selected for this specific prosthesis.

Discussion

It is important to inform patients that immediately postoperatively they may have some numbness in the mid-upper lip giving them the sensation of a speech impediment. Motor nerve injuries have not been a problem. It has primarily been the temporary lip numbness that has been inferred to be an improper speech mechanism.

Augmenting the zygomatic arch by cutting it anteriorly, springing the bone laterally, and placing an interpositional cranial bone graft has not proven successful in the laboratory. In monkeys followed for 3 years, the zygomatic arch position has gradually changed to the preoperative contour.

CHEEK AND ZYGOMATIC ARCH: REDUCTION

Cheek and zygomatic arch reduction for excessive prominence is rarely requested. In the four cases that I have completed (three males and one female), three have been Orientals and one an American Indian. The largest published series is three cases from the Japanese literature.

In addition to hereditary factors, this condition may be related in some manner to sinus hyperpneumatization and possibly also to benign masseteric hypertrophy. In the latter condition, the origin end of the masseteric muscle may cause a bony overgrowth similar to that occurring at the angle of the mandible; various factors may be involved, possibly including clenching of the teeth while weight lifting.

Method

Whitaker and Onizuka and colleagues have both used an inferior approach dissecting upward from the buccal sulcus. I find this to be a difficult approach; the exposure is not nearly as great and I am concerned that the reduction may not be as symmetrical, as complete, or as smooth at the upper margin as when a superior approach is utilized.

The bicoronal incision can be utilized to obtain complete exposure of the zygomatic arch with visualization around and onto the anterior margin of the cheek to the infraorbital neurovascular bundle. The hypertrophy often extends posteriorly to the beginning of the zygomatic process of the temporal bone. By the superior approach, one can see exactly the position of the temporalis muscle going deep to the arch. The arch remaining after contouring should probably be at least 2 to 3 mm thick. The masseter muscle needs to be partially dissected from the bone in order to develop the inferior margin contour. By using the superior approach, one can check on symmetry far better than through an inferior approach. In those cases with anterior cheek prominence alone, combined osteotomy and ostectomy can be used to reduce the deformity.

Discussion

Radiographic evaluation of the zygomatic arch is extremely important prior to surgery. The bowing of the zygomatic arch is in part related to the thickness of the temporalis muscle. With a thick temporalis muscle, the zygomatic arch may be bowed around the muscle, but is not necessarily of increased thickness. No attempt has been made to reduce the thickness of the muscle as one does in masseteric hypertrophy. This might be possible, but I would be concerned about an adhesion developing between the muscle and the inner surface of the zygomatic arch that could cause limitation of mandibular movement.

MANDIBULAR ANGLE: AUGMENTATION

An occasional patient requests augmentation of the mandibular angle. The common denominator in these cases has been a broad neck with a relatively narrow bimandibular angle width that causes a less obvious demarcation between the mandible and the upper neck. These patients are requesting more definition in this area.

Methods

Through an intraoral incision, only the upper portion of the masseter muscle is dissected from the side of the proximal ramus of the mandible. Using a reciprocating saw, the outer table of bone is cut from the side of the angle without detaching the remaining muscle. By carefully watching the bone cut, one can cut superficially and thus avoid nerve injury. The pterygomasseteric sling is not cut, but may be scored to allow a width increase. A cranial bone graft is then inserted between the layers of bone. No fixation of the bony segments has been used, but a fixed pressure dressing has been applied.

Results

Patient satisfaction has been excellent and there have been no complications. Although the changes are subtle, the results seem to be permanent at 2 years postsurgery.

Discussion

Onlay bone grafts under the masseter muscle show a high percentage of resorption. In monkey studies, bone grafts under the masseter muscle have shown a high percentage of resorption. Bone graft augmentation on the lateral border of the mandibular body anterior to the masseter muscle has not proved successful because the grafts are rapidly resorbed. Whitaker has tried to place implants along the lateral margin, but his few cases apparently all became infected and the implants had to be removed. To split the body of the mandible and place an interpositional bone graft would probably be extremely difficult without injury to the inferior alveolar neurovascular bundle.

MANDIBULAR ANGLE: REDUCTION

The treatment of benign masseteric hypertrophy is well established. Reduction of the resulting bony flaring and associated excess muscle has been well documented. The long-term results are satisfying. Occasionally, patients without true benign masseteric hypertrophy request a reduction in bimandibular width.

Methods

This procedure is best completed through an intraoral approach where the masseter muscle is first reduced by excising a portion of the inferior inner muscle mass, followed by recontouring of the inferior lateral bone at the angle. An occasional patient will also have a posterior bony projection that is most easily removed using a small, right-angle, power-driven oscillating blade.

Results

These patients all have a significant amount of postsurgery swelling and must be warned that it will take some weeks for their final result to be appreciated. The results are pleasing in these cases. If the individual is a weight lifter, it is recommended that they stop their weight lifting if they wish a permanent result.

CHIN: AUGMENTATION

Chin augmentation is a well-accepted surgical procedure. The chin-implant is generally extremely successful for small augmentations. However, chin implants do have the potential complication of migration to an asymmetrical position, migration into the bone (sometimes markedly so), possible infection, and extrusion. Sliding genioplasties are particularly useful in implant failures, in the larger augmentations, when the chin is asymmetrical, or when a vertical reduction is combined with an advancement. Various osteotomy designs are useful for correcting unusual chin contours.

It must be recognized that there is a marked difference between the male and the female chin. Figure 5 shows the typical male and female chin.

In advancing the chin, there is the possibility of causing the chin to become wide secondary to the flaring of the advanced lateral segments. Splitting of the chin with the removal of a small posterior wedge will allow for advancement of the chin while maintaining a more feminine appearance. This can be utilized to develop a feminine chin if so desired (Fig. 6).

Sliding genioplasties can be completed under general or local anesthesia. I prefer general anesthesia as there is considerably more time available to develop the result. This is particularly important if the planned procedure is more than a simple advancement.

Discussion

The results of sliding genioplasties seem to be permanent, are esthetically pleasing, and the complication rate is low. Of major importance is the potential problem of a mental nerve injury with resulting numbness of half or the entire lower lip. It is important that the osteotomies are in most cases at least 7 to 8 mm below the inferior border of the mental nerve foramen.

Vertical augmentation can also be completed with a sliding genioplasty. Cranial bone may be interposed as necessary to obtain the desired result. Although in

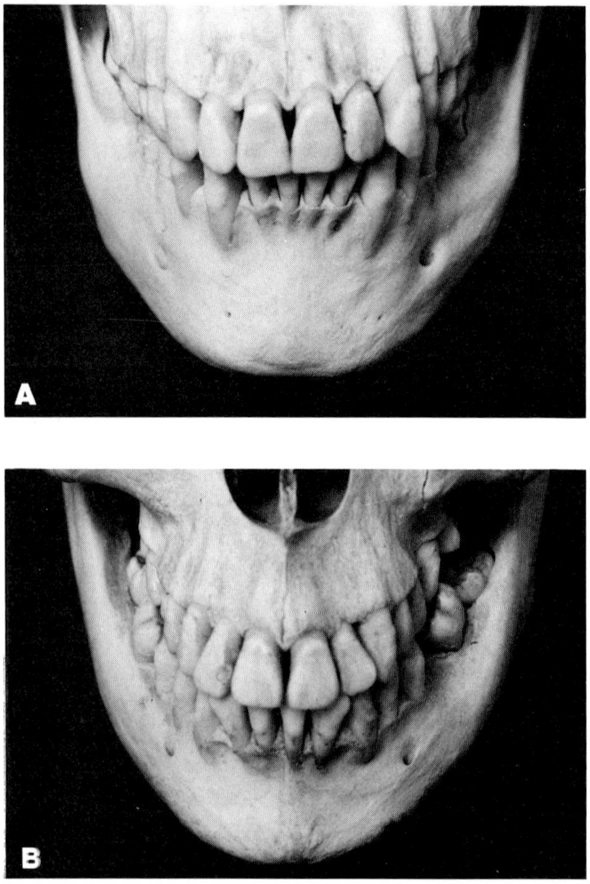

Figure 5 *A*, Normal male chin; *B*, Normal female chin. (Atkinson Skull Collection)

general I use wire fixation in these cases, angled K wires or internal fixation plates can be utilized.

CHIN: REDUCTION

Chin reduction is, in general, a much more difficult procedure than advancement to obtain a desired result. With reduction by the sliding genioplasty technique in either the vertical or the horizontal directions, there is a possibility of producing a significant cosmetic deformity of the "witch's chin" type. A "witch's chin" is even more likely to occur if the chin is reduced by degloving and then the outer circumference of the bone is reduced.

Chin reduction is completed in the same manner as described for chin augmentation—the sliding genioplasty technique—but through a tunneling procedure in which the periosteum is not elevated from the inferior segment. The reduction must be limited in both the posterior and the vertical movement. When a "witch's chin" results from a chin reduction, the problem is extremely difficult to correct, if correctable at all. In some cases, it may be totally resistant to reconstruction. Reducing a chin too much also tends to cause a broad, boxy appearance.

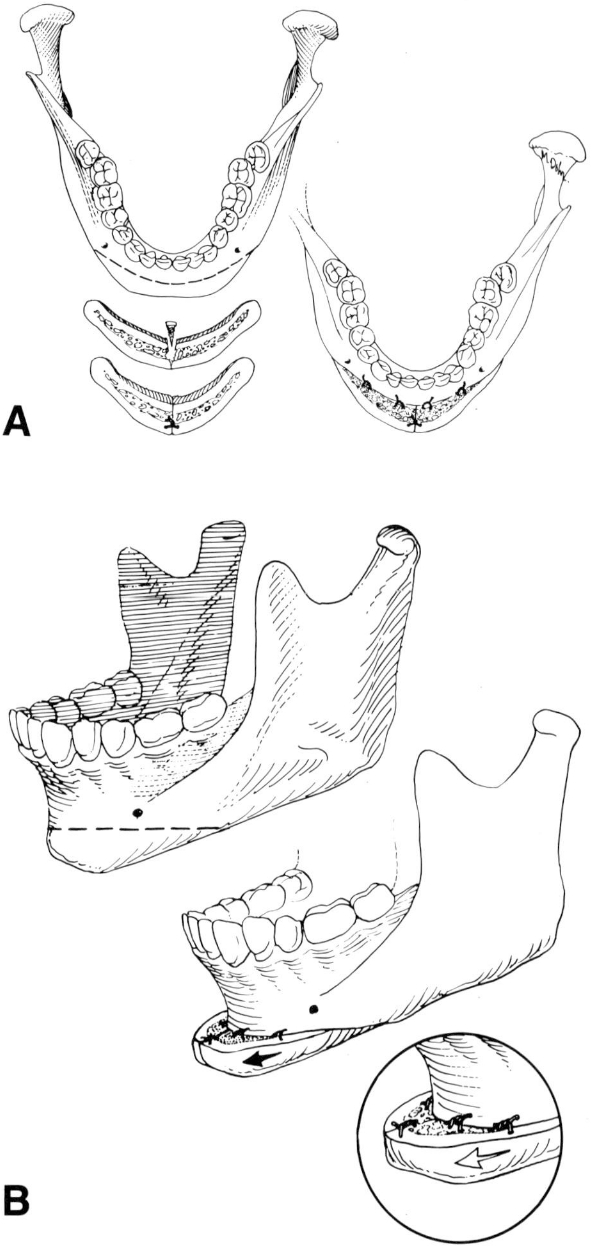

Figure 6 *A* and *B*, Design of procedure used in advancing the chin to preserve or obtain feminine contour.

A submental, suction-assisted lipectomy is indicated with most chin reductions since there is a tendency to develop some submental fullness when the chin is moved back even slightly.

SUGGESTED READING

Millard DR Jr. Chin implants. Plast Reconstr Surg 1954; 13:70-74.
Onizuka T, Watanabe K, Takasu K, Keyama A. Reduction malar plasty. Aesthetic Plast Surg 1983; 7:121-125.

Ousterhout DK. Feminization of the forehead: contour changing to improve female aesthetics. Plast Reconstr Surg 1987; 79:701-711.

Ousterhout DK, Baker S, Zlotolow I. Methyl-methacrylate onlay implants in the treatment of forehead deformities secondary to craniosynostosis. J Maxillofac Surg 1980; 8:228-233.

Ousterhout DK, Penoff JH. Surgical treatment of facial deformity secondary to acromegaly. Ann Plast Surg 1981; 7:68-74.

Roncevic R. Masseter muscle hypertrophy, aetiology and therapy. J Maxillofac Surg 1986; 14:344-346.

Spears SL, Mausner ME, Kawamoto HK. Sliding genioplasty as a local anesthetic outpatient procedure: a prospective two center trial. Plast Reconstr Surg 1987; 80:55-66.

Thieme FP, Schull WJ. Sex determination from the skeleton. Hum Biol 1957; 29:242-273.

Thompson ERE. Sagittal genioplasty: a new technique of genioplasty. Br J Plast Surg 1985; 38:70-74.

Whitaker LA, Morales L, Farkas LG. Aesthetic surgery of the supraorbital ridge and forehead structures. Plast Reconstr Surg 1986; 78:23-32.

Whitaker LA, Pertschuk M. Facial skeletal contouring for aesthetic purposes. Plast Reconstr Surg 1982; 69:245-253.

White JC. Late complications following cranioplasty with alloplastic plates. Ann Surg 1948; 128:743-755.

Wolfe SA. Aesthetic procedures on the chin. In: Regnault P, Daniel R, eds. Aesthetic plastic surgery. Boston: Little, Brown, 1984.

INDEX